Color Atlas of Canine and Feline Surgical Oncology

Color Atlas of Canine and Feline Surgical Oncology

Julius M. Liptak, BVSc, MVetClinStud, FANZCVS, DACVS-SA, DECVS
ACVS Founding Fellow, Surgical Oncology
ACVS Founding Fellow, Oral and Maxillofacial Surgery
RCVS Specialist in Surgical Oncology
Capital City Specialty & Emergency Animal Hospital
Kanata, Ontario
Canada

Paolo Buracco, DVM, DECVS
EBVS European Specialist in Small Animal Surgery
Full Professor of Veterinary Surgery (retired)
University of Turin
Turin, Italy

William T. N. Culp, VMD, DACVS
ACVS Founding Fellow, Surgical Oncology
ACVS Founding Fellow, Minimally Invasive Surgery
ACVS Founding Fellow, Oral and Maxillofacial Surgery
University of California, Davis
School of Veterinary Medicine
Davis, California

Nicholas J. Bacon, MA, VetMB, CertVR, CertSAS, DECVS, DACVS, FRCVS
ACVS Founding Fellow, Surgical Oncology
RCVS Specialist in Small Animal Surgery (Oncology)
Professor, Surgical Oncology
University of Surrey School of Veterinary Medicine
AURA Veterinary
Guildford, Surrey
United Kingdom

WILEY

Published by John Wiley & Sons, Inc., Hoboken, New Jersey.
Published simultaneously in Canada.

Library of Congress Cataloging-in-Publication Data Applied for:

Hardback ISBN: 9781119630753

Cover Design: Wiley
Cover Images: © Nicholas J. Bacon

Set in 9.5/12.5pt STIXTwoText by Straive, Pondicherry, India

Printed in Singapore
M102045290425

Dedications

To my wife, Allison, and son, Ollie, for their understanding and support. To Drs. Stephen Withrow, Bill Dernell, and Nicole Ehrhart for their guidance, training, and support, and continuing to be a source of inspiration for the teaching and dissemination of knowledge and skills of surgical oncology. To our colleagues, especially those within the Veterinary Society of Surgical Oncology, for their advice, support, innovation, inspiration, and pursuit of excellence in the treatment of dogs and cats with cancer.

Julius M. Liptak

To my wife, Monica, for her understanding and support during all these years of my professional career, and to my sons, Emiliano and Nahuel, now grown-up adults. To professor Ralph Richardson, who, when I was at Purdue University in 1987–1988, introduced me to the field of veterinary oncology. To professor Stephen Withrow, one of the fathers of veterinary surgical oncology, who I had the chance to work with for a while at Colorado State University Teaching Hospital; he showed me a new professional reality that I later developed in my own country, Italy. To all my Italian and foreign colleagues with whom I have worked in the veterinary oncological field. Finally, to the Veterinary Society of Surgical Oncology, a continuous source of inspiration.

Paolo Buracco

To my girls, Carrie, Sienna, and Rylie, for being a constant source of inspiration. To my mentors, for their time, training, and dedication. To all the amazing students, interns, residents, and fellows whom I have been fortunate enough to work with and learn from. And to my colleagues who are continuing to push the boundaries of what we can offer in the treatment of cancer so that we can help our patients to achieve better and longer lives.

William T. N. Culp

To those who helped lay the pioneering foundation of veterinary surgical oncology. Appreciation to the AURA Veterinary team, whose dedication to patients and families is an ongoing source of inspiration and knowledge. A respectful nod to the mentor who shared the wisdom: “There are no brave surgeons, only brave patients.” Finally, sending love and gratitude to Rebecca, Will, and Amelie for bringing joy and making everything better.

Nicholas J. Bacon

Contents

Foreword

It is an honor to write the foreword for this textbook. All four authors are former trainees and valued colleagues and friends. Surgical oncology has been a rapidly evolving specialty discipline with application to the general practitioner and specialty surgeon. This textbook complements existing oncology literature with excellent graphics and technique descriptions. The emphasis is on tumor site rather than tumor type, but both apply. Both tumor resection and reconstruction are included. Many variables apply when making a decision on the best oncologic procedure for each pet and owner. Surgeon experience and owner goals (such as curative-intent versus palliation) vary widely. Not all procedures described will be applicable to all surgeons given the specialty nature of some of the equipment and techniques, such as staples, “cautery,” scoping, stenting, sentinel lymph node sampling, and embolization. Making all surgeons aware of possible interventions is important, however. This textbook will be a valuable addition to both the general surgeon and the specialist.

Stephen Withrow, DVM, DACVS,
ACVS Founding Fellow in Surgical Oncology
University Distinguished Professor
Stuart Chair in Oncology – Emeritus
Founding Director, Flint Animal Cancer Center
Colorado State University
Fort Collins, CO

Preface

Dr. Stephen Withrow, one of the forefathers of veterinary surgical oncology, started a fellowship training program, the first of its kind, at Colorado State University with the aim of training surgeons in the art of surgical oncology. Euphemistically, he wanted to "spread the word." Since his pioneering vision, his surgical oncology fellows have gone on to develop their own fellowship programs in other academic institutions, establish the Veterinary Society of Surgical Oncology, be instrumental in the American College of Veterinary Surgeons recognizing surgical oncology as a subdiscipline, and publishing a dedicated surgical oncology textbook, *Veterinary Surgical Oncology*. This textbook is another step in "spreading the word" of surgical oncology to all veterinarians, from general practitioners to residents and specialists. In the same vein as Dr. Kirpensteijn and Dr. Haar's *Reconstructive Surgery and Wound Management of the Dog and Cat*, we wanted to provide a step-by-step guide on how to perform a comprehensive list of oncologic and reconstructive surgeries using high-quality images of clinical cases. We felt it was important to use images from clinical cases to provide as realistic a representation of the intraoperative exposure and visualization as possible. With the aim of providing an overview of the pertinent information for each surgical procedure, especially for communication with owners and colleagues, we also included brief summaries of suggested diagnostic and clinical staging tests, postoperative management, postoperative complications, suggested adjuvant treatment options, and oncologic prognosis for each of the surgical procedures; however, this information is presented in lists and tables and is based on published studies. For more comprehensive information on the clinical staging tests, pathophysiology, treatment options, postoperative complications and their management, and prognosis for each tumor type, we recommend referring to textbooks such as *Withrow & MacEwen's Small Animal Clinical Oncology*, *Veterinary Surgical Oncology*, *Tumors in Domestic Animals, Atlas of Small Animal Wound Management and Reconstructive Surgery*, and *Complications in Small Animal Surgery*. We hope that our readers find this book a practical and informative addition to their library and a valuable reference for performing oncologic and reconstructive procedures in their practice.

Acknowledgments

We thank and acknowledge all of our colleagues who have contributed images to this textbook: Drs. Takeshi Aikawa, Josep Aisa, Pierre Amsellem, Maurizio Annoni, Stephen Bilbrey, Jonathan Bray, Herve Brissot, Dan Brockman, Roberto Bussadori, Brad Case, Ben Clarke, Leandro Crivellenti, Dario Druri, Laurent Findji, Bart Van Goethem, Adolfo Guandalini, Martin Kessler, Dan Linden, Mischa McDonald-Lynch, Phil Mayhew, Milan Milovancev, Eric Monnet, Ryohei Nishimura, Manuel Jiménez Peláez, Bernard Séguin, James Simcock, Lucinda Van Stee, Maurine Thomson, Brian Trumpatori, and Rosario Vallefuoco.

We also thank the team at Wiley for making this textbook possible, especially Erica Judisch, Vallikkannu Narayanan, and Merryl Le Roux.

Section 1
Surgical Oncology Principles

Chapter 1: Surgical Resection of Cutaneous and Subcutaneous Tumors

There are two basic surgical approaches for tumor resection: marginal and wide surgical resection. With a wide surgical resection, a certain width of normal tissue is resected lateral and deep to the tumor to account for microscopic extension from the tumor. There are two proposed margin systems: metric and proportional. The metric width of normal tissue depends on the tumor type and varies from 1 cm for benign tumors and malignant carcinomas to 2 cm for mast cell tumors and soft tissue sarcomas and up to 5 cm for vaccine-associated sarcomas in cats. Alternatively, when using the proportional margin system, the width of the lateral margins is equal to the maximum dimension of the tumor. Note that both the metric [1] and proportional margin systems [2] have been validated for only a subset of cutaneous mast cell tumors in dogs, and all other margin recommendations are based on anecdotal evidence. For both margin systems, the deep margin includes an anatomic barrier, an uninvolved fascial layer, rather than a metric measurement.

The advantage of wide surgical resection is that risk of local tumor recurrence is significantly decreased. Although the majority of wounds after wide surgical resection can be closed primarily, occasionally they cannot. If the wound cannot be closed, then the wound can be managed with second intention healing (see *46. Second Intention Healing*), random subdermal or axial pattern flaps (see *39. Advancement Flap*, *40. Rotation Flap*, *41. Transposition Flap*, *42. Flank Fold Flaps*, *43. Axial Pattern Flaps*, and *44. Distant Indirect Flap*), or free-meshed skin grafts (see *45. Skin Grafts*). Although these reconstructive techniques are usually successful in the long term, they are more expensive and are associated with higher postoperative complication rates.

Marginal tumor resection is an option for the curative-intent management of benign and malignant tumors or for the palliative management of certain tumors, such as tumors that are having a negative impact on quality of life of the patient (e.g. ulcerated tumor causing pain and secondary infection in a patient with metastatic disease). By definition, marginal surgical resection is resection of a tumor with lateral margins less than recommended for the tumor type and/or not including an uninvolved fascial layer for deep margins. The advantage of marginal surgical resection is that the defect is more likely to be able to be closed primarily with a lower risk of wound healing complications; however, the disadvantage is that there may be an increased risk of incomplete histologic excision and local tumor recurrence. Marginal surgical resection should not be recommended solely because primary wound closure would not be possible after a wide surgical resection; however, it should be considered following consent from owners who have been informed of the increased risk of local tumor recurrence after marginal surgical resection, as well as the increased risk of postoperative complications associated with reconstructive surgery following wide surgical resection.

Suggested Diagnostic Workup and Clinical Staging

- Complete blood count, serum biochemistry, and urinalysis
- Fine-needle aspirate, core aspirate, or core needle biopsy
- ± Sentinel lymph node mapping (see *50.1. Sentinel Lymph Node Mapping*) or regional lymph node fine-needle aspirate cytology, dependent on tumor type
- ± Abdominal ultrasound or computed tomography (CT) scan, dependent on tumor type
- ± Ultrasound-guided fine-needle aspirate cytology of spleen ± liver for localized histiocytic sarcomas and high-grade mast cell tumors
- ± Three-view thoracic radiographs or thoracic CT scan for assessment of lung metastasis, dependent on tumor type

Surgical Technique – Wide Surgical Resection (See Plate 1A–D)

A) A sterile marker pen can be used to mark appropriate metric or proportional lateral margins around the tumor.
B) Skin incisions are made along the marked margins.

Color Atlas of Canine and Feline Surgical Oncology, First Edition. Julius M. Liptak, Paolo Buracco, William T. N. Culp, and Nicholas J. Bacon.

Plate 1

Surgical Resection of Cutaneous and Subcutaneous Tumors

A)

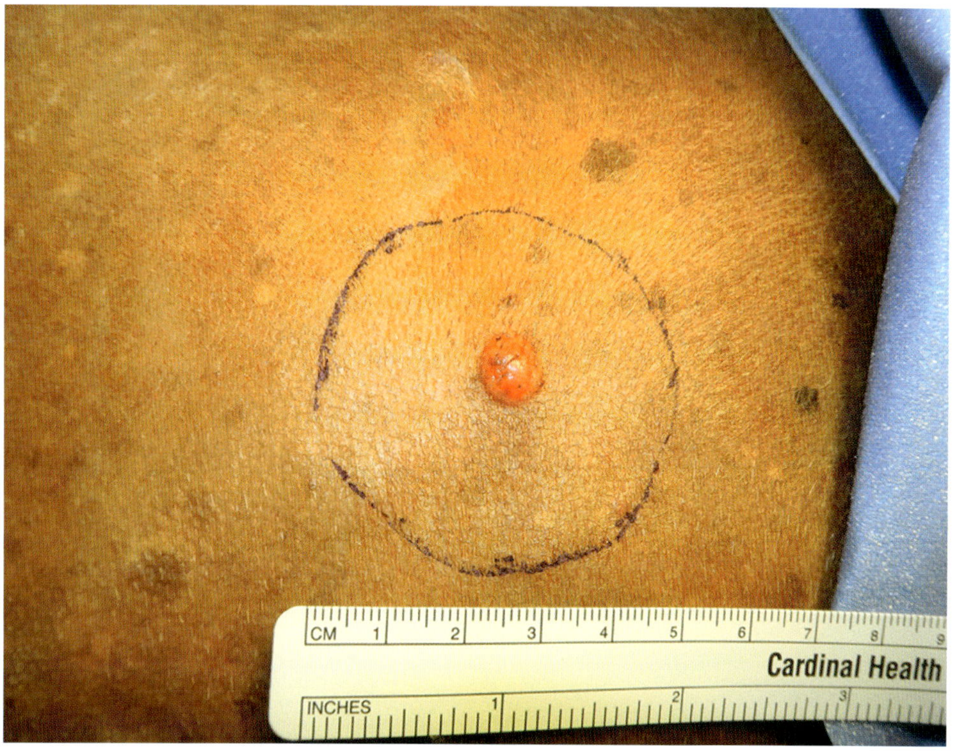

B)

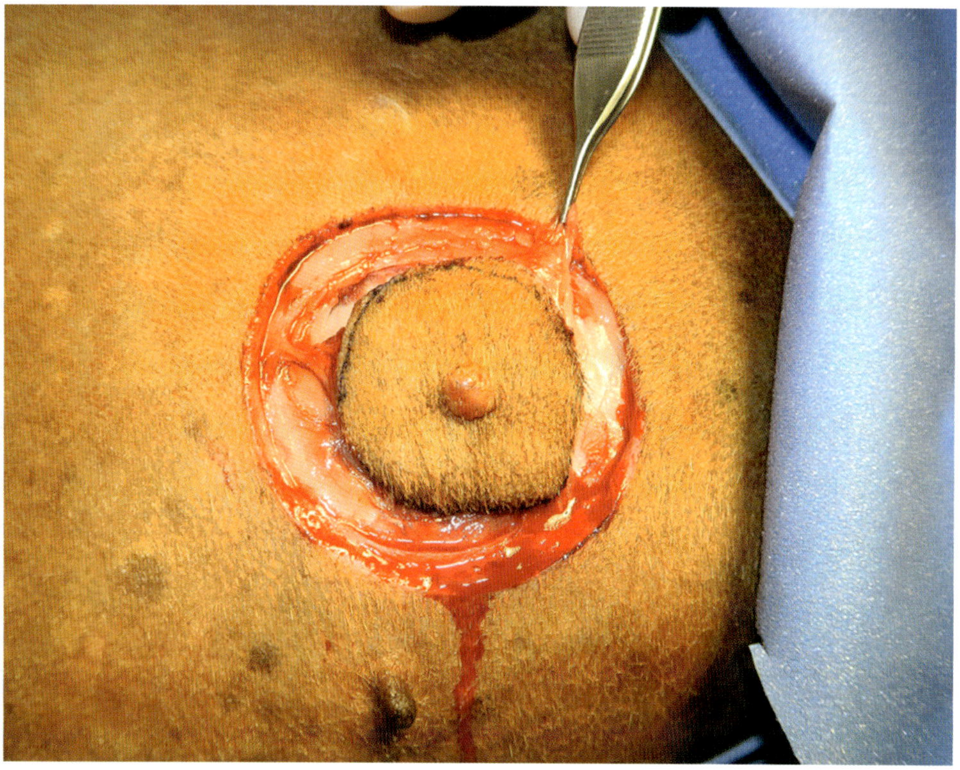

Surgical Technique – Wide Surgical Resection (See Plate 1A–D) *continued*

C) The dissection is continued deeply through the subcutaneous tissue perpendicular to the skin incision and through the deep fascial layer (i–iii).

D) The deep fascial layer may include fascia (i), or partial (ii, iii) or full thickness muscle deep to the tumor. Inclusion of this layer very rarely results in functional deficits following surgery.

Plate 1

Surgical Resection of Cutaneous and Subcutaneous Tumors *continued*

C-i)

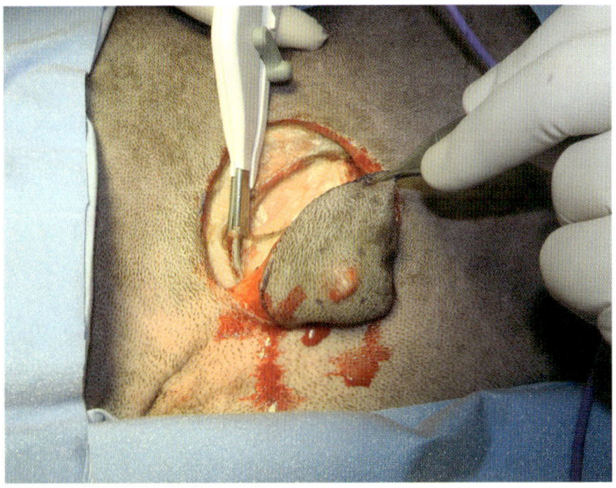

C-ii)

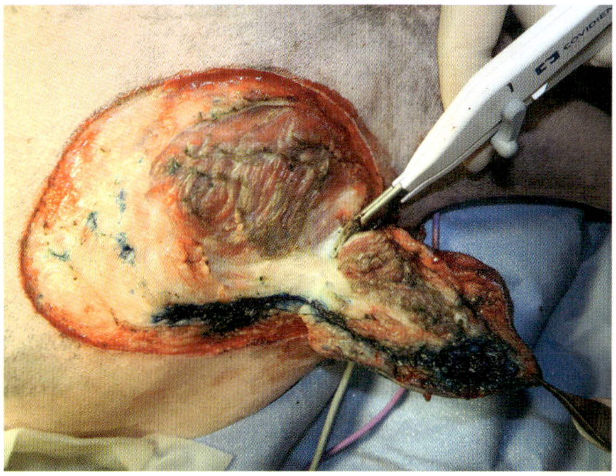

C-iii)

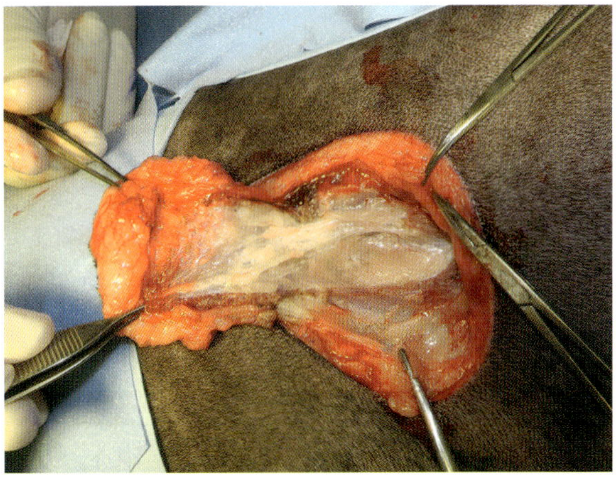

D-i)

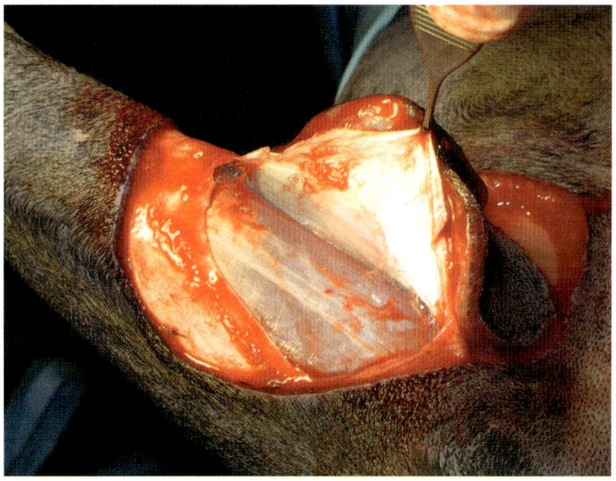

D-ii)

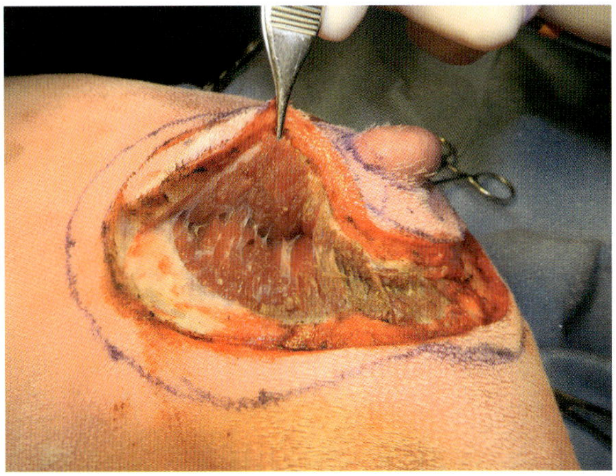

D-iii)

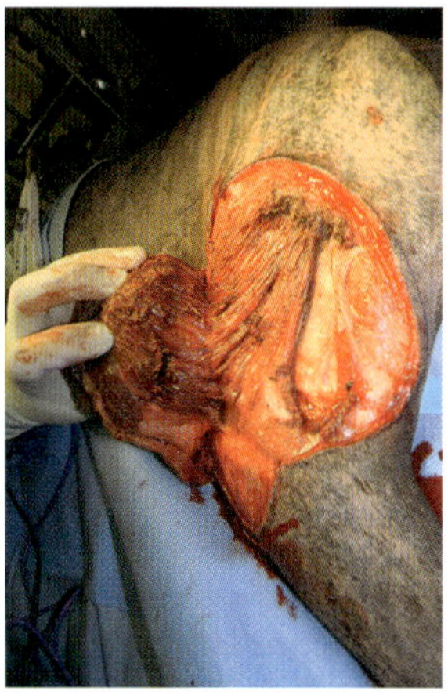

Surgical Technique – Marginal Surgical Resection (See Plate 1E–H)

E) A sterile marker pen can be used to mark appropriate lateral margins around the tumor (i). If marginal resection of a subcutaneous tumor is planned and the skin is freely movable over the subcutaneous mass (ii), then this skin can be preserved to allow primary closure of the subsequent defect (iii); however, en bloc resection of the skin overlying the tumor is preferred because the tumor can extend microscopically into the overlying skin [3].

F) Skin incisions are made along the marked margins (i). If a skin incision is being made in freely movable skin over a subcutaneous tumor, then this incision should be done very carefully to prevent compromising the tumor capsule (ii). This can be done by undermining the freely movable skin (iii) and then, once undermined, continuing to incise over the tumor with scissors (iv).

Plate 1

Surgical Resection of Cutaneous and Subcutaneous Tumors *continued*

E-i)

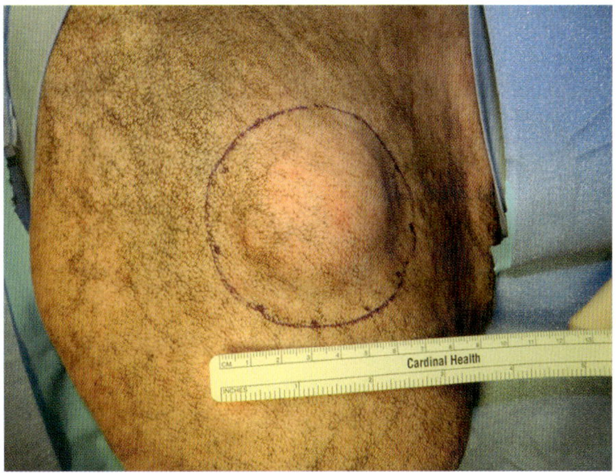

E-ii)

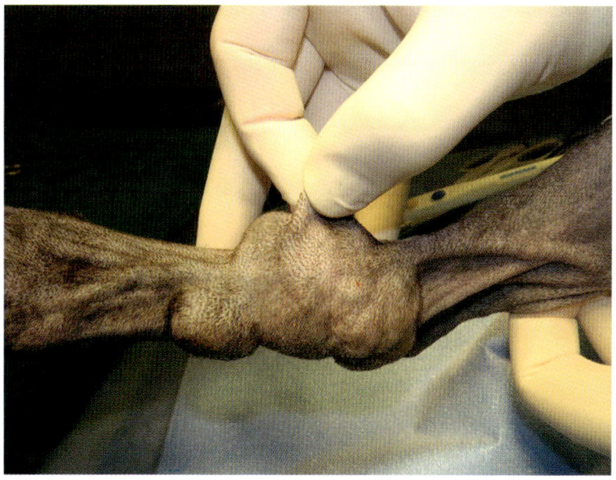

E-iii)

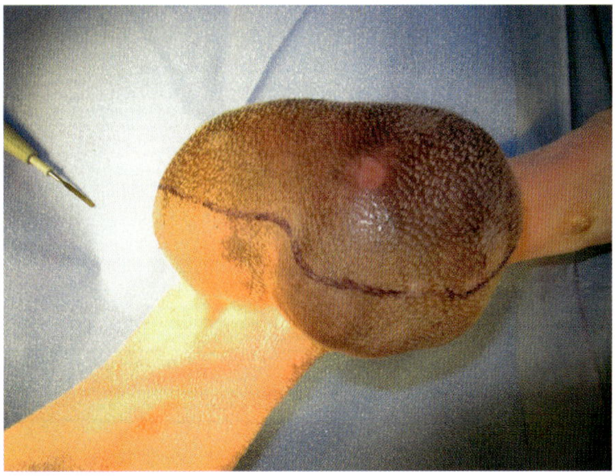

F-i)

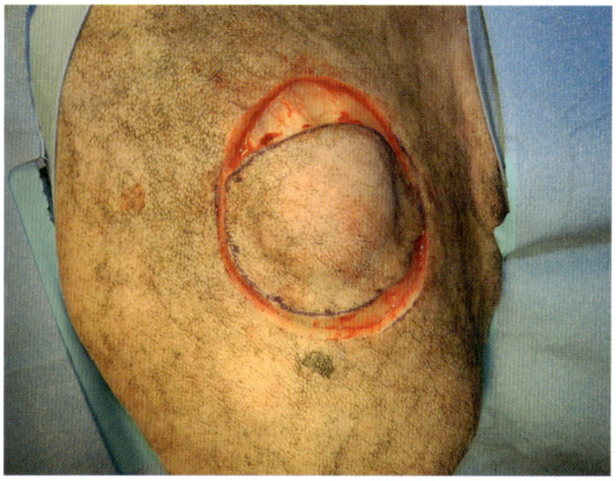

F-ii)

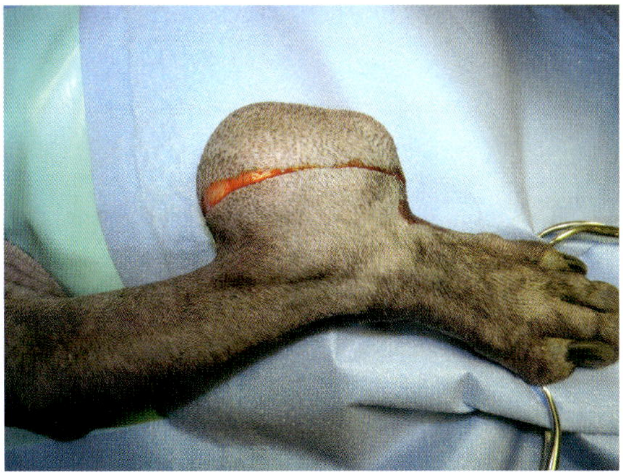

F-iii)

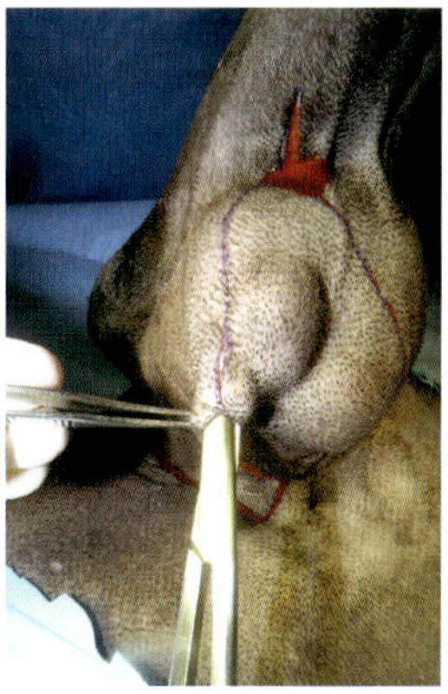

F-iv)

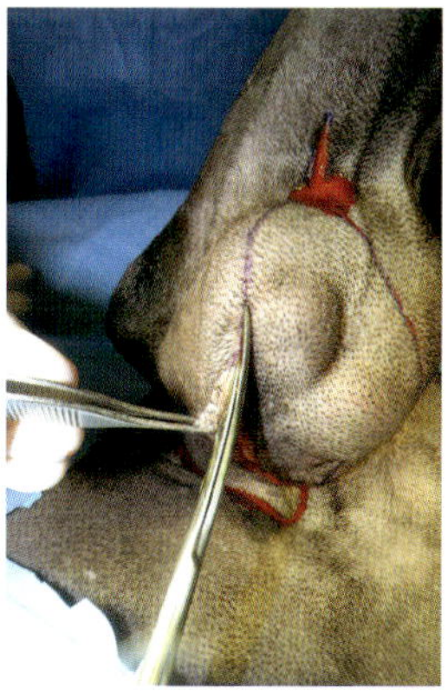

Surgical Technique – Marginal Surgical Resection (See Plate 1E–H) *continued*

G) The dissection is continued deeply through the subcutaneous tissue perpendicular to the skin incision. If the incision has been made in the movable skin over a subcutaneous tumor, then the freely movable skin should be carefully dissected off the tumor to minimize the risk of compromising the tumor capsule (i–iii).

H) If a deep fascial layer is planned to be included in the resection, then this may include partial or full-thickness muscle deep to the tumor (i, ii). Inclusion of this layer rarely results in functional deficits postsurgery. If a deep fascial layer is not planned to be included in the resection, then the deep aspect of the tumor should be dissected very carefully off the deeper normal tissue to prevent compromising the tumor capsule (iii, iv).

Plate 1

Surgical Resection of Cutaneous and Subcutaneous Tumors *continued*

G-i)

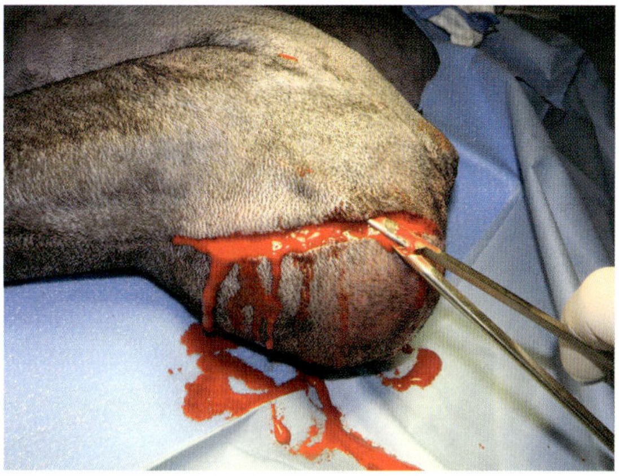

G-ii)

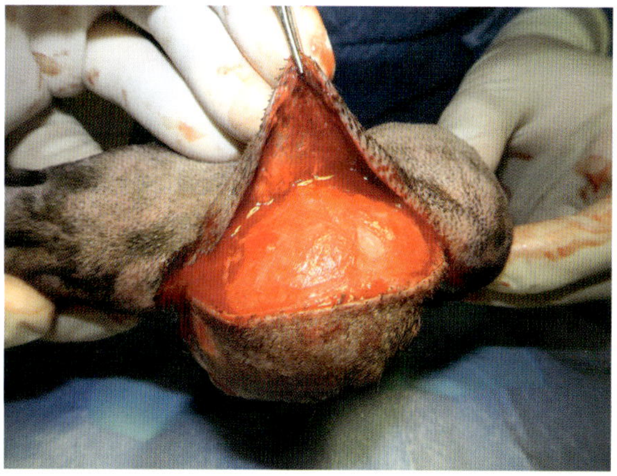

G-iii)

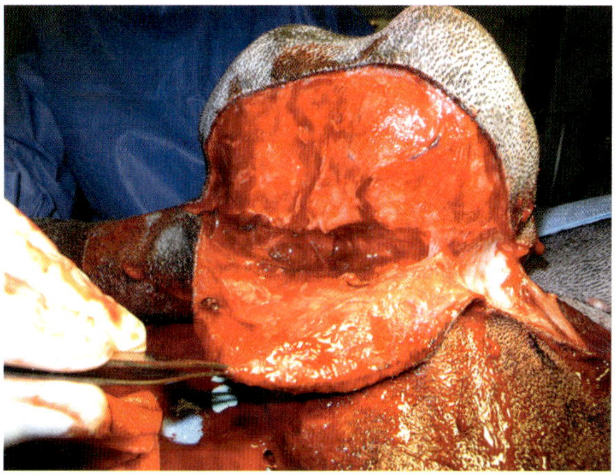

H-i)

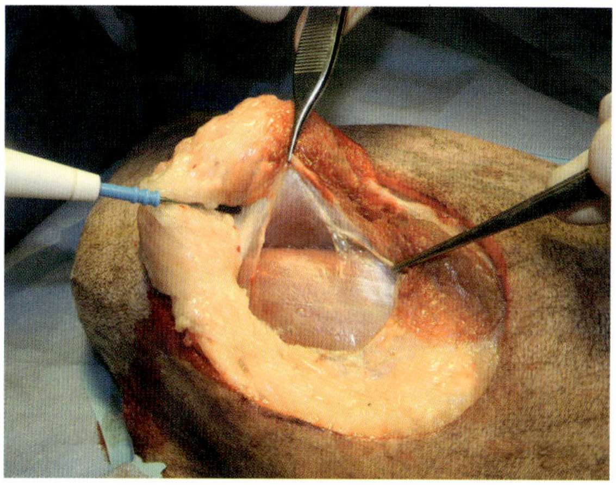

H-ii)

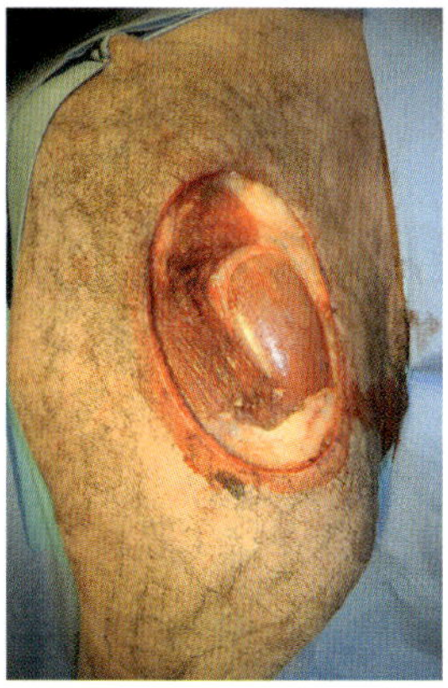

H-iii)

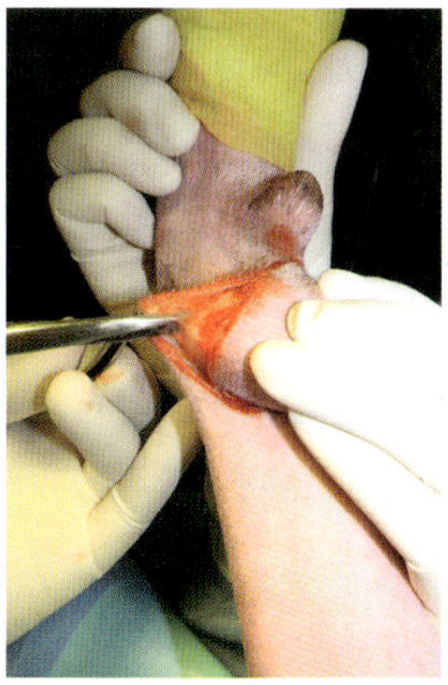

H-iv)

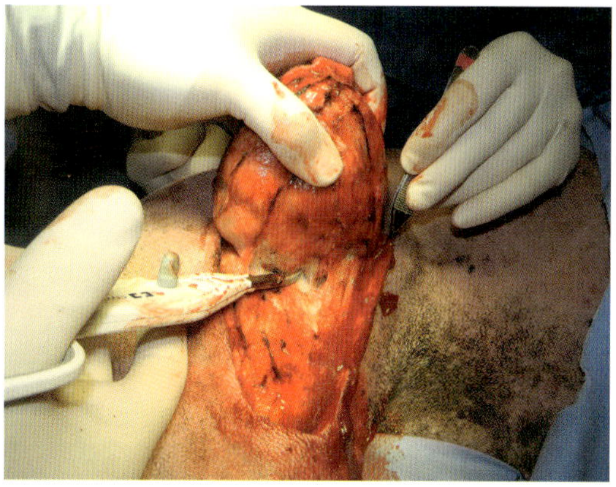

Closure (See Plate 1I)

I) For primary closure, the deep aspect of the defect can be closed, if required, using 0 to 3-0 absorbable monofilament suture material in a simple interrupted or continuous suture pattern (i, ii). The skin incision is closed routinely in two layers with a simple continuous suture pattern using monofilament absorbable suture material in the subcutis and either an interrupted or continuous suture pattern using monofilament nonabsorbable suture material in the skin (iii–vi).

Postoperative Management

1) Multimodal analgesia
2) Elizabethan collar

Complications in Dogs [4, 5]

- Overall: 13%–24%
- Surgical-site infection
- Incisional dehiscence
- Seroma

Suggested Adjuvant Treatments

Treatment is dependent on histologic margins, tumor type, and histologic grade.

References

1 Simpson, A.M., Ludwig, L.L., Newman, S.J. et al. (2004). Evaluation of surgical margins required for complete excision of cutaneous mast cell tumors in dogs. *J. Am. Vet. Med. Assoc.* 224 (2): 236–240.

2 Pratschke, K.M., Atherton, M.J., Sillito, J.A. et al. (2013). Evaluation of a modified proportional margins approach for surgical resection of mast cell tumors in dogs: 40 cases (2008-2012). *J. Am. Vet. Med. Assoc.* 243 (10): 1436–1441.

3 Del Magno, S., Morello, E., Iussich, S. et al. (2021). Evaluation of the neoplastic infiltration of the skin overlying canine subcutaneous soft tissue sarcomas: an explorative study. *Vet. Comp. Oncol.* 19 (2): 304–310.

4 Iodence, A.E., Wallace, M.L., Grimes, J.A. et al. (2021). Dogs undergoing surgical excision of mast cell tumors are not at increased risk of incisional complications. *J. Am. Vet. Med. Assoc.* 260 (suppl 1): S88–S95.

5 Cockburn, E., Jonovec, J., Solano, M.A. et al. (2022). Marginal excision of cutaneous mast cell tumors in dogs was not associated with a higher rate of complications or prolonged wound healing than marginal excision of soft tissue sarcomas. *J. Am. Vet. Med. Assoc.* 260 (7): 741–746.

Plate 1

Surgical Resection of Cutaneous and Subcutaneous Tumors *continued*

I-i)

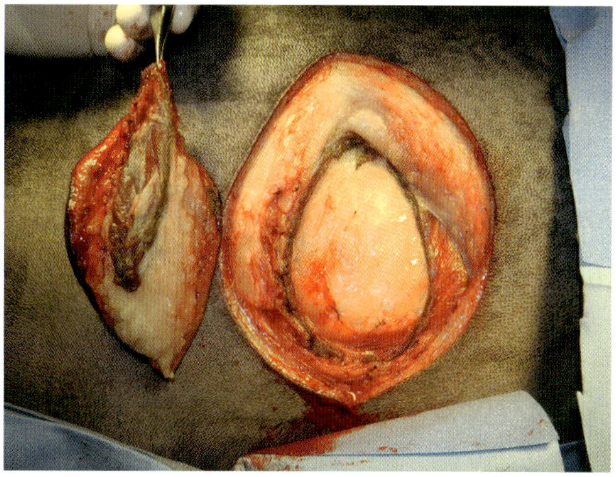

I-ii)

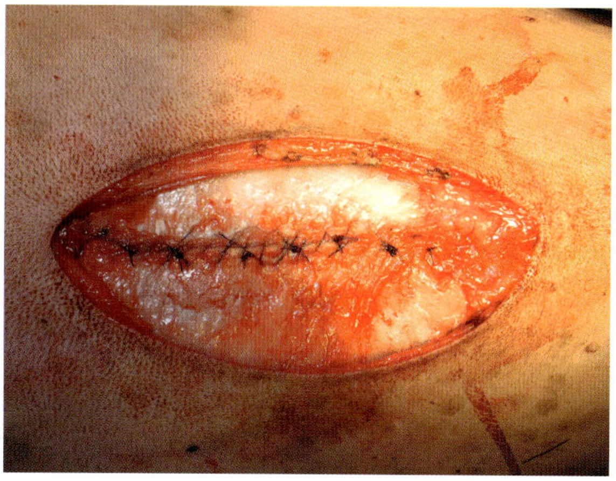

I-iii)

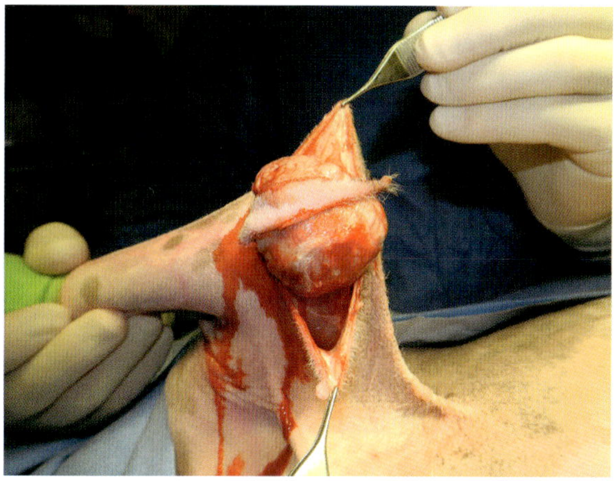

I-iv)

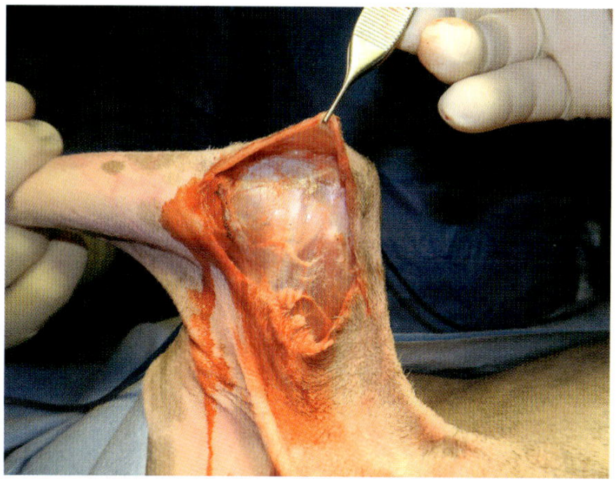

I-v)

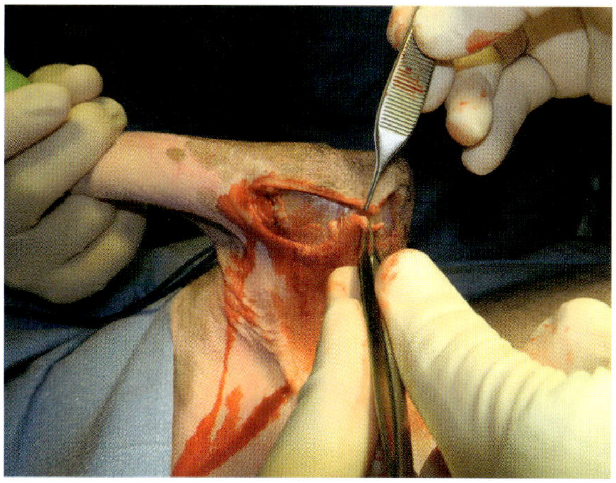

I-vi)

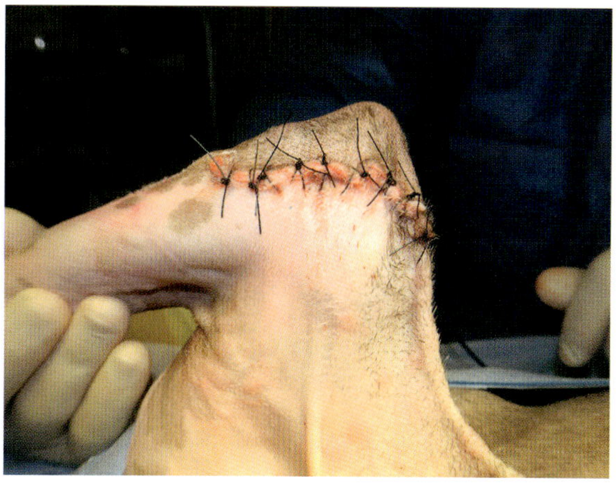

Section 2

Head and Neck

Chapter 2: Eyes and Orbit

2.1 Enucleation

Indications

1) Resection of primary intraocular tumors
2) Palliation for exophthalmos secondary to retrobulbar or orbital tumors
3) Treatment of primary intraocular disease or trauma or prolapsed eye

Suggested Diagnostic Workup and Clinical Staging

- Complete blood count, serum biochemistry, and urinalysis
- ± Ultrasound, computed tomography (CT) scan, or magnetic resonance imaging of the affected eye
- ± Ultrasound-guided fine-needle aspiration and cytology
- ± Ultrasound-guided aspiration of the regional lymph nodes (parotid and medial retropharyngeal) for clinical staging if a malignant tumor is suspected
- ± Three-view thoracic radiographs or CT scan for clinical staging if a malignant tumor is suspected

Patient Positioning

The patient is positioned in lateral recumbency with the affected side uppermost.

Surgical Technique – Subconjunctival Approach (See Plate 2.1A–E)

A) A 1- to 2-cm lateral canthotomy can be performed to increase exposure.
B) The upper (i) and lower eyelids (ii), third eyelid (iii), and third eyelid gland (iv) are excised either before (pictured) or after excision of the globe (see step E).

Color Atlas of Canine and Feline Surgical Oncology, First Edition. Julius M. Liptak, Paolo Buracco, William T. N. Culp, and Nicholas J. Bacon.

Plate 2.1

Enucleation

A)

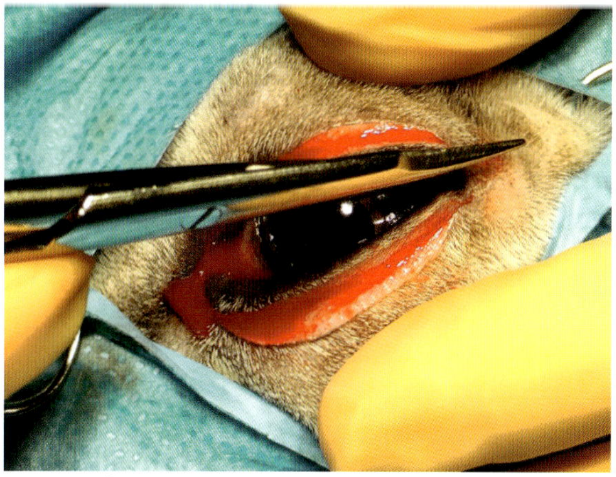

Courtesy of Dr. Adolfo Guandalini

B-i)

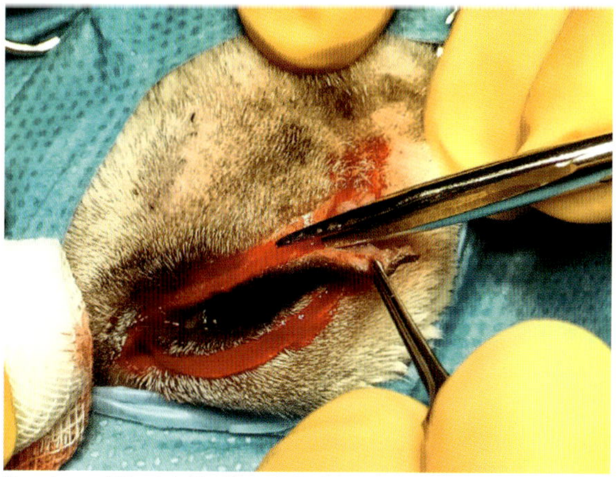

Courtesy of Dr. Adolfo Guandalini

B-ii)

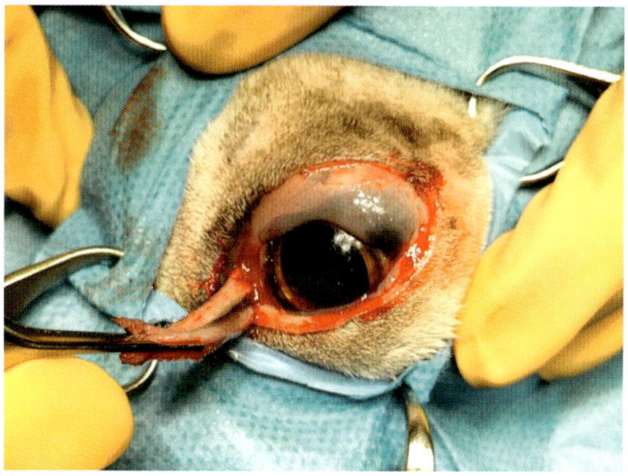

Courtesy of Dr. Adolfo Guandalini

B-iii)

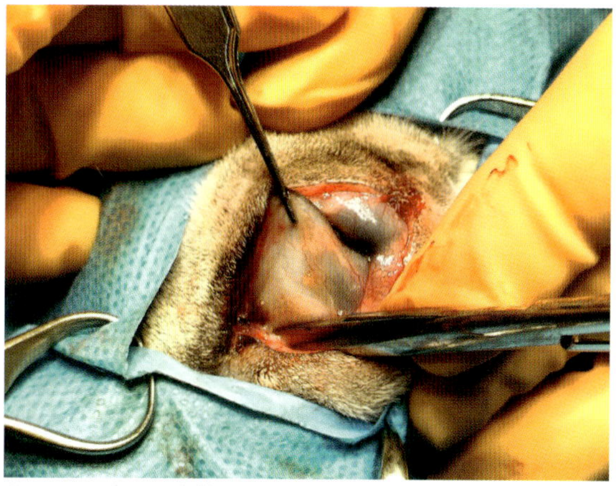

Courtesy of Dr. Adolfo Guandalini

B-iv)

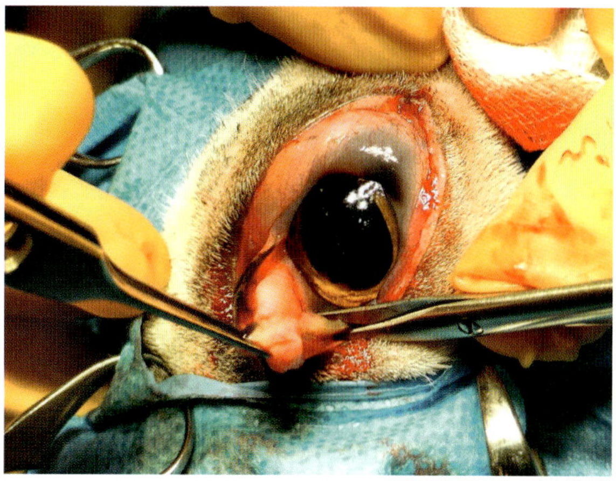

Courtesy of Dr. Adolfo Guandalini

Surgical Technique – Subconjunctival Approach (See Plate 2.1A–E) *continued*

C) Grasp the conjunctiva adjacent to the limbus and perform a 360-degree perilimbal incision with iris scissors (i–iii).
D) Progressively elevate and transect conjunctival, fascial, and extraocular muscle attachments to the sclera with Metzenbaum scissors.
E) The third eyelid (i, ii) and lower (iii, iv) and upper eyelids (v) are excised.

Plate 2.1

Enucleation *continued*

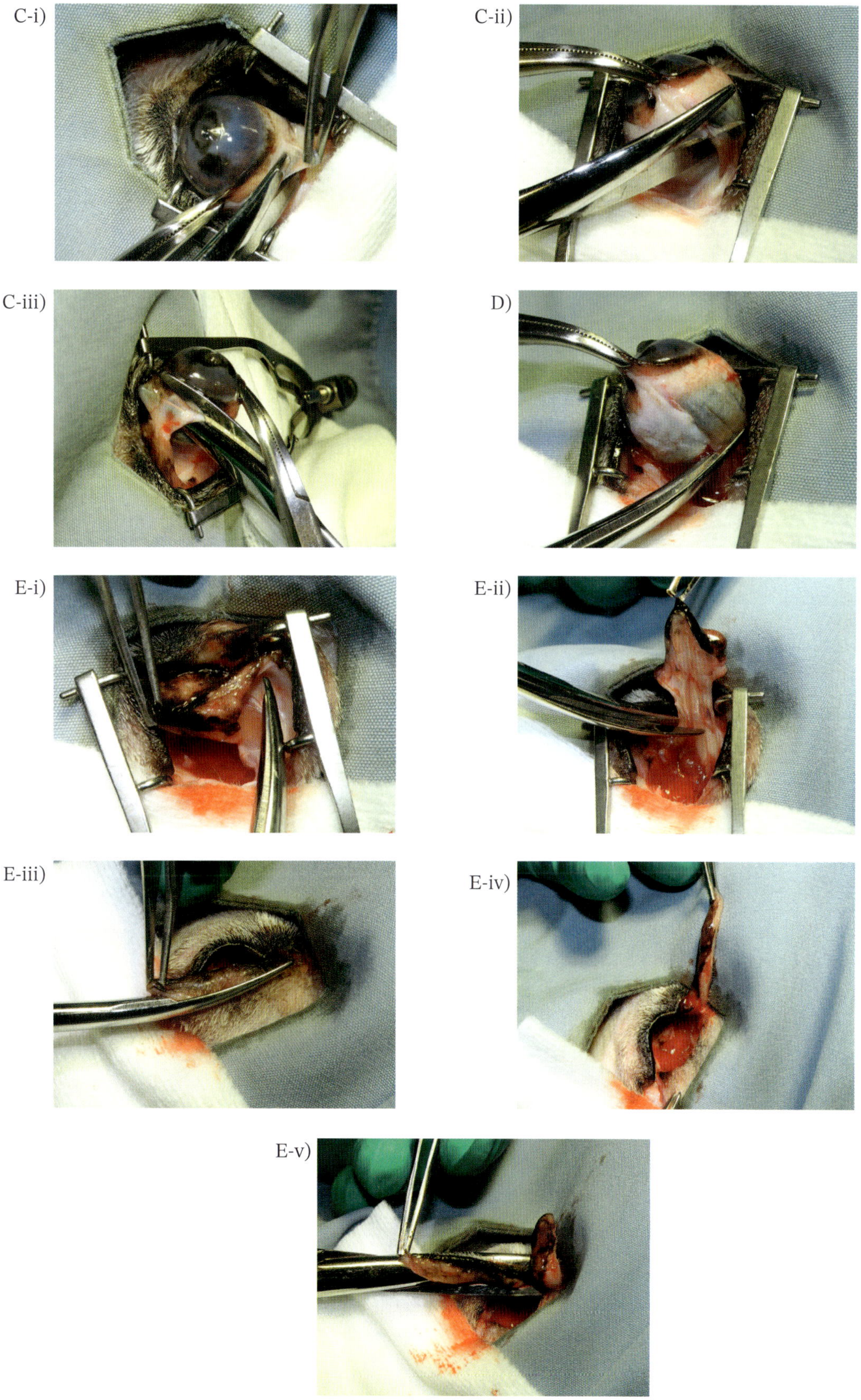

Surgical Technique – Transpalpebral Approach (See Plate 2.1F–H)

F) Suture the eyelid margins using a continuous suture pattern. The ends of the suture may be used as stay sutures for manipulation/traction (i). Perform an elliptical periocular incision around the eyelids (ii).
G) Continue the dissection circumferentially down to, but not perforating, the conjunctiva (i) and transect the orbital septum at the level of the orbital rim (ii).
H) Progressively elevate and transect fascial and extraocular muscle attachments to the sclera with Metzenbaum scissors (i, ii).

Surgical Technique Common to Both Approaches – Optic Nerve Transection (See Plate 2.1I–K)

I) Apply a clamp to the optic nerve and associated vessels and wait for 3–5 minutes.
J) Transect the optic nerve while avoiding excessive traction to avoid damage to the optic chiasma. Transection can be done with either Metzenbaum or Mayo (i) scissors or a vessel sealing device. The enucleated globe is then removed from the surgical field (ii).

Plate 2.1

Enucleation *continued*

F-i)

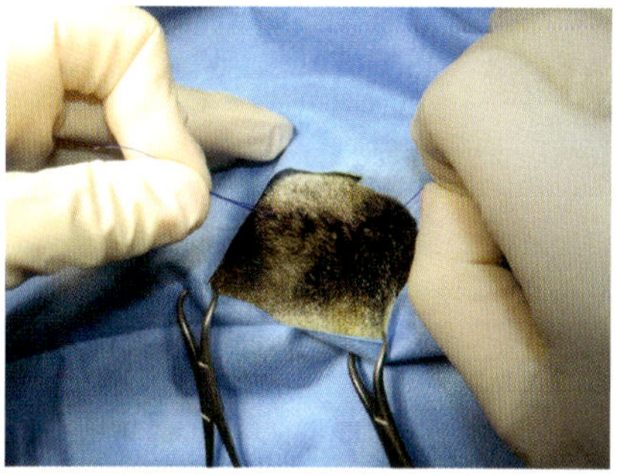

F-ii)

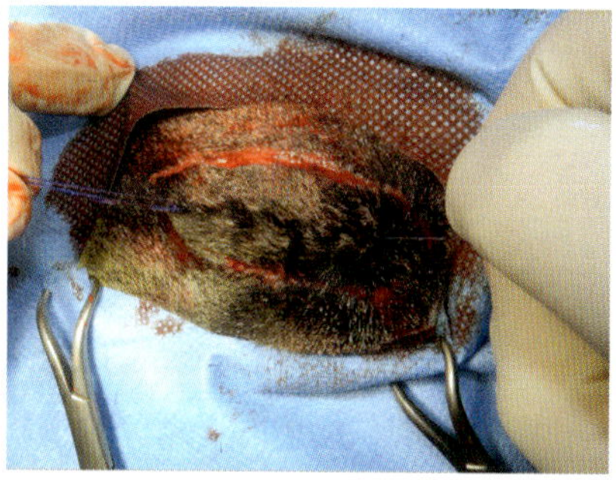

G-i)

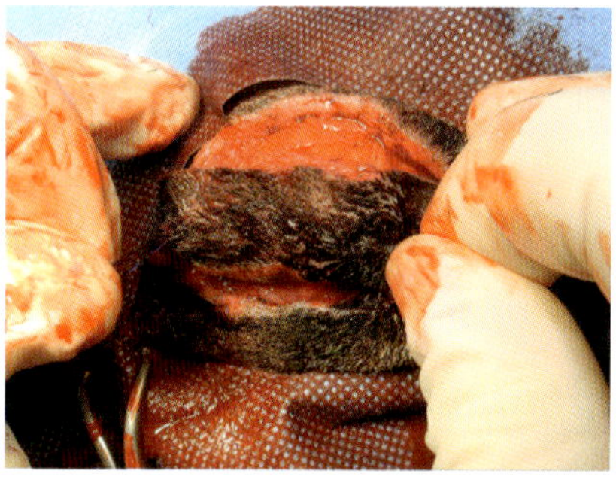

G-ii)

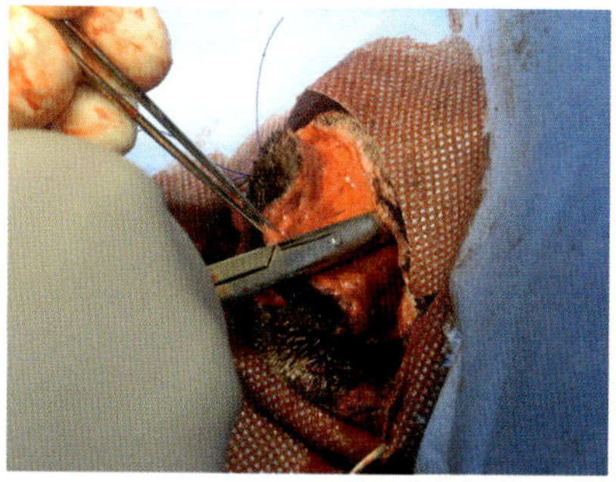

H-i)

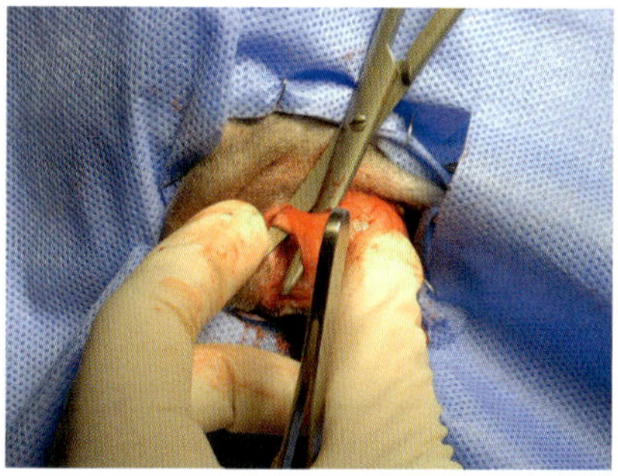

Courtesy of Dr. Mischa McDonald-Lynch

H-ii)

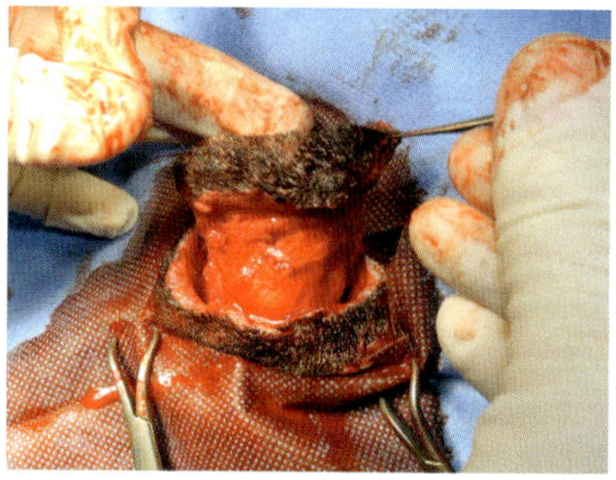

I)

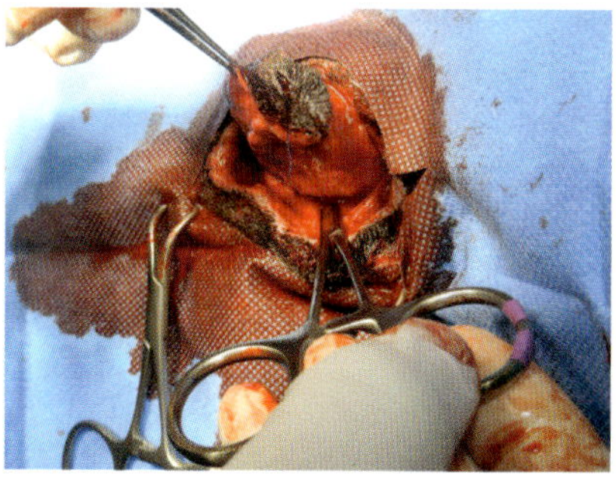

J-i)

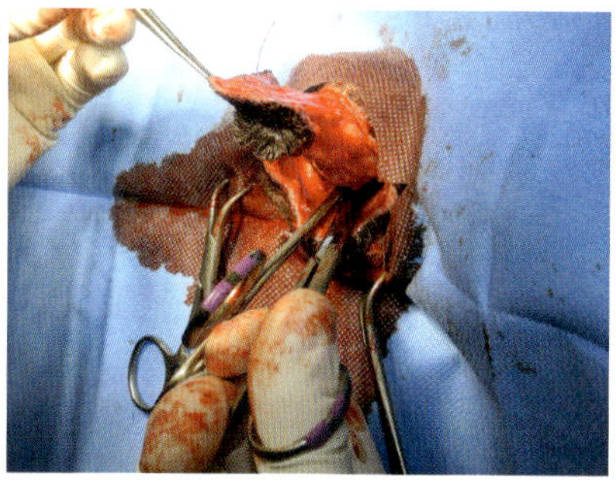

J-ii)

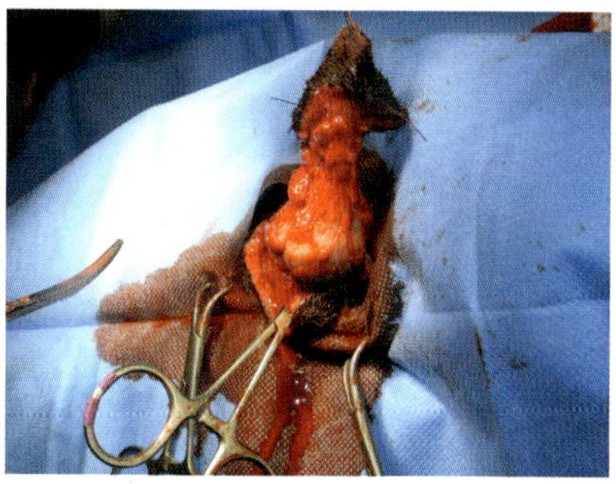

Surgical Technique Common to Both Approaches – Optic Nerve Transection (See Plate 2.1I–K) *continued*

K) Alternatively, the optic nerve can be transected without clamping. If not performed with a vessel sealing device, then the transected end of the optic nerve can be clamped for 3–5 minutes (pictured). If bleeding persists, then the orbit can be packed with gauze swabs for 3–5 minutes to compress the vessel, the orbit can be packed with absorbable hemostatic sponges, or the vessel can be ligated, cauterized, or sealed. Additional analgesia can be provided with either a bupivacaine splash block or packing the orbit with an absorbable gelatin hemostatic sponge soaked with 1% ropivacaine solution [1].

Closure (See Plate 2.1L)

L) The wound is closed routinely in three layers. A simple continuous suture pattern using monofilament absorbable suture material is used to close the orbital fascia and subcutis (i). An interrupted or continuous suture pattern using monofilament nonabsorbable suture material is used to close the skin (ii).

Postoperative Management

1) Multimodal analgesia
2) Elizabethan collar

Complications

- Bleeding
- Swelling/seroma
- Infection
- Contralateral blindness if excessive traction is applied to the optic nerve with subsequent damage to the optic chiasma
- Chronic drainage secondary to infraorbital mucocele/cyst formation if all the conjunctival tissue and glandular tissue are not excised [2]
- Emphysema in brachycephalic dogs if the nasolacrimal duct is not ligated or removed [3]

Suggested Adjuvant Treatments

- ± Chemotherapy, depending on tumor type and histologic grade
- ± Radiation therapy, depending on tumor type and completeness of excision

Plate 2.1

Enucleation *continued*

K)

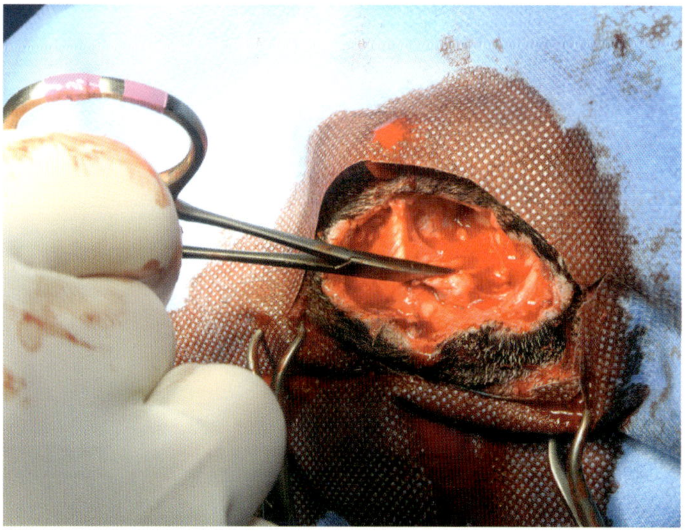

L-i)

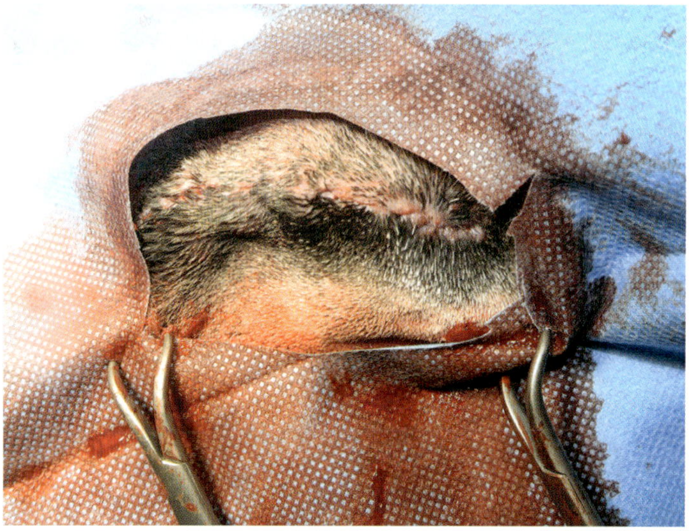

L-ii)

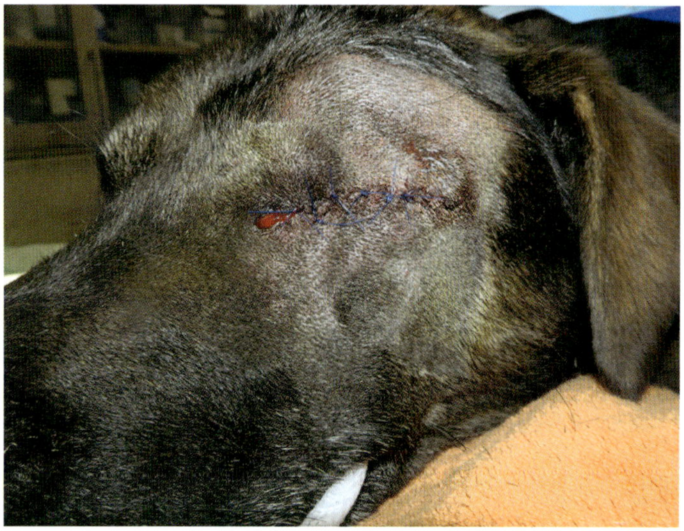

Prognosis and Oncologic Outcome

Tumor Type	Local Recurrence Rate	Metastatic Rate	Disease-Free Interval (d)	Median Survival Time (d)	1-Year Survival Rate	2-Year Survival Rate
Lymphoma – dog [4]						
• Intraocular	–	–	178	178	–	–
• Conjunctival	–	–	221	549	–	–
Lymphoma – cat [5]						
• Intraocular	–	–	–	154	–	–
• Intraocular/systemic	–	–	–	69	–	–
Iris melanoma – cat [6]	–	19%–24%	–	1095	–	–
Ocular posttraumatic sarcoma – cat [7]	–	Rare	–	213–335	–	–
Iridociliary adenoma/ adenocarcinoma – dog [8]	57%	–	–	–	–	–
Orbital meningioma – dog [9]	35%	0%	–	NR	–	–

NR, not reached.

References

1 Shilo-Benjamini, Y., Slav, S.A., Kahane, N. et al. (2019). Analgesic effects of intraorbital insertion of an absorbable gelatin hemostatic sponge soaked with 1% ropivacaine solution following enucleation in dogs. *J. Am. Vet. Med. Assoc.* 255 (11): 1255–1262.

2 Ward, A.A. and Neaderland, M.H. (2011). Complications from residual adnexal structures following enucleation in three dogs. *J. Am. Vet. Med. Assoc.* 239 (12): 1580–1583.

3 Cho, J. (2008). Surgery of the globe and orbit. *Top. Companion Anim. Med.* 23 (1): 23–37.

4 Wiggans, K.T., Skorupski, K.A., Reilly, C.M. et al. (2014). Presumed solitary intraocular or conjunctival lymphoma in dogs and cats: 9 cases (1985-2013). *J. Am. Vet. Med. Assoc.* 244 (4): 460–470.

5 Musciano, A.R., Lanza, M.R., Dubielzig, R.R. et al. (2020). Clinical and histopathological classification of feline intraocular lymphoma. *Vet. Ophthalmol.* 23 (1): 77–89.

6 Wiggans, K.T., Reilly, C.M., Kass, P.H. et al. (2016). Histologic and immunohistochemical predictors of clinical behavior for feline diffuse iris melanoma. *Vet. Ophthalmol.* 19 (suppl 1): 44–55.

7 Wood, C. and Scott, E.M. (2019). Feline ocular post-traumatic sarcomas: current understanding, treatment and monitoring. *J. Feline Med. Surg.* 21 (9): 835–842.

8 Beckwith-Cohen, B., Bentley, E., and Dubielzig, R.R. (2015). Outcome of iridociliary epithelial tumour biopsies in dogs: a retrospective study. *Vet. Rec.* 176 (6): 147.

9 Mauldin, E.A., Deehr, A.J., Hertzke, D. et al. (2000). Canine orbital meningiomas: a review of 22 cases. *Vet. Ophthalmol.* 3 (1): 11–16.

2.2 Exenteration

Indications

1) Resection of primary ocular tumors with extraocular extension
2) Resection of primary extensive or infiltrative infraorbital tumors
3) Resection of extensive or infiltrative eyelid, third eyelid, or lacrimal gland tumors

Suggested Diagnostic Workup and Clinical Staging

- Complete blood count, serum biochemistry, and urinalysis
- Fine-needle aspirate cytology or incisional biopsy of eyelid, third eyelid, or lacrimal gland tumors.
- ± Ultrasound, computed tomography (CT) scan, or magnetic resonance imaging of the affected eye
- ± Ultrasound-guided fine-needle aspiration and cytology
- ± Ultrasound-guided aspiration of the regional lymph nodes (parotid and retropharyngeal) for clinical staging if a malignant tumor is suspected.
- ± Three-view thoracic radiographs or CT scan for clinical staging if a malignant tumor is suspected.

Patient Positioning

The patient is positioned in lateral recumbency with the affected side uppermost.

Surgical Technique (See Plate 2.2A–C)

A) Make an elliptical incision around the periorbital mass with appropriate lateral margins for the tumor type (pictured), or suture the eyelids closed with a continuous suture pattern and then perform an elliptical periorbital incision around the eyelids if an ocular or infraorbital tumor is being resected.
B) Continue the dissection circumferentially and deeply to include the extraocular muscle attachments to the orbit (i); the globe, third eyelid, and all periorbital tissue (ii); and the orbital periosteum, if indicated (iii, arrows).
C) Transect the optic nerve while avoiding excessive traction to avoid damage to the optic chiasma. Transection can be done with either Metzenbaum or Mayo scissors or a vessel sealing device (pictured).

Color Atlas of Canine and Feline Surgical Oncology, First Edition. Julius M. Liptak, Paolo Buracco, William T. N. Culp, and Nicholas J. Bacon.

Plate 2.2

Exenteration

A)

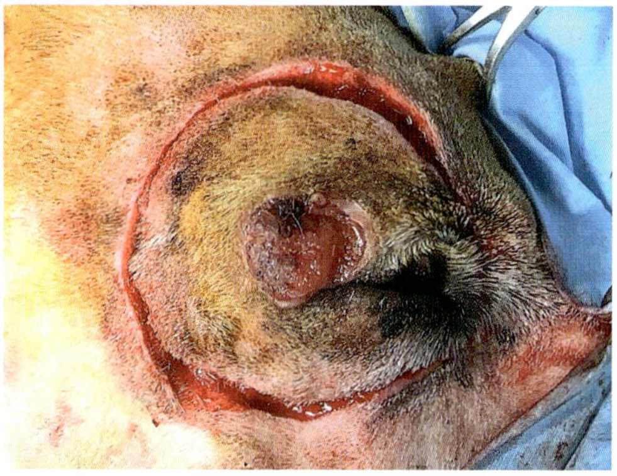

B-i)

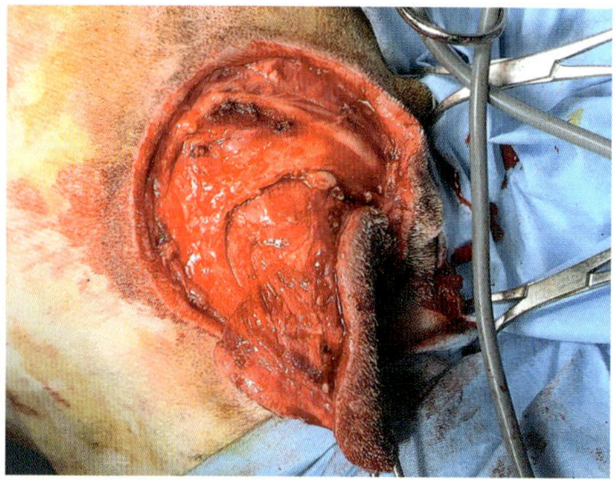

B-i)

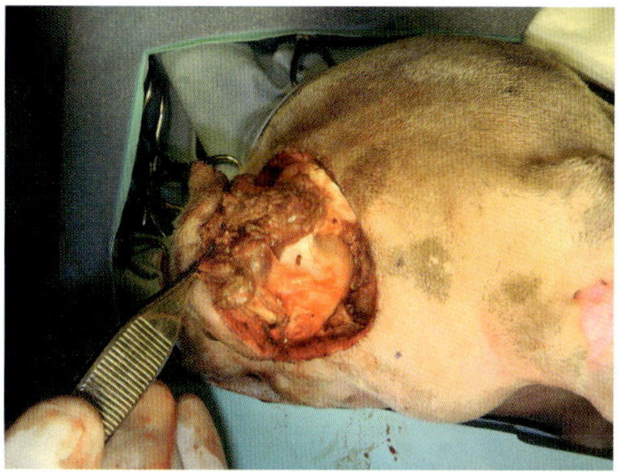

B-ii)

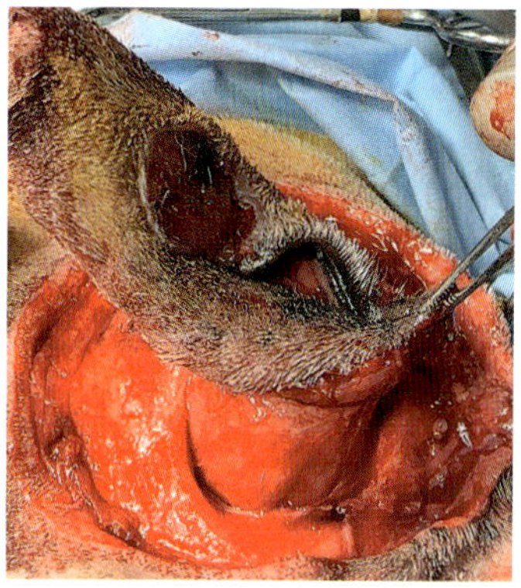

B-ii)

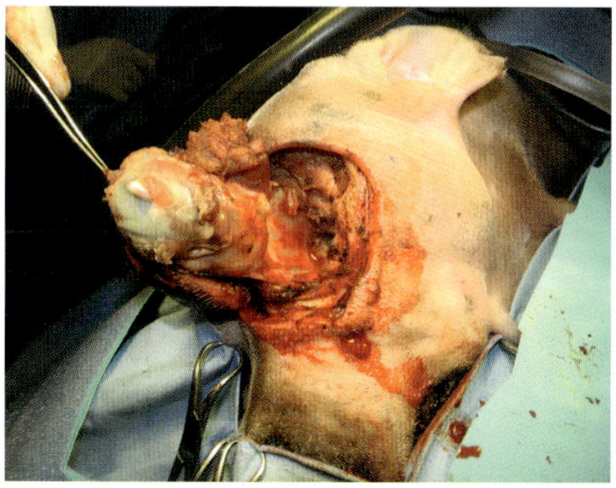

B-iii)

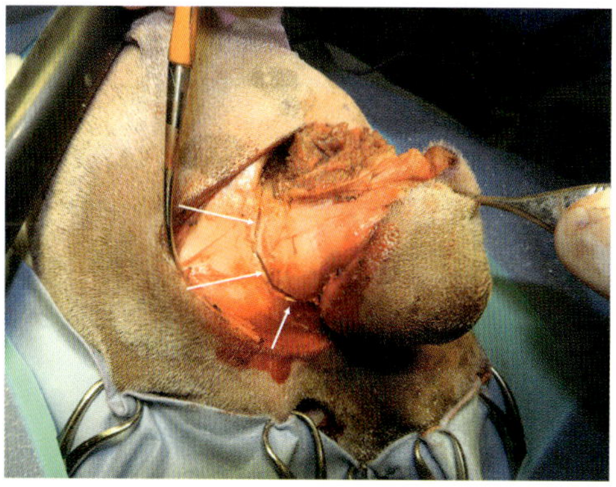

C)

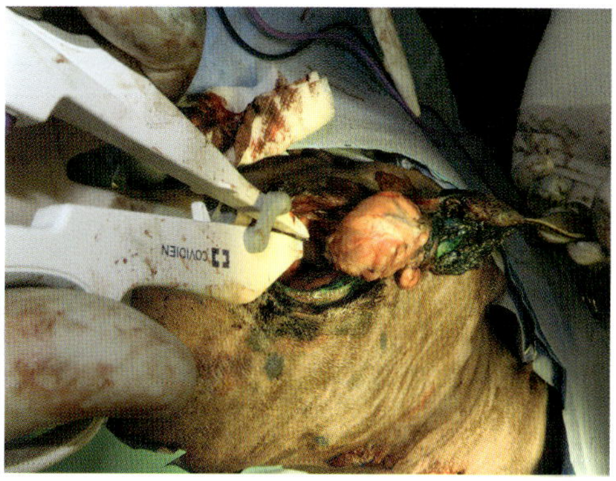

Closure (See Plate 2.2D)

D) To avoid concavity of skin over the orbit, consider placement of a mesh of nonabsorbable suture material placed through predrilled holes in the ventral and dorsal orbital rims (i) in a simple interrupted or cruciate suture pattern (ii). The wound is then closed routinely in two layers. A simple continuous suture pattern using monofilament absorbable suture material is used to close the subcutis. An interrupted or continuous suture pattern using monofilament nonabsorbable suture material is used to close the skin (iii). Following wide resection of some eyelid tumors, the resulting wound may not be able to be closed primarily. In these cases, reconstructive surgery may be required for wound closure. Options for closure of periocular defects include an advancement flap (see *39. Advancement Flap*), rotation flap (see *40. Rotation Flap*), transposition flap (see *41. Transposition Flap*), facial axial pattern flap (see *43.1. Facial Axial Pattern Flap*), or caudal auricular axial pattern flap (see *43.3. Caudal Auricular Axial Pattern Flap*).

Postoperative Management

1) Multimodal analgesia
2) Elizabethan collar

Complications

- Bleeding
- Swelling/seroma
- Infection
- Contralateral blindness if excessive traction is applied to the optic nerve with subsequent damage to the optic chiasma
- Chronic drainage secondary to infraorbital mucocele/cyst formation if all the conjunctival tissue and glandular tissue are not excised [1]
- Emphysema in brachycephalic dogs if the nasolacrimal duct is not ligated or removed [2]

Suggested Adjuvant Treatments

- ± Chemotherapy, depending on tumor type and histologic grade
- ± Radiation therapy, depending on tumor type and completeness of excision

Plate 2.2

Exenteration *continued*

D-i)

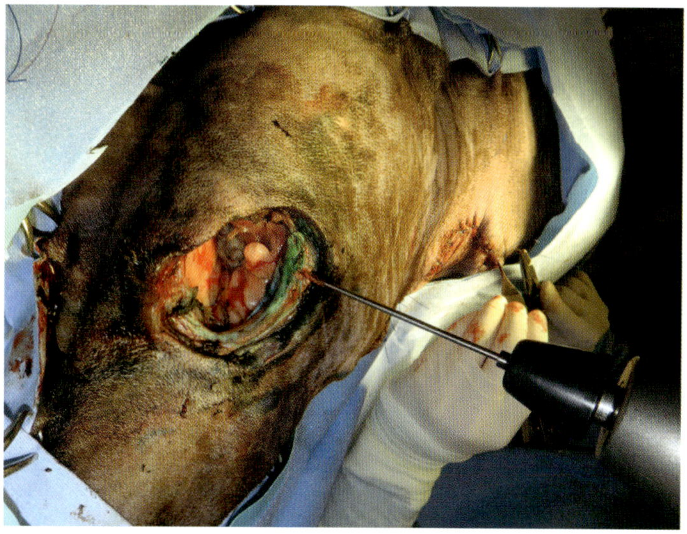

D-ii)

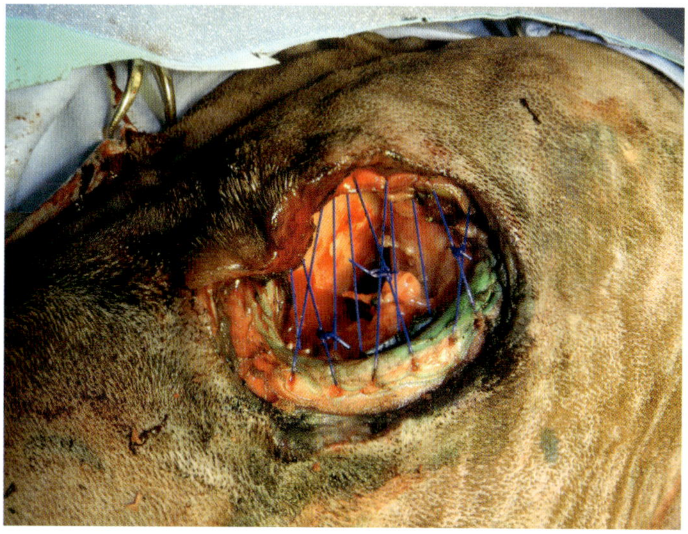

D-iii)

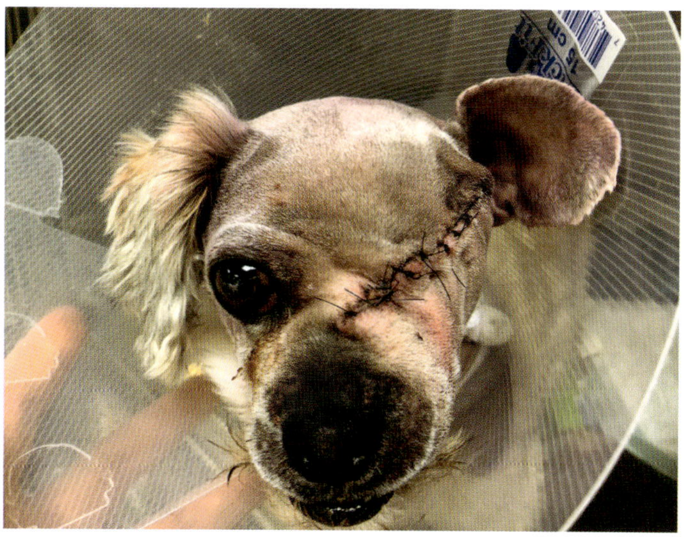

Prognosis and Oncologic Outcome

Tumor Type	Local Recurrence Rate	Metastatic Rate	Disease-Free Interval (d)	Median Survival Time (d)	1-Year Survival Rate	2-Year Survival Rate
Orbital lobular adenoma – dog [3]	33%	0%	–	–	–	–
Conjunctival melanoma – cat [4]	30%	23%	–	–	–	–
Conjunctival mast cell tumor – dog [5]	8%	0%	–	NR	–	–
Third eyelid gland adenocarcinoma [6]						
• Dog	13%	9%	–	671	–	–
• Cat	25%	50%	–	335	–	–
Orbital rhabdomyosarcoma – dog [7]						
• ≤4 years	56%	56%	–	–	–	–
• ≥6 years	0%	0%	–	–	–	–
Optic nerve meningioma – dog [8]	35%	0%	–	NR	–	–

NR, not reached.

References

1 Ward, A.A. and Neaderland, M.H. (2011). Complications from residual adnexal structures following enucleation in three dogs. *J. Am. Vet. Med. Assoc.* 239 (12): 1580–1583.

2 Cho, J. (2008). Surgery of the globe and orbit. *Top. Companion Anim. Med.* 23 (1): 23–37.

3 Headrick, J.F., Bentley, E., and Dubielzig, R.R. (2004). Canine lobular orbital adenoma: a report of 15 cases with distinctive features. *Vet. Ophthalmol.* 7 (1): 47–51.

4 Schobert, C.S., Labelle, P., and Dubielzig, R.R. (2010). Feline conjunctival melanoma: histopathological characteristics and clinical outcomes. *Vet. Ophthalmol.* 13 (1): 43–46.

5 Fife, M., Blocker, T., Fife, T. et al. (2011). Canine conjunctival mast cell tumors: a retrospective study. *Vet. Ophthalmol.* 14 (3): 153–160.

6 Dees, D.D., Schobert, C.S., Dubielzig, R.R. et al. (2016). Third eyelid gland neoplasms of dogs and cats: a retrospective histopathologic study of 145 cases. *Vet. Ophthalmol.* 19 (2): 138–143.

7 Scott, E.M., Teixeira, L.B.C., Flanders, D.J. et al. (2016). Canine orbital rhabdomyosarcoma: a report of 18 cases. *Vet. Ophthalmol.* 19 (2): 130–137.

8 Mauldin, E.A., Deehr, A.J., Hertzke, D. et al. (2000). Canine orbital meningiomas: a review of 22 cases. *Vet. Ophthalmol.* 3 (1): 11–16.

2.3 Lateral Orbitotomy

Indications

1) Approach for resection of benign or malignant retrobulbar tumors
2) This explorative approach can be converted, if necessary, to an exenteration (see *2.2. Exenteration*)
3) Lateral orbitotomy can be combined with a caudal mandibulectomy (see *6.6. Caudal Mandibulectomy*) for additional exposure

Suggested Diagnostic Workup and Clinical Staging

- Complete blood count, serum biochemistry, and urinalysis
- Ultrasound-guided aspirate or biopsy, if possible
- Regional imaging, such as ultrasound, computed tomography scan, or magnetic resonance imaging

Patient Positioning

The patient is positioned in either sternal recumbency or lateral recumbency with the affected eye uppermost.

Surgical Technique – Modified Lateral Approach [1, 2] (See Plate 2.3A–F)

A) Make a skin incision along the dorsal border of the zygomatic arch from ventral to the lateral canthus to 2–3 cm rostral to the base of the ear. Identify the palpebral nerve immediately dorsal to the incision and retract it dorsally.
B) Incise the insertion of the temporalis (TM) and masseter muscles (MM) on the dorsal and ventral aspects of the zygomatic arch (ZA), respectively, and elevate these muscles to retract them away from the zygomatic arch. Transect the orbital ligament at its midpoint and apply a suture to each end to allow identification of the ends for apposition after completion of the procedure. In select cases, the orbital ligament can be preserved.
C) Rostral (i) and caudal (ii) osteotomies of the zygomatic arch are then performed with an oscillating or sagittal saw or Gigli wire. The soft tissues medial to the zygomatic arch are protected with periosteal elevators or malleable retractors when performing the osteotomies. The zygomatic branch of the infraorbital artery and facial vein should be preserved along the rostral aspect of the zygomatic arch. The zygomatic arch is commonly discarded after resection (iii, iv); however, if the zygomatic arch is to be preserved, then two holes can be predrilled on either side of the proposed rostral and caudal osteotomies for later reconstruction with hemicerclage wires.

Color Atlas of Canine and Feline Surgical Oncology, First Edition. Julius M. Liptak, Paolo Buracco, William T. N. Culp, and Nicholas J. Bacon.

Plate 2.3

Lateral Orbitotomy

A)

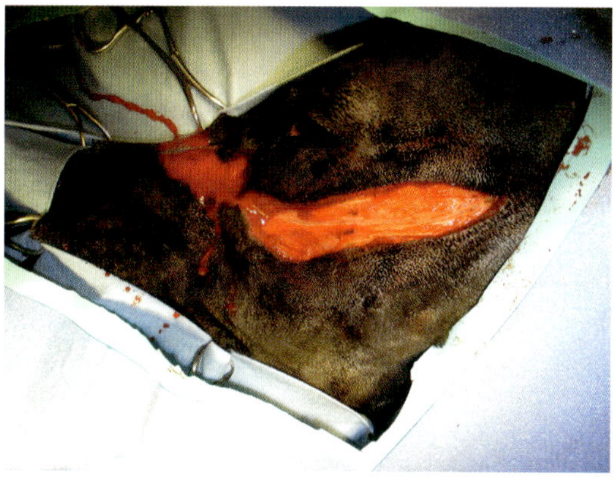

B)

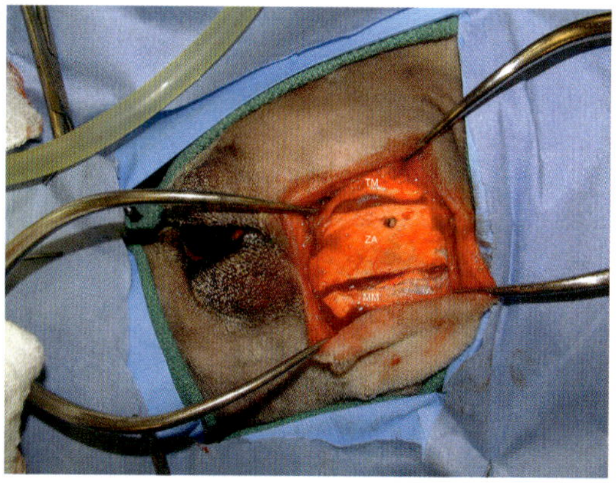

B)

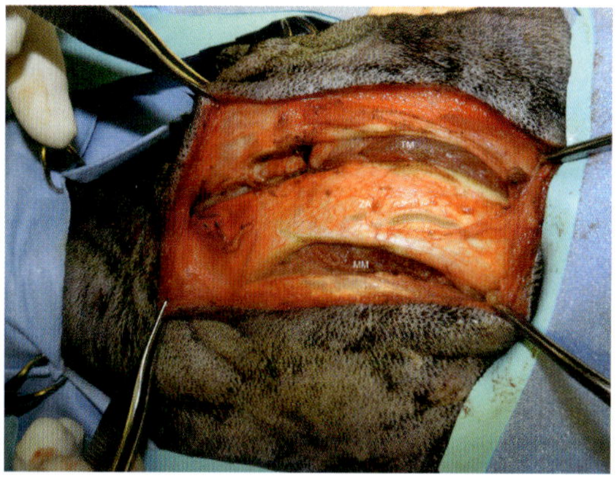

C-i)

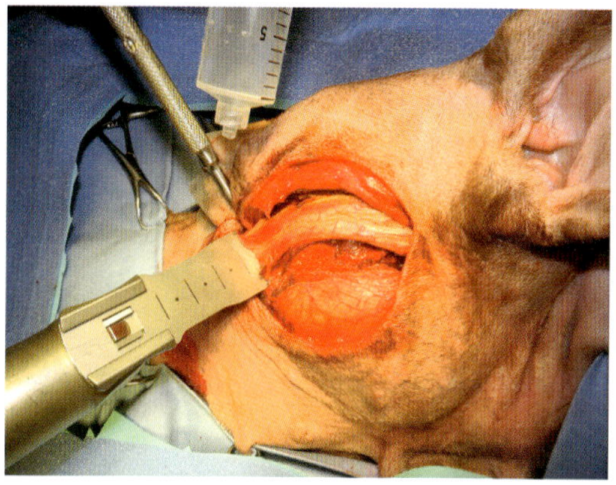

C-ii)

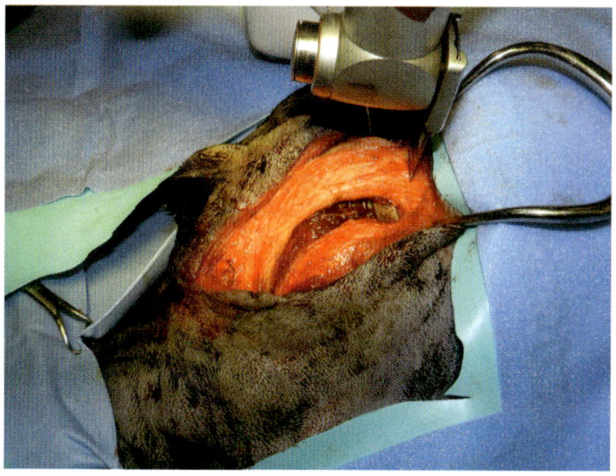

C-iii)

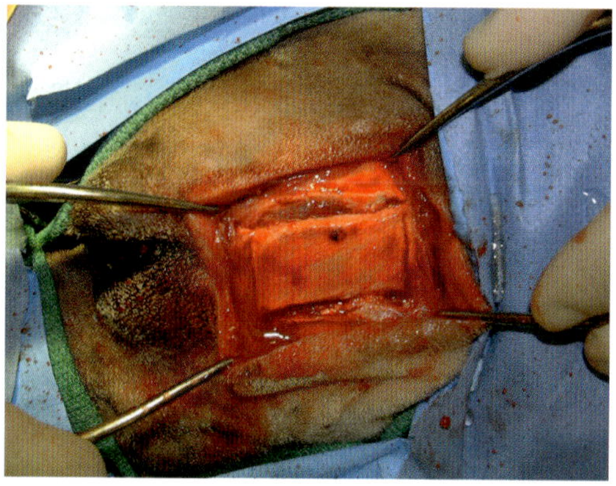

C-iv)

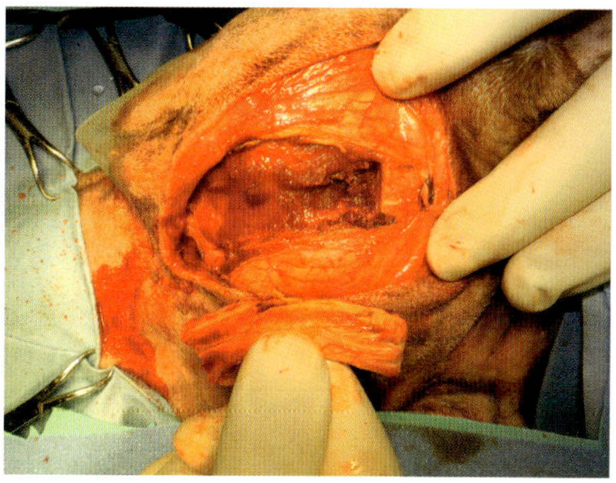

Surgical Technique – Modified Lateral Approach [1, 2] (See Plate 2.3A–F) *continued*

D) A caudal mandibulectomy (see *6.6. Caudal Mandibulectomy*) can be performed to increase exposure of the caudal aspect of the orbit for resection of larger retrobulbar masses. The masseter is transected along the planned osteotomy site, and an osteotomy of the ramus of the mandible is performed proximal to the temporomandibular joint with an oscillating or sagittal saw (i, ii, arrows). Note the increased exposure of the orbit after caudal mandibulectomy (iii).

E) The periorbital tissues are retracted to expose the retrobulbar mass (leiomyoma in this case).

Plate 2.3

Lateral Orbitotomy *continued*

D-i)

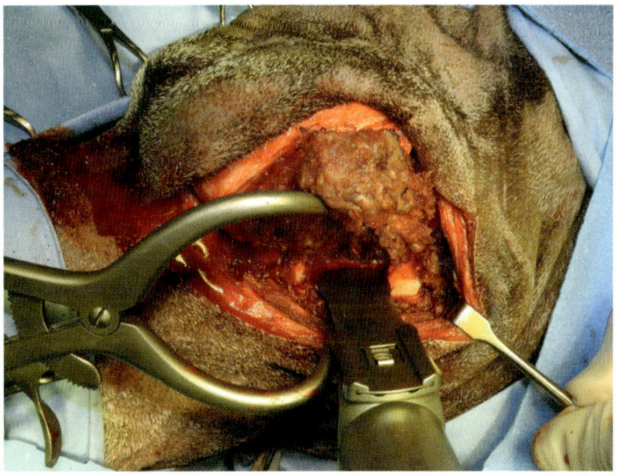

D-ii)

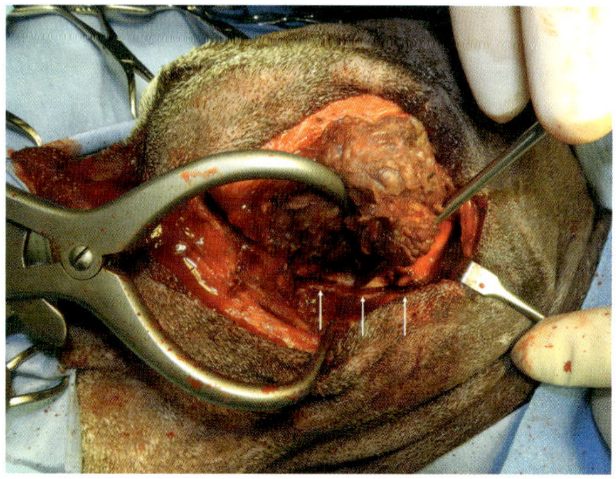

D-iii)

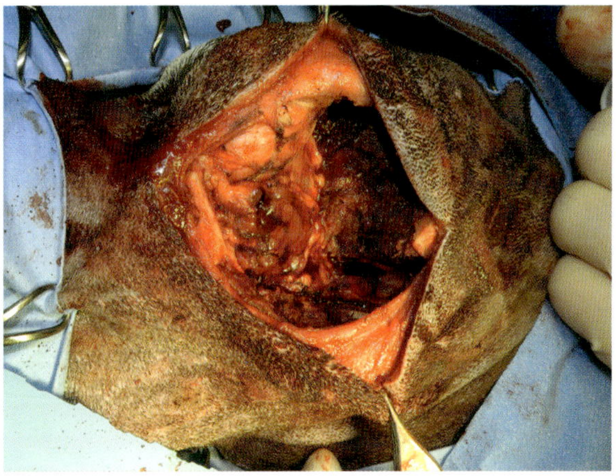

E)

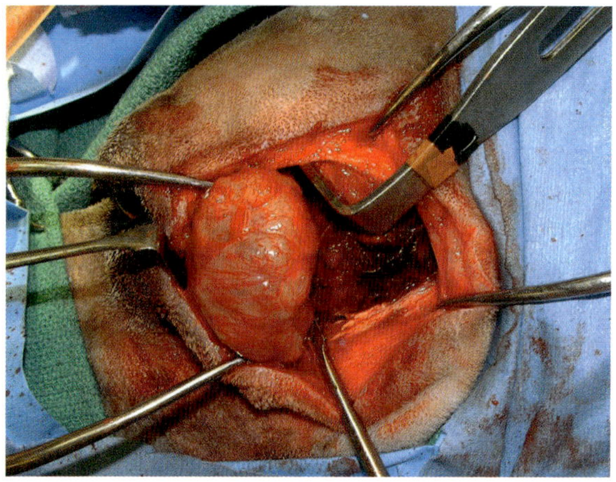

Surgical Technique – Modified Lateral Approach [1, 2] (See Plate 2.3A–F) *continued*

F) The retrobulbar mass is then either extirpated (i, retrobulbar lymphoma in a cat; ii and iii, lacrimal gland adenocarcinoma in a dog) or resected in combination with an exenteration (iv and v, grade III myxosarcoma adhered to the caudal aspect of the globe [arrows]; vi, rhabdomyosarcoma adhered to the caudal aspect of the globe; see *2.2. Exenteration*). The choice between extirpation and exenteration depends on whether the retrobulbar mass invades or is deeply adhered to the globe or optic nerve.

Plate 2.3

Lateral Orbitotomy *continued*

F-i)

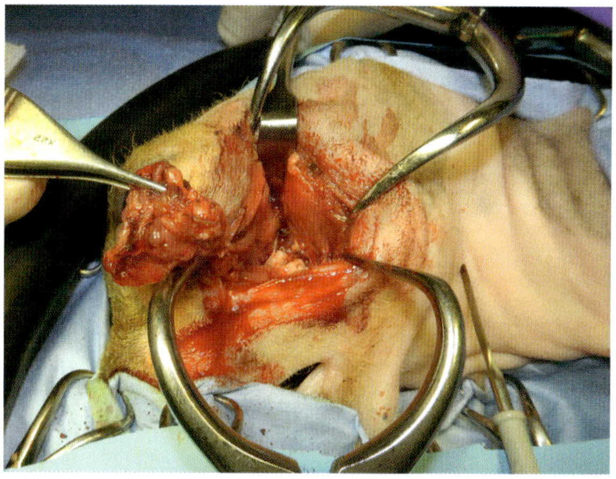

F-ii)

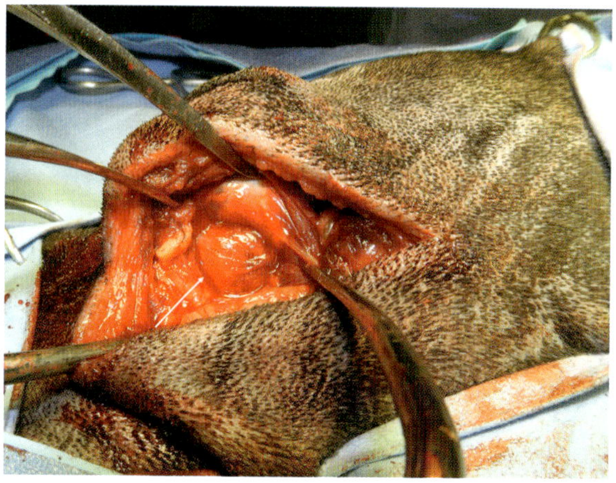

F-iii)

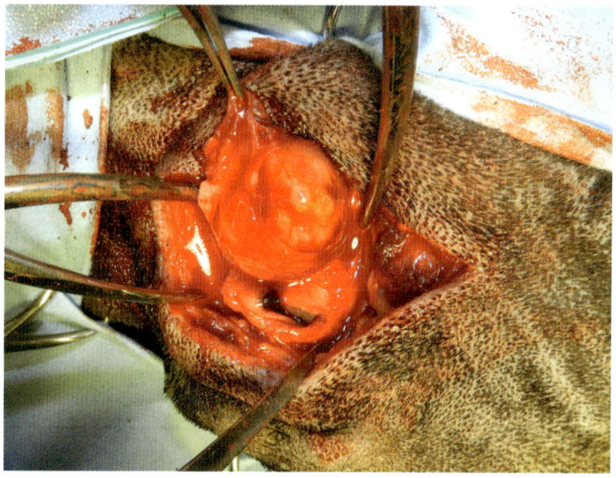

F-iv)

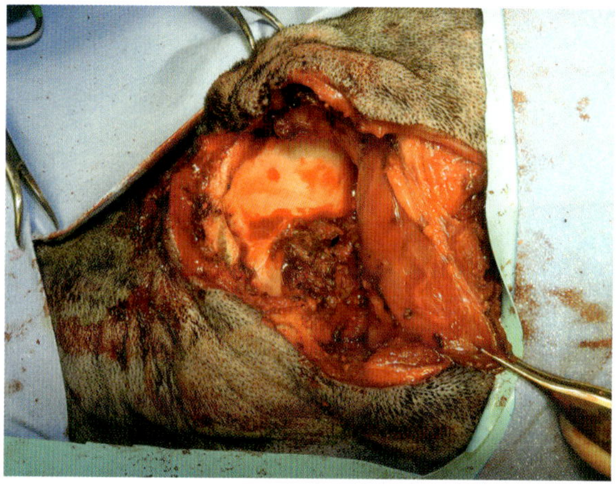

F-v)

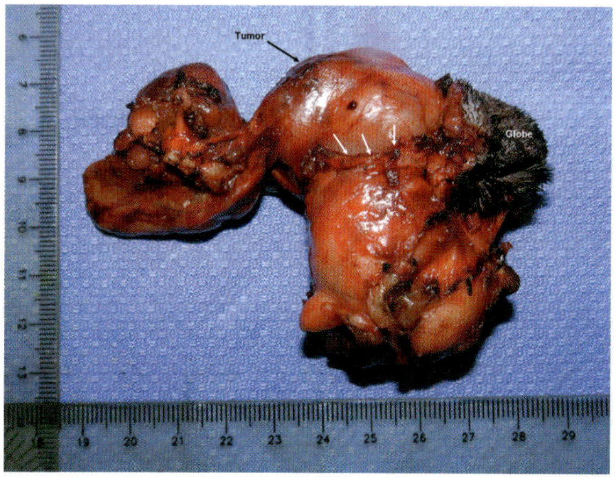

F-vi)

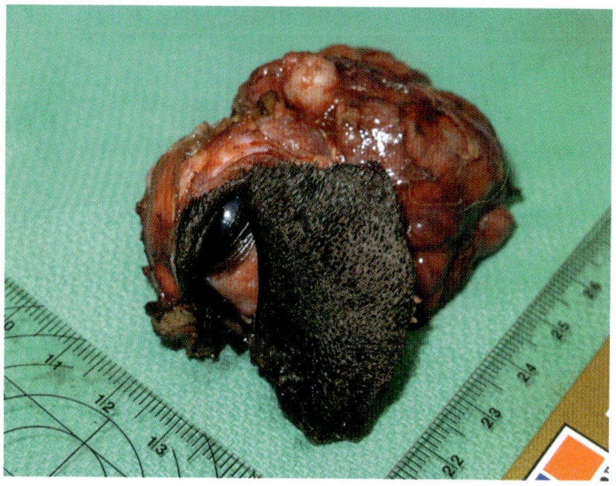

Closure (See Plate 2.3G, H)

G) If the zygomatic arch is discarded, then the transected ends of the temporalis and masseter muscles and the orbital ligament are apposed with absorbable suture material in an interrupted pattern (i, ii). The wound is then closed routinely in two layers. A simple continuous suture pattern using monofilament absorbable suture material is used to close the subcutis. An interrupted or continuous suture pattern using monofilament nonabsorbable suture material is used to close the skin (iii, 6-hour postoperative appearance after extirpation of the retrobulbar mass; iv, 11-day postoperative appearance following exenteration).
H) If the zygomatic arch is preserved, then this can be reattached with either bone plates (pictured) or with either wire or heavy suture material through predrilled holes on either side of the rostral and caudal osteotomies.

Postoperative Management

1) Multimodal analgesia
2) Elizabethan collar

Complications

- Transient swelling/edema
- Lack of eyelid movement if the palpebral nerve has been severed
- Seroma

Suggested Adjuvant Treatments

- ± Chemotherapy, depending on tumor type and histologic grade
- ± Radiation therapy, depending on tumor type and completeness of excision

Prognosis and Oncologic Outcome

Tumor Type	Local Recurrence Rate	Metastatic Rate	Disease-Free Interval (d)	Median Survival Time (d)	1-Year Survival Rate	2-Year Survival Rate
Orbital lobular adenoma – dog [3]	33%	0%	–	–	–	–
Orbital rhabdomyosarcoma – dog [4]						
• ≤4 years	56%	56%	–	–	–	–
• ≥6 years	0%	0%	–	–	–	–
Optic nerve meningioma – dog [5]	35%	0%	–	NR	–	–

NR, not reached.

References

1 Tremolada, G., Milovancev, M., Culp, W.T.N. et al. (2015). Surgical management of canine refractory retrobulbar abscesses: six cases. *J. Small Anim. Pract.* 56 (11): 667–670.
2 Selmic, L.E., Cray, M.T., Good, J.G. et al. (2019). Modified lateral orbitotomy with combined partial zygomatic arch and vertical ramus ostectomies for excision of a frontal and parietal bone osteoma in a dog. *Vet. Surg.* 48 (2): 257–262.
3 Headrick, J.F., Bentley, E., and Dubielzig, R.R. (2004). Canine lobular orbital adenoma: a report of 15 cases with distinctive features. *Vet. Ophthalmol.* 7 (1): 47–51.
4 Scott, E.M., Teixeira, L.B.C., Flanders, D.J. et al. (2016). Canine orbital rhabdomyosarcoma: a report of 18 cases. *Vet. Ophthalmol.* 19 (2): 130–137.
5 Mauldin, E.A., Deehr, A.J., Hertzke, D. et al. (2000). Canine orbital meningiomas: a review of 22 cases. *Vet. Ophthalmol.* 3 (1): 11–16.

Plate 2.3

Lateral Orbitotomy *continued*

G-i)

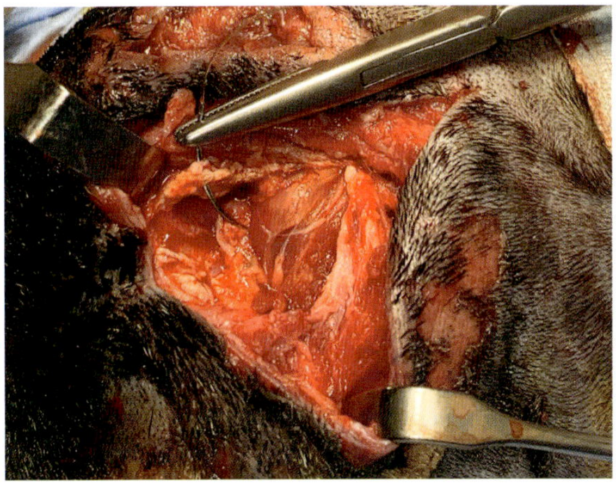

G-ii)

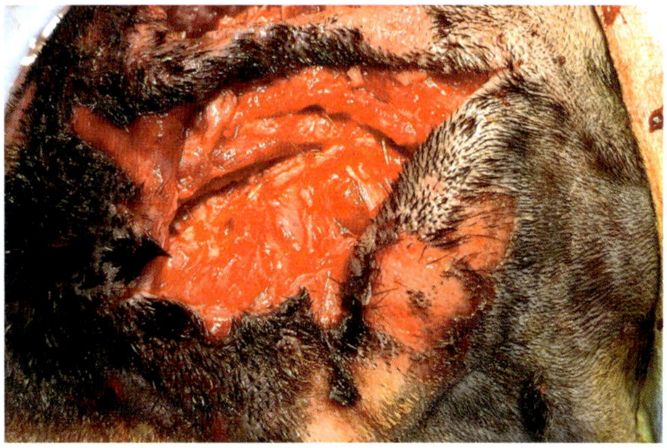

G-iii)

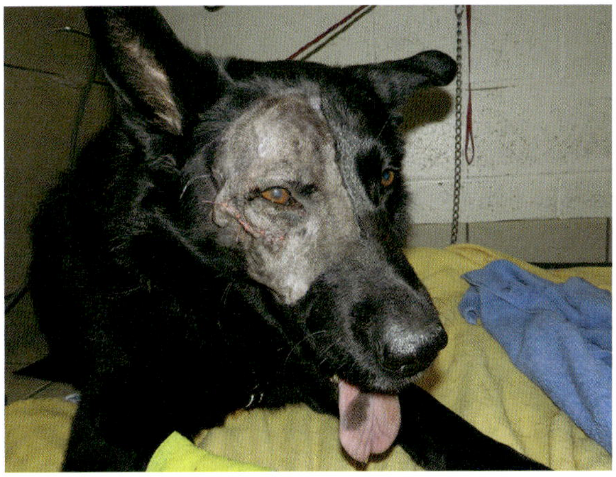

G-iv)

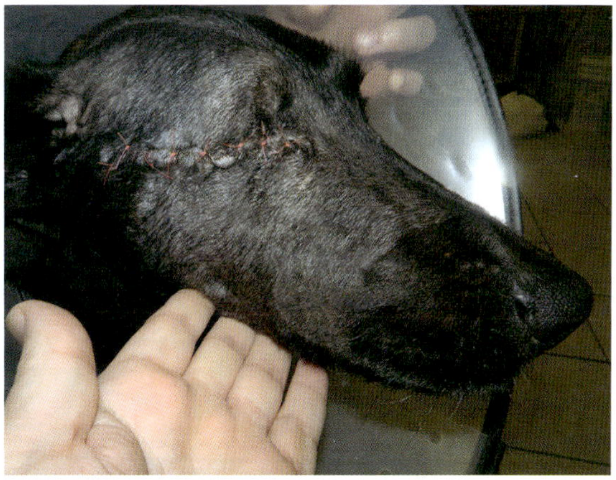

H)

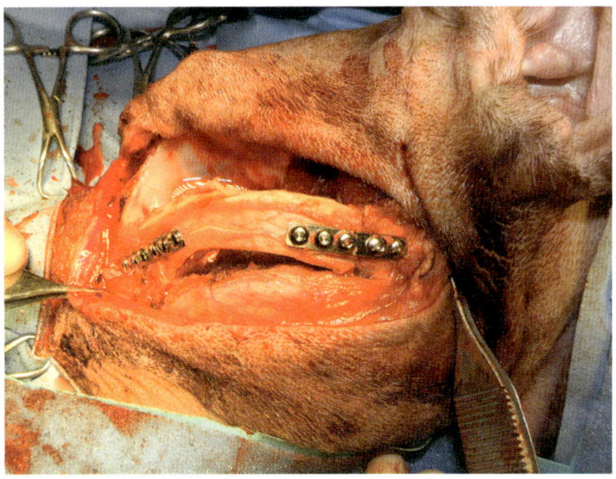

Chapter 3: Ear

3.1 Pinnectomy

Indications

1) Resection of tumors of the skin or cartilage of the pinna
2) Complete or partial pinnectomy (transverse or longitudinal) can be performed; this is dependent on the location of the tumor, the extent of the tumor, and the tumor type

Suggested Diagnostic Workup and Clinical Staging

- Complete blood count, serum biochemistry, and urinalysis
- Preoperative biopsy
- ± Sentinel lymph node mapping (see *50.1. Sentinel Lymph Node Mapping*) or ultrasound-guided aspirate cytology of the parotid, medial retropharyngeal, and superficial cervical (prescapular) lymph nodes
- ± Three-view thoracic radiographs or thoracic computed tomography, depending on tumor type

Patient Positioning

The patient is positioned in lateral recumbency with the affected ear uppermost, and the nose is slightly elevated so it is parallel to the table and the external auditory opening is facing the surgeon vertically. The mandibles should be overlying each other, and the thoracic limbs can be retracted caudally to make a comfortable space for the surgeon.

Surgical Technique (See Plate 3.1A–E)

A) A sterile marker pen is used to mark the level of pinnectomy on both the convex (thicker mobile skin, i) and concave (thinner fixed skin, ii) surfaces. For squamous cell carcinoma/carcinoma in situ/actinic keratosis in cats, a margin of at least 10 mm of visibly normal skin is taken. For other tumors of the pinna, the margin will be dictated by tumor type (e.g. mast cell tumor, soft tissue sarcoma, adenoma, etc.).
B) The skin incision on the convex surface should be made with a scalpel in a continuous smooth action. It is normal for the skin to retract along the pinna cartilage by 5–10 mm. In cats, the incision may be at the very base of the pinna. In dogs, larger vessels will be encountered on the convex surface and will need to be ligated or cauterized.
C) The cartilage and closely adherent concave skin should be cut with Mayo scissors along the previously marked line. The crushing action of the scissors will reduce the capillary oozing from the cut surfaces. As long cuts as possible should be made to keep the cut edge smooth without a jagged edge. Any bleeding along the cut cartilage edge in larger ears should have pressure applied to it. Avoid using cautery on the cartilage where possible.

Color Atlas of Canine and Feline Surgical Oncology, First Edition. Julius M. Liptak, Paolo Buracco, William T. N. Culp, and Nicholas J. Bacon.

Plate 3.1

Pinnectomy

A-i)

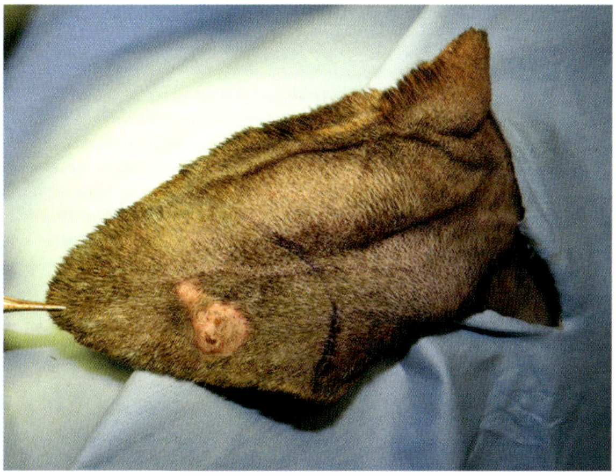

A-ii)

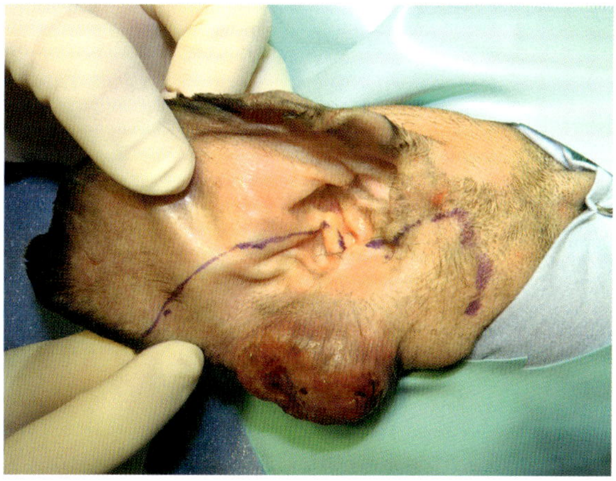

B)

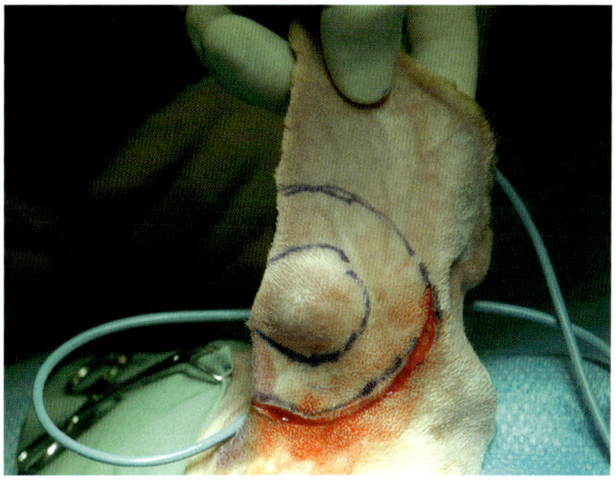

C)

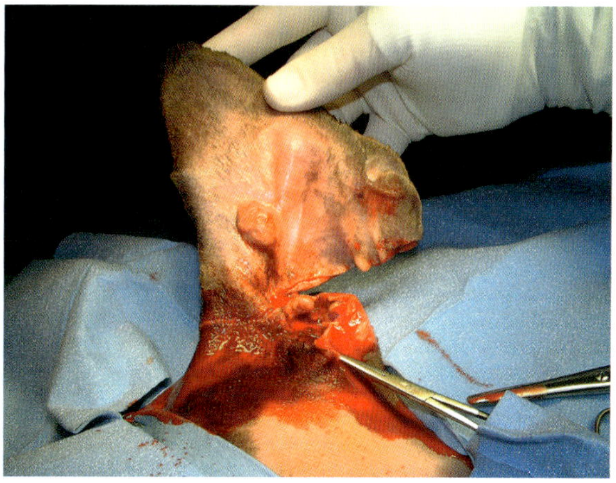

Surgical Technique (See Plate 3.1A–E) *continued*

D) When the tumor involves only the thin concave skin (i), it is possible to resect an island of skin and underlying cartilage as a circular disc with the tumor in the center (ii). The exposed dermis of the convex skin can be managed as an open wound, or a foam-based primary layer can be sutured over the defect to protect the wound. The foam will require changing every few days until a mature granulation bed is present.

E) When the mass involves the rostral or caudal edge, then a longitudinal strip of pinna can be resected, leaving a thinner pinnal remnant (i, ii).

Plate 3.1

Pinnectomy *continued*

D-i)

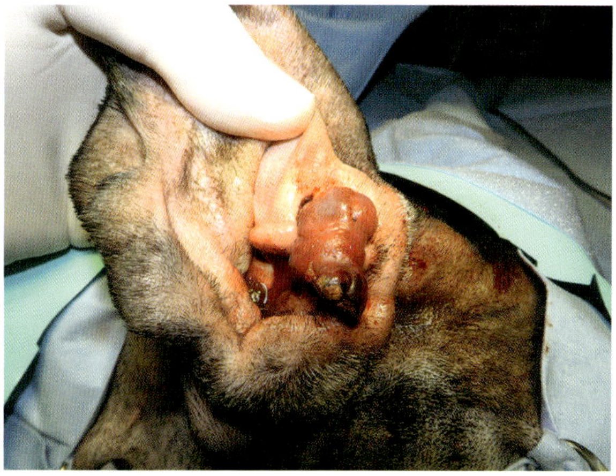

D ii)

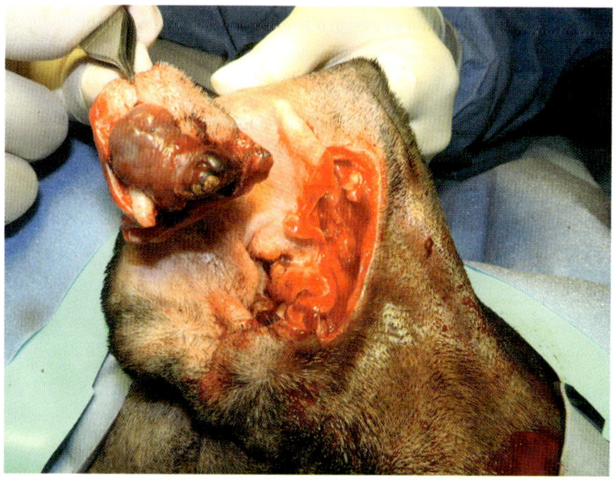

E-i)

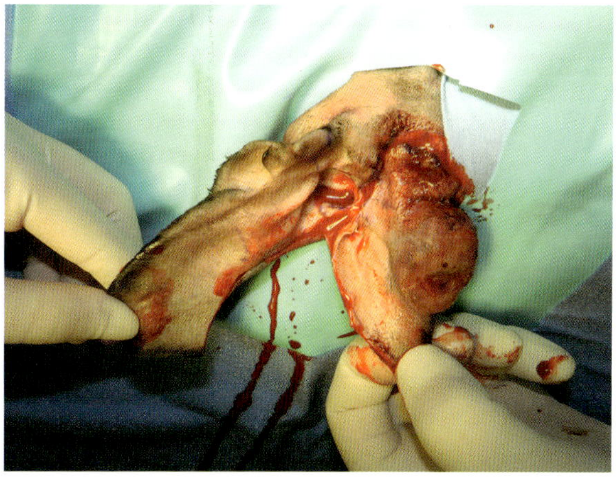

E-ii)

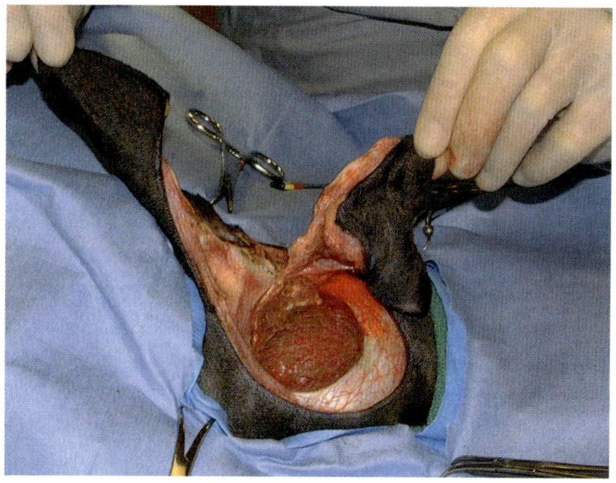

Closure (See Plate 3.1F)

F) The more mobile convex skin should be pulled over the cut cartilage edge and sutured to the concave skin in a simple interrupted or continuous pattern of nonabsorbable suture material (i, partial transverse pinnectomy in a cat with a squamous cell carcinoma, immediate postoperative appearance; ii, bilateral partial transverse pinnectomy in a cat with squamous cell carcinoma, 6 months postoperative appearance; iii, partial transverse pinnectomy in a dog with a low grade II mast cell tumor [see A – i]; partial longitudinal pinnectomy in a dog with a high grade II mast cell tumor [see A – ii and E – i]; iv, immediate postoperative appearance; v, 1-day postoperative appearance; vi, partial longitudinal pinnectomy in a dog with a grade II soft tissue sarcoma [see E – ii]; total pinnectomy in a dog with a low grade II mast cell tumor;

Plate 3.1

Pinnectomy *continued*

F-i)

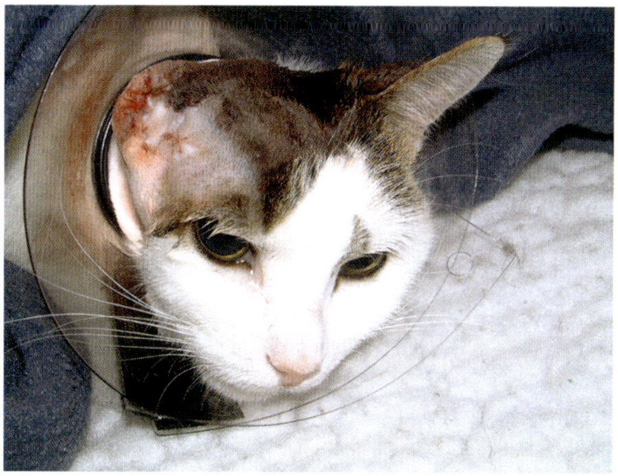

F-ii)

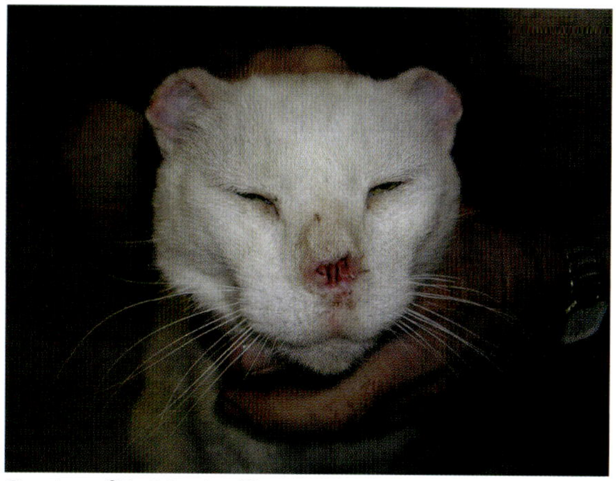

Courtesy of Dr. Maurine Thomson

F-iii)

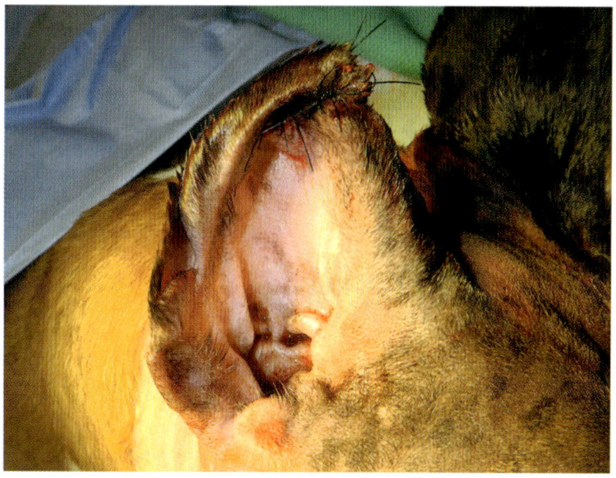

F-iv)

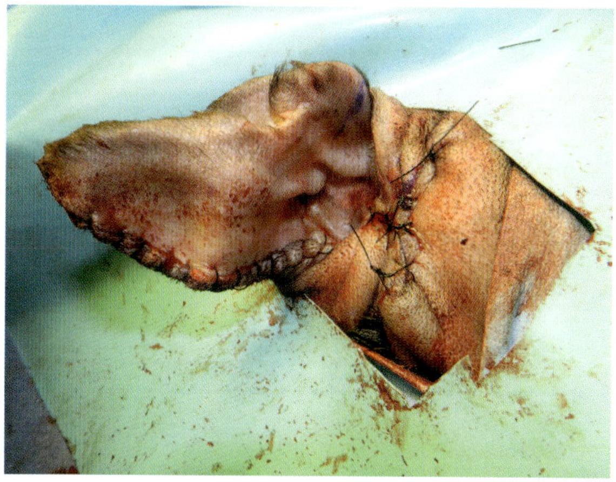

F-v)

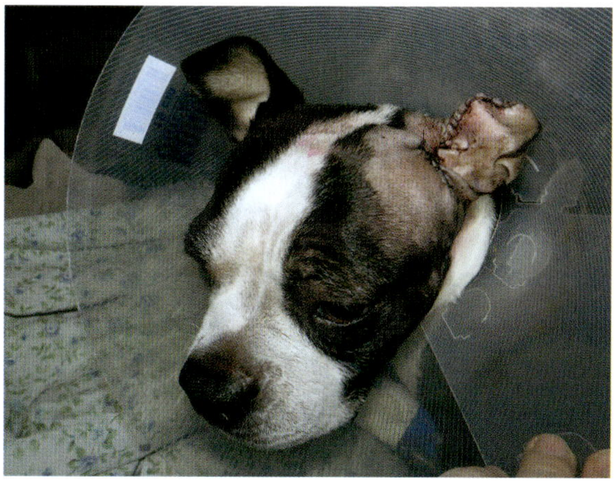

F-vi)

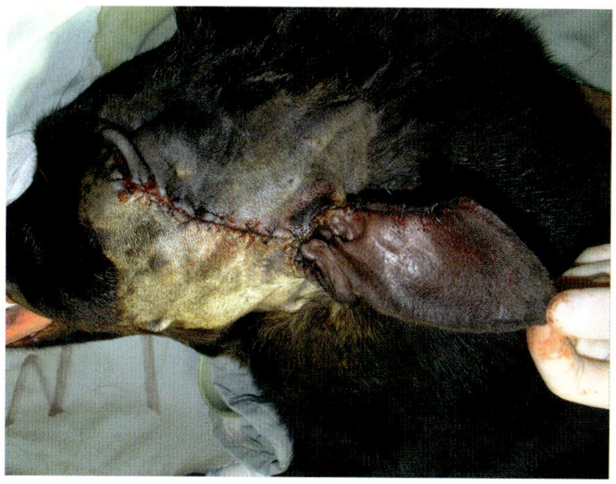

Closure (See Plate 3.1F) *continued*

vii, immediate postoperative appearance; viii, 1-day postoperative appearance; ix, total pinnectomy in a dog with a malignant melanoma, 14-day postoperative appearance).

Postoperative Management

1) Multimodal analgesia, including ring block around the base of the pinna
2) Elizabethan collar

Complications

- Hemorrhage in the immediate postoperative period
- Pain
- Incisional dehiscence
- Self-trauma

Suggested Adjuvant Treatments

- None for cats with squamous cell carcinoma or mast cell tumor
- Chemotherapy ± radiation therapy for dogs with high-grade mast cell tumors ± HN_3 lymph node metastasis

Prognosis and Oncologic Outcome

Tumor Type	Local Recurrence Rate	Metastatic Rate	Disease-Free Interval (d)	Median Survival Time (d)	1-Year Survival Rate	2-Year Survival Rate
Squamous cell carcinoma – cat [1]	0%	0%	681[a]	799[a]	–	–
Mast cell tumor – dog [2]						
• Grade I/II	20%	–	–	NR	–	–
• Grade III	88%	–	–	304	–	–

[a] Disease-free interval and median survival time includes cats treated with surgery, cryosurgery, or radiation therapy.
NR, not reached.

References

1 Lana, S.E., Ogilvie, G.K., Withrow, S.J. et al. (1997). Feline cutaneous squamous cell carcinoma of the nasal planum and the pinnae: 61 cases. *J. Am. Anim. Hosp. Assoc.* 33 (4): 329–332.
2 Schwab, T.M., Popovitch, C., DeBiasio, J. et al. (2014). Clinical outcome for MCTs of canine pinnae treated with surgical excision (2004-2008). *J. Am. Anim. Hosp. Assoc.* 50 (3): 187–191.

Plate 3.1

Pinnectomy *continued*

F-vii)

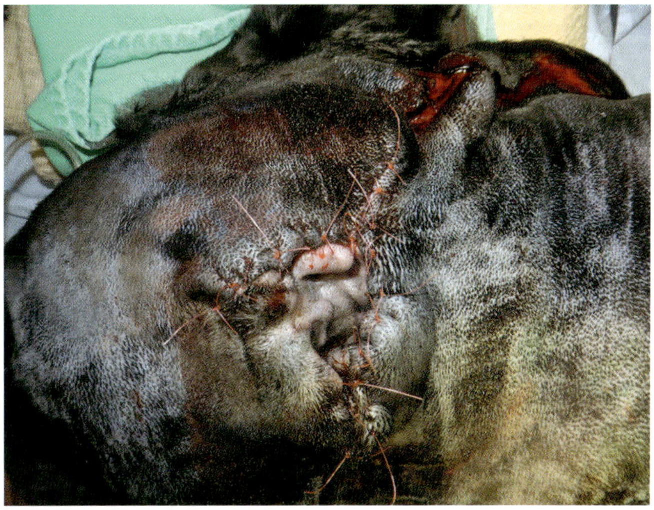

F-viii)

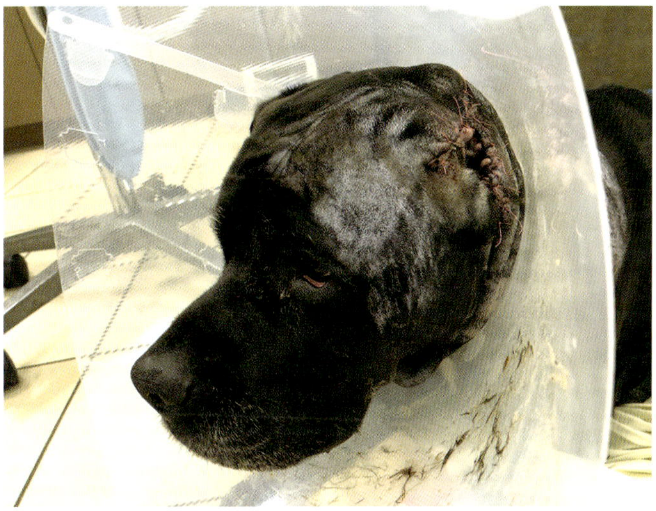

F-ix)

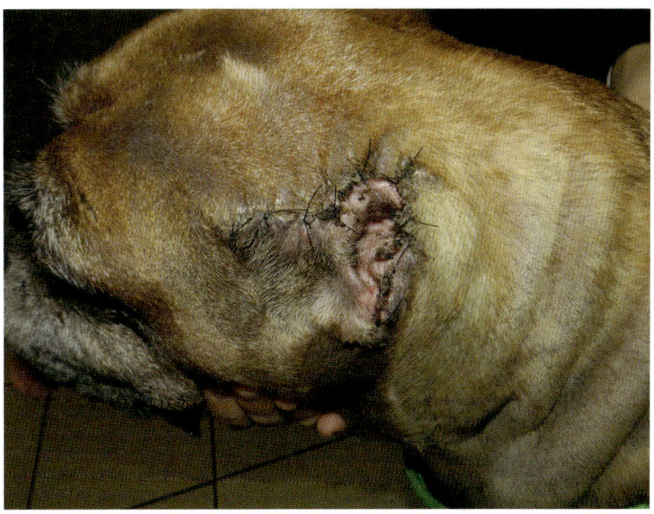

3.2 Total Ear Canal Ablation – Lateral Bulla Osteotomy

Indications

1) Resection of tumors involving the vertical and horizontal ear canals (HECs)
2) Resection of tumors involving only the HEC
3) Resection or cytoreduction of tumors affecting the middle ear

Suggested Diagnostic Workup and Clinical Staging

- Complete blood count, serum biochemistry, and urinalysis
- Otoscopy
- Otic fine-needle aspirate cytology or grab biopsy
- ± Sentinel lymph node mapping (see *50.1. Sentinel Lymph Node Mapping*) or ultrasound-guided aspirate cytology of the parotid, medial retropharyngeal, and superficial cervical (prescapular) lymph nodes
- Skull computed tomography (CT)
- ± Three-view thoracic radiographs or thoracic CT, depending on tumor type

Patient Positioning

The patient is positioned in lateral recumbency with the affected ear uppermost and the nose slightly elevated so it is parallel to the table and the external auditory opening is facing the surgeon vertically. The mandibles should be overlying each other, and the thoracic limbs can be retracted caudally to make a comfortable space for the surgeon.

Surgical Technique (See Plate 3.2A–F)

A) A skin incision is made around the external auditory meatus keeping as close to the base of the pinna as possible. This includes incising through the underlying cartilage to free up the proximal canal entirely. The incision is then continued over the vertical ear canal (VEC) from the tragus ventrally to the level of the junction with the HEC to result in a T-shaped incision (i). Alternatively, an incision around the external auditory meatus without extending the incision over the VEC affords similar exposure as the more extensive approach (ii).
B) The freed VEC is grasped with Allis tissue forceps, and the muscles and soft tissues inserting and attached to the VEC are sharply incised as close to the cartilage as possible. Visibility is improved by using two pairs of Gelpi retractors deeply placed at 90 degrees to each other (i) or a Lonestar retractor (ii).

Color Atlas of Canine and Feline Surgical Oncology, First Edition. Julius M. Liptak, Paolo Buracco, William T. N. Culp, and Nicholas J. Bacon.

Plate 3.2

Total Ear Canal Ablation – Lateral Bulla Osteotomy

A-i)

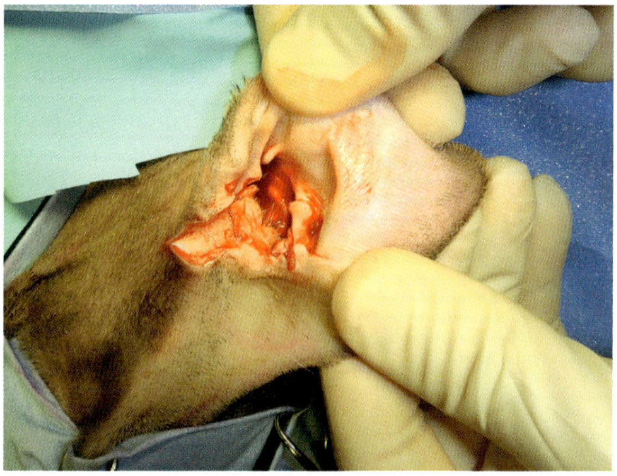

A-ii)

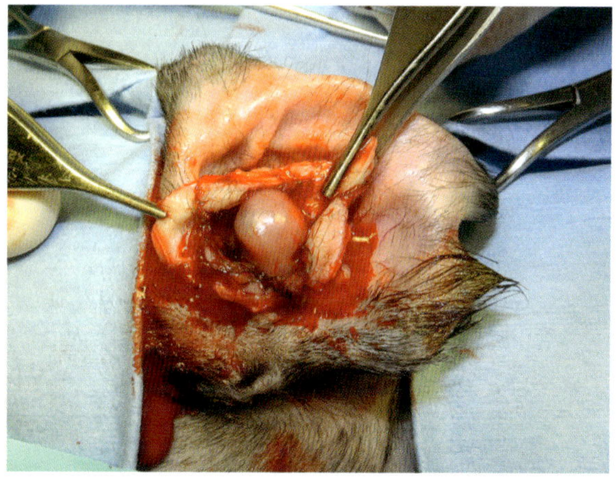

B-i)

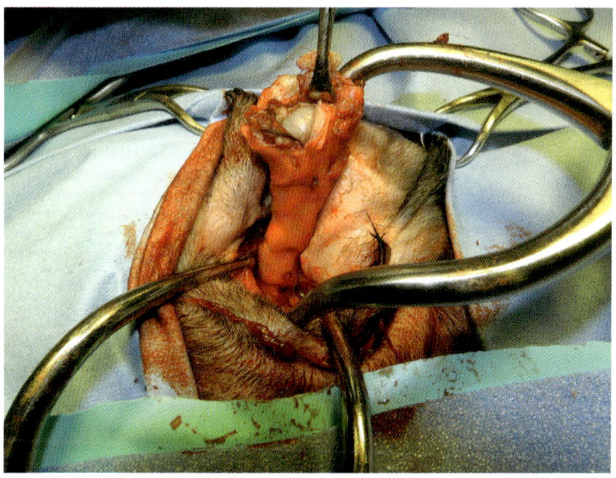

B-ii)

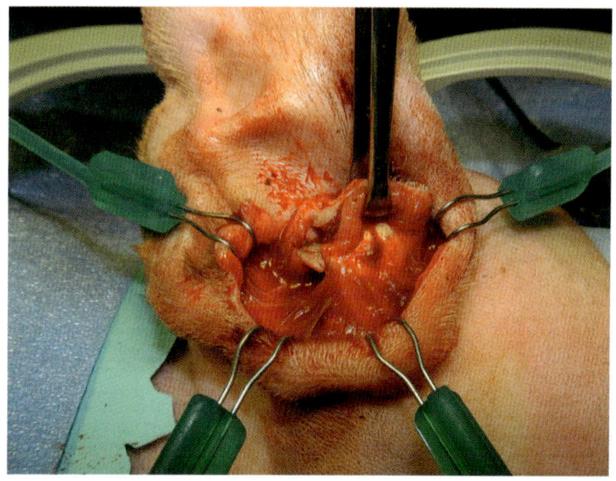

Surgical Technique (See Plate 3.2A–F) *continued*

C) Dissection is continued deeply along the HEC watching for the facial nerve as it runs caudoventral to the ear and then curving rostrally (arrow). The facial nerve may not be encountered if the dissection is kept as close to the ear cartilage as possible.

D) At the level of the osseous foramen, the HEC is amputated with either scissors or a scalpel blade (pictured) in a ventral-to-dorsal direction to protect the facial nerve.

E) Curettes (i) are then used to debride the epithelium from the lining of the osseus meatus to define the opening of the tympanic bulla (ii). Soft tissues below the osseus meatus are gently retracted or elevated ventrally with a periosteal elevator, taking care to avoid the retroglenoid vein rostrally and carotid artery and maxillary vein ventromedially to the osseous bulla.

F) A lateral bulla osteotomy is performed with either rongeurs or a pneumatic burr (i). If using a pneumatic burr, the adjacent soft tissues should be protected with a periosteal elevator or similar instrument (arrow). This results in greater exposure (ii) of the middle ear to debride the epithelium (iii) or remove neoplastic tissue. The bulla is lavaged with warm sterile saline, and a splash block of local anesthesia is applied to the soft tissues before closure.

Plate 3.2

Total Ear Canal Ablation – Lateral Bulla Osteotomy *continued*

C)

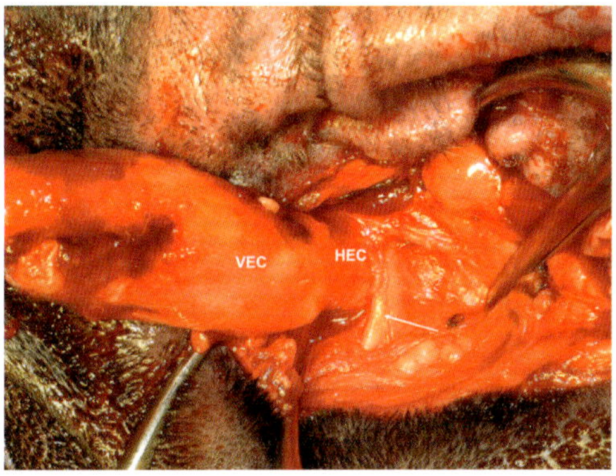

D)

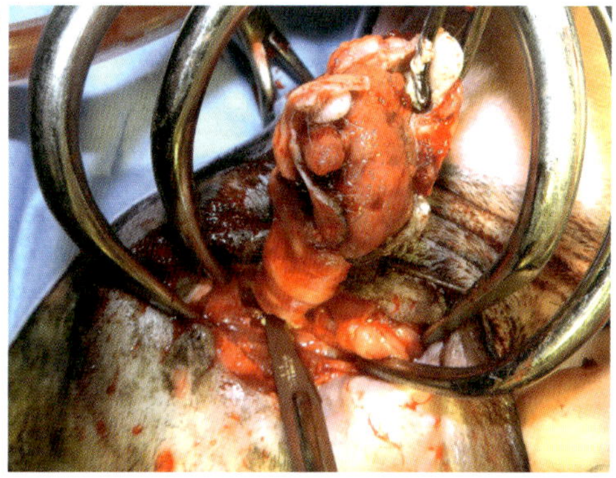

E-i)

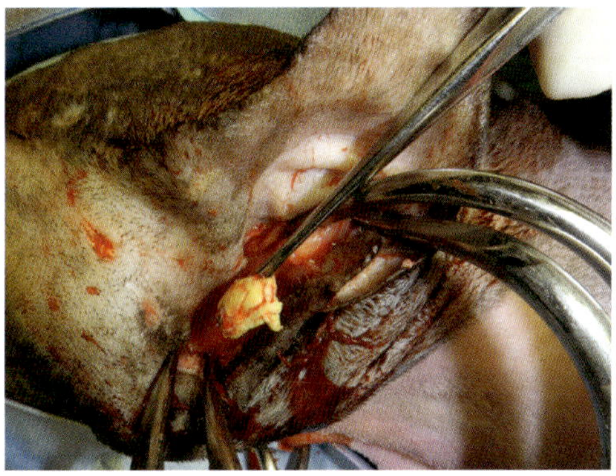

E-ii)

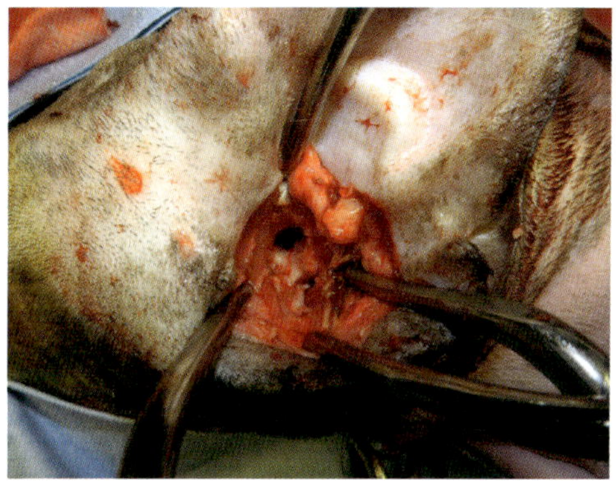

F-i)

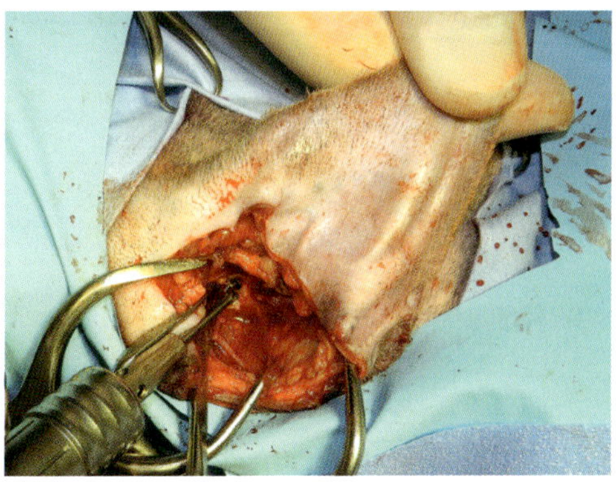

F-ii)

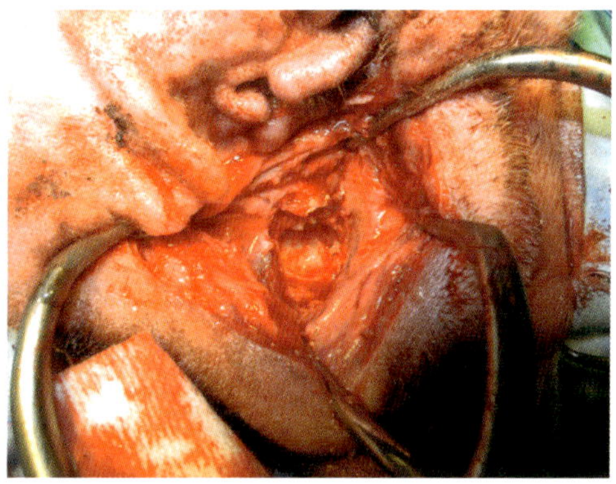

F-iii)

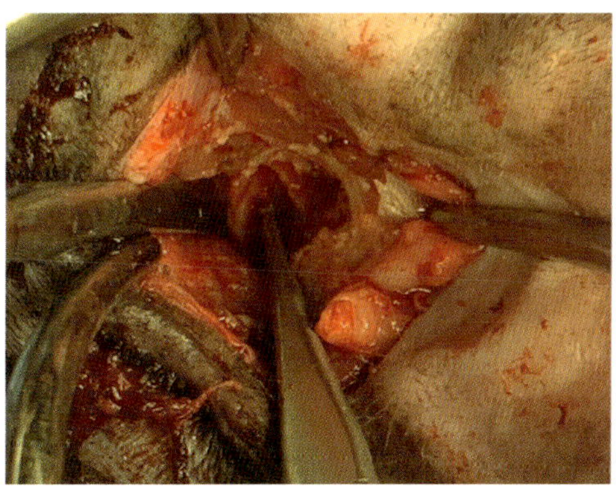

Closure (See Plate 3.2G)

G) The wound is then closed routinely in two to three layers. The deeper subcutaneous tissue can be closed with absorbable monofilament suture material in an interrupted or continuous suture pattern. A simple continuous suture pattern using monofilament absorbable suture material is used to close the subcutis. An interrupted or continuous suture pattern using monofilament nonabsorbable suture material is used to close the skin. The incision is closed in a T shape (i) if an incision was performed along the VEC or as a linear wound if this approach was not made (ii).

To preserve ear carriage in dogs with upright ears, the above technique can be modified so the most superficial 1–2 cm of ear canal is left in situ attached to the pinna and is then turned into a blind-ending pouch. The ventral wound is then closed routinely.

To preserve upright ear carriage in cats, a single pedicle advancement flap is created with 2-cm-long incisions directed ventrally at the rostral and caudal aspects of the encircling incision around the external auditory meatus (iii). The flap is undermined to its ventral base (iv). After completion of the total ear canal ablation and lateral bulla osteotomy, the flap is advanced into the defect at the base of the pinna (v, vi) [1].

Postoperative Management

1) Multimodal analgesia, including ring block around the base of the pinna
2) Cold packing (10 minutes twice daily for the first 2–3 days)
3) Elizabethan collar
4) Gentle wound cleaning every 24 hours for the first 3 days; conscious if possible, but under light sedation if necessary

Complications – Dogs [2–4]

Intraoperative Complications

- Hemorrhage (from the retroglenoid artery, 4.3%–5.2%)

Postoperative Complications

- Pain
- Facial nerve paresis/paralysis (22%–47%; 27% paresis and 20% paralysis)
- Horner's syndrome (3%–6%)
- Vestibular disease/head tilt (11%–19.0%* with 53% of these being transient)
- Hearing loss (49% partial hearing loss and 48% deaf*)
- Incisional complications (5%–28% overall)
  - Seroma (17%)
  - Infection (5%)
  - Drainage (10%)
- Surgical-site infection, late (2%–14%) [5]

Complications – Cats [2, 6]

Intraoperative Complications

- Hemorrhage (from the retroglenoid artery)

* Includes both dogs and cats.

Plate 3.2

Total Ear Canal Ablation – Lateral Bulla Osteotomy *continued*

G-i)
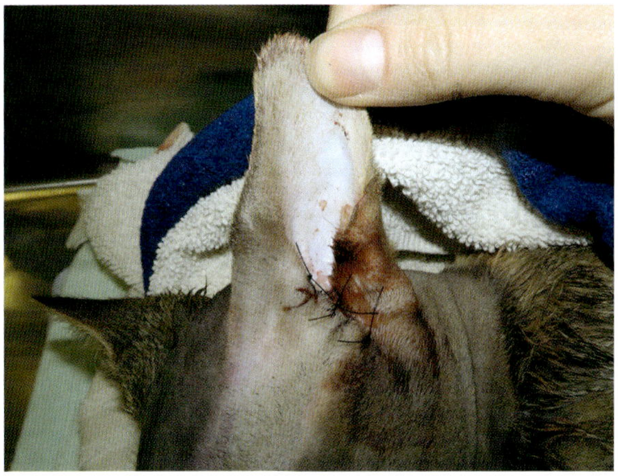

G-ii)
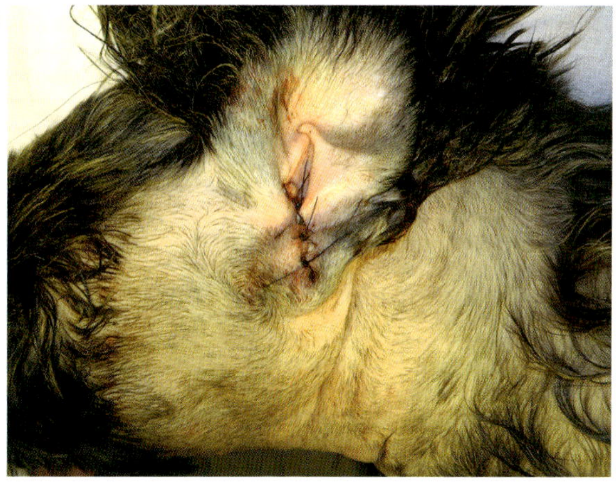

G-iii)
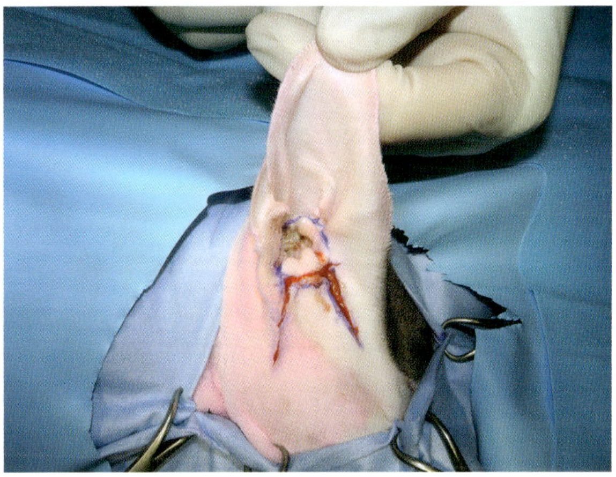

G-iv)
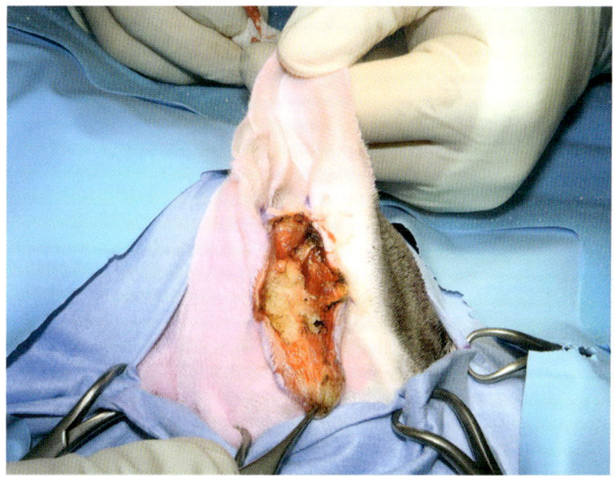

G-v)
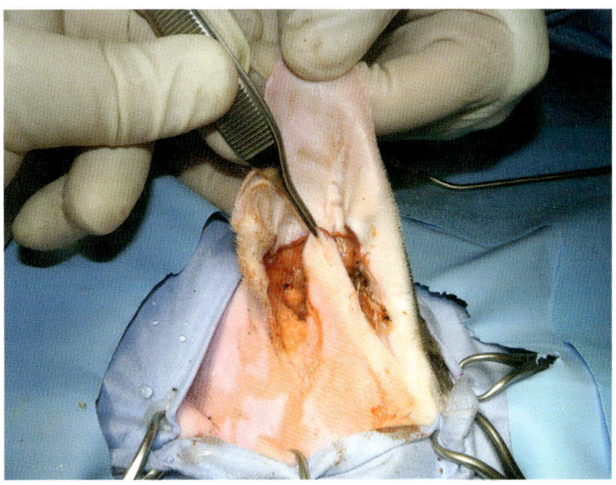

G-vi)
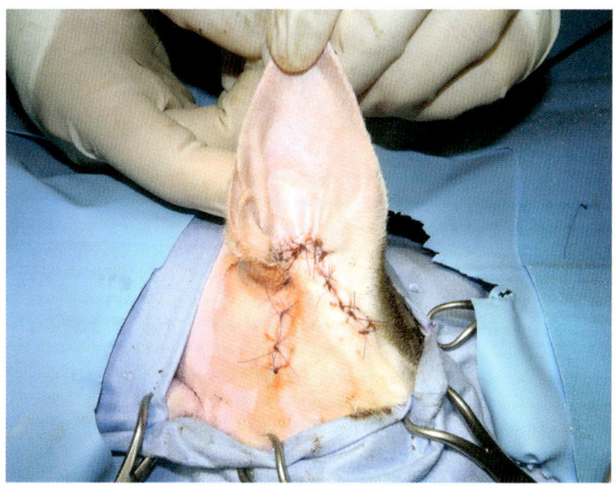

Postoperative Complications

- Pain
- Incisional dehiscence
- Self-trauma
- Facial nerve paresis/paralysis (54%–67% overall with 72% transient and 28% permanent)
- Horner's syndrome (42%–58% with 86% transient and 14% permanent)
- Vestibular disease/head tilt (19%*)
- Hearing loss (49% partial hearing loss and 48% deaf*)
- Surgical-site infection, early
- Surgical-site infection, late

Suggested Adjuvant Treatments

- ± Chemotherapy, depending on tumor type and histologic grade
- ± Radiation therapy, depending on tumor type and completeness of excision

Prognosis and Oncologic Outcome – Dogs

Tumor Type	Local Recurrence Rate	Metastatic Rate	Disease-Free Interval (d)	Median Survival Time (d)
Malignant ear canal tumors [7]	–	–	–	>1764
Tumor type				
Ceruminous gland adenocarcinoma [8]	0%	0%	NR	–
Tumor extension [7]				
Tumor confined to ear canal	–	–	–	>913
Tumor extended beyond ear canal	–	–	–	161

NR, not reached.

Prognosis and Oncologic Outcome – Cats

Tumor Type	Local Recurrence Rate	Metastatic Rate	Disease-Free Interval (d)	Median Survival Time (d)
Malignant ear canal tumors [7]	–	–	–	356
Tumor type				
Ceruminous gland adenocarcinoma [6, 7, 9]	25%	–	1278	>1490–1530
Squamous cell carcinoma	–	–	–	116
Undifferentiated carcinoma	–	–	–	173
Neurologic signs [7]				
No	–	–	–	471
Yes	–	–	–	46
Tumor extension [7]				
Tumor confined to ear canal	–	–	–	660
Tumor extended beyond ear canal	–	–	–	122

References

1 McNabb, A.H. and Flanders, J.A. (2004). Cosmetic results of a ventrally based advancement flap for closure of total ear canal ablations in 6 cats: 2002-2003. *Vet. Surg.* 33 (5): 435–439.

2 Spivack, R.E., Elkins, A.D., Moore, G.E. et al. (2013). Postoperative complications following TECA-LBO in the dog and cat. *J. Am. Anim. Hosp. Assoc.* 49 (3): 160–168.

3 Mason, L.K., Harvey, C.E., and Orsher, R.J. (1988). Total ear canal ablation combined with lateral bulla osteotomy for end-stage otitis in dogs. Results in thirty dogs. *Vet. Surg.* 17 (5): 263–268.

4 Coleman, K.A. and Smeak, D.D. (2016). Complication rates after bilateral versus unilateral total ear canal ablation with lateral bulla osteotomy for end-stage inflammatory ear disease in dogs: 79 ears. *Vet. Surg.* 45 (5): 659–663.

5 Smeak, D.D. (2016). Treatment of persistent deep infection after total ear canal ablation and lateral bulla osteotomy. *Vet. Clin. North Am. Small Anim. Pract.* 46 (4): 609–621.

6 Bacon, N.J., Gilbert, R.L., Bostock, D.E. et al. (2003). Total ear canal ablation in the cat: indications, morbidity and long-term survival. *J. Small Anim. Pract.* 44 (10): 430–434.

7 London, C.A., Dubilzeig, R.R., Vail, D.M. et al. (1996). Evaluation of dogs and cats with tumors of the ear canal: 145 cases (1978-1992). *J. Am. Vet. Med. Assoc.* 208 (9): 1413–1418.

8 Marino, D.J., MacDonald, J.M., Matthiesen, D.T. et al. (1993). Results of surgery and long-term follow-up in dogs with ceruminous gland adenocarcinoma. *J. Am. Anim. Hosp. Assoc.* 29: 560–563.

9 Marino, D.J., MacDonald, J.M., and Matthiesen, D.T. (1994). Results of surgery in cats with ceruminous gland adenocarcinoma. *J. Am. Anim. Hosp. Assoc.* 30: 54–58.

3.3 Ventral Bulla Osteotomy

Indications

1) Resection of inflammatory polyps, benign tumors, and malignant tumors involving the middle ear. Note that single-session, bilateral ventral bulla osteotomies should not be done in cats because of a significantly increased risk of respiratory-related deaths [1].
2) Ventral bulla osteotomy can be combined with a total ear canal ablation and lateral bulla osteotomy (see *3.2. Total Ear Canal Ablation – Lateral Bulla Osteotomy*).

Suggested Diagnostic Workup and Clinical Staging

- Complete blood count, serum biochemistry, and urinalysis
- ± Precontrast and postcontrast computed tomography (CT) scan of the head and neck
- ± Three-view thoracic radiographs or thoracic CT scan, depending on tumor type

Patient Positioning

The patient is positioned in dorsal recumbency with the neck extended over a padded structure and the head secured to the surgical table with adhesive tape over the chin.

Surgical Technique [2] (See Plate 3.3A–E)

A) The osseous bulla is palpated caudal and slightly medial to the vertical ramus of the mandible. An ipsilateral paramedian skin incision is performed over the osseous bulla, medial to the mandibular salivary gland and extending from the angular process of the mandible rostrally to the wing of the atlas caudally. The skin incision is continued deeply through the platysma muscle.
B) The digastricus muscle belly is bluntly dissected away from the mylohyoideus muscle in dogs and the masseter muscle in cats. These respective muscles are retracted to identify and protect the lingual artery and vein (i), hypoglossal nerve on the lateral aspect of the hypoglossal muscle (ii), and stylohyoid bone. The blunt dissection is continued deeply between the jugular process of the skull and mandible to expose the osseous bulla (iii).

Color Atlas of Canine and Feline Surgical Oncology, First Edition. Julius M. Liptak, Paolo Buracco, William T. N. Culp, and Nicholas J. Bacon.

Plate 3.3

Ventral Bulla Osteotomy

A)

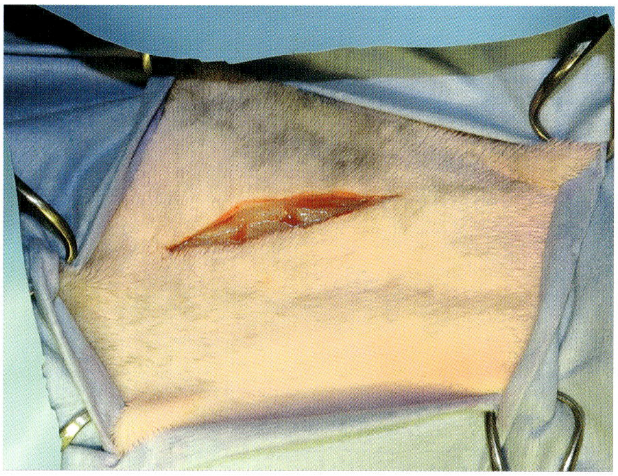

B-i)

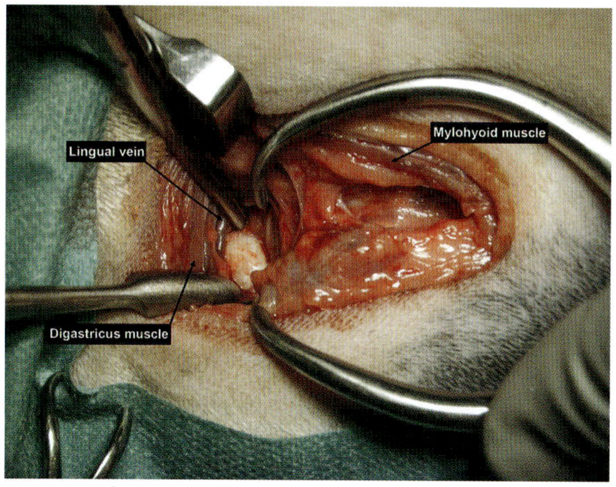

Courtesy of Dr. Manuel Jiménez Peláez

B-ii)

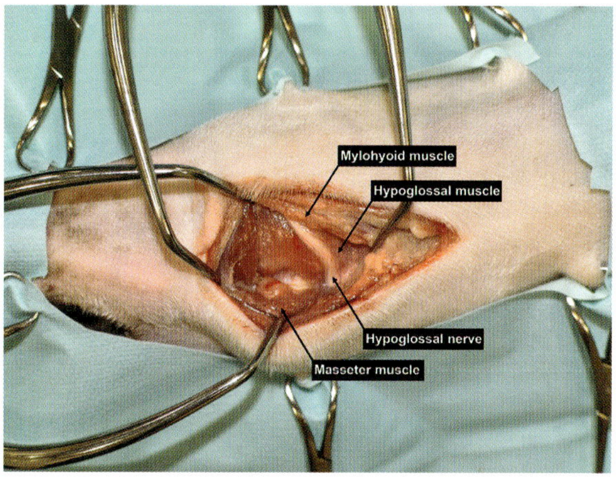

B-iii)

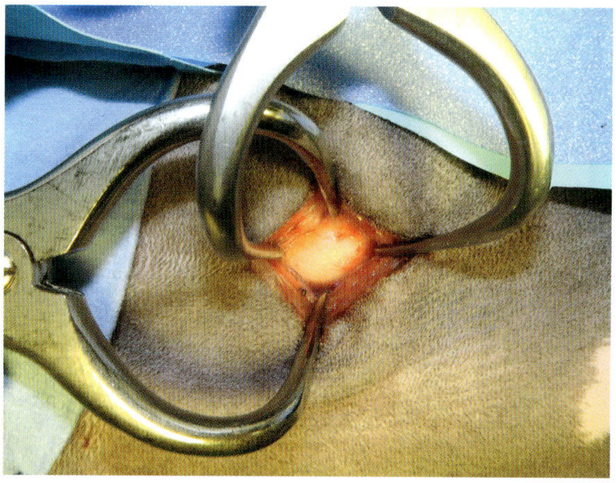

Surgical Technique [2] (See Plate 3.3A–E) *continued*

C) The osseous bulla is entered with a Steinmann pin (i) or a pneumatic drill (ii) and widened with either a pneumatic drill (iii) or rongeurs.
D) In cats, the middle ear is divided into a larger ventromedial compartment and a smaller dorsolateral compartment by a thin bony septum. This bony septum should also be removed with either a pneumatic drill or rongeurs to expose the entirety of the middle ear.
E) The inflammatory polyp (i, ii) or tumor is removed. If possible, the mass should be removed intact, but piecemeal removal may be necessary.
F) Once the mass is removed, the epithelial lining of the bulla and inflammatory debris within the bulla are removed with a bone curette (see step D). The tympanic cavity is flushed and suctioned until there is no evidence of residual debris.
G) The use of a drain can be considered, but this is usually unnecessary.

Closure

The wound is closed routinely in three layers. A simple continuous suture pattern using monofilament absorbable suture material is used in the platysma muscle and subcutis. An interrupted or continuous suture pattern using monofilament nonabsorbable suture material is used to close the skin. The ipsilateral ear canal and nasopharynx should be checked for residual inflammatory polyp in cats; if present, the residual polyp should be tractioned [1].

Postoperative Management

1) Multimodal analgesia
2) Elizabethan collar

Suggested Adjuvant Treatments

- Radiation therapy for incompletely excised tumors

Plate 3.3

Ventral Bulla Osteotomy *continued*

C-i)

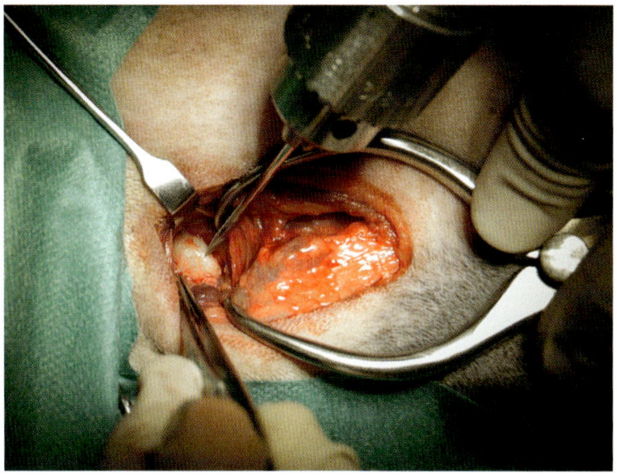

Courtesy of Dr. Manuel Jiménez Peláez

C-ii)

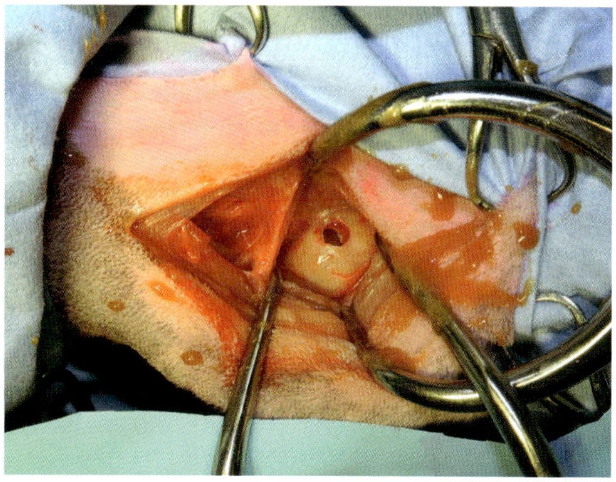

C-iii)

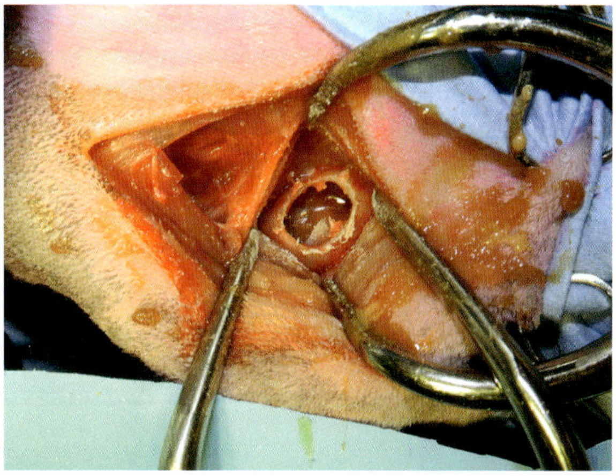

D)

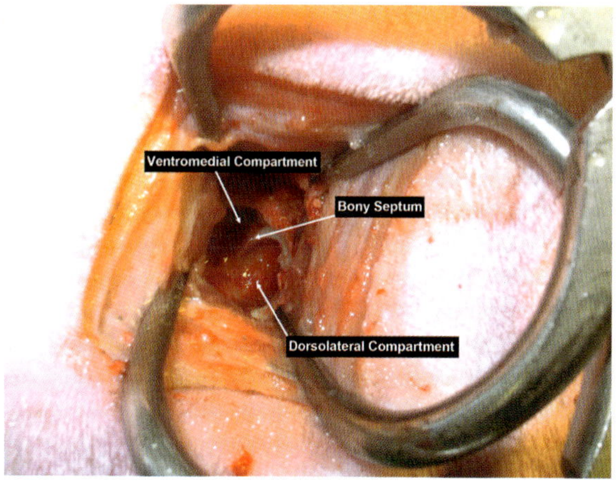

E-i)

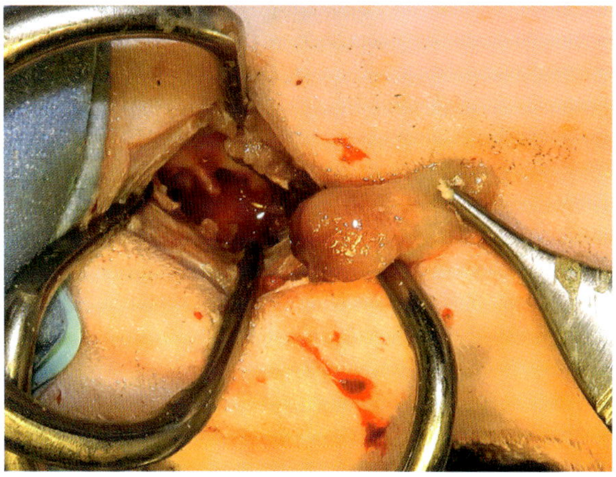

E-ii)

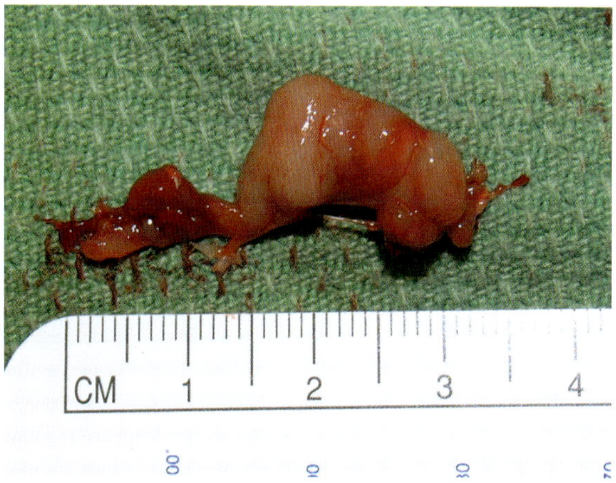

Complications in Cats [1] (See Plate 3.3H, I)

	Inflammatory Polyp	Benign Tumor	Malignant Tumor
Horner's syndrome (H)			
• 0–24 h	69%	80%	58%
• 1–14 d	65%	80%	58%
• >14 d	45%	100%	36%
Head tilt (I)			
• 0–24 h	26%	20%	33%
• 1–14 d	25%	20%	33%
• >14 d	19%	20%	18%
Facial nerve paralysis			
• 0–24 h	9%	20%	50%
• 1–14 d	8%	20%	42%
• >14 d	8%	20%	27%
Respiratory signs			
• 0–24 h	7%	0%	0%
• 1–14 d	6%	0%	0%
• >14 d	3%	0%	9%
Dysphagia			
• 0–24 h	0%	0%	0%
• 1–14 d	6%	20%	50%
• >14 d	3%	0%	18%
Otitis externa or media			
• 0–24 h	0%	0%	0%
• 1–14 d	5%	20%	8%
• >14 d	6%	20%	0%
Incisional complications			
• 0–24 h	2%	0%	0%
• 1–14 d	5%	20%	8%
• >14 d	1%	0%	0%
Overall			
• 0–24 h	80%	100%	83%
• 1–14 d	78%	100%	67%
• >14 d	62%	100%	82%

Prognosis and Oncologic Outcome – Cats [1]

Tumor Type	Local Recurrence Rate	Metastatic Rate	Disease-Free Interval (d)	Median Survival Time (d)	1-Year Survival Rate	2-Year Survival Rate
Inflammatory polyp	5%	–	NR	1322	89%	74%
Benign tumor	21%	–	NR	1244	60%	33%
Malignant Tumor	44%	0%	638	855	75%	50%

NR, not reached.

References

1 Wainberg, S.H., Selmic, L.E., Haagsman, A.N. et al. (2019). Comparison of complications and outcome following unilateral, staged bilateral, and single-stage bilateral ventral bulla osteotomy in cats. *J. Am. Vet. Med. Assoc.* 255 (7): 828–836.

2 Smith, M. and Waldron, D. (1993). *Atlas of Approaches for General Surgery of the Dog and Cat*, 1e. Philadelphia, PA: W.B. Saunders.

Plate 3.3

Ventral Bulla Osteotomy *continued*

H)

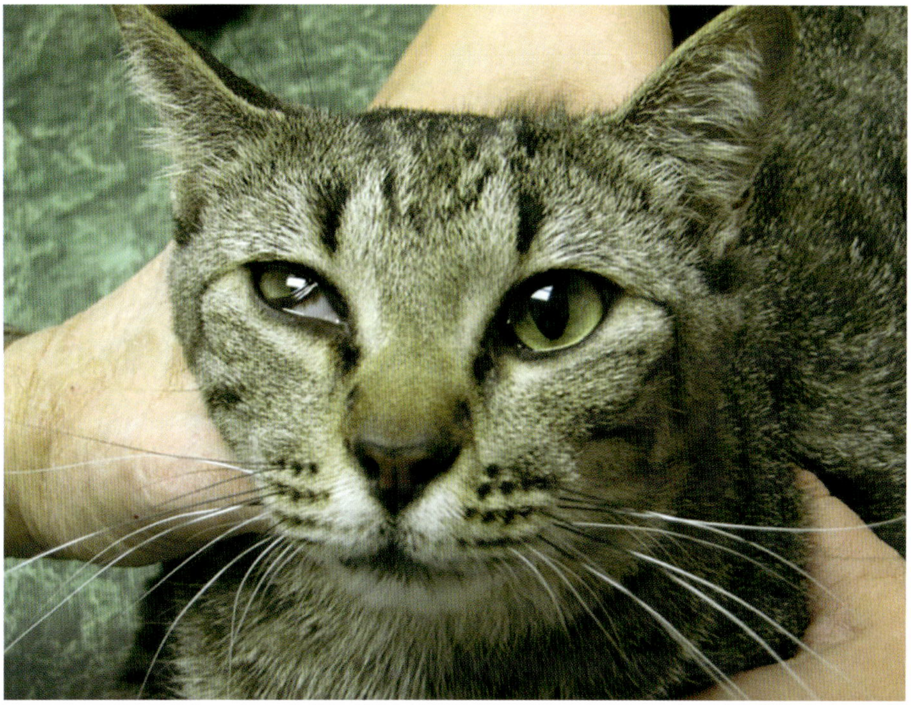

I)

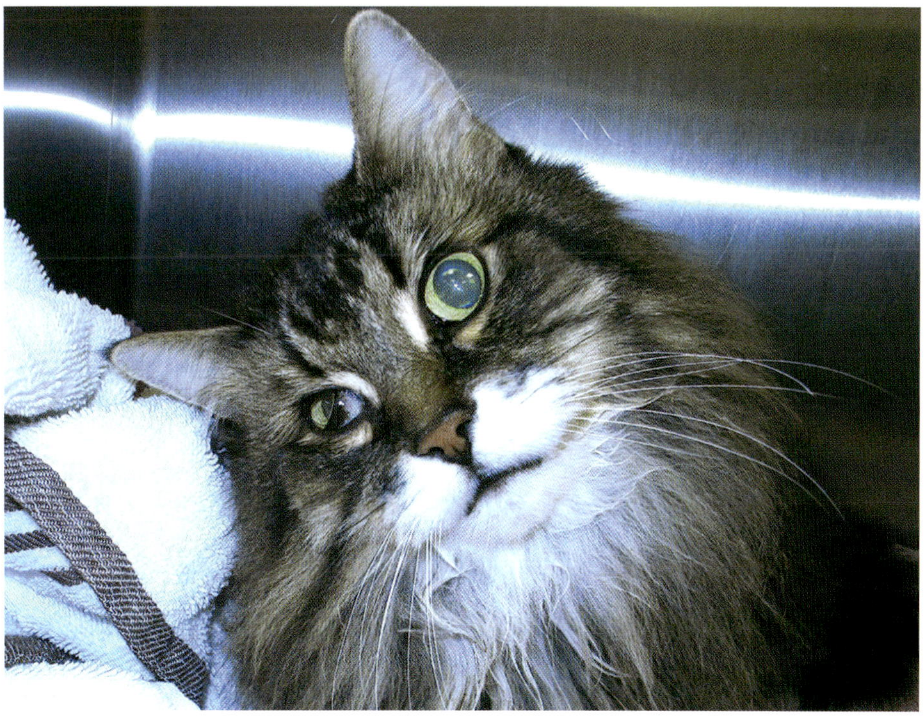

3.4 Vertical Ear Canal Resection

Indications

1) Resection of tumors affecting only the vertical ear canal
2) Resection of extensive tumors involving the base of the convex pinna
3) Resection of extensive tumors involving the external auditory meatus

Suggested Diagnostic Workup and Clinical Staging

- Complete blood count, serum biochemistry, and urinalysis
- Otoscopy
- Otic fine-needle aspirate cytology or grab biopsy
- ± Sentinel lymph node mapping (see *50.1. Sentinel Lymph Node Mapping*) or ultrasound-guided aspirate cytology of the parotid, medial retropharyngeal, and superficial cervical (prescapular) lymph nodes
- ± Skull computed tomography (CT)
- ± Three-view thoracic radiographs or thoracic CT, depending on tumor type

Patient Positioning

The patient is positioned in lateral recumbency with the affected ear uppermost and the nose slightly elevated so it is parallel to the table and the external auditory opening is facing the surgeon vertically. The mandibles should be overlying each other, and the thoracic limbs can be retracted caudally to make a comfortable space for the surgeon.

Surgical Technique (See Plate 3.4A–D)

A) The surgical approach depends on the tumor location and tumor type. If the tumor involves the vertical ear canal, then an incision is made around the external auditory meatus keeping as close to the base of the pinna as possible (pictured). If the tumor involves the base of the pinna (convex or concave surface), a skin incision is made around the pinna and external auditory meatus and then continued in a ventral direction over the palpable vertical ear canal to the predetermined resection margins or to the junction with the horizontal canal. The entire pinna and vertical ear canal will be resected with this latter approach.
B) The freed vertical ear canal is grasped with Allis tissue forceps, and the muscles and soft tissues inserting and attached to the vertical ear canal are sharply incised as close to the cartilage as possible to the level of the junction with the horizontal ear canal (arrow). Visibility is improved by using two pairs of Gelpi retractors deeply placed at 90 degrees to each other (pictured) or a Lonestar retractor.

Color Atlas of Canine and Feline Surgical Oncology, First Edition. Julius M. Liptak, Paolo Buracco, William T. N. Culp, and Nicholas J. Bacon.

Plate 3.4

Vertical Ear Canal Resection

A)

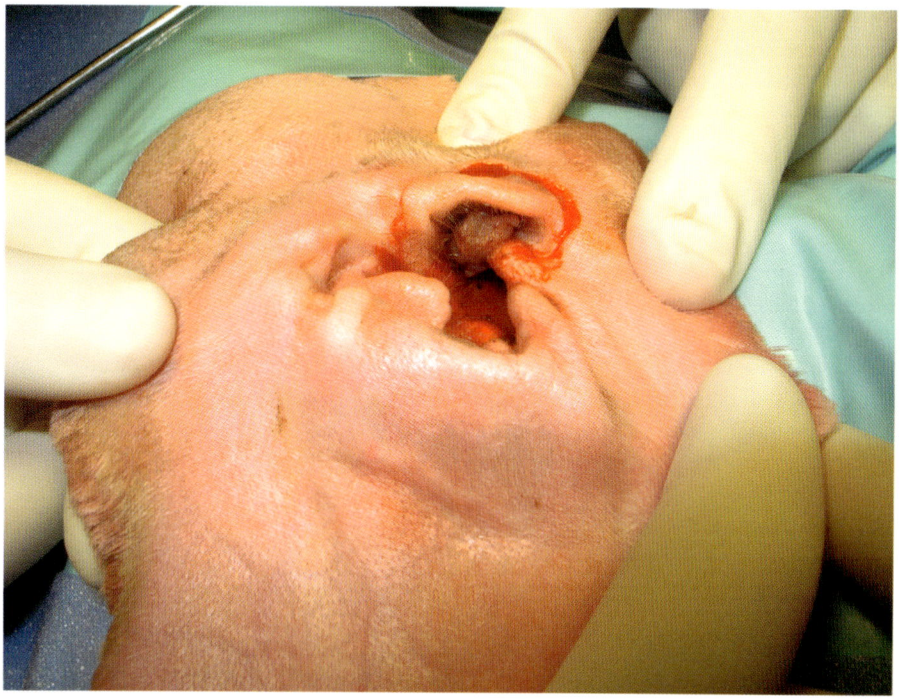

B)

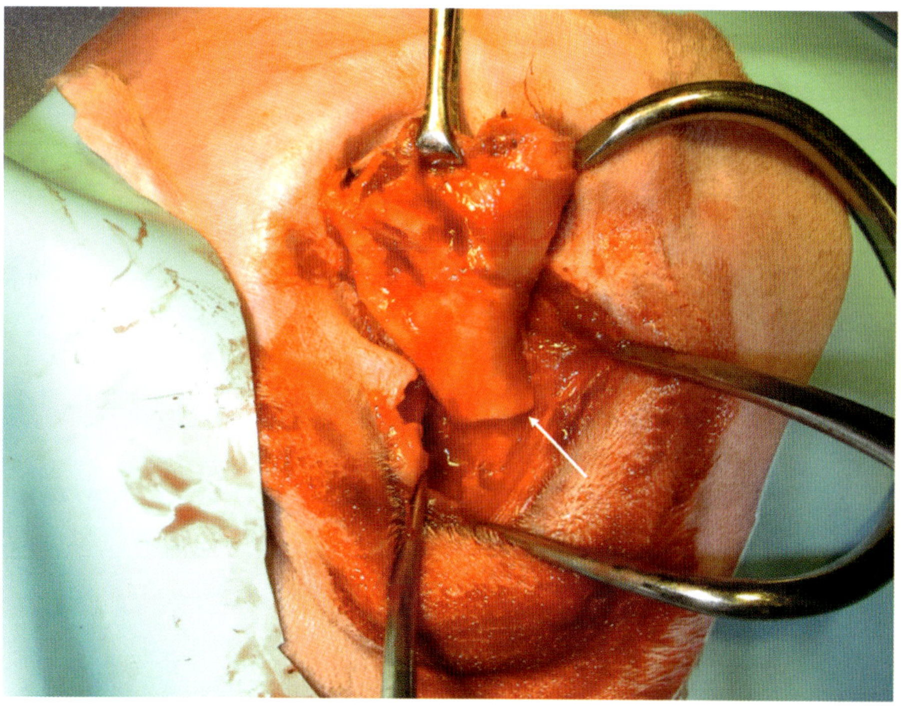

Surgical Technique (See Plate 3.4A–D) *continued*

C) The freed-up proximal ear canal is folded ventrally and the ear canal amputated with a scalpel parallel with the skin surface in its new position.

D) An incision is made ventrally at the level of the horizontal ear canal (i) if the horizontal ear canal is not positioned within the defect (see step C). If possible, short 5- to 10-mm vertical incisions are made at the rostral and caudal edge of the horizontal ear canal to create small dorsal and ventral drainage boards to allow for a large stoma (ii). If this is not possible, then the horizontal ear canal can be sutured directly to the skin (iii).

Closure

The mucosa of the horizontal ear canal is sutured to the ventral skin incision with nonabsorbable monofilament suture material in a simple interrupted suture pattern (see D – ii, iii). The mucosal lining of the horizontal ear canal retracts from the cartilage edge, and hence it is important to identify the mucosa to minimize the risk of stenosis of the horizontal ear canal stoma. The dorsal wound is then closed routinely in two layers. A simple continuous suture pattern using monofilament absorbable suture material is used to close the subcutis. An interrupted or continuous suture pattern using monofilament nonabsorbable suture material is used to close the skin.

Postoperative Management

1) Multimodal analgesia, including ring block around the base of the pinna
2) Cold packing (10 minutes twice daily for the first 2–3 days)
3) Elizabethan collar
4) Gentle wound cleaning every 24 hours for the first 3 days; conscious if possible, but under light sedation if necessary

Complications [1–3]

- Hemorrhage in the immediate postoperative period
- Pain
- Incisional dehiscence
- Self-trauma
- Surgical-site infection
- Stenosis and stricture of the stoma

Suggested Adjuvant Treatments

- ± Chemotherapy, depending on tumor type and histologic grade
- ± Radiation therapy, depending on tumor type and completeness of excision

References

1 Tigari, M. and Pinniger, R.S. (1986). Pull-through technique for vertical canal ablation for the treatment of otitis externa in dogs and cats. *J. Small Anim. Pract.* 27: 123–131.

2 Tirgari, M. (1988). Long-term evaluation of the pull-through technique for vertical canal ablation for the treatment of otitis externa in dogs and cats. *J. Small Anim. Pract.* 29: 165–175.

3 Bacon, N.J. (2018). Pinna and external ear canal. In: *Veterinary Surgery: Small Animal*, 2e (ed. K.M. Tobias and S.A. Johnston), 2309–2328. St. Louis: Elsevier.

Plate 3.4

Vertical Ear Canal Resection *continued*

C)

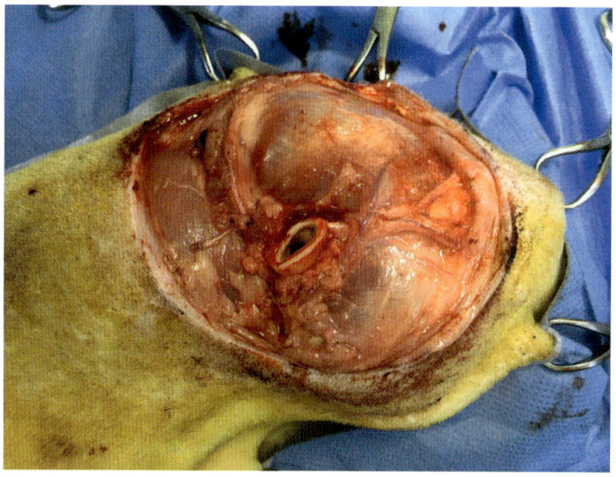

Courtesy of Dr. Josep Aisa

D-i)

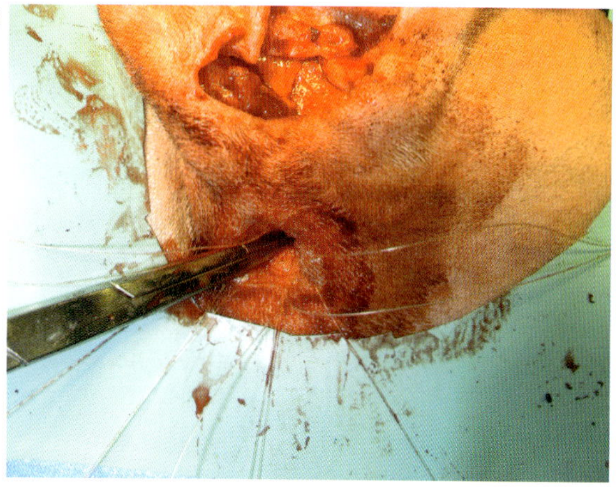

D-ii)

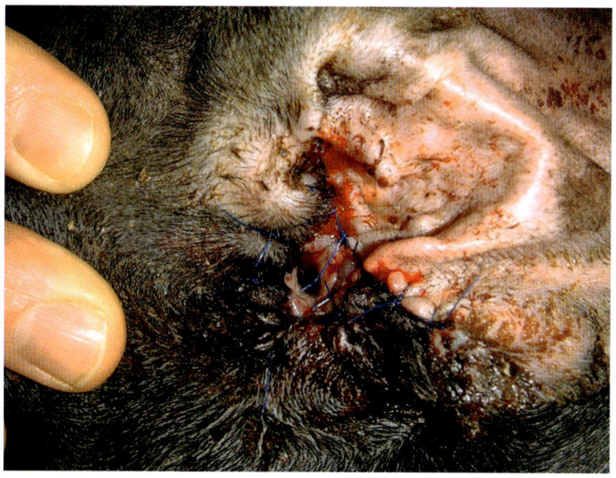

D-iii)

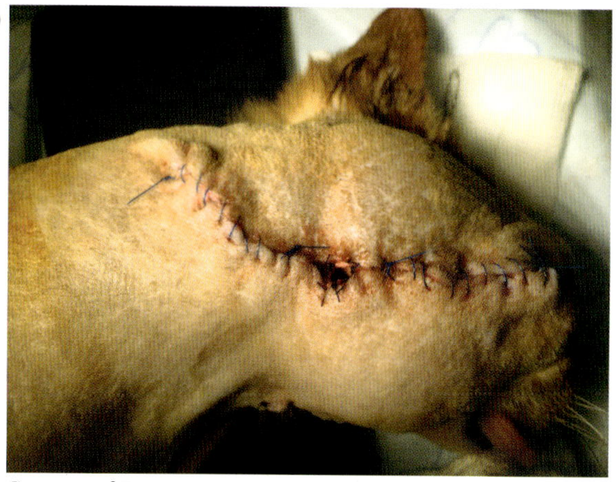

Courtesy of Dr. Josep Aisa

3.5 Lateral Ear Canal Resection

Indications (See Plate 3.5 – 1)

1) Resection of tumors affecting only the lateral cartilage of the vertical ear canal (1, confined ceruminous gland adenocarcinoma).
2) Resection of cutaneous or subcutaneous tumors overlying the vertical ear canal where the vertical ear canal acts as a deep margin.

Suggested Diagnostic Workup and Clinical Staging

- Complete blood count, serum biochemistry, and urinalysis
- Otoscopy
- Otic fine-needle aspirate cytology or grab biopsy
- ± Sentinel lymph node mapping (see *50.1. Sentinel Lymph Node Mapping*) or ultrasound-guided aspirate cytology of the parotid, medial retropharyngeal, and superficial cervical (prescapular) lymph nodes
- ± Skull computed tomography (CT)
- ± Three-view thoracic radiographs or thoracic CT, depending on tumor type

Patient Positioning

The patient is positioned in lateral recumbency with the affected ear uppermost and the nose slightly elevated so it is parallel to the table and the external auditory opening is facing the surgeon vertically. The mandibles should be overlying each other, and the thoracic limbs can be retracted caudally to make a comfortable space for the surgeon.

Surgical Technique (See Plate 3.5A–D)

A) The margin around the mass is marked on the skin with a surgical pen (dotted line). This might also include the rectangular aural tragus (Tr) at the lateral margin of the external auditory meatus.
B) Sharp dissection is continued around the marked perimeter and extended to the appropriate fascial depth. Care should be taken distally as the parotid salivary gland, a nonencapsulated poorly marginated V-shaped structure, is located over the distal end of the vertical ear canal, where it becomes the horizontal canal.

Color Atlas of Canine and Feline Surgical Oncology, First Edition. Julius M. Liptak, Paolo Buracco, William T. N. Culp, and Nicholas J. Bacon.

Plate 3.5

Lateral Ear Canal Resection

1)

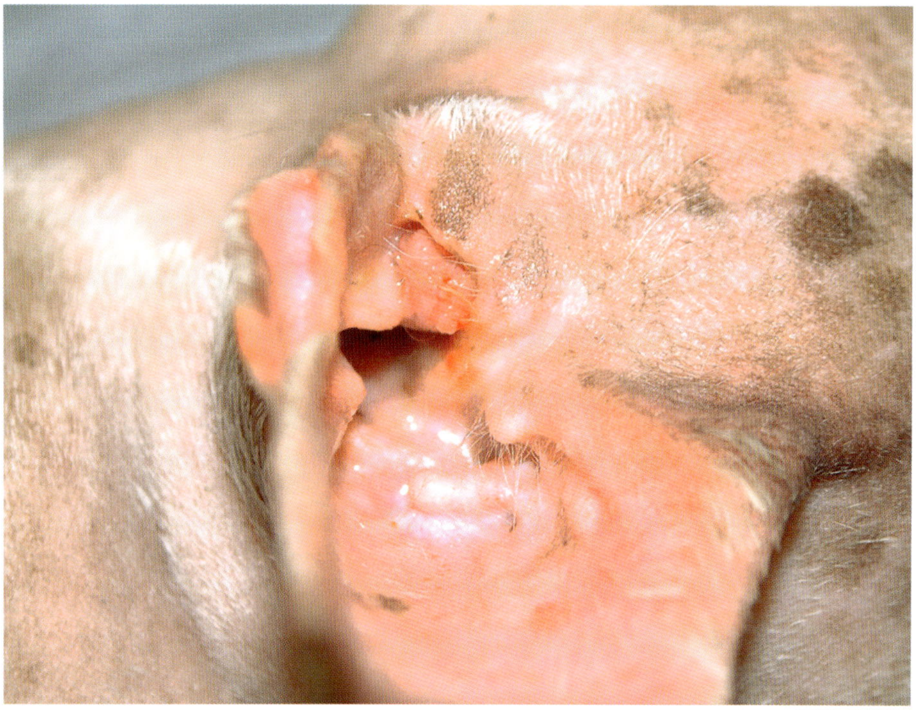

A)

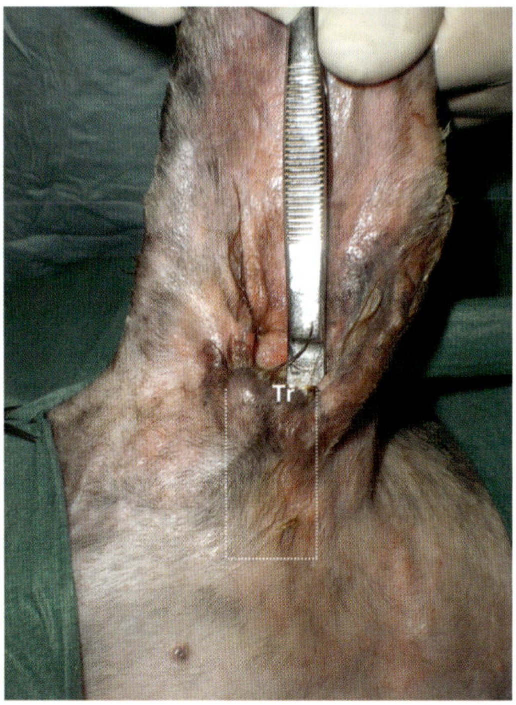

Courtesy of Dr. Roberto Bussadori

B)

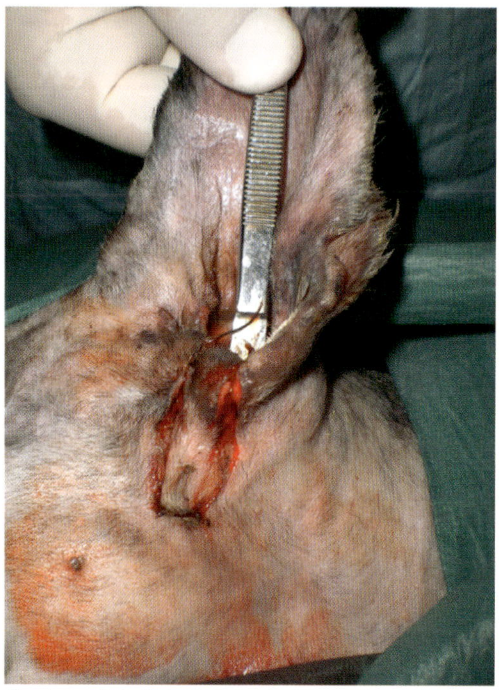

Courtesy of Dr. Roberto Bussadori

Surgical Technique (See Plate 3.4A–D) *continued*

C) The soft tissues overlying the cartilage to be incised are resected, and the rostral and caudal borders of the vertical canal are exposed. Gelpi retractors are useful to maximize exposure.

D) One blade of a straight Mayo scissor is inserted into the ear canal and then rotated 90 degrees so the surgeon's palm faces the tabletop, ensuring the cut edge of the cartilage is parallel with the skin surface. A rostral and caudal straight cut allows 50% of the vertical ear canal circumference to be resected. An incision is done connecting the distal ends of the rostral and caudal incisions, again with the surgeon's palm face down toward the tabletop.

Closure (See Plate 3.5E)

E) The dead space from the soft tissue resection either side of the now-visible medial wall of the vertical ear canal is closed with absorbable sutures. This closure also advances the leading skin edge toward the cut edge of the cartilage. Simple interrupted sutures of monofilament absorbable material are used to appose the mucosa of the vertical ear canal to the skin (i, ii). The needle should pass through the cut edge of the cartilage for security and to reduce tension. The deepest mucosal sutures are placed first, typically the most distal near the junction with the horizontal canal, before moving proximally toward the pinna, alternating between the rostral and caudal edges of the remaining vertical ear canal.

Postoperative Management

1) Multimodal analgesia, including ring block around the base of the pinna
2) Elizabethan collar
3) Gentle wound cleaning every 24 hours for the first 3 days; conscious if possible, but under light sedation if necessary

Complications

- Hemorrhage in the immediate postoperative period
- Pain
- Incisional dehiscence
- Self-trauma
- Surgical-site infection

Suggested Adjuvant Treatment

- ± Chemotherapy, depending on tumor type and histologic grade
- ± Radiation therapy, depending on tumor type and completeness of excision

Prognosis and Oncologic Outcome – Dogs

Tumor Type	Local Recurrence Rate	Metastatic Rate	Disease-Free Interval (d)	Median Survival Time (d)
Ceruminous gland adenocarcinoma [1]	75%	0%	–	–

Reference

1 Marino, D.J., MacDonald, J.M., Matthiesen, D.T. et al. (1993). Results of surgery and long-term follow-up in dogs with ceruminous gland adenocarcinoma. *J. Am. Anim. Hosp. Assoc.* 29: 560–563.

Plate 3.5

Lateral Ear Canal Resection *continued*

C)

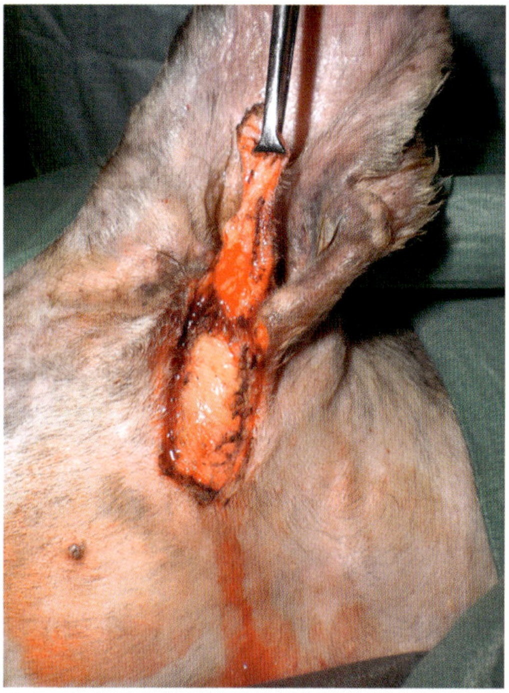

Courtesy of Dr. Roberto Bussadori

D)

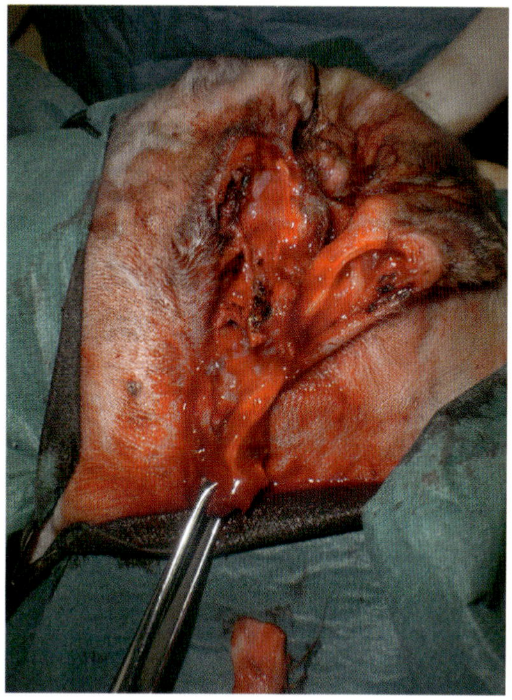

Courtesy of Dr. Roberto Bussadori

E-i)

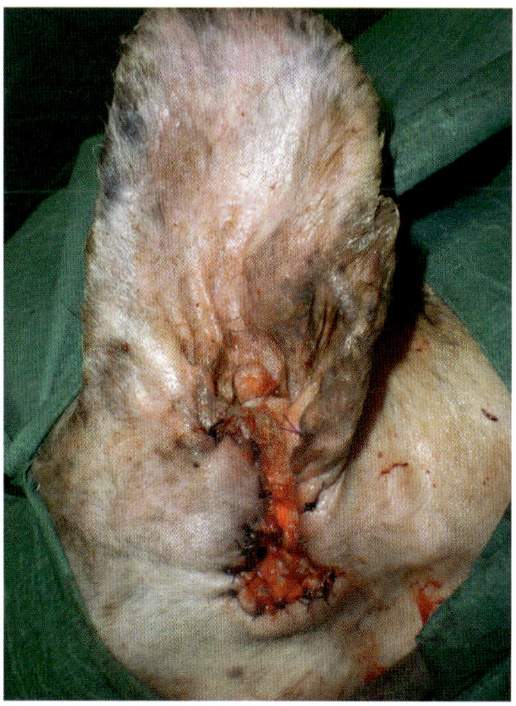

Courtesy of Dr. Roberto Bussadori

E-ii)

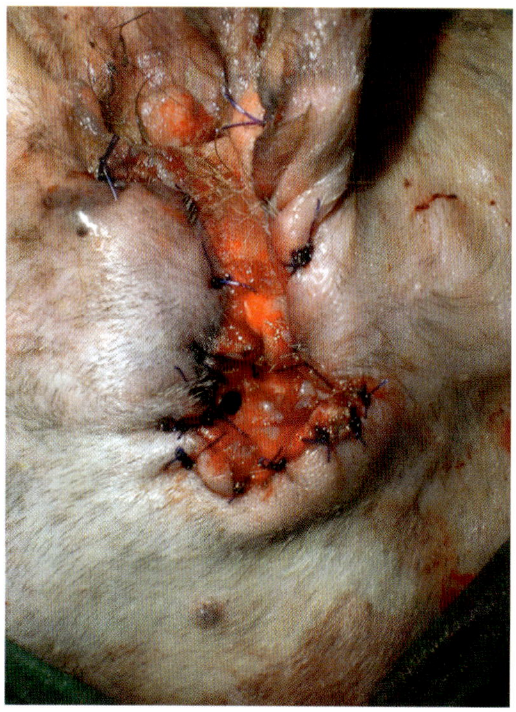

Courtesy of Dr. Roberto Bussadori

Chapter 4: Nasal Planum Resection

4.1 Nasal Planum Resection – Feline

Indications

1) Resection of nasal planum tumors. The most common nasal planum tumor in cats is a squamous cell carcinoma (SCC). These are generally thought to be sunlight induced and may represent a malignant transformation from keratosis or carcinoma in situ to SCC. Although surgical removal is reasonable in many cats with nasal planum neoplasia, other treatment modalities include strontium plesiotherapy, curettage and diathermy, cryosurgery, and intralesional chemotherapy.
2) Nasal planum resection can be combined with a maxillary incisivectomy (see *6.10. Maxillary Incisivectomy*) for greater caudal margins.
3) Nasal planum resection can be combined with an upper lip advancement flap (see *39.2. Upper Lip Advancement Flap*) if the nasal planum defect is also associated with a rostral lip defect.

Suggested Diagnostic Workup and Clinical Staging

- Complete blood count, serum biochemistry, and urinalysis
- Preoperative biopsy
- ± Sentinel lymph node mapping (see *50.1. Sentinel Lymph Node Mapping*) or ultrasound-guided aspirate cytology of the mandibular, medial retropharyngeal, and parotid lymph nodes bilaterally
- ± Skull computed tomography (CT), although this is likely a low-yield staging test because the majority of nasal planum SCCs are locally confined and rarely metastatic
- ± Three-view thoracic radiographs or thoracic CT, depending on tumor type

Patient Positioning

The patient is positioned in sternal recumbency with head elevated to allow for access to the nasal planum.

Surgical Technique (See Plate 4.1A–D)

A) When surgically treating nasal planum tumors in cats, the entire nasal planum will need to be removed, and this region can be isolated within the sterile field. A region including approximately 0.5 cm of margin (whenever possible) around the tumor is denoted and marked with a sterile marker to guide the surgical incision.
B) Once the surgical margin has been clearly identified, a scalpel blade is used to make a full-thickness incision through the skin and down through the cartilage of the nasal turbinates (i). This incision is continued ventrally until the incisive bones are encountered, and laterally through the skin on the left and right side immediately caudal to the nasal planum (ii).

Color Atlas of Canine and Feline Surgical Oncology, First Edition. Julius M. Liptak, Paolo Buracco, William T. N. Culp, and Nicholas J. Bacon.

Plate 4.1

Nasal Planum Resection – Feline

A)

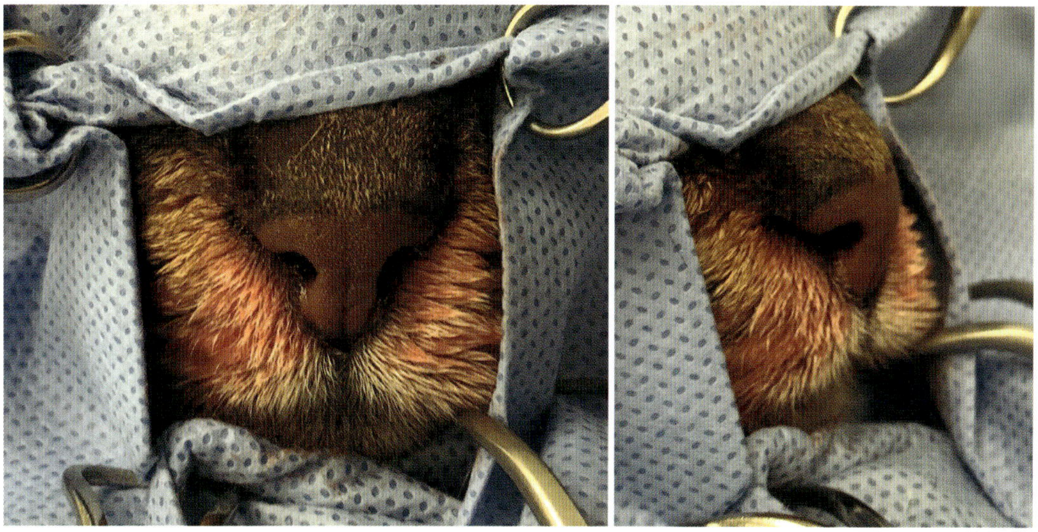

B-i)

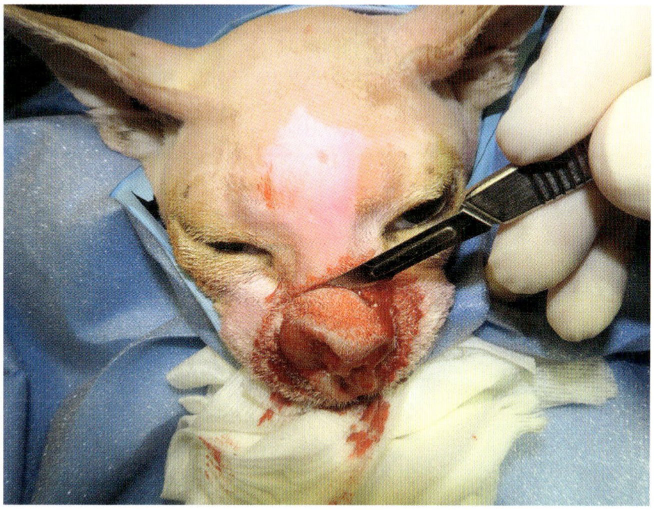

B-ii)

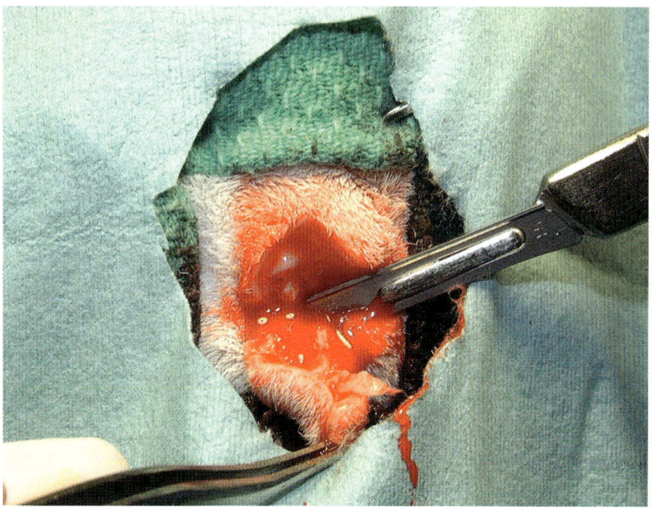

Surgical Technique (See Plate 4.1A–D) *continued*

C) Removal of the lip margin on the midline is determined by the extent of the tumor and the margin that the surgeon is attempting to achieve. Any remaining ventral attachments to the incisive bones can be removed with a scalpel blade or sharp dissecting scissors.
D) The left and right alar folds are grasped and excised. This may improve airflow through the nasal aperture after nasal planum resection. Bleeding from the nasal turbinates can be brisk. Hemostasis should be attempted with a combination of pressure and electrosurgery.

Closure (See Plate 4.1E, F)

E) Two closure techniques have been described: purse-string suture [1] and mucocutaneous apposition [2]. The purse-string suture technique should be avoided because of a higher risk of stenosis of the nasal aperture. If the resection extends ventrally through the margin of the superior lip (exposing the incisive bones), then closure of the skin and mucosa in the region of the palate should commence first. For the mucocutaneous apposition technique, the skin is sutured directly to the cartilaginous tissues of the nasal passage using 4-0 or 5-0 nonabsorbable suture, or absorbable suture is used in a simple interrupted pattern.
F) For more caudal resections where there will be limited cartilaginous tissue, especially nasal planum resections combined with maxillary incisivectomy, bone tunnels will need to be drilled into the maxillary and incisive bone; the skin is then sutured using the same technique to these bone tunnels.

Postoperative Management

1) Multimodal analgesia
2) Allow blood clot to form in region of nasal aperture and do not remove the clot unless marked difficulty with airflow is noted
3) Elizabethan collar

Complications

Intraoperative Complications

- Bleeding: controlled with gentle application of gauze sponges or cotton-tipped applicators to regions of bleeding or electrosurgery

Postoperative Complications (0–14 Days)

- Bleeding
- Sneezing and nasal discharge; this generally resolves by 14 days postoperatively
- Poor appetite; this may be reduced by using infraorbital blocks
- Dehiscence (rare)
- Although not technically a complication, a crust of blood and nasal discharge material can form over the nasal aperture after surgery. This can be gently removed at approximately 14 days postoperatively.

Postoperative Complications (>14 Days)

- Stenosis of nasal aperture (after purse-string suture closure)

Plate 4.1

Nasal Planum Resection – Feline *continued*

C)

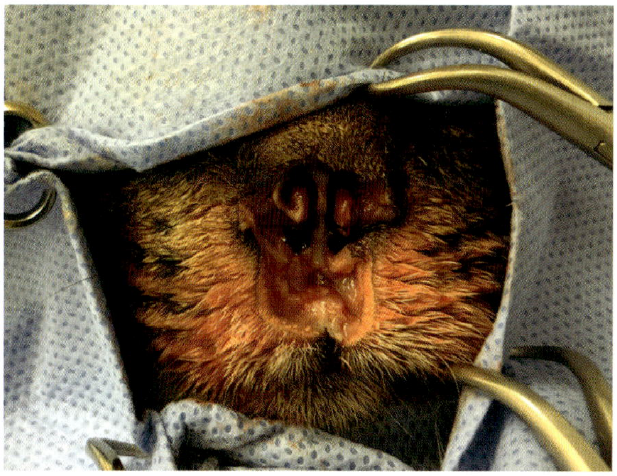

D)

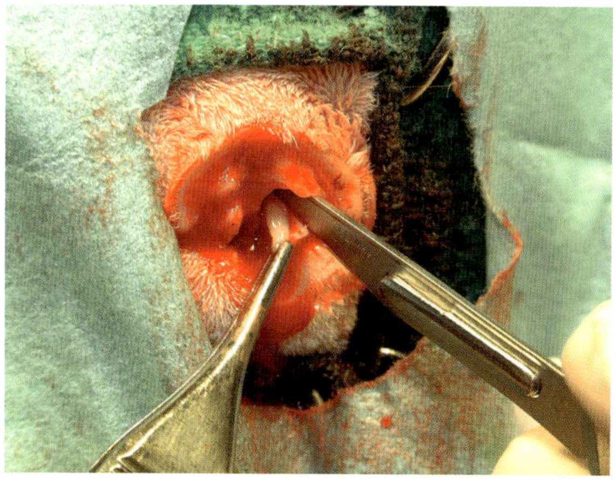

E)

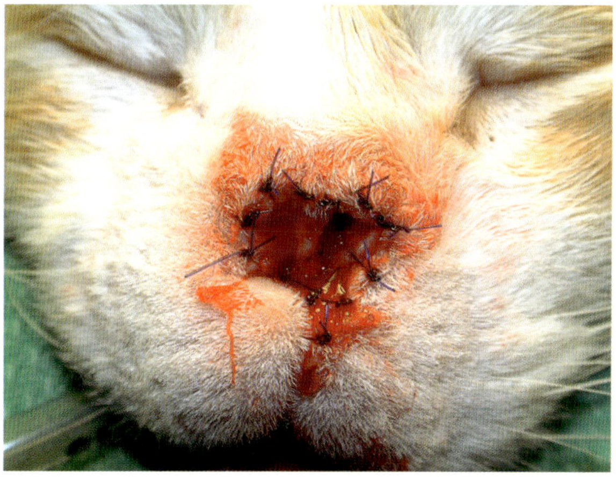

F)

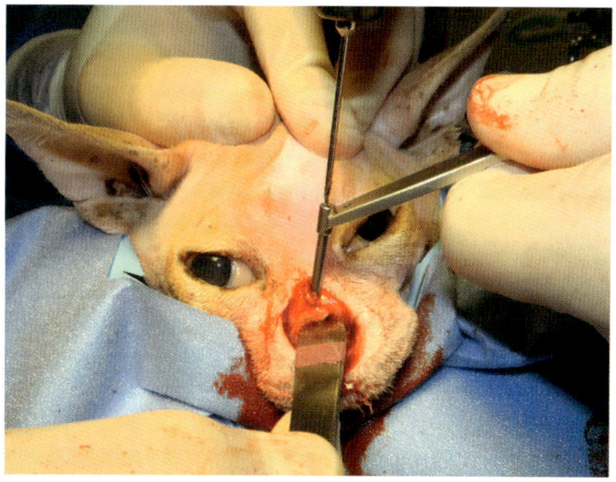

Suggested Adjuvant Treatments

- External beam radiation therapy, strontium plesiotherapy, intralesional chemotherapy, photodynamic therapy, or cryosurgery should be considered if surgical resection results in incomplete histologic margins
- Systemic chemotherapy should be considered if there is documented metastasis to the regional lymph nodes.

Prognosis and Oncologic Outcome [1–3]

Tumor Type	Local Recurrence Rate	Metastatic Rate	Median Disease-Free Interval (d)	Median Survival Time (d)
Squamous cell carcinoma	29%–33%	<5%	524	675

References

1 Withrow, S.J. and Straw, R.C. (1990). Resection of the nasal planum in nine cats and five dogs. *J. Am. Anim. Hosp. Assoc.* 26: 219–222.

2 Thomson, M. (2007). Squamous cell carcinoma of the nasal planum in cats and dogs. *Clin. Tech. Small Anim. Pract.* 22 (2): 42–45.

3 Lana, S.E., Ogilvie, G.K., Withrow, S.J. et al. (1997). Feline cutaneous squamous cell carcinoma of the nasal planum and the pinnae: 61 cases. *J. Am. Anim. Hosp. Assoc.* 33: 329–332.

4.2 Nasal Planum Resection – Canine

Indications

1) Resection of malignant tumors of the nasal planum
2) Nasal planum resection can be combined with a maxillary (see *6.10. Maxillary Incisivectomy*) for greater caudal margins
3) Nasal planum resection can be combined with an upper lip advancement flap (see *39.2. Upper Lip Advancement Flap*) if the nasal planum defect is also associated with a rostral lip defect

Suggested Diagnostic Workup and Clinical Staging

- Complete blood count, serum biochemistry, and urinalysis
- Preoperative biopsy
- Sentinel lymph node mapping (see *50.1. Sentinel Lymph Node Mapping*) or ultrasound-guided aspirate cytology of the mandibular, medial retropharyngeal, and parotid lymph nodes bilaterally
- Skull computed tomography (CT)
- Three-view thoracic radiographs or thoracic CT scan for assessment of lung metastasis

Patient Positioning

The patient is positioned in sternal recumbency with head elevated to allow for access to the nasal planum.

Surgical Technique (See Plate 4.2A–D)

A) A region including approximately 2 cm of margin around the tumor is marked with a sterile marker to guide the surgical resection. In most dogs, the goal of excision is to remove the entire nasal planum with the caudal aspect of the incision on the dorsal and lateral aspects extending to the junction between the cartilaginous tissue and the bones of the maxilla. In cases where only removal of part of the nasal planum is needed (rare), the nasal planum cartilage can be reapposed primarily by suturing the cut edges together, being sure to allow for appropriate opening of the nares.
B) Once the surgical margin has been clearly identified, a scalpel blade is used to make a full-thickness incision through the skin on the dorsal aspect of the nose and caudal to the nasal planum (i), and then extending ventrally through the cartilage of the nasal turbinates (ii). This incision is continued ventrally until the incisive bones are encountered, and laterally through the skin on the left and right side, immediately caudal to the nasal planum (iii). Some authors recommend incising ventrally at an angle of 45 degrees to the hard palate to decrease tension on the closure [1]. Occasionally, an incisivectomy will need to be performed for achieving adequate caudal margins (iv) (see *6.10. Maxillary Incisivectomy*).

Color Atlas of Canine and Feline Surgical Oncology, First Edition. Julius M. Liptak, Paolo Buracco, William T. N. Culp, and Nicholas J. Bacon.

Plate 4.2

Nasal Planum Resection – Canine

A)

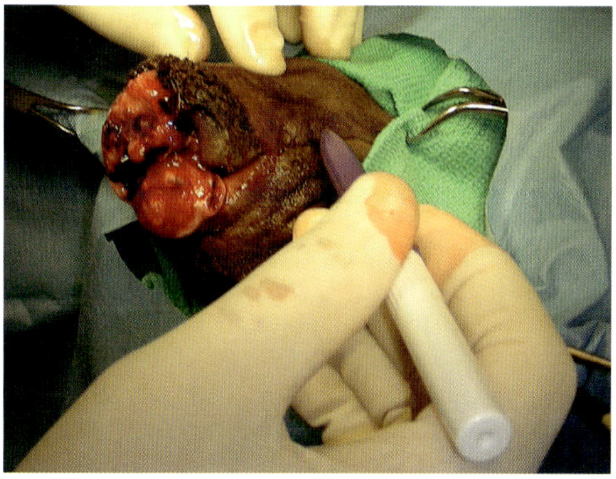

B-i)

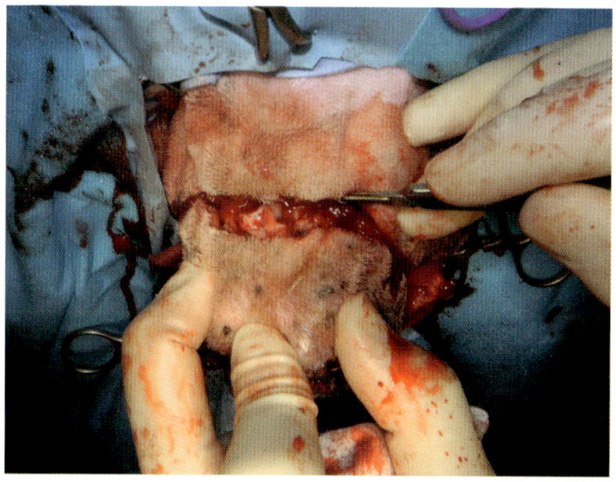

B-ii)

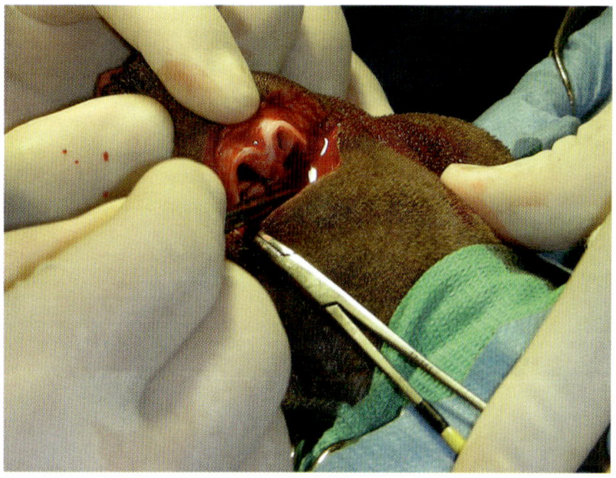

B-iii)

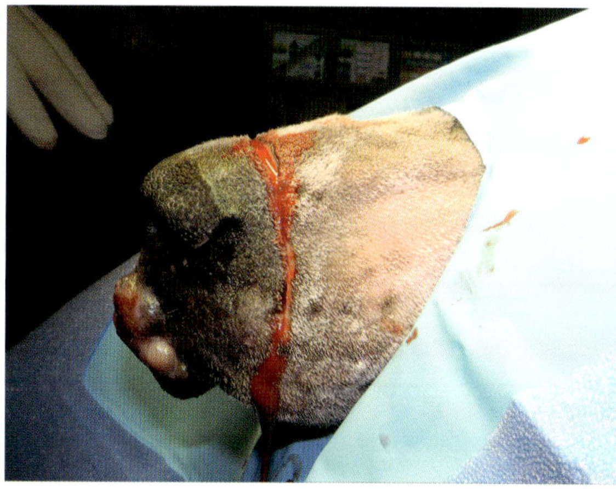

B-iv)

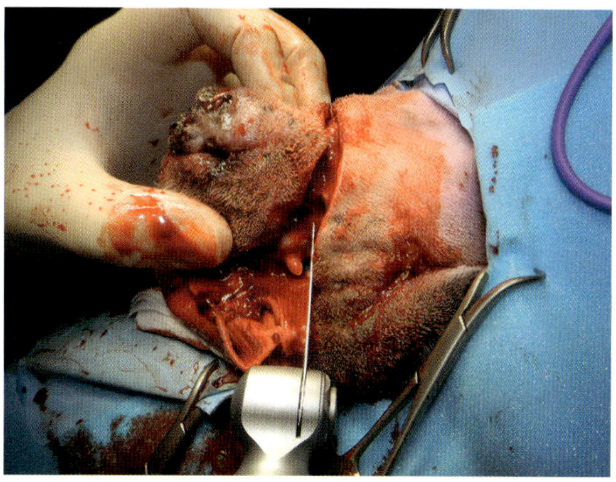

Surgical Technique (See Plate 4.2A–D) *continued*

C) Removal of the lip margin on midline is determined by the extent of the tumor and margin that the surgeon is attempting to achieve. Any remaining ventral attachments to the incisive bones can be removed with a scalpel blade or sharp dissecting scissors. Alar folds can also be removed to allow for increased opening into the nasal passages (pictured).
D) Bleeding from the nasal turbinates tends to be significant. Hemostasis should be attempted with a combination of pressure and electrosurgery or the use of hemostatic sponges (pictured, arrows).

Closure (See Plate 4.2E–J)

E) The three most commonly described closure techniques are a purse-string suture [1], mucocutaneous apposition [2], and bilateral mucocutaneous rotation-advancement flaps [3]. The purse-string suture technique is the least preferred of the closure techniques because of a higher rate of stenosis of the nasal aperture. If the resection extends ventrally through the margin of the superior lip (exposing the incisive bones), closure of the skin and mucosa in the region of the palate should commence first when performing a purse-string suture or mucocutaneous appositional closure (i, arrow; ii).
F) The surgeon can consider drilling bone tunnels through the incisive bone to allow for more secure attachment of the overlying lip (i, ii). Absorbable suture material is preplaced through the bone tunnels and submucosa/subcutaneous of the lips (iii) and then secured (iv).

Plate 4.2

Nasal Planum Resection – Canine *continued*

C)

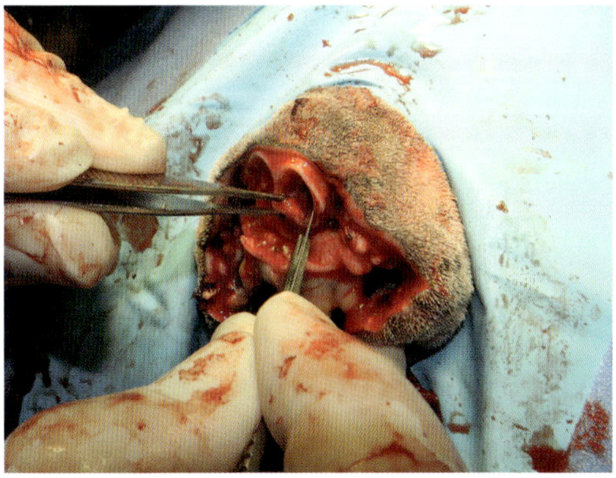

D)

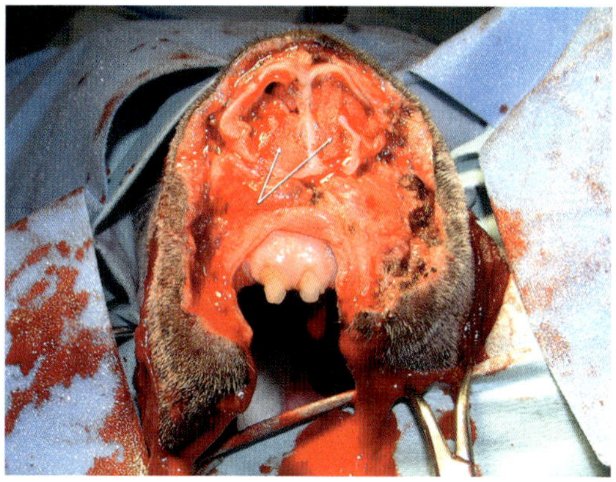

E-i)

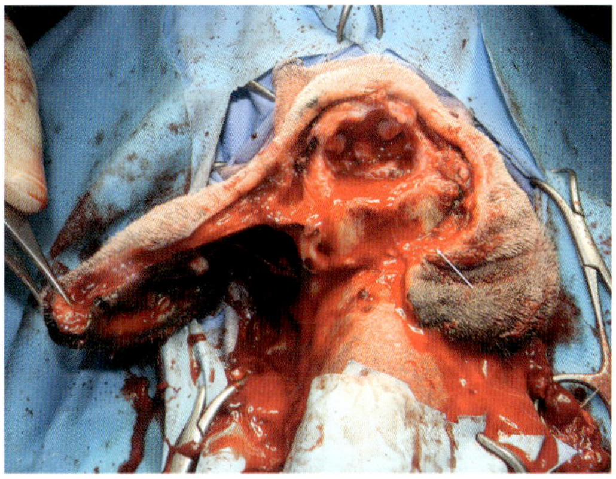

E-ii)

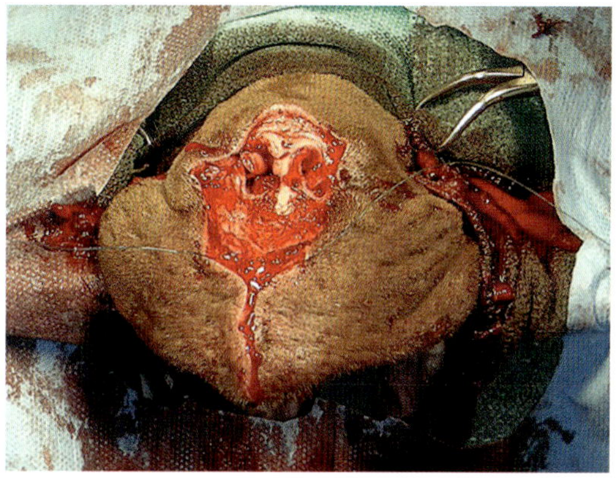

F-i)

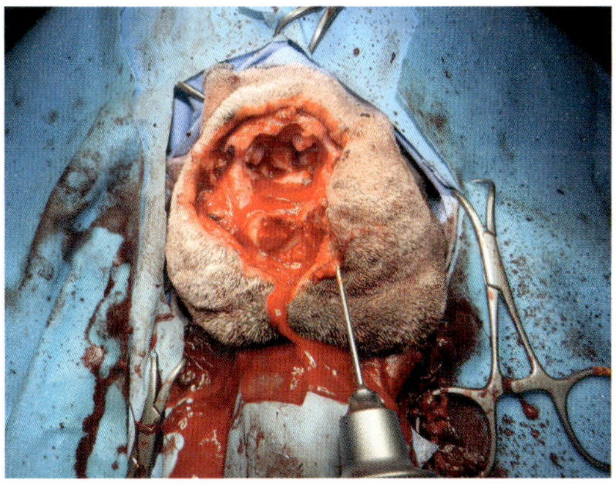

F-ii)

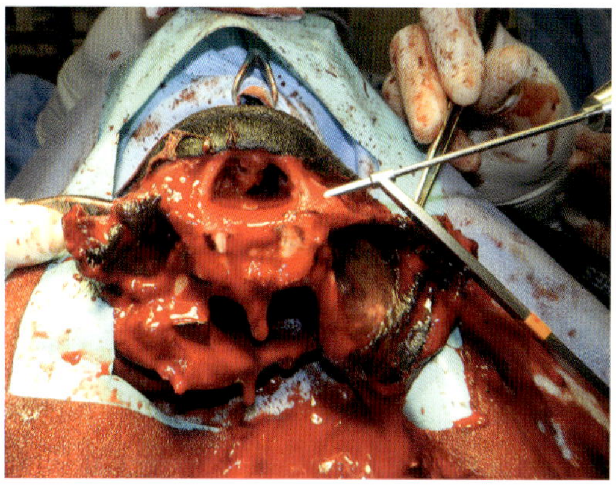

F-iii)

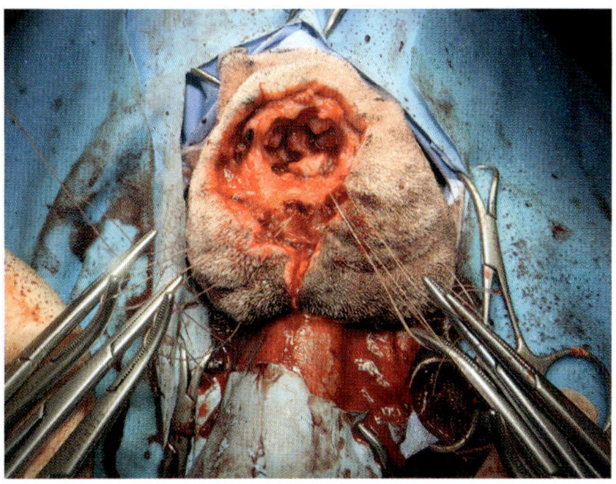

F-iv)

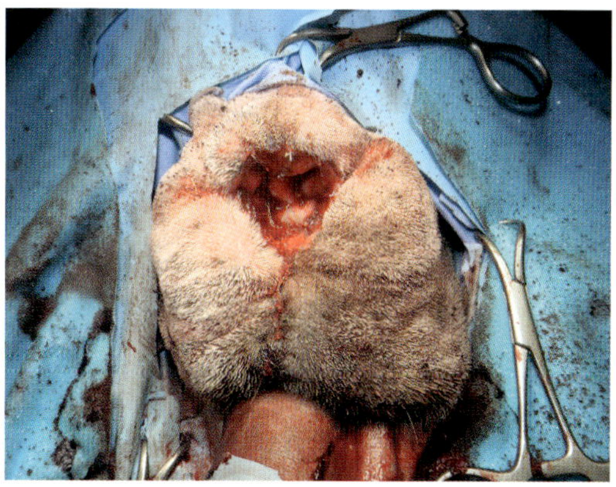

Closure (See Plate 4.2E–J) *continued*

G) For mucocutaneous apposition, the skin is sutured directly to the cartilaginous tissues of the nasal passage using 3-0 to 5-0 nonabsorbable suture, or absorbable suture is used in a simple interrupted pattern (i, ii). If possible, the cartilaginous structures should be pulled out laterally away from the nasal passages to allow for improved airflow.

H) The bilateral labial mucocutaneous rotation-advancement flap [2, 4] was developed in an attempt to improve the cosmetic outcome after nasal planum resection. After resection of the nasal planum, the alar fold and nasal septal cartilage are debrided to create a larger nasal aperture (see step C). The labial mucosa of the left and right rostral lip is then sutured to the ipsilateral nasal mucosa in a continuous or simple interrupted suture pattern using 4-0 to 3-0 monofilament absorbable suture.

I) This is performed bilaterally to allow the labial mucosa to be sutured completely around the nasal opening, including over the cut edge of the incisive bone (preplaced sutures through bone tunnels are pictured).

J) The lip margins are then used to create a philtrum by excising a section of the mucocutaneous margin of the lip bilaterally (i, ii). The floor of the rostral nasal passage is created by incising through the labial mucosa, and the labial mucosa is apposed intraorally with 4-0 to 3-0 monofilament absorbable suture in a continuous pattern (iii).

Postoperative Management

1) Multimodal analgesia
2) Allow blood clot to form in region of nasal aperture and do not remove unless marked difficulty with airflow is noted
3) Elizabethan collar

Complications

Intraoperative Complications

- Bleeding

Postoperative Complications (0–14 Days)

- Bleeding
- Sneezing and nasal discharge; this generally resolves by 14 days postoperatively
- Poor appetite
- Dehiscence (50% after reconstruction with the bilateral labial mucocutaneous rotation-advancement flaps technique) [3]
- Although not technically a complication, a crust of blood and nasal discharge material can form over the nasal aperture after surgery; this can be gently removed at approximately 14 days postoperatively

Postoperative Complications (>14 Days)

- Stenosis (19% after reconstruction with the bilateral labial mucocutaneous rotation-advancement flaps technique) [3]
- Cosmesis is generally well tolerated; however, owners should be counseled preoperatively for the altered postoperative appearance (3 months postoperatively)

Suggested Adjuvant Treatments

- External beam radiation therapy, strontium plesiotherapy, intralesional chemotherapy, photodynamic therapy, or cryosurgery should be considered if surgical resection results in incomplete histologic margins.
- Systemic chemotherapy should be considered if there is documented metastasis to the regional lymph nodes.

Plate 4.2

Nasal Planum Resection – Canine *continued*

G-i)

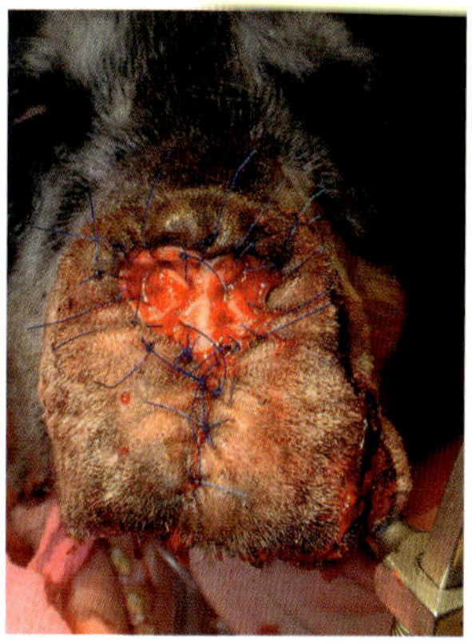

G-ii)

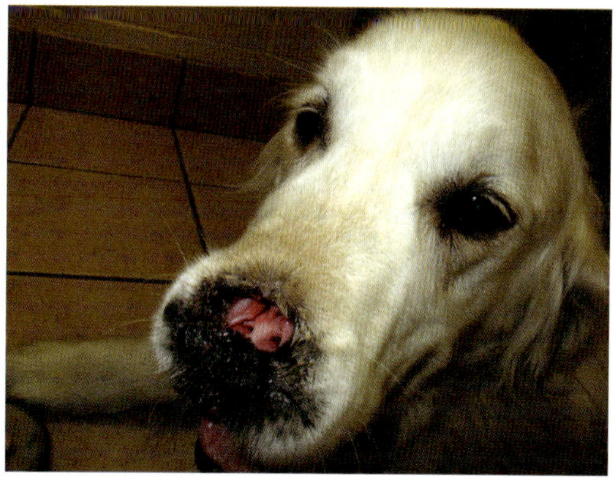

H)

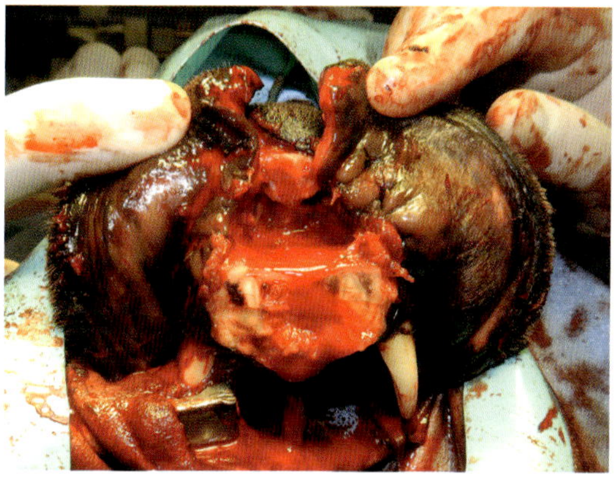

I)

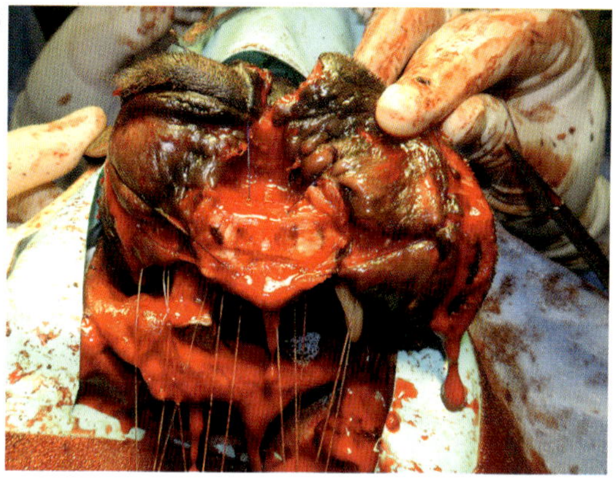

J-i)

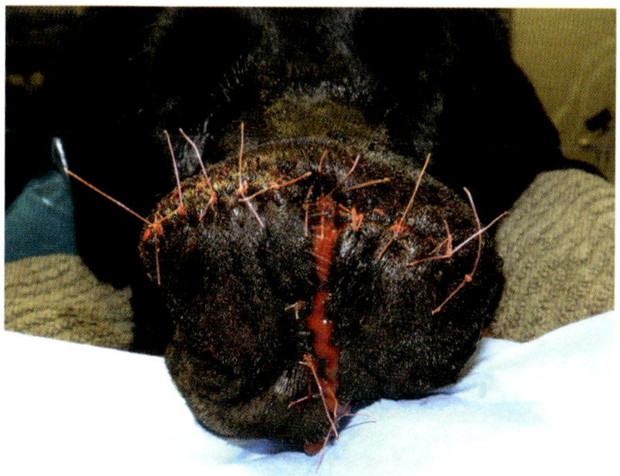

J-iii)

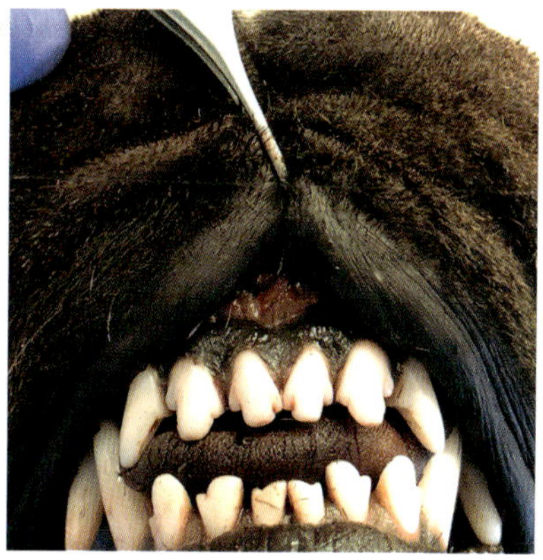

J-ii)

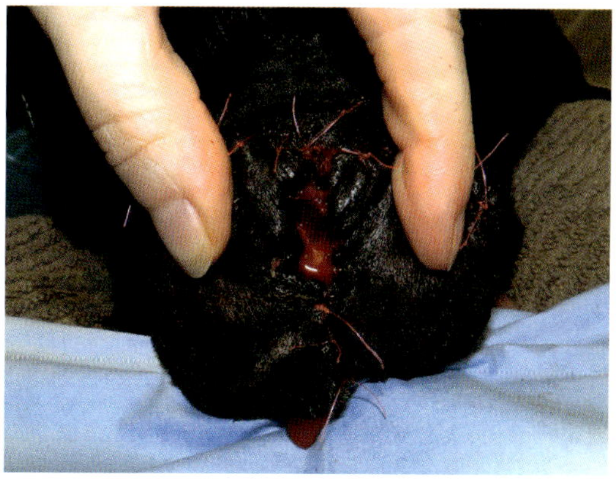

Prognosis and Oncologic Outcome [1–5]

Tumor Type	Local Recurrence Rate	Metastatic Rate	Median Survival Time (d)
SCC			
Overall	–	0%–9%	1542
Complete excision	0%	–	–
Incomplete excision	8%–33%	–	–

References

1 Withrow, S.J. and Straw, R.C. (1990). Resection of the nasal planum in nine cats and five dogs. *J. Am. Anim. Hosp. Assoc.* 26: 219–222.

2 Lascelles, B.D., Parry, A.T., Stidworthy, M.F. et al. (2000). Squamous cell carcinoma of the nasal planum in 17 dogs. *Vet. Rec.* 147 (17): 473–476.

3 Dickerson, V.M., Grimes, J.A., Vetter, C.A. et al. (2019). Outcome following cosmetic rostral nasal reconstruction after planectomy in 26 dogs. *Vet. Surg.* 48 (1): 64–69.

4 Rogers, K.S., Helman, R.G., and Walker, M.A. (1995). Squamous cell carcinoma of the canine nasal planum: eight cases (1988–1994). *J. Am. Anim. Hosp. Assoc.* 31 (5): 373–378.

5 Lascelles, B.D., Henderson, R.A., Seguin, B. et al. (2004). Bilateral rostral maxillectomy and nasal planectomy for large rostral maxillofacial neoplasms in six dogs and one cat. *J. Am. Anim. Hosp. Assoc.* 40 (2): 137–146.

Chapter 5: Tonsillectomy

Indications

1) Resection of malignant tonsillar tumors
2) Clinical staging for malignant oropharyngeal tumors
3) Management of persistent or recurrent tonsillitis

Suggested Diagnostic Workup and Clinical Staging (See Plate 1)

- Oropharyngeal examination under heavy sedation or light general anesthesia
- Preoperative biopsy
- Sentinel lymph node mapping (1; see *50.1. Sentinel Lymph Node Mapping*) or ultrasound-guided aspirate cytology of the mandibular, medial retropharyngeal, and parotid lymph nodes bilaterally
- ± Skull computed tomography (CT)
- Three-view thoracic radiographs or thoracic CT

Patient Positioning

The patient is positioned in sternal recumbency with the head at the end of the table and the maxilla hanging by a length of tape suspended from an over-the-table stand. A small pharyngeal pack should be placed to protect the airway. A mouth gag will assist with additional exposure, although this should be used with caution in cats to avoid blindness [1].

Surgical Technique – Small Tonsillar Mass (See Plate 5A–E)

A) The affected tonsil should be tractioned into the oropharynx with DeBakey forceps (i). A curved long-armed clamp should then be placed along the base of the tonsil (ii). Care should be taken not to include excess oral mucosa from the wall of the pharynx caudal to the tonsil because this tissue is often loose and mobile.
B) A scalpel blade is run along the surface of the clamp to complete the tonsillectomy.

Color Atlas of Canine and Feline Surgical Oncology, First Edition. Julius M. Liptak, Paolo Buracco, William T. N. Culp, and Nicholas J. Bacon.

Plate 5

Tonsillectomy

1)

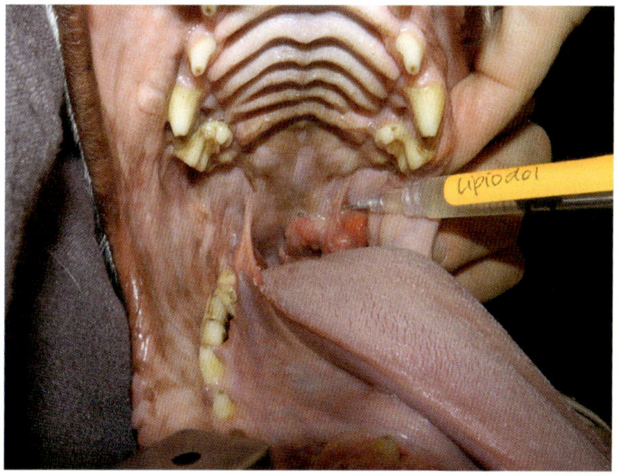

A-i)

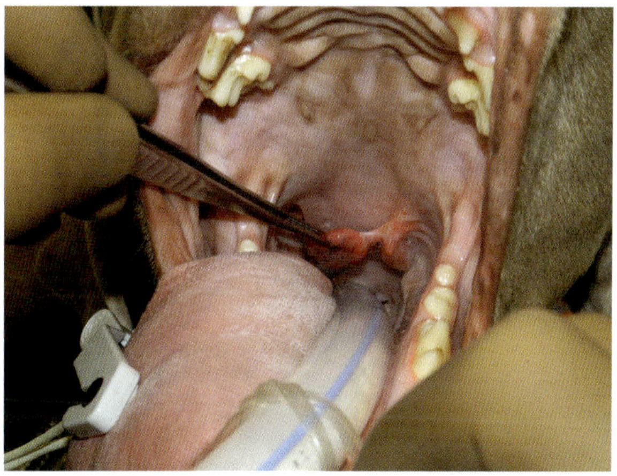

A-ii)

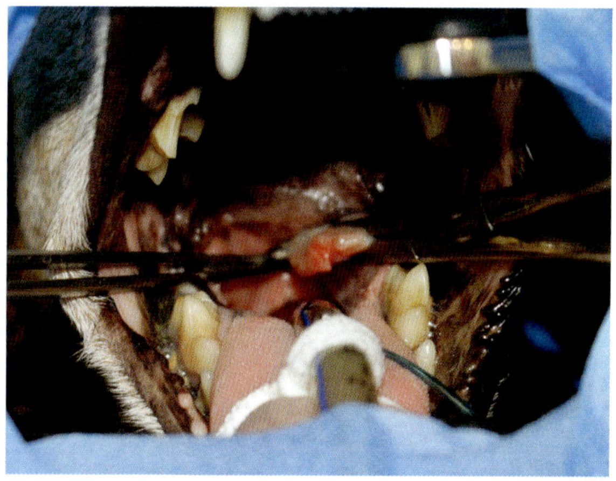

B)

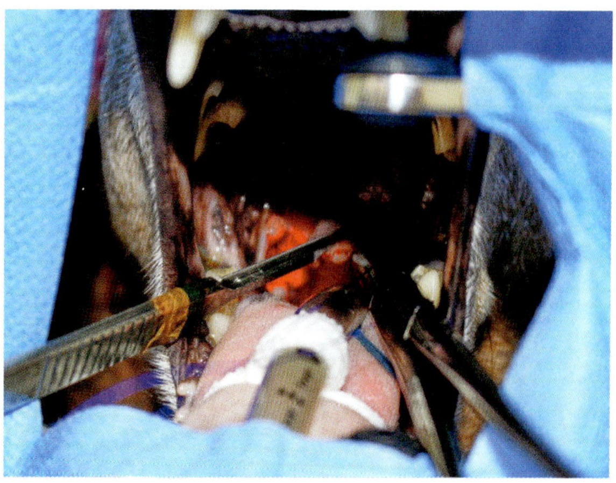

Surgical Technique – Small Tonsillar Mass (See Plate 5A–E) *continued*

C) A Parker-Kerr suture pattern using 3-0 monofilament absorbable suture material is started at the caudal end of the pedicle (i). The ears on the caudal suture knot initially should be left long. The Parker-Kerr suture pattern is loosely continued over the clamp with 2–3 mm between suture passes along the length of the pedicle until the rostral end of the pedicle is reached. A mosquito forcep should be placed on the ears of the caudal suture knot. The jaws of the clamp are gently opened and the clamp is withdrawn (ii). The oversewn suture is to be tightened by tractioning the caudal and rostral ends of the suture to provide immediate hemostasis (iii), and then the rostral knot is secured and the ears on the caudal knot are trimmed to a shorter length (iv).

D) If a vessel sealing device is available, the tonsil is tractioned medially as outlined in A. Rather than clamping and oversewing the tonsil, the base is sealed within the tonsillar crypt from a rostral to caudal direction in multiple small steps (i). No suture material is required for closure (ii).

E) The contralateral tonsil should be removed for staging purposes, using the steps outlined above (A–C or D), because bilateral disease is reported (see G-v).

Plate 5

Tonsillectomy *continued*

C-i)

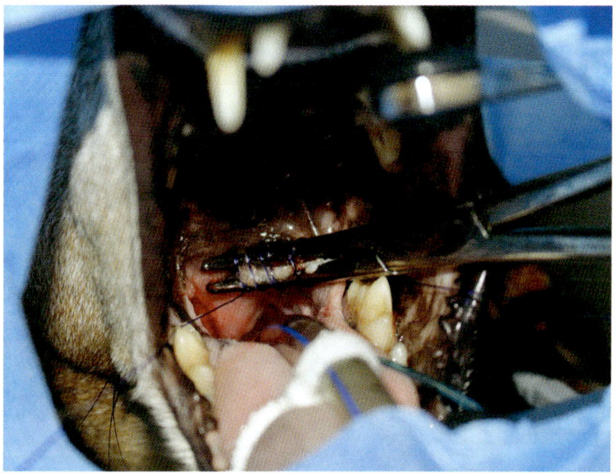

C-ii)

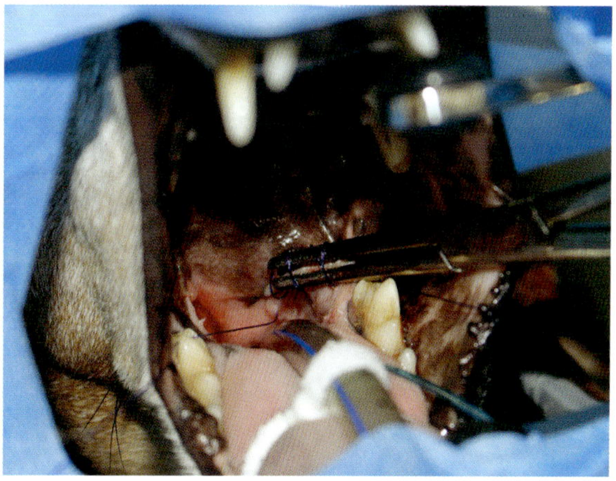

C-iii)

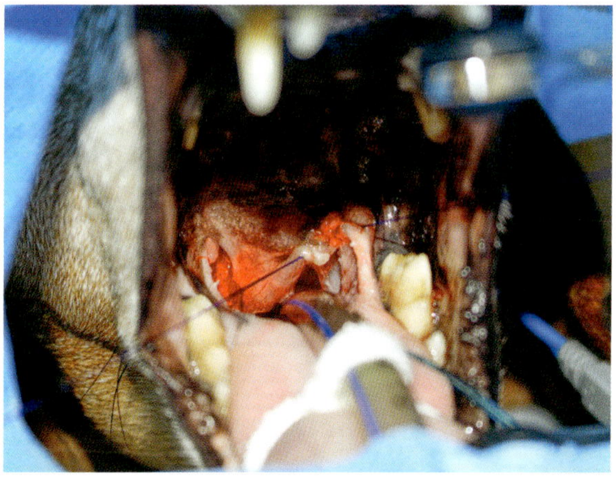

C-iv)

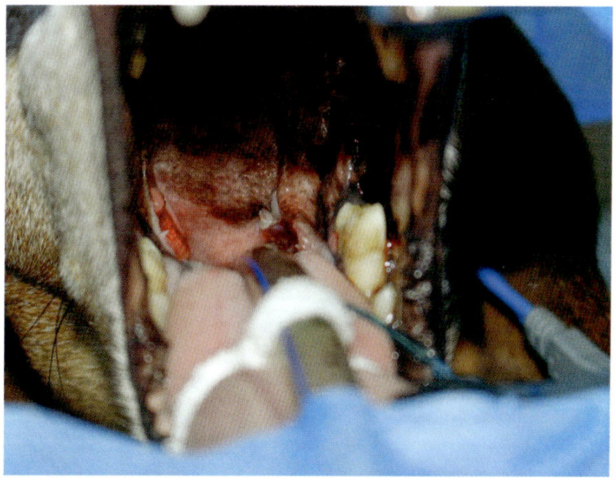

D-i)

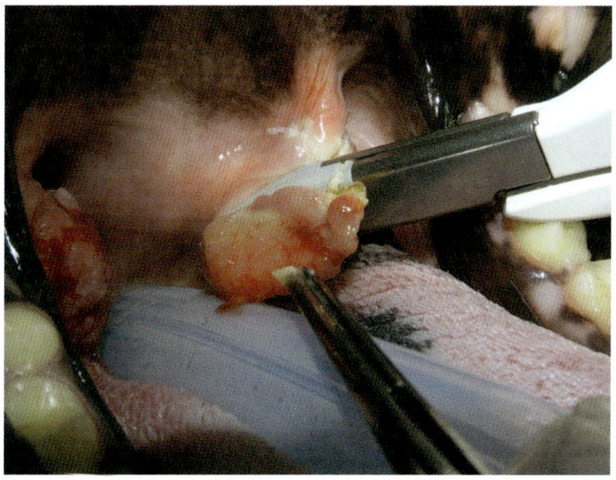

D-ii)

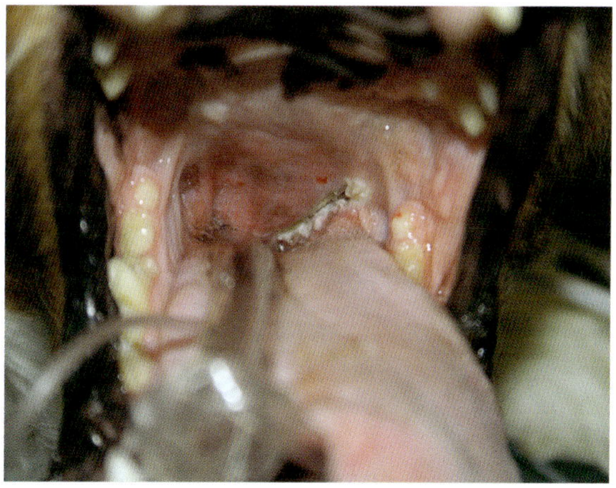

Surgical Technique – Large Tonsillar Mass (See Plate 5F–H)

F) When the tonsillar mass has grown into the pedicle (i), it is necessary to resect the adjacent oral mucosa to allow dissection deep to the mass. An openmouthed CT of the skull with contrast will delineate the deep extent of the tumor before surgery. The oral mucosa adjacent to the mass is incised 5–10 mm around the visible tumor (ii), starting rostrally and encircling the entire tonsillar crypt if access permits. The mobility of the local mucosa is helpful in obtaining a slightly wider surgical margin. Resection of the entire tonsillar bed and crypt is performed with a combination of sharp and electrosurgery dissection (iii) or a vessel sealing device (iii). This results in a large pharyngeal wall defect (iv, v).

Plate 5

Tonsillectomy *continued*

F-i)

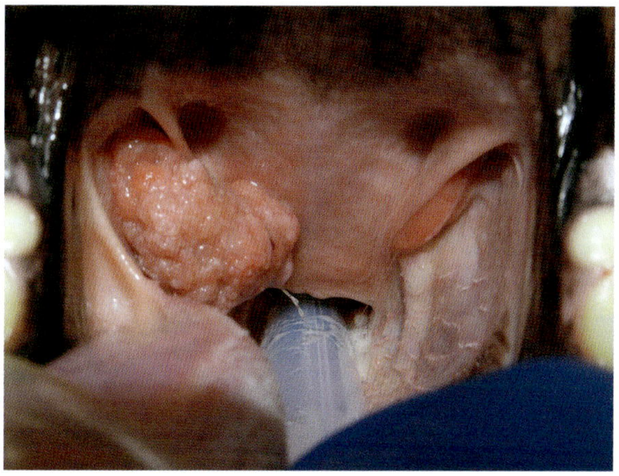

F-ii)

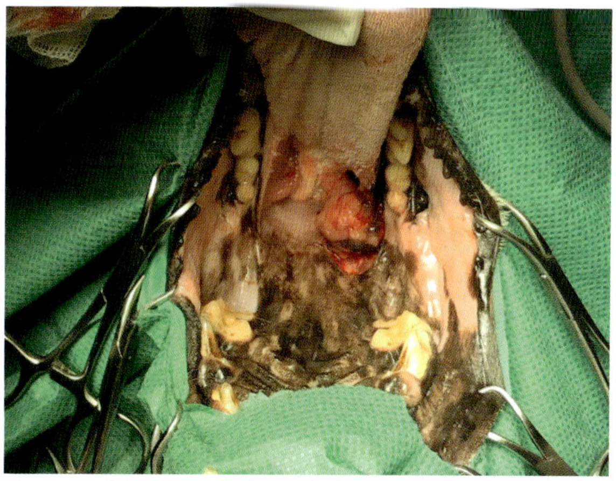

Courtesy of Dr. Maurizio Annoni

F-iii)

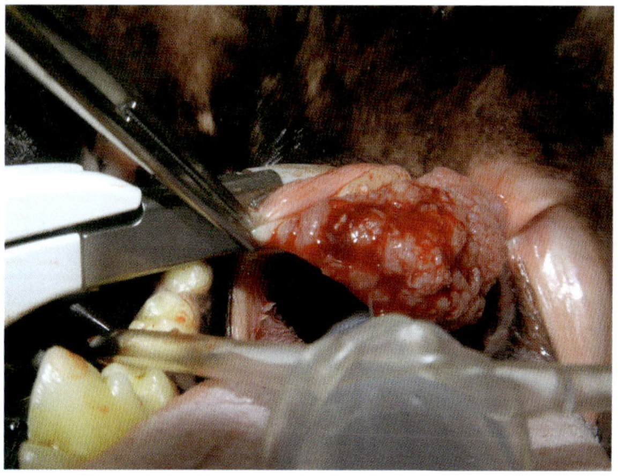

F-iv)

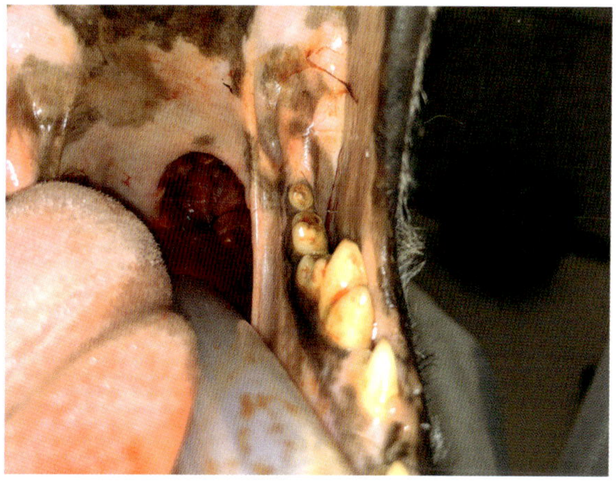

F-v)

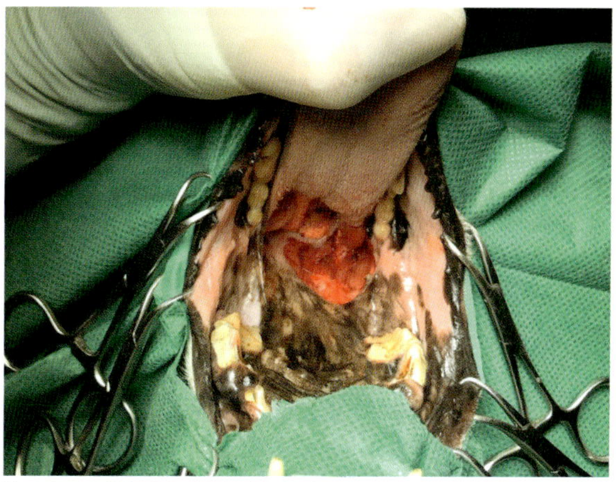

Courtesy of Dr. Maurizio Annoni

Surgical Technique – Large Tonsillar Mass (See Plate 5F–H) *continued*

G) The surrounding oral mucosa is gently undermined. The mucosa is closed primarily with simple interrupted or continuous suture pattern using 3-0 to 4-0 absorbable suture material (i, ii); reconstructed with an angularis oris axial pattern flap (iii, iv); or the open wound can be left to heal by second intention if primary closure is not possible (v).
H) The contralateral tonsil should be removed for staging purposes, using the steps outlined earlier (A–C or D), because bilateral disease is reported (see G-v).

Postoperative Management

1) Multimodal analgesia

Complications

Intraoperative Complications

- Bleeding

Postoperative Complications

- Pain
- Bleeding
- Poor appetite
- Pharyngeal swelling
- Aspiration pneumonia

Suggested Adjuvant Treatments

Systemic chemotherapy should be considered for dogs and cats with tonsillar squamous cell carcinoma or malignant melanoma because of high rates of metastasis to the regional lymph nodes and lungs.

Prognosis and Oncologic Outcome – Dogs

Tumor Type	Local Recurrence Rate	Metastatic Rate	Disease-Free Interval (d)	Median Survival Time (d)	1-Year Survival Rate	2-Year Survival Rate
Squamous cell carcinoma [2–5]	–	58%–67%	91	179–243	11%–40%	11%–20%
Clinical signs at diagnosis [5]						
No	–	–	–	185	–	–
Yes	–	–	–	113	–	–
Clinical stage [2, 4, 5]						
No metastasis	–	–	–	365–638	50%	25%
Lymph node metastasis	–	–	–	122–153	9%	0%
Distant metastasis	–	–	–	75–88	–	–
Treatment [5]						
Surgery	–	–	–	196	–	–
No surgery	–	–	–	88	–	–

Plate 5

Tonsillectomy *continued*

G-i)

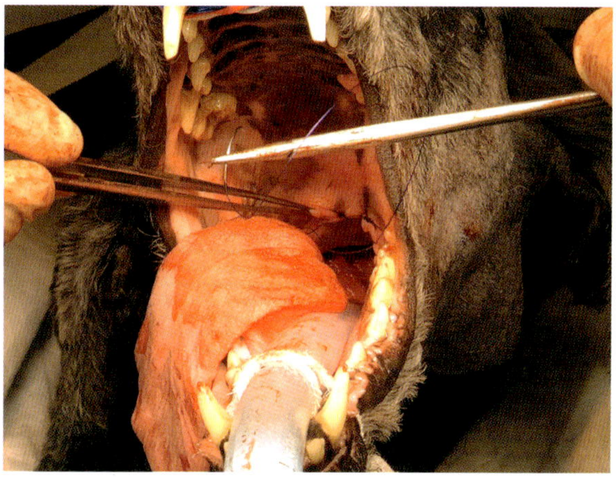

G-ii)

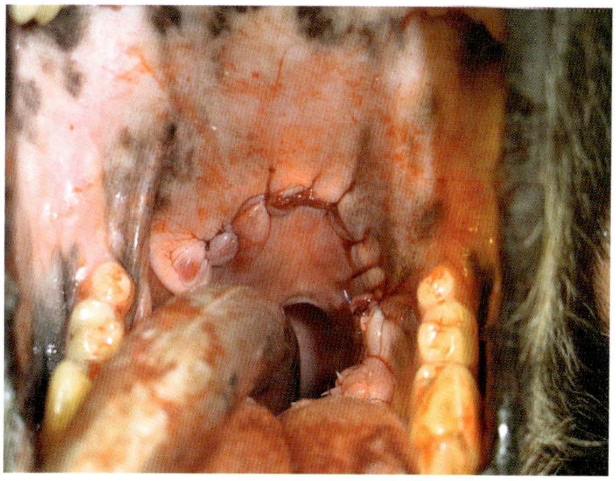

G-iii)

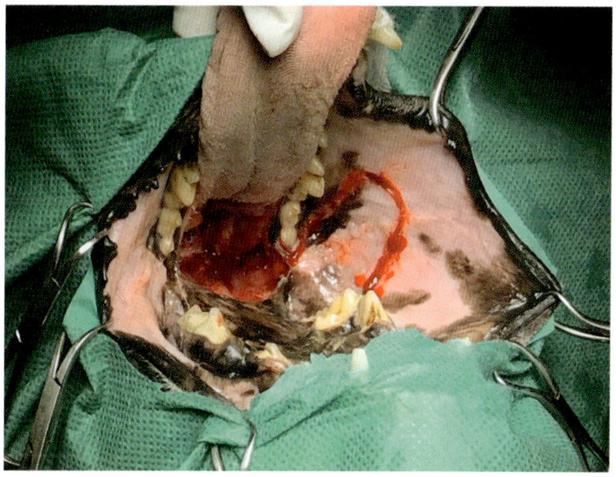

Courtesy of Dr. Maurizio Annoni

G-iv)

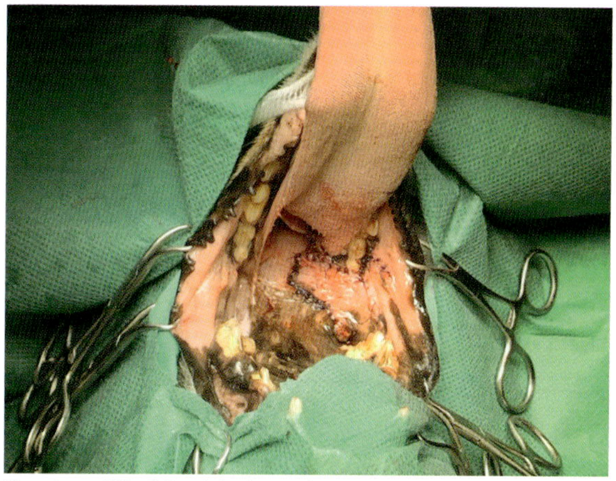

Courtesy of Dr. Maurizio Annoni

G-v)

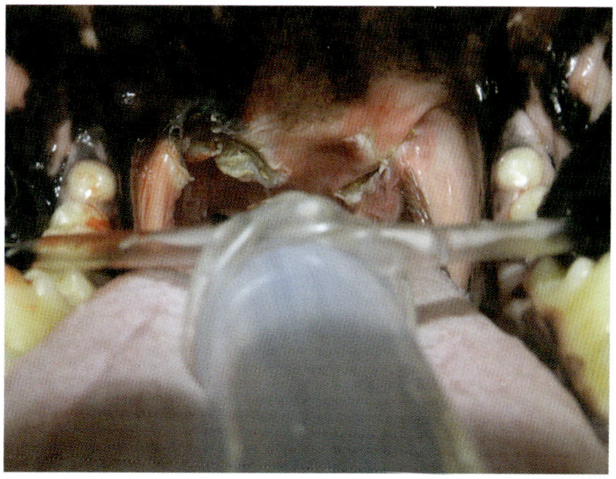

References

1 Stiles, J., Weil, A.B., Packer, R.A. et al. (2012). Post-anesthetic cortical blindness in cats: twenty cases. *Vet. J.* 193 (2): 367–373.

2 Kühnel, S. and Kessler, M. (2010). Tonsillar squamous cell carcinoma in the dog. A retrospective study of 33 cases. *Tierarztl. Prax.* 38 (6): 367–373.

3 Mas, A., Blackwood, L., Cripps, P. et al. (2011). Canine tonsillar squamous cell carcinoma - a multi-Centre retrospective review of 44 clinical cases. *J. Small Anim. Pract.* 52 (7): 359–364.

4 Grant, J. and North, S. (2016). Evaluation of the factors contributing to long-term survival in canine tonsillar squamous cell carcinoma. *Aust. Vet. J.* 94 (6): 197–202.

5 Treggiari, E., Pellin, M.A., Romanelli, G. et al. (2023). Tonsillar carcinoma in dogs: treatment outcome and potential prognostic factors in 123 cases. *J. Vet. Intern. Med.* 37 (1): 247–257.

Chapter 6: Mandibulectomy and Maxillectomy

Mandibulectomy and maxillectomy are indicated for surgical resection of benign and malignant oral tumors; however, the majority of peripheral odontogenic fibromas can be managed with less aggressive surgical approaches that do not require the resection of bone. Surgery is the most effective treatment modality for the management of oral tumors in cats and dogs. Alternative treatment options are available for certain tumor types, including radiation therapy [1] or intralesional bleomycin [2] for acanthomatous ameloblastomas, and radiation therapy for malignant melanomas [3].

Suggested Adjuvant Treatments

- Radiation therapy for incompletely excised malignant oral tumors
- Melanoma vaccine for cats and dogs with high-grade ± all melanomas
- Chemotherapy for dogs with oral osteosarcomas

Prognosis and Oncologic Outcome

Prognosis and Oncologic Outcome After Mandibulectomy or Maxillectomy – Dogs

	Local Recurrence Rate	Metastatic Rate	Disease-Free Interval (d)	Median Survival Time (d)	1-Year Survival Rate	2-Year Survival Rate
			Malignant Melanoma [4]			
Overall	17%	36%	>567	874	–	–
Clinical stage						
• Stage I	–	–	>567	874	–	–
• Stage II	–	–	>187	818	–	–
• Stage III	–	–	245	207	–	–
• Stage IV	–	–	–	–	–	–
			Squamous Cell Carcinoma [5, 6]			
Overall	23%	5%	NR	NR	79%–94%	76%
Clinical stage						
• Stage I	–	–	–	NR	–	–
• Stage II	–	–	–	420	–	–
• Stage III	–	–	–	365	–	–
• Stage IV	–	–	–	50	–	–

Color Atlas of Canine and Feline Surgical Oncology, First Edition. Julius M. Liptak, Paolo Buracco, William T. N. Culp, and Nicholas J. Bacon.

	Local Recurrence Rate	Metastatic Rate	Disease-Free Interval (d)	Median Survival Time (d)	1-Year Survival Rate	2-Year Survival Rate
			Fibrosarcoma [5, 7]			
Overall	38%	15%	>653	557–743	61%–88%	42%–58%
			Osteosarcoma			
Overall[a] [8]	44%	39%	239	329	–	–
Mandible [9]	18%	58%	627[b]	525	–	–
			Acanthomatous Ameloblastoma [10]			
Overall	0%	–	NR	NR	–	–
			Extramedullary Plasmacytoma [11]			
Overall	31%	11%	–	973	–	–

[a] Includes calvarial osteosarcomas.
[b] Metastasis-free interval.
NR, not reached.

Prognosis and Oncologic Outcome After Mandibulectomy – Cats [12]

	Local Recurrence Rate	Metastatic Rate	Disease-Free Interval (d)	Median Survival Time (d)	1-Year Survival Rate	2-Year Survival Rate
			Squamous Cell Carcinoma			
Overall	38%	–	–	217	43%	43%
			Fibrosarcoma			
Overall	67%	–	–	NR	67%	67%
			Osteosarcoma			
Overall	17%	–	–	NR	83%	83%

NR, not reached.

Prognosis and Oncologic Outcome After Maxillectomy – Cats [13]

	Local Recurrence Rate	Metastatic Rate	Disease-Free Interval (d)	Median Survival Time (d)	1-Year Survival Rate	2-Year Survival Rate
			Squamous Cell Carcinoma			
Overall	20%	20%	–	2657	83%	83%
			Fibrosarcoma			
Overall	23%	0%	–	NR	94%	94%
			Osteosarcoma			
Overall	40%	0%	–	NR	80%	80%

NR, not reached.

References

1 Thrall, D.E. (1984). Orthovoltage radiotherapy of acanthomatous epulides in 39 dogs. *J. Am. Vet. Med. Assoc.* 184 (7): 826–829.

2 Kelly, J.M., Belding, B.A., and Schaefer, A.K. (2010). Acanthomatous ameloblastoma in dogs treated with intralesional bleomycin. *Vet. Comp. Oncol.* 8 (2): 81–86.

3 Kawabe, M., Mori, T., Ito, Y. et al. (2015). Outcomes of dogs undergoing radiotherapy for treatment of oral malignant melanoma: 111 cases (2006-2012). *J. Am. Vet. Med. Assoc.* 247 (10): 1146–1153.

4 Tuohy, J.L., Selmic, L.E., Worley, D.R. et al. (2014). Outcome following curative-intent surgery for oral melanoma in dogs: 70 cases (1998–2011). *J. Am. Vet. Med. Assoc.* 245 (11): 1266–1273.

5 Riggs, J., Adams, V.J., Hermer, J.V. et al. (2018). Outcomes following surgical excision or surgical excision combined with adjunctive, hypofractionated radiotherapy in dogs with oral squamous cell carcinoma or fibrosarcoma. *J. Am. Vet. Med. Assoc.* 253 (1): 73–83.

6 Fulton, A.J., Nemec, A., Murphy, B.G. et al. (2013). Risk factors associated with survival in dogs with nontonsillar oral squamous cell carcinoma 31 cases (1990-2010). *J. Am. Vet. Med. Assoc.* 243 (5): 696–702.

7 Frazier, S.A., Johns, S.M., Ortega, J. et al. (2012). Outcome in dogs with surgically resected oral fibrosarcoma (1997-2008). *Vet. Comp. Oncol.* 10 (1): 33–43.

8 Selmic, L.E., Lafferty, M.H., Kamstock, D.A. et al. (2014). Outcome and prognostic factors for osteosarcoma of the maxilla, mandible, or calvarium in dogs: 183 cases (1986-2012). *J. Am. Vet. Med. Assoc.* 245 (8): 930–938.

9 Coyle, V.J., Rassnick, K.M., Borst, L.B. et al. (2015). Biological behaviour of canine mandibular osteosarcoma. A retrospective study of 50 cases (1999-2007). *Vet. Comp. Oncol.* 13 (2): 89–97.

10 Goldschmidt, S.L., Bell, C.M., Hetzel, S. et al. (2017). Clinical characterization of canine acanthomatous ameloblastoma (CAA) in 263 dogs and the influence of postsurgical histopathological margin on local recurrence. *J. Vet. Dent.* 34 (4): 241–247.

11 Evenhuis, J.V., Oates, A., Hoyer, N. et al. (2023). A retrospective study of canine oral extramedullary plasmacytoma over a 15-year period (July 2004-July 2019): treatment, histologic parameters and clinical outcomes. *Vet. Comp. Oncol.* 21 (2): 302–314.

12 Northrup, N.C., Selting, K.A., Rassnick, K.M. et al. (2006). Outcomes of cats with oral tumors treated with mandibulectomy: 42 cases. *J. Am. Anim. Hosp. Assoc.* 42 (5): 350–360.

13 Liptak, J.M., Thatcher, G.P., Mestrinho, L.A. et al. (2021). Outcomes of cats treated with maxillectomy: 60 cases. A Veterinary Society of Surgical Oncology retrospective study. *Vet. Comp. Oncol.* 19 (4): 641–650.

6.1 Mandibular Incisivectomy

Indications (See Plate 6.1 – 1)

1) Resection of benign oral tumors (pictured, acanthomatous ameloblastoma) and small or low-grade malignant oral tumors confined to the incisive bone and associated incisor teeth.
2) Incisivectomy can combined with a lower lip advancement flap (see *39.3. Lower Lip Advancement Flap*) if the incisivectomy is also associated with a rostral lip defect.

Suggested Diagnostic Workup and Clinical Staging for Benign Mandibular Tumors

- Complete blood count, serum biochemistry, and urinalysis
- Preoperative biopsy
- ± Precontrast and postcontrast computed tomography (CT) scan of the head for surgical planning

Suggested Diagnostic Workup and Clinical Staging for Malignant Mandibular Tumors

- Complete blood count, serum biochemistry, and urinalysis
- Preoperative biopsy
- Regional lymph node assessment for evaluation of lymph node metastasis
  - Fine-needle aspirate cytology of the mandibular lymph nodes
  - Sentinel lymph node mapping and excision of the sentinel lymph node (see *50.1. Sentinel Lymph Node Mapping*)
  - Nonselective excision of the bilateral mandibular and medial retropharyngeal lymph nodes through a ventral midline cervical approach (see *50.3. Combined Mandibular and Medial Retropharyngeal Lymph Node Excision*), or excision of the ipsilateral mandibular, medial retropharyngeal, and parotid lymph nodes through a lateral approach (see *50.4. Combined Parotid, Mandibular, and Medial Retropharyngeal Lymph Node Excision*)
- ± Radiographs or precontrast and postcontrast CT scan of the head and neck for surgical planning
- Three-view thoracic radiographs or thoracic CT scan for assessment of lung metastasis

Patient Positioning

The patient is positioned in either dorsal or sternal recumbency. The pharynx should be packed with gauze sponges to minimize the risk of aspirating lavage fluid and blood.

Color Atlas of Canine and Feline Surgical Oncology, First Edition. Julius M. Liptak, Paolo Buracco, William T. N. Culp, and Nicholas J. Bacon.

Plate 6.1

Mandibular Incisivectomy

1)

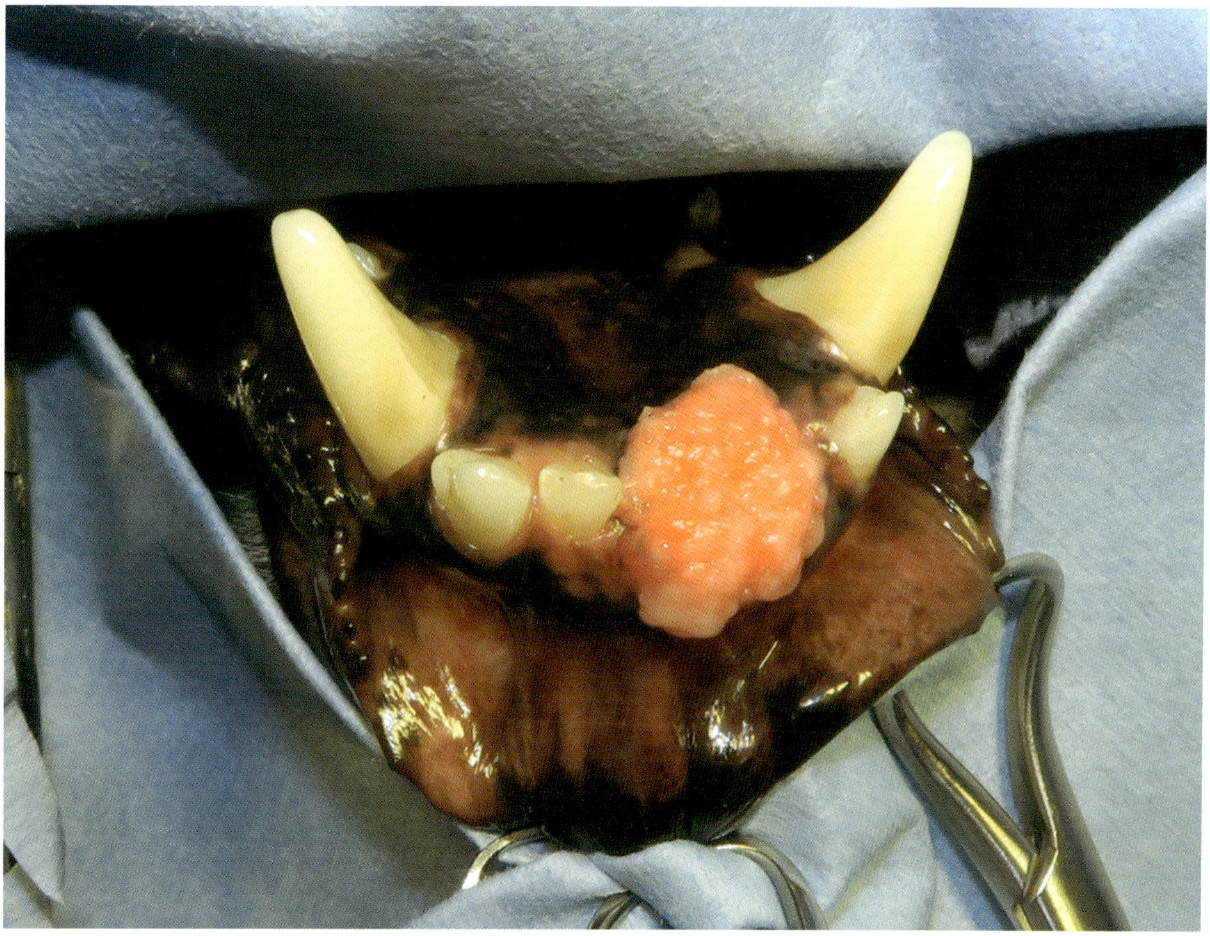

Surgical Technique (See Plate 6.1A–C)

A) The rostral labial and lingual aspects of the gingival mucosa are incised with a scalpel blade with a minimum of 5- to 10-mm margins around the oral mass. The mucosa is then elevated with a periosteal elevator to expose the mandibular bone in preparation for the osteotomy.
B) An osteotomy is performed with a minimum of 1-cm bone margins along the mucosal incision. This osteotomy can be performed with an oscillating, sagittal (i), or biradial saw (ii), pneumatic drill, or piezoelectric instruments. Bleeding is generally minor.
C) Exposed tooth roots are extracted with a dental elevator.

Closure (See Plate 6.1D)

D) The mucosa and submucosa of the adjacent rostral lip are elevated with a combination of blunt and sharp dissection toward the lip margin to create a labial mucosal-submucosal flap (i). The labial mucosal-submucosal flap is then advanced into the oral defect and sutured to the lingual gingival mucosa using 3-0 to 4-0 monofilament absorbable material on a reverse cutting needle in a simple interrupted or far-near-near-far suture pattern (ii–iv). If necessary, the labial mucosa-submucosal flap can be sutured to bone tunnels drilled into the rostral mandible with a 1.5- or 2.0-mm drill bit (v).

Postoperative Management

1) Multimodal analgesia
2) Soft foods for 4 weeks
3) No chewing on hard objects or playing with toys for 4 weeks
4) Elizabethan collar

Complications

- Dehiscence

Plate 6.1

Mandibular Incisivectomy *continued*

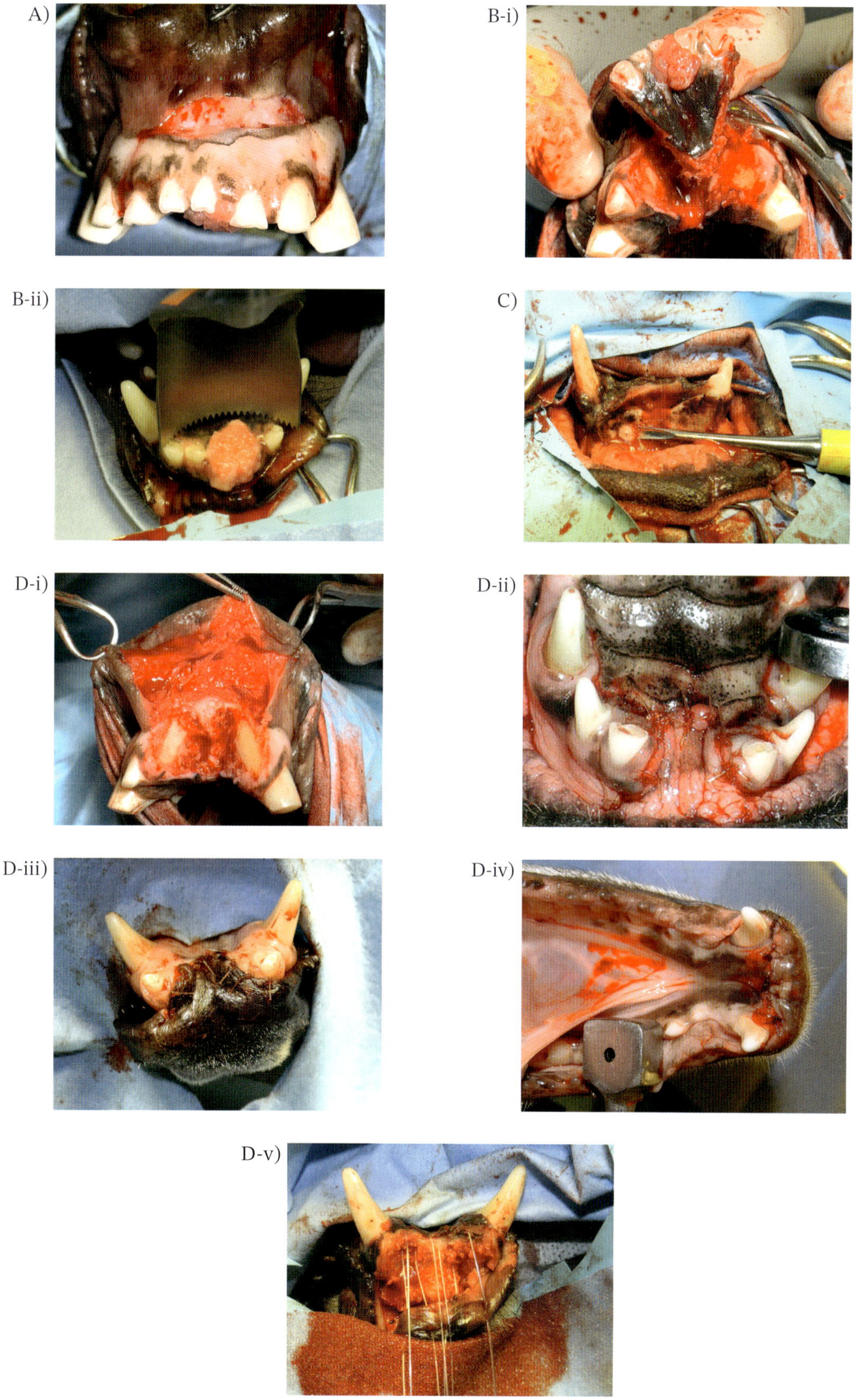

Cosmetic Appearance (See Plate 6.1E)

- No to minimal effects on cosmesis (E – i, immediate postoperatively; E – ii, 1 day postoperatively)

Suggested Adjuvant Treatments

- See *6. Mandibulectomy and Maxillectomy*.

Prognosis and Oncologic Outcome

- See *6. Mandibulectomy and Maxillectomy*.

Plate 6.1

Mandibular Incisivectomy *continued*

E-i)

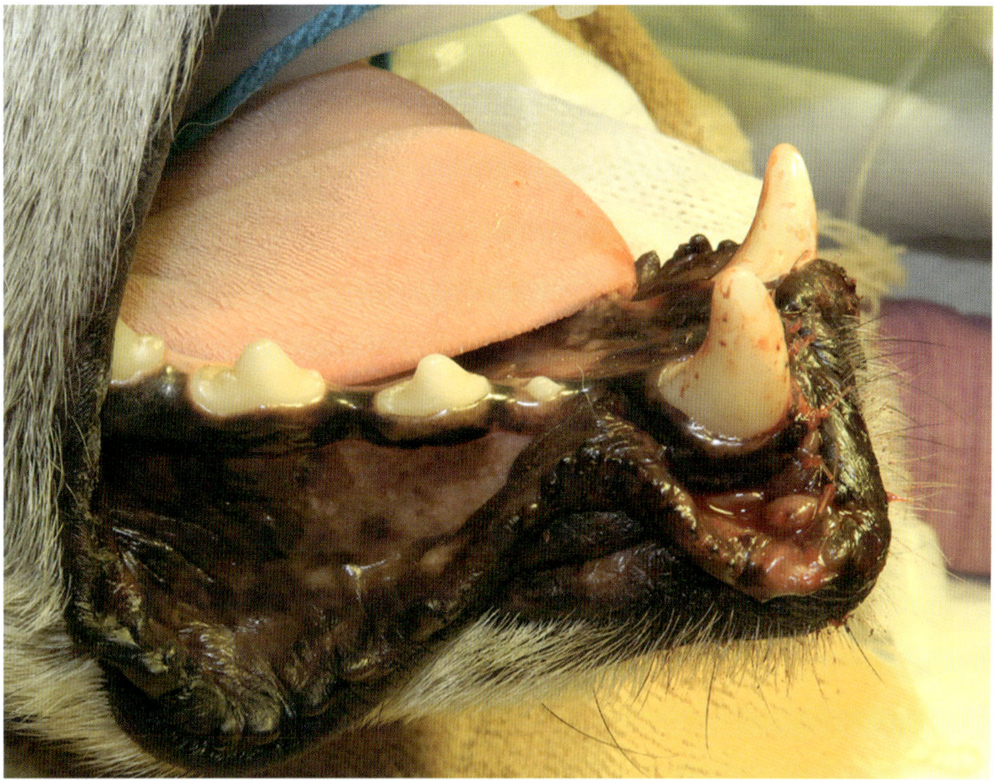

E-ii)

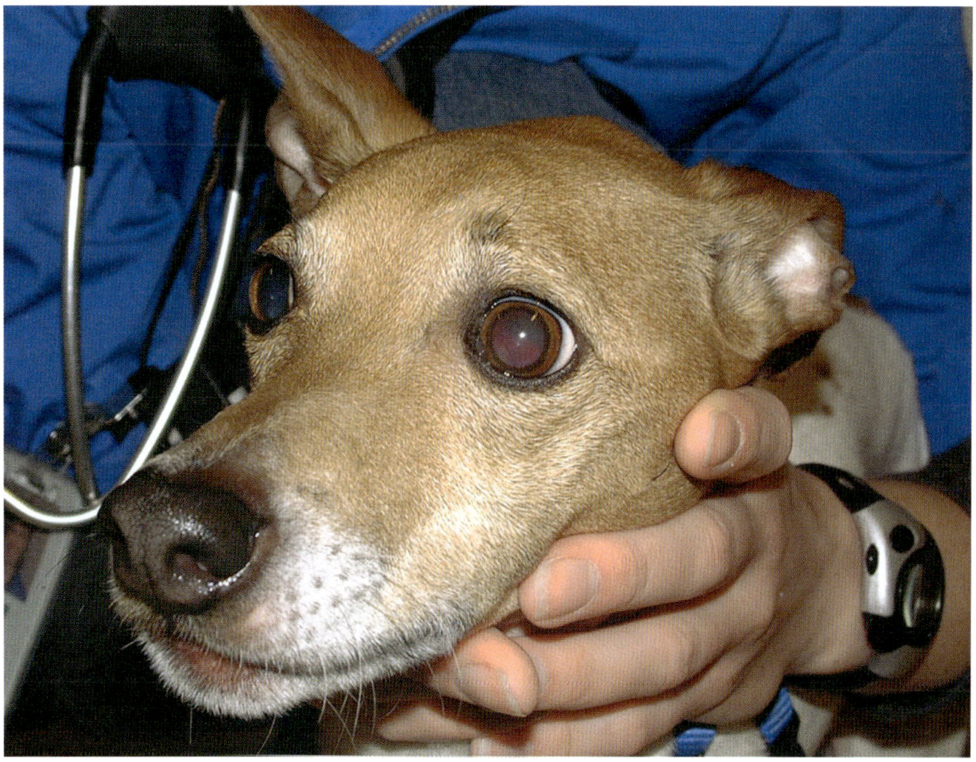

6.2 Unilateral Rostral Mandibulectomy

Indications (See Plate 6.2 – 1)

1) Resection of benign oral tumors, particularly acanthomatous ameloblastoma (pictured), or small or low-grade malignant oral tumors adjacent to the mandibular canine tooth and that do not cross the midline or extend further caudally than the second premolar tooth.
2) Unilateral rostral mandibulectomy can combined with a lower lip advancement flap (see *39.3. Lower Lip Advancement Flap*) if the mandibulectomy is also associated with a rostral lip defect.

Suggested Diagnostic Workup and Clinical Staging for Benign Mandibular Tumors

- Complete blood count, serum biochemistry, and urinalysis
- Preoperative biopsy
- ± Precontrast and postcontrast computed tomography (CT) scan of the head for surgical planning

Suggested Diagnostic Workup and Clinical Staging for Malignant Mandibular Tumors

- Complete blood count, serum biochemistry, and urinalysis
- Preoperative biopsy
- Regional lymph node assessment for evaluation of lymph node metastasis
  - Fine-needle aspirate cytology of the mandibular lymph nodes
  - Sentinel lymph node mapping and excision of the sentinel lymph node (see *50.1. Sentinel Lymph Node Mapping*)
  - Nonselective excision of the bilateral mandibular and medial retropharyngeal lymph nodes through a ventral midline cervical approach (see *50.3. Combined Mandibular and Medial Retropharyngeal Lymph Node Excision*), or excision of the ipsilateral mandibular, medial retropharyngeal, and parotid lymph nodes through a lateral approach (see *50.4. Combined Parotid, Mandibular, and Medial Retropharyngeal Lymph Node Excision*)
- ± Radiographs or precontrast and postcontrast CT scan of the head and neck for surgical planning
- Three-view thoracic radiographs or thoracic CT scan for assessment of lung metastasis

Patient Positioning

The patient is positioned in either dorsal or lateral recumbency. If positioned in lateral recumbency, the affected side should be uppermost. The pharynx should be packed with gauze sponges to minimize the risk of aspirating lavage fluid and blood.

Color Atlas of Canine and Feline Surgical Oncology, First Edition. Julius M. Liptak, Paolo Buracco, William T. N. Culp, and Nicholas J. Bacon.

Plate 6.2

Unilateral Rostral Mandibulectomy

1)

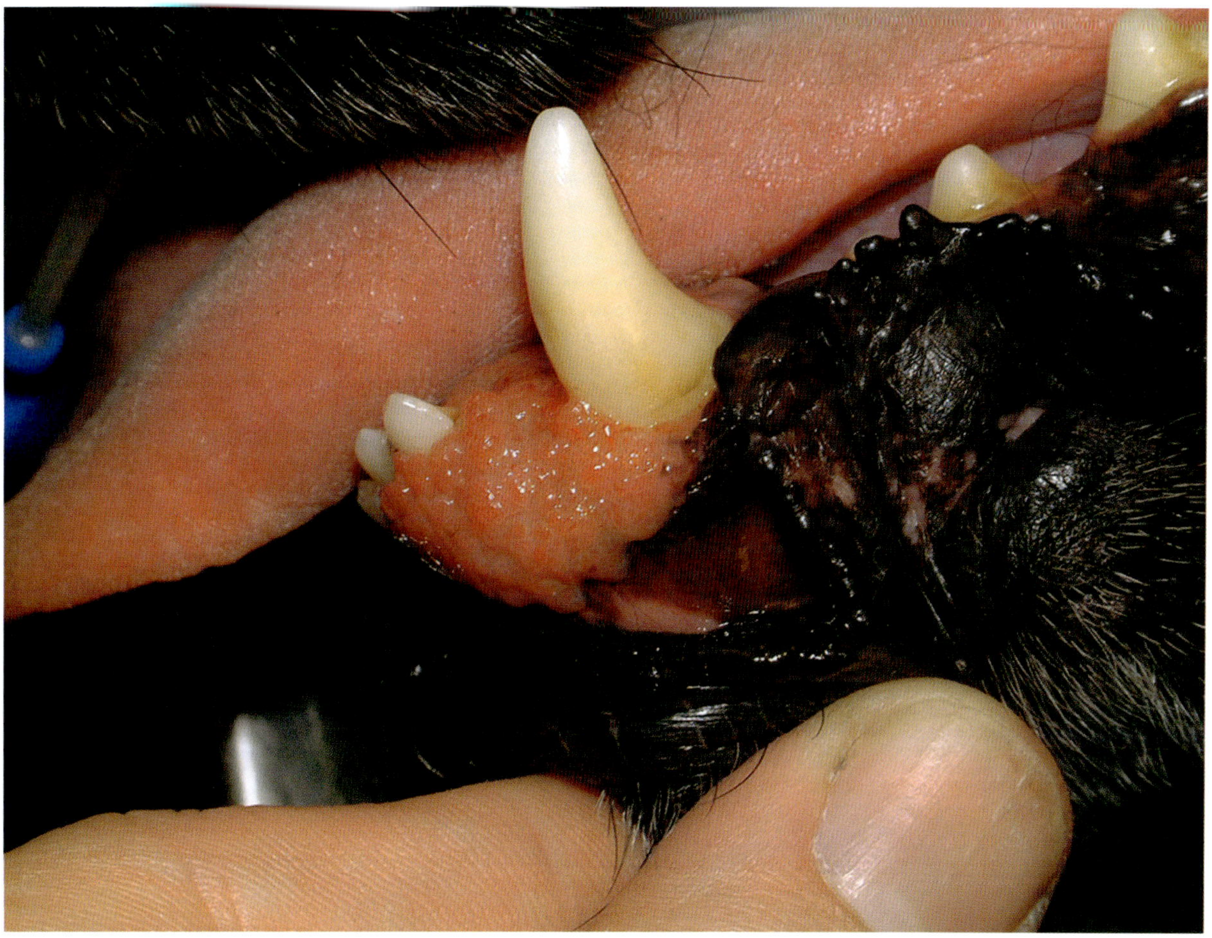

Surgical Technique (See Plate 6.2A–D)

A) The labial and lingual aspects of the gingival mucosa are incised with a scalpel blade (i) with a minimum of 5- to 10-mm margins around the oral mass and extending to the planned osteotomy sites. The mucosa is then elevated with a periosteal elevator to expose the mandibular bone in preparation for the osteotomies (ii).

B) The rostral osteotomy is performed with a minimum of 1-cm bone margins, but medial to the contralateral mandibular canine tooth. Ideally, this should include the mandibular symphysis because this may act as a physical barrier to tumor invasion. This osteotomy can be performed with an oscillating or sagittal (pictured) saw, pneumatic drill, piezoelectric instruments, or osteotome and mallet. Bleeding is generally minor.

C) The caudal osteotomy is performed with a minimum of 1-cm bone margins. This osteotomy can be performed with an oscillating, sagittal (i, pictured), or biradial saw, pneumatic drill, piezoelectric instruments, or Gigli wire. Bleeding is generally minor if the caudal osteotomy is performed rostral to the caudal extent of the mandibular symphysis (ii). If the caudal osteotomy is performed caudal to the caudal extent of the mandibular symphysis, then bleeding from the inferior alveolar artery within the mandibular canal should be expected. Hemostasis can be achieved by clamping the artery and then either cauterizing (iii, arrow) or ligating the artery, or packing of bone wax into the mandibular canal (iv, arrow).

D) Exposed tooth roots are extracted with a dental elevator.

Plate 6.2

Unilateral Rostral Mandibulectomy *continued*

A-i)

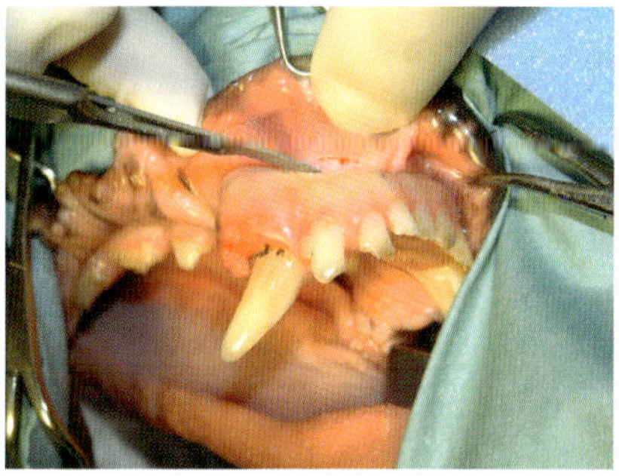

A-ii)

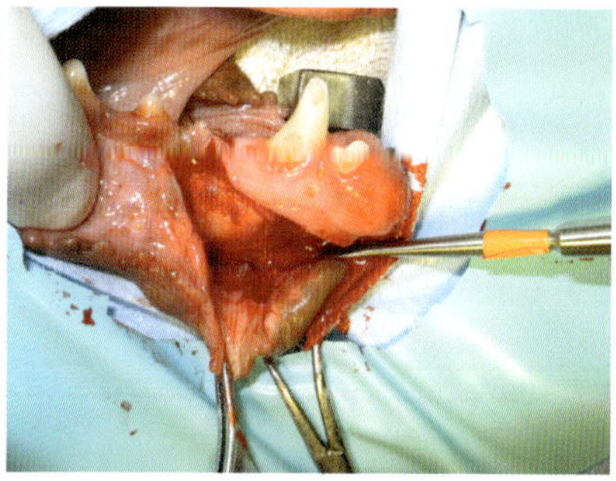

B)

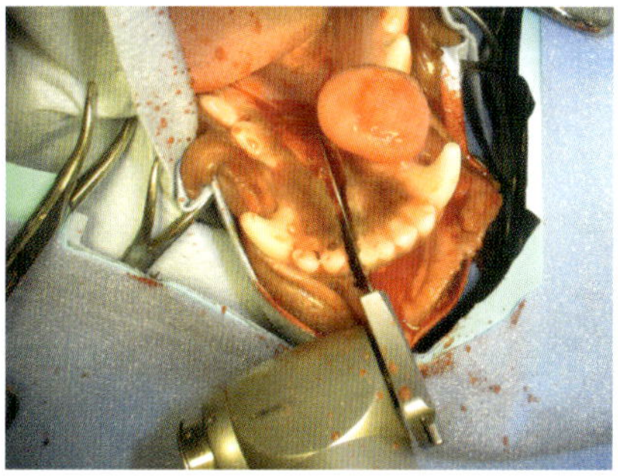

C-i)

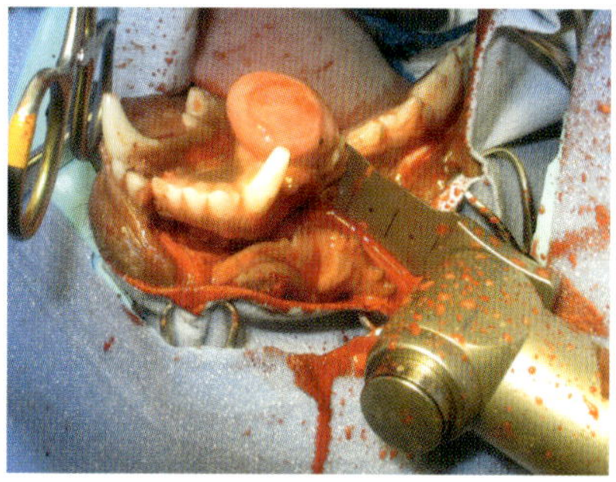

C-ii)

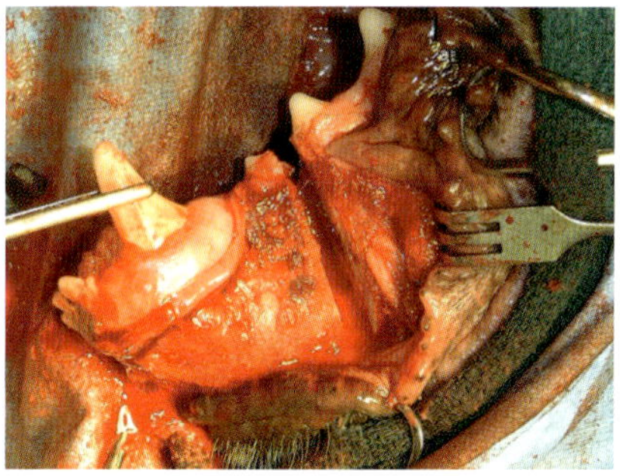

C-ii)

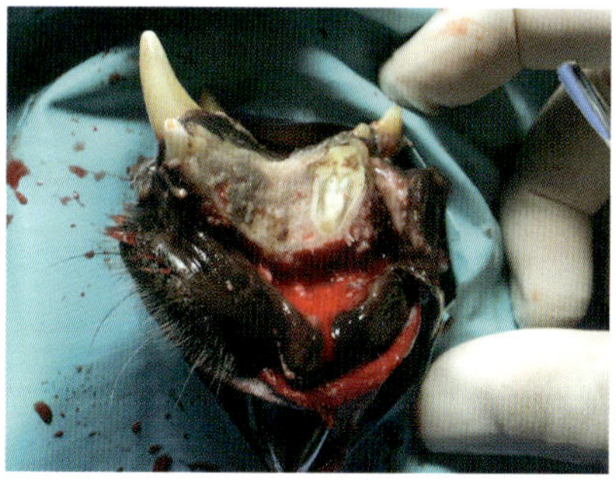

C-iii)

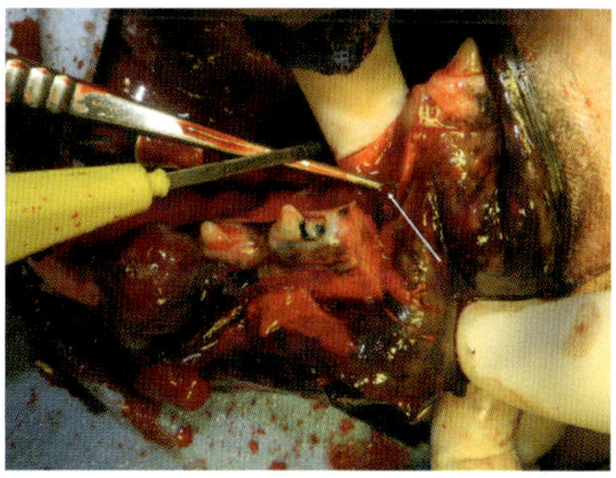

C-iv)

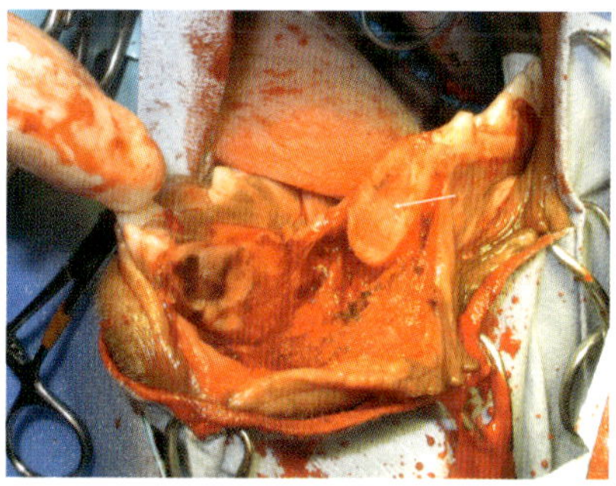

D)

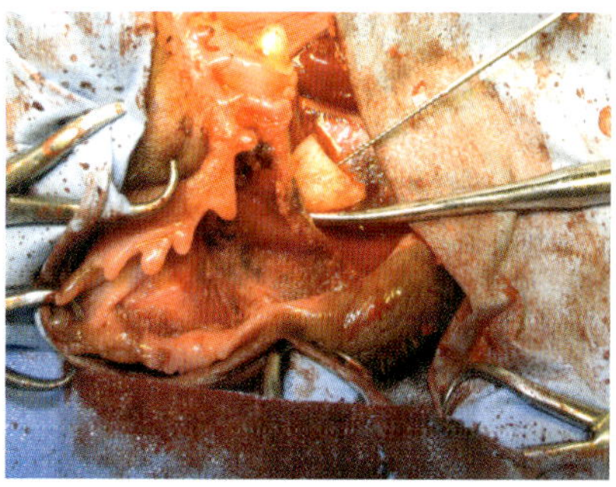

Closure (See Plate 6.2E)

E) The mucosa and submucosa of the adjacent rostral lip is elevated with a combination of blunt and sharp dissection toward the lip margin to create a labial mucosal-submucosal flap. The labial mucosal-submucosal flap is then advanced into the oral defect and sutured to the lingual gingival mucosa using 3-0 to 4-0 monofilament absorbable material on a reverse cutting needle in a simple interrupted or far-near-near-far suture pattern.

Postoperative Management

1) Multimodal analgesia
2) Soft foods for 4 weeks
3) No chewing on hard objects or playing with toys for 4 weeks
4) Elizabethan collar
5) ± Esophagostomy tube and supplemental feeding in cats

Complications – Dogs [1, 2]

Intraoperative Complications

- Blood loss from the inferior alveolar artery

Postoperative Complications (See Plate 6.2F, G)

- Overall: 12%
- Prehension/eating difficulties (rare, median time to eating is 1 day)
- Ranula formation (rare; F, 1 day postoperative, arrow)
- Incisional dehiscence (0%–4%; G, 6 days postoperative)
- Excessive drooling (4%)
- Mandibular drift (rare)

Plate 6.2

Unilateral Rostral Mandibulectomy *continued*

E)

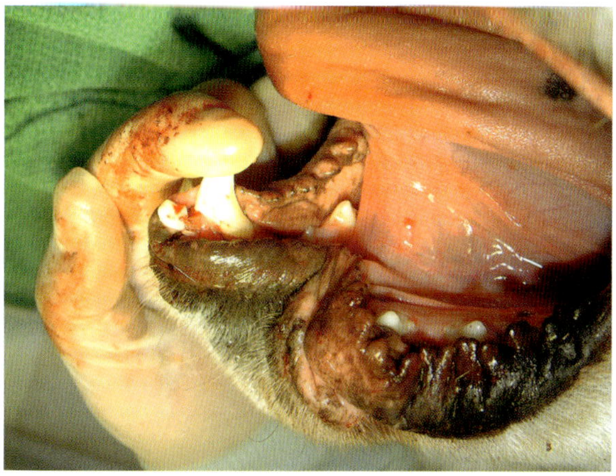

E)

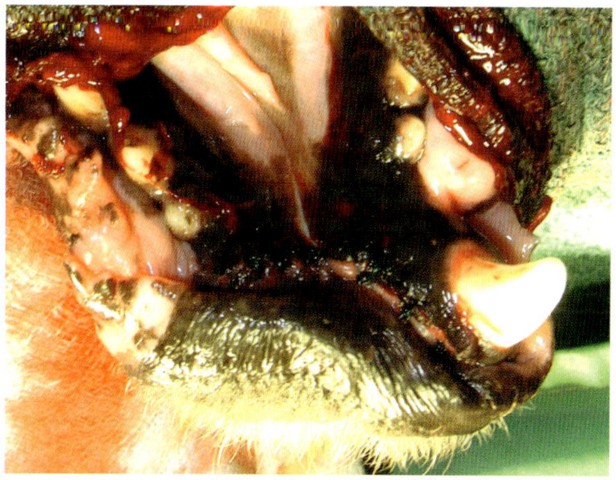

F)

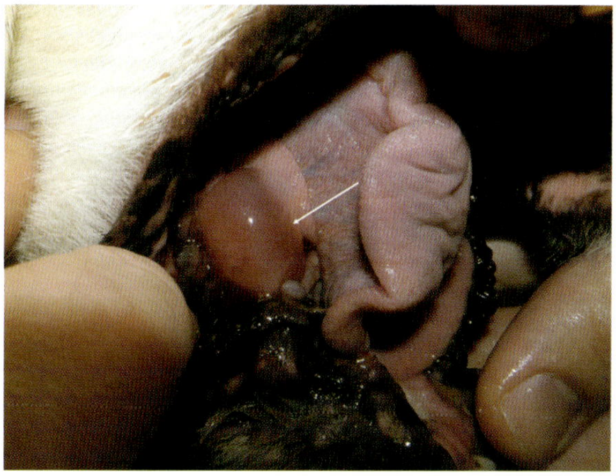

G)

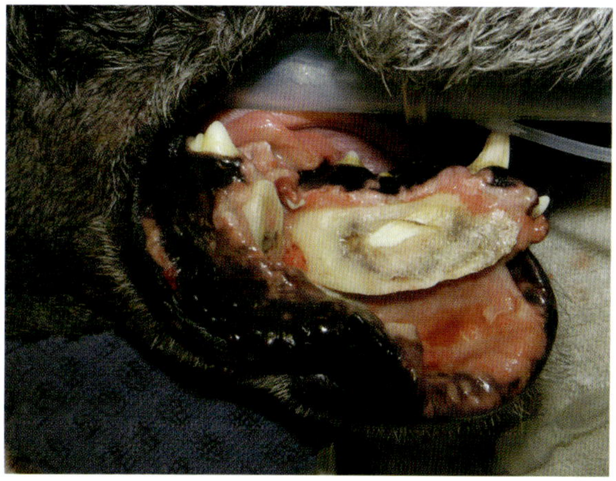

Cosmetic Appearance (See Plate 6.2H)

- No to minimal effects on cosmesis with occasional tongue lag on the resected side (H – i–vi, all images taken 1 day postoperatively).

Suggested Adjuvant Treatments

- See *6. Mandibulectomy and Maxillectomy*.

Prognosis and Oncologic Outcome

- See *6. Mandibulectomy and Maxillectomy*.

References

1 Salisbury, S.K. and Lantz, G.C. (1988). Long-term results of partial mandibulectomy for treatment of oral tumors in 30 dogs. *J. Am. Anim. Hosp. Assoc.* 24: 285–294.

2 Schwarz, P.D., Withrow, S.J., Curtis, C.R. et al. (1991). Mandibular resection as a treatment for oral cancer in 81 dogs. *J. Am. Anim. Hosp. Assoc.* 27: 601–610.

Plate 6.2

Unilateral Rostral Mandibulectomy *continued*

H-i)

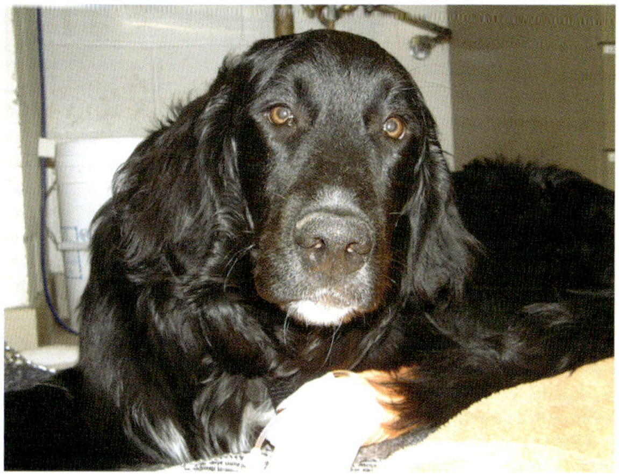

H-ii)

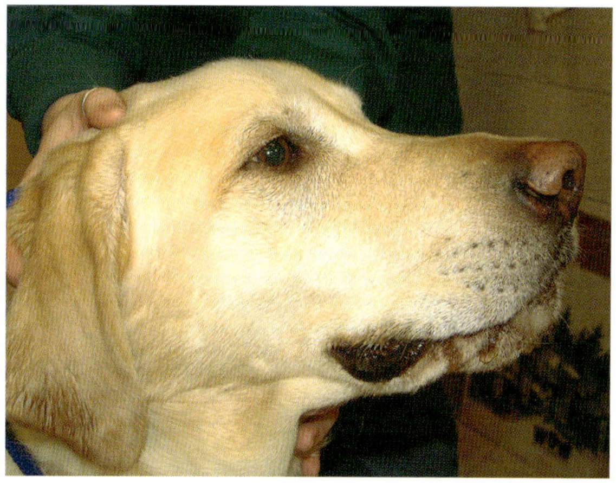

H-iii)

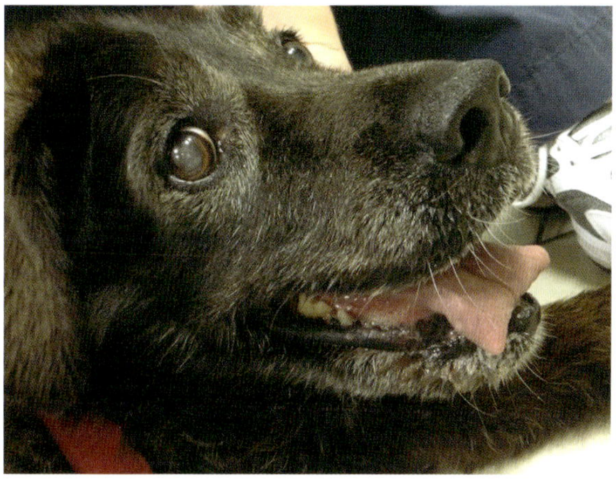

H-iv)

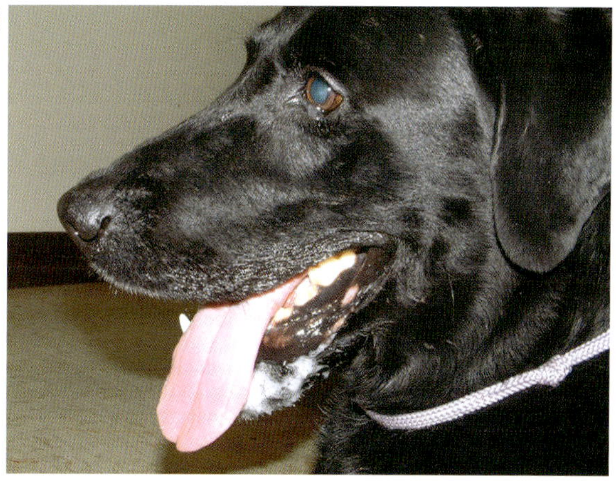

H-v)

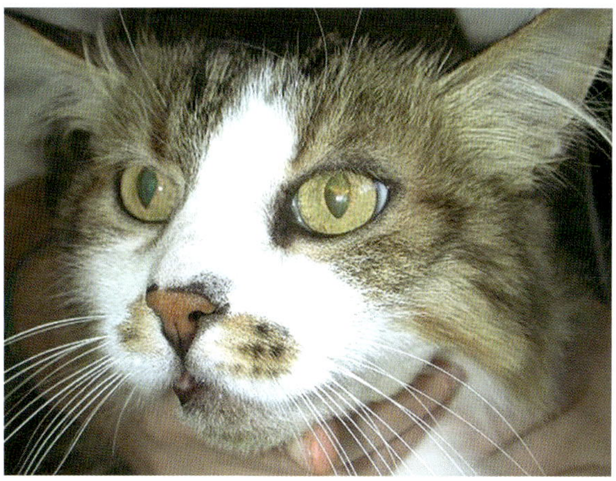

H-vi)

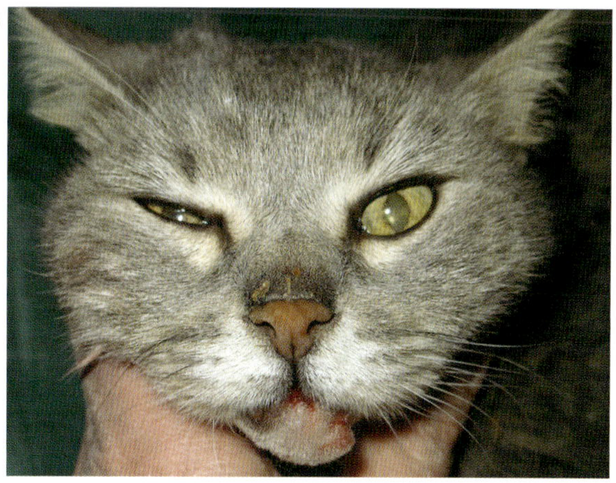

6.3 Bilateral Rostral Mandibulectomy

Indications (See Plate 6.3 – 1)

1) Resection of benign oral tumors, particularly acanthomatous ameloblastomas, or malignant oral tumors rostral to the second premolar tooth (pictured, malignant melanoma), but as far caudally as the fourth premolar tooth, and that have crossed the midline.
2) Bilateral rostral mandibulectomy can be combined with a lower lip advancement flap (see *39.3. Lower Lip Advancement Flap*) if the mandibulectomy is also associated with a rostral lip defect.

Suggested Diagnostic Workup and Clinical Staging for Benign Mandibular Tumors

- Complete blood count, serum biochemistry, and urinalysis
- Preoperative biopsy
- ± Precontrast and postcontrast computed tomography (CT) scan of the head for surgical planning

Suggested Diagnostic Workup and Clinical Staging for Malignant Mandibular Tumors

- Complete blood count, serum biochemistry, and urinalysis
- Preoperative biopsy
- Regional lymph node assessment for evaluation of lymph node metastasis
  - Fine-needle aspirate cytology of the mandibular lymph nodes
  - Sentinel lymph node mapping and excision of the sentinel lymph node (see *50.1. Sentinel Lymph Node Mapping*)
  - Nonselective excision of the bilateral mandibular and medial retropharyngeal lymph nodes through a ventral midline cervical approach (see *50.3. Combined Mandibular and Medial Retropharyngeal Lymph Node Excision*), or excision of the ipsilateral mandibular, medial retropharyngeal, and parotid lymph nodes through a lateral approach (see *50.4. Combined Parotid, Mandibular, and Medial Retropharyngeal Lymph Node Excision*)
- ± Radiographs or precontrast and postcontrast CT scan of the head and neck for surgical planning
- Three-view thoracic radiographs or thoracic CT scan for assessment of lung metastasis

Patient Positioning

The patient is positioned in either dorsal or sternal recumbency. Surgical exposure and resection are superior when the patient is in dorsal recumbency, but closure of the defect after resection is superior when the patient is in sternal recumbency. When positioned in sternal recumbency, the head is elevated and the maxilla is suspended by perforating the canine maxillary teeth with a long strip of adhesive tape whose ends are fixed laterally to over-the-table stands. The pharynx should be packed with gauze sponges to minimize the risk of aspirating lavage fluid and blood.

Color Atlas of Canine and Feline Surgical Oncology, First Edition. Julius M. Liptak, Paolo Buracco, William T. N. Culp, and Nicholas J. Bacon.

Plate 6.3

Bilateral Rostral Mandibulectomy

1)

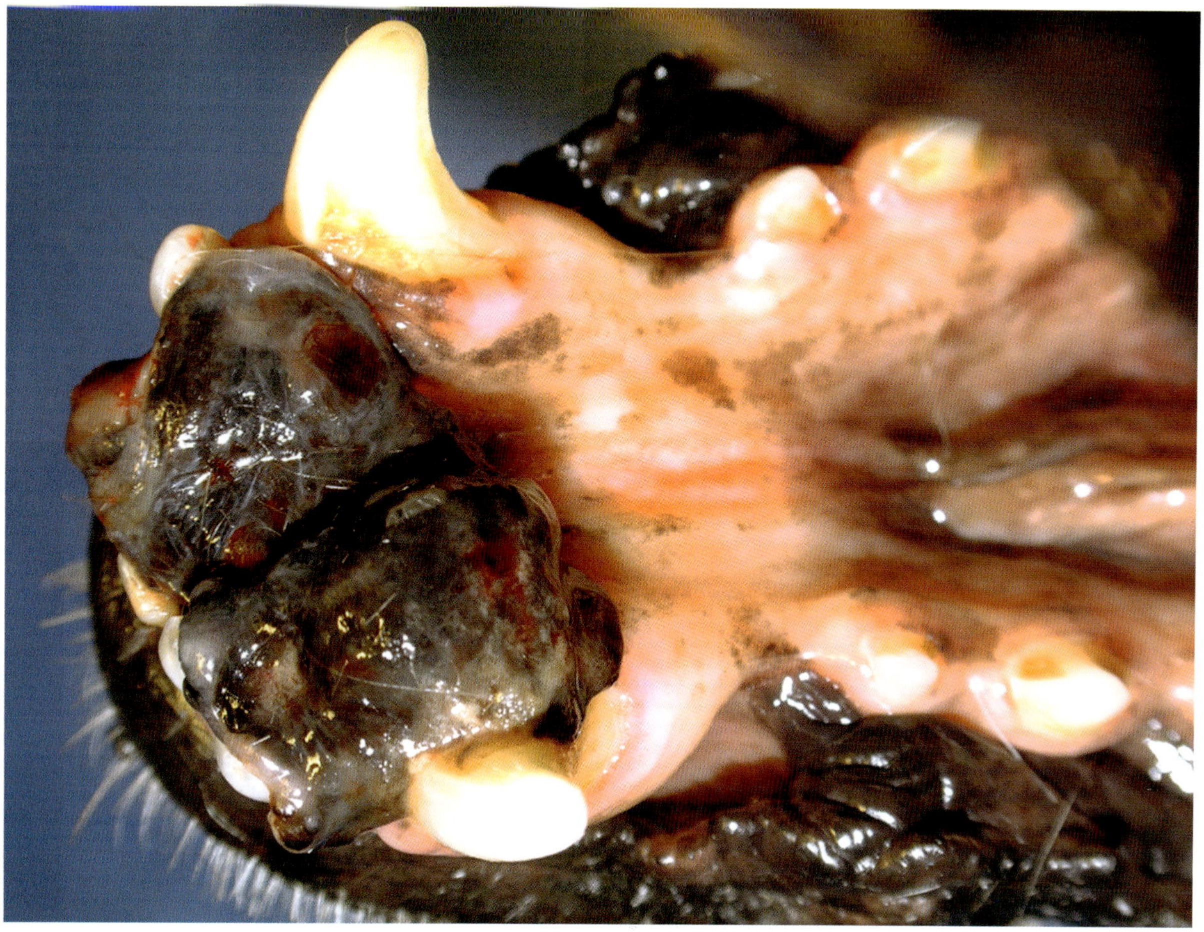

Surgical Technique (See Plate 6.3A–D)

A) The labial and lingual aspects of the gingival mucosa are incised with a scalpel blade with a minimum of 5- to 10-mm margins around the oral mass and extending to the planned osteotomy sites. The mucosa is then elevated with a periosteal elevator to expose the mandibular bone in preparation for the osteotomies.

B) The osteotomies are performed with a minimum of 1-cm bone margins. These osteotomies can be performed with an oscillating (i) or sagittal saw (ii), pneumatic drill, piezoelectric instruments, or Gigli wire.

C) Bleeding is generally minor if the osteotomies are performed rostral to the caudal extent of the mandibular symphysis (i). If the osteotomies are performed caudal to the caudal extent of the mandibular symphysis, then bleeding from the inferior alveolar arteries within the mandibular canals should be expected. Hemostasis can be achieved by clamping these arteries and then either cauterizing or ligating the arteries, or packing of bone wax into the mandibular canals (ii, arrows).

D) Exposed tooth roots are extracted with a dental elevator.

E) Stabilization of the two mandibular bodies is not necessary.

Plate 6.3

Bilateral Rostral Mandibulectomy *continued*

A)

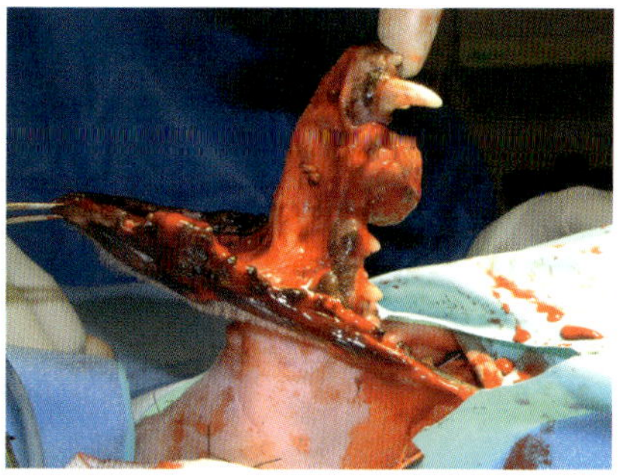

A)

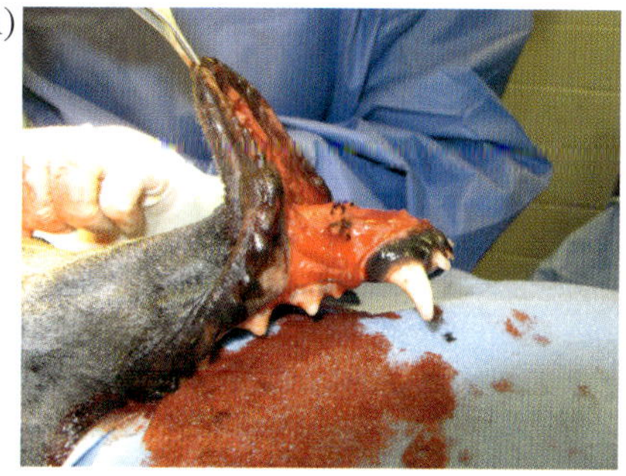

A)

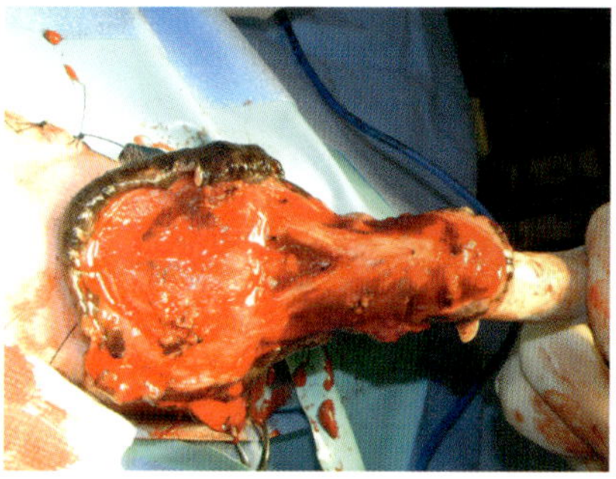

B-i)

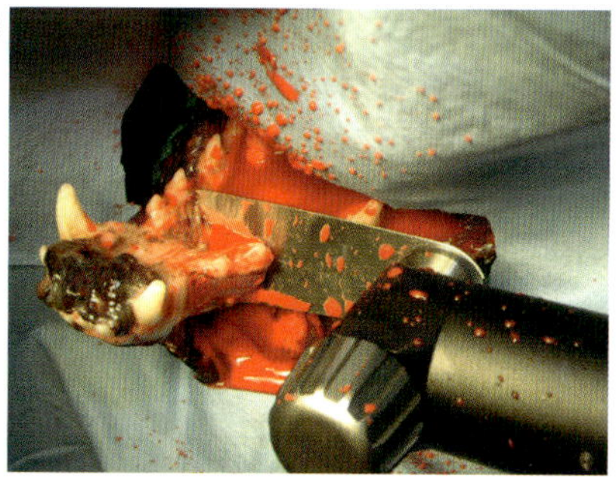

B-i)

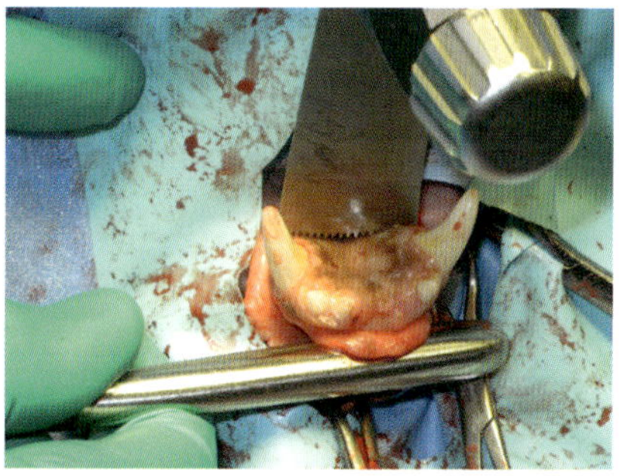

B-ii)

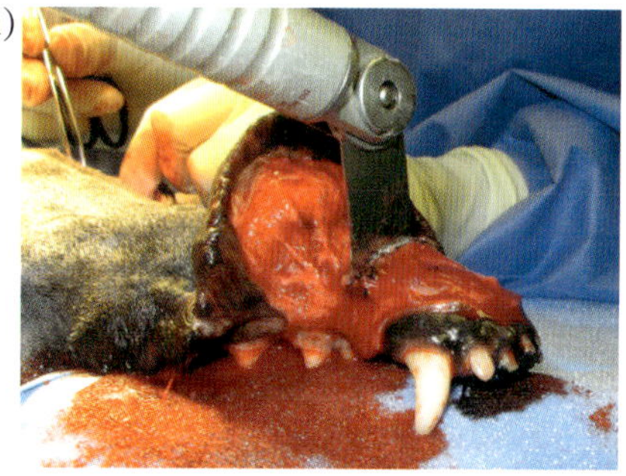

C-i)

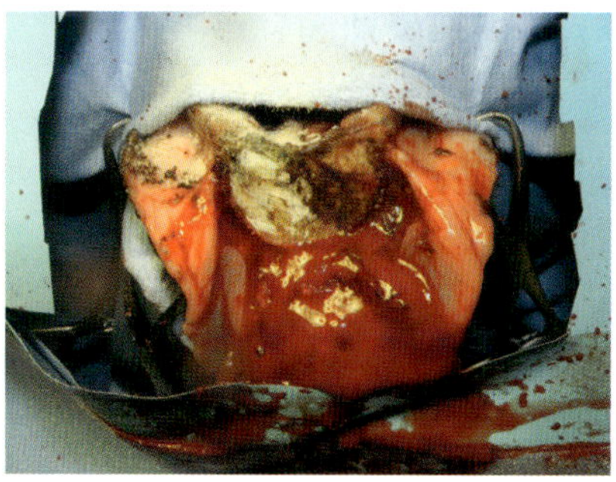

C-ii)

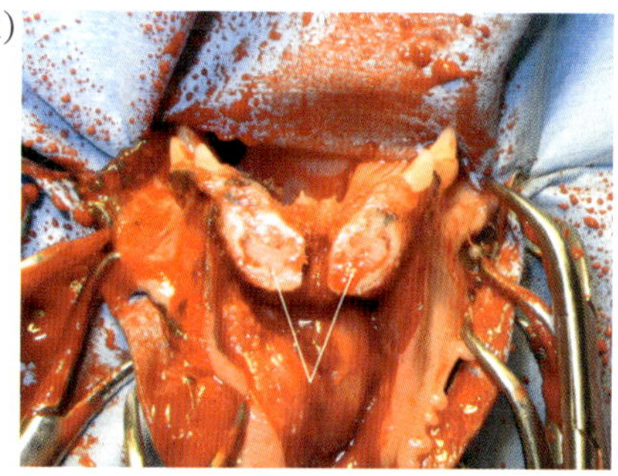

D)

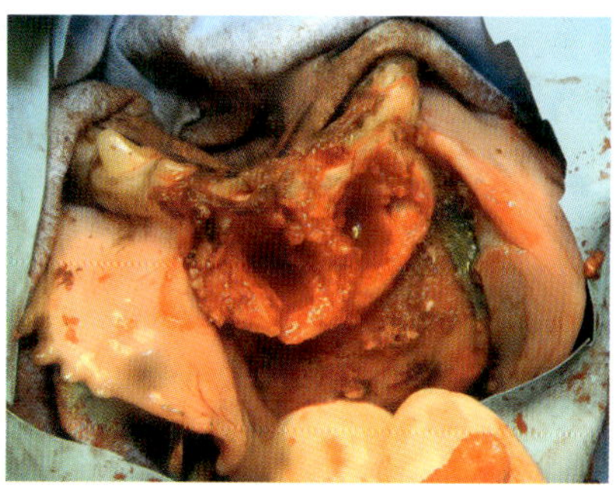

Closure (See Plate 6.3F–I)

Excessive skin may need to be resected, depending on the length of the mandibular resection (F – i–iii).

If the osteotomies were performed caudal to the mandibular symphysis, then the intermandibular soft tissues may need to be apposed with absorbable monofilament suture material in either an interrupted or continuous suture pattern (G).

A cheiloplasty may be required to create a dam to limit excessive drooling. This can either be done with a single dam created in the midline on the rostral aspect of the mandible (H – i–iii) or two dams created bilaterally at the rostral aspect of the mandible (I – i, ii).

The skin of the ventral mandible is sutured to the lingual gingival mucosa using 3-0 to 4-0 monofilament absorbable material on a reverse cutting needle in a simple interrupted or far-near-near-far suture pattern (H, I).

Plate 6.3

Bilateral Rostral Mandibulectomy *continued*

F-i)

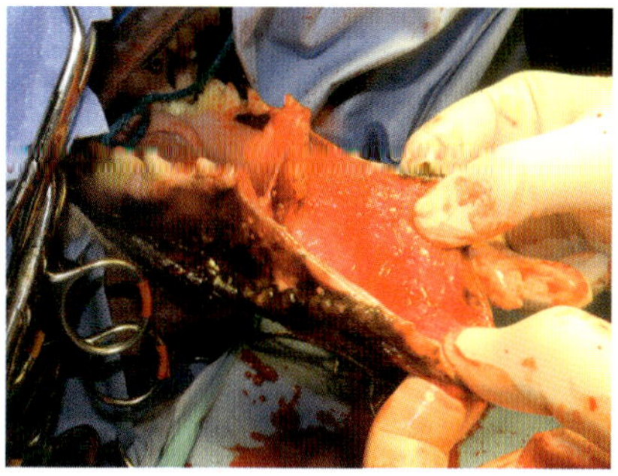

F-ii)

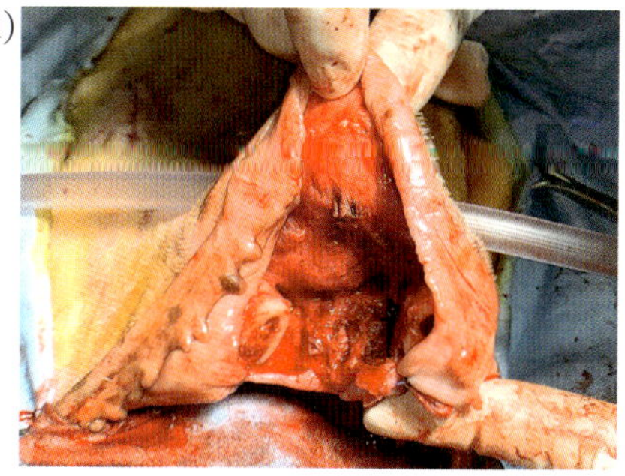

F-iii)

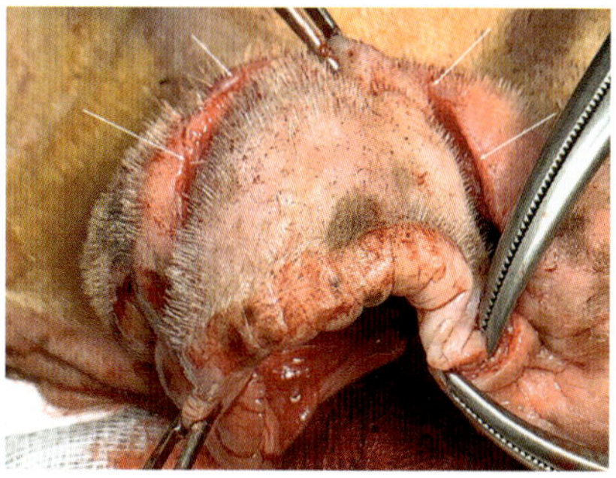

G)

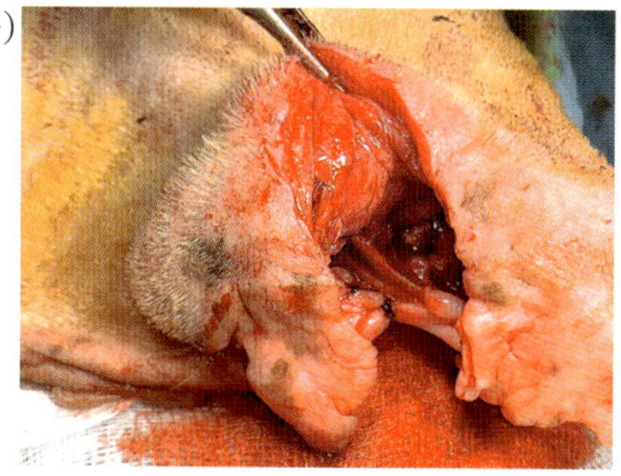

H-i)

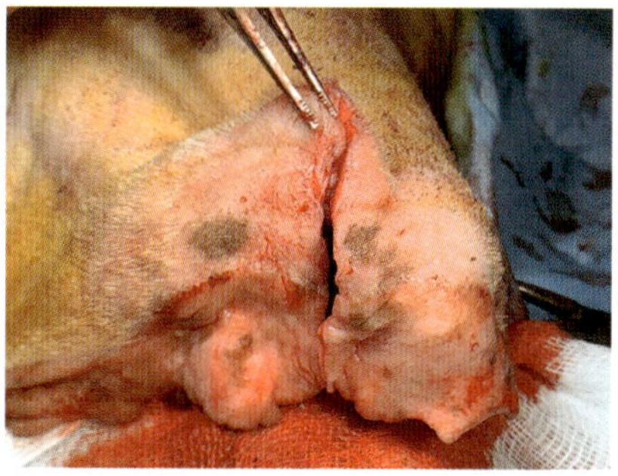

H-ii)

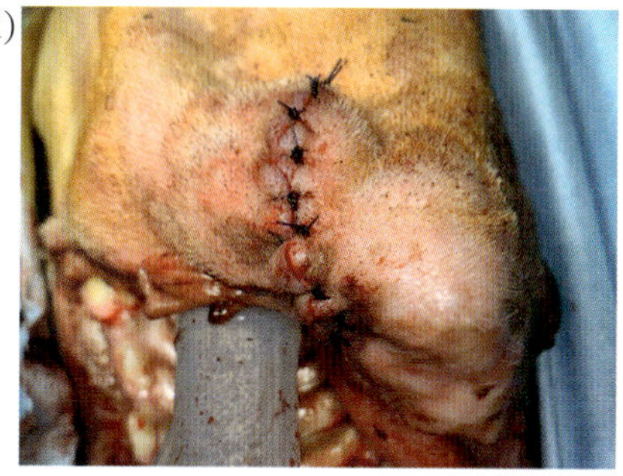

H-iii)

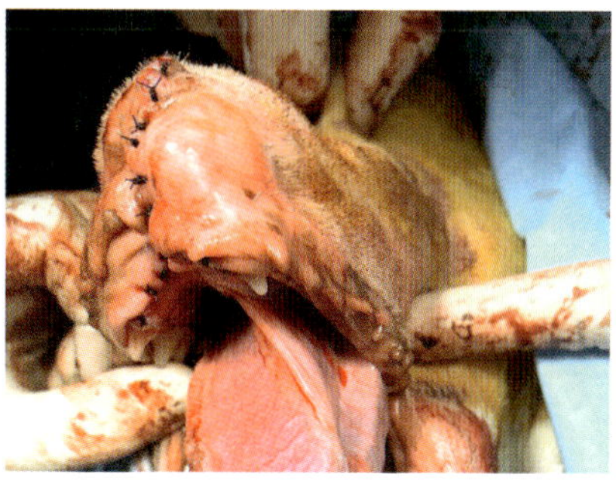

I-i)

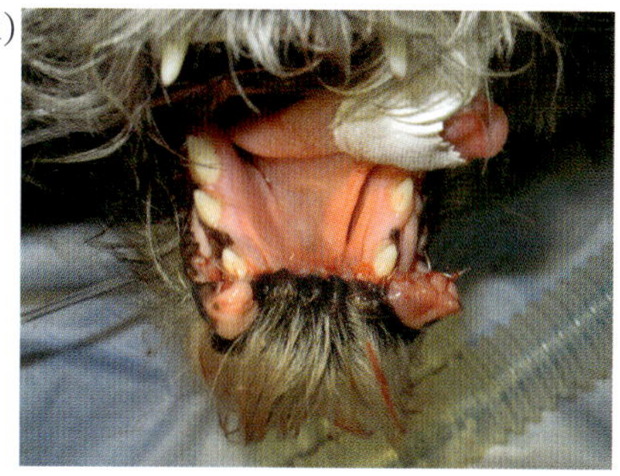

I-ii)

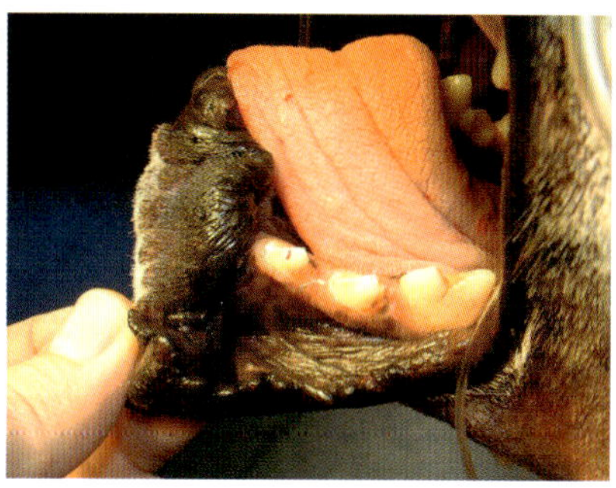

Postoperative Management (See Plate 6.3J)

1) Multimodal analgesia
2) Soft foods for 4 weeks
3) No chewing on hard objects or playing with toys for 4 weeks
4) Elizabethan collar
5) Esophagostomy tube and supplemental feeding in cats (J)

Complications – Dogs [1, 2]

Intraoperative Complications

- Blood loss from the inferior alveolar artery

Postoperative Complications (See Plate 6.3K, L)

- Overall: 19%
- Prehension/eating difficulties (6.3% median time to eating is 2 days)
- Ranula formation (14%)
- Incisional dehiscence (0%–29%; K, 7 days postoperative)
- Excessive drooling (L – i, 21 days postoperative; L – ii, 14 days postoperative)
- Mandibular drift (rare)

Complications – Cats [3]

Postoperative Complications (0–28 Days)

- Overall: 92%
- Dysphagia/inappetence (83%)
- Excessive drooling (50%)
- Mandibular drift (17%)
- Tongue protrusion (33%)
- Pain (17%)
- Grooming difficulties (17%)
- Incisional dehiscence (17%)

Postoperative Complications (>28 Days)

- Overall: 50%
- Dysphagia/inappetence (10%)
- Excessive drooling (30%)
- Mandibular drift (20%)
- Tongue protrusion (30%)
- Grooming difficulties (10%)

Plate 6.3

Bilateral Rostral Mandibulectomy *continued*

J)

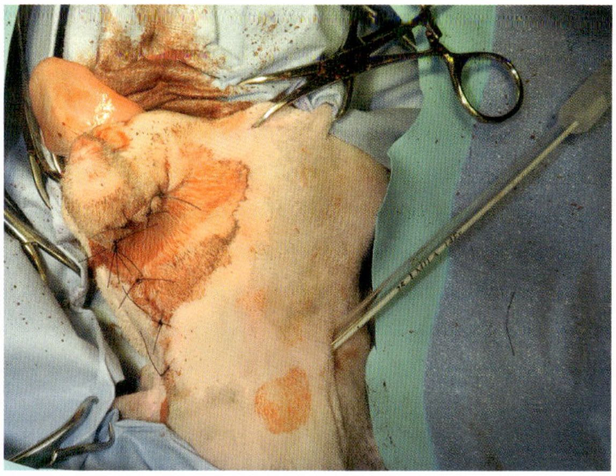

K)

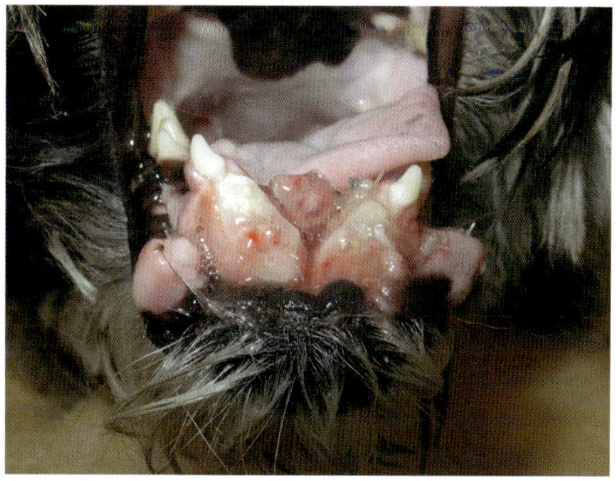

L-i)

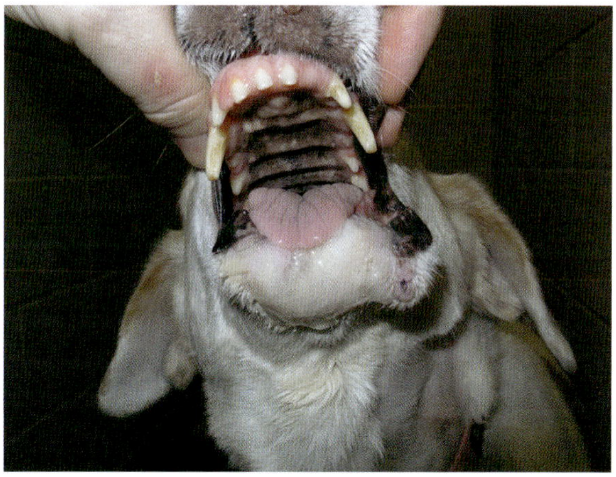

L-ii)

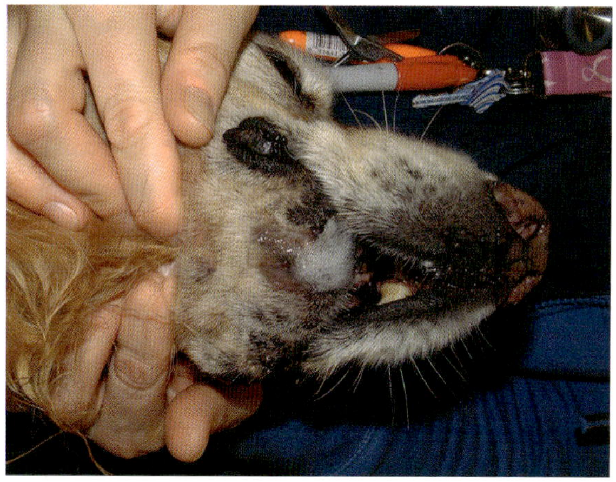

Cosmetic Appearance (See Plate 6.3M, N)

- Mandibular shortening, which is most evident in a mouth-open position (M – i, ii)
- Depending on the length of rostral mandible resected, a variable length of the tongue can hang rostrally (N – i–v)

Suggested Adjuvant Treatments

- See *6. Mandibulectomy and Maxillectomy*.

Prognosis and Oncologic Outcome

- See *6. Mandibulectomy and Maxillectomy*.

References

1 Salisbury, S.K. and Lantz, G.C. (1988). Long-term results of partial mandibulectomy for treatment of oral tumors in 30 dogs. *J. Am. Anim. Hosp. Assoc.* 24: 285–294.

2 Schwarz, P.D., Withrow, S.J., Curtis, C.R. et al. (1991). Mandibular resection as a treatment for oral cancer in 81 dogs. *J. Am. Anim. Hosp. Assoc.* 27: 601–610.

3 Northrup, N.C., Selting, K.A., Rassnick, K.M. et al. (2006). Outcomes of cats with oral tumors treated with mandibulectomy: 42 cases. *J. Am. Anim. Hosp. Assoc.* 42 (5): 350–360.

Plate 6.3

Bilateral Rostral Mandibulectomy *continued*

M-i)

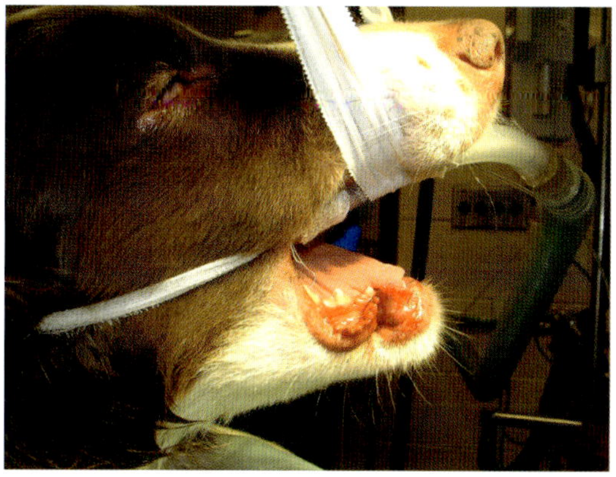

M-ii)

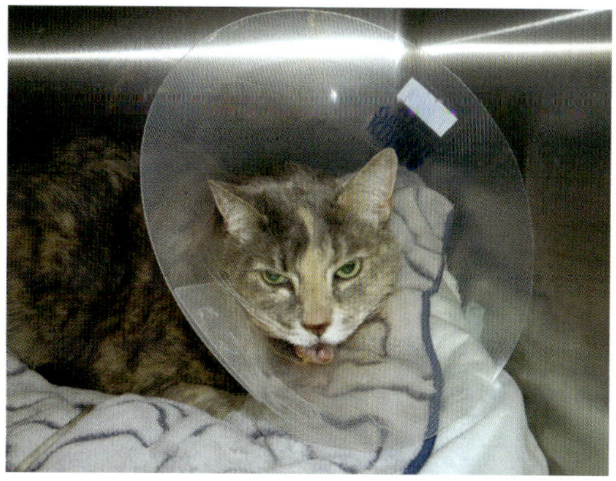

N-i)

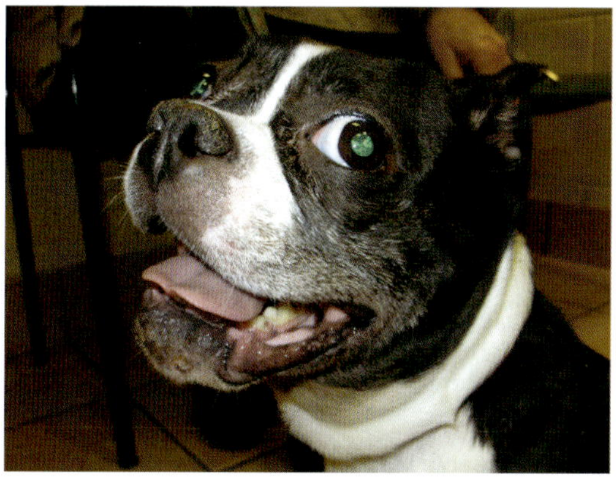

N-ii)

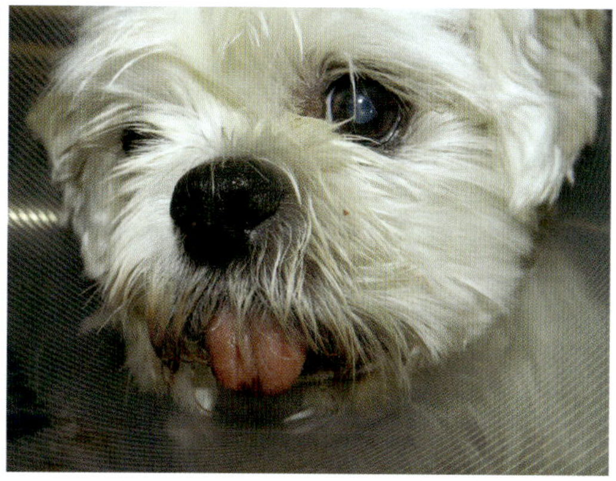

N-iii)

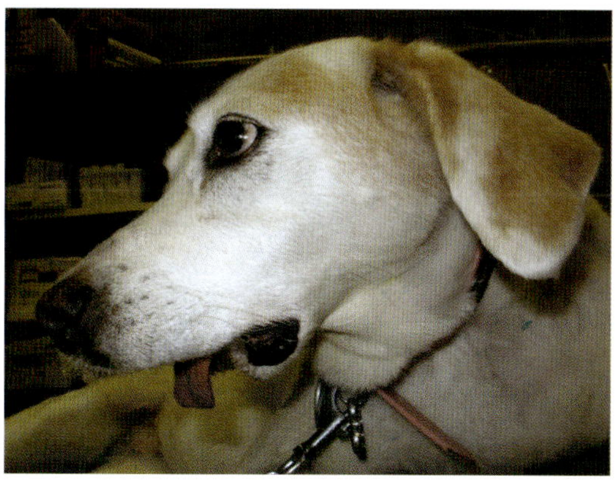

N-iv)

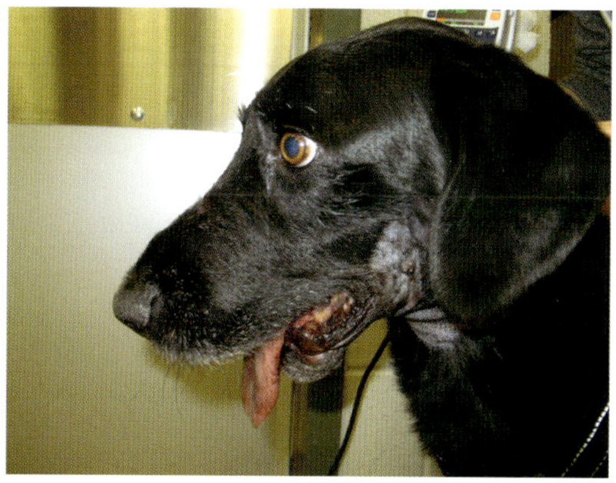

N-v)

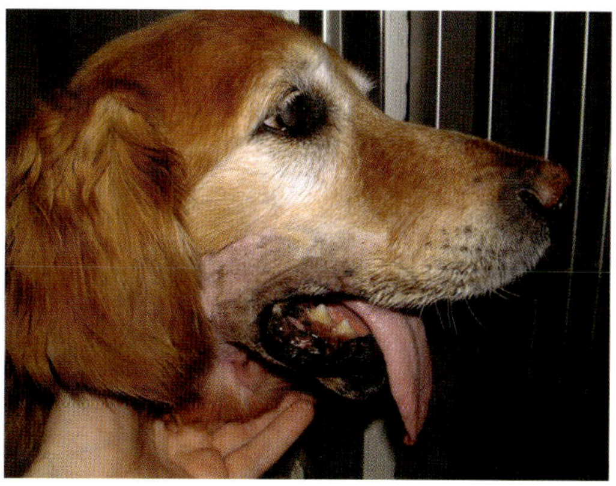

6.4 Segmental Mandibulectomy

Indications (See Plate 6.4 – 1, 2)

1) Resection of benign oral tumors (pictured, extramedullary plasmacytoma)
2) Resection of small malignant oral tumors (pictured, fibrosarcoma) of the mandibular body with no evidence of bone invasion

Suggested Diagnostic Workup and Clinical Staging for Benign Mandibular Tumors

- Complete blood count, serum biochemistry, and urinalysis
- Preoperative biopsy
- ± Precontrast and postcontrast computed tomography (CT) scan of the head for surgical planning

Suggested Diagnostic Workup and Clinical Staging for Malignant Mandibular Tumors

- Complete blood count, serum biochemistry, and urinalysis
- Preoperative biopsy
- Regional lymph node assessment for evaluation of lymph node metastasis
  - Fine-needle aspirate cytology of the mandibular lymph nodes
  - Sentinel lymph node mapping and excision of the sentinel lymph node (see *50.1. Sentinel Lymph Node Mapping*)
  - Nonselective excision of the bilateral mandibular and medial retropharyngeal lymph nodes through a ventral midline cervical approach (see *50.3. Combined Mandibular and Medial Retropharyngeal Lymph Node Excision*), or excision of the ipsilateral mandibular, medial retropharyngeal, and parotid lymph nodes through a lateral approach (see *50.4. Combined Parotid, Mandibular, and Medial Retropharyngeal Lymph Node Excision*)
- ± Radiographs or precontrast and postcontrast CT scan of the head and neck for surgical planning
- Three-view thoracic radiographs or thoracic CT scan for assessment of lung metastasis

Patient Positioning

The patient is positioned in lateral recumbency with the affected side uppermost. Segmental mandibulectomy can also be performed through a ventral approach (see *6.7. Ventral Approach for Mandibulectomy*), in which case the patient is position in dorsal recumbency with a towel or sandbag under the neck so the mandible is parallel to the table. The pharynx should be packed with gauze sponges to minimize the risk of aspirating lavage fluid and blood.

Color Atlas of Canine and Feline Surgical Oncology, First Edition. Julius M. Liptak, Paolo Buracco, William T. N. Culp, and Nicholas J. Bacon.

Plate 6.4

Segmental Mandibulectomy

1)

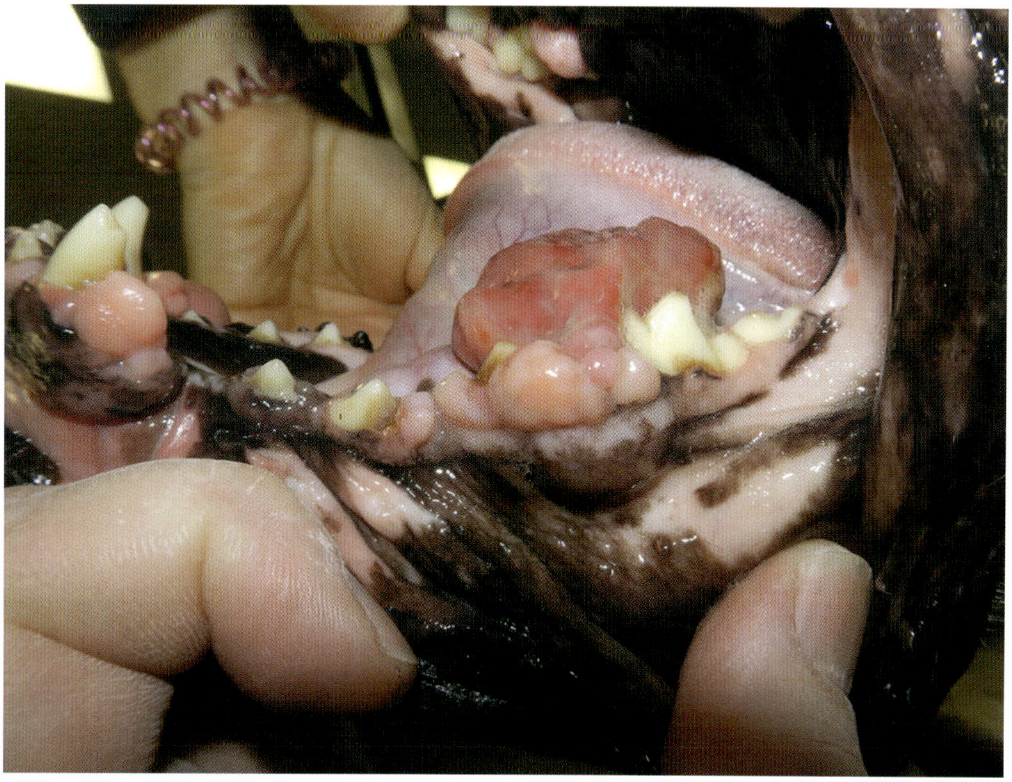

2)

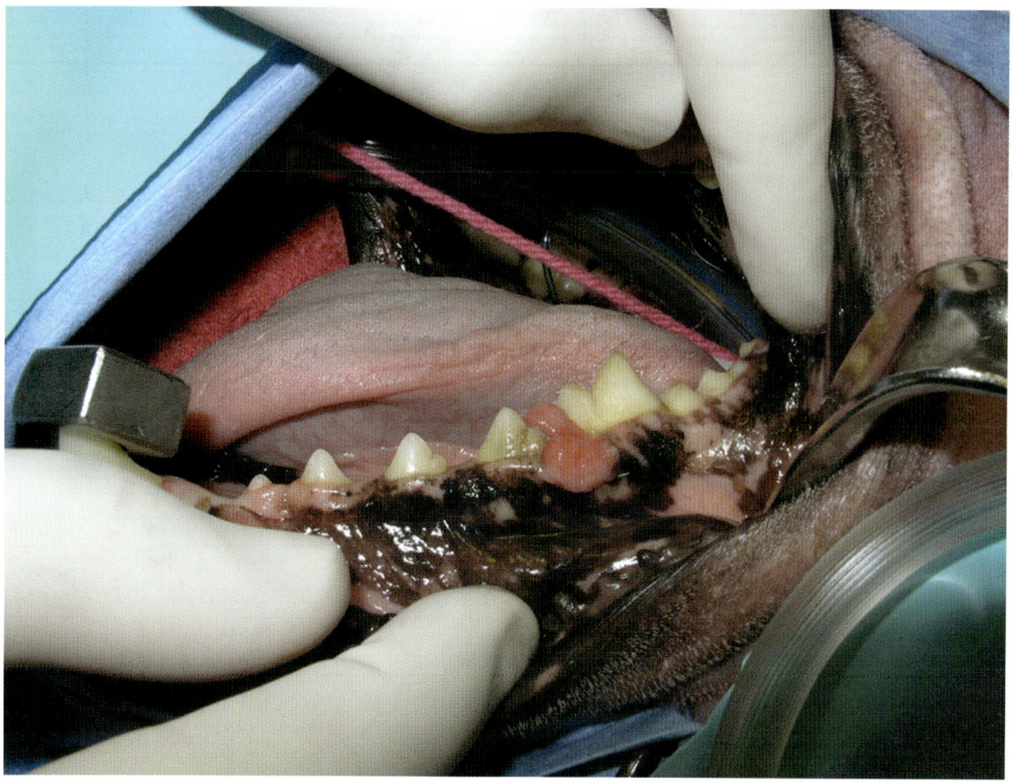

Surgical Technique (See Plate 6.4A–E)

A) If additional caudal exposure is necessary, a full-thickness incision extending caudally from the caudal commissure of the lips can be made.
B) The gingival mucosa on the labial and lingual aspects of the mandibular body are incised with a scalpel blade with a minimum of 5- to 10-mm margins around the oral mass and extending to the planned osteotomy sites. The mucosa and muscle insertions are then elevated with a periosteal elevator to expose the mandibular bone in preparation for the osteotomies.
C) The osteotomies are performed rostral (i, intraoral approach; ii, ventral approach with stabilization of mandible with preplaced string of pearls plate) and caudal (iii, intraoral approach, arrow; iv, ventral approach with stabilization of mandible with preplaced string-of-pearls plate) to the tumor with margins appropriate for the tumor type. These osteotomies can be performed with an oscillating or sagittal saw (pictured), pneumatic drill, piezoelectric instruments, or Gigli wire.
D) After the caudal osteotomy, bleeding from the inferior alveolar artery within the mandibular canal should be controlled by clamping the artery and then either cauterizing (i) or ligating the artery, or packing of bone wax into the mandibular alveolar canal (ii, arrow).
E) Exposed tooth roots are removed with a dental elevator (not pictured).

Plate 6.4

Segmental Mandibulectomy *continued*

A)

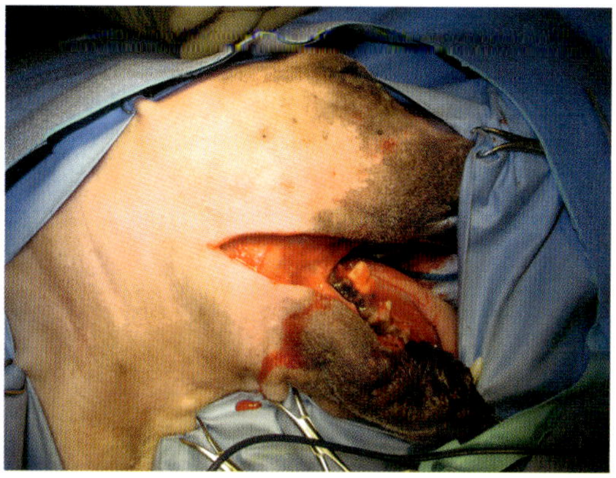

B)

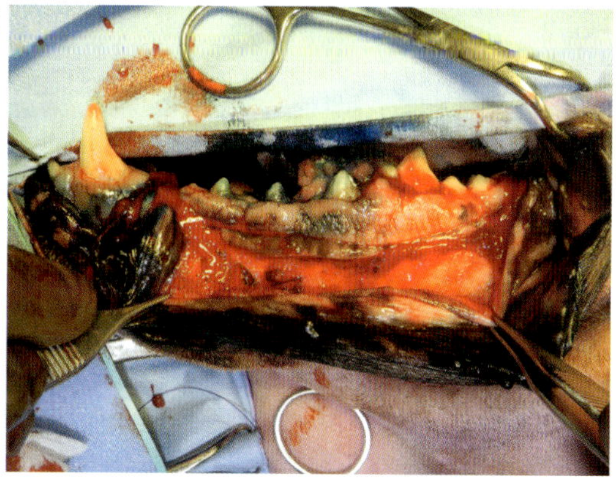

C-i)

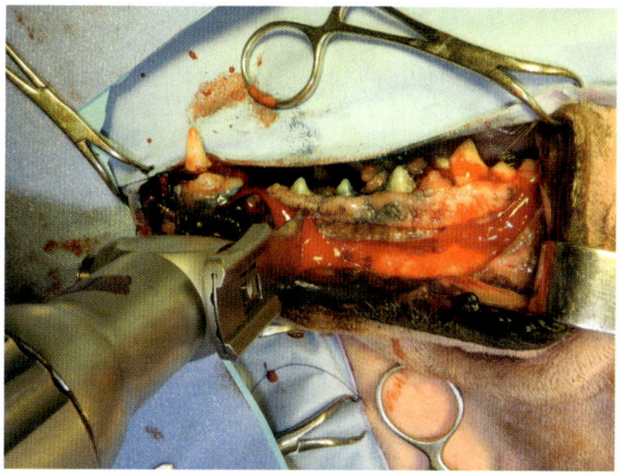

C-ii)

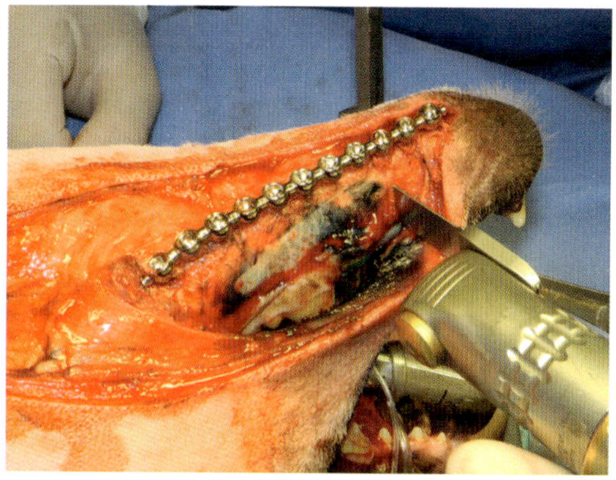

C-iii)

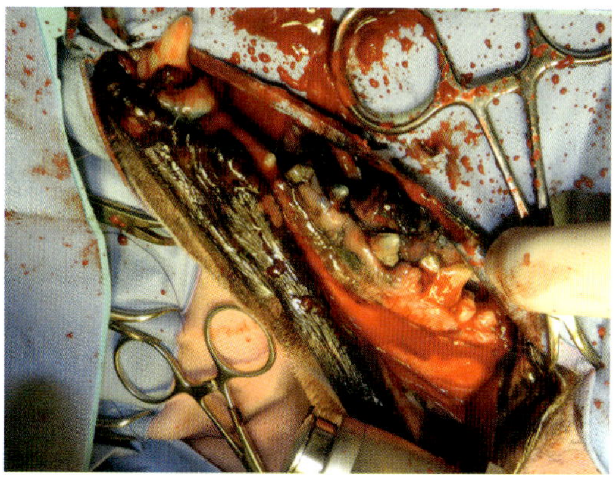

C-iv)

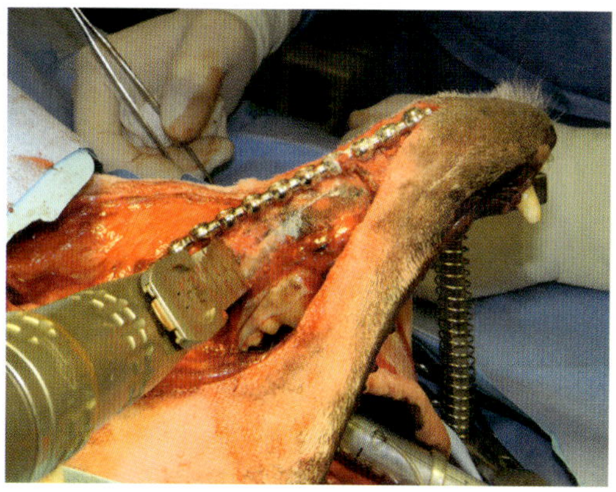

D-i)

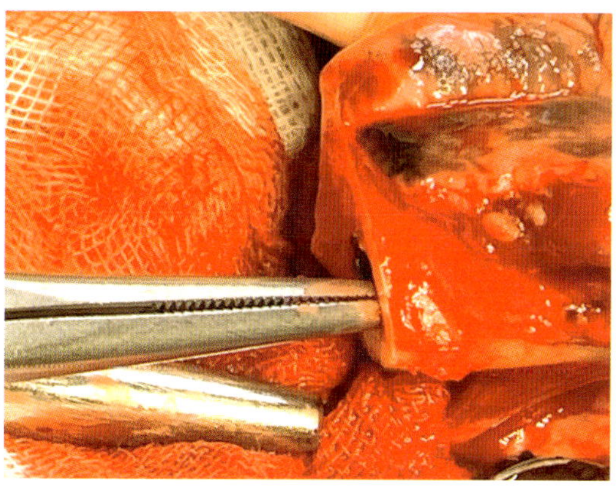

D-ii)

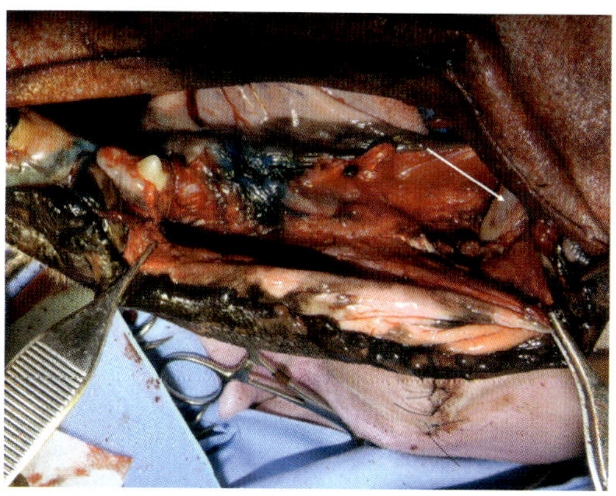

Closure (See Plate 6.4F, G)

F) The defect is closed in two layers. The lingual and labial gingival submucosa are sutured with 3-0 to 4-0 monofilament absorbable suture material in a simple continuous suture pattern. The lingual and labial gingival mucosa are also sutured with 3-0 to 4-0 monofilament absorbable suture material in a simple continuous or interrupted suture pattern.

G) If a commissurotomy has been performed (i), then this is closed in three layers. The labial mucosa (ii) and then submucosa are sutured with 3-0 to 4-0 monofilament absorbable suture material in a simple continuous suture pattern. The skin is closed with 3-0 to 4-0 monofilament nonabsorbable suture material in a simple interrupted or continuous suture pattern (iii, iv).

Postoperative Management

1) Multimodal analgesia
2) Soft foods for 4 weeks
3) No chewing on hard objects or playing with toys for 4 weeks
4) Elizabethan collar
5) Esophagostomy tube and supplemental feeding in cats

Complications – Dogs [1, 2]

Intraoperative Complications

- Blood loss from the inferior alveolar artery

Postoperative Complications (See Plate 6.4H, I)

- Overall: 0%–33%
- Prehension/eating difficulties (rare)
- Ranula formation (rare; H, arrow)
- Incisional dehiscence (33%)
- Mandibular drift (33%; I)

Complications – Cats [3]

Postoperative Complications (0–28 Days)

- Overall: 67%
- Mandibular drift (33%)
- Tongue protrusion (33%)
- Incisional dehiscence (33%)
- Malocclusion with palatine trauma (33%)

Postoperative Complications (>28 Days)

- Overall: 67%
- Mandibular drift (33%)
- Malocclusion with palatine trauma (67%)

Plate 6.4

Segmental Mandibulectomy *continued*

F)

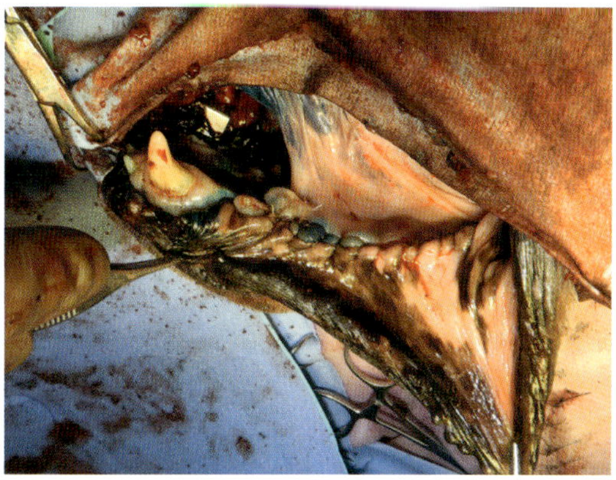

G-i)

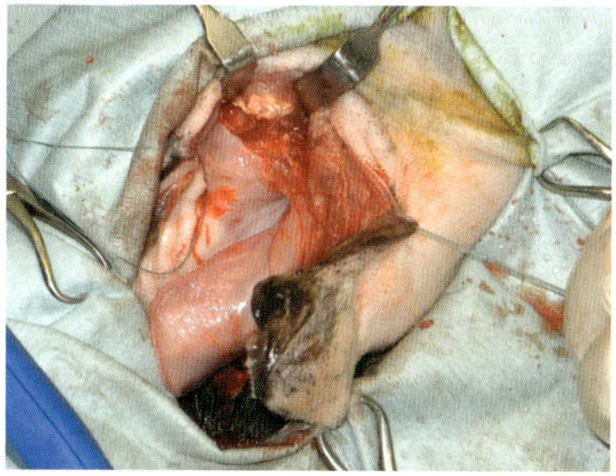

G-ii)

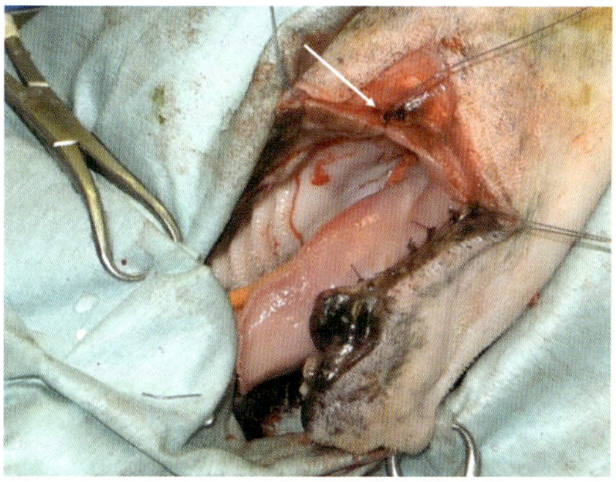

G-iii)

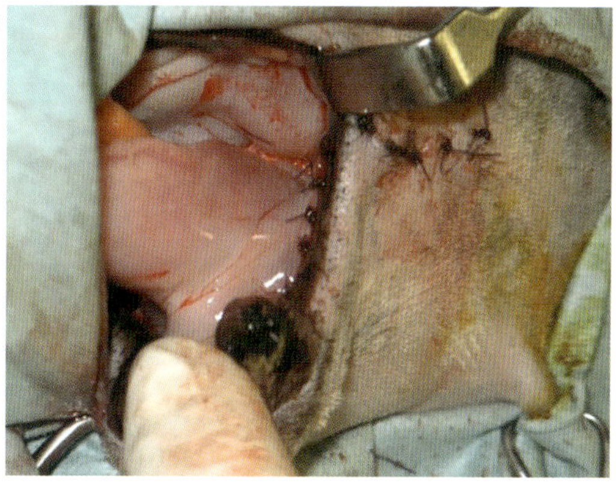

G-iv)

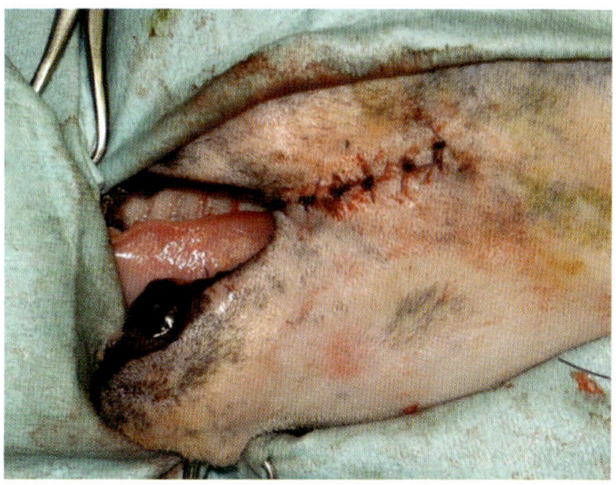

H)

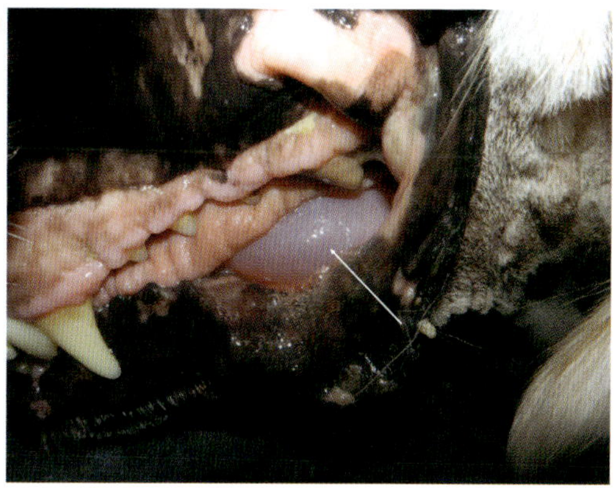

I)

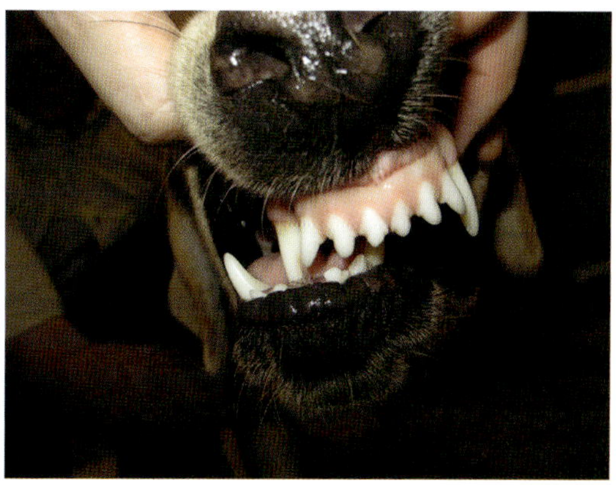

Cosmetic Appearance (See Plate 6.4J, K)

- No to minimal effects on cosmesis (J – i–iii) with occasional tongue lag on the resected side (K, 1 day postoperatively)

Suggested Adjuvant Treatments

- See *6. Mandibulectomy and Maxillectomy*.

Prognosis and Oncologic Outcome

- See *6. Mandibulectomy and Maxillectomy*.

References

1 Salisbury, S.K. and Lantz, G.C. (1988). Long-term results of partial mandibulectomy for treatment of oral tumors in 30 dogs. *J. Am. Anim. Hosp. Assoc.* 24: 285–294.

2 Schwarz, P.D., Withrow, S.J., Curtis, C.R. et al. (1991). Mandibular resection as a treatment for oral cancer in 81 dogs. *J. Am. Anim. Hosp. Assoc.* 27: 601–610.

3 Northrup, N.C., Selting, K.A., Rassnick, K.M. et al. (2006). Outcomes of cats with oral tumors treated with mandibulectomy: 42 cases. *J. Am. Anim. Hosp. Assoc.* 42 (5): 350–360.

Plate 6.4

Segmental Mandibulectomy *continued*

J-i)

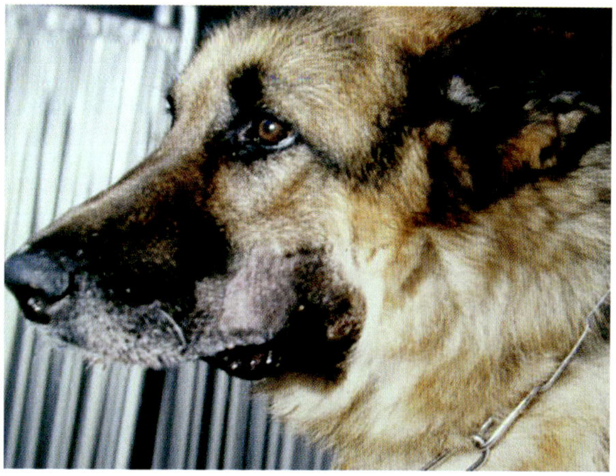

J-ii)

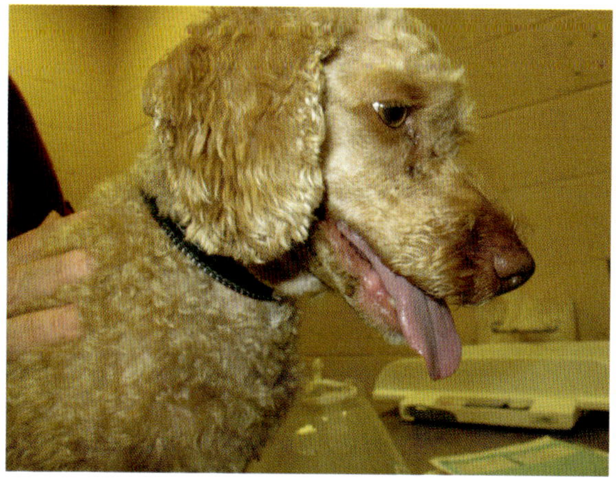

J-iii)

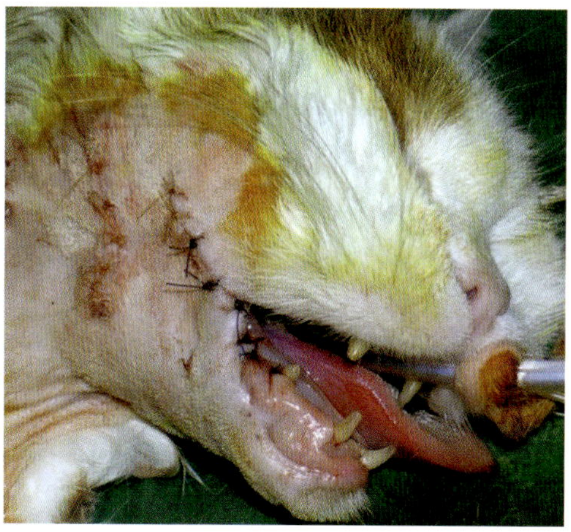

K)

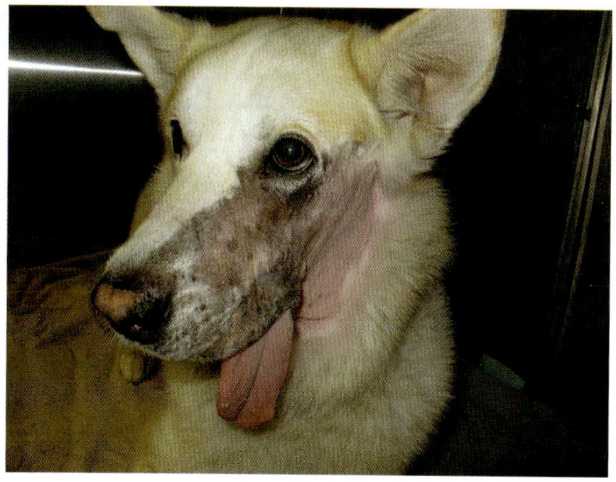

6.5 Rim Mandibulectomy

Indication (See Plate 6.5 – 1)

1) Resection of benign (pictured, peripheral odontogenic fibroma) or small, low-grade malignant tumors, confined to the alveolar margin of the mandibular body and not invasive into the mandibular canal; this procedure is usually performed in large-breed dogs

Suggested Diagnostic Workup and Clinical Staging for Benign Mandibular Tumors

- Complete blood count, serum biochemistry, and urinalysis
- Preoperative biopsy
- ± Precontrast and postcontrast computed tomography (CT) scan of the head for surgical planning

Suggested Diagnostic Workup and Clinical Staging for Malignant Mandibular Tumors

- Complete blood count, serum biochemistry, and urinalysis
- Preoperative biopsy
- Regional lymph node assessment for evaluation of lymph node metastasis
  - Fine-needle aspirate cytology of the mandibular lymph nodes
  - Sentinel lymph node mapping and excision of the sentinel lymph node (see *50.1. Sentinel Lymph Node Mapping*)
  - Nonselective excision of the bilateral mandibular and medial retropharyngeal lymph nodes through a ventral midline cervical approach (see *50.3. Combined Mandibular and Medial Retropharyngeal Lymph Node Excision*), or excision of the ipsilateral mandibular, medial retropharyngeal, and parotid lymph nodes through a lateral approach (see *50.4. Combined Parotid, Mandibular, and Medial Retropharyngeal Lymph Node Excision*)
- ± Radiographs or precontrast and postcontrast CT scan of the head and neck for surgical planning
- Three-view thoracic radiographs or thoracic CT scan for assessment of lung metastasis

Patient Positioning

The patient is positioned in lateral recumbency with the affected side uppermost. The pharynx should be packed with gauze sponges to minimize the risk of aspirating lavage fluid and blood.

Color Atlas of Canine and Feline Surgical Oncology, First Edition. Julius M. Liptak, Paolo Buracco, William T. N. Culp, and Nicholas J. Bacon.

Plate 6.5

Rim Mandibulectomy

1) 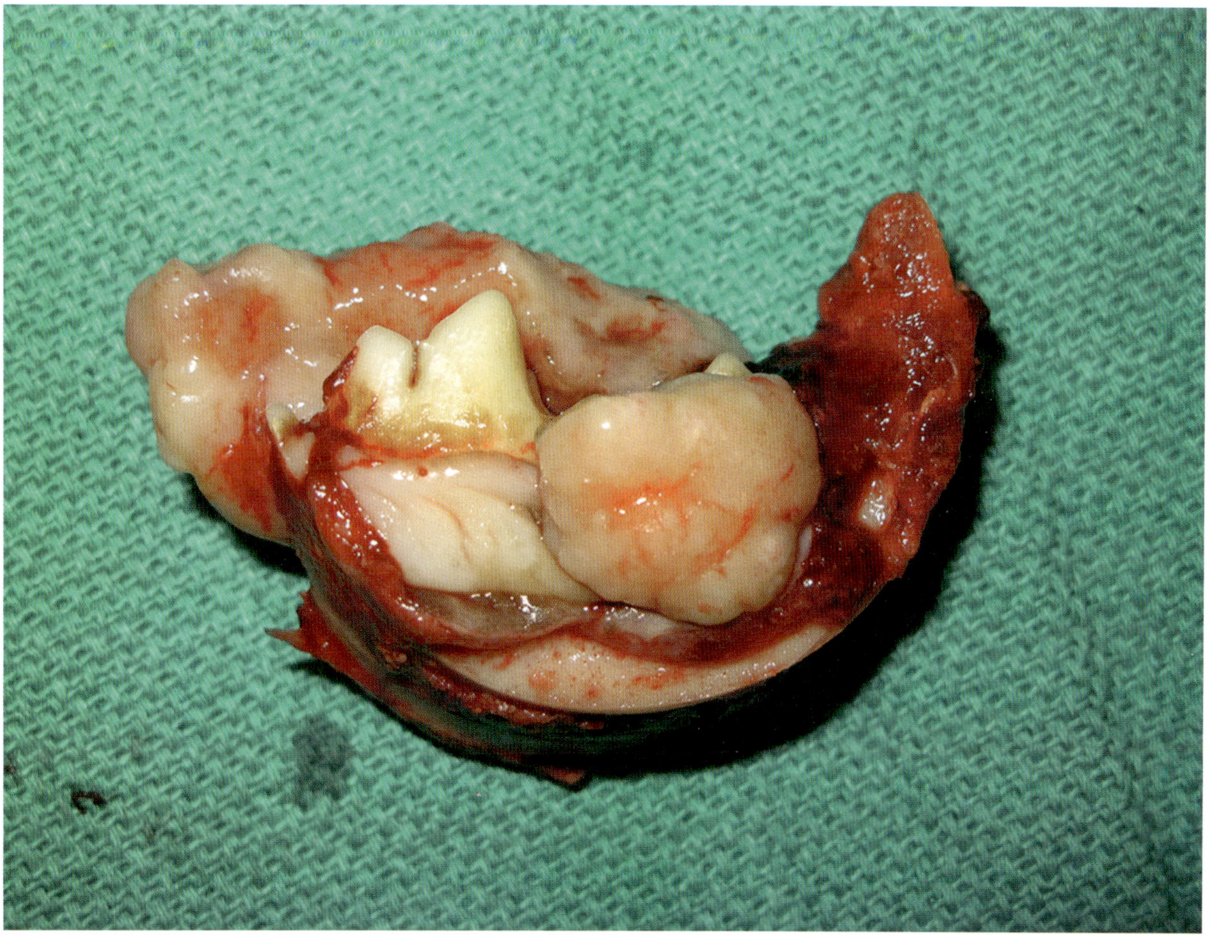

Surgical Technique [1] (See Plate 6.5A–C)

A) The gingival mucosa on the labial and lingual aspects of the mandibular body are incised with a scalpel blade with a minimum of 5- to 10-mm margins around the oral mass and extending to the planned osteotomy sites. The mucosa and muscle insertions are then elevated with a periosteal elevator to expose the mandibular body in preparation for the osteotomy.
B) An osteotomy is performed with an appropriately sized biradial saw (i), pneumatic drill, or piezoelectric instruments such that the mass is resected with a minimum of 1-cm bone margins and a minimum of 1 cm of the ventral cortex of the mandible is preserved (ii). Care is taken to preserve the mandibular alveolar neurovascular bundle.
C) Exposed tooth roots (i) are removed (ii) with a dental elevator.

Closure (See Plate 6.5D)

D) The mucosa and submucosa of the adjacent lip are elevated with a combination of blunt and sharp dissection toward the lip margin to create a labial mucosal-submucosal flap. The labial mucosal-submucosal flap is then advanced into the oral defect and sutured to the lingual mucosa using 3-0 to 4-0 monofilament absorbable material on a reverse cutting needle in a simple interrupted or continuous suture pattern.

Postoperative Management

1) Multimodal analgesia
2) Soft foods for 28 days
3) No chewing on hard objects or playing with toys for 28 days
4) Elizabethan collar

Complications (See Plate 6.5E)

- Incisional dehiscence (rare; E)

Cosmetic Appearance (See Plate 6.5F)

- Normal (F, 2 hours postoperatively)

Suggested Adjuvant Treatments

- See *6. Mandibulectomy and Maxillectomy*.

Prognosis and Oncologic Outcome

- See *6. Mandibulectomy and Maxillectomy*.

Reference

1 Arzi, B. and Verstraete, F.J.M. (2010). Mandibular rim excision in seven dogs. *Vet. Surg.* 39 (2): 226–231.

Plate 6.5

Rim Mandibulectomy *continued*

A)

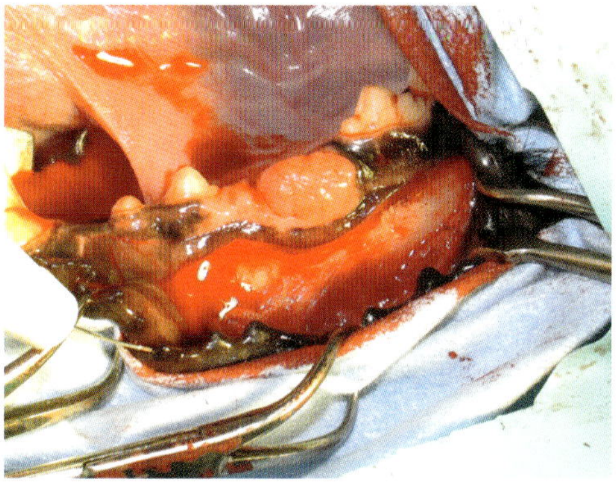

B i)

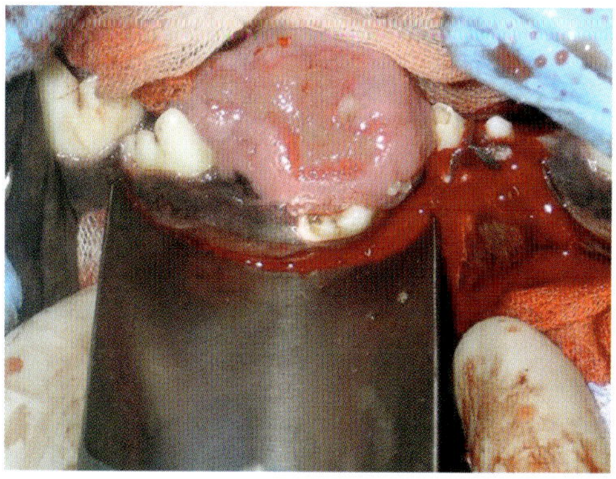

B-ii)

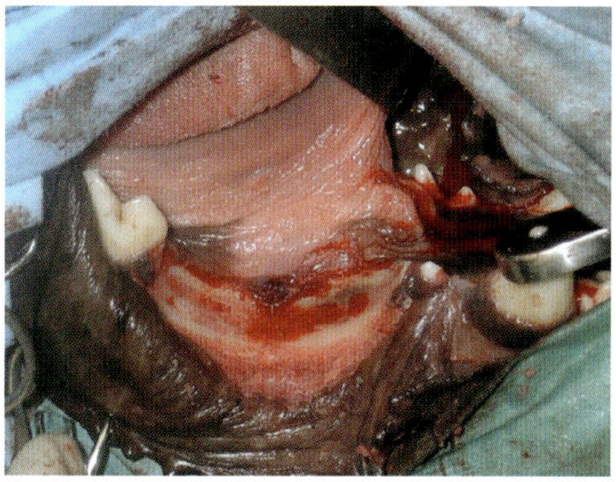

C-i)

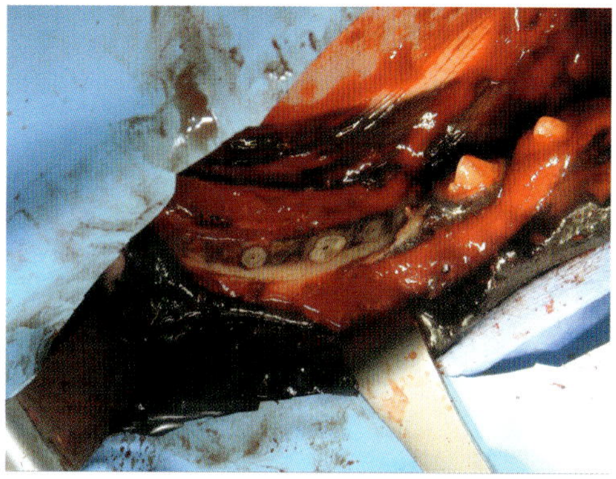

C-ii)

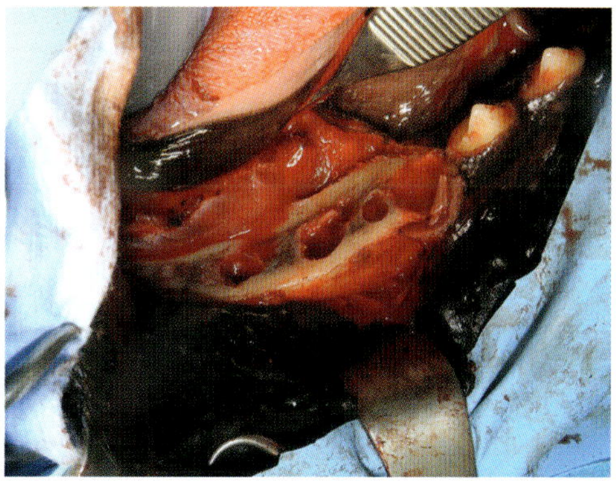

D)

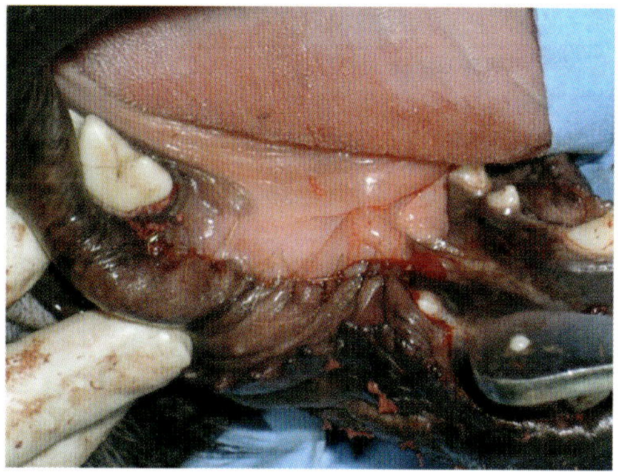

E)

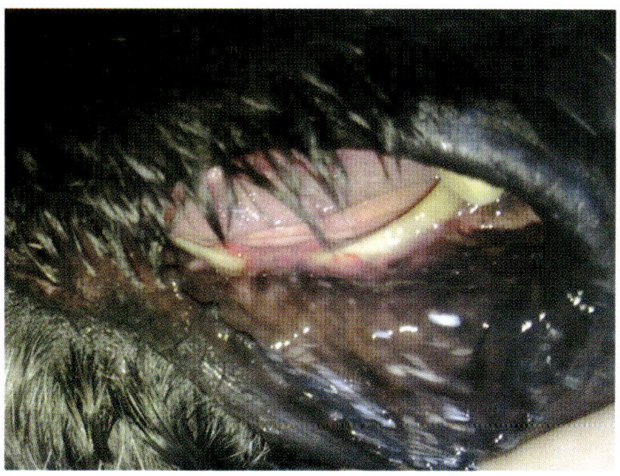

F)

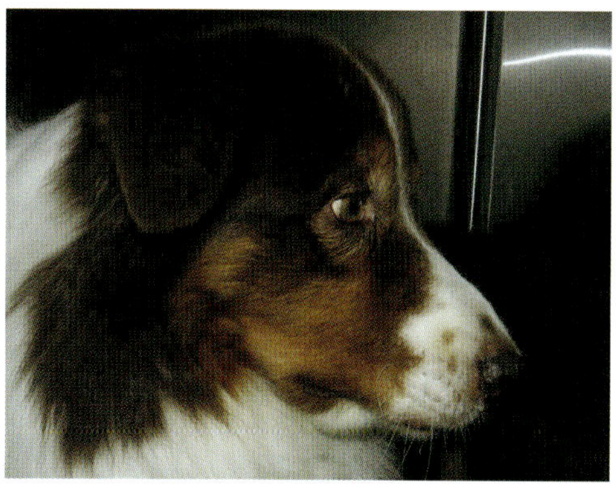

6.6 Caudal Mandibulectomy

Indications (See Plate 6.6 – 1)

1) Resection of malignant bone tumors of the ramus of the mandible
2) Resection of soft tissue tumors with invasion into the ramus of the mandible

Suggested Diagnostic Workup and Clinical Staging for Benign Mandibular Tumors

- Complete blood count, serum biochemistry, and urinalysis
- Preoperative biopsy
- Precontrast and postcontrast computed tomography (CT) scan of the head for surgical planning

Suggested Diagnostic Workup and Clinical Staging for Malignant Mandibular Tumors

- Complete blood count, serum biochemistry, and urinalysis
- Preoperative biopsy
- Regional lymph node assessment for evaluation of lymph node metastasis
  - Fine-needle aspirate cytology of the mandibular lymph nodes
  - Sentinel lymph node mapping and excision of the sentinel lymph node (see *50.1. Sentinel Lymph Node Mapping*)
  - Nonselective excision of the bilateral mandibular and medial retropharyngeal lymph nodes through a ventral midline cervical approach (see *50.3. Combined Mandibular and Medial Retropharyngeal Lymph Node Excision*), or excision of the ipsilateral mandibular, medial retropharyngeal, and parotid lymph nodes through a lateral approach (see *50.4. Combined Parotid, Mandibular, and Medial Retropharyngeal Lymph Node Excision*)
- Precontrast and postcontrast CT scan of the head and neck for surgical planning (1, multilobular osteochondrosarcoma)
- Thoracic CT scan for assessment of lung metastasis

Patient Positioning

The patient is positioned in lateral recumbency with the affected side uppermost. The pharynx should be packed with gauze sponges to minimize the risk of aspirating lavage fluid and blood.

Color Atlas of Canine and Feline Surgical Oncology, First Edition. Julius M. Liptak, Paolo Buracco, William T. N. Culp, and Nicholas J. Bacon.

Plate 6.6

Caudal Mandibulectomy

1) 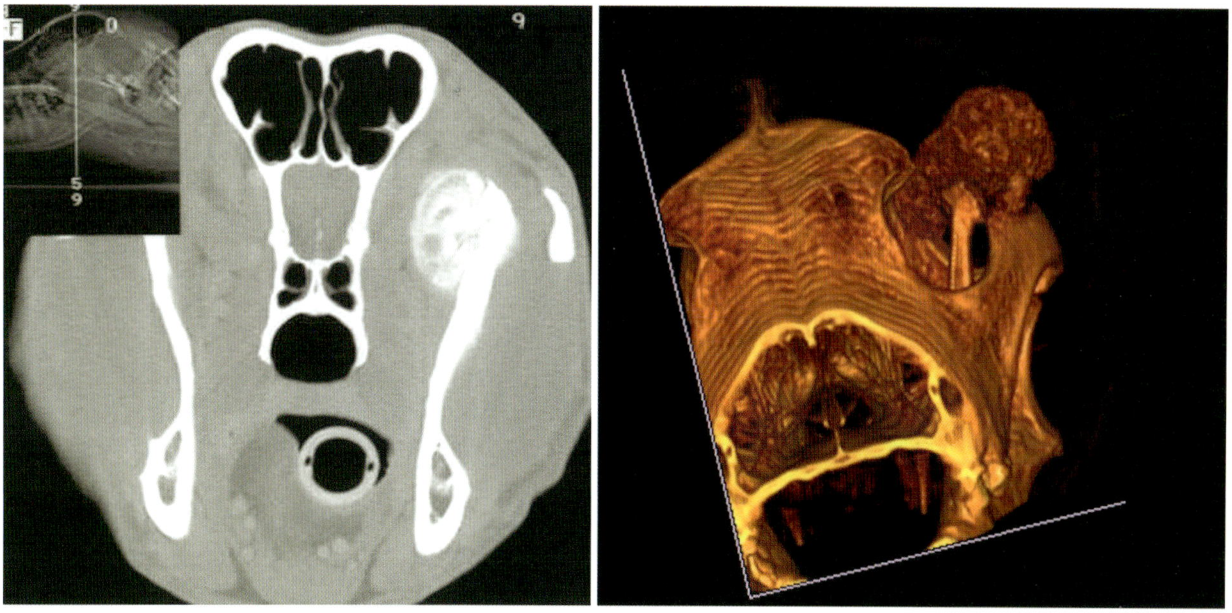

Surgical Technique (See Plate 6.6A–F)

A) Make a skin incision along the dorsal border of the zygomatic arch from ventral to the lateral canthus (LC) to 2–3 cm rostral to the base of the ear. Identify the palpebral nerve immediately dorsal to the incision and retract it dorsally.

B) Incise the insertion of the temporalis (TM) and masseter muscles (MM) on the dorsal and ventral aspects of the zygomatic arch (ZA), respectively, and elevate these muscles to retract them away from the zygomatic arch.

C) Rostral (i) and caudal (ii) osteotomies of the zygomatic arch are then performed with an oscillating or sagittal saw or Gigli wire. The soft tissues medial to the zygomatic arch are protected with periosteal elevators or malleable retractors when performing the osteotomies. The zygomatic branch of the infraorbital artery and facial vein should be preserved along the rostral aspect of the zygomatic arch. The zygomatic arch is commonly discarded after resection (iii, arrow).

D) The facial nerve (FN), coursing over the lateral aspect of the masseter muscle, should be preserved.

Plate 6.6

Caudal Mandibulectomy *continued*

A)

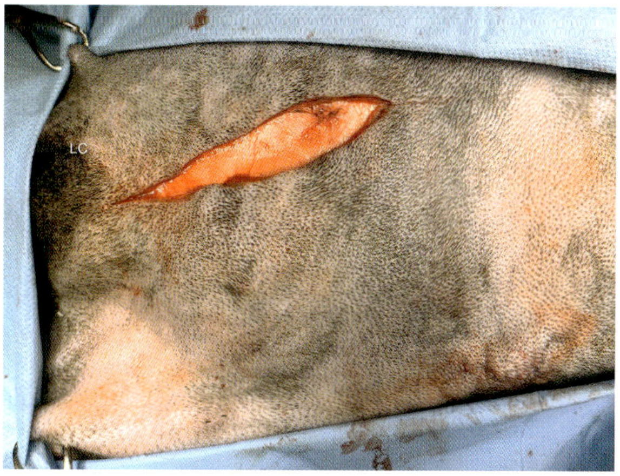

B)

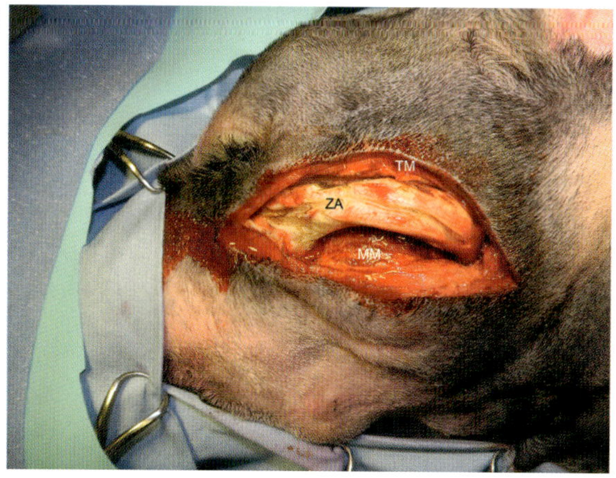

C-i)

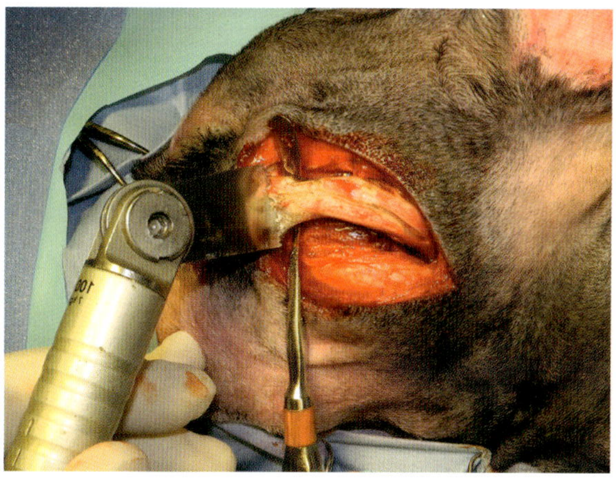

C-ii)

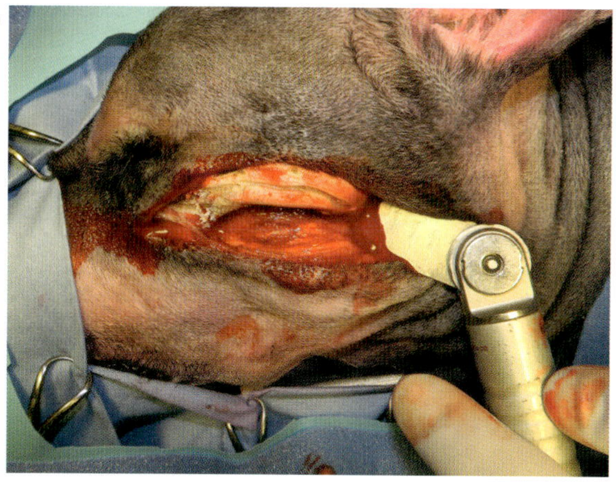

C-iii)

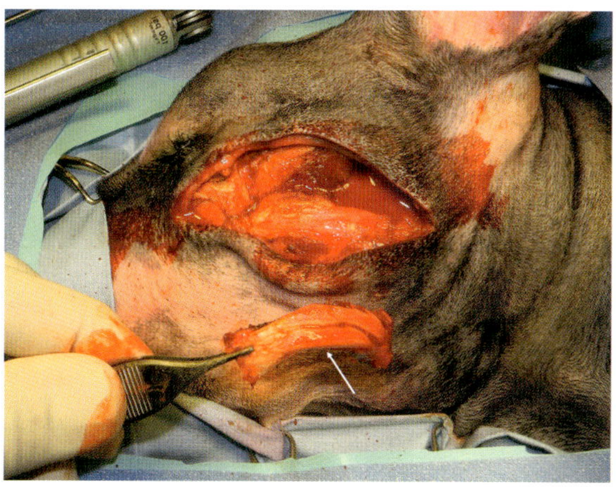

D)

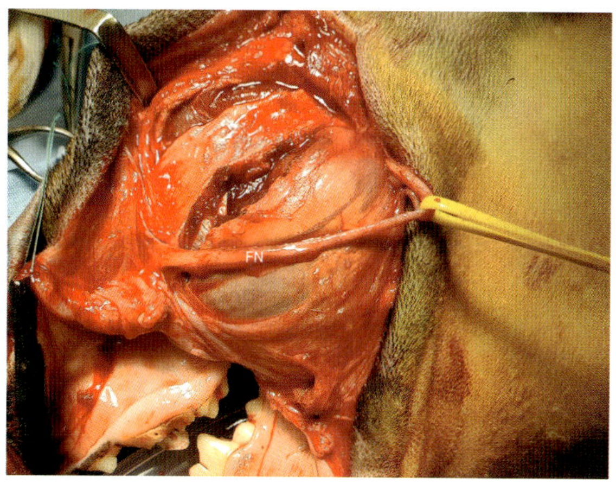

Surgical Technique (See Plate 6.6A–F) *continued*

E) The masseter muscle (MM) is transected along the planned osteotomy site (dashed line) and retracted (i), and an osteotomy of the ramus of the mandible is performed with 2-cm bone margins, either proximal or distal to the temporomandibular joint (TMJ) depending on these margins, with an oscillating or sagittal saw (ii, iii), pneumatic drill, or piezoelectric instruments. If the caudal mandibulectomy is performed distal to the TMJ, then the TMJ is disarticulated with either a scalpel blade or cautery (iv, arrow). This dissection is performed as close as possible to the condyloid process, especially medially and caudally, to avoid iatrogenic damage to the maxillary artery and its branches (v, arrow). Alternatively, if the tumor is in close proximity to the TMJ, then the TMJ can be resected en bloc with the caudal mandible (vi). If the osteotomy is to be performed distal to the TMJ and includes the condyloid process, then the inferior alveolar vessels (vii, arrow) are ligated, cauterized or sealed, and transected as they course over the lateral aspect of the medial pterygoid muscle. The inferior alveolar nerve is transected as close as possible to the mandibular foramen to preserve the lingual nerve (viii).

F) The temporalis muscle (TM) is detached (or transected) from its lateral and medial insertions on the ramus of the mandible and coronoid process.

Plate 6.6

Caudal Mandibulectomy *continued*

E-i)

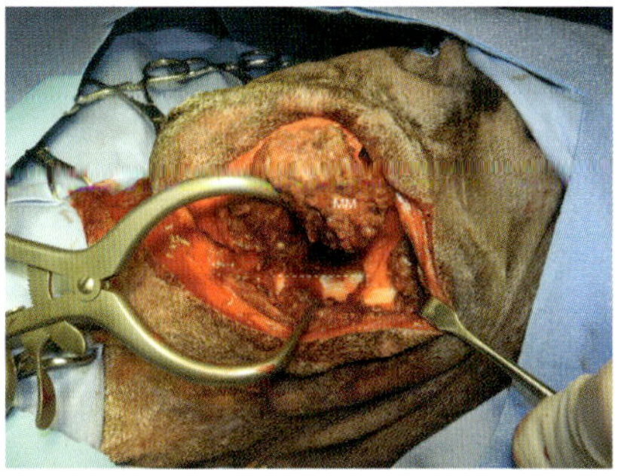

E-ii)

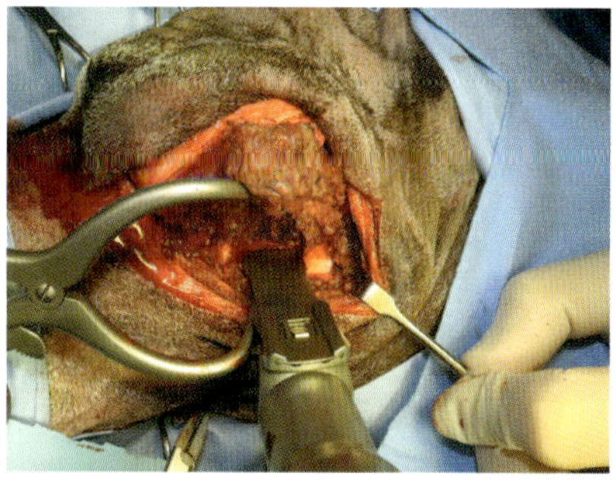

E-iii)

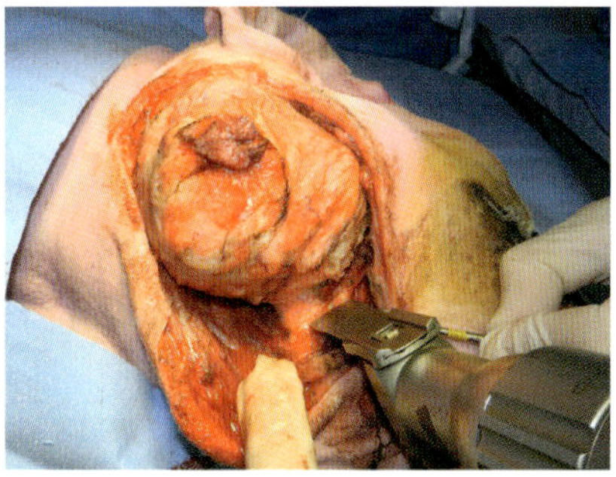

E-iv)

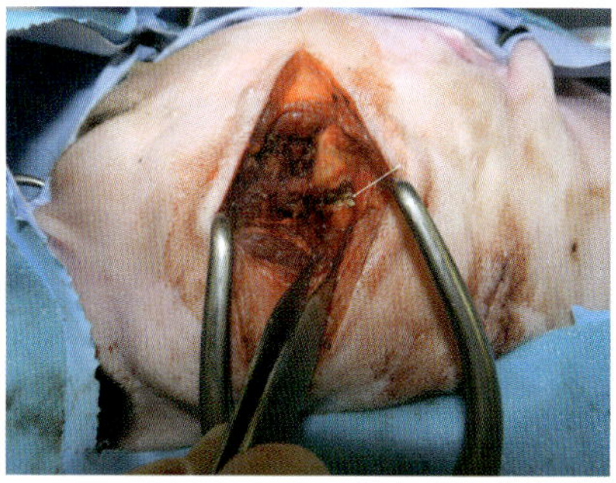

E-v)

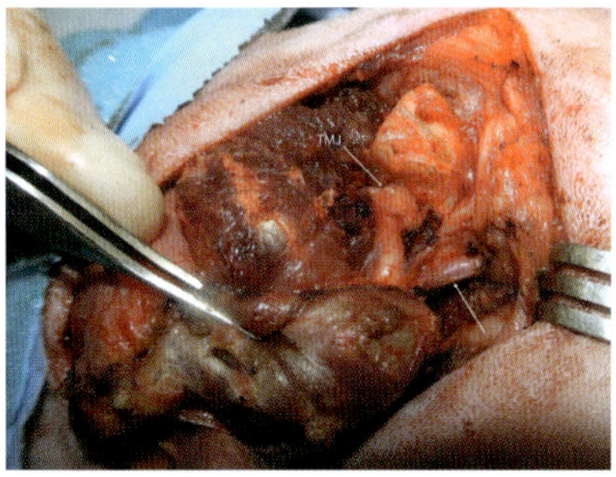

E-vi)

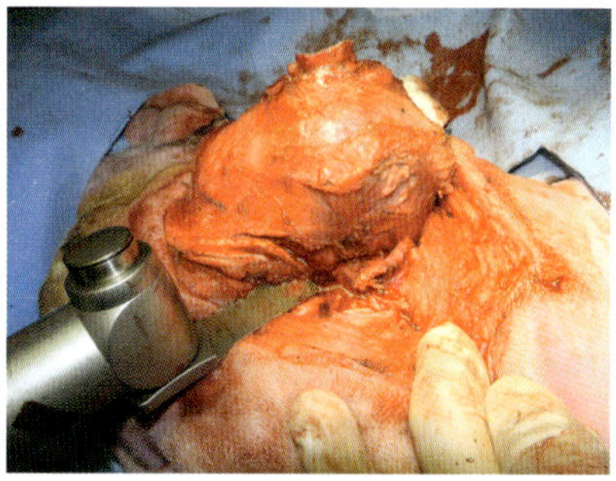

E-vii)

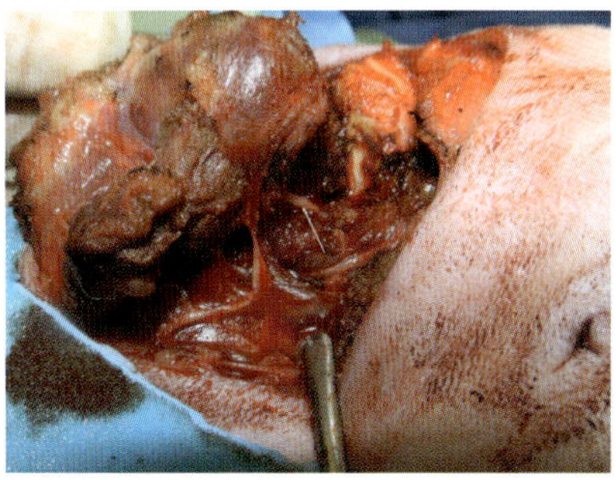

E-viii)

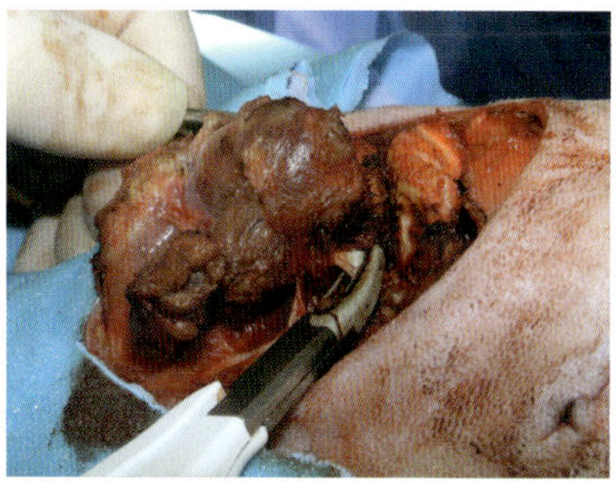

F)

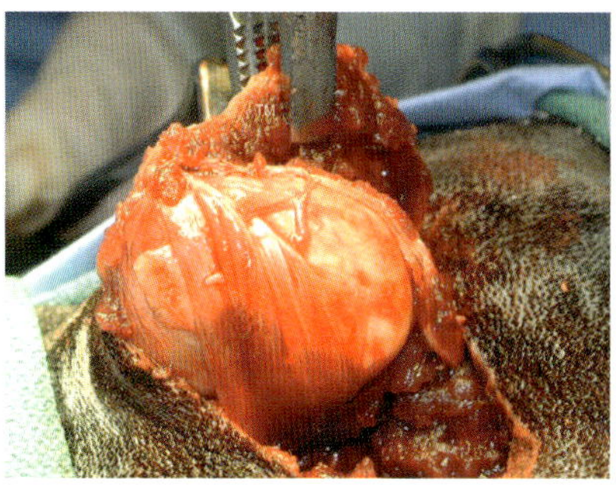

Closure (See Plate 6.6G)

The temporalis and masseter muscles are apposed with absorbable suture material in an interrupted pattern (i). The wound is then closed routinely in two layers. A simple continuous suture pattern using monofilament absorbable suture material is used to close the subcutis. An interrupted or continuous suture pattern using monofilament nonabsorbable suture material is used to close the skin (ii). The oral cavity is not usually entered with this approach, but intraoral mucosal defects should be checked and closed if present (iii).

Postoperative Management

1) Multimodal analgesia
2) Soft foods for 4 weeks
3) No chewing on hard objects or playing with toys for 4 weeks
4) Elizabethan collar

Complications – Dogs [1]

Intraoperative Complications

- Blood loss

Postoperative Complications

- Overall: 0%
- Incisional swelling (rare)
- Incisional dehiscence (rare)

Cosmetic Appearance (See Plate 6.6H)

- No to minimal effects on cosmesis (H – i, ii, 1 day postoperative)

Suggested Adjuvant Treatments

- See *6. Mandibulectomy and Maxillectomy*.

Prognosis and Oncologic Outcome

- See *6. Mandibulectomy and Maxillectomy*.

Reference

1 Schwarz, P.D., Withrow, S.J., Curtis, C.R. et al. (1991). Mandibular resection as a treatment for oral cancer in 81 dogs. *J. Am. Anim. Hosp. Assoc.* 27: 601–610.

Plate 6.6

Caudal Mandibulectomy *continued*

G-i)

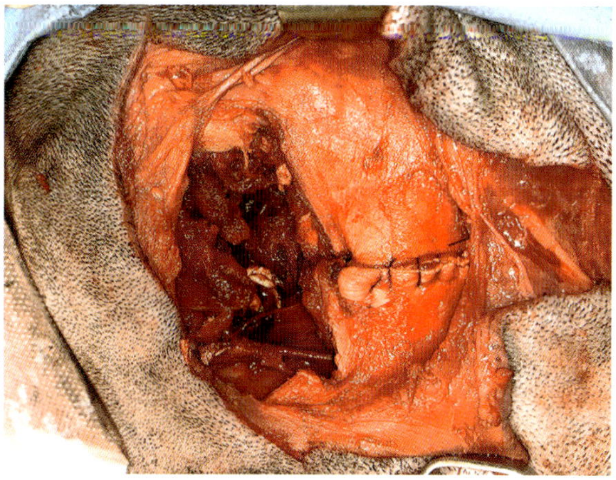

G-ii)

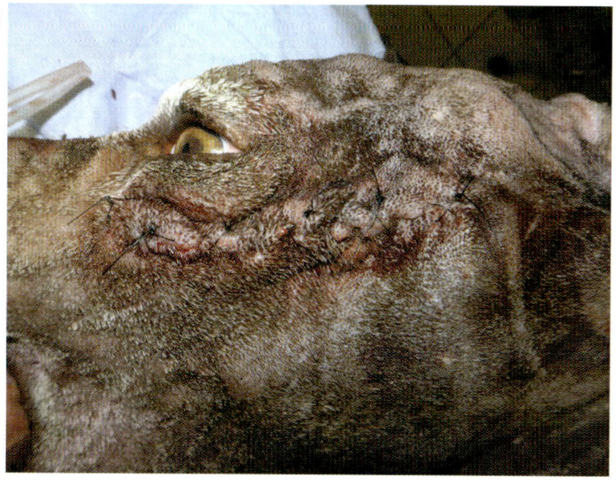

G-iii)

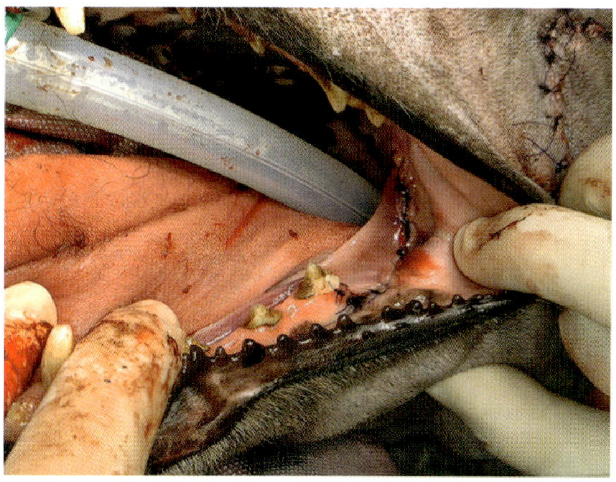

H-i)

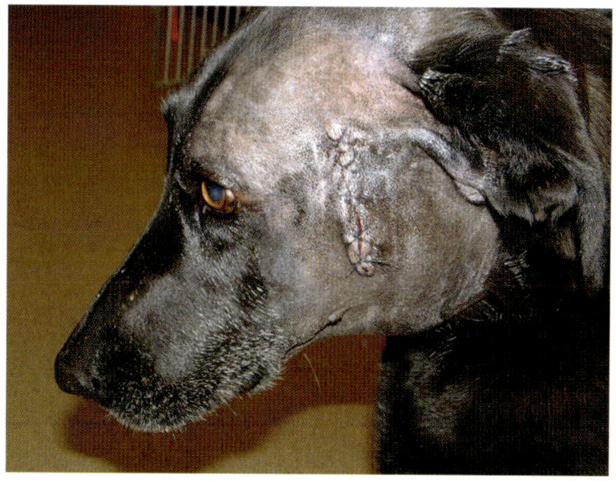

H-ii)

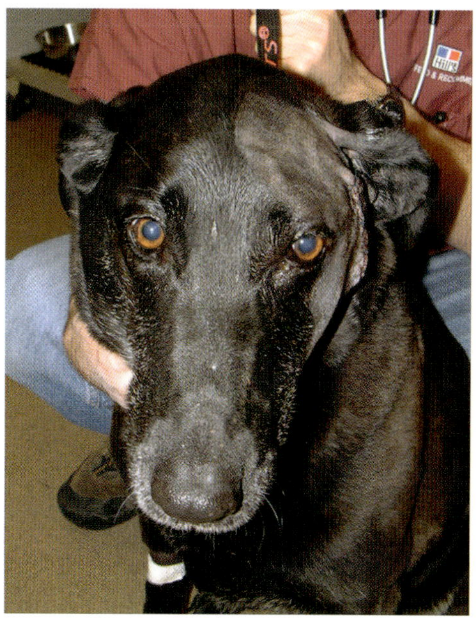

6.7 Ventral Approach for Mandibulectomy

Indications

1) Resection of tumors involving the mid to caudal mandibular body to the ramus of the mandible

Suggested Diagnostic Workup and Clinical Staging for Benign Mandibular Tumors

- Complete blood count, serum biochemistry, and urinalysis
- Preoperative biopsy
- ± Precontrast and postcontrast computed tomography (CT) scan of the head for surgical planning

Suggested Diagnostic Workup and Clinical Staging for Malignant Mandibular Tumors

- Complete blood count, serum biochemistry, and urinalysis
- Preoperative biopsy
- Regional lymph node assessment for evaluation of lymph node metastasis
  - Fine-needle aspirate cytology of the mandibular lymph nodes
  - Sentinel lymph node mapping and excision of the sentinel lymph node (see *50.1. Sentinel Lymph Node Mapping*)
  - Nonselective excision of the bilateral mandibular and medial retropharyngeal lymph nodes through a ventral midline cervical approach (see *50.3. Combined Mandibular and Medial Retropharyngeal Lymph Node Excision*), or excision of the ipsilateral mandibular, medial retropharyngeal, and parotid lymph nodes through a lateral approach (see *50.4. Combined Parotid, Mandibular, and Medial Retropharyngeal Lymph Node Excision*)
- ± Radiographs or precontrast and postcontrast CT scan of the head and neck for surgical planning
- Three-view thoracic radiographs or thoracic CT scan for assessment of lung metastasis

Patient Positioning

The patient is positioned in dorsal recumbency with a towel or sandbag under the neck so the mandible is parallel to the table. A pharyngeal pack is placed to protect the airway. The thoracic limbs are pulled caudally and tied in position. The skull is fixed in position by passing adhesive tape from the edge of the table through the oral cavity immediately caudal to the canine teeth and over the endotracheal tube, to the other side of the table. A mouth gag can be used on the unaffected side, but the mouth should be only partially opened.

Surgical Technique [1] (See Plate 6.7A–J)

A) A skin incision is made along the ventral border of the mandible 2–3 cm longer than the section of mandible to be removed. The skin incision is extended caudally to the angular process of the mandible if performing a caudal or total unilateral mandibulectomy.

B) If the regional lymph nodes are to be removed, this is performed at this stage by extending the skin incision farther caudally to allow for excision of the mandibular and medial retropharyngeal lymph nodes. The mandibular lymph nodes are located superficially beneath the platysma at the junction of the lingual and facial veins uniting to become the jugular vein (i, ii, arrow). The medial retropharyngeal lymph node is located medial, dorsal, and caudal to the mandibular salivary gland and is approached by gentle blunt dissection (iii).

Color Atlas of Canine and Feline Surgical Oncology, First Edition. Julius M. Liptak, Paolo Buracco, William T. N. Culp, and Nicholas J. Bacon.

Plate 6.7

Ventral Approach for Mandibulectomy

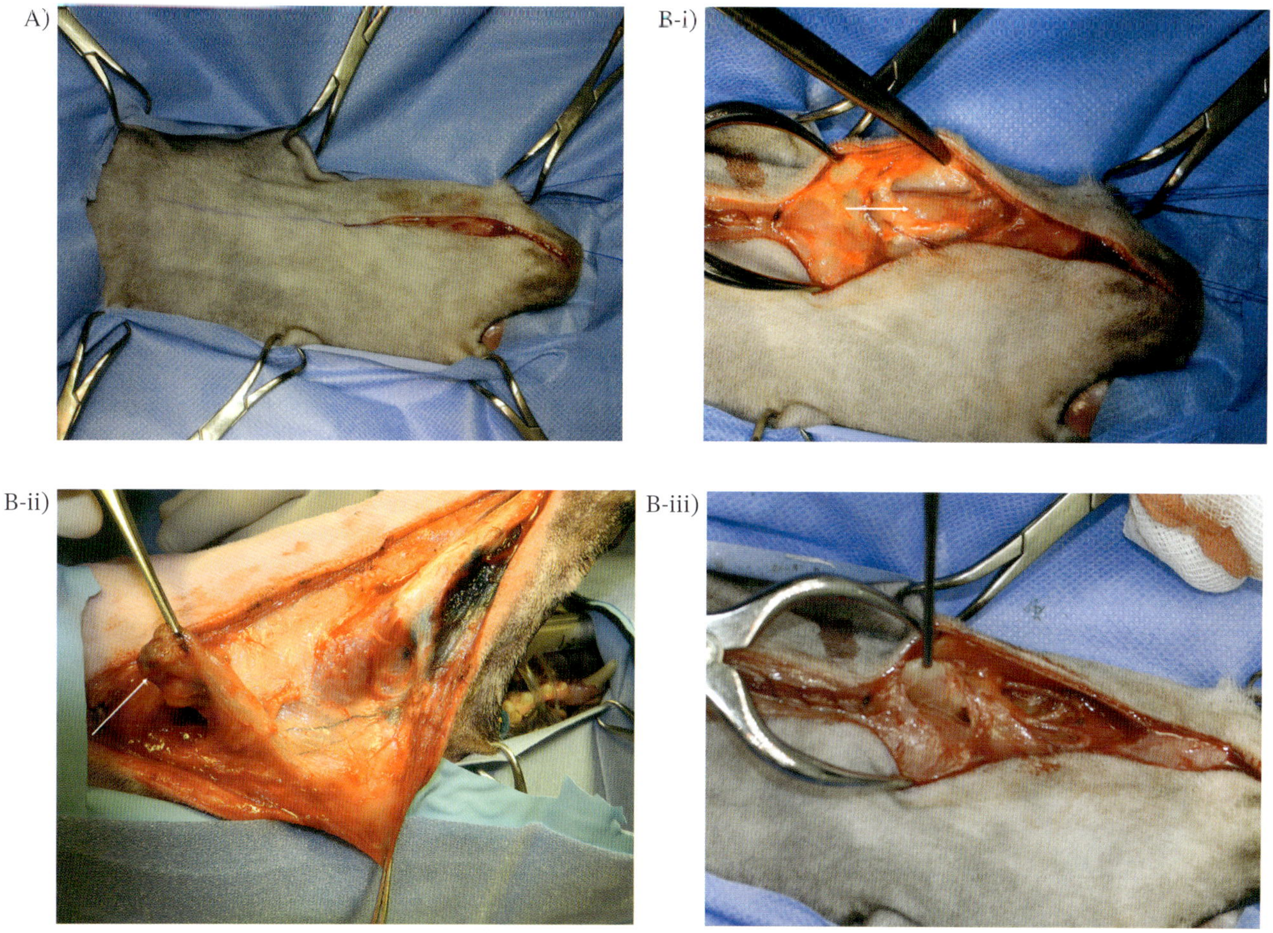

Surgical Technique [1] (See Plate 6.7A–J) *continued*

C) The platysma is excised to expose the bone of the ventral mandible. The insertions of digastricus (DG, ventromedial border of the mid-mandible) and masseter muscles (MM, ventrolateral border of mid-mandible) are transected at the level of the bone. The mylohyoideus (MH) muscle inserting on the medial surface of the mandible is elevated along the length of the mandibular body. The mylohyoideus muscle and tongue are retracted medially to expose the ventral aspect of the lingual mucosa. The soft tissues on the lateral aspect of the mandible are elevated along the lateral aspect of the mandible with a periosteal elevator to expose the ventral aspect of the buccal mucosa.

D) A stab incision is made into the lingual and buccal mucosa (i) either side of the mandible with a scalpel blade, and then these incisions are carefully extended with Metzenbaum scissors in both directions, frequently checking the orientation from both the wound and the oral sides of the approach (ii).

E) The rostral osteotomy is performed with an oscillating or sagittal saw (i, ii), pneumatic drill, or piezoelectric instruments in a ventral-to-intraoral direction. If performed caudal to the mandibular symphysis, then the inferior alveolar artery is ligated or cauterized; however, the rostral osteotomy is often performed through the mandibular symphysis.

F) Once freed, the rostral mandible is exteriorized through the ventral skin incision. This helps with subsequent caudal dissection as the mandible can now be moved from side to side.

G) The freed mandibular body is lateralized to expose the caudal aspect of the medial mandible and the inferior alveolar vessels entering the mandibular canal. The inferior alveolar vessels are ligated, cauterized (pictured), or sealed, and then transected.

H) The mucosa in the oral fornix directly over the length of the palpable ramus of the mandible is sharply incised to reveal the rostral border of the vertical ramus (arrow). The muscle insertions are then transected using either electrosurgery or a scalpel blade.

Plate 6.7

Ventral Approach for Mandibulectomy *continued*

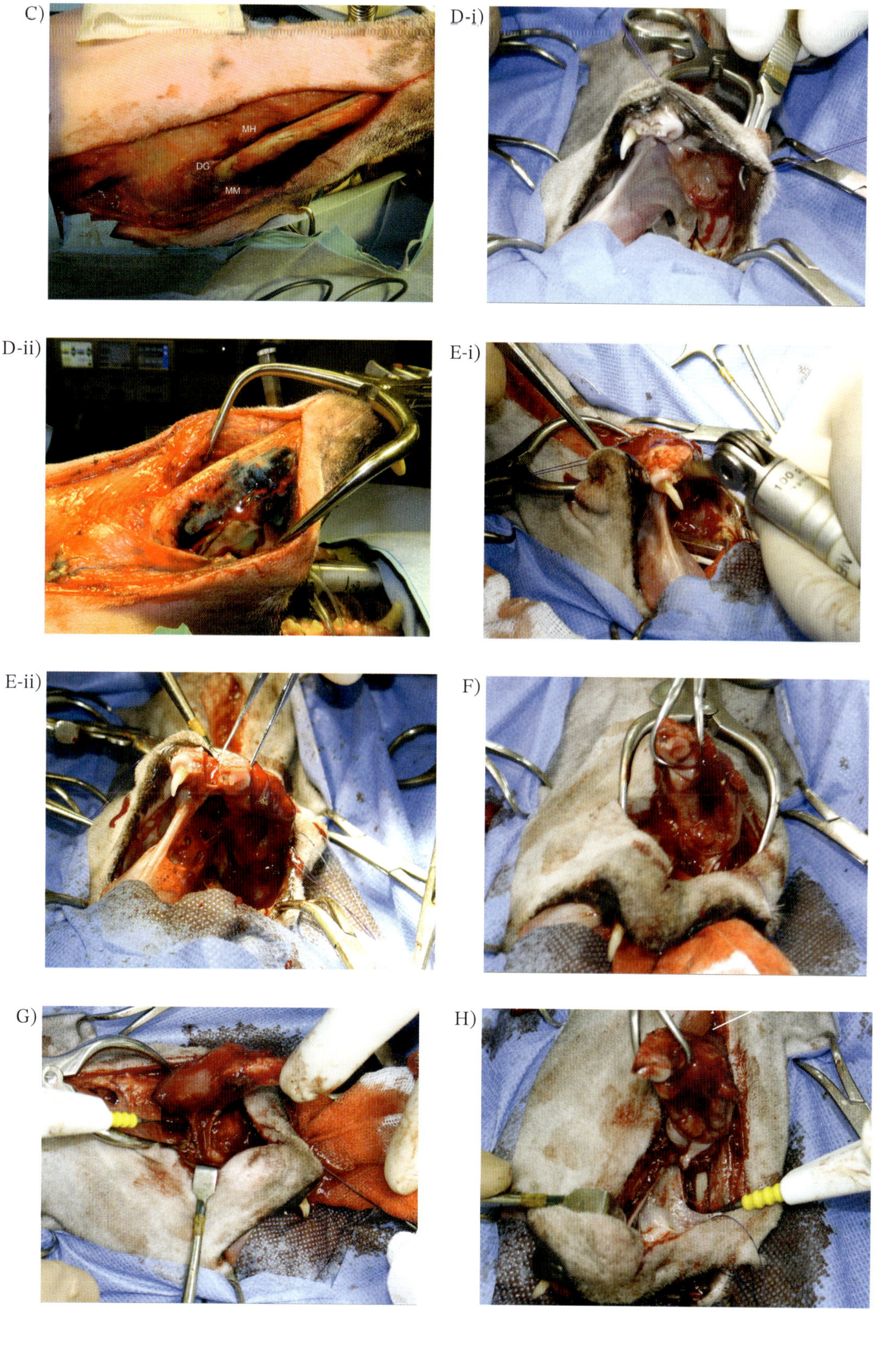

Surgical Technique [1] (See Plate 6.7A–J) *continued*

I) The mandible is then rotated medially to elevate the masseter muscle from the masseteric fossa with a periosteal elevator (i, arrow) or electrosurgery. The pterygoid muscles are transected from the condyloid process (ii, arrow).
J) The temporomandibular joint is identified and disarticulated by incising the joint capsule with a scalpel blade or electrosurgery. Once disarticulated, the remaining soft tissues are transected to complete the mandibulectomy.

Closure (See Plate 6.7K)

The oral mucosa is closed from the wound side with a simple continuous pattern of absorbable monofilament suture material (i–iv). The midbody (e.g. digastricus, mylohyoideus, masseter) and caudal muscles (e.g. masseter, temporal, pterygoid) are sutured to reduce the dead space. The subcutaneous tissue is closed in a simple continuous pattern (v), and the skin is closed with either a continuous or an interrupted suture pattern (vi).

Plate 6.7

Ventral Approach for Mandibulectomy *continued*

I-i)

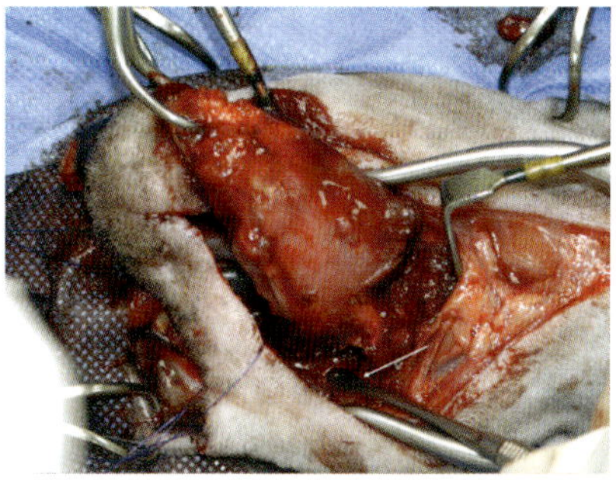

I-ii)

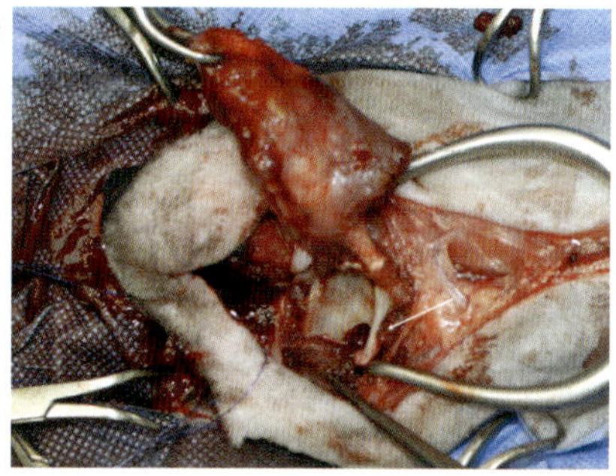

J)

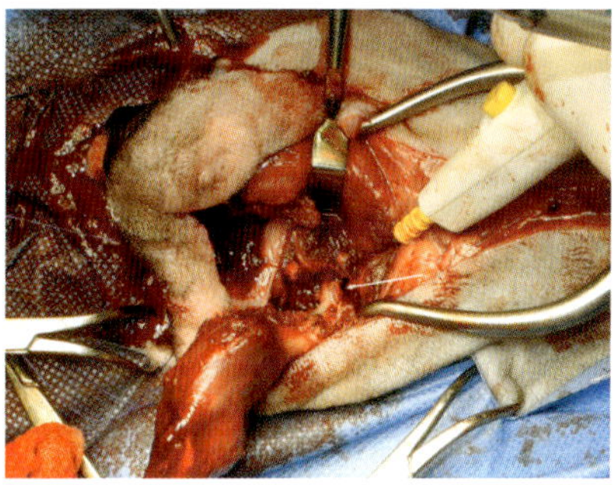

K-i)

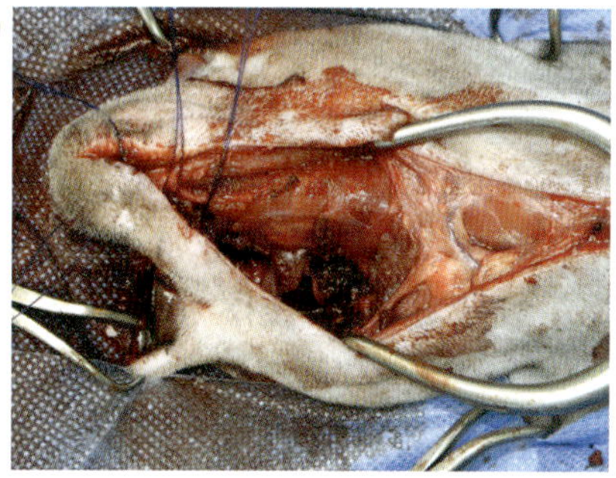

K-ii)

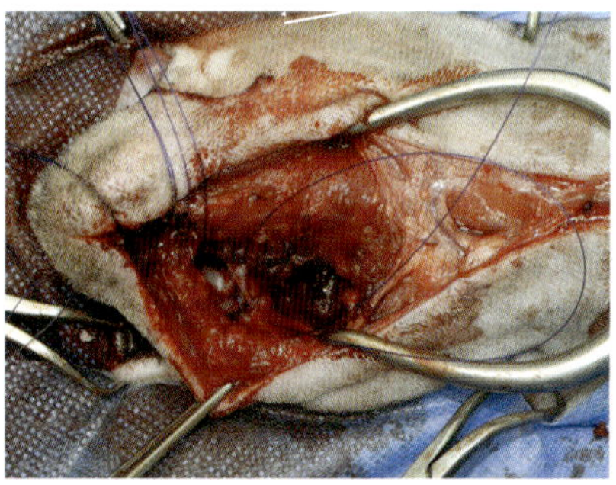

K-iii)

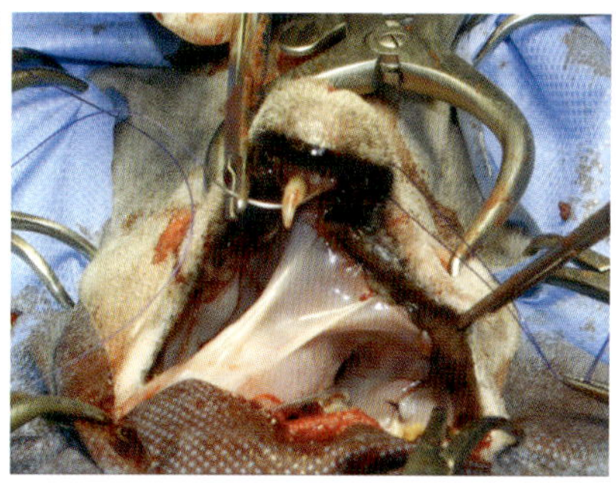

K-iv)

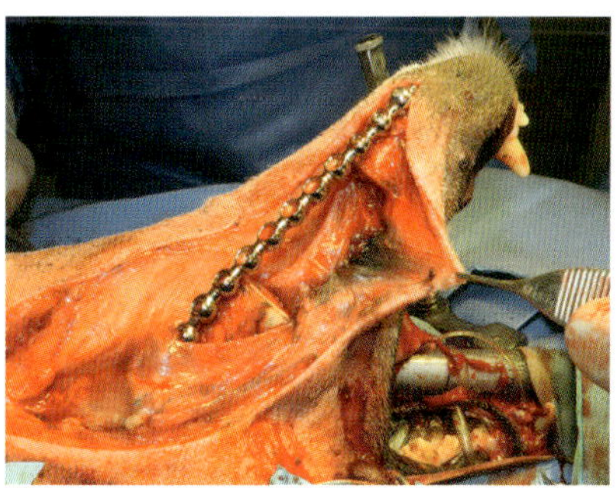

K-v)

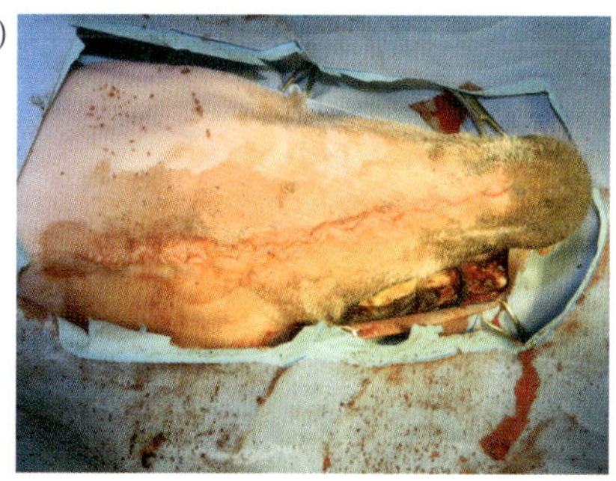

K-vi)

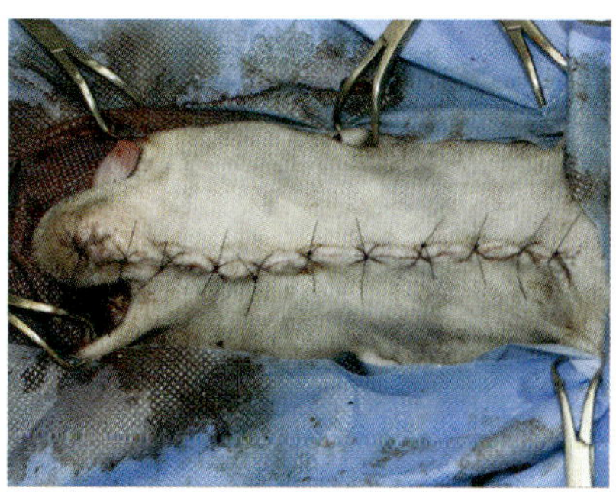

Postoperative Management (See Plate 6.7L)

1) Multimodal analgesia
2) Soft foods for 4 weeks
3) No chewing on hard objects or playing with toys for 4 weeks
4) Elizabethan collar
5) Esophagostomy tube and supplemental feeding in cats (L – i, ii)

Complications – Dogs [1]

Intraoperative Complications

- Blood loss (6%)

Postoperative Complications

- Incisional swelling/edema (76%, more common with concurrent lymph node excision)
- Ranula (rare)
- Incisional dehiscence (rare)

Suggested Adjuvant Treatments

- See *6. Mandibulectomy and Maxillectomy.*

Prognosis and Oncologic Outcome

- See *6. Mandibulectomy and Maxillectomy.*

Reference

1 de Mello Souza, C.H., Bacon, N., Boston, S. et al. (2019). Ventral mandibulectomy for removal of oral tumours in the dog: surgical technique and results in 19 cases. *Vet. Comp. Oncol.* 17 (3): 271–275.

Plate 6.7

Ventral Approach for Mandibulectomy *continued*

L-i)

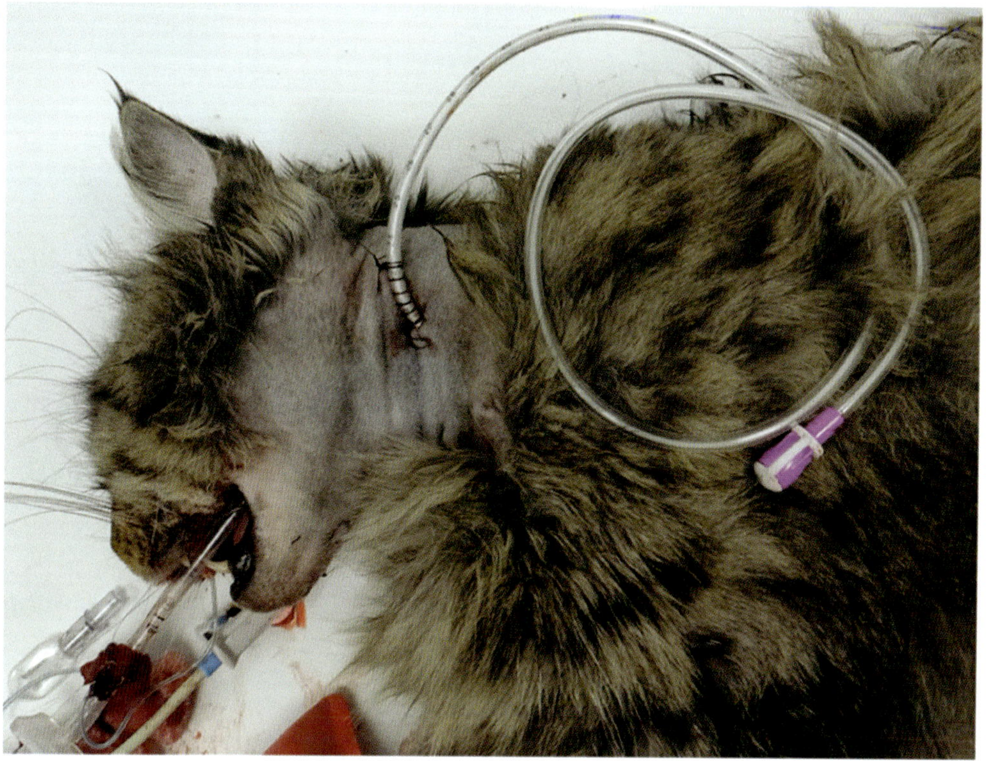

L-ii)

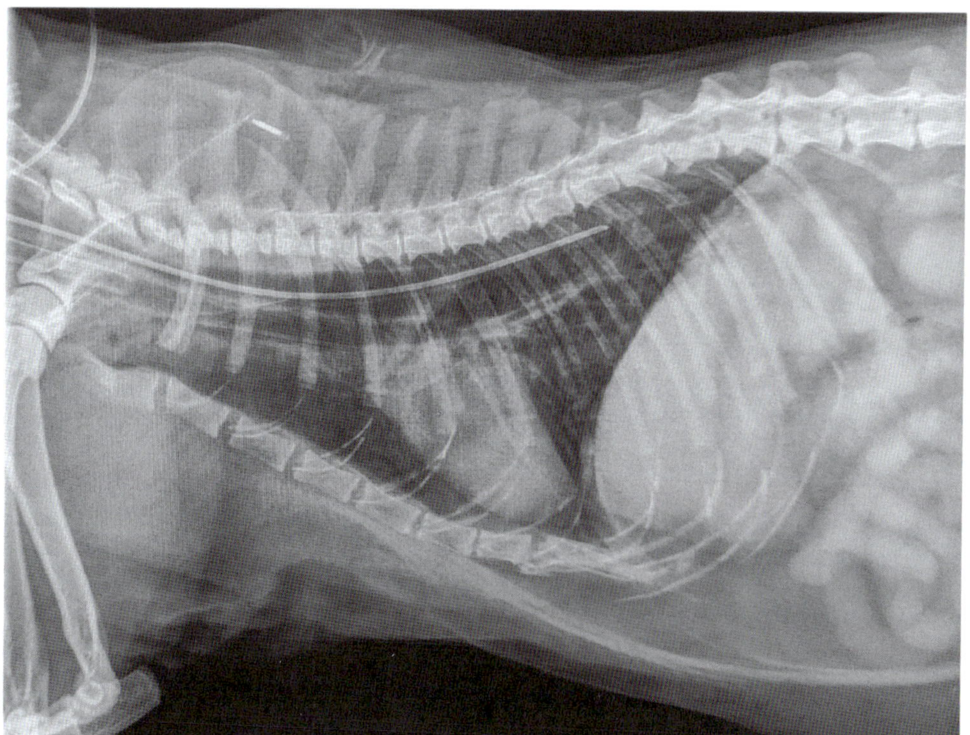

6.8 Unilateral Subtotal Mandibulectomy

Indications (See Plate 6.8 – 1)

1) Resection of extensive or large oral tumors of the mandibular body rostral to the ramus of the mandible (pictured, osteosarcoma)
2) Unilateral subtotal mandibulectomy can be combined with contralateral unilateral rostral mandibulectomy (see *6.2. Unilateral Rostral Mandibulectomy*) if the tumor extends rostrally across the midline

Suggested Diagnostic Workup and Clinical Staging for Benign Mandibular Tumors

- Complete blood count, serum biochemistry, and urinalysis
- Preoperative biopsy
- ± Precontrast and postcontrast computed tomography (CT) scan of the head for surgical planning

Suggested Diagnostic Workup and Clinical Staging for Malignant Mandibular Tumors

- Complete blood count, serum biochemistry, and urinalysis
- Preoperative biopsy
- Regional lymph node assessment for evaluation of lymph node metastasis
  - Fine-needle aspirate cytology of the mandibular lymph nodes
  - Sentinel lymph node mapping and excision of the sentinel lymph node (see *50.1. Sentinel Lymph Node Mapping*)
  - Nonselective excision of the bilateral mandibular and medial retropharyngeal lymph nodes through a ventral midline cervical approach (see *50.3. Combined Mandibular and Medial Retropharyngeal Lymph Node Excision*), or excision of the ipsilateral mandibular, medial retropharyngeal, and parotid lymph nodes through a lateral approach (see *50.4. Combined Parotid, Mandibular, and Medial Retropharyngeal Lymph Node Excision*)
- ± Radiographs or precontrast and postcontrast CT scan of the head and neck for surgical planning
- Three-view thoracic radiographs or thoracic CT scan for assessment of lung metastasis

Patient Positioning

The patient is positioned in lateral recumbency with the affected side uppermost. Unilateral subtotal mandibulectomy can also be performed through a ventral approach (see *6.7. Ventral Approach for Mandibulectomy*), in which case the patient is positioned in dorsal recumbency with a towel or sandbag under the neck so the mandible is parallel to the table. The pharynx should be packed with gauze sponges to minimize the risk of aspirating lavage fluid and blood.

Color Atlas of Canine and Feline Surgical Oncology, First Edition. Julius M. Liptak, Paolo Buracco, William T. N. Culp, and Nicholas J. Bacon.

Plate 6.8

Unilateral Subtotal Mandibulectomy

1)

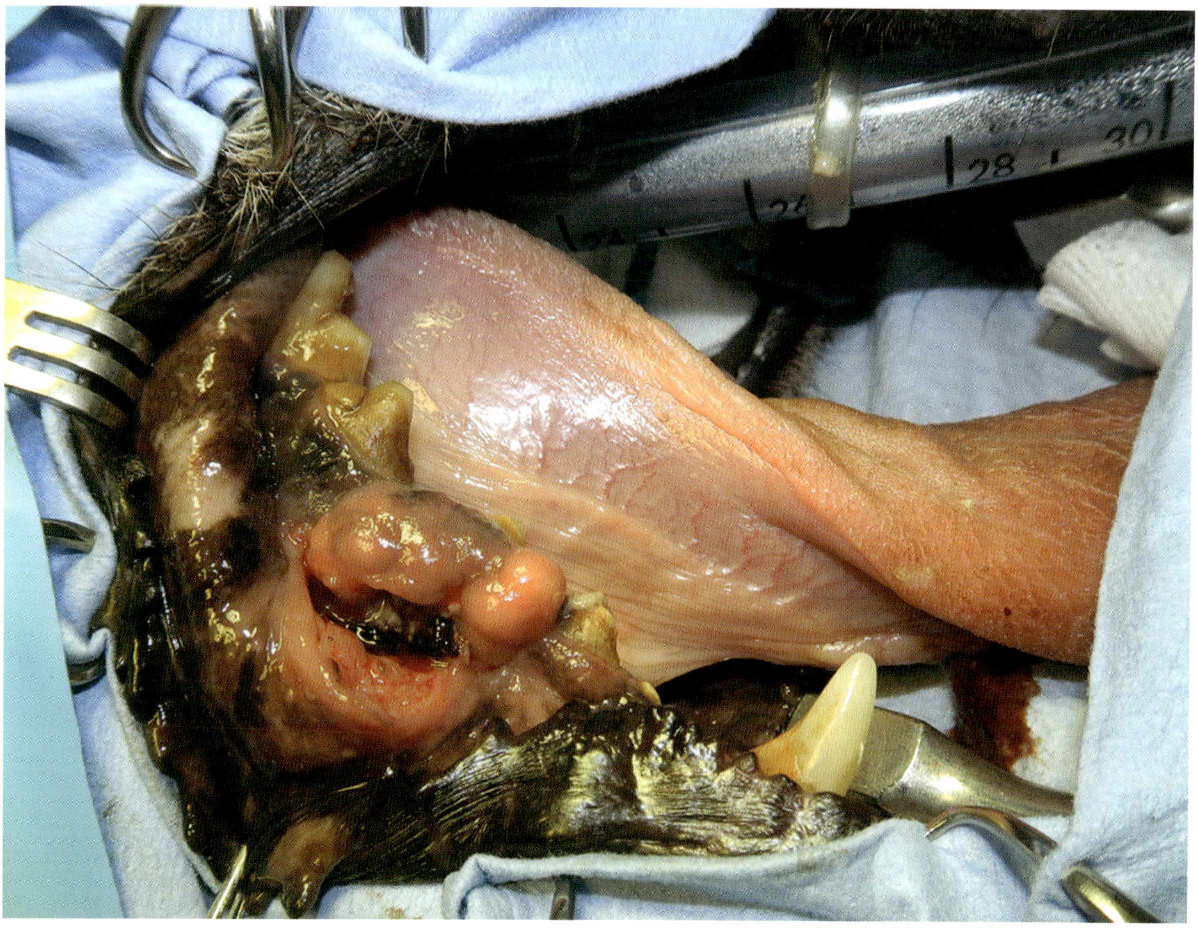

Surgical Technique (See Plate 6.8A–D)

A) The gingival mucosa on the buccal and lingual aspects of the mandibular body and labial aspect of the rostral mandible are incised with a scalpel blade (i, buccal) or Metzenbaum scissors (ii, lingual) with a minimum of 1-cm margins around the oral mass and extending to the planned osteotomy sites. The mucosa (laterally) and genioglossus, geniohyoideus, and mylohyoideus muscle insertions (medially) are then elevated with a periosteal elevator to expose the mandibular bone in preparation for the osteotomies.

B) The rostral osteotomy site is planned with appropriate bone margins for the tumor type and can be performed with an oscillating or sagittal saw (i), pneumatic drill, piezoelectric instruments, or, if at the mandibular symphysis, osteotome and mallet. A unilateral subtotal mandibulectomy can be combined with a contralateral unilateral rostral mandibulectomy (see *6.2. Unilateral Rostral Mandibulectomy*) if the tumor extends rostrally across the midline (ii).

C) The caudal osteotomy site is planned with appropriate bone margins for the tumor type and can be performed with an oscillating or sagittal saw (i, ii), pneumatic drill, piezoelectric instruments, or Gigli wire.

D) After the caudal osteotomy, bleeding from the inferior alveolar artery within the mandibular canal should be controlled by clamping the artery and then either cauterizing (pictured) or ligating the artery, or packing of bone wax into the mandibular alveolar canal.

Plate 6.8

Unilateral Subtotal Mandibulectomy *continued*

A-i)

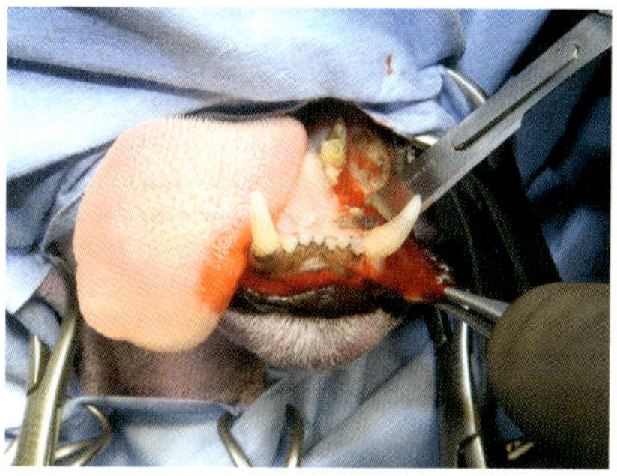

A-i)

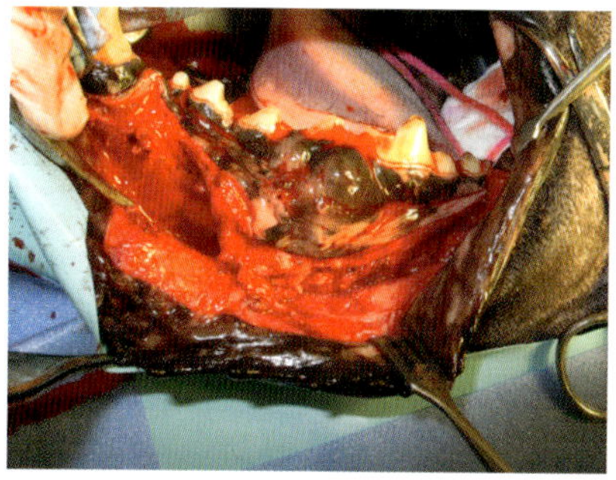

A-ii)

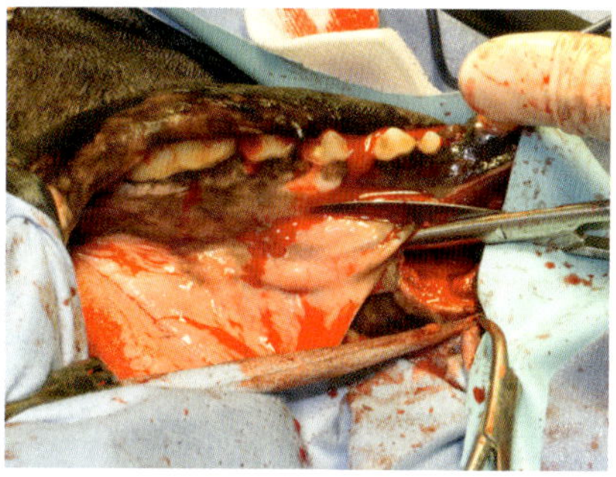

A-ii)

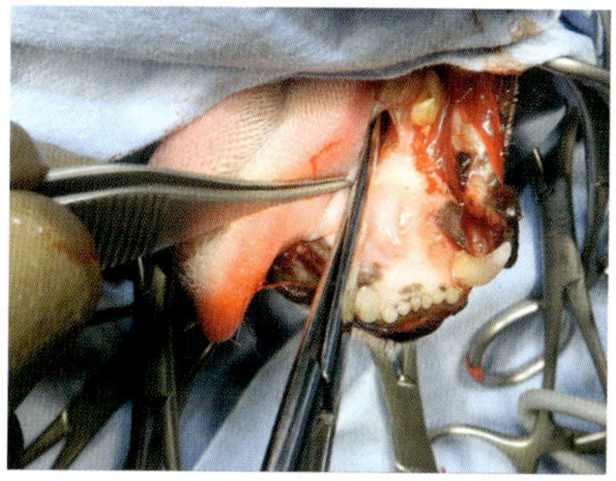

B-i)

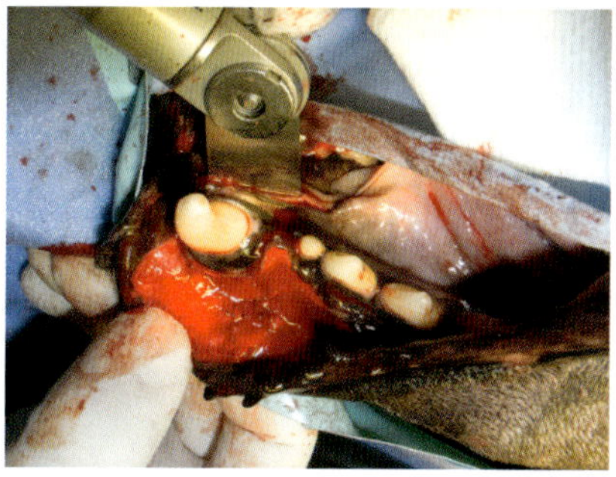

B-ii)

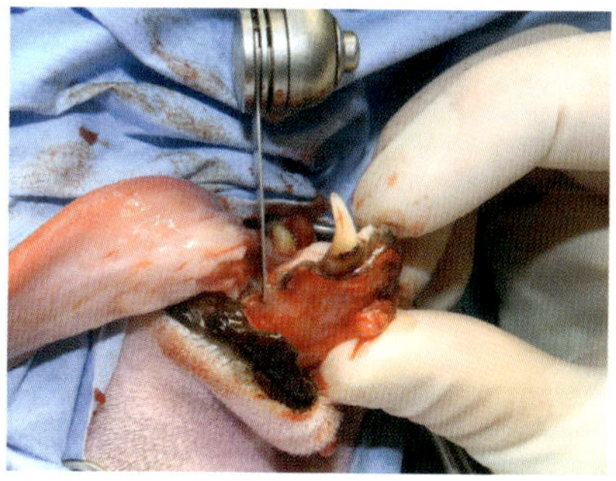

C-i)

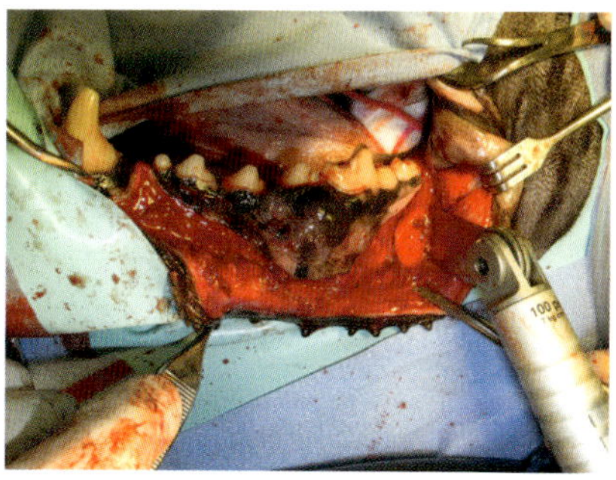

C-ii)

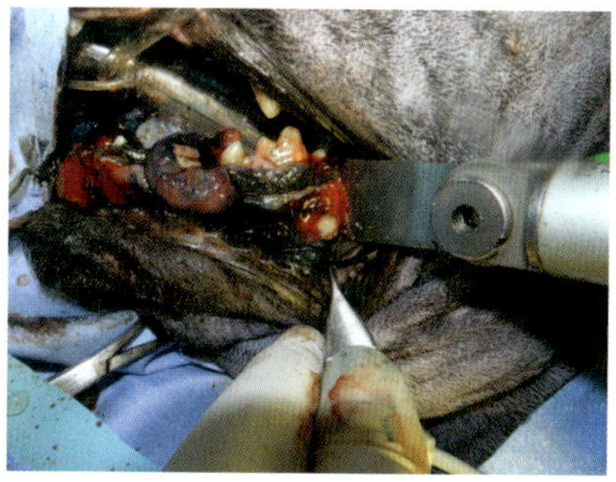

D)

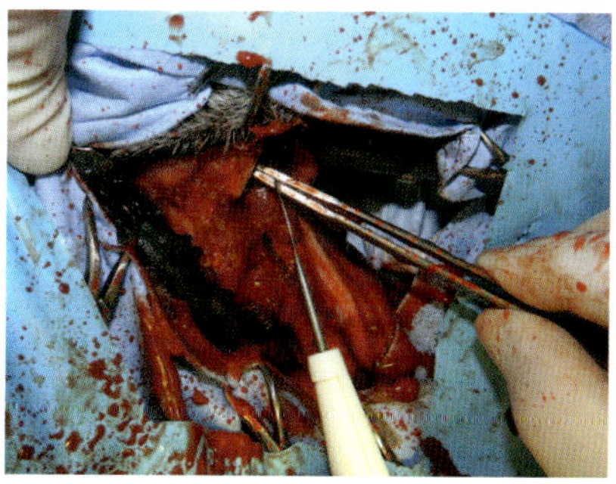

Closure (See Plate 6.8E)

E) The intraoral defect is closed in two to three layers. The lingual and labial/buccal gingival submucosa are sutured with 3-0 to 4-0 monofilament absorbable suture material in a simple continuous suture pattern. The lingual and labial/buccal gingival mucosa are also sutured with 3-0 to 4-0 monofilament absorbable suture material in a simple continuous suture pattern (i, ii).

Postoperative Management

1) Multimodal analgesia
2) Soft foods for 4 weeks
3) No chewing on hard objects or playing with toys for 4 weeks
4) Elizabethan collar
5) Esophagostomy tube and supplemental feeding in cats

Complications – Dogs* [1, 2]

Intraoperative Complications

- Blood loss from the inferior alveolar artery

Postoperative Complications (See Plate 6.8F)

- Overall: 38%
- Prehension/eating difficulties (12%, median time to eating is 2.5 days)
- Incisional swelling (common)
- Ranula formation (6%; F – i, ii, arrow)
- Incisional dehiscence (19%–35%)
- Excessive drooling (4%)
- Mandibular drift (4%)

Complications – Cats† [3]

Intraoperative Complications

- Blood loss

Postoperative Complications (0–28 Days) (See Plate 6.8G)

- Overall: 100%
- Dysphagia/inappetence (76%)
- Excessive drooling (48%)
- Mandibular drift (56%)
- Tongue protrusion (44%)
- Pain (24%)
- Grooming difficulties (24%)
- Incisional dehiscence (8%)
- Malocclusion with palatine trauma (12%; G)
- Temporomandibular joint crepitus (8%)

* Combined complications for unilateral subtotal and total mandibulectomy.
† Combined complications for unilateral subtotal and total mandibulectomy.

Plate 6.8

Unilateral Subtotal Mandibulectomy *continued*

E-i)

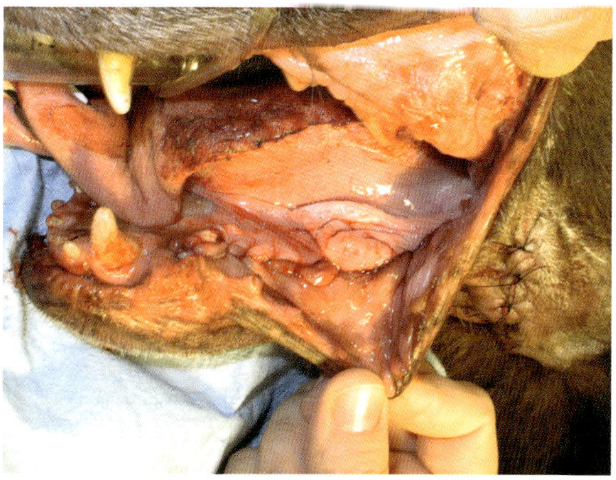

E-ii)

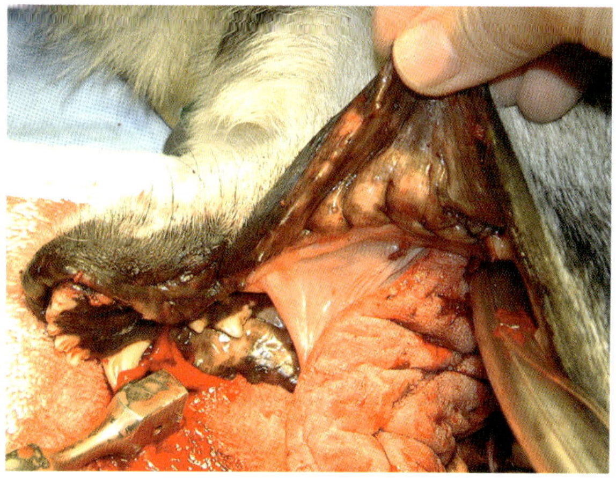

F-i)

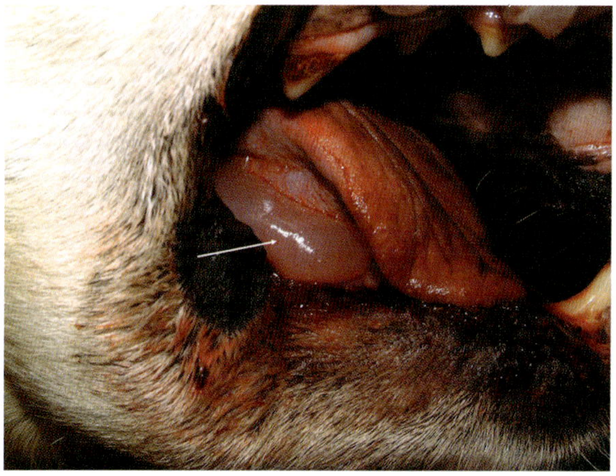

F-ii)

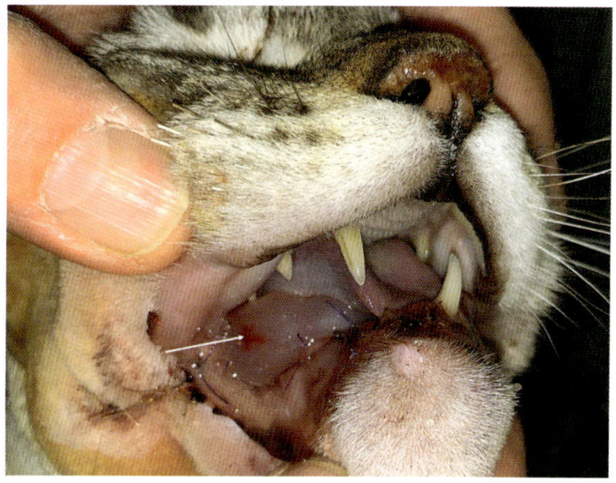

G)

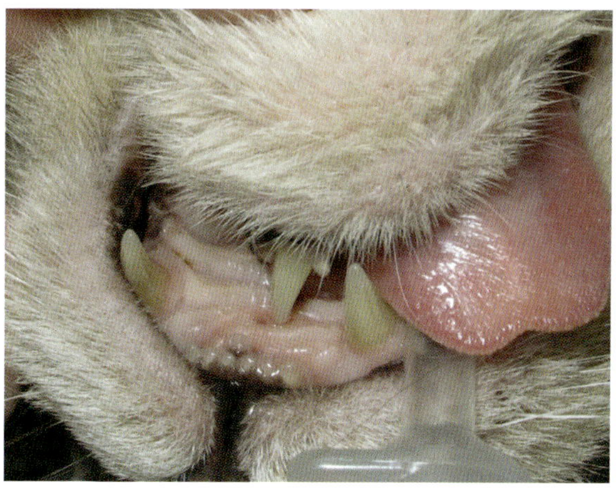

Postoperative Complications (>28 Days)

- Overall: 88%
- Dysphagia/inappetence (60%)
- Excessive drooling (24%)
- Mandibular drift (44%)
- Tongue protrusion (32%)
- Grooming difficulties (24%)
- Malocclusion with palatine trauma (20%)
- Temporomandibular joint crepitus (4%)

Cosmetic Appearance (See Plate 6.8H, I)

- No to minimal effects on cosmesis (H – i, ii)
- Tongue lag on the resected side (I – i, i)

Suggested Adjuvant Treatments

- See 6. *Mandibulectomy and Maxillectomy*.

Prognosis and Oncologic Outcome

- See 6. *Mandibulectomy and Maxillectomy*.

References

1 Salisbury, S.K. and Lantz, G.C. (1988). Long-term results of partial mandibulectomy for treatment of oral tumors in 30 dogs. *J. Am. Anim. Hosp. Assoc.* 24: 285–294.
2 Schwarz, P.D., Withrow, S.J., Curtis, C.R. et al. (1991). Mandibular resection as a treatment for oral cancer in 81 dogs. *J. Am. Anim. Hosp. Assoc.* 27: 601–610.
3 Northrup, N.C., Selting, K.A., Rassnick, K.M. et al. (2006). Outcomes of cats with oral tumors treated with mandibulectomy: 42 cases. *J. Am. Anim. Hosp. Assoc.* 42 (5): 350–360.

Plate 6.8

Unilateral Subtotal Mandibulectomy *continued*

H-i)

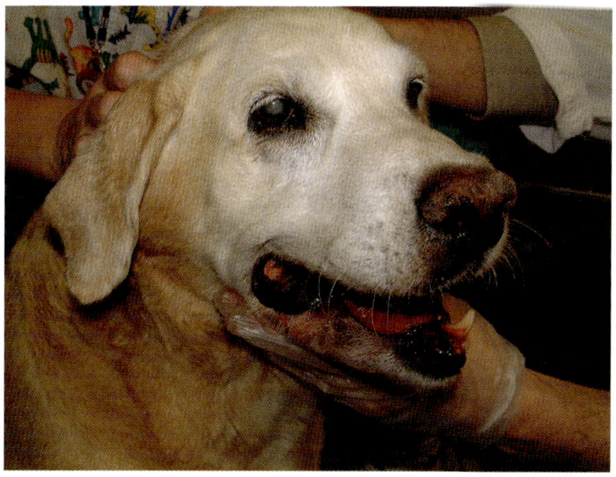

H-ii)

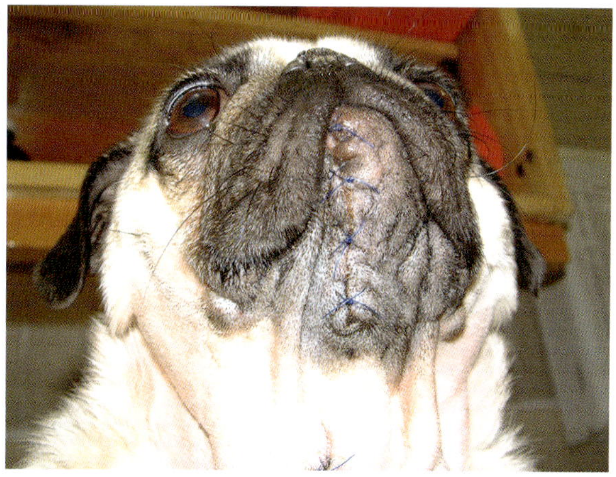

I-i)

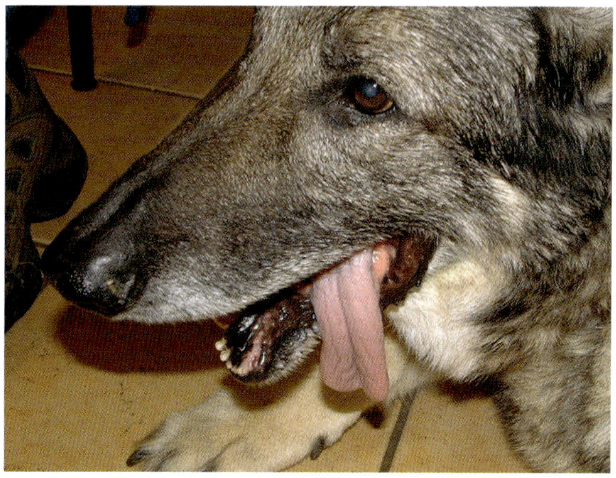

I-ii)

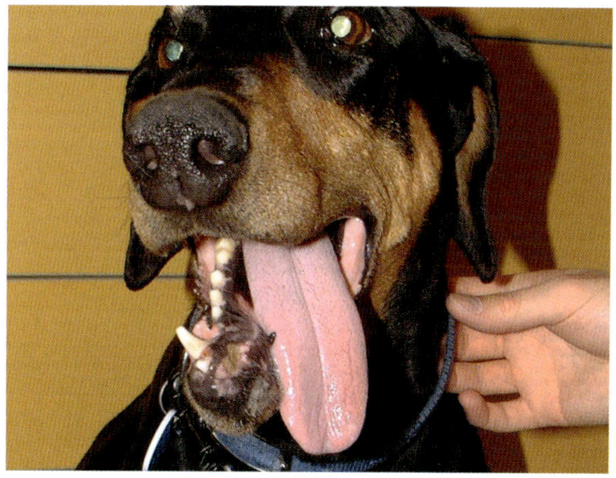

6.9 Unilateral Total Mandibulectomy

Indications (See Plate 6.9 – 1)

1) Resection of extensive or large oral tumors involving the mandibular body and/or ramus of the mandible (pictured, fibrosarcoma)
2) Unilateral total mandibulectomy can be combined with contralateral unilateral rostral mandibulectomy (see *6.2. Unilateral Rostral Mandibulectomy*) if the tumor extends rostrally across the midline

Suggested Diagnostic Workup and Clinical Staging for Benign Mandibular Tumors

- Complete blood count, serum biochemistry, and urinalysis
- Preoperative biopsy
- ± Precontrast and postcontrast computed tomography (CT) scan of the head for surgical planning

Suggested Diagnostic Workup and Clinical Staging for Malignant Mandibular Tumors

- Complete blood count, serum biochemistry, and urinalysis
- Preoperative biopsy
- Regional lymph node assessment for evaluation of lymph node metastasis
  - Fine-needle aspirate cytology of the mandibular lymph nodes
  - Sentinel lymph node mapping and excision of the sentinel lymph node (see *50.1. Sentinel Lymph Node Mapping*)
  - Nonselective excision of the bilateral mandibular and medial retropharyngeal lymph nodes through a ventral midline cervical approach (see *50.3. Combined Mandibular and Medial Retropharyngeal Lymph Node Excision*), or excision of the ipsilateral mandibular, medial retropharyngeal, and parotid lymph nodes through a lateral approach (see *50.4. Combined Parotid, Mandibular, and Medial Retropharyngeal Lymph Node Excision*)
- ± Radiographs or precontrast and postcontrast CT scan of the head and neck for surgical planning
- Three-view thoracic radiographs or thoracic CT scan for assessment of lung metastasis

Patient Positioning

The patient is positioned in lateral recumbency with the affected side uppermost. Unilateral total mandibulectomy can also be performed through a ventral approach (see *6.7. Ventral Approach for Mandibulectomy*), in which case the patient is positioned in dorsal recumbency with a towel or sandbag under the neck so the mandible is parallel to the table. The pharynx should be packed with gauze sponges to minimize the risk of aspirating lavage fluid and blood.

Color Atlas of Canine and Feline Surgical Oncology, First Edition. Julius M. Liptak, Paolo Buracco, William T. N. Culp, and Nicholas J. Bacon.

Plate 6.9

Unilateral Total Mandibulectomy

1)

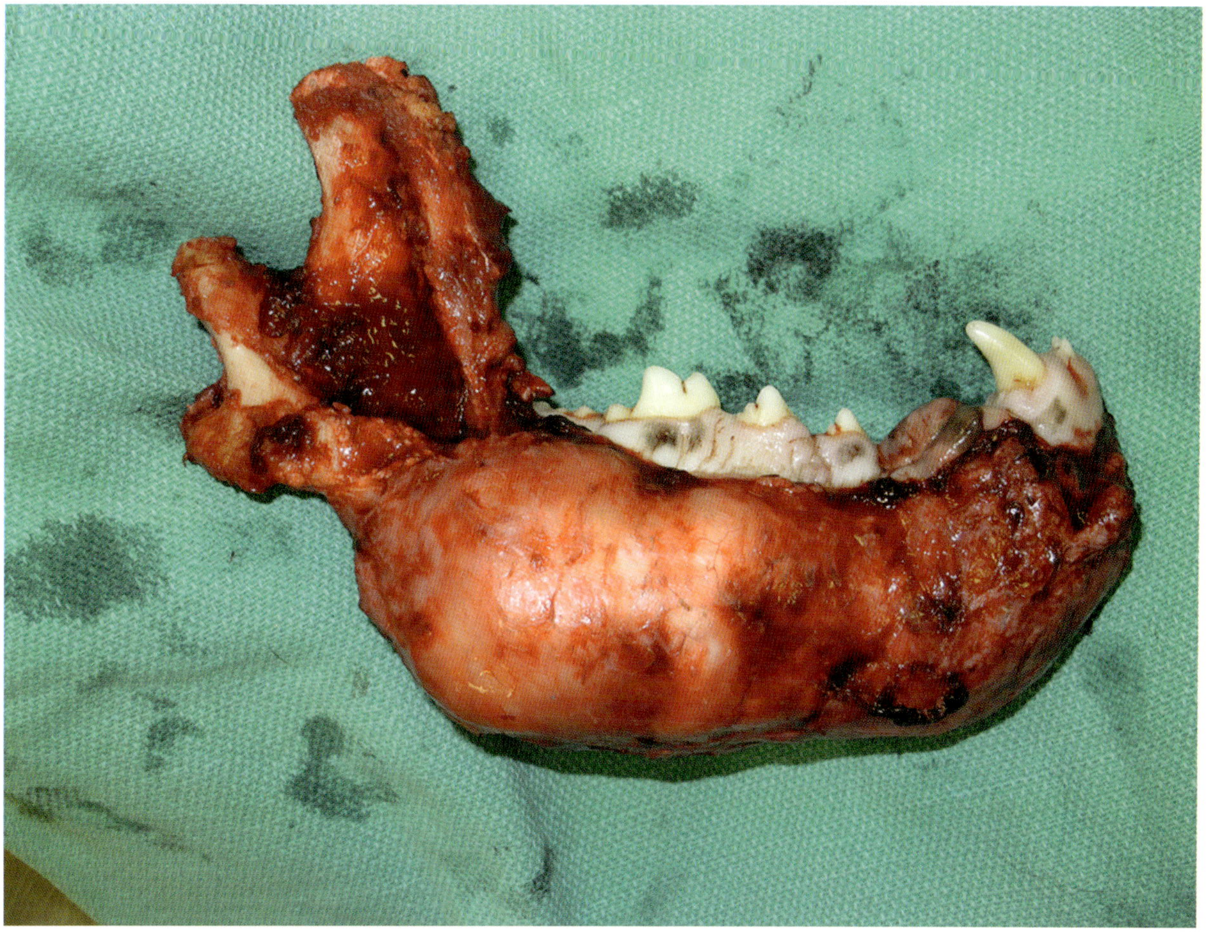

Surgical Technique (See Plate 6.9A–G)

A) A full-thickness incision is made extending caudally from the caudal commissure of the lips.

B) The gingival mucosa on the buccal and lingual (i) aspects of the mandibular body and labial aspect of the rostral mandible are incised with a scalpel blade or Metzenbaum scissors with a minimum of 1-cm margins around the oral mass and extending to the planned osteotomy sites. The mucosa (laterally) and genioglossus, geniohyoideus, and mylohyoideus muscle insertions (medially) are then elevated with a periosteal elevator to isolate the mandibular body (ii–vii, multiple cases showing progressive isolation of the mandibular body).

Plate 6.9

Unilateral Total Mandibulectomy *continued*

A)

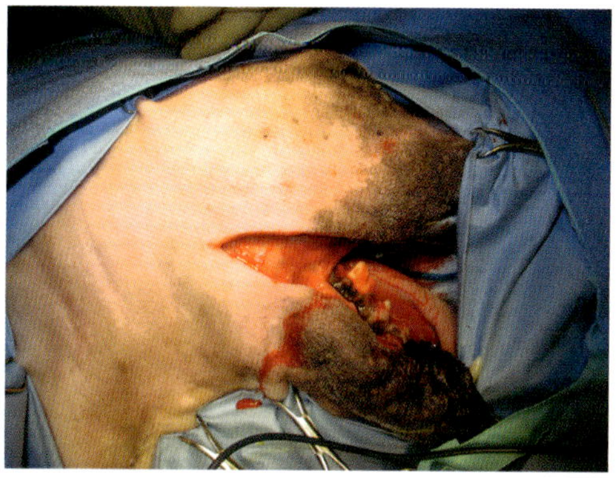

B-i)

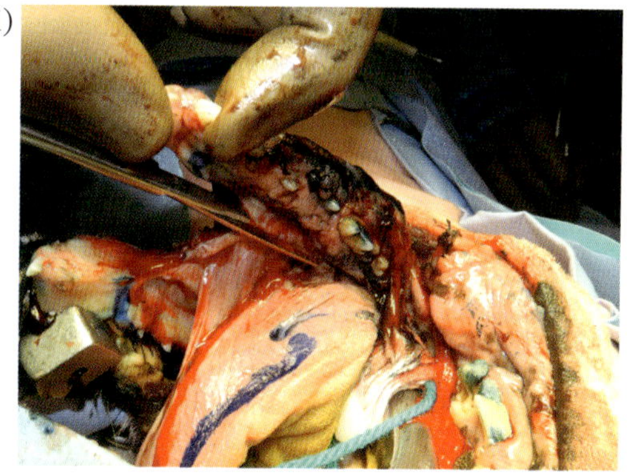

B-ii)

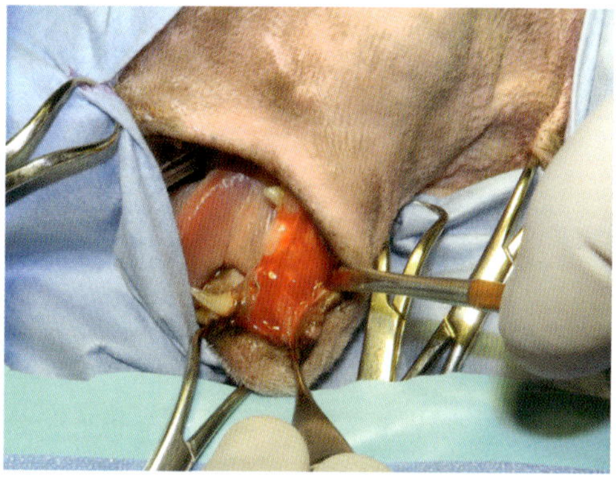

B-iii)

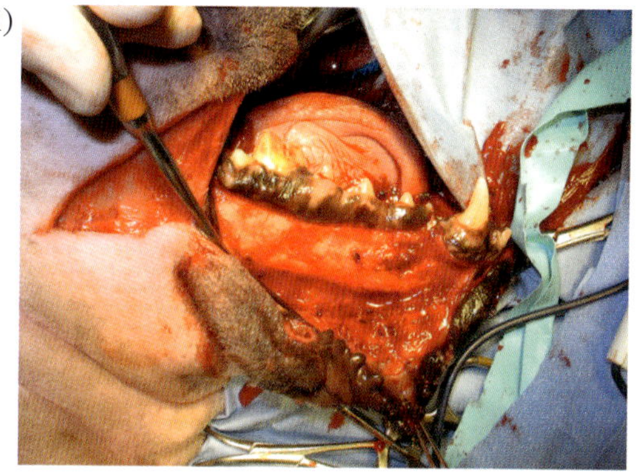

B-iv)

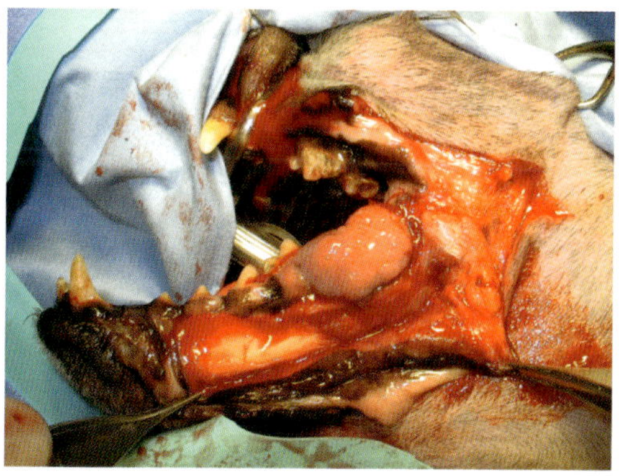

B-v)

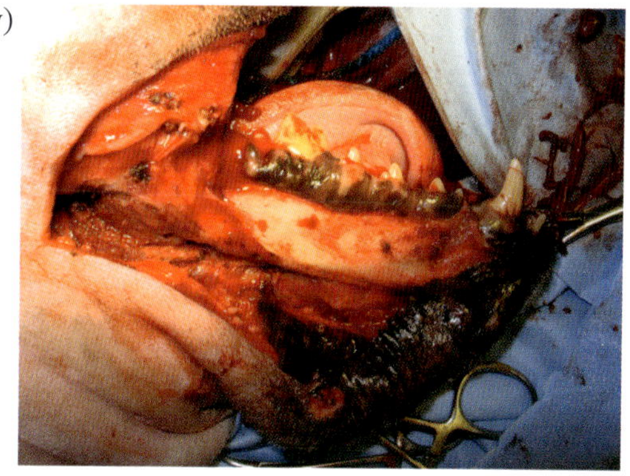

B-vi)

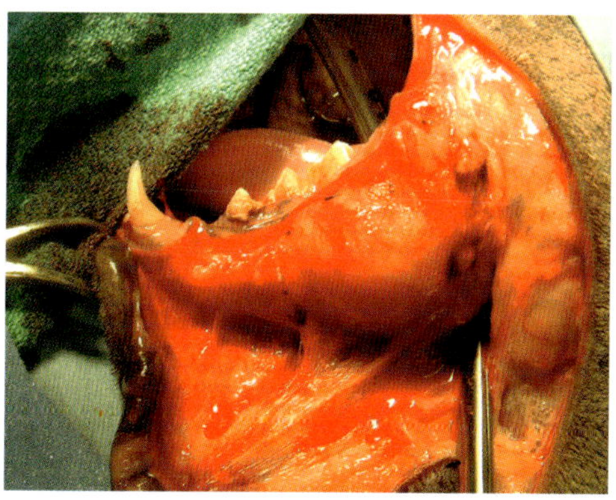

B-vii)

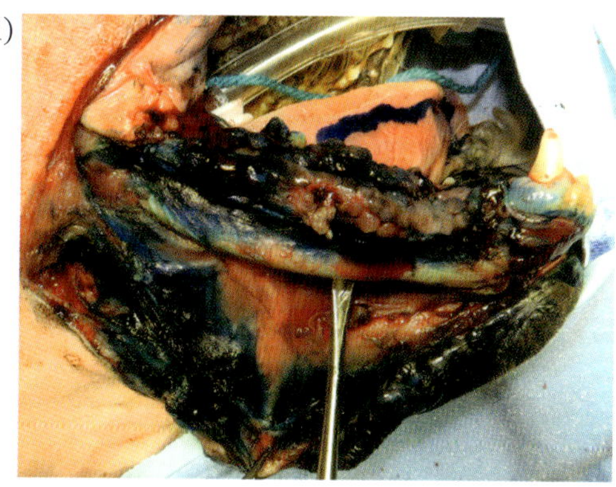

Surgical Technique (See Plate 6.9A–G) *continued*

C) The rostral osteotomy site is planned with appropriate bone margins for the tumor type and can be performed with an oscillating or sagittal saw (i, mandibular symphysis; ii, rostral mandibular body), pneumatic drill, piezoelectric instruments, or, if at the mandibular symphysis, osteotome and mallet (iii), bone cutters (iv), or Gigli wire. A unilateral total mandibulectomy can be combined with a contralateral unilateral rostral mandibulectomy (see *6.2. Unilateral Rostral Mandibulectomy*) if the tumor extends rostrally across the midline (v, arrow).

D) The freed mandibular body is lateralized to expose the caudal aspect of the medial mandible and the inferior alveolar vessels entering the mandibular canal. The inferior alveolar vessels are ligated (i), cauterized, or sealed (ii), and then transected.

Plate 6.9

Unilateral Total Mandibulectomy *continued*

C-i)

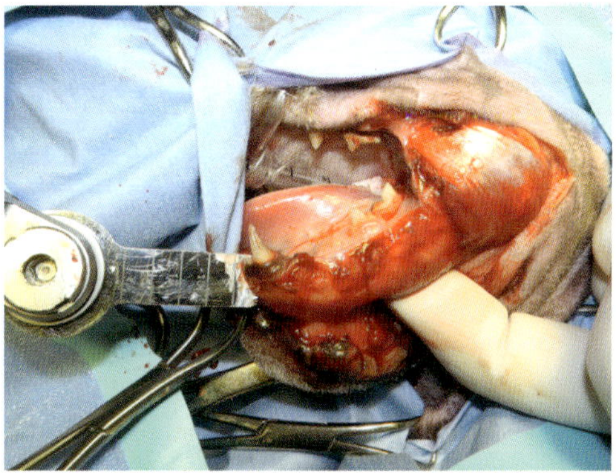

C-ii)

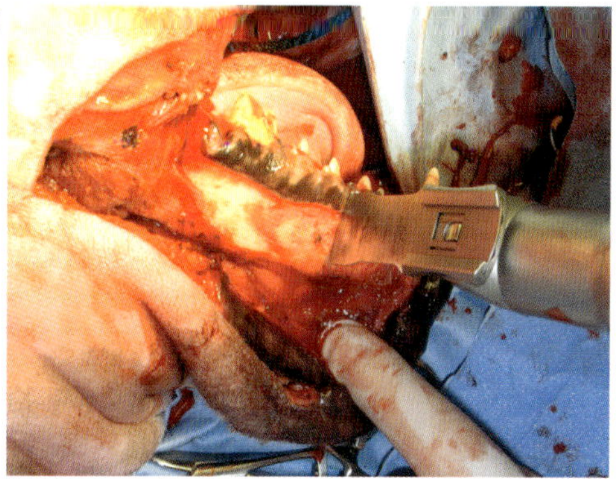

C-iii)

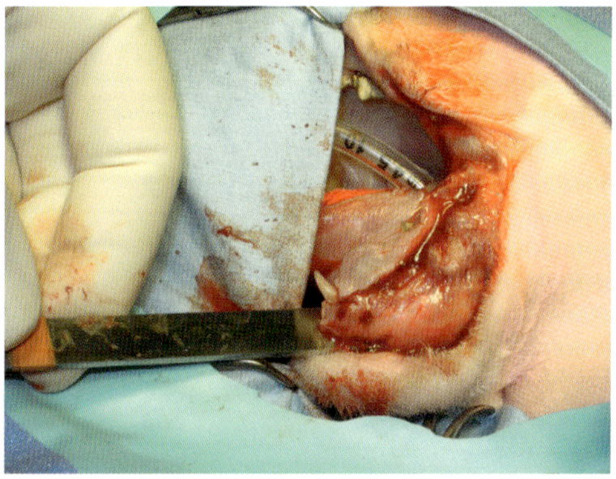

C-iv)

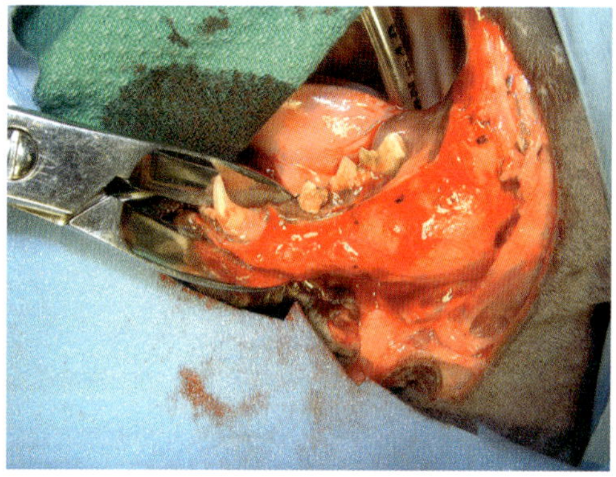

C-v)

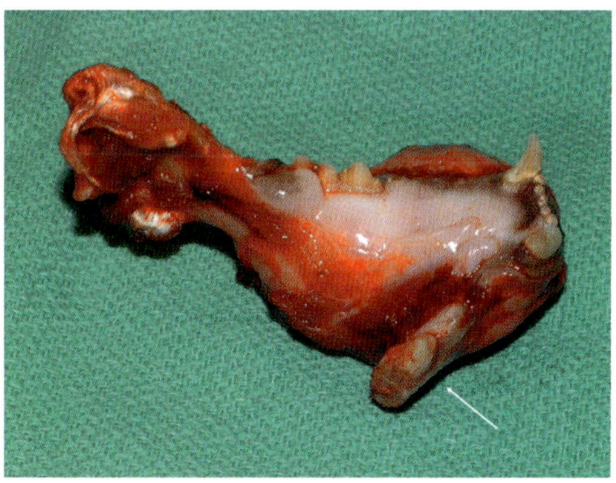

D-i)

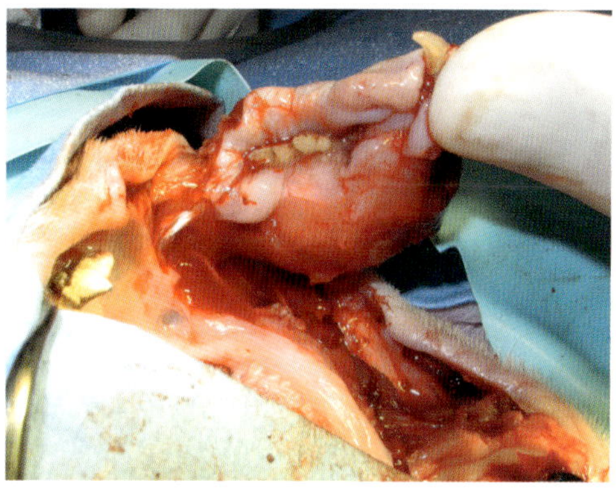

D-i)

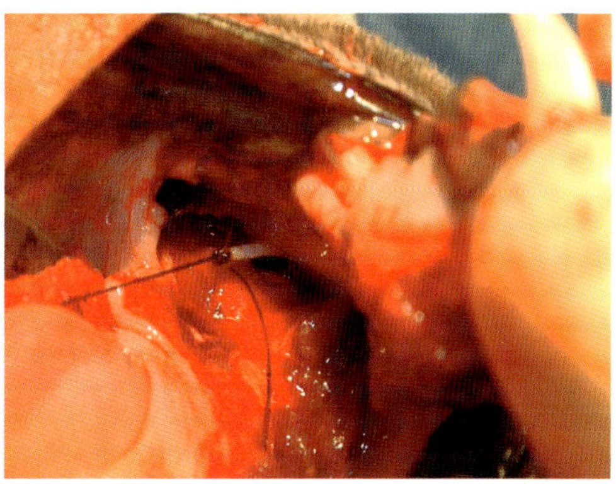

D-ii)

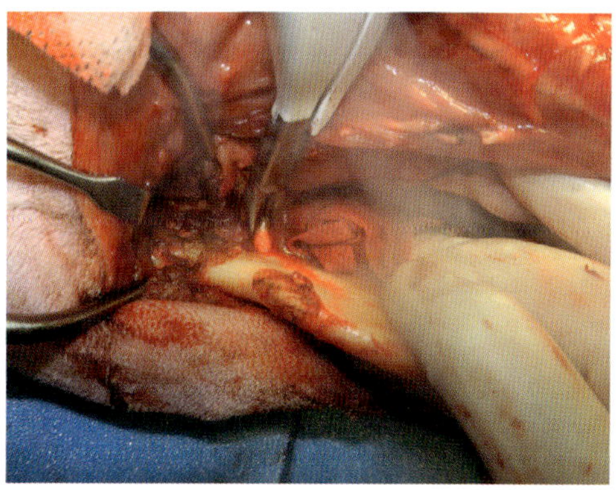

Surgical Technique (See Plate 6.9A–G) *continued*

E) The muscle insertions on the caudal mandible and ramus of the mandible are either transected or elevated with a periosteal elevator. This includes the masseter muscle (MM) from the ventrolateral aspect of the caudal mandible, taking care to preserve the facial nerve (i, arrow) coursing over the lateral aspect of the muscle; the digastricus muscle (DG) from the caudoventral aspect of the mandibular body (ii); and the pterygoid muscles (PG) from the medial aspect of the angular process of the mandible (iii).

F) The temporomandibular joint (TMJ; arrow) is identified and then disarticulated by incising the joint capsule with a scalpel blade or electrosurgery (i). This dissection is performed as close as possible to the condyloid process, especially medially and caudally, to avoid iatrogenic damage to the maxillary artery and its branches (ii, arrows).

G) The insertion of the temporalis muscle (TM) on the coronoid process of the ramus of the mandible is transected or elevated, and the mandible is removed from the surgical field.

Closure (See Plate 6.9H–K)

H) The midbody (e.g. digastricus, mylohyoideus, masseter) and caudal muscles (e.g. masseter, temporalis, pterygoid) are sutured to reduce the dead space.

I) The intraoral defect is then closed in two layers. The lingual and labial mucosa are sutured with 3-0 to 4-0 monofilament absorbable suture material in a simple interrupted or continuous suture pattern.

J) The lingual and labial submucosa are also sutured with 3-0 to 4-0 monofilament absorbable suture material in a simple continuous or interrupted suture pattern.

Plate 6.9

Unilateral Total Mandibulectomy *continued*

E-i)

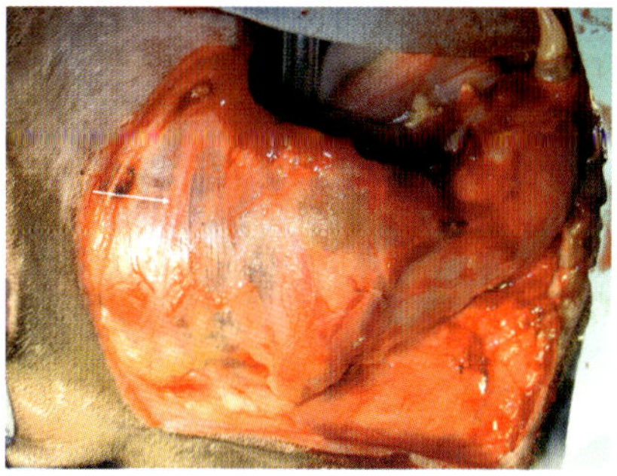

E-ii)

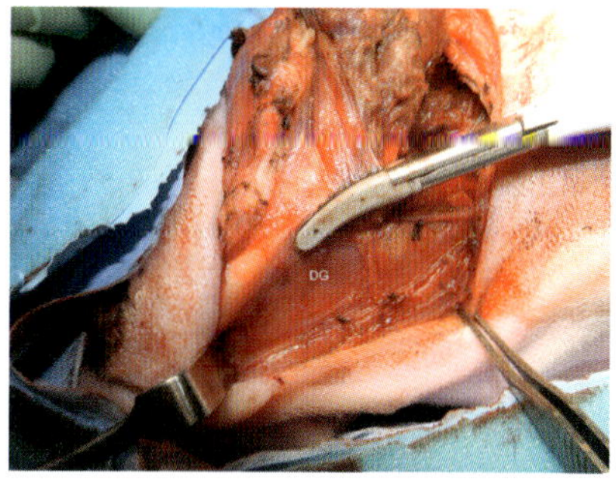

E-iii)

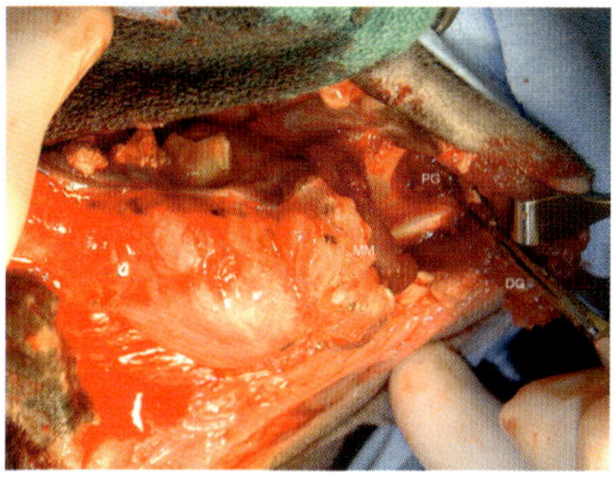

F-i)

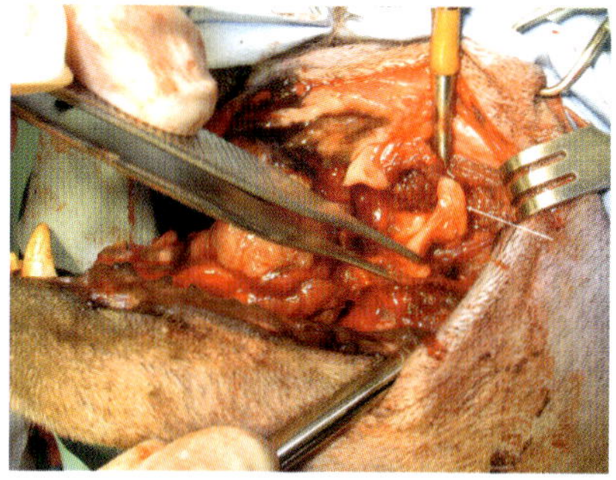

F-ii)

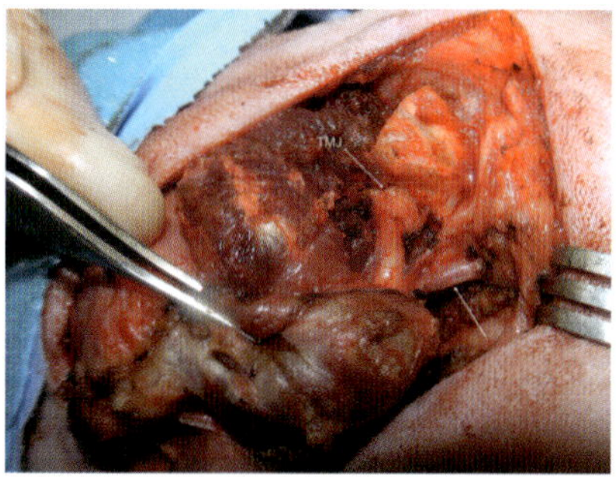

G)

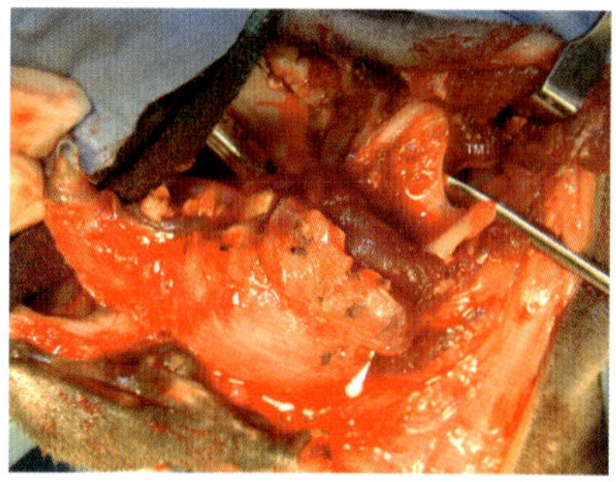

H)

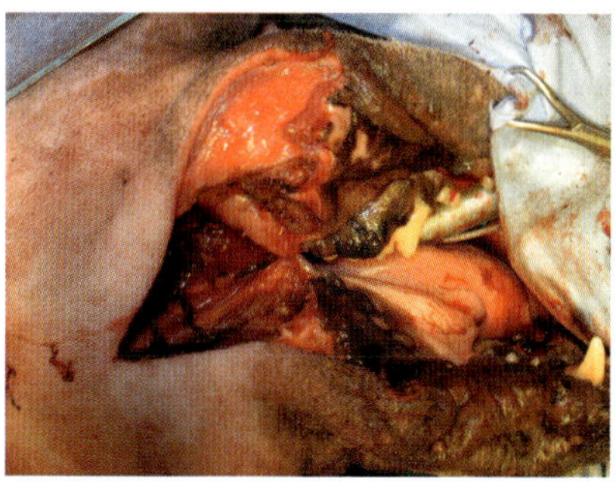

I)

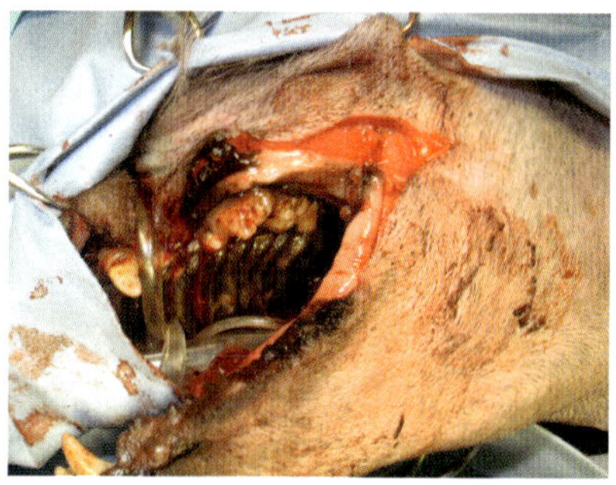

J)

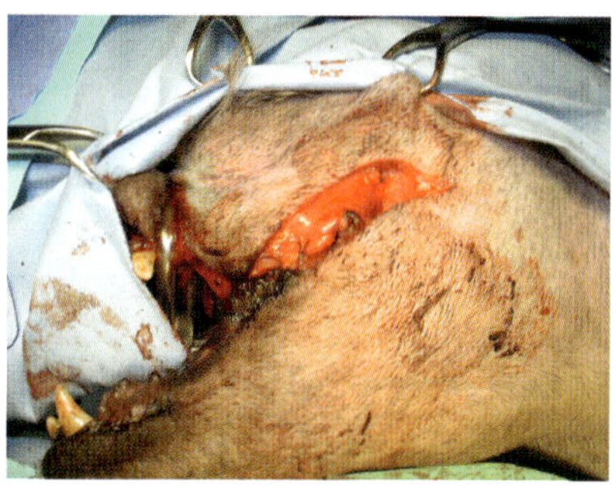

Closure (See Plate 6.9H–K) *continued*

K) The commissurotomy is modified by resecting a third to a half of the caudal aspect of the upper (i) and lower lips (ii) with either Mayo scissors or a scalpel blade to advance the caudal commissure of the lips. The commissurotomy (iii) is closed in three layers. Starting at the rostral margin (iv, arrow), the labial mucosa (v) and then submucosa are sutured with 3-0 to 4-0 monofilament absorbable suture material in a simple interrupted or continuous suture pattern. The skin is closed with 3-0 to 4-0 monofilament nonabsorbable suture material in a simple interrupted suture pattern (vi).

Postoperative Management (See Plate 6.9L)

1) Multimodal analgesia
2) Soft foods for 4 weeks
3) No chewing on hard objects or playing with toys for 4 weeks
4) Elizabethan collar
5) Esophagostomy tube and supplemental feeding in cats (L)

Complications – Dogs* [1, 2]

Intraoperative Complications

- Blood loss from the inferior alveolar artery

* Combined complications for unilateral subtotal and total mandibulectomy.

Plate 6.9

Unilateral Total Mandibulectomy *continued*

K-i)

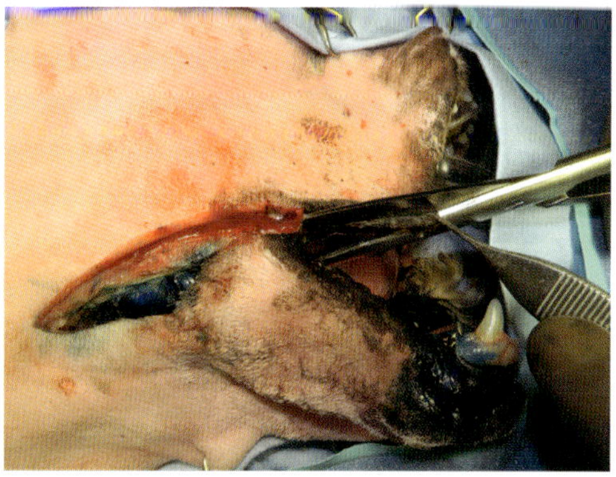

K-ii)

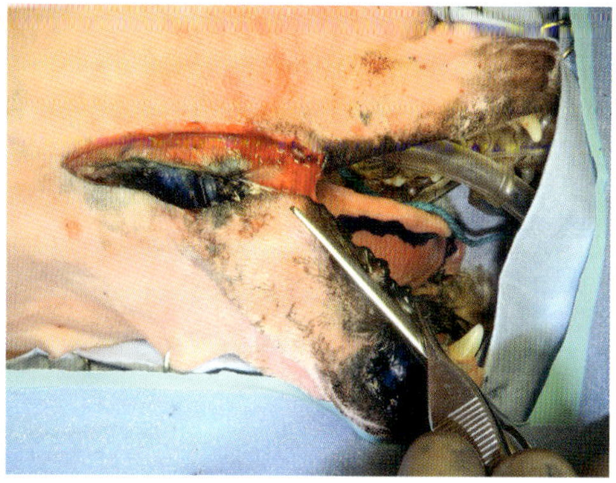

K-iii)

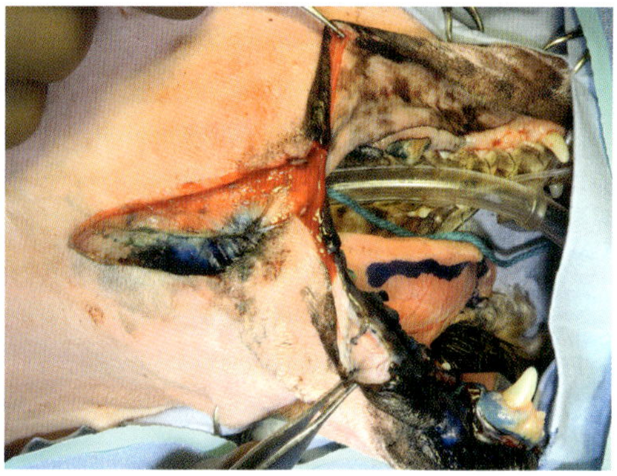

K-iv)

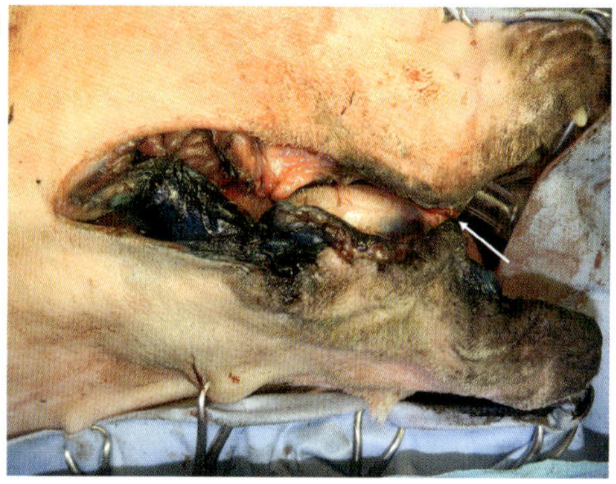

K-v)

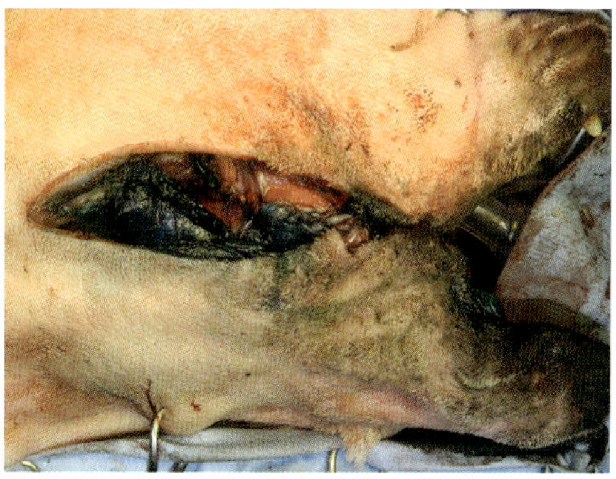

K-vi)

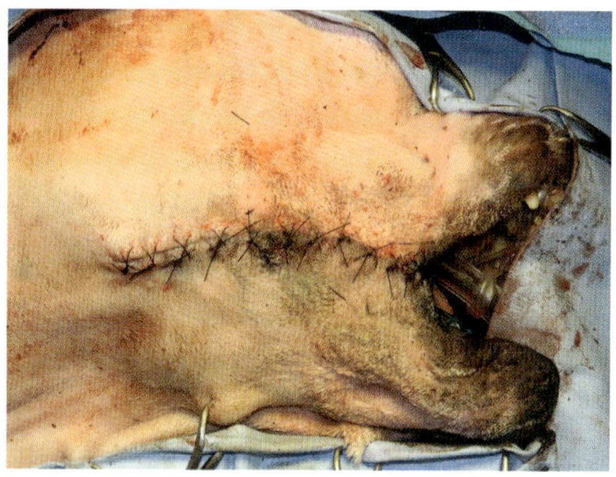

L)

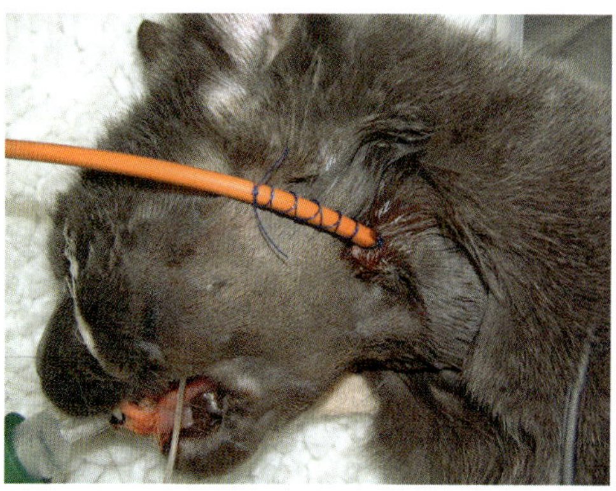

Postoperative Complications (See Plate 6.9M–O)

- Overall: 38%
- Prehension/eating difficulties (12%, median time to eating is 2.5 days)
- Incisional swelling (common; M – i–iii)
- Ranula formation (6%)
- Incisional dehiscence (19%–35%; N)
- Excessive drooling (4%)
- Mandibular drift (4%; O – i, ii)

Complications – Cats† [3]

Intraoperative Complications

- Blood loss

Postoperative Complications (0–28 Days)

- Overall: 100%
- Dysphagia/inappetence (76%)
- Excessive drooling (48%)
- Mandibular drift (56%)
- Tongue protrusion (44%)
- Pain (24%)
- Grooming difficulties (24%)
- Incisional dehiscence (8%)
- Malocclusion with palatine trauma (12%)
- TMJ crepitus (8%)

Postoperative Complications (>28 Days)

- Overall: 88%
- Dysphagia/inappetence (60%)
- Excessive drooling (24%)
- Mandibular drift (44%)
- Tongue protrusion (32%)
- Grooming difficulties (24%)
- Malocclusion with palatine trauma (20%)
- TMJ crepitus (4%)

Cosmetic Appearance (See Plate 6.9P, Q)

- No to minimal effects on facial cosmesis (P – i, ii)
- Tongue lag on the resected side (Q)

---

† Combined complications for unilateral subtotal and total mandibulectomy.

Plate 6.9

Unilateral Total Mandibulectomy *continued*

M-i)

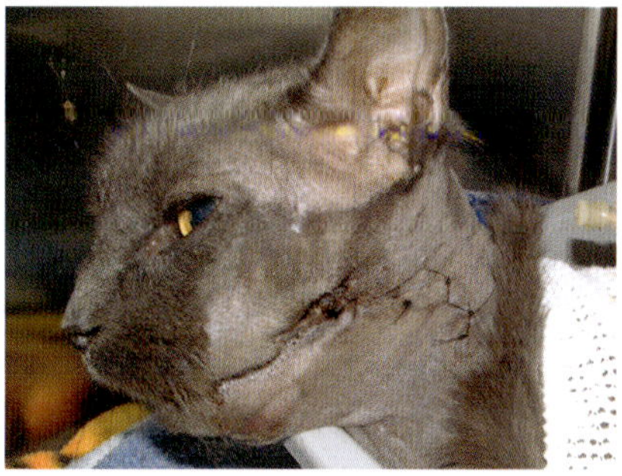

M-ii)

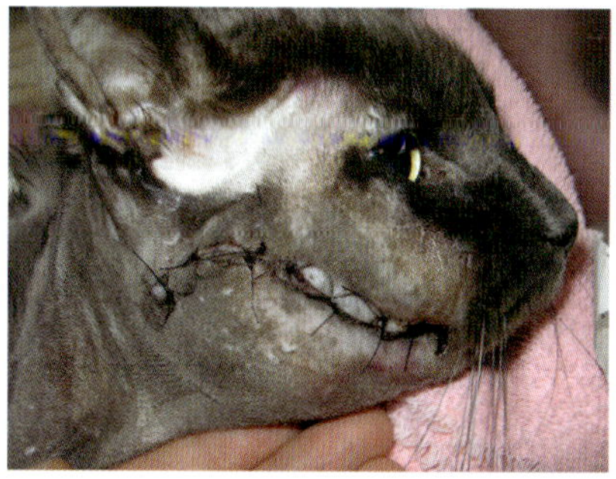

M-iii)

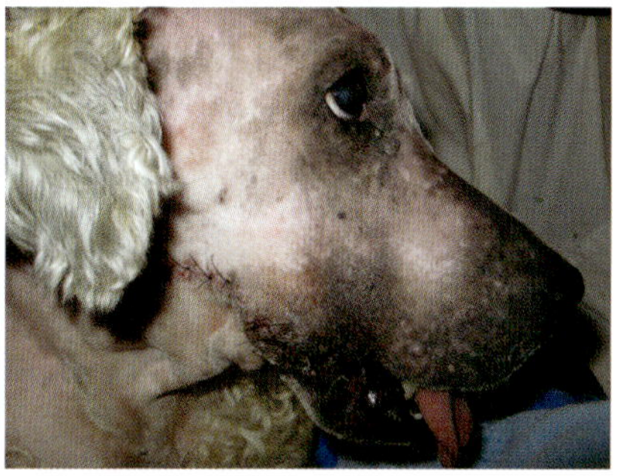

N)

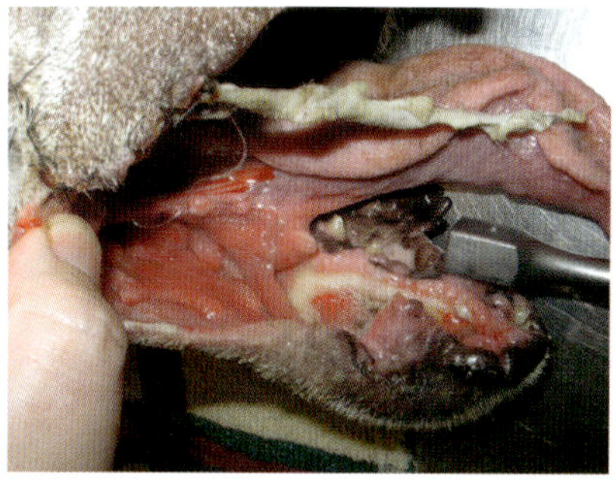

O-i)

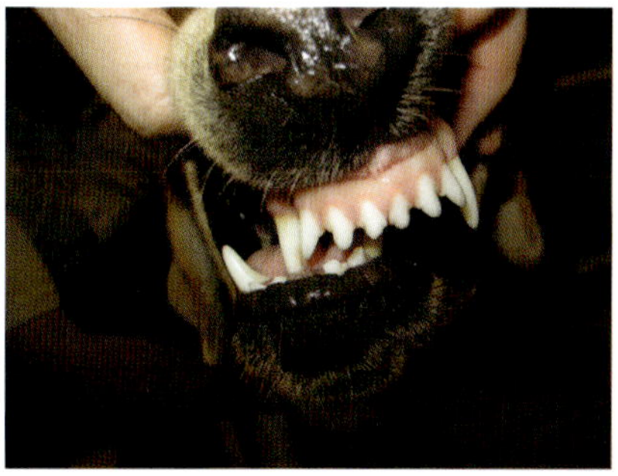

O-ii)

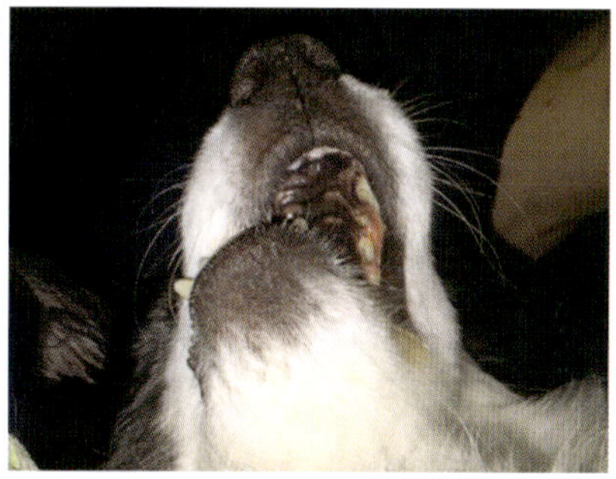

P-i)

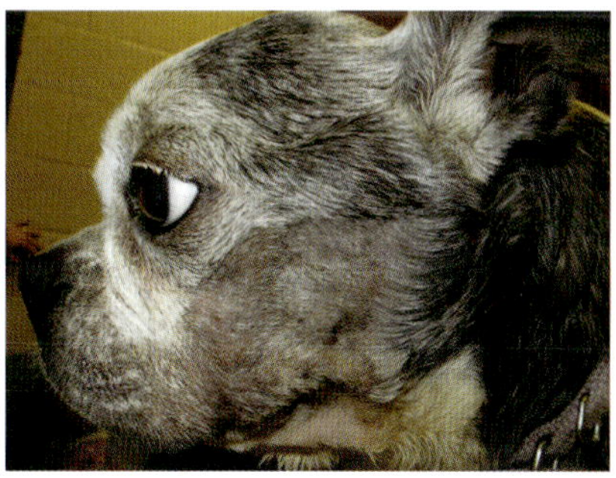

P-ii)

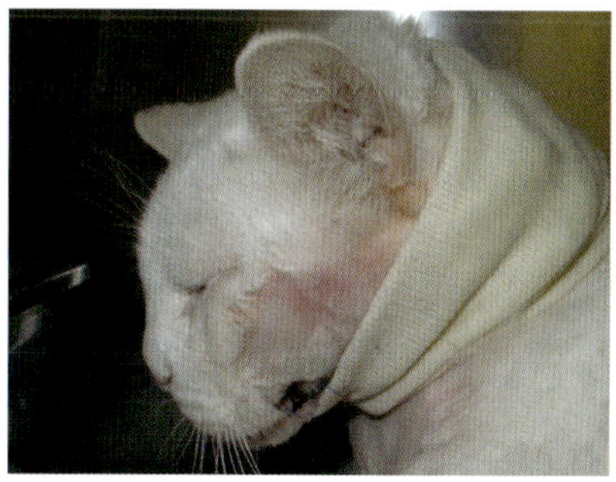

Q)

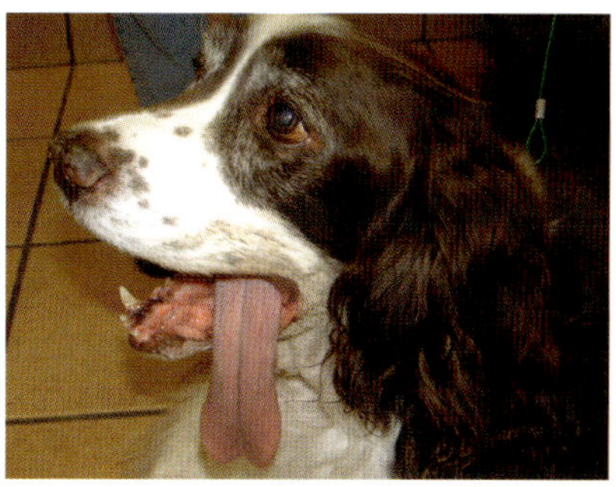

Suggested Adjuvant Treatments

- See 6. *Mandibulectomy and Maxillectomy*.

Prognosis and Oncologic Outcome

- See 6. *Mandibulectomy and Maxillectomy*.

References

1. Salisbury, S.K. and Lantz, G.C. (1988). Long-term results of partial mandibulectomy for treatment of oral tumors in 30 dogs. *J. Am. Anim. Hosp. Assoc.* 24: 285–294.
2. Schwarz, P.D., Withrow, S.J., Curtis, C.R. et al. (1991). Mandibular resection as a treatment for oral cancer in 81 dogs. *J. Am. Anim. Hosp. Assoc.* 27: 601–610.
3. Northrup, N.C., Selting, K.A., Rassnick, K.M. et al. (2006). Outcomes of cats with oral tumors treated with mandibulectomy: 42 cases. *J. Am. Anim. Hosp. Assoc.* 42 (5): 350–360.

6.10 Maxillary Incisivectomy

Indications

1) Resection of benign oral tumors (pictured, acanthomatous ameloblastoma) and small or low-grade malignant oral tumors confined to the incisive bone and associated incisor teeth.
2) Incisivectomy can be combined with nasal planum resection for tumors involving the nasal planum with invasion into the incisive bone (see *4.1. Nasal Planum Resection – Feline* and *4.2. Nasal Planum Resection – Canine*, respectively).
3) Incisivectomy can be combined with an upper lip advancement flap (see *39.2. Upper Lip Advancement Flap*) if the maxillectomy is also associated with a rostral lip defect.

Suggested Diagnostic Workup and Clinical Staging for Benign Maxillary Tumors

- Complete blood count, serum biochemistry, and urinalysis
- Preoperative biopsy
- ± Precontrast and postcontrast computed tomography (CT) scan of the head for surgical planning

Suggested Diagnostic Workup and Clinical Staging for Malignant Maxillary Tumors

- Complete blood count, serum biochemistry, and urinalysis
- Preoperative biopsy
- Regional lymph node assessment for evaluation of lymph node metastasis
  - Fine-needle aspirate cytology of the mandibular lymph nodes
  - Sentinel lymph node mapping and excision of the sentinel lymph node (see *50.1. Sentinel Lymph Node Mapping*)
  - Nonselective excision of the bilateral mandibular and medial retropharyngeal lymph nodes through a ventral midline cervical approach (see *50.3. Combined Mandibular and Medial Retropharyngeal Lymph Node Excision*), or excision of the ipsilateral mandibular, medial retropharyngeal, and parotid lymph nodes through a lateral approach (see *50.4. Combined Parotid, Mandibular, and Medial Retropharyngeal Lymph Node Excision*)
- Precontrast and postcontrast CT scan of the head and neck for surgical planning
- Thoracic CT scan for assessment of lung metastasis

Patient Positioning

The patient is positioned in dorsal recumbency. A mouth gag should be placed on the mandibular and maxillary canine teeth to improve exposure. Mouth gags should be used with caution in cats because of the risk of cortical blindness secondary to compression of the maxillary artery; 20- or 30-mm plastic gags are preferred to spring-loaded gags [1]. The pharynx should be packed with gauze sponges to minimize the risk of aspirating lavage fluid and blood.

Surgical Technique (See Plate 6.10A–C)

A) The labial mucosa (i) and palatine mucoperiosteum are incised with a scalpel blade with a minimum of 5- to 10-mm margins around the oral mass. The palatine mucoperiosteum should be incised rostral to the maxillary canine teeth. The mucosa (ii) and mucoperiosteum are then elevated with a periosteal elevator to prepare for the osteotomy and protect soft tissues from iatrogenic damage during the osteotomy.

Plate 6.10

Maxillary Incisivectomy

1)

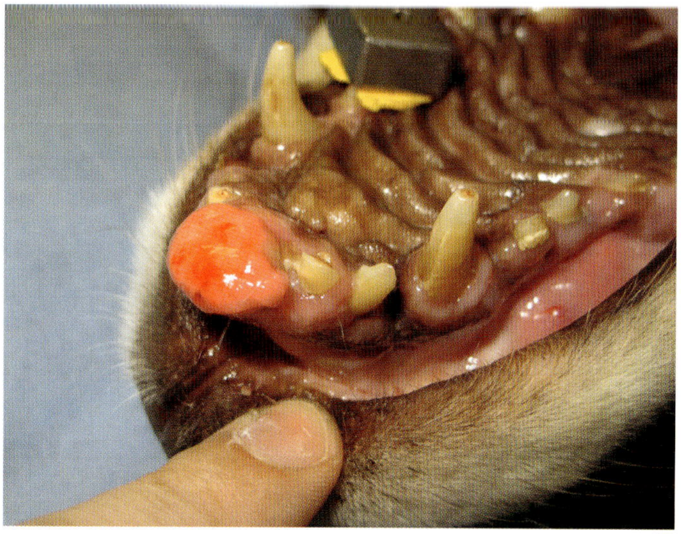

A-i)

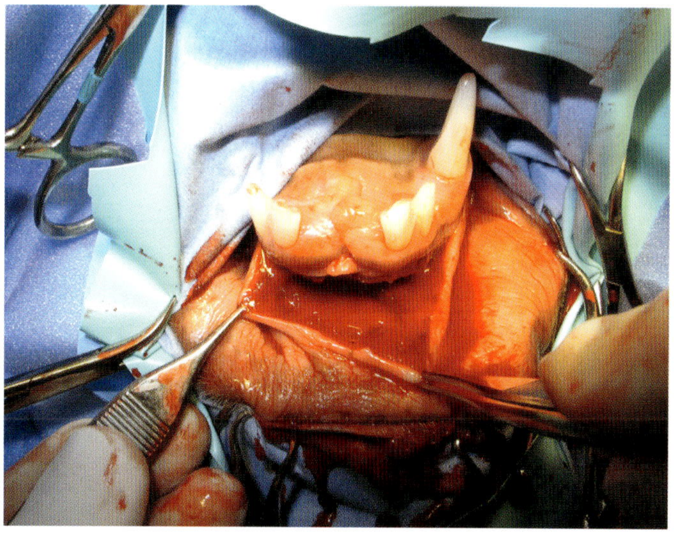

A-ii)

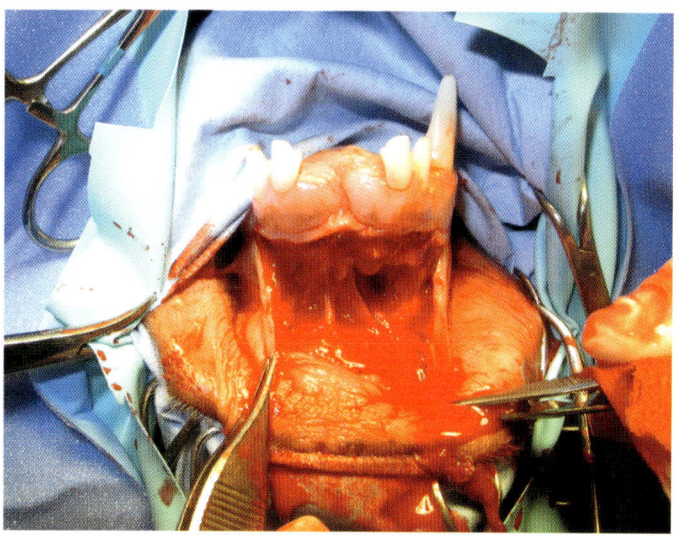

Surgical Technique (See Plate 6.10A–C) *continued*

B) An osteotomy is performed, with a minimum of 1-cm bone margins, caudal to the mass along the mucoperiosteal incision. This osteotomy can be performed with an oscillating, sagittal, or biradial saw (i), pneumatic drill, or piezoelectric instruments. The extent of the bone resection will depend on whether, or how much, bone is involved in the neoplastic process (ii). The nasal cavity is not usually entered in this procedure, but the ventrolateral nasal cartilages are exposed. Bleeding is generally minor and is controlled by a combination of cautery, ligation, and direct pressure.
C) Exposed tooth roots (i) are extracted with a dental elevator (ii, iii).

Closure (See Plate 6.10D, E)

A labial mucosal-submucosal flap is raised by undermining the labial mucosa and submucosa with Metzenbaum scissors from the incised edge of the labial mucosa toward the labial margins (D). The labial mucosal-submucosal flap is advanced into the oral defect and closed in two layers using monofilament absorbable suture material on a reverse cutting needle. Vertical releasing incisions are used if necessary. The submucosa of the labial mucosal-submucosal flap is sutured to either predrilled holes in the hard palate using an interrupted suture pattern or to the submucosa of the mucoperiosteum in a simple continuous suture pattern. The mucosa of the labial mucosal-submucosal flap is then sutured to the mucosa of the mucoperiosteum in either an interrupted or simple continuous suture pattern (E).

Postoperative Management

1) Multimodal analgesia
2) Soft foods for 28 days
3) No chewing on hard objects or playing with toys for 28 days.
4) Elizabethan collar
5) Note that feeding tubes are rarely required in either dogs or cats after incisivectomy.

Complications – Dogs [2]

Postoperative Complications (<48 Hours)

- Epistaxis (30%)

Postoperative Complications (48 Hours to 4 Weeks)

- None

Cosmetic Appearance (See Plate 6.10F)

- There are typically no cosmetic defects after incisivectomy (F, 1 day postoperatively).

Plate 6.10

Maxillary Incisivectomy *continued*

B-i)

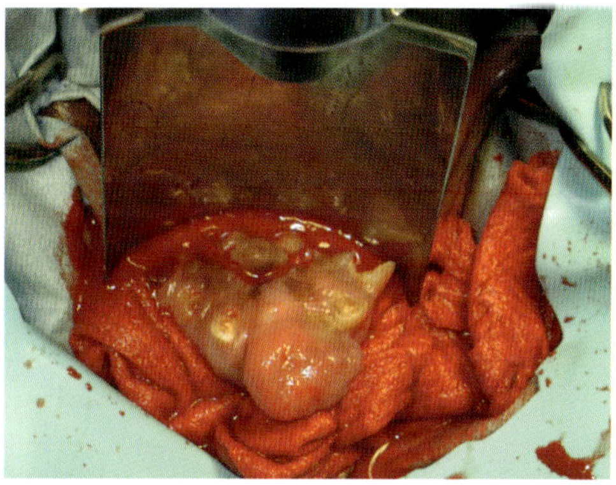

B-ii)

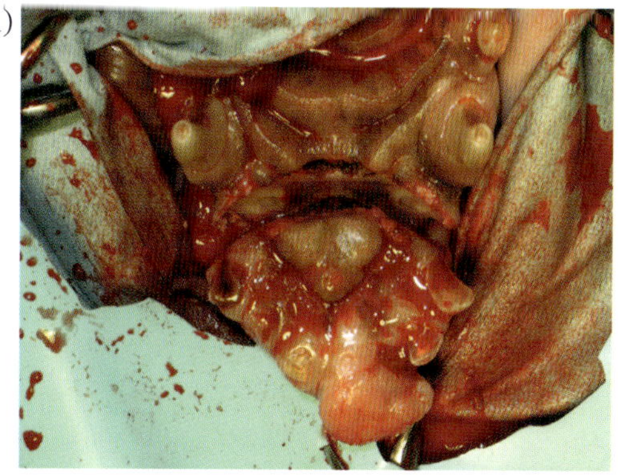

C-i)

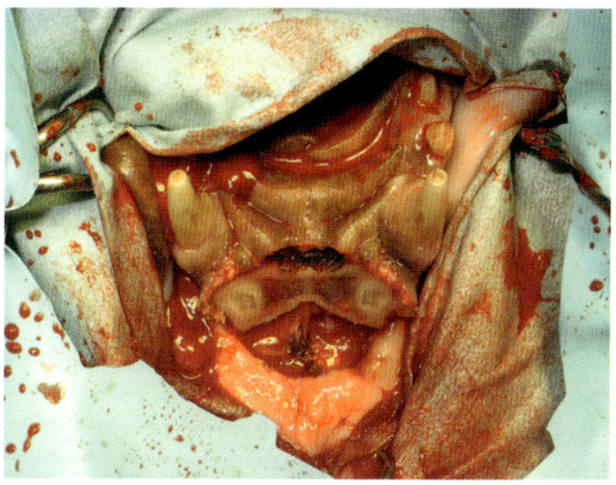

C-ii)

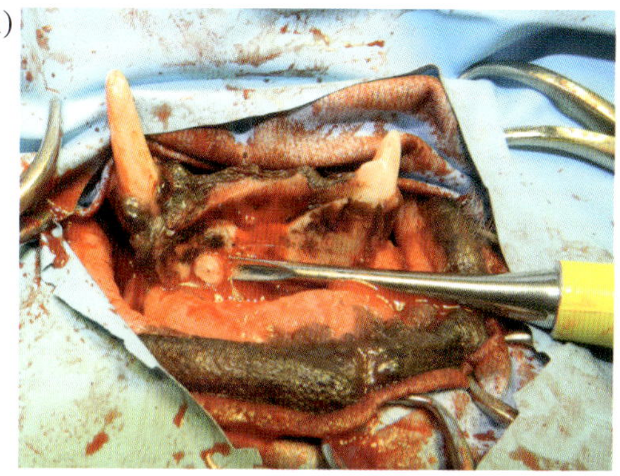

C-iii)

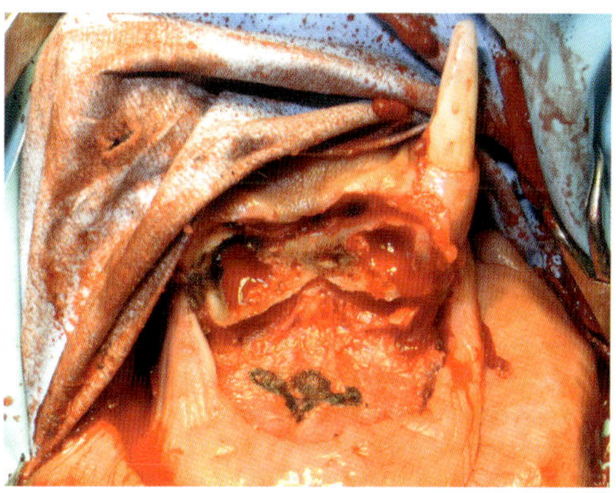

D)

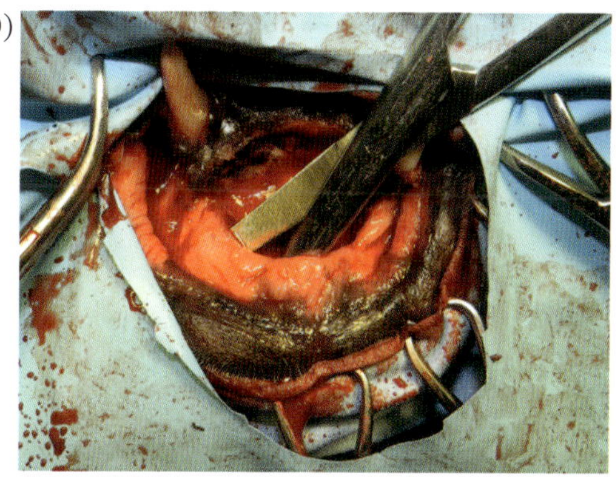

E)

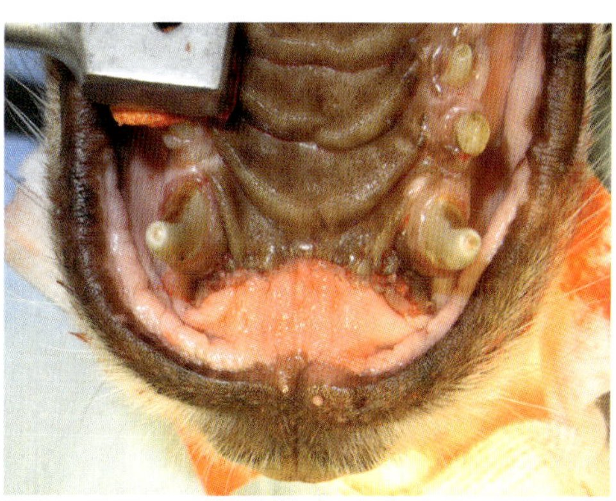

F)

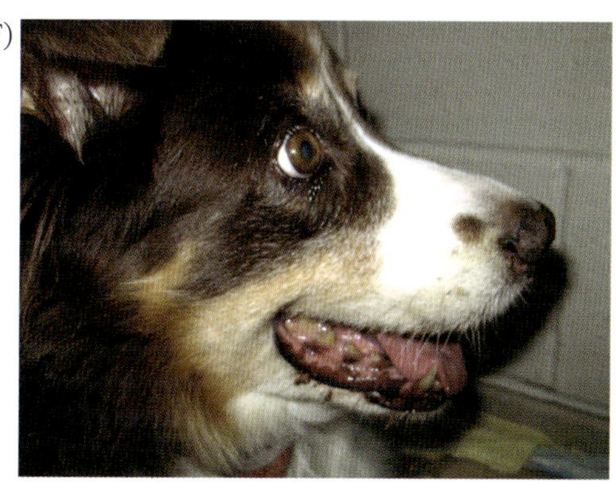

Suggested Adjuvant Treatments

- See *6. Mandibulectomy and Maxillectomy*.

Prognosis and Oncologic Outcome

- See *6. Mandibulectomy and Maxillectomy*.

References

1 Reiter, A.M. (2014). Open wide: blindness in cats after the use of mouth gags. *Vet. J.* 201: 5–6.
2 MacLellan, R.H., Rawlinson, J.E., Rao, S. et al. (2018). Intraoperative and postoperative complications of partial maxillectomy for the treatment of oral tumors in dogs. *J. Am. Vet. Med. Assoc.* 252 (12): 1538–1547.

6.11 Unilateral Rostral Maxillectomy

Indications (See Plate 6.11 – 1)

1) Resection of benign oral tumors, particularly acanthomatous ameloblastomas (pictured), or small or low-grade malignant oral tumors located adjacent to the maxillary canine tooth and that do not cross the palatine midline or extend farther caudally than the second premolar tooth
2) Unilateral rostral maxillectomy can be combined with an upper lip advancement flap (see *39.2. Upper Lip Advancement Flap*) if the maxillectomy is also associated with a rostral lip defect

Suggested Diagnostic Workup and Clinical Staging for Benign Maxillary Tumors

- Complete blood count, serum biochemistry, and urinalysis
- Preoperative biopsy
- Precontrast and postcontrast computed tomography (CT) scan of the head for surgical planning

Suggested Diagnostic Workup and Clinical Staging for Malignant Maxillary Tumors

- Complete blood count, serum biochemistry, and urinalysis
- Preoperative biopsy
- Regional lymph node assessment for evaluation of lymph node metastasis
  - Fine-needle aspirate cytology of the mandibular lymph nodes
  - Sentinel lymph node mapping and excision of the sentinel lymph node (see *50.1. Sentinel Lymph Node Mapping*)
  - Nonselective excision of the bilateral mandibular and medial retropharyngeal lymph nodes through a ventral midline cervical approach (see *50.3. Combined Mandibular and Medial Retropharyngeal Lymph Node Excision*), or excision of the ipsilateral mandibular, medial retropharyngeal, and parotid lymph nodes through a lateral approach (see *50.4. Combined Parotid, Mandibular, and Medial Retropharyngeal Lymph Node Excision*)
- Precontrast and postcontrast CT scan of the head and neck for surgical planning
- Thoracic CT scan for assessment of lung metastasis

Patient Positioning

The patient can be positioned in either lateral recumbency with the affected side uppermost or in dorsal recumbency. A mouth gag should be placed on the contralateral mandibular and maxillary canine teeth to improve exposure. Mouth gags should be used with caution in cats because of the risk of cortical blindness secondary to compression of the maxillary artery; 20- or 30-mm plastic gags are preferred to spring-loaded gags [1]. The pharynx should be packed with gauze sponges to minimize the risk of aspirating lavage fluid and blood.

Color Atlas of Canine and Feline Surgical Oncology, First Edition. Julius M. Liptak, Paolo Buracco, William T. N. Culp, and Nicholas J. Bacon.

Plate 6.11

Unilateral Rostral Maxillectomy

1)
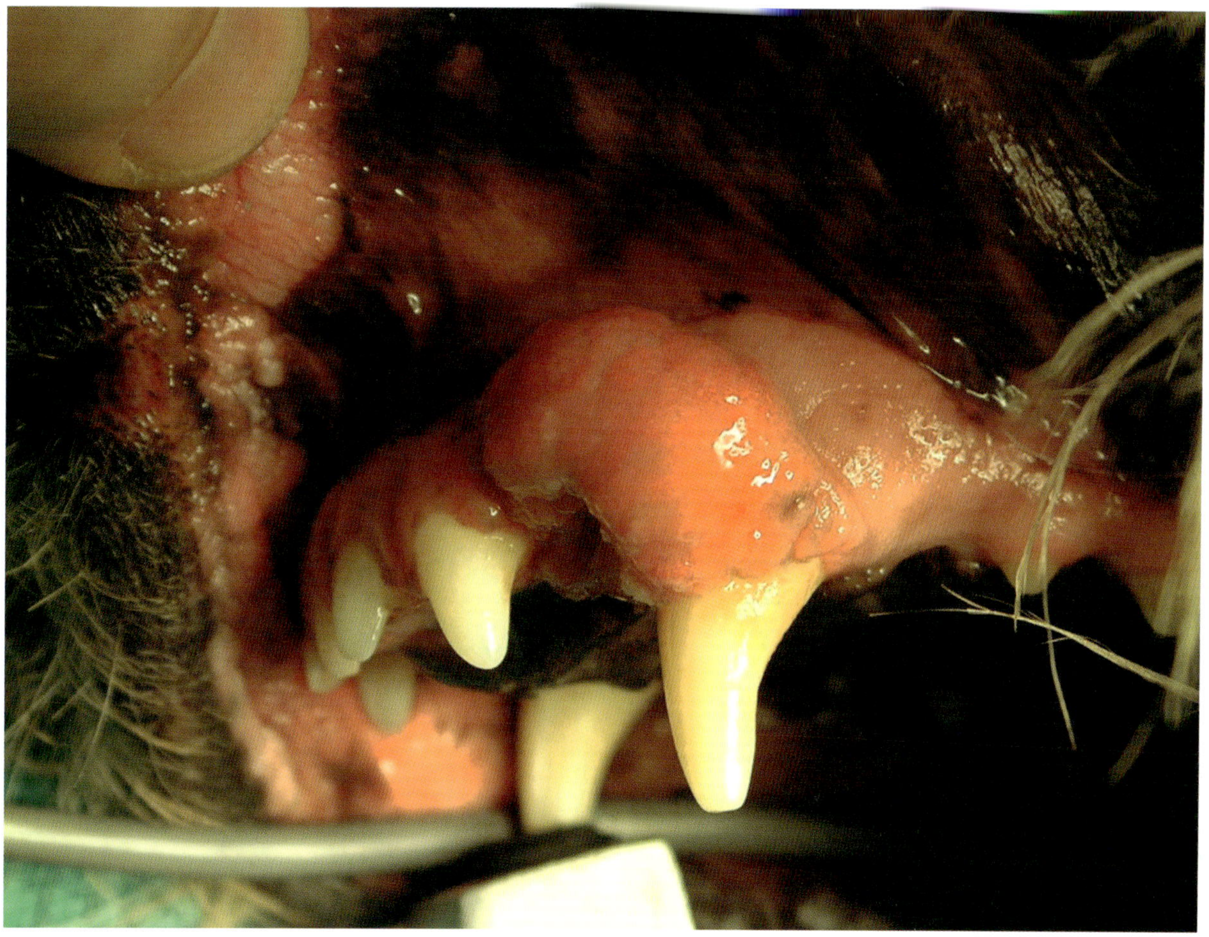

Surgical Technique (See Plate 6.11A–C)

A) The labial and buccal gingival mucosa and palatine mucoperiosteum are incised with a scalpel blade with a minimum of 5- to 10-mm margins, and the mucosa and mucoperiosteum are then elevated with a periosteal elevator to prepare for the osteotomies and protect soft tissues from iatrogenic damage during the osteotomies. Bleeding from the transected major palatine artery can typically be controlled with digital pressure, but ligation or cautery may be required.
B) Osteotomies are performed, with a minimum of 1-cm bone margins for benign tumors and 2-cm bone margins for malignant tumors, in the maxillary bone laterally (i) and caudally (ii), incisive bone rostrally, and hard palate medially (iii, arrow). These osteotomies can be performed with an oscillating, sagittal (i–iii), or biradial saw (iv), pneumatic drill, or piezoelectric instruments. The caudal osteotomy should be performed last so that bleeding from the sphenopalatine, major palatine, and infraorbital vessels can be quickly controlled after removal of the maxillary bone segment. Bleeding from the exposed nasal turbinates can be controlled with tamponade, ice-cold saline, 0.05% oxymetazoline spray, or thrombin-impregnated sponges [2, 3].
C) Exposed tooth roots (pictured, arrows) are extracted with a dental elevator (not pictured).

Closure (See Plate 6.11D, E)

A labial mucosal-submucosal flap is raised by undermining the labial and buccal mucosa and submucosa with Metzenbaum scissors from the incised edge of the labial and buccal mucosa toward the ventral margins of the lips (D). The labial mucosal-submucosal flap is advanced into the oral defect and closed in two layers using monofilament absorbable suture material on a reverse cutting needle. The submucosa of the labial mucosal-submucosal flap is sutured to either predrilled holes in the hard palate using an interrupted suture pattern or to the submucosa of the mucoperiosteum in a simple continuous suture pattern. The mucosa of the labial mucosal-submucosal flap is then sutured to the mucosa of the mucoperiosteum in either an interrupted or simple continuous suture pattern (E – i, ii).

Postoperative Management

1) Multimodal analgesia
2) Soft foods for 28 days
3) No chewing on hard objects or playing with toys for 28 days
4) Elizabethan collar
5) Note that feeding tubes are rarely required in either dogs or cats after unilateral rostral maxillectomy

Complications – Dogs [3]

Intraoperative Complications

- Intraoperative blood loss (36%) with 25% of these dogs requiring a blood transfusion

Postoperative Complications (<48 Hours)

- Epistaxis (47%)
- Facial swelling (27%)
- Facial pawing (7%)
- Eating difficulties (7%)

Plate 6.11

Unilateral Rostral Maxillectomy *continued*

A)

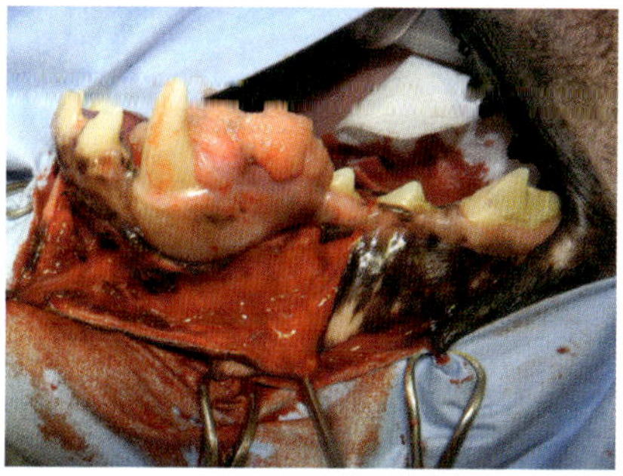

B-i)

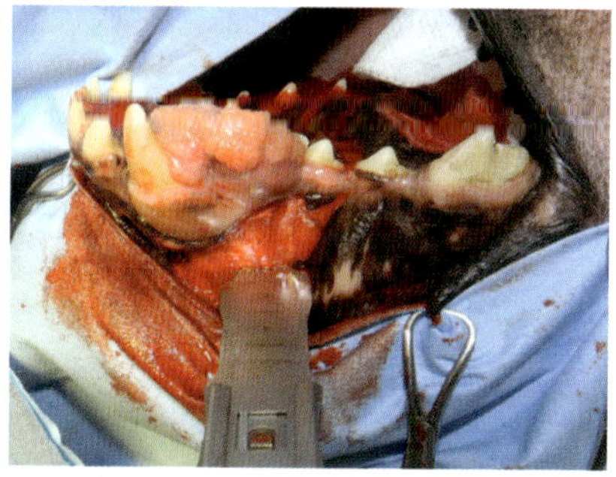

B-ii)

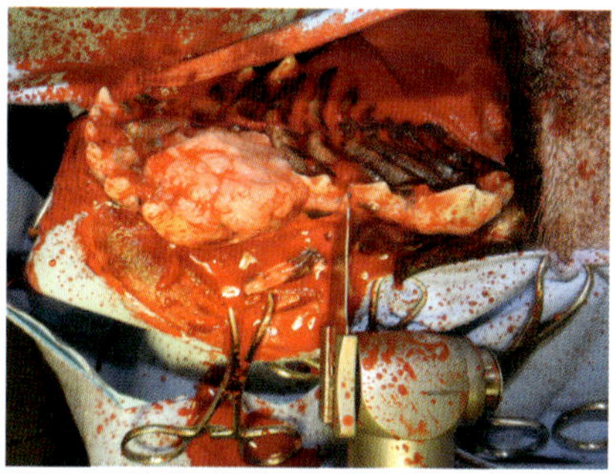

B-iii)

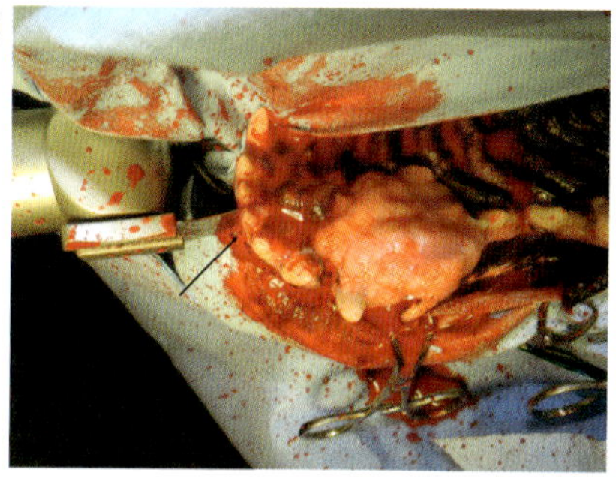

B-iv)

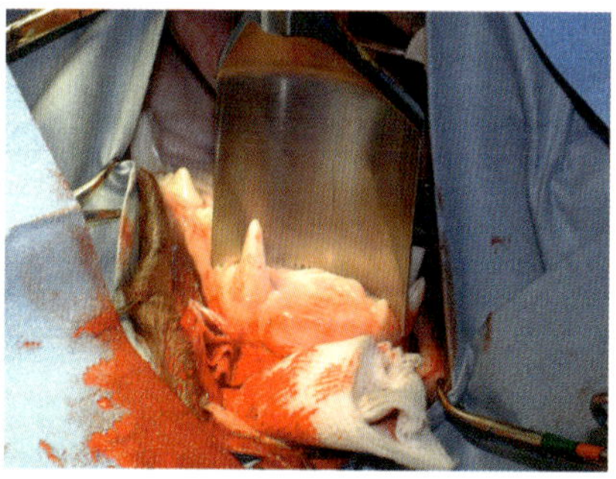

C)

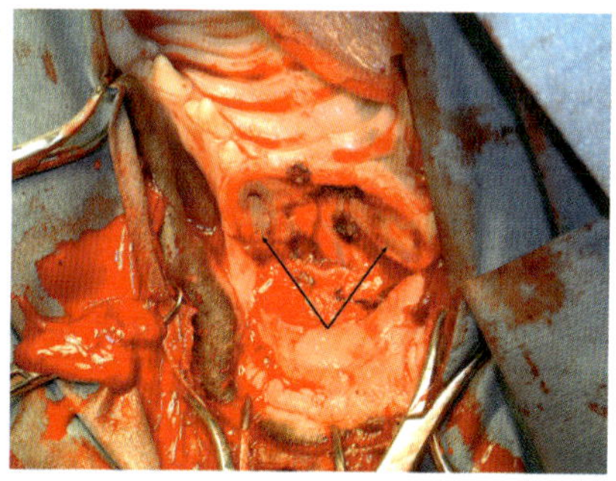

D)

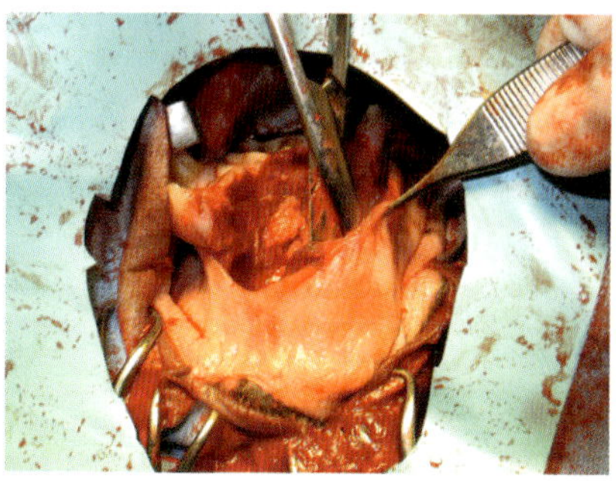

E-i)

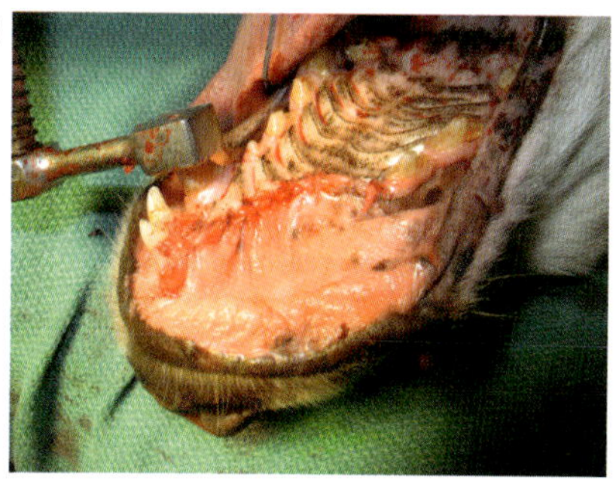

E-ii)

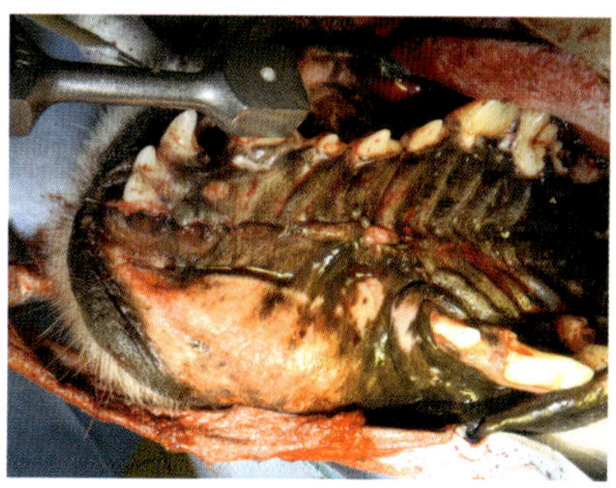

Postoperative Complications (48 Hours to 4 Weeks)

- Trauma to the upper lip as a result of the lip being drawn into the occlusal plane of the ipsilateral mandibular canine tooth (21%)
- Incisional dehiscence (8%)
- Oronasal fistula (3%)
- Surgical site infection (3%)
- Epiphora (3%)

Complications – Cats* [4] (See Plate 6.11F)

- Epistaxis (13%)
- Wound dehiscence and oronasal fistula (20%)
- Trauma to the upper lip as a result of the lip being drawn into the occlusal plane of the ipsilateral mandibular canine tooth (15%; F)
- Eating difficulties (15%)
- Facial swelling (10%)
- Subcutaneous emphysema (2%)
- Hypersalivation and drooling (2%)

Cosmetic Appearance (See Plate 6.11G, H)

The lip can be drawn toward the midline because of the use of the labial mucosal-submucosal flap for reconstruction of the intraoral defect (G – i, ii). The extent of this medialization of the lip depends on the medial extent of the resection, the width of the lip, and the length of the labial mucosal-submucosal flap. Provided that the labial mucosal-submucosal flap is sufficiently undermined, the cosmetic appearance is usually very good (H – i–vi).

Suggested Adjuvant Treatments

- See *6. Mandibulectomy and Maxillectomy*.

Prognosis and Oncologic Outcome

- See *6. Mandibulectomy and Maxillectomy*.

References

1 Reiter, A.M. (2014). Open wide: blindness in cats after the use of mouth gags. *Vet. J.* 201: 5–6.
2 Liptak, J.M. and Lascelles, B.D.X. (2012). Oral tumors. In: *Veterinary Surgical Oncology*, 1e (ed. S.T. Kudnig and B. Séguin), 119–178. Wiley-Blackwell.
3 MacLellan, R.H., Rawlinson, J.E., Rao, S. et al. (2018). Intraoperative and postoperative complications of partial maxillectomy for the treatment of oral tumors in dogs. *J. Am. Vet. Med. Assoc.* 252 (12): 1538–1547.
4 Liptak, J.M., Thatcher, G.P., Mestrinho, L.A. et al. (2021). Outcomes of cats treated with maxillectomy: 60 cases. A veterinary society of surgical oncology retrospective study. *Vet. Comp. Oncol.* 19 (4): 641–650.

* These complications are for all maxillectomy procedures and not specifically for unilateral rostral maxillectomy.

Plate 6.11

Unilateral Rostral Maxillectomy *continued*

F)

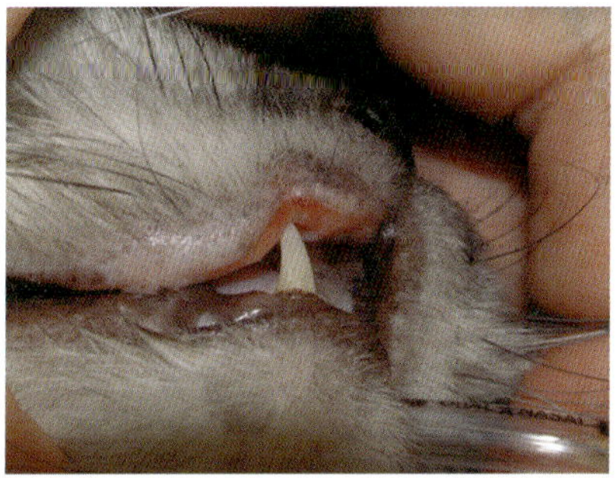

G-i)

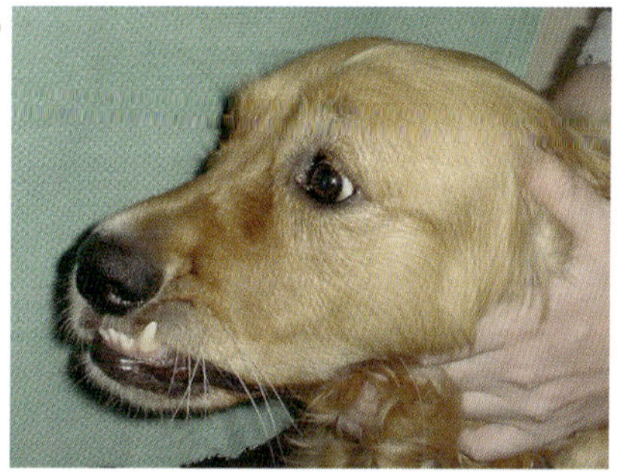

G-ii)

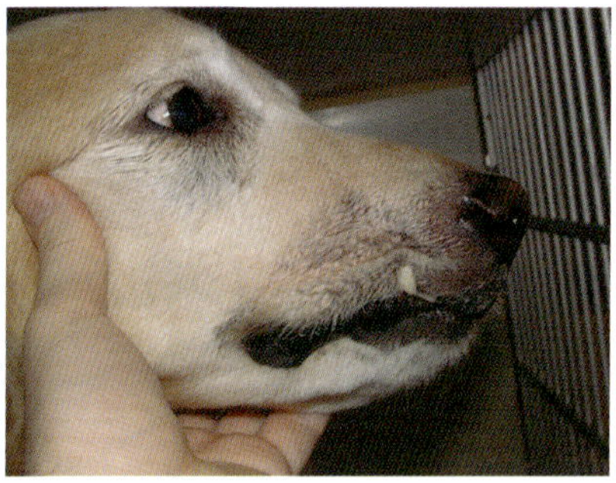

H-i)

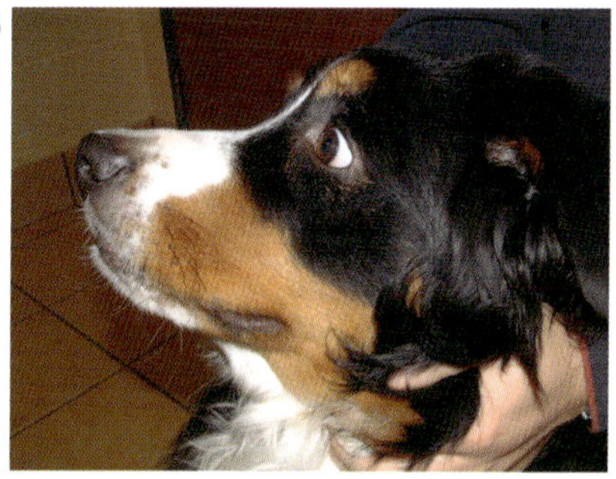

H-ii)

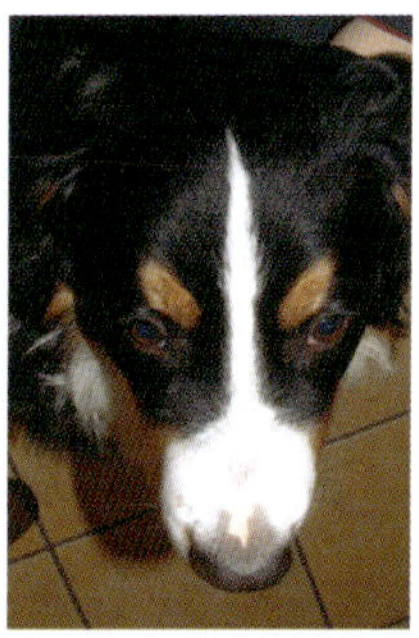

H-iii)

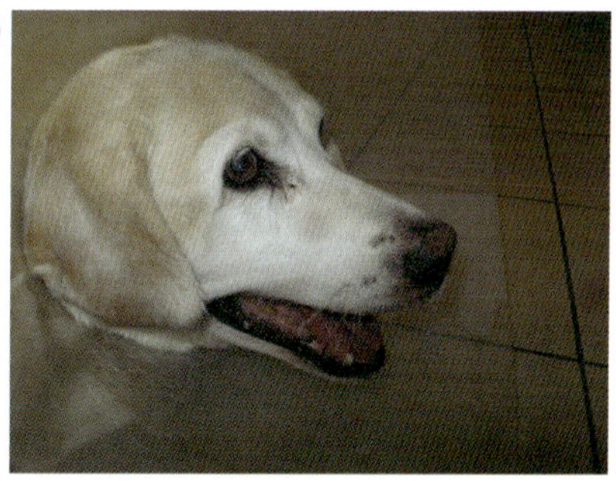

H-iv)

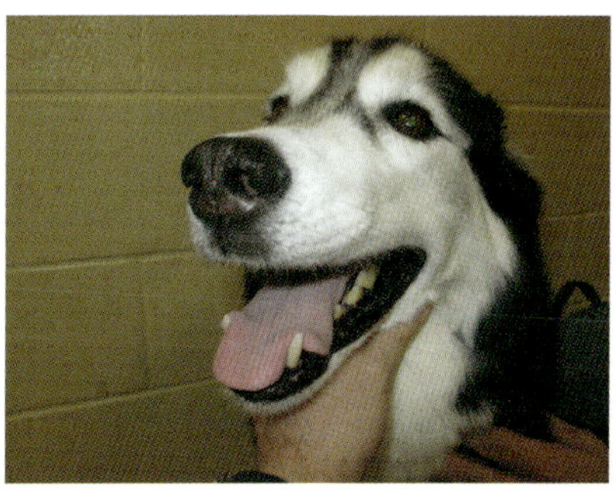

H-v)

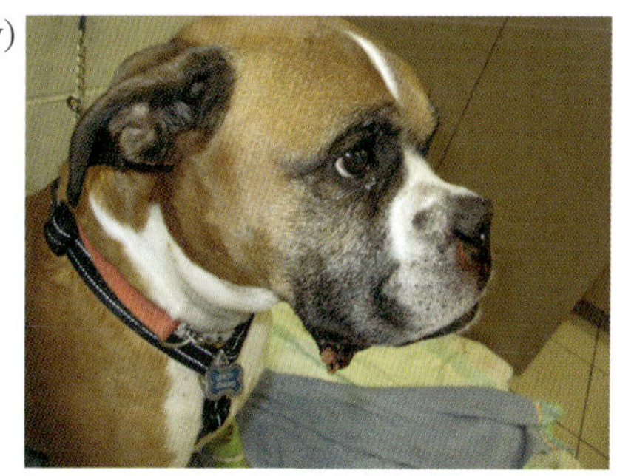

H-vi)

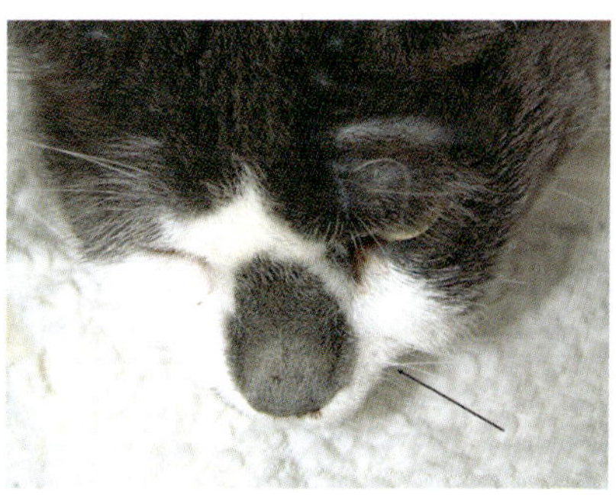

6.12 Bilateral Rostral Maxillectomy

Indications (See Plate 6.12 – 1)

1) Resection of benign oral tumors (i, acanthomatous ameloblastoma) or small or low-grade malignant oral tumors rostral to the second premolar tooth and that have crossed the midline (ii, fibrosarcoma).
2) Bilateral rostral maxillectomy can be combined with nasal planum resection for tumors involving the nasal planum with invasion into the incisive bone (see *4.1. Nasal Planum Resection – Feline* and *4.2. Nasal Planum Resection – Canine*).
3) Bilateral rostral maxillectomy can be combined with an upper lip advancement flap (see *39.2. Upper Lip Advancement Flap*) if the maxillectomy is also associated with a rostral lip defect.
4) Bilateral rostral maxillectomy can be combined with a cantilever suture technique to correct postoperative nasal droop (see *6.13. Cantilever Suture Technique*).

Suggested Diagnostic Workup and Clinical Staging for Benign Maxillary Tumors

- Complete blood count, serum biochemistry, and urinalysis
- Preoperative biopsy
- Precontrast and postcontrast computed tomography (CT) scan of the head for surgical planning

Suggested Diagnostic Workup and Clinical Staging for Malignant Maxillary Tumors

- Complete blood count, serum biochemistry, and urinalysis
- Preoperative biopsy
- Regional lymph node assessment for evaluation of lymph node metastasis
  - Fine-needle aspirate cytology of the mandibular lymph nodes
  - Sentinel lymph node mapping and excision of the sentinel lymph node (see *50.1. Sentinel Lymph Node Mapping*)
  - Nonselective excision of the bilateral mandibular and medial retropharyngeal lymph nodes through a ventral midline cervical approach (see *50.3. Combined Mandibular and Medial Retropharyngeal Lymph Node Excision*), or excision of the ipsilateral mandibular, medial retropharyngeal, and parotid lymph nodes through a lateral approach (see *50.4. Combined Parotid, Mandibular, and Medial Retropharyngeal Lymph Node Excision*)
- Precontrast and postcontrast CT scan of the head and neck for surgical planning
- Thoracic CT scan for assessment of lung metastasis

Color Atlas of Canine and Feline Surgical Oncology, First Edition. Julius M. Liptak, Paolo Buracco, William T. N. Culp, and Nicholas J. Bacon.

Plate 6.12

Bilateral Rostral Maxillectomy

1-i)

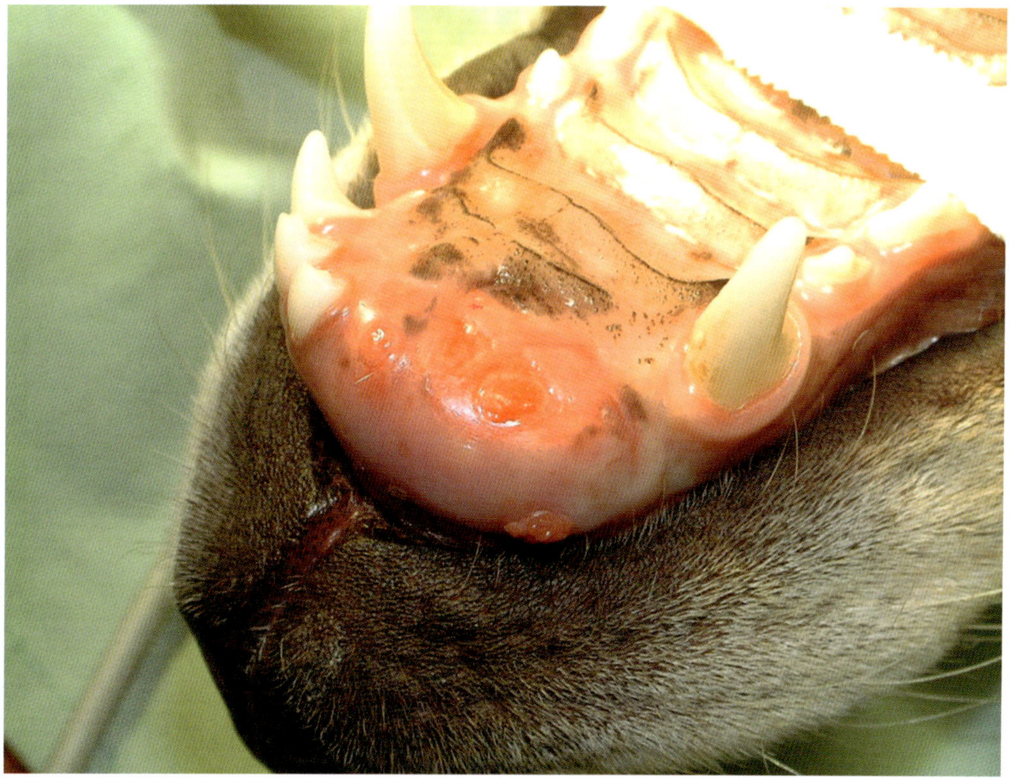

1-ii)

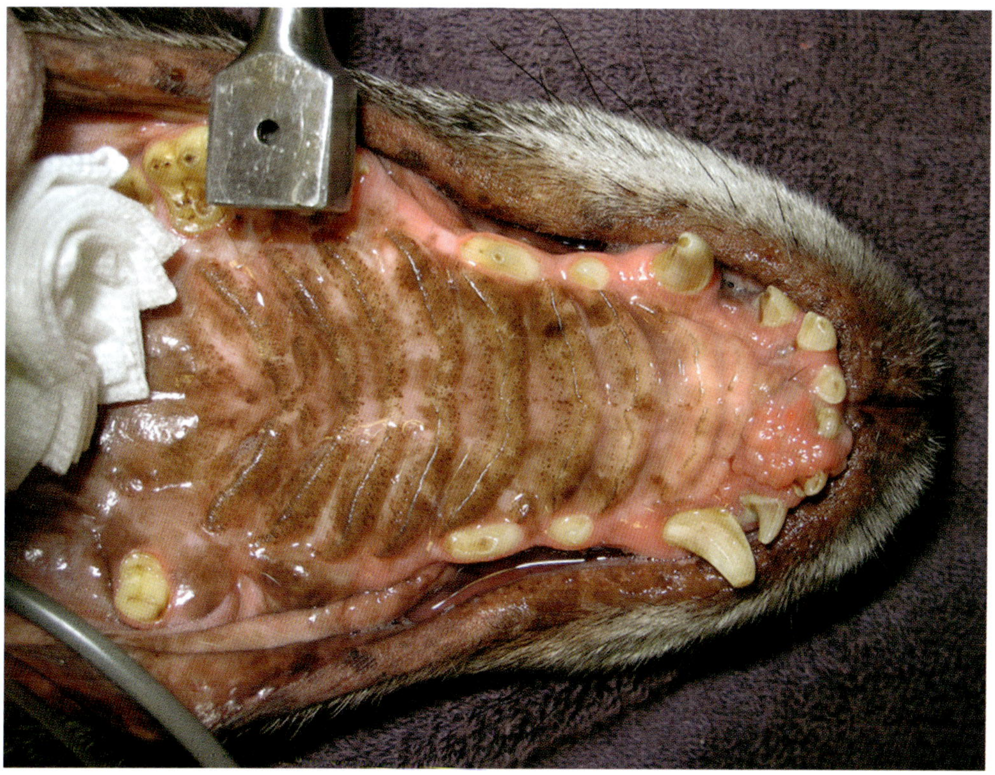

Patient Positioning

The patient is positioned in dorsal recumbency. A mouth gag should be placed to improve exposure. Mouth gags should be used with caution in cats because of the risk of cortical blindness secondary to compression of the maxillary artery; 20- or 30-mm plastic gags are preferred to spring-loaded gags [1]. The pharynx should be packed with gauze sponges to minimize the risk of aspirating lavage fluid and blood.

Surgical Technique (See Plate 6.12A–C)

A) The labial gingival mucosa (i) and palatine mucoperiosteum are incised with a scalpel blade with a minimum of 5-mm margins, and the mucosa (ii) and mucoperiosteum are then elevated with a periosteal elevator to prepare for the osteotomy and protect soft tissues from iatrogenic damage during the osteotomy. Bleeding from the transected major palatine artery can typically be controlled with digital pressure, but ligation or cautery may be required.
B) Osteotomies are performed, with a minimum of 1-cm bone margins for benign tumors and 2-cm bone margins for malignant tumors, in the maxillary bone lateral (i) and caudal (ii) to the mass along the mucoperiosteal incision. This osteotomy can be performed with an oscillating, sagittal, or biradial saw (ii), pneumatic drill, or piezoelectric instruments. Bleeding from the exposed nasal turbinates can be controlled with tamponade, ice-cold saline, 0.05% oxymetazoline spray, or thrombin-impregnated sponges (iii, arrows) [2, 3].
C) Exposed tooth roots are extracted with a dental elevator.

Closure (See Plate 6.12D–H)

Bilateral rostral labial mucosal-submucosal flaps are raised by undermining the left and right rostral labial mucosa and submucosa with Metzenbaum scissors from the incised edge of the labial mucosa toward the labial margins (D). The labial mucosal-submucosal flaps are advanced into the oral defect and closed in a T-shape in two layers using monofilament absorbable suture material on a reverse cutting needle. The submucosa of the labial mucosal-submucosal flaps is sutured to either predrilled holes in the hard palate (E) using an interrupted suture pattern (F) or to the submucosa of the

Plate 6.12

Bilateral Rostral Maxillectomy *continued*

A-i)

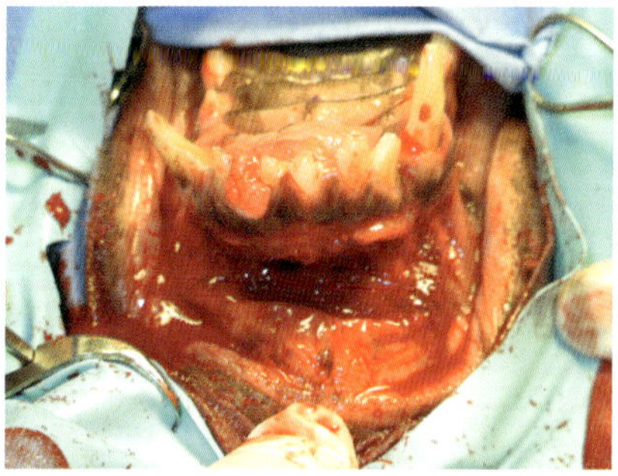

A-ii)

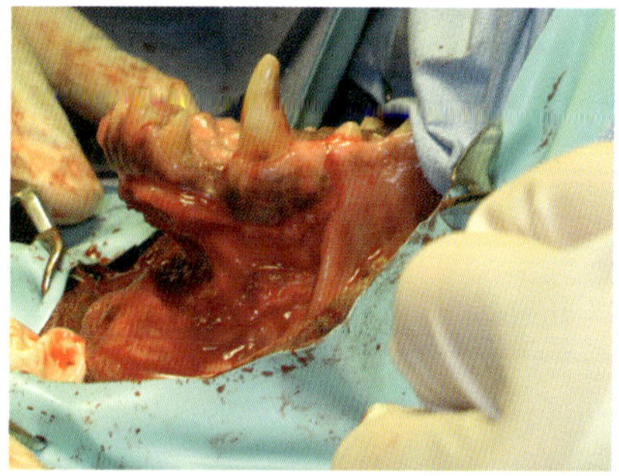

B-i)

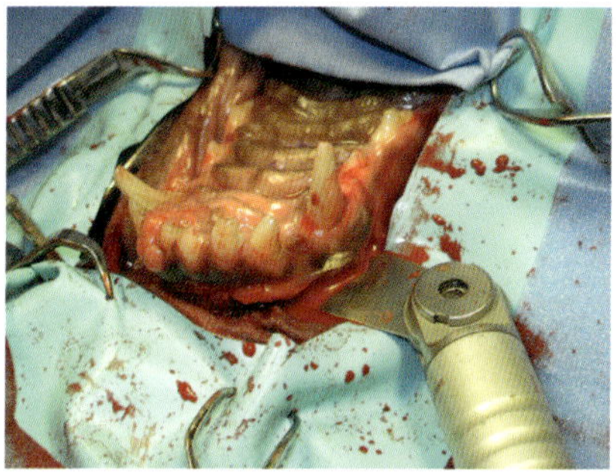

B-ii)

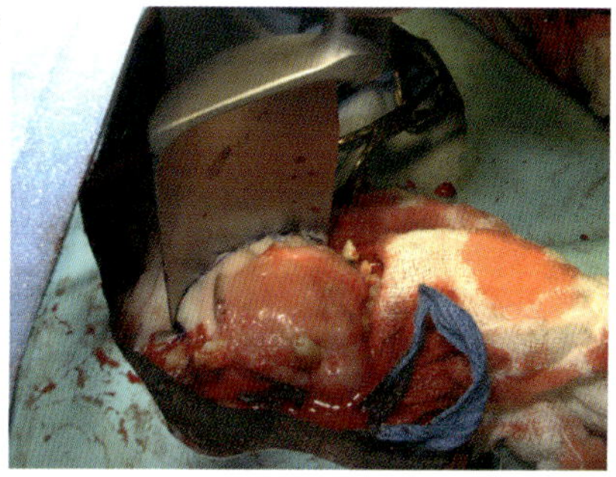

B-iii)

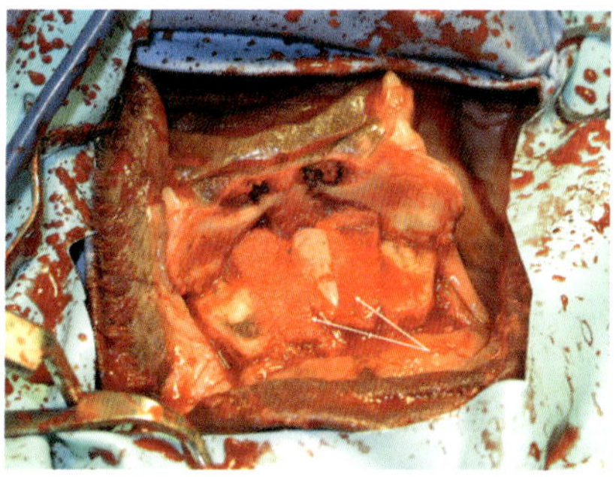

C)

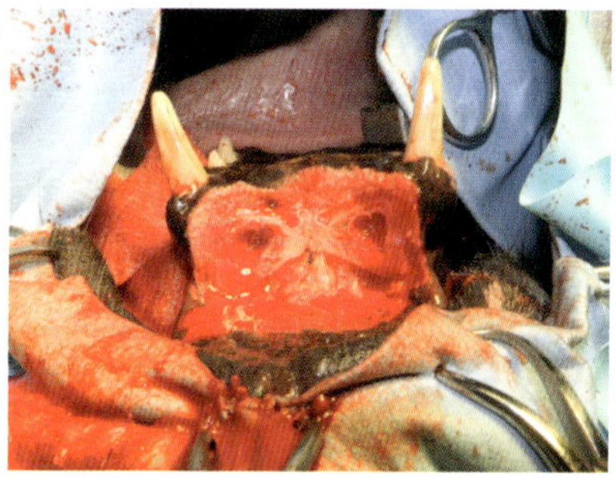

D)

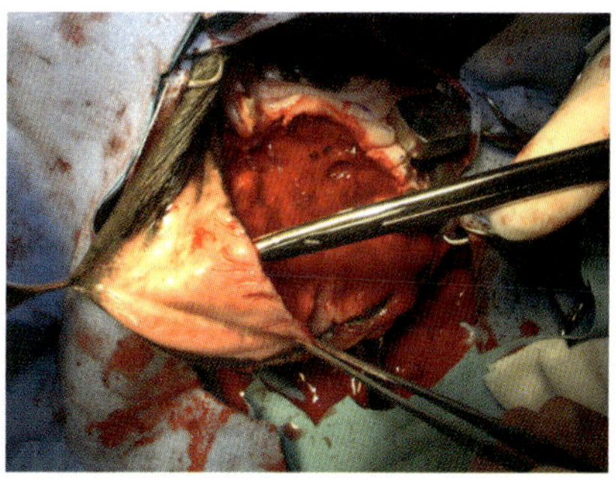

E)

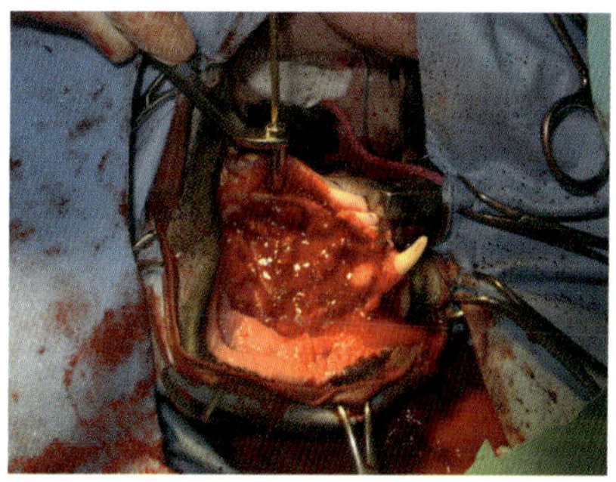

F)

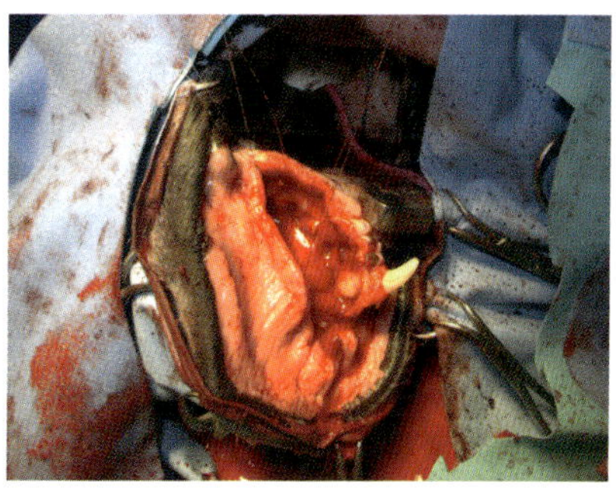

Closure (See Plate 6.12D–H) *continued*

mucoperiosteum in a simple continuous suture pattern (G). The mucosa of the labial mucosal-submucosal flaps is sutured to the mucosa of the mucoperiosteum in either an interrupted or simple continuous suture pattern (H – i–iii).

Postoperative Management

1) Multimodal analgesia
2) Soft foods for 28 days
3) No chewing on hard objects or playing with toys for 28 days
4) Elizabethan collar
5) Note that feeding tubes are rarely required in either dogs or cats after bilateral rostral maxillectomy

Complications – Dogs [3]

Intraoperative Complications

- Intraoperative blood loss (38%) with 30% of these dogs requiring a blood transfusion

Postoperative Complications (<48 Hours)

- Epistaxis (46%)
- Facial swelling (19%)
- Facial pawing (12%)
- Eating difficulties (4%)

Postoperative Complications (48 Hours to 4 Weeks) (See Plate 6.12I)

- Trauma to the upper lip as a result of the lips being drawn into the occlusal plane of the mandibular canine teeth (17%)
- Incisional dehiscence and oronasal fistula (6%; I)
- Surgical-site infection (6%)
- Epiphora (6%)

Complications – Cats* [4]

- Epistaxis (13%)
- Wound dehiscence and oronasal fistula (19.6%)
- Trauma to the upper lip as a result of the lip being drawn into the occlusal plane of the ipsilateral mandibular canine tooth (15%)
- Eating difficulties (15%)
- Facial swelling (10%)
- Subcutaneous emphysema (2%)
- Hypersalivation and drooling (2%)

* These complications are for all maxillectomy procedures and not specifically for bilateral rostral maxillectomy.

Plate 6.12

Bilateral Rostral Maxillectomy *continued*

G)

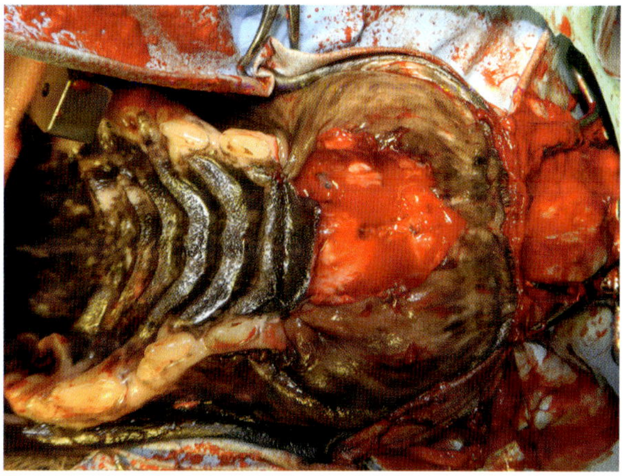

H-i)

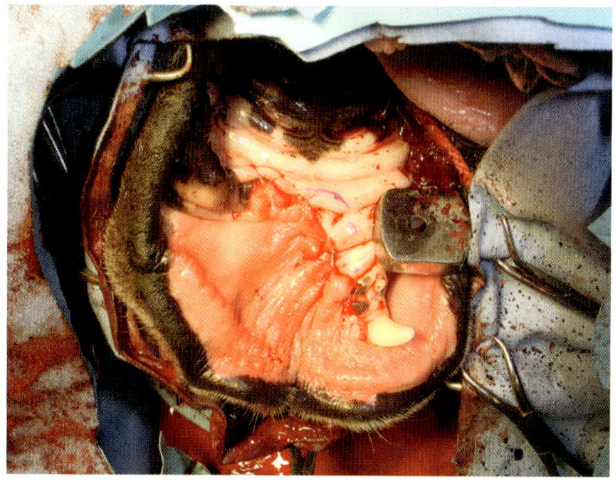

H-ii)

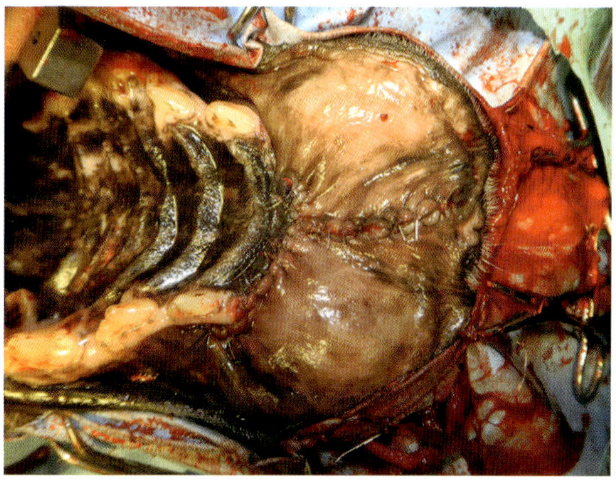

H-iii)

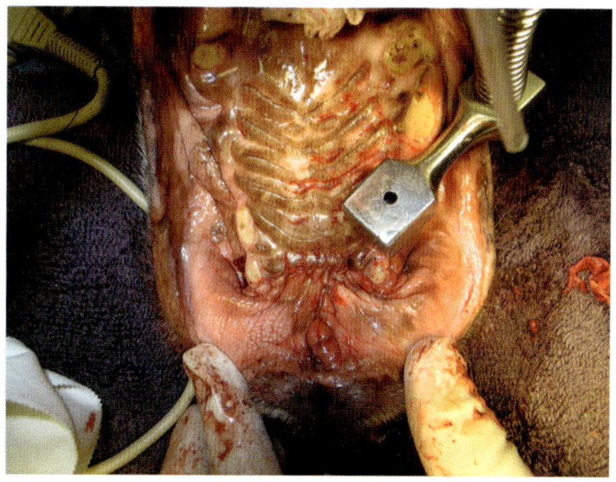

I)

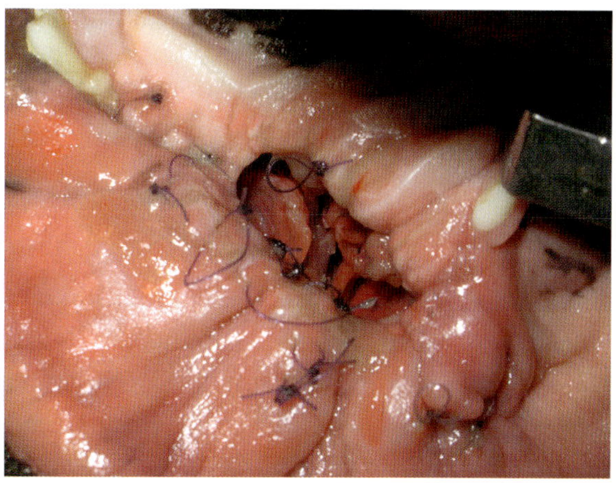

Cosmetic Appearance (See Plate 6.12J)

Drooping of the nose (J – i, ii) as a result of loss of rostroventral bone support can occur after bilateral rostral maxillectomy. The extent of this droop depends on the length of the nose and the extent of the bilateral rostral maxillectomy and is more pronounced when the head is in an elevated position (J – ii). This droop may partially obstruct the common nasal meati and respiratory difficulties. Nasal drooping can be corrected using a cantilever suture technique (see *6.13. Cantilever Suture Technique*).

Suggested Adjuvant Treatments

- See *6. Mandibulectomy and Maxillectomy*.

Prognosis and Oncologic Outcome

- See *6. Mandibulectomy and Maxillectomy*.

References

1 Reiter, A.M. (2014). Open wide: blindness in cats after the use of mouth gags. *Vet. J.* 201: 5–6.
2 Liptak, J.M. and Lascelles, B.D.X. (2012). Oral tumors. In: *Veterinary Surgical Oncology*, 1e (ed. S.T. Kudnig and B. Séguin), 119–178. Wiley-Blackwell.
3 MacLellan, R.H., Rawlinson, J.E., Rao, S. et al. (2018). Intraoperative and postoperative complications of partial maxillectomy for the treatment of oral tumors in dogs. *J. Am. Vet. Med. Assoc.* 252 (12): 1538–1547.
4 Liptak, J.M., Thatcher, G.P., Mestrinho, L.A. et al. (2021). Outcomes of cats treated with maxillectomy: 60 cases. A veterinary society of surgical oncology retrospective study. *Vet. Comp. Oncol.* 19 (4): 641–650.

Plate 6.12

Bilateral Rostral Maxillectomy *continued*

J-i)

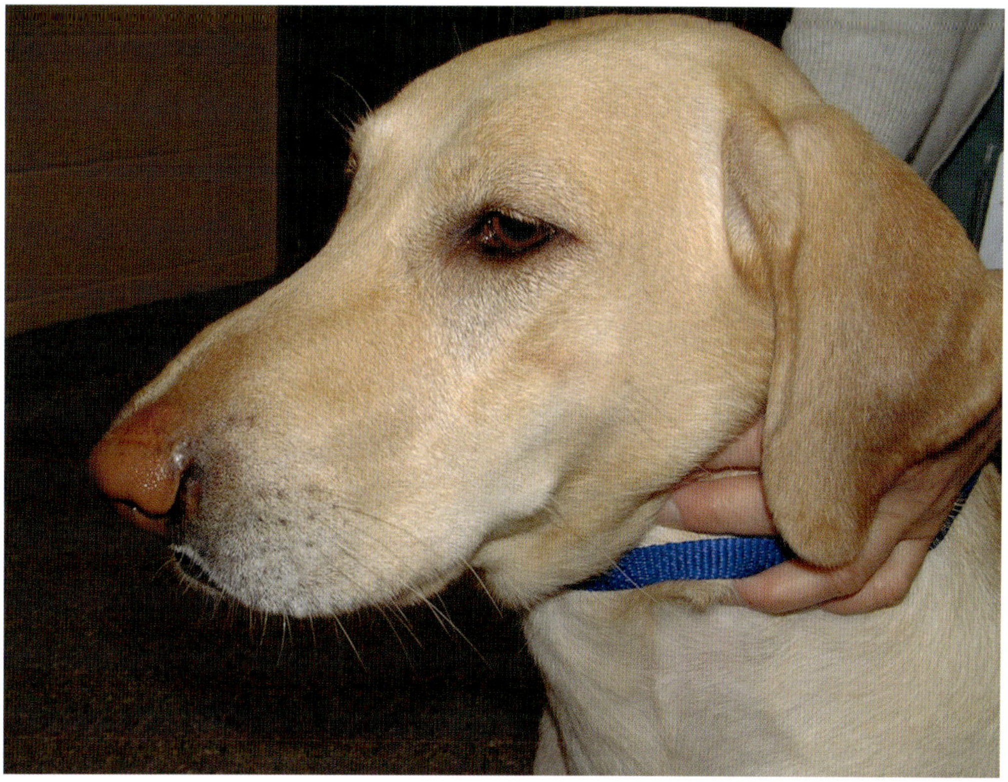

J-ii)

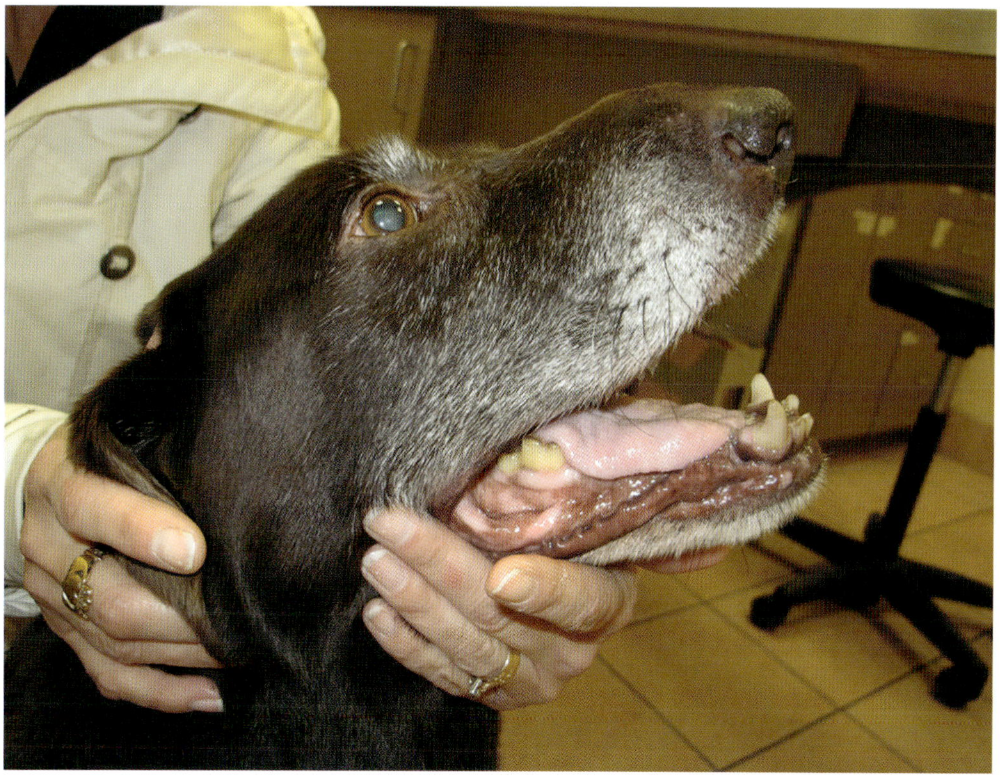

6.13 Cantilever Suture Technique

Indications (See Plate 6.13 – 1)

1) Correction of nasal droop after bilateral rostral maxillectomy.

Patient Positioning

The patient is positioned in sternal recumbency with the head in an elevated position.

Surgical Technique [1] (See Plate 6.13A–C)

A) A midline skin incision is made along the dorsal midline of the muzzle from the medial canthi to just caudal to the nasal planum. The skin is undermined and the edges retracted to expose the underlying nasal and maxillary bones. A small hole is drilled, using either a 1/16-inch Steinmann pin (i, ii) or 2.0-mm drill bit, transversely across the maxillary bones immediately ventral to the nasal bones.
B) Suture material is passed through the drill hole, using either a swaged on straight needle (pictured) or suture material passed through a 16- or 18-gauge hypodermic needle inserted into the drill hole; 0 or 1 nonabsorbable monofilament suture material is recommended.
C) Five-millimeter incisions are made in the dorsolateral aspect of each lateral cartilage of the nasal planum (i, ii, arrows). The swaged on straight needle is passed rostrally and subcutaneously through the dorsal muzzle skin incision and exits out of the incision in the dorsolateral aspect of the ipsilateral lateral cartilage of the nasal planum. The needle is then redirected transversely across the nasal cartilage from the ipsilateral to contralateral incisions in the dorsolateral aspects of the lateral cartilages of the nasal planum. Finally, the needle is passed caudally through the incision in the dorsolateral aspect of the contralateral lateral cartilage of the nasal planum and subcutaneously exits through the dorsal muzzle incision. The first throw of the surgeon's knot is used to assess the most appropriate tension on the cantilever suture to correct the nasal droop.

Closure (See Plate 6.13D, E)

The dorsal muzzle incision is closed routinely in two layers with a simple continuous suture pattern using monofilament absorbable suture material in the subcutis and either an interrupted or continuous suture pattern using monofilament nonabsorbable suture material in the skin (D). The incisions in the lateral cartilages of the nasal planum do not require closure because the cantilever suture recesses into the cartilage below the epithelial surface and partially collapses these incisions (E).

Color Atlas of Canine and Feline Surgical Oncology, First Edition. Julius M. Liptak, Paolo Buracco, William T. N. Culp, and Nicholas J. Bacon.

Plate 6.13

Cantilever Suture Technique

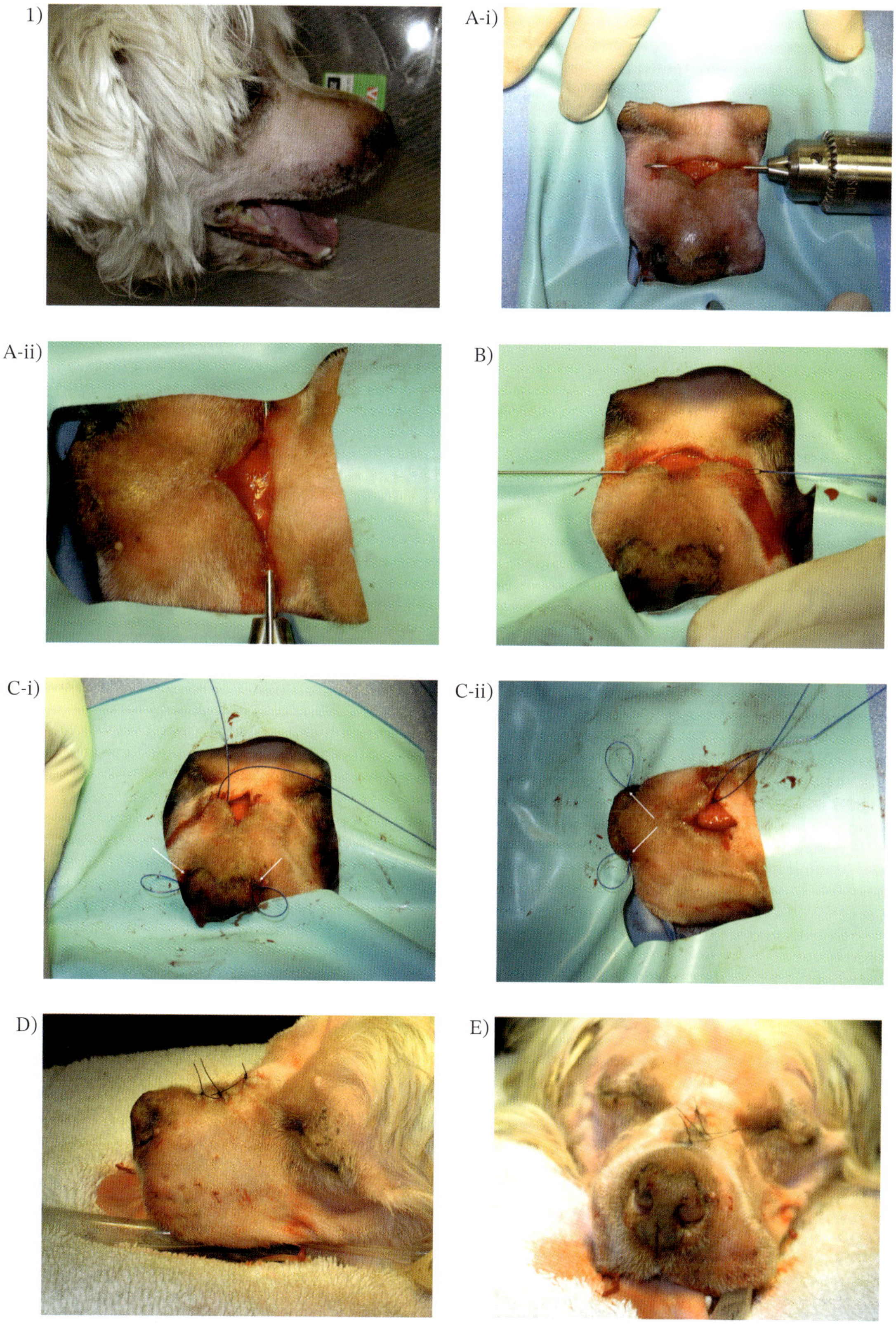

Postoperative Management

1) Multimodal analgesia
2) Elizabethan collar

Complications

1) Incisional complications (e.g. infection, dehiscence, seroma)
2) Overtightening of the cantilever suture resulting in a depression or dimple in the lateral nasal cartilages

Reference

1 Pavletic, M.M. (ed.) (2010). Cantilever suture technique. In: *Atlas of Small Animal Wound Management & Reconstructive Surgery*, 3e, 596–599. Wiley-Blackwell.

6.14 Radical Bilateral Rostral Maxillectomy

Indications (See Plate 6.14 – 1)

1) Resection of malignant tumors (pictured, squamous cell carcinoma) of the rostral maxilla, which extend dorsally into the nasal cavity
2) Resection of malignant tumors that extend caudal to the second premolar teeth and across the midline of the hard palate

Suggested Diagnostic Workup and Clinical Staging for Malignant Maxillary Tumors

- Complete blood count, serum biochemistry, and urinalysis
- Preoperative biopsy
- Regional lymph node assessment for evaluation of lymph node metastasis
  - Fine-needle aspirate cytology of the mandibular lymph nodes
  - Sentinel lymph node mapping and excision of the sentinel lymph node (see *50.1. Sentinel Lymph Node Mapping*)
  - Nonselective excision of the bilateral mandibular and medial retropharyngeal lymph nodes through a ventral midline cervical approach (see *50.3. Combined Mandibular and Medial Retropharyngeal Lymph Node Excision*), or excision of the ipsilateral mandibular, medial retropharyngeal, and parotid lymph nodes through a lateral approach (see *50.4. Combined Parotid, Mandibular, and Medial Retropharyngeal Lymph Node Excision*)
- Precontrast and postcontrast computed tomography (CT) scan of the head and neck for surgical planning
- Thoracic CT scan for assessment of lung metastasis

Patient Positioning

The patient is positioned in dorsal recumbency. A mouth gag should be placed to improve exposure. Mouth gags should be used with caution in cats because of the risk of cortical blindness secondary to compression of the maxillary artery; 20- or 30-mm plastic gags are preferred to spring-loaded gags [1]. The pharynx should be packed with gauze sponges to minimize the risk of aspirating lavage fluid and blood.

Surgical Technique [2] (See Plate 6.14A, B)

A) The skin, buccal, and gingival mucosa and palatine mucoperiosteum are incised with a minimum of 2-cm margins. The skin is incised full thickness through the lips (i), perpendicular to the buccal margins, and extending dorsally (ii) and transversely across the maxilla and full thickness through the contralateral lips. The skin incision is continued deeply through the subcutaneous tissue and nasolabial muscles to the bone (iii). The infraorbital neurovascular bundle should be ligated or sealed and transected (arrow).
B) The gingival mucosa is incised at the same level as the full-thickness lip incisions, and this incision is extended transversely across the palatine mucoperiosteum to join the full-thickness lip incisions. Bleeding from the transected major palatine arteries can typically be controlled with digital pressure, but ligation or cautery may be required. An osteotomy is performed from a dorsal approach with an oscillating or sagittal saw perpendicular to the maxilla (pictured). This osteotomy should be performed slightly caudal to the level of the skin and mucosal incisions to facilitate reconstruction.

Color Atlas of Canine and Feline Surgical Oncology, First Edition. Julius M. Liptak, Paolo Buracco, William T. N. Culp, and Nicholas J. Bacon.

Plate 6.14

Radical Bilateral Rostral Maxillectomy

1)

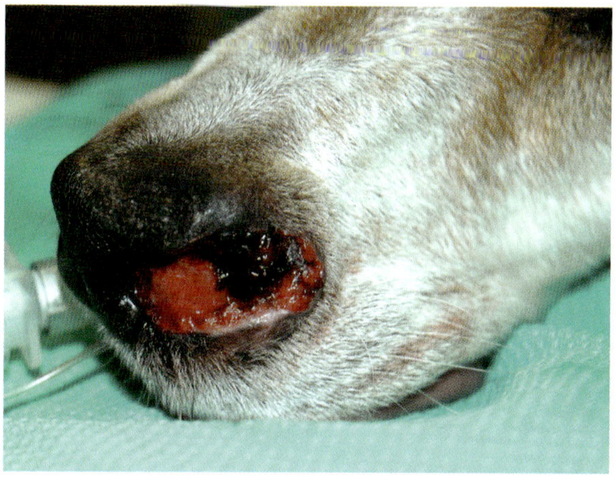

A i)

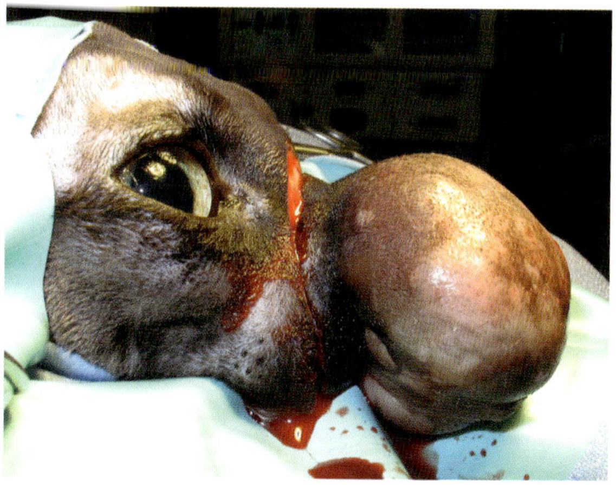

A-ii)

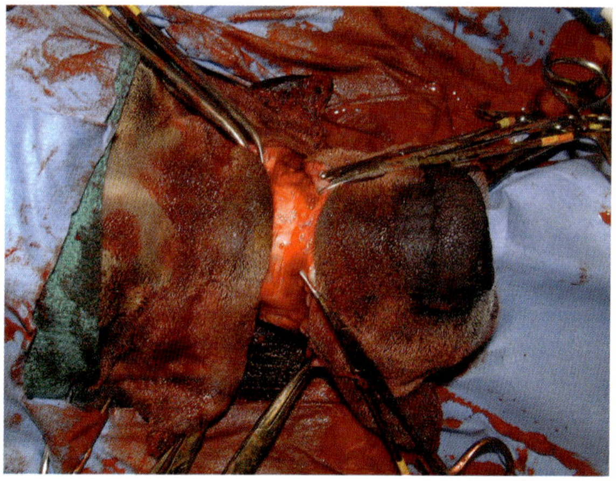

A-iii)

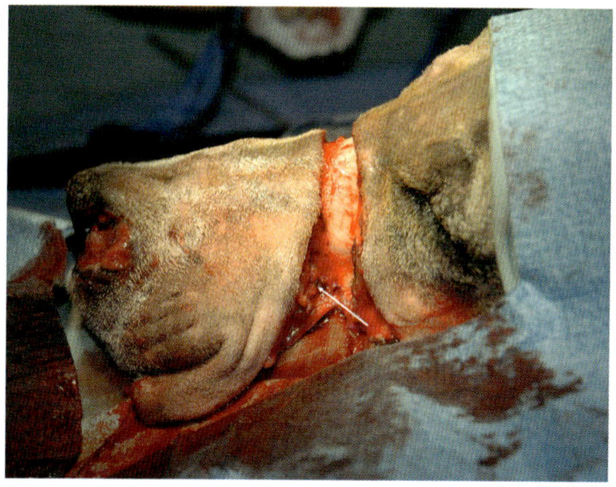

B)

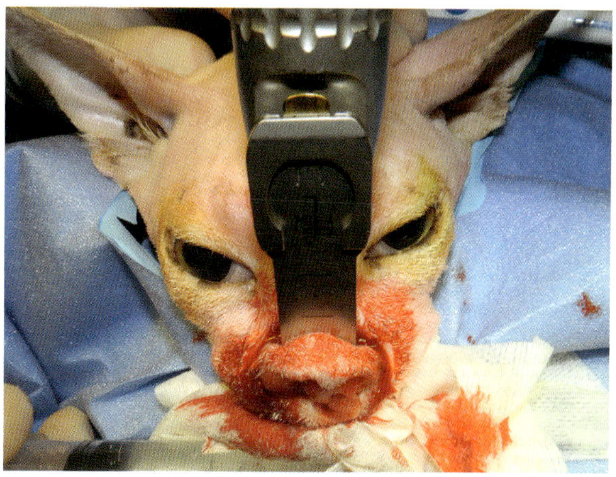

Closure (See Plate 6.14C–F)

C) The defect is reconstructed by drawing the free edges of the lips to the rostral maxilla so that the left and right lips meet in the midline of the rostral extent of the excised palate (arrows indicating where the free edges of the lips should meet). This creates a continuous rostral lip and new nasal orifice, and divides the nasal and oral cavities (see steps D and E).
D) The buccal mucosa is sutured to the palatine mucoperiosteum using monofilament absorbable suture material in either an interrupted or simple continuous suture pattern, and then buccal submucosa is sutured to either predrilled bone tunnels in the hard palate using monofilament absorbable suture material in a simple interrupted pattern or the submucosa of the palatine mucoperiosteum using monofilament absorbable suture material in either an interrupted or simple continuous suture pattern (arrow).
E) To reconstruct the nasal orifice, the skin edges are sutured to predrilled bone tunnels (i) in the maxillary bone using monofilament nonabsorbable suture material in either a rolling figure-of-eight or simple interrupted suture pattern (ii).
F) The skin of the lips is sutured using monofilament nonabsorbable suture material in an interrupted suture pattern (i, ii).

Postoperative Management

1) Multimodal analgesia
2) Soft foods for 28 days
3) No chewing on hard objects or playing with toys for 28 days
4) Elizabethan collar
5) Note that feeding tubes are rarely required in either dogs or cats after radical bilateral rostral maxillectomys

Complications – Dogs (<3 Weeks) [2]

- Serosanguineous discharge from the nasal turbinates resulting in crusting and contamination with food and saliva (100%)
- Eating difficulties (33%)
- Dehiscence (33%)
- Nasal stenosis (17%)
- Excessive free rostral lip resulting in interference with eating (17%)

Cosmetic Appearance (See Plate 6.14G)

The cosmetic appearance after radical bilateral rostral maxillectomy can be challenging. The maxilla is shortened relative to the mandible, and the nasal turbinates are exposed (G – i, ii, 1 day postoperatively; G – iii, 28 days postoperatively).

Suggested Adjuvant Treatments

- See 6. *Mandibulectomy and Maxillectomy*.

Prognosis and Oncologic Outcome

- See 6. *Mandibulectomy and Maxillectomy*.

References

1 Reiter, A.M. (2014). Open wide: blindness in cats after the use of mouth gags. *Vet. J.* 201: 5–6.
2 Lascelles, B.D.X., Henderson, R.A., Seguin, B. et al. (2004). Bilateral rostral maxillectomy and nasal planectomy for large rostral maxillofacial neoplasms in six dogs and one cat. *J. Am. Anim. Hosp. Assoc.* 40 (2): 137–146.

Plate 6.14

Radical Bilateral Rostral Maxillectomy *continued*

C-i)

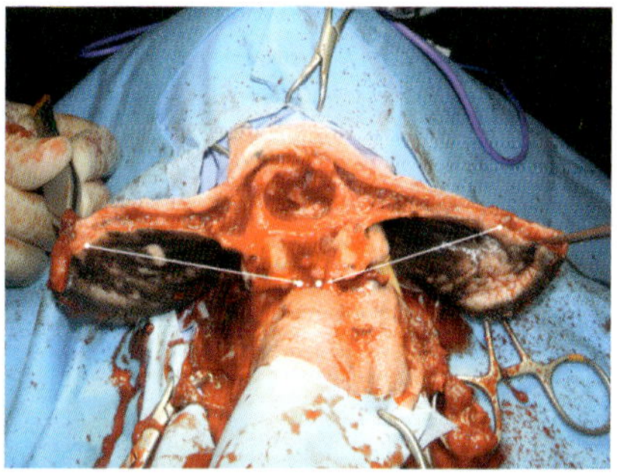

D)

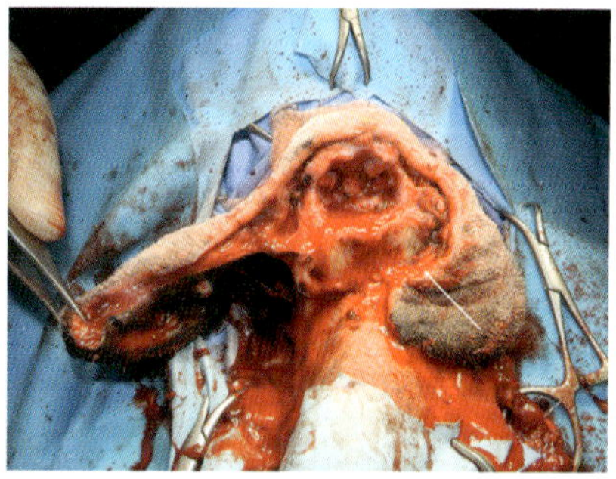

E-i)

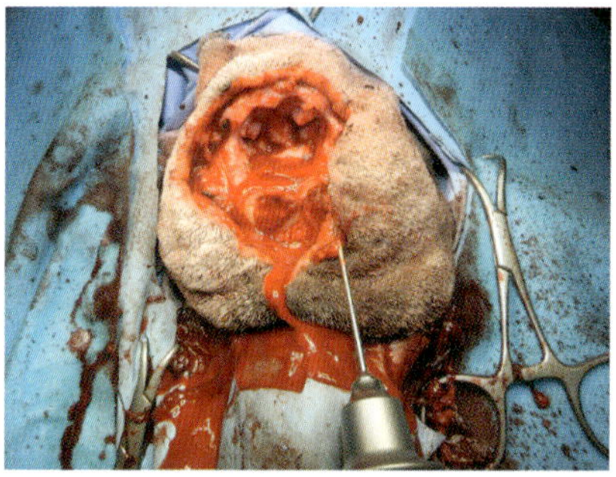

E-ii)

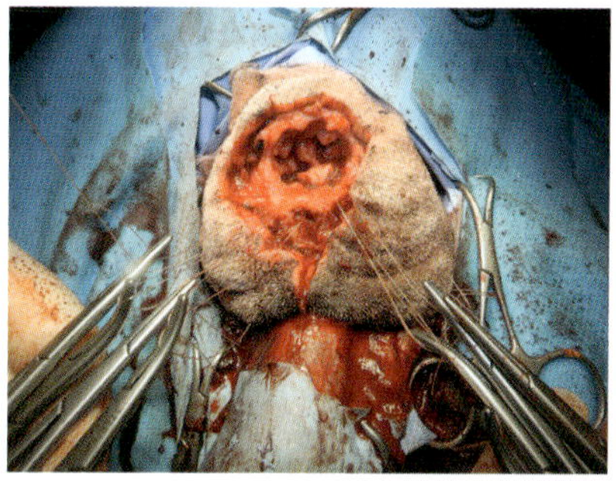

F-i)

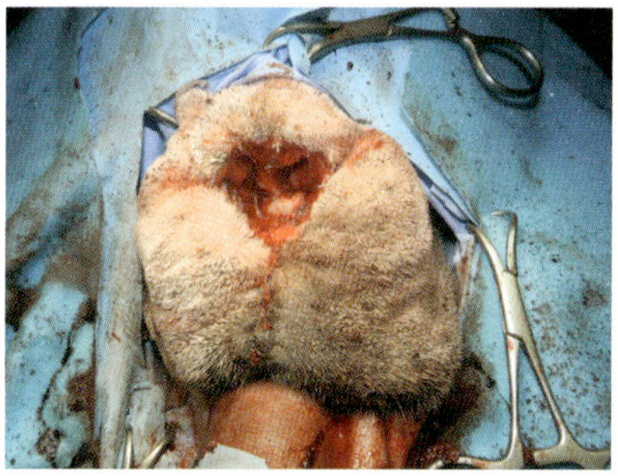

F-ii)

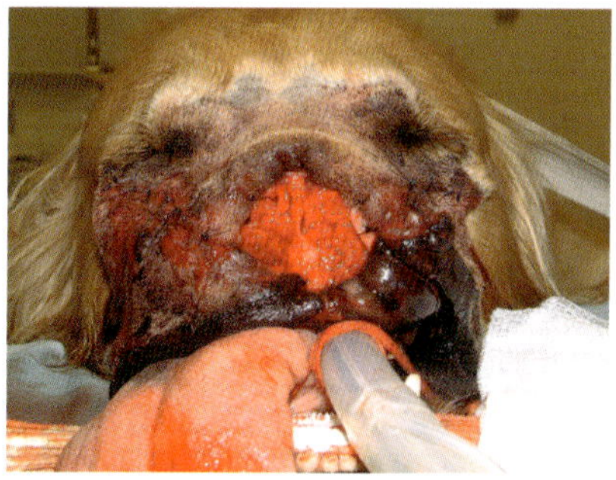

G-i)

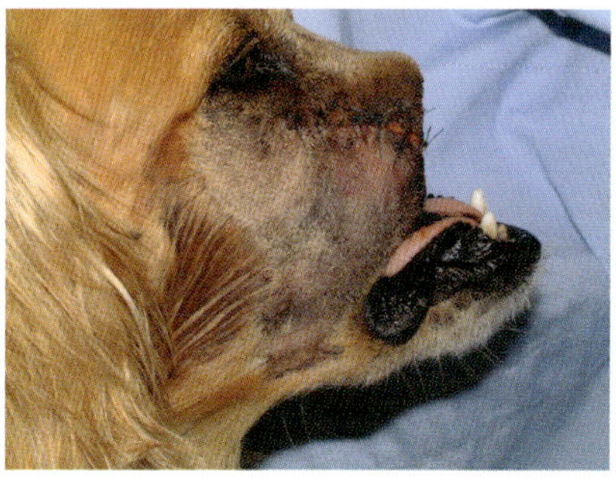

G-ii)

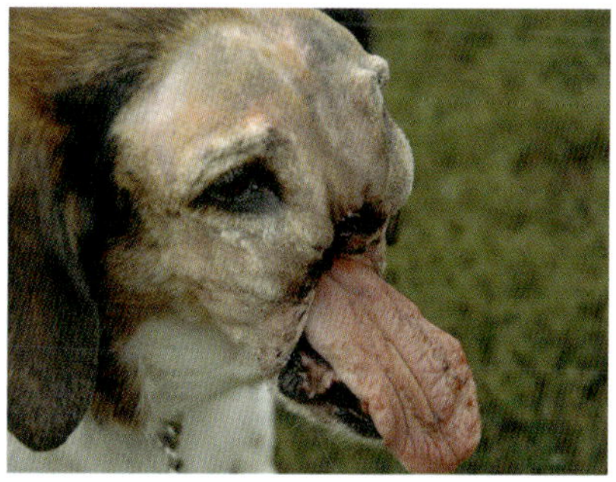

G-iii)

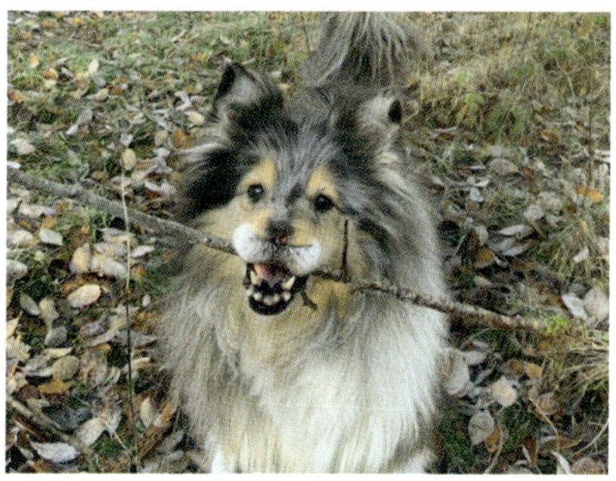

6.15 Intraoral Approach for Caudal and Total Unilateral Maxillectomy

Indications (See Plate 6.15 – 1)

1) Resection of benign, particularly acanthomatous ameloblastomas, and malignant oral tumors (A, melanotic melanoma; B, amelanotic melanoma; C, fibrosarcoma) located on the alveolar margins of the mid-to-caudal maxilla
2) The intraoral approach can be combined with a dorsolateral skin incision for resection of more extensive maxillary tumors (see *6.16. Combined Approach for Caudal and Total Unilateral Maxillectomy*)

Suggested Diagnostic Workup and Clinical Staging for Malignant Maxillary Tumors

- Complete blood count, serum biochemistry, and urinalysis
- Preoperative biopsy
- Regional lymph node assessment for evaluation of lymph node metastasis
  - Fine-needle aspirate cytology of the mandibular lymph nodes
  - Sentinel lymph node mapping and excision of the sentinel lymph node (see *50.1. Sentinel Lymph Node Mapping*).
  - Nonselective excision of the bilateral mandibular and medial retropharyngeal lymph nodes through a ventral midline cervical approach (see *50.3. Combined Mandibular and Medial Retropharyngeal Lymph Node Excision*), or excision of the ipsilateral mandibular, medial retropharyngeal, and parotid lymph nodes through a lateral approach (see *50.4. Combined Parotid, Mandibular, and Medial Retropharyngeal Lymph Node Excision*).
- Precontrast and postcontrast computed tomography (CT) scan of the head and neck for surgical planning
- Thoracic CT scan for assessment of lung metastasis

Patient Positioning

The patient is positioned in lateral, dorsolateral, or dorsal recumbency. A mouth gag should be placed on the contralateral mandibular and maxillary canine teeth to improve exposure. Mouth gags should be used with caution in cats because of the risk of cortical blindness secondary to compression of the maxillary artery; 20- or 30-mm plastic gags are preferred to spring-loaded gags [1]. The pharynx should be packed with gauze sponges to minimize the risk of aspirating lavage fluid and blood.

Surgical Technique (See Plate 6.15A, B)

A) The labial and buccal aspects of the gingival mucosa and palatine mucoperiosteum are incised with a scalpel blade (i) with a minimum of 5- to 10-mm margins, and the mucosa (ii, iii) and mucoperiosteum (iv, arrows) are then elevated with a periosteal elevator (v, vi) to prepare for the osteotomy and protect soft tissues from iatrogenic damage during the osteotomies. Bleeding from the transected major palatine artery can typically be controlled with digital pressure, but ligation or cautery may be required.

Color Atlas of Canine and Feline Surgical Oncology, First Edition. Julius M. Liptak, Paolo Buracco, William T. N. Culp, and Nicholas J. Bacon.

Plate 6.15

Intraoral Approach for Caudal and Total Unilateral Maxillectomy

1A)

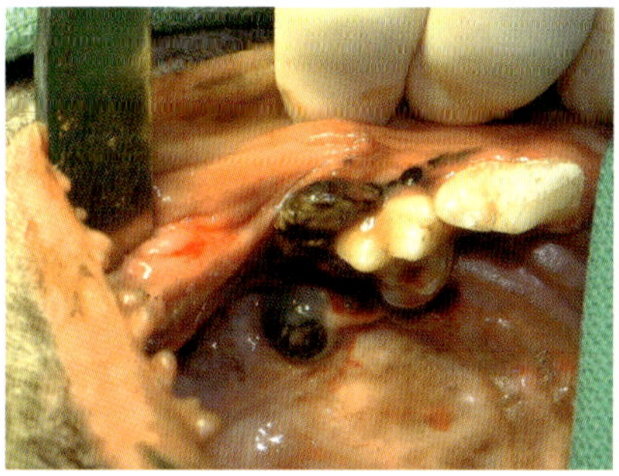

1B)

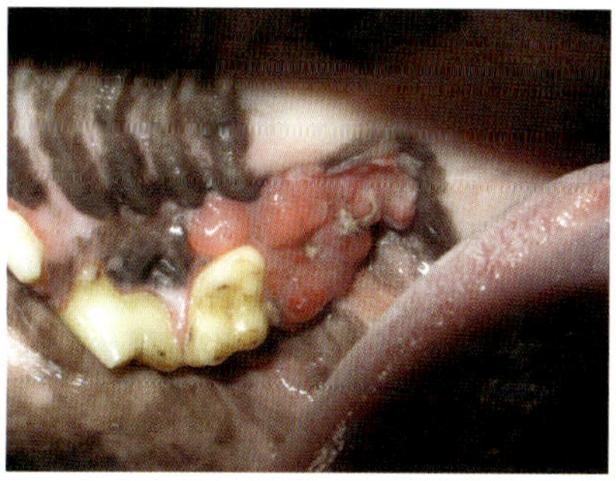

1C)

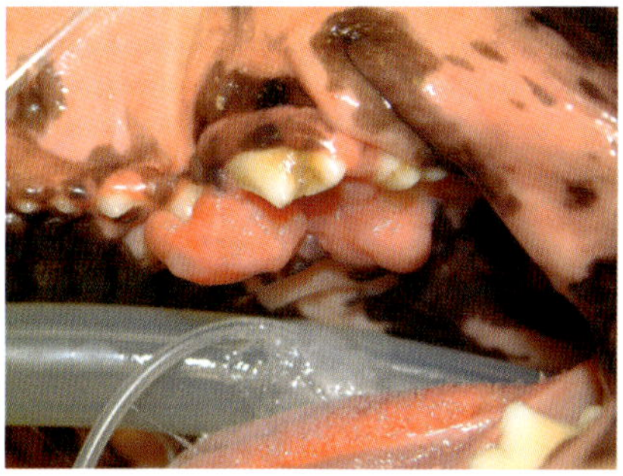

A-i)

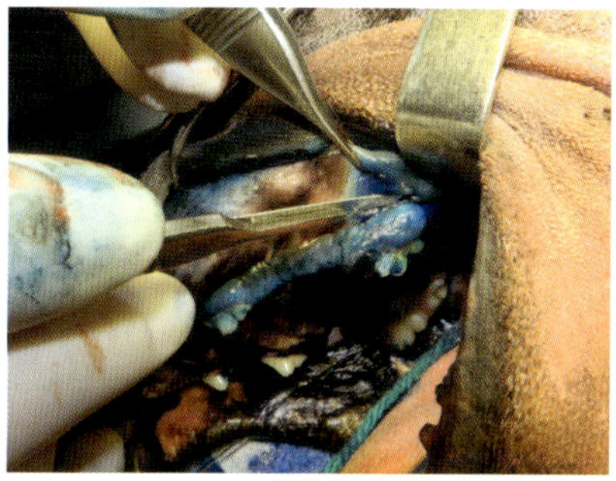

A-ii)

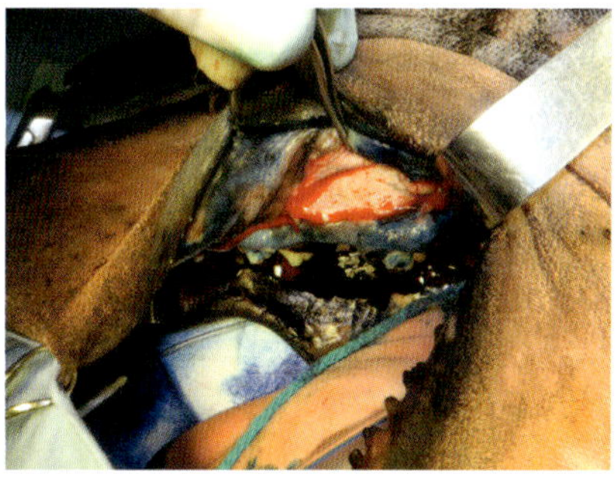

A-iii)

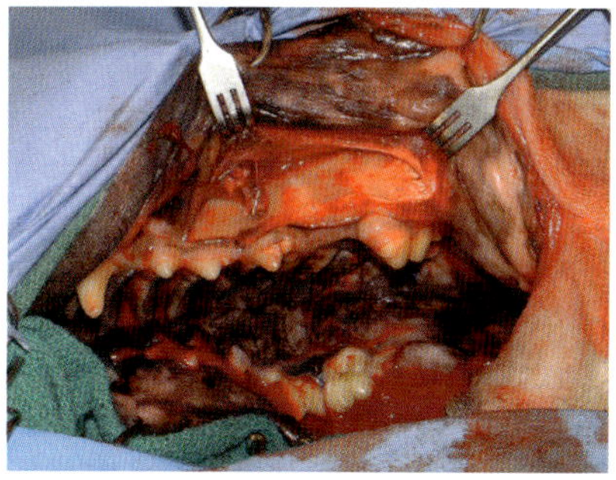

A-iv)

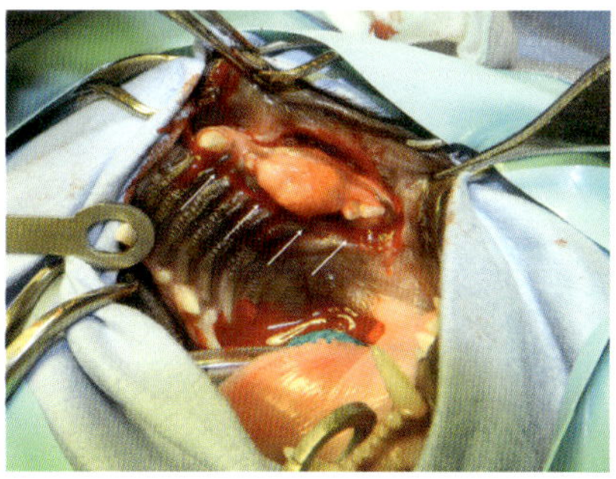

A-v)

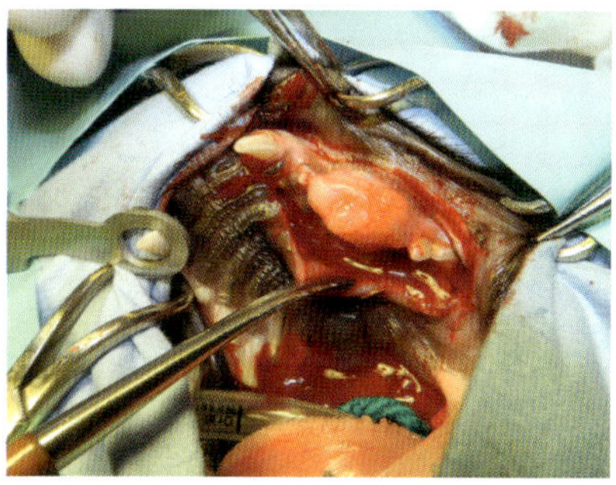

A-vi)

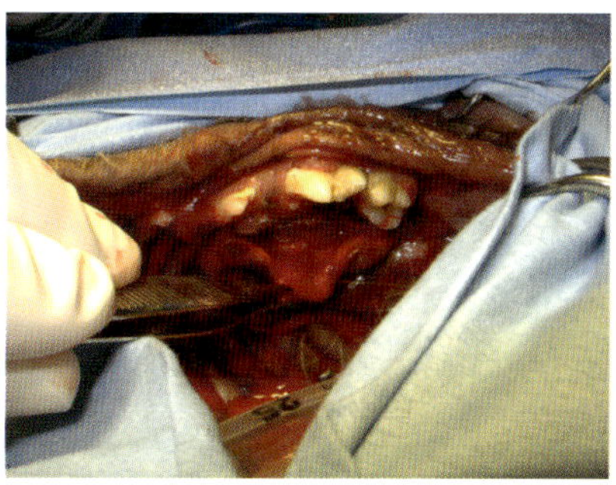

Surgical Technique (See Plate 6.15A, B) *continued*

B) Osteotomies are performed, with a minimum of 1-cm bone margins for benign tumors and 2-cm bone margins for malignant tumors, in the following order: rostral (i), lateral (ii, iii), palatine (iv, v), and caudal (vi–viii). The palatine and caudal osteotomies are performed last because these have the greatest potential for bleeding; the degree of blood loss can be minimized by reducing the interval between these osteotomies and removal of the maxillary bone segment to be able to identify and control the transected vessels. Alternatively, ligation of the maxillary artery before caudal maxillectomy has been described to reduce intraoperative blood loss from transection of this vessel during the caudal osteotomy [2].

Plate 6.15

Intraoral Approach for Caudal and Total Unilateral Maxillectomy *continued*

B-i)
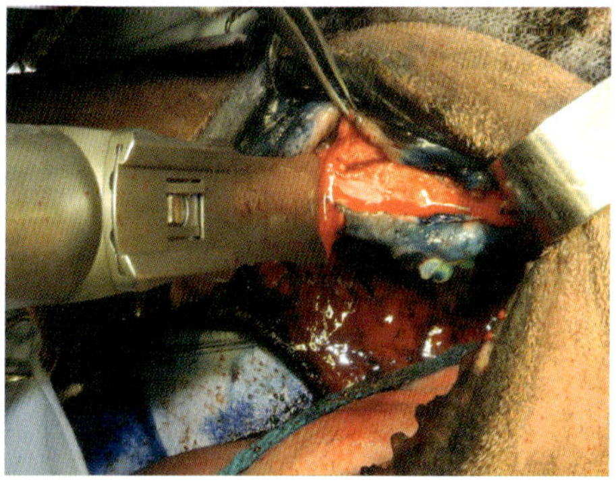

B-ii)
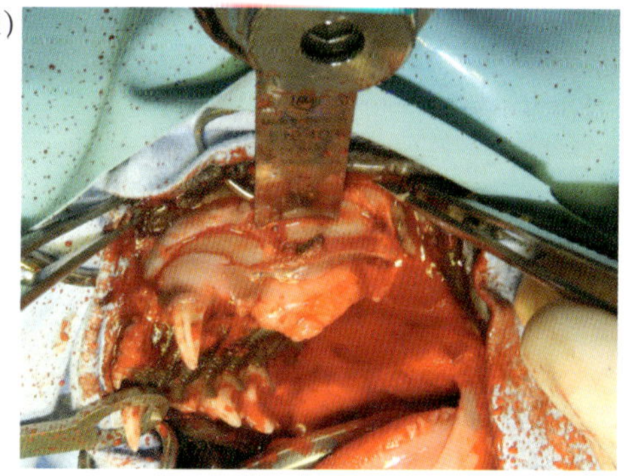

B-iii)
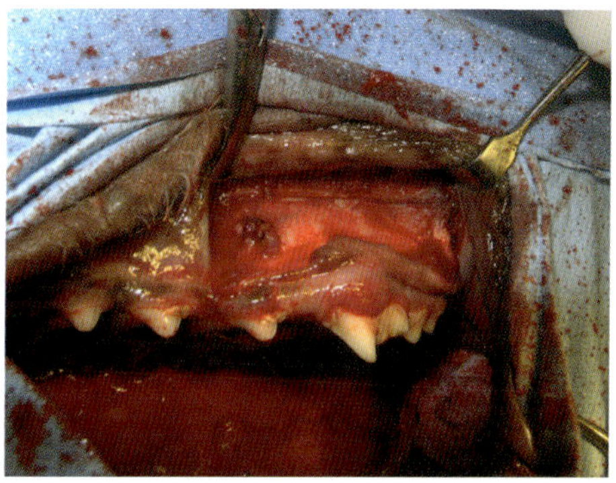

B-iv)
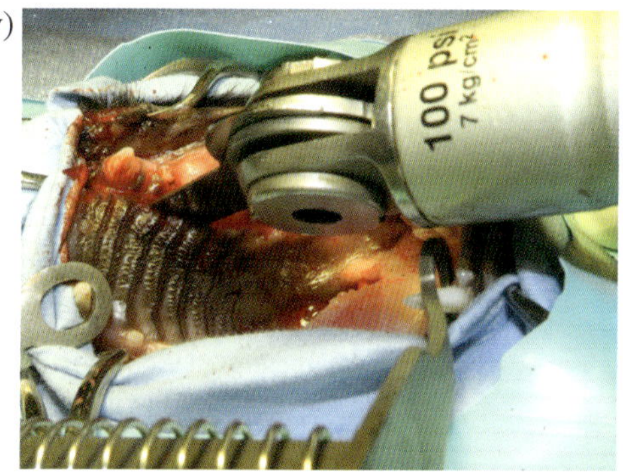

B-v)
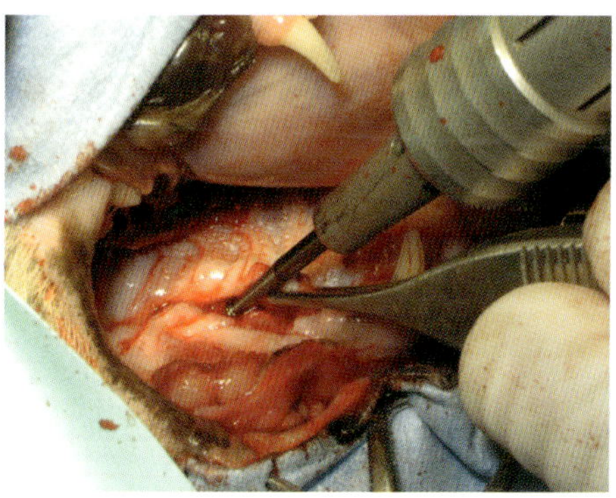

B-vi)
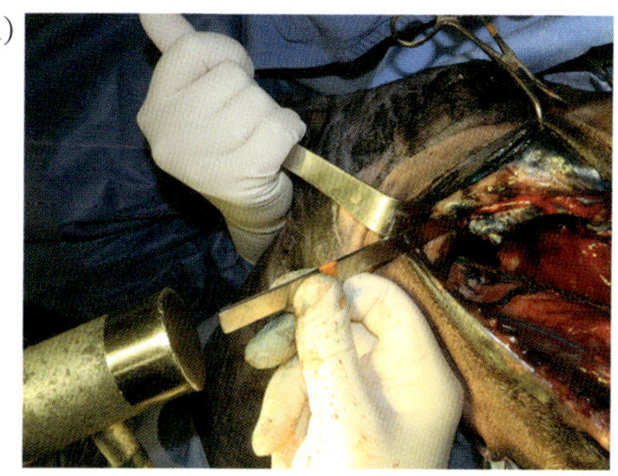

B-vii)
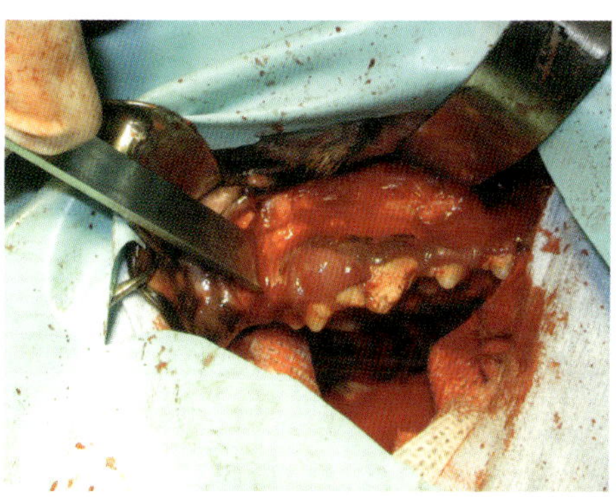

B-viii)
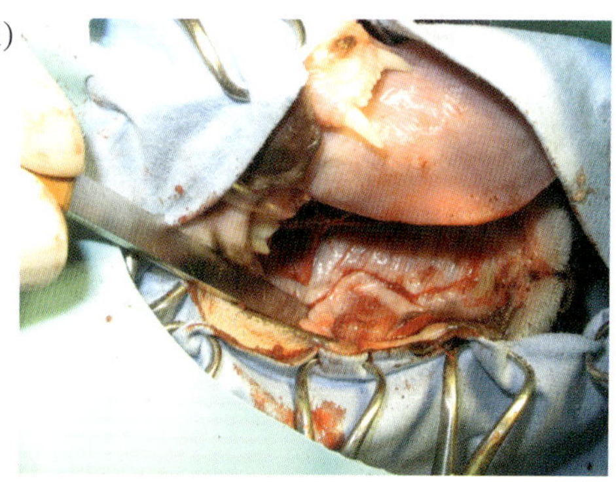

Surgical Technique (See Plate 6.15A, B) *continued*

These osteotomies can be performed with an oscillating or sagittal saw, pneumatic drill, piezoelectric instruments, or osteotome and mallet. After completion of the osteotomies, the free bone segment should be gently elevated and removed from the surgical field (ix, x). If the bone segment is not free, then an osteotome and mallet should be used along each of the osteotomies to ensure that these osteotomies are full thickness through the bone and that they connect at each of the intersections between each of the osteotomies. The maxillary artery should be identified and ligated after removal of the free bone segment. Bleeding from the exposed nasal turbinates can be controlled with tamponade, ice-cold saline, 0.05% oxymetazoline spray, or thrombin-impregnated sponges [3, 4].

C) Exposed tooth roots are extracted with a dental elevator (not pictured).

Closure (See Plate 6.15D–F)

D) A labial mucosal-submucosal flap is raised by undermining the labial and buccal mucosa and submucosa with Metzenbaum scissors from the incised edge of the labial and buccal mucosa toward the ventral margins of the lips.
E) The labial mucosal-submucosal flap is advanced into the oral defect and closed in two layers using monofilament absorbable suture material on a reverse cutting needle. The submucosa of the labial mucosal-submucosal flap is sutured to either predrilled holes in the hard palate (i) using an interrupted suture pattern (ii) or to the submucosa of the mucoperiosteum in a simple continuous suture pattern.
F) The mucosa of the labial mucosal-submucosal flap is then sutured to the mucosa of the mucoperiosteum in either an interrupted (i) or simple continuous suture pattern (ii).

Postoperative Management

1) Multimodal analgesia
2) Soft foods for 28 days
3) No chewing on hard objects or playing with toys for 28 days
4) Elizabethan collar
5) Note that feeding tubes are rarely required in either dogs or cats after intraoral caudal or total unilateral maxillectomy

Complications – Dogs [4]

Intraoperative Complications

- Intraoperative blood loss (54%) with 24% of these dogs requiring a blood transfusion

Postoperative Complications (<48 Hours)* (See Plate 6.15G, H)

- Epistaxis (56–67%; G, 1 day postoperative)
- Facial swelling (44%–58%; H, 1 day postoperative)
- Facial pawing (14%–17%)
- Eating difficulties (16%–22%)

---

* These complications are for all caudal maxillectomy and total unilateral maxillectomy procedures regardless of the surgical approach (intraoral or combined).

Plate 6.15

Intraoral Approach for Caudal and Total Unilateral Maxillectomy *continued*

B-ix)

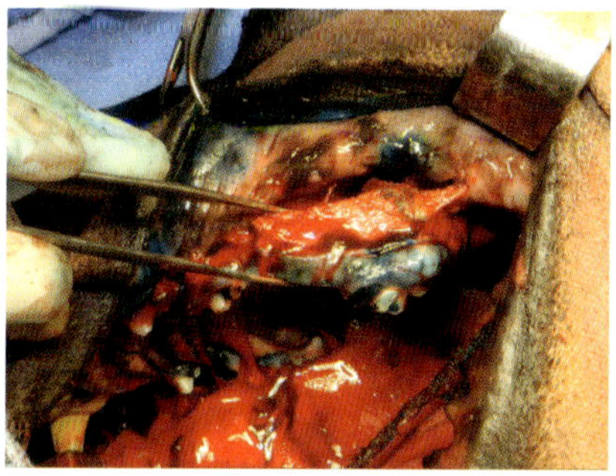

B-x)

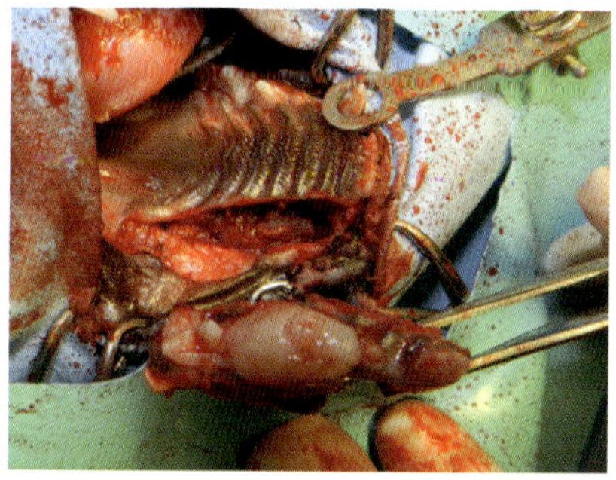

D)

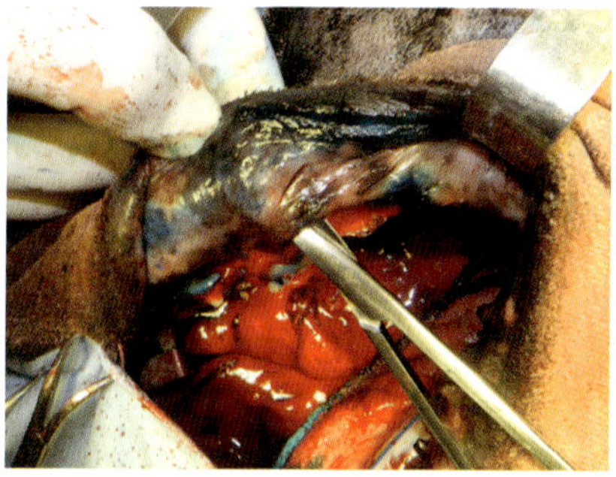

E-i)

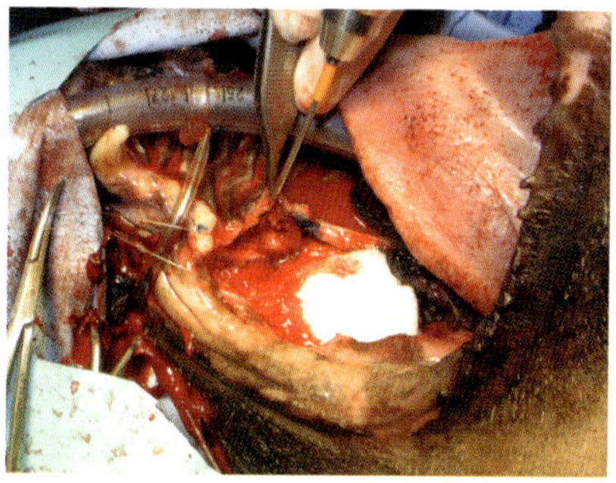

E-ii)

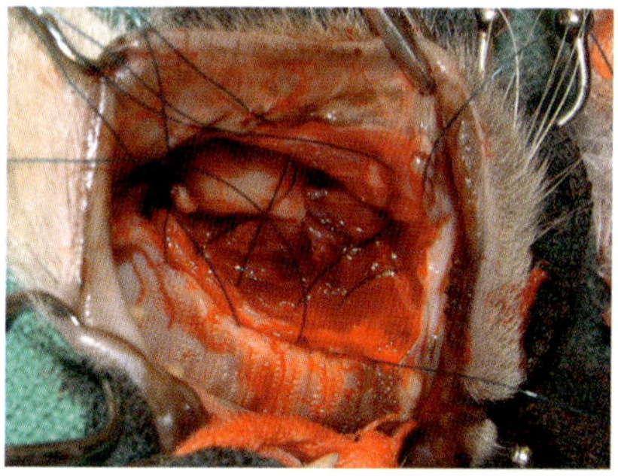

F-i)

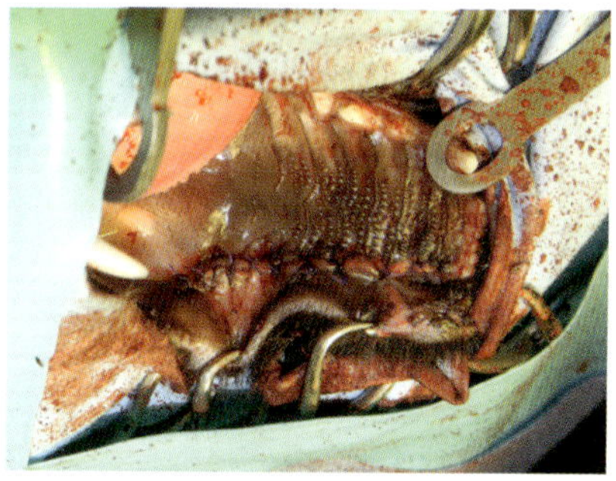

F-ii)

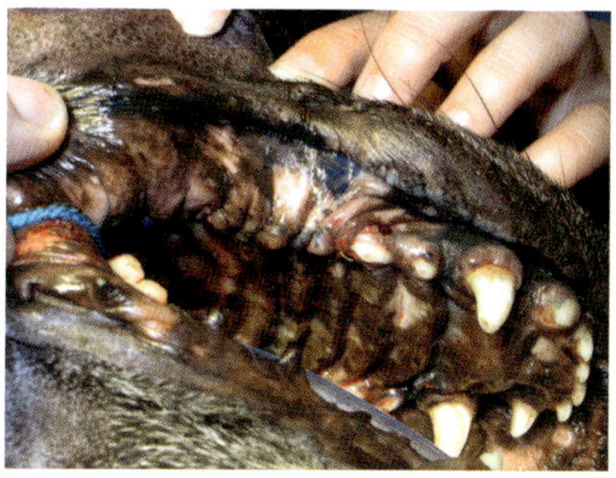

G)

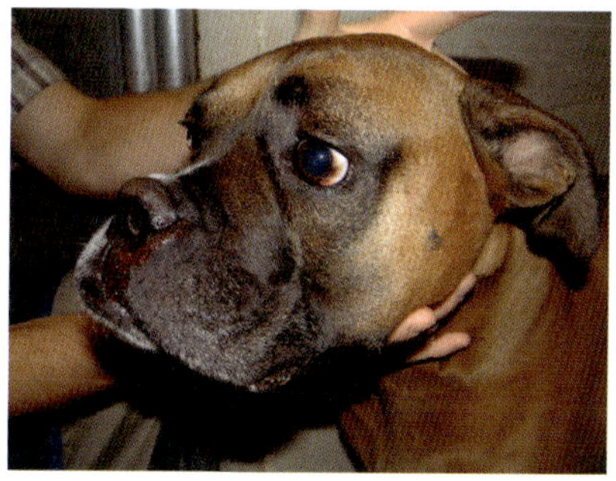

H)

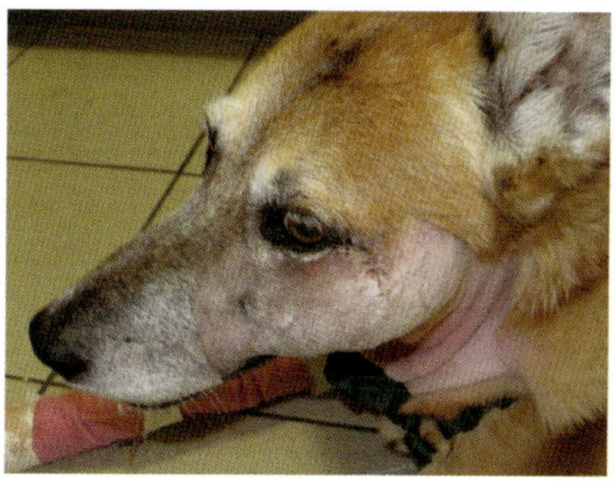

Postoperative Complications (48 Hours to 4 Weeks)[†] (See Plate 6.15I)

- Trauma to the upper lip as a result of the lip being drawn into the occlusal plane of the ipsilateral mandibular canine tooth (10%–18%)
- Incisional dehiscence (13%–18%)
- Oronasal fistula (16%–18%; I, 14 days postoperatively)
- Surgical-site infection (10%–12%)
- Epiphora (13%–24%)

Complications – Cats[‡] [5] (See Plate 6.15J, K)

- Epistaxis (13%; J, 1 day postoperative)
- Wound dehiscence and oronasal fistula (29%; K, 21 days postoperatively)
- Trauma to the upper lip as a result of the lip being drawn into the occlusal plane of the ipsilateral mandibular canine tooth (15%)
- Eating difficulties (15%)
- Facial swelling (10%)
- Subcutaneous emphysema (2%)
- Hypersalivation and drooling (2%)

Cosmetic Appearance (See Plate 6.15L, M)

The lip can be drawn toward the midline because of the use of the labial mucosal-submucosal flap for reconstruction of the intraoral defect. This results in a scalloping of the lateral muzzle (L). The extent of this scalloping and medialization of the lip depends on the medial extent of the resection, the width of the lip, and the length of the labial mucosal-submucosal flap (M).

Suggested Adjuvant Treatments

- See *6. Mandibulectomy and Maxillectomy*.

Prognosis and Oncologic Outcome

- See *6. Mandibulectomy and Maxillectomy*.

References

1 Reiter, A.M. (2014). Open wide: blindness in cats after the use of mouth gags. *Vet. J.* 201: 5–6.

2 Carrol, K.A. and Mathews, K.G. (2020). Ligation of the maxillary artery prior to caudal maxillectomy in the dog – a description of the technique, retrospective evaluation of blood loss, and cadaveric evaluation of maxillary artery anatomy. *Front. Vet. Sci.* 7: 588945.

3 Liptak, J.M. and Lascelles, B.D.X. (2012). Oral tumors. In: *Veterinary Surgical Oncology*, 1e (ed. S.T. Kudnig and B. Séguin), 119–178. Wiley-Blackwell.

4 MacLellan, R.H., Rawlinson, J.E., Rao, S. et al. (2018). Intraoperative and postoperative complications of partial maxillectomy for the treatment of oral tumors in dogs. *J. Am. Vet. Med. Assoc.* 252 (12): 1538–1547.

5 Liptak, J.M., Thatcher, G.P., Mestrinho, L.A. et al. (2021). Outcomes of cats treated with maxillectomy: 60 cases. A veterinary society of surgical oncology retrospective study. *Vet. Comp. Oncol.* 19 (4): 641–650.

---

† These complications are for all caudal maxillectomy and total unilateral maxillectomy procedures regardless of the surgical approach (intraoral or combined).

‡ These complications are for all maxillectomy procedures and not specifically for caudal maxillectomy and total unilateral maxillectomy through an intraoral approach.

Plate 6.15

Intraoral Approach for Caudal and Total Unilateral Maxillectomy *continued*

I)
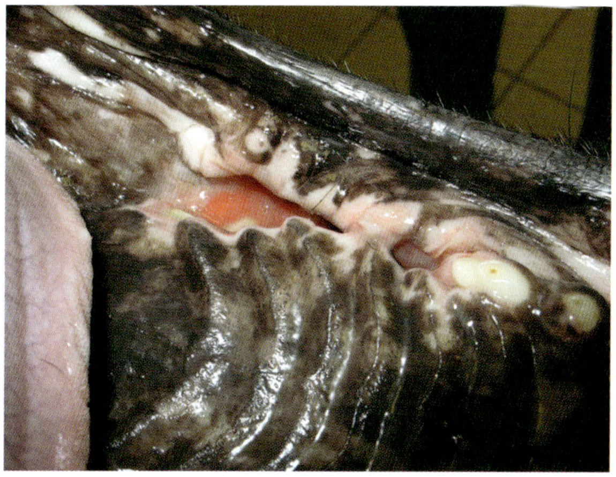

J)
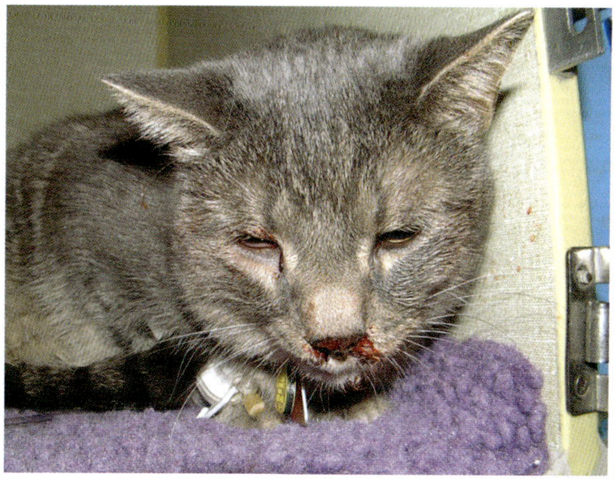

K)
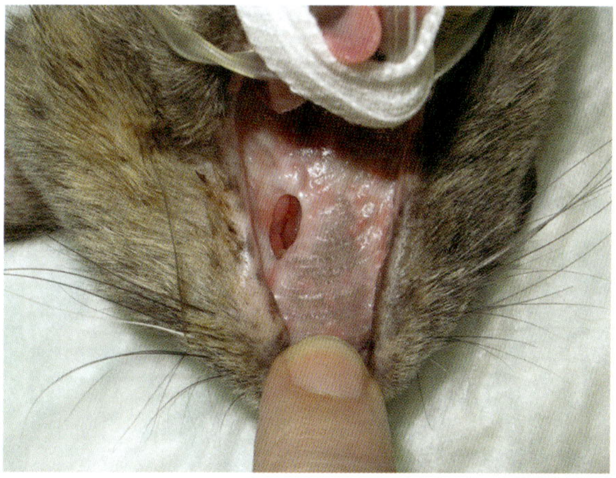

L)
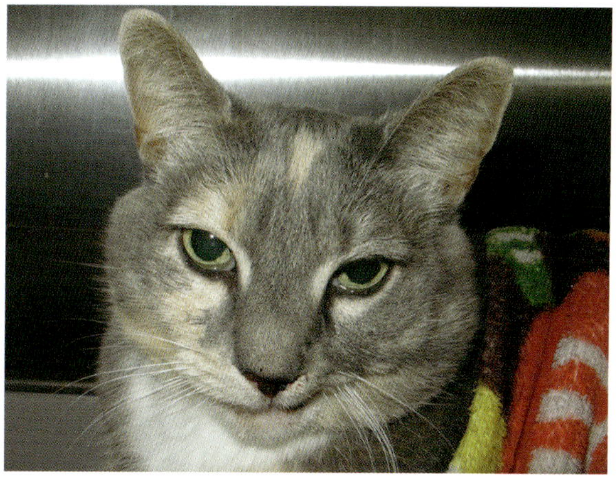

M)
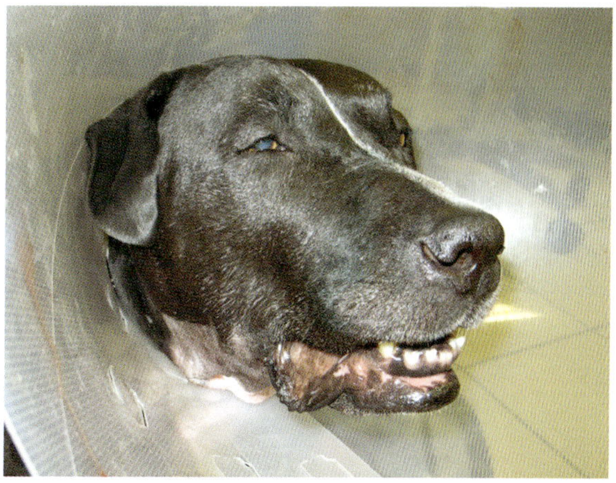

6.16 Combined Approach for Caudal and Total Unilateral Maxillectomy

Indications (See Plate 6.16 – 1, 2)

1) Resection of benign (i, acanthomatous ameloblastoma) and malignant oral tumors (ii, squamous cell carcinoma) located in the mid-to-caudal maxilla and either arise or extend dorsolaterally and/or caudally to the alveolar margin. The combined approach provides better exposure, with better ability to achieve hemostasis and completely excise the tumor, compared with the intraoral approach for more extensive caudal maxillary tumors.
2) The combined approach can be combined with either an inferior or subtotal orbitectomy (pictured, postoperative orbitectomy specimen), enucleation (see *2.1. Enucleation*) or exenteration (see *2.2. Exenteration*), or a craniectomy.

Suggested Diagnostic Workup and Clinical Staging for Malignant Maxillary Tumors

- Complete blood count, serum biochemistry, and urinalysis
- Preoperative biopsy
- Regional lymph node assessment for evaluation of lymph node metastasis
  - Fine-needle aspirate cytology of the mandibular lymph nodes
  - Sentinel lymph node mapping and excision of the sentinel lymph node (see *50.1. Sentinel Lymph Node Mapping*)
  - Nonselective excision of the bilateral mandibular and medial retropharyngeal lymph nodes through a ventral midline cervical approach (see *50.3. Combined Mandibular and Medial Retropharyngeal Lymph Node Excision*), or excision of the ipsilateral mandibular, medial retropharyngeal, and parotid lymph nodes through a lateral approach (see *50.4. Combined Parotid, Mandibular, and Medial Retropharyngeal Lymph Node Excision*)
- Precontrast and postcontrast computed tomography (CT) scan of the head and neck for surgical planning
- Thoracic CT scan for assessment of lung metastasis

Patient Positioning

The patient is positioned in lateral recumbency. A mouth gag should be placed on the contralateral mandibular and maxillary canine teeth to improve exposure. Mouth gags should be used with caution in cats because of the risk of cortical blindness secondary to compression of the maxillary artery; 20- or 30-mm plastic gags are preferred to spring-loaded gags [1]. The pharynx should be packed with gauze sponges to minimize the risk of aspirating lavage fluid and blood.

Color Atlas of Canine and Feline Surgical Oncology, First Edition. Julius M. Liptak, Paolo Buracco, William T. N. Culp, and Nicholas J. Bacon.

Plate 6.16

Combined Approach for Caudal and Total Unilateral Maxillectomy

1-i)

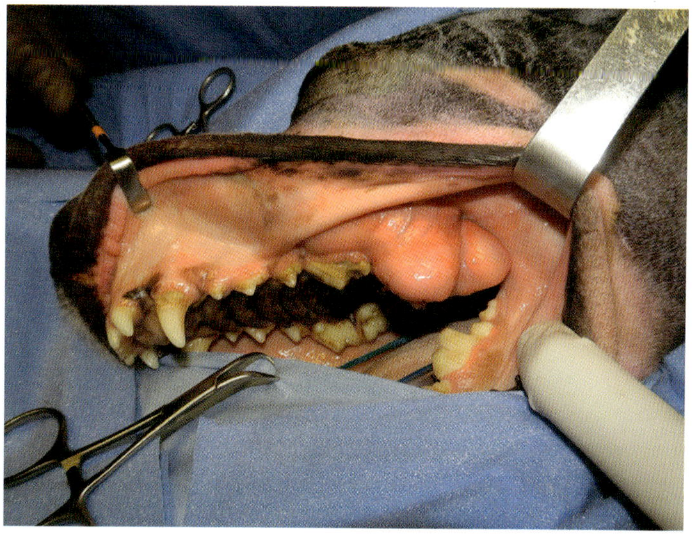

1-ii)

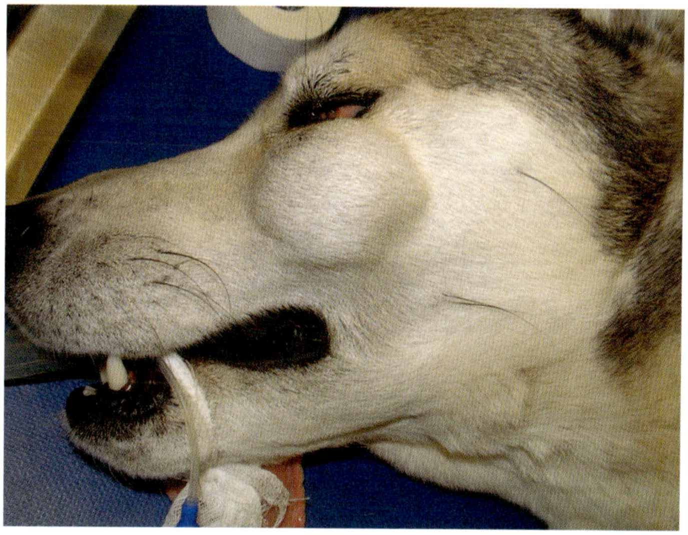

2)

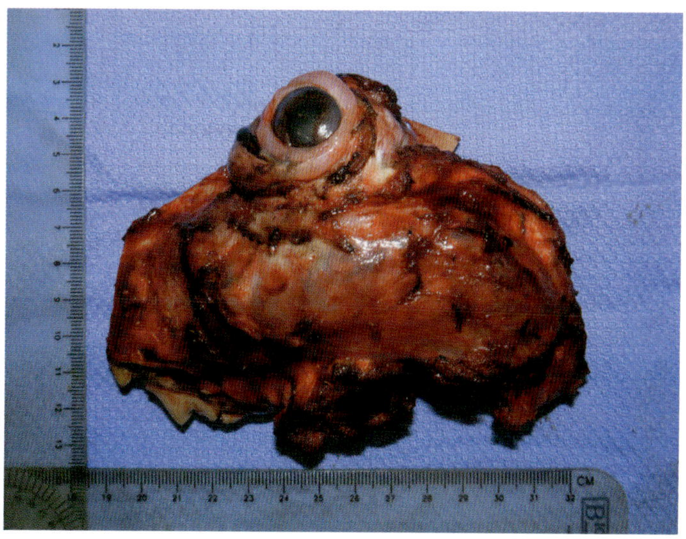

Surgical Technique [2] (See Plate 6.16A, B, D–H)

A) A skin incision is made on or lateral to the dorsal midline of the muzzle and extended caudally and ventrally to the eye along the zygomatic bone (i). The skin incision is continued deeply through the subcutaneous tissue, between the paired levator nasolabialis muscles, and down to bone (ii). The dorsal margins are prepared by reflecting the periosteum and associated soft tissues with a periosteal elevator. The ventral aspect of the globe is separated from the dorsal aspect of the rostral zygomatic arch (ZA) with a combination of sharp and blunt dissection. The conjunctival sac should be preserved.

B) The ZA is isolated by incising and elevating the masseter muscle (MM) from the ventral aspect of the ZA and the temporalis muscle (TM) from the dorsal aspect of the ZA.

C) If possible, the maxillary artery should be ligated and divided before performing the osteotomies for resection of the maxillary tumor [3]. The maxillary artery courses along the ventral aspect of the orbit. Identification and subsequent ligation of the maxillary artery should be attempted by gently retracting the globe dorsally. If identified and accessible, the maxillary artery can be ligated with suture material, metallic clips, or a vessel sealing device (not pictured).

D) The labial and buccal aspects of the gingival mucosa are incised with a scalpel blade with a minimum of 5- to 10-mm margins (i). The mucosal incision is continued down to the bone and undermined with periosteal elevators (ii) and scissors (iii) to connect the mucosal and dorsal skin incisions and create a bipedicle flap (iv). This bipedicle flap can be retracted dorsally to improve intraoral exposure (v) and ventrally to improve dorsal and caudal exposure (vi). The infraorbital artery and vein, which will be encountered during this dissection along with the infraorbital nerve, should be individually ligated, cauterized, or sealed. The facial vein should also be ligated at the most dorsocaudal aspect of the incision, but the facial vein should be preserved, if possible, at the level of the dorsal nasal tributary to facilitate venous drainage from the muzzle.

Plate 6.16

Combined Approach for Caudal and Total Unilateral Maxillectomy *continued*

A-i)

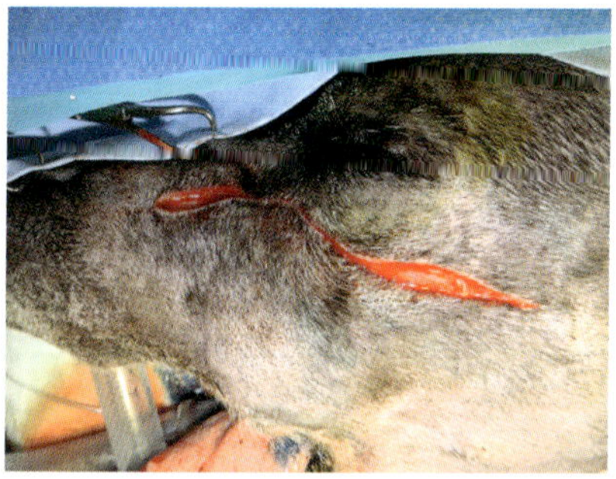

A-ii)

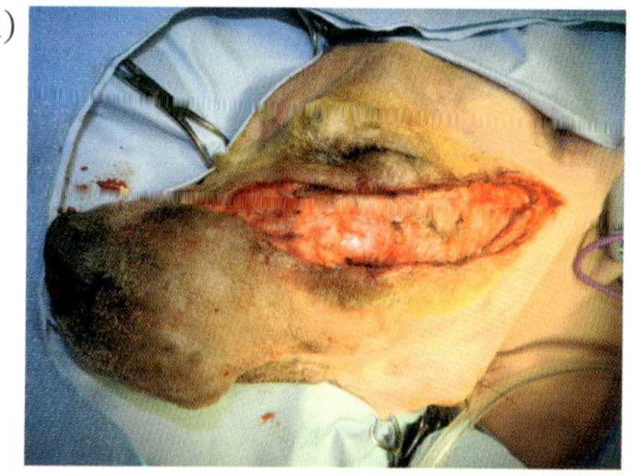

B)

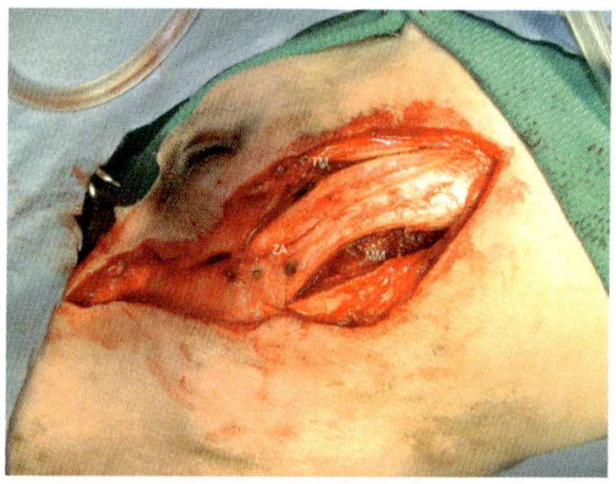

D-i)

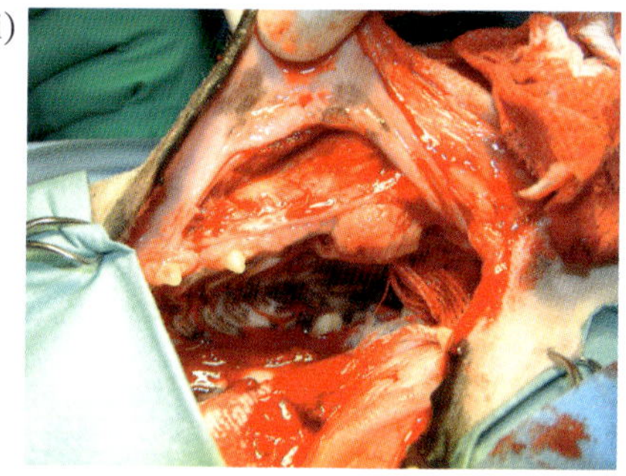

D-ii)

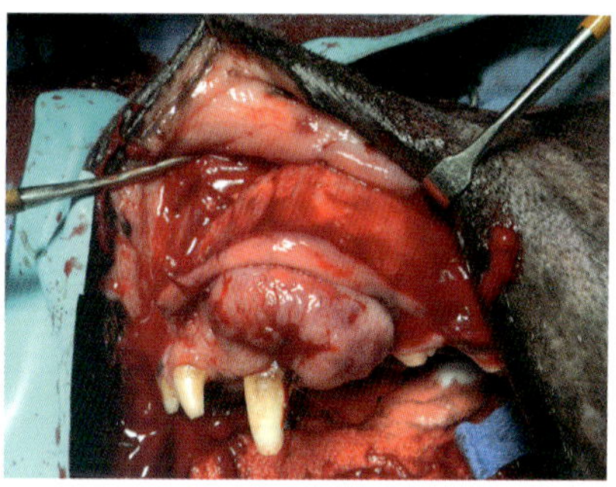

D-iii)

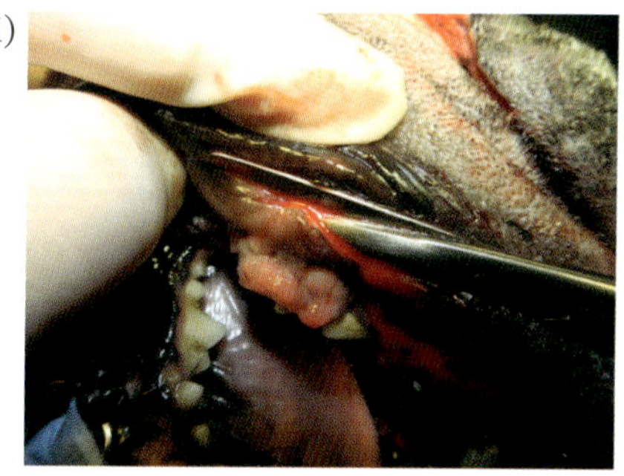

D-iv)

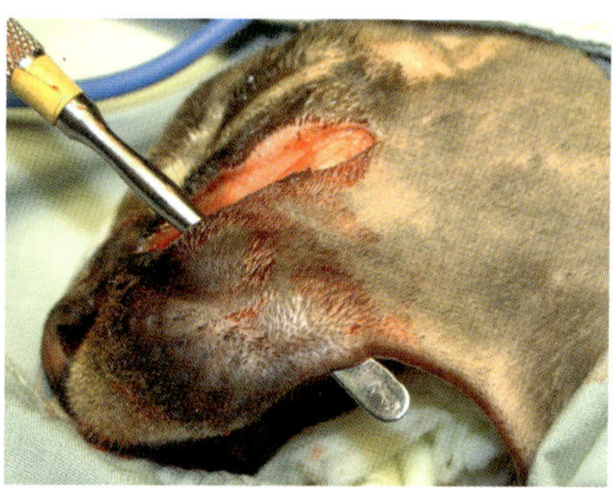

D-v)

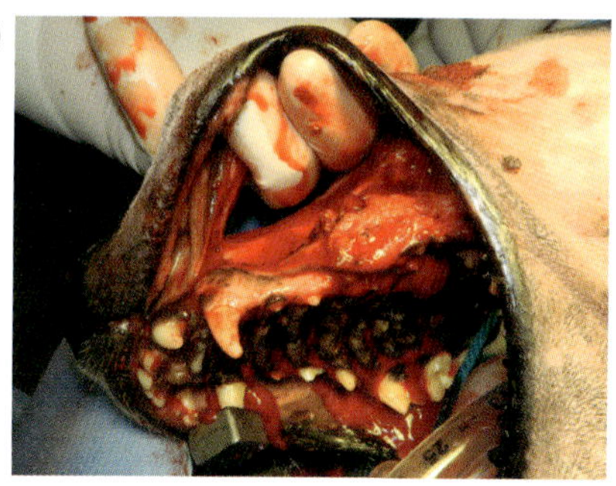

D-vi)

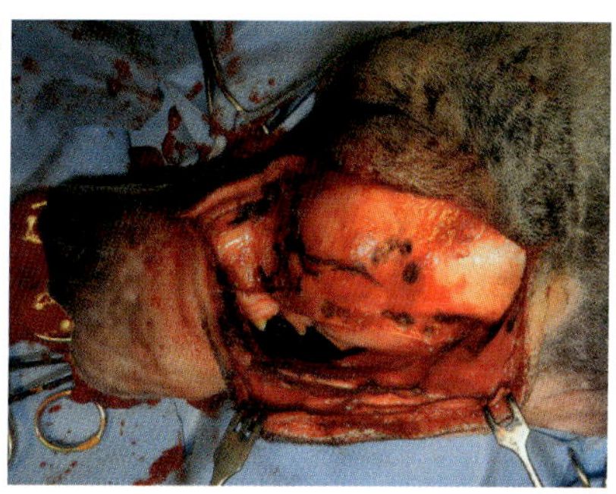

Surgical Technique [2] (See Plate 6.16A, B, D–H) *continued*

E) The palatine mucoperiosteum is incised with a scalpel blade with a minimum of 5- to 10-mm margins. The mucoperiosteum is then elevated with a periosteal elevator (pictured) to prepare for the palatine osteotomy and protect the mucoperiosteum from iatrogenic damage during the palatine osteotomy. Bleeding from the transected major palatine artery can typically be controlled with digital pressure, but ligation or cautery may be required.

F) Osteotomies are performed, with a minimum of 1-cm bone margins for benign tumors and 2-cm bone margins for malignant tumors, in the following order: ZA (i, ii), rostral (iii), dorsolateral (iv) to dorsal (v), palatine (vi, vii), and caudal. For a combined maxillectomy-orbitectomy, the ZA osteotomy typically needs to be positioned more caudally (viii). The palatine and caudal osteotomies are performed last because these have the greatest potential for bleeding; the degree of blood loss can be minimized by reducing the interval between these osteotomies and removal of the maxillary bone segment to be able to identify and control the transected maxillary artery. These osteotomies can be performed with an oscillating, sagittal, or biradial saw, pneumatic drill, piezoelectric instruments, or osteotome and mallet.

Plate 6.16

Combined Approach for Caudal and Total Unilateral Maxillectomy *continued*

F)

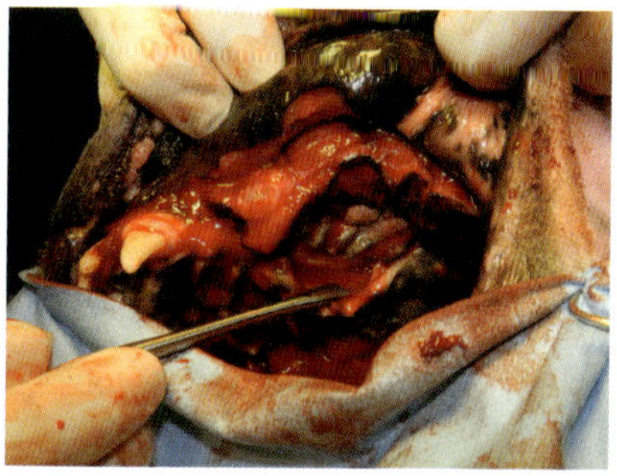

F-i)

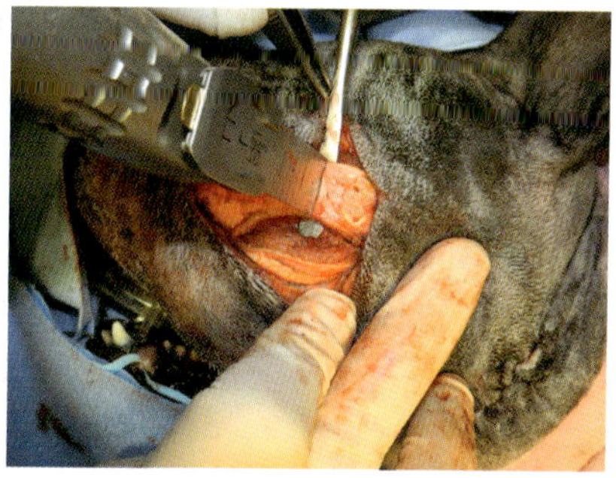

F-ii)

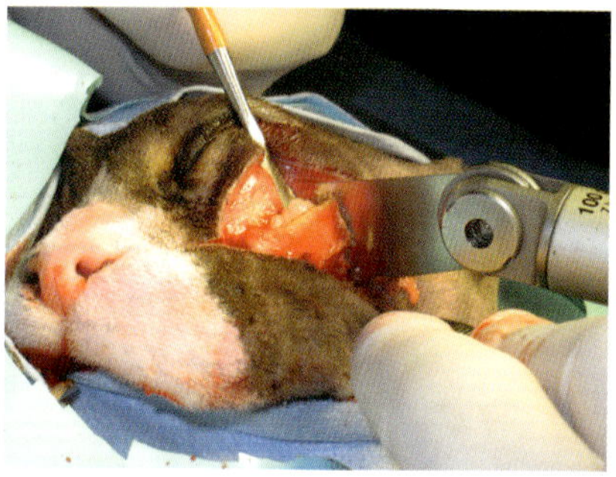

F-iii)

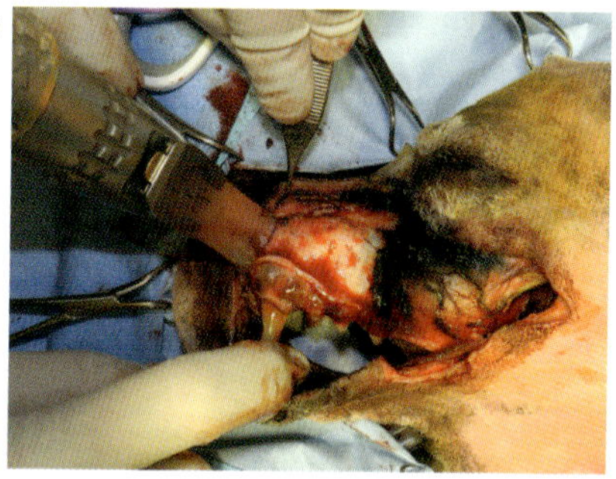

F-iv)

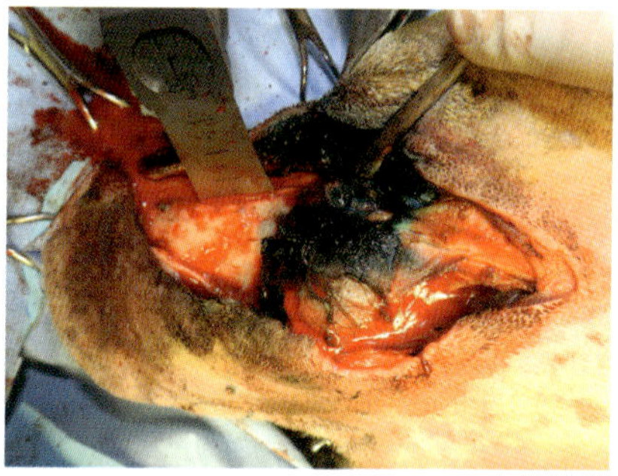

F-v)

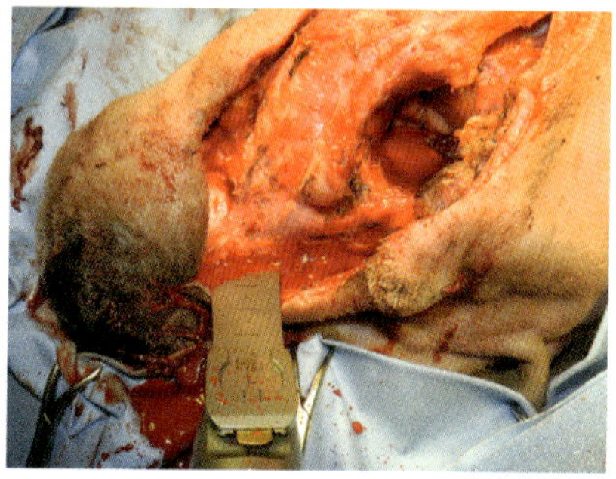

F-vi)

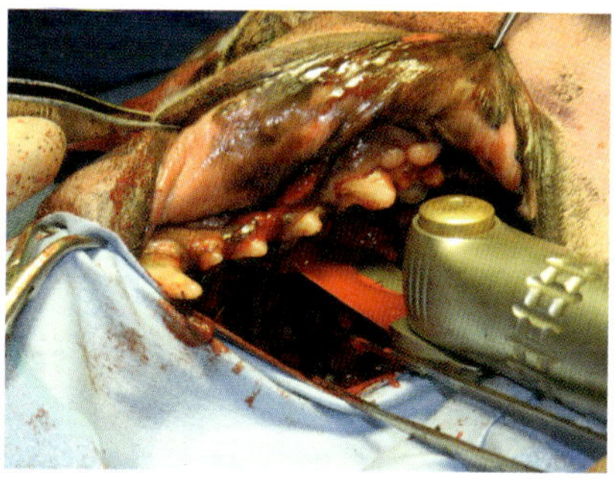

F-vii)

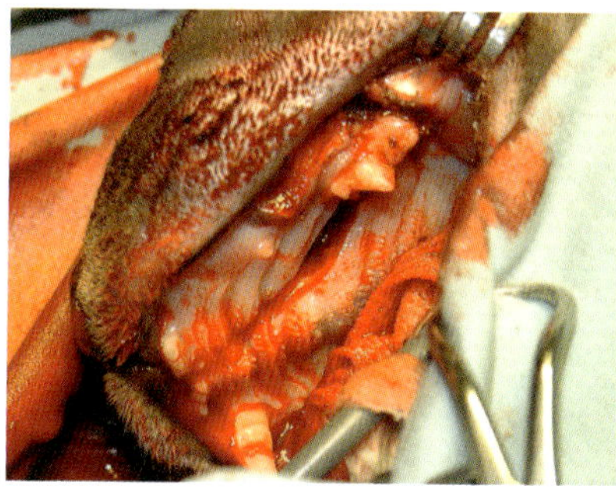

F-viii)

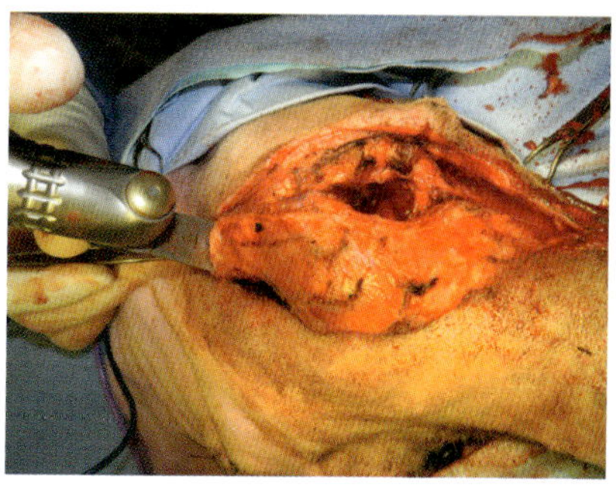

Surgical Technique [2] (See Plate 6.16A, B, D–H) *continued*

G) The caudal osteotomy is often performed within the inferior orbit (i), but this caudal margin may be rostral to the orbit (ii) or can be extended farther caudally to include an orbitectomy (iii, iv) or craniectomy if required. If the caudal osteotomy is performed at the level of the inferior orbit, then the globe is gently retracted caudally and dorsally, and an osteotomy is performed infraorbitally with an osteotome and mallet (i) or, if there is adequate exposure, an oscillating or sagittal saw (v). The osteotome is positioned at the junction between the inferior orbit and caudal maxilla, caudal to the molar teeth, and directed ventrally within the inferior orbit to connect the lateral maxillary and palatine osteotomies. If the caudal osteotomy has to be positioned farther caudally to achieve adequate surgical margins, then an enucleation (see *2.1. Enucleation*) or exenteration (see *2.2. Exenteration*) will likely be required for adequate exposure of the orbit to be able to perform the en bloc orbitectomy. Once the enucleation or exenteration has been completed, the caudal osteotomy is then completed as described earlier (iii, iv). After completion of the osteotomies, the free bone segment should be gently elevated and removed from the surgical field (vi). If the bone segment is not free, then an osteotome and mallet should be used along each of the osteotomies to ensure that these osteotomies are full thickness through the bone and that they connect at each of the intersections between each of the osteotomies.

H) If not done previously, the maxillary artery should be identified and ligated, cauterized, or sealed (pictured) after removal of the free bone segment. Bleeding from the exposed nasal turbinates can be controlled with tamponade, ice-cold saline, 0.05% oxymetazoline spray, or thrombin-impregnated sponges, although this is often unnecessary [4, 5].

I) Exposed tooth roots are extracted with a dental elevator (not pictured).

Closure (See Plate 6.16J–M)

J) A labial mucosal-submucosal flap is raised by undermining the buccal mucosa and submucosa with Metzenbaum scissors from the incised edge of the buccal mucosa toward the labial margins.

Plate 6.16

Combined Approach for Caudal and Total Unilateral Maxillectomy *continued*

G-i)

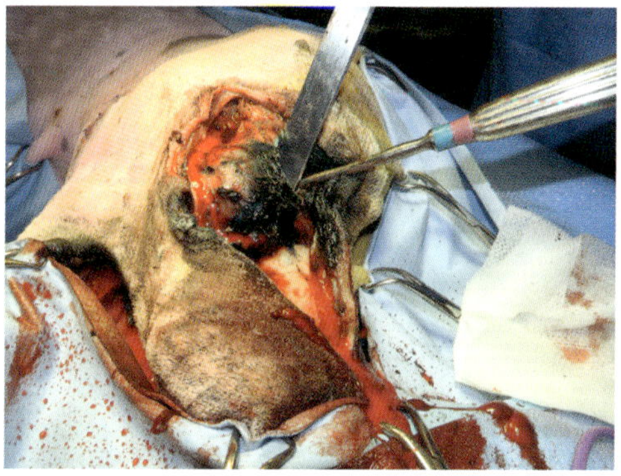

G-ii)

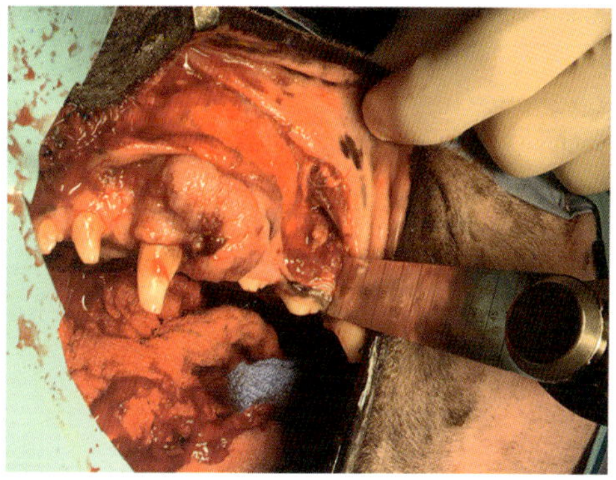

G-iii)

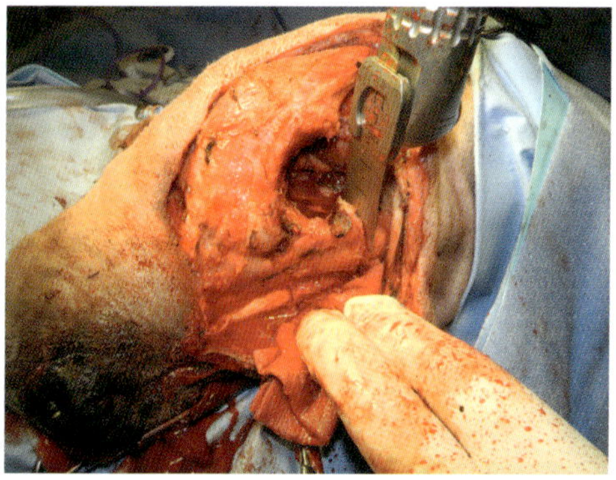

G-iv)

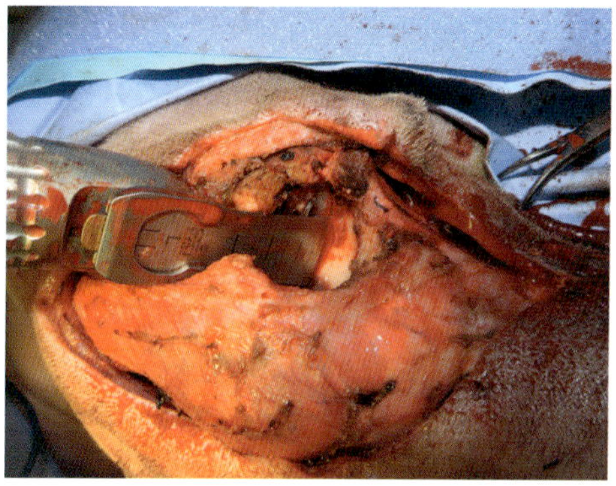

G-v)

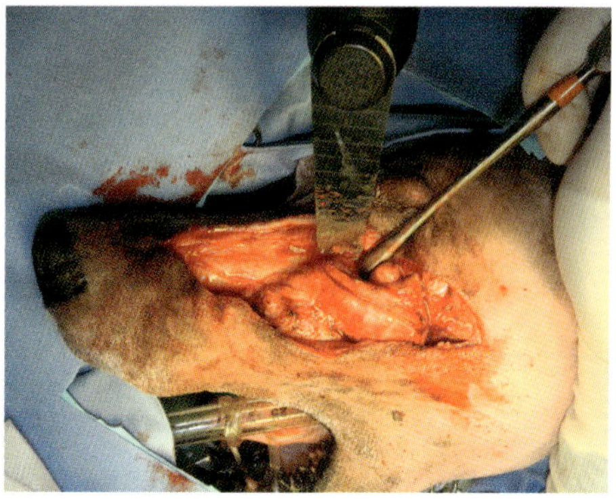

G-vi)

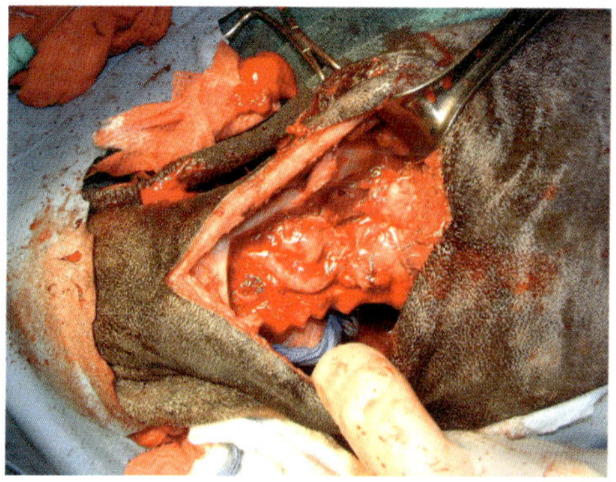

H)

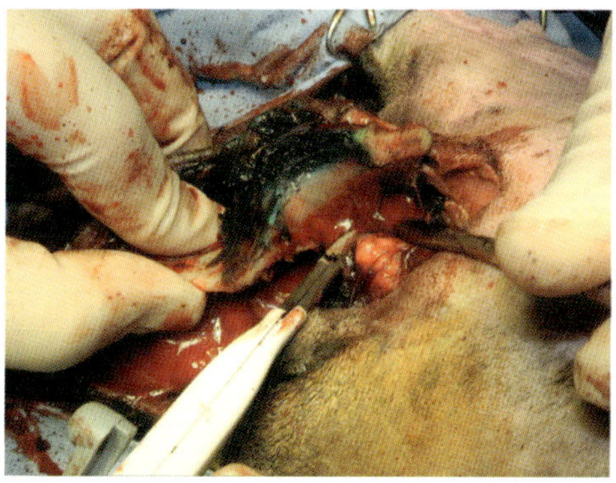

J)

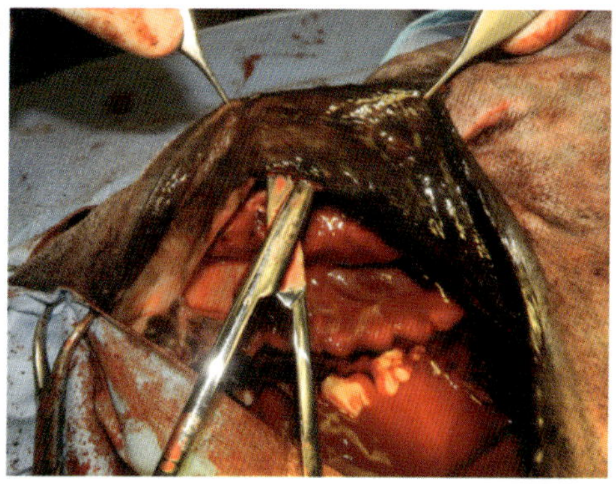

Closure (See Plate 6.16J–M) *continued*

K) The labial mucosal-submucosal flap (i, ii) is advanced into the oral defect and closed in two layers using monofilament absorbable suture material on a reverse cutting needle. This is best approached from a dorsal direction through the bipedicle flap (i, ii). If this closure is performed through the dorsal skin incision, then the buccal mucosa and mucoperiosteum of the hard palate are opposed using either an interrupted or continuous suture pattern (iii). The thick fibrovascular free edge of the lip is sutured to predrilled holes in the bone of the hard palate in an interrupted pattern.

L) If this closure is performed through an intraoral approach, which tends to be more awkward, then the submucosa of the labial mucosal-submucosal flap is sutured to either predrilled holes in the hard palate using an interrupted suture pattern (i) or to the submucosa of the mucoperiosteum in a simple continuous suture pattern. The mucosa of the labial mucosal-submucosal flap is then sutured to the mucosa of the mucoperiosteum in either an interrupted (ii) or simple continuous suture pattern (iii).

M) The dorsolateral skin incision is closed routinely in two layers with a simple continuous suture pattern using monofilament absorbable suture material in the subcutis and either an interrupted (pictured) or continuous suture pattern using monofilament nonabsorbable suture material in the skin.

Postoperative Management

1) Multimodal analgesia
2) Soft foods for 28 days
3) No chewing on hard objects or playing with toys for 28 days
4) Elizabethan collar
5) Note that feeding tubes are rarely required in either dogs or cats after a combined approach for caudal or total unilateral maxillectomy

Complications – Dogs [5]

Intraoperative Complications

- Intraoperative blood loss (83%) with 63% of these dogs requiring a blood transfusion

Postoperative Complications (<48 Hours)* (See Plate 6.16N, O)

- Epistaxis (56%–67%; N)
- Facial swelling (44%–58%; O)
- Facial pawing (14%–17%)
- Eating difficulties (16%–22%)

* These complications are for all caudal maxillectomy and total unilateral maxillectomy procedures regardless of the surgical approach (intraoral or combined).

Plate 6.16

Combined Approach for Caudal and Total Unilateral Maxillectomy *continued*

K-i)

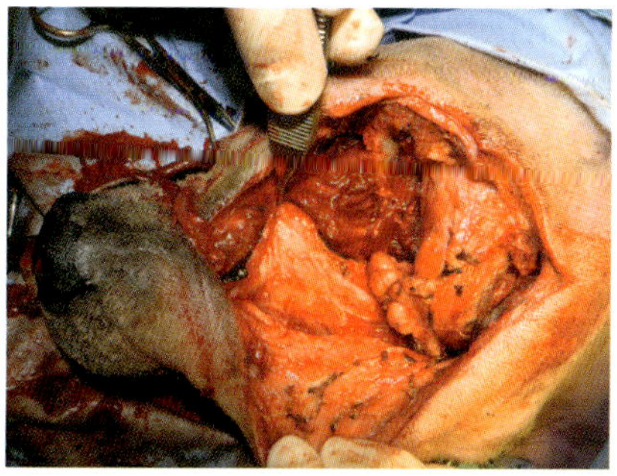

K-ii)

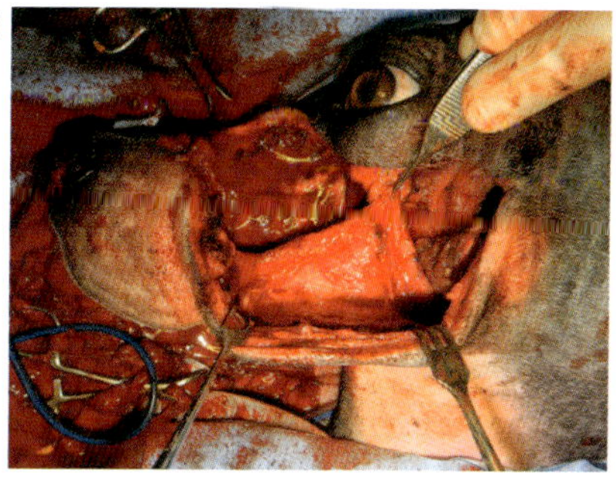

K-iii)

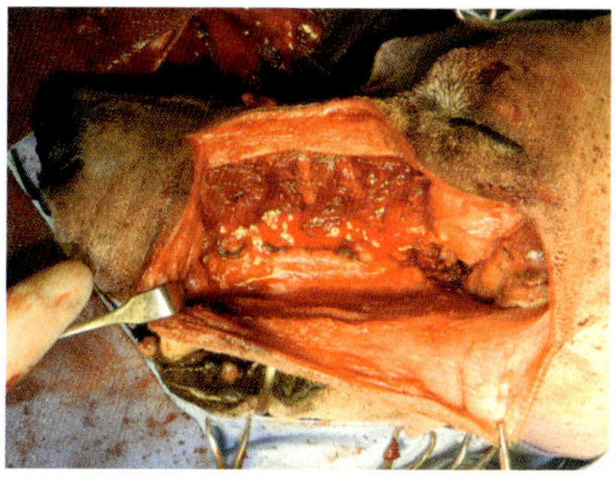

L-i)

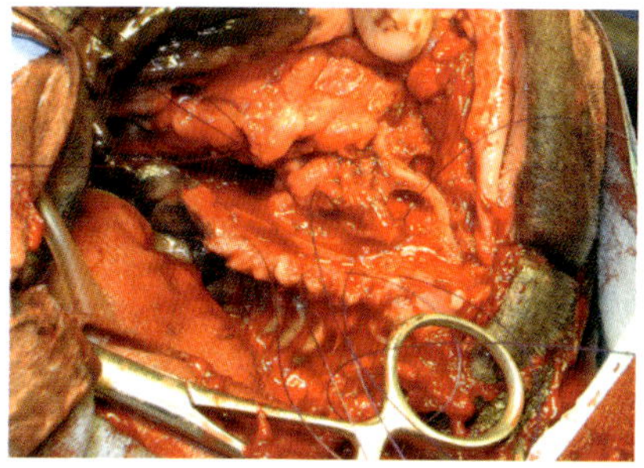

L-ii)

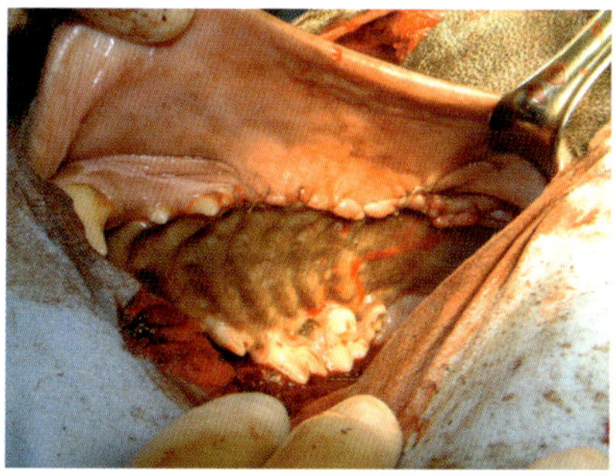

L-iii)

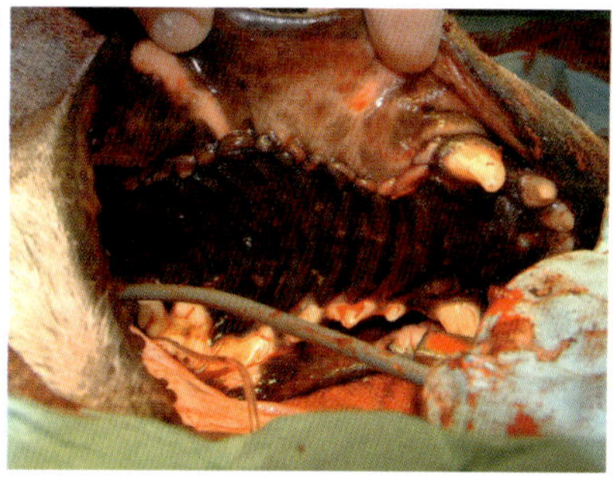

M)

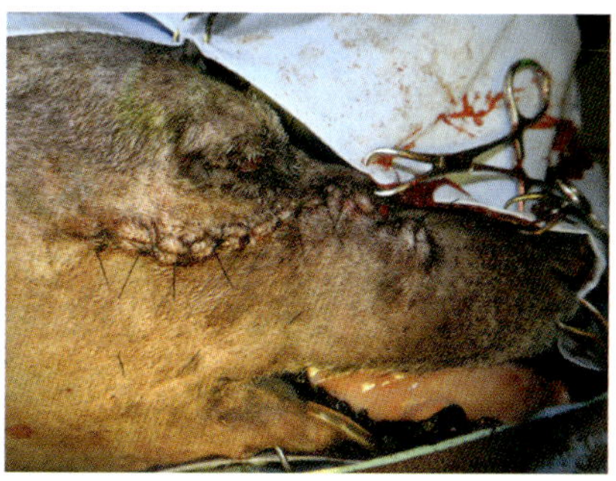

N)

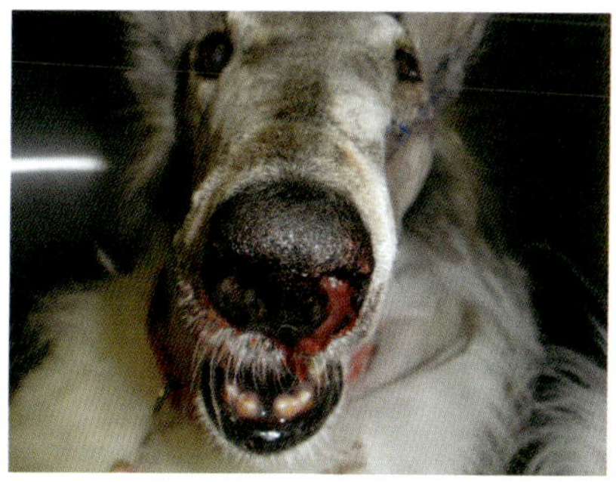

O)

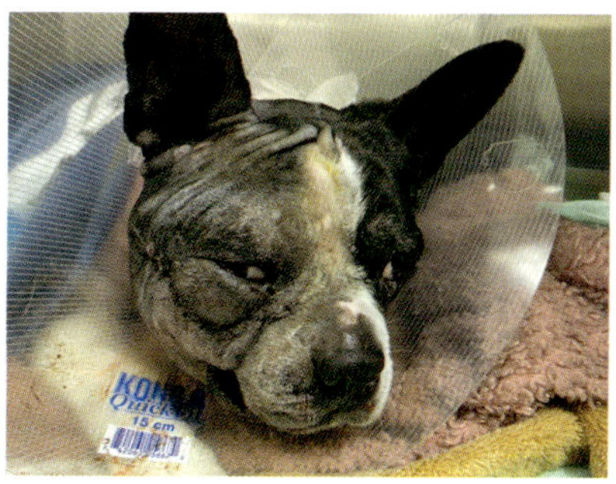

Postoperative Complications (48 Hours to 4 Weeks)† (See Plate 6.16P–R)

- Trauma to the upper lip as a result of the lip being drawn into the occlusal plane of the ipsilateral mandibular canine tooth (10%–18%; P, arrow)
- Incisional dehiscence (13%–18%; Q, 7 days postoperatively)
- Oronasal fistula (16%–18%; R, 105 days postoperatively)
- Surgical-site infection (10%–12%)
- Epiphora (13%–24%)

Complications – Cats‡ [6]

- Epistaxis (13%)
- Wound dehiscence and oronasal fistula (20%)
- Trauma to the upper lip as a result of the lip being drawn into the occlusal plane of the ipsilateral mandibular canine tooth (15%)
- Eating difficulties (15%)
- Facial swelling (10%)
- Subcutaneous emphysema (2%)
- Hypersalivation and drooling (2%)

† These complications are for all caudal maxillectomy and total unilateral maxillectomy procedures regardless of the surgical approach (intraoral or combined).

‡ These complications are for all maxillectomy procedures and not specifically for caudal maxillectomy and total unilateral maxillectomy through an intraoral approach.

Plate 6.16

Combined Approach for Caudal and Total Unilateral Maxillectomy *continued*

P)

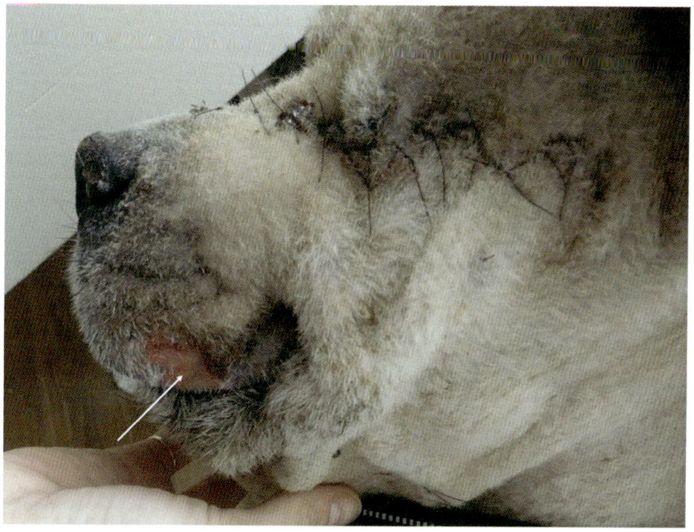

Q)

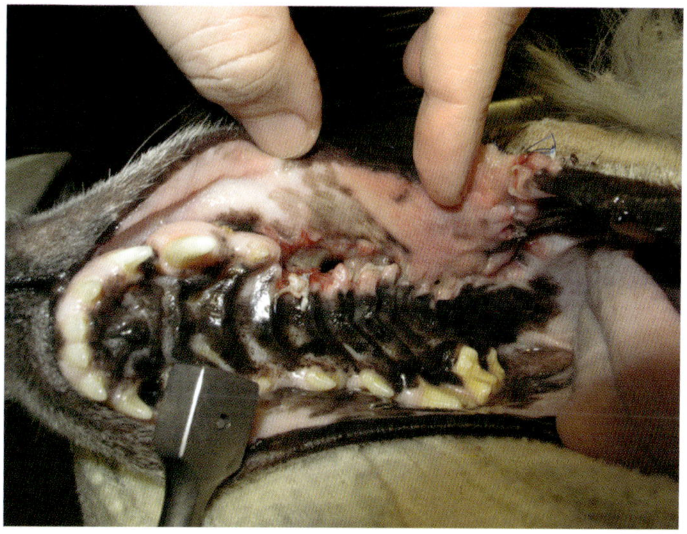

R)

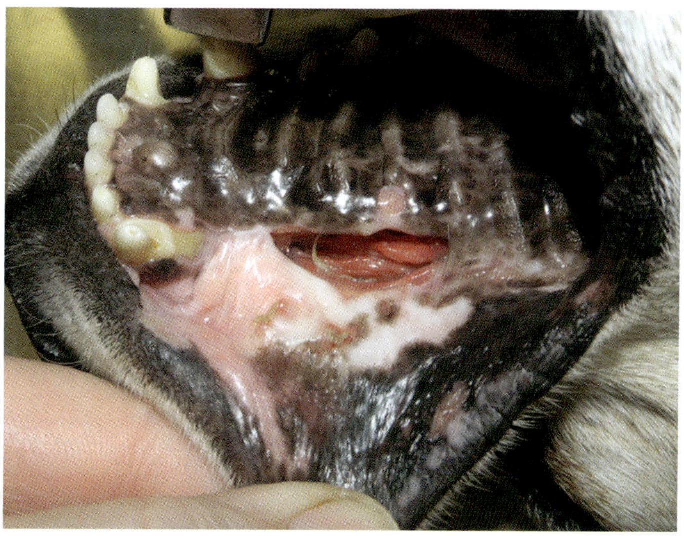

Cosmetic Appearance (See Plate 6.16S)

The lip can be drawn toward the midline because of the use of the labial mucosal-submucosal flap for reconstruction of the intraoral defect. This results in a scalloping of the lateral muzzle. The extent of this scalloping and medialization of the lip depends on the medial extent of the resection, the width of the lip, and the length of the labial mucosal-submucosal flap (S – i–vii).

The skin overlying the maxillary defect will often move paradoxically with respiration. This typically resolves within 7 days of surgery.

Suggested Adjuvant Treatments

- See 6. *Mandibulectomy and Maxillectomy*.

Prognosis and Oncologic Outcome

- See 6. *Mandibulectomy and Maxillectomy*.

References

1 Reiter, A.M. (2014). Open wide: blindness in cats after the use of mouth gags. *Vet. J.* 201: 5–6.
2 Thomson, M.J., Dernell, W.S., Lafferty, M. et al. (2003). Combined dorsolateral and intraoral approach for the resection of tumors of the maxilla in the dog. *J. Am. Anim. Hosp. Assoc.* 39 (3): 294–305.
3 Carrol, K.A. and Mathews, K.G. (2020). Ligation of the maxillary artery prior to caudal maxillectomy in the dog – a description of the technique, retrospective evaluation of blood loss, and cadaveric evaluation of maxillary artery anatomy. *Front. Vet. Sci.* 7: 588945.
4 Liptak, J.M. and Lascelles, B.D.X. (2012). Oral tumors. In: *Veterinary Surgical Oncology*, 1e (ed. S.T. Kudnig and B. Séguin), 119–178. Wiley-Blackwell.
5 MacLellan, R.H., Rawlinson, J.E., Rao, S. et al. (2018). Intraoperative and postoperative complications of partial maxillectomy for the treatment of oral tumors in dogs. *J. Am. Vet. Med. Assoc.* 252 (12): 1538–1547.
6 Liptak, J.M., Thatcher, G.P., Mestrinho, L.A. et al. (2021). Outcomes of cats treated with maxillectomy: 60 cases. A veterinary society of surgical oncology retrospective study. *Vet. Comp. Oncol.* 19 (4): 641–650.

Plate 6.16

Combined Approach for Caudal and Total Unilateral Maxillectomy *continued*

S-i)

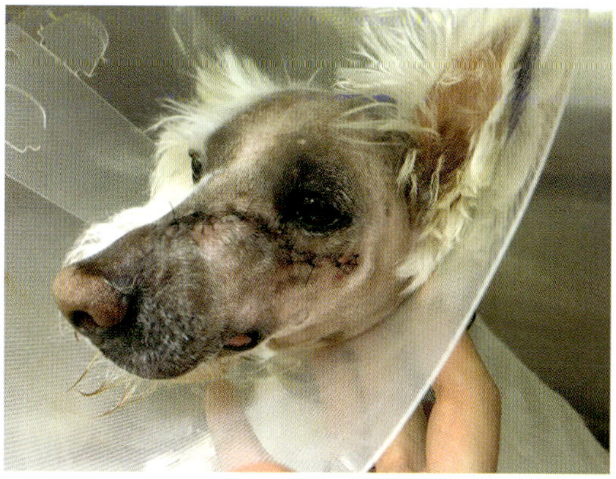

S-ii)

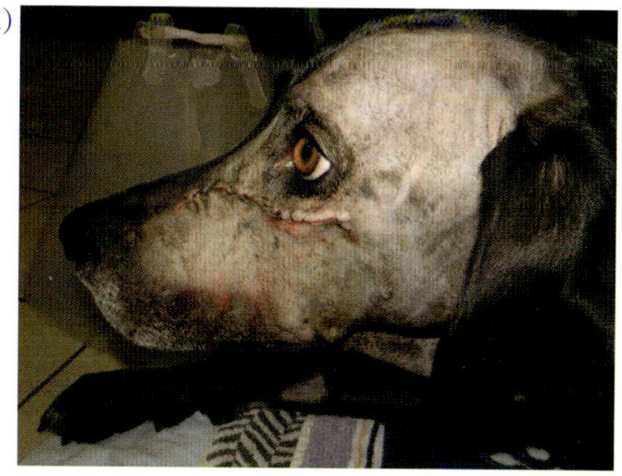

S-iii)

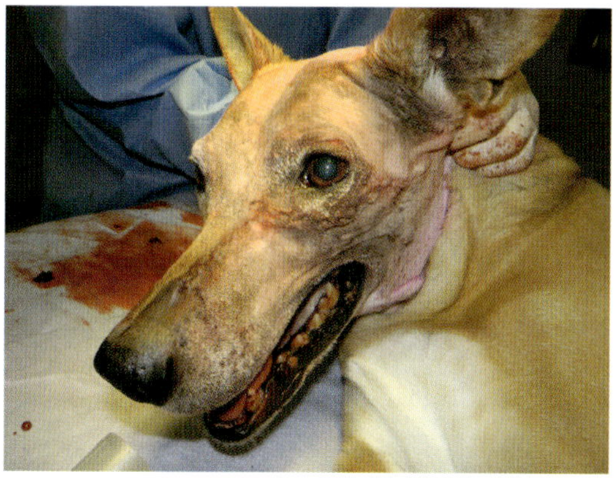

S-iv)

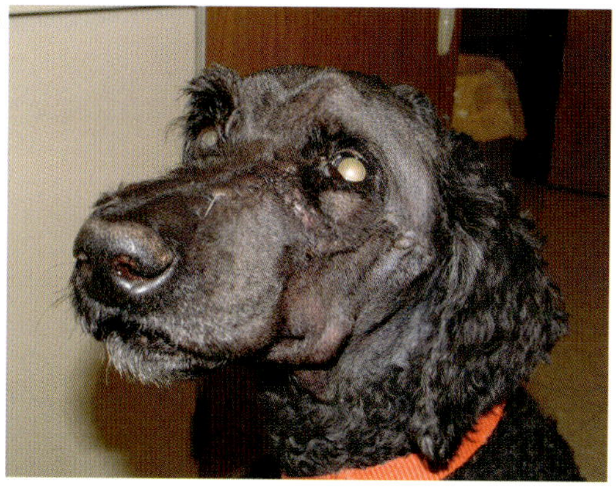

S-v)

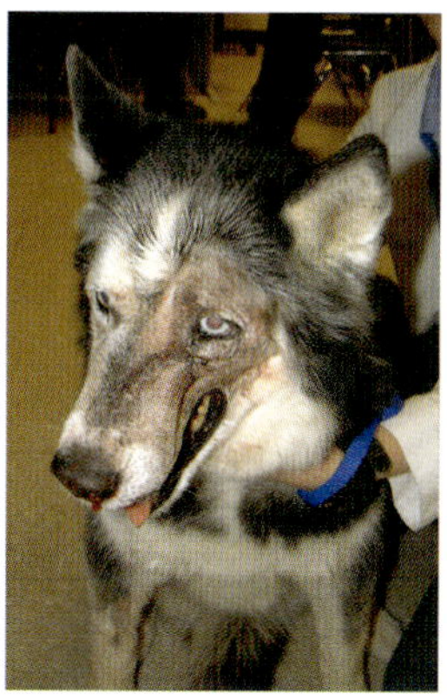

S-vi)

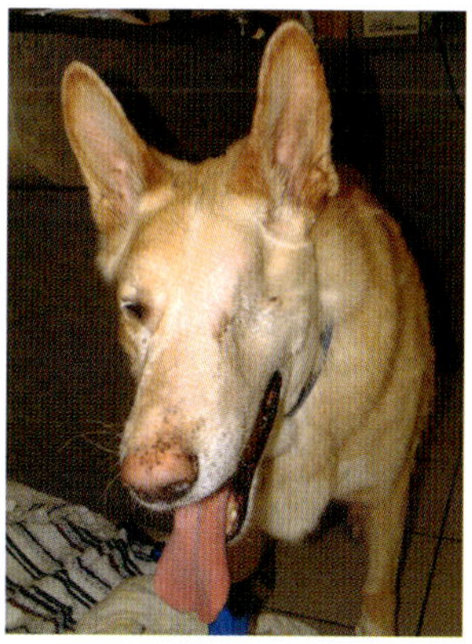

S-vii)

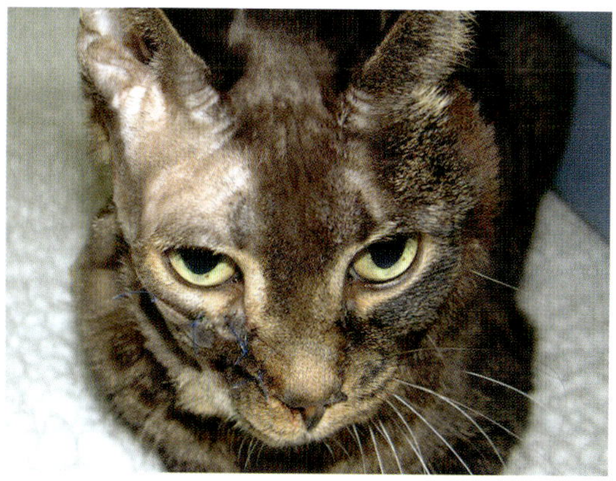

Chapter 7: Partial and Total Glossectomy

Indications

1) Resection of benign and malignant tumors of the tongue
2) Management of tongue trauma, thermal injury, glossitis, or chronic linear foreign bodies (in cats)
3) Partial glossectomy is defined as full-thickness resection of any portion of the free tongue rostral to the frenulum; subtotal glossectomy is defined as resection of the free tongue and a portion of tongue caudal to the frenulum; near-total glossectomy is defined as resection of ≥75% of the tongue; total glossectomy is defined as resection of the entire tongue [1, 2]

Suggested Diagnostic Workup and Clinical Staging

- Complete blood count, serum biochemistry, and urinalysis
- Preoperative biopsy
- Regional lymph node assessment for evaluation of lymph node metastasis
  - Fine-needle aspirate cytology of the mandibular lymph nodes
  - Sentinel lymph node mapping and excision of the sentinel lymph node (see *50.1. Sentinel Lymph Node Mapping*)
  - Nonselective excision of the bilateral mandibular and medial retropharyngeal lymph nodes through a ventral midline cervical approach (see *50.3. Combined Mandibular and Medial Retropharyngeal Lymph Node Excision*), or excision of the ipsilateral mandibular, medial retropharyngeal, and parotid lymph nodes through a lateral approach (see *50.4. Combined Parotid, Mandibular, and Medial Retropharyngeal Lymph Node Excision*)
- ± Radiographs or precontrast and postcontrast CT scan of the head and neck for surgical planning
- Three-view thoracic radiographs or thoracic CT scan for assessment of lung metastasis

Patient Positioning

The patient is positioned in either sternal or lateral recumbency, depending on the location of the tongue tumor. If in lateral recumbency, the patient is positioned with the side of the tongue tumor uppermost. A small pharyngeal pack should be placed to protect the airway. A mouth gag will assist with additional exposure, although this should be used with caution in cats to avoid blindness [3].

Surgical Technique (See Plate 7A–E)

A) The tongue should be tractioned rostrally to provide better exposure of the tongue and tongue tumor, especially for more caudally located tumors (arrow, mast cell tumor).
B) The tongue tumor should be resected with appropriate lateral margins based on the tumor type (a minimum of 1 cm is recommended) [2]. Resection is typically performed with a scalpel blade (i, partial glossectomy for an extramedullary plasmacytoma; ii, near-total glossectomy for a squamous cell carcinoma).

Color Atlas of Canine and Feline Surgical Oncology, First Edition. Julius M. Liptak, Paolo Buracco, William T. N. Culp, and Nicholas J. Bacon.

Plate 7

Partial and Total Glossectomy

A)

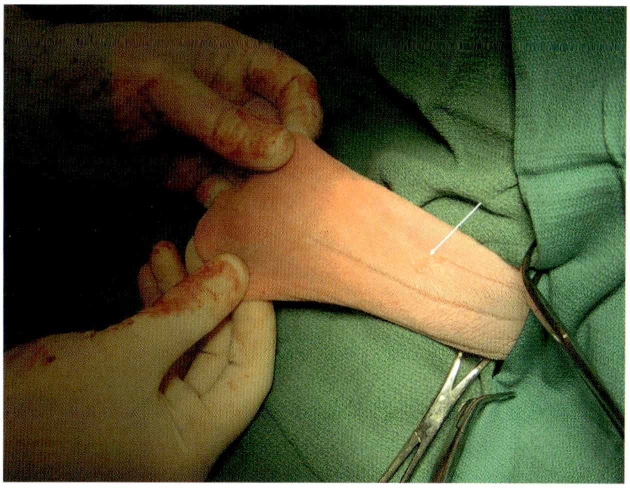

B-i)

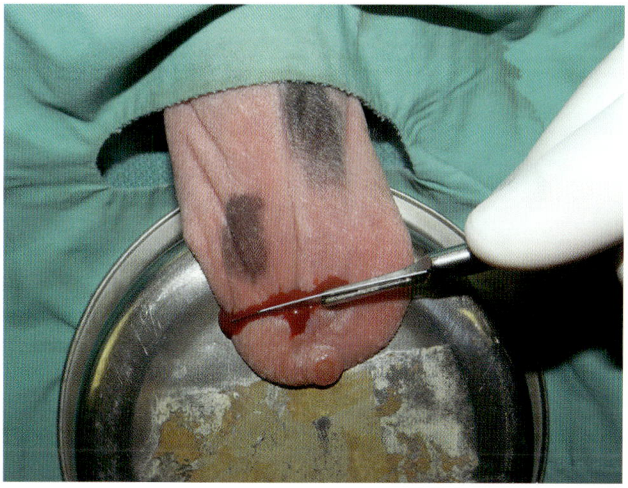

B-ii)

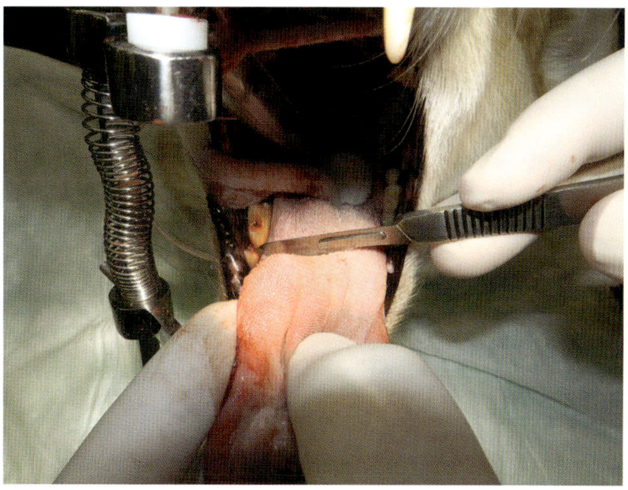

Surgical Technique (See Plate 7A–E) *continued*

C) Deep margins are typically full-thickness tongue (i and ii, soft tissue sarcoma; iii, fibrosarcoma); however, for benign tumors and small, low-grade malignant tumors, a portion of the tongue can be preserved deep to the tumor (iv, dorsal tongue, extramedullary plasmacytoma; v, frenulum, squamous cell carcinoma). The incision through the body of the tongue can be done with scalpel blade, Metzenbaum or Mayo scissors, or a vessel sealing device (vi). For partial lateral glossectomies, one of the left or right lingual vessels should be preserved. Ligation of both the left and the right lingual vessels will result in partial necrosis of the tongue rostral to the ligated vessels (vii).

Plate 7

Partial and Total Glossectomy *continued*

C-i)

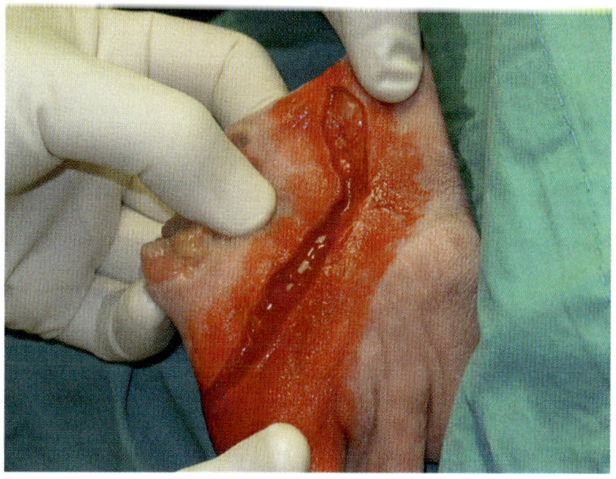

C-ii)

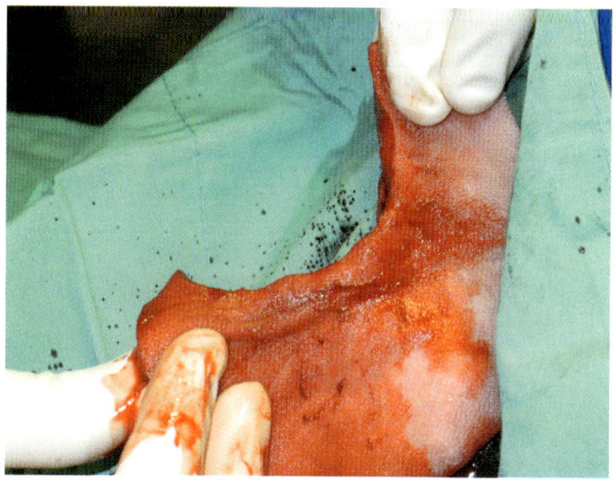

C-iii)

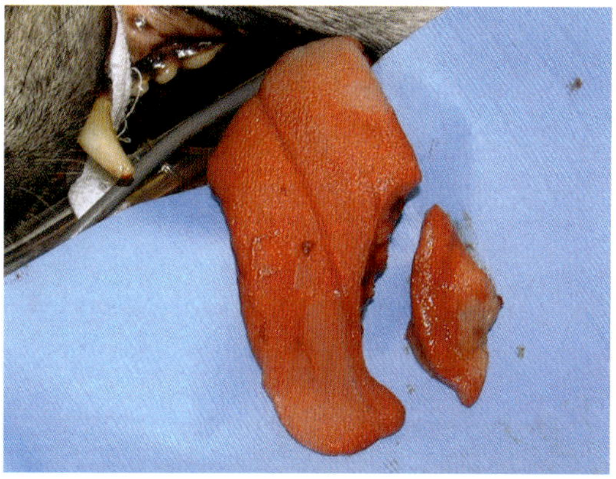

C-iv)

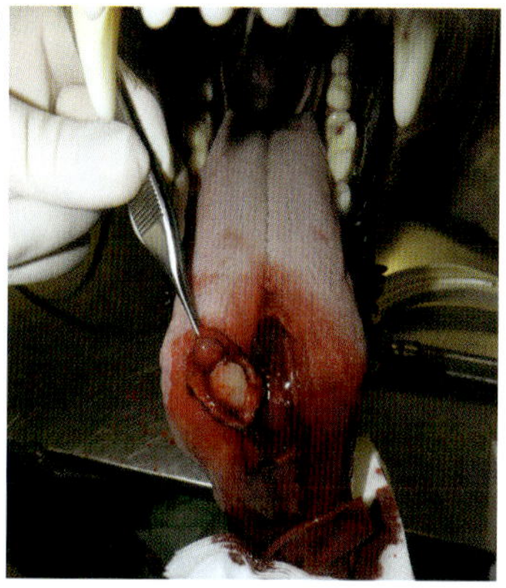

C-v)

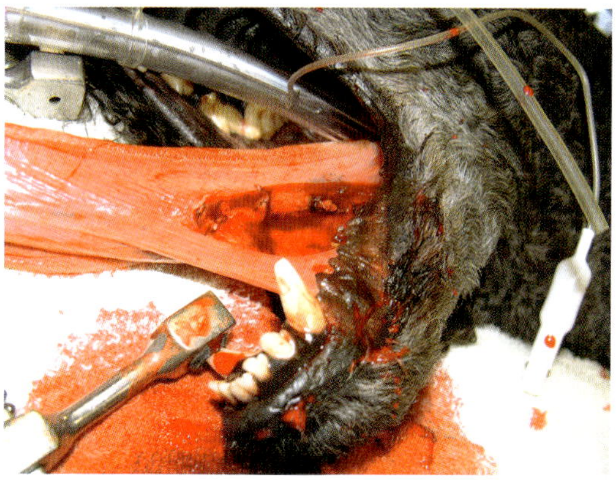

C-vi)

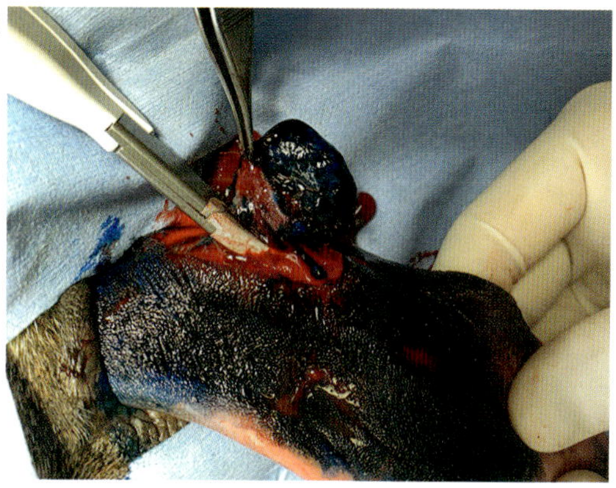

C-vii)

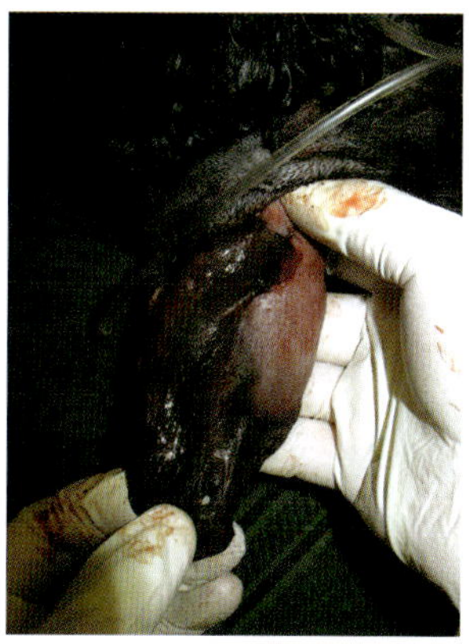

Surgical Technique (See Plate 7A–E) *continued*

D) For total or near-total glossectomies, the frenulum is incised along the floor of the intermandibular space (i), and transection of the glossal muscles is continued caudally with either scissors or a vessel sealing device (ii–iv) to the level of the planned caudal margins. The dorsal aspect of the root of the tongue is then incised along the planned caudal margins (v) with a scalpel blade (see B – ii),

Plate 7

Partial and Total Glossectomy *continued*

D-i)

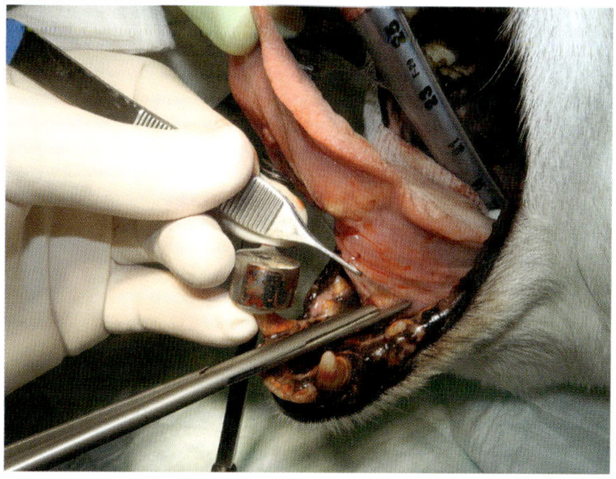

D-ii)

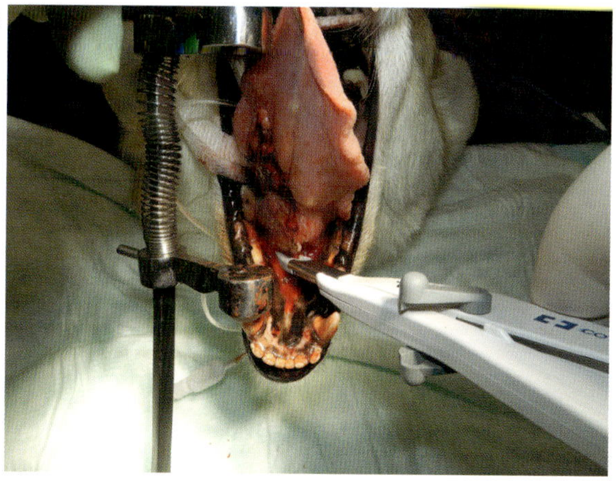

D-iii)

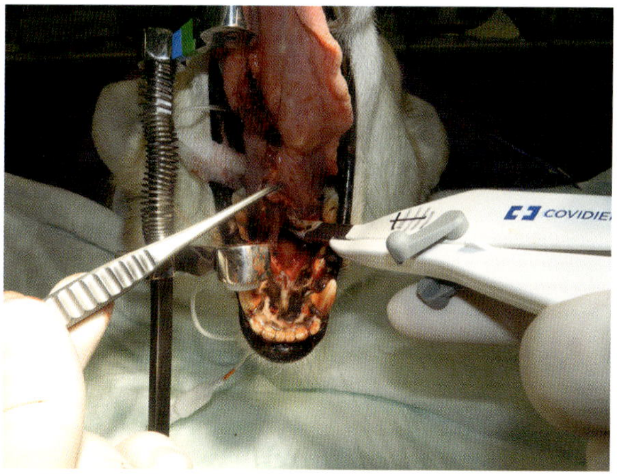

D-iv)

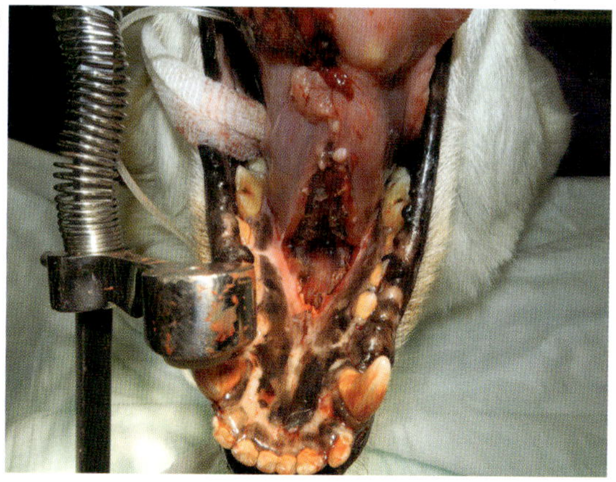

D-v)

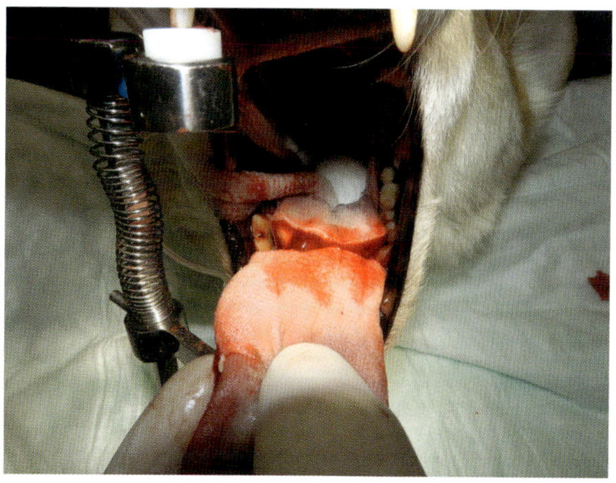

Surgical Technique (See Plate 7A–E) *continued*

and this is continued laterally on both the left and right sides of the tongue (vi, vii). The dorsal and lateral incisions are connected to the ventral dissection with either scissors or a vessel-sealing device (viii–x) to complete the glossectomy. A vessel sealing device is preferred for this part of the glossectomy because of superior hemostasis and less blood loss.

Plate 7

Partial and Total Glossectomy *continued*

D-vi)
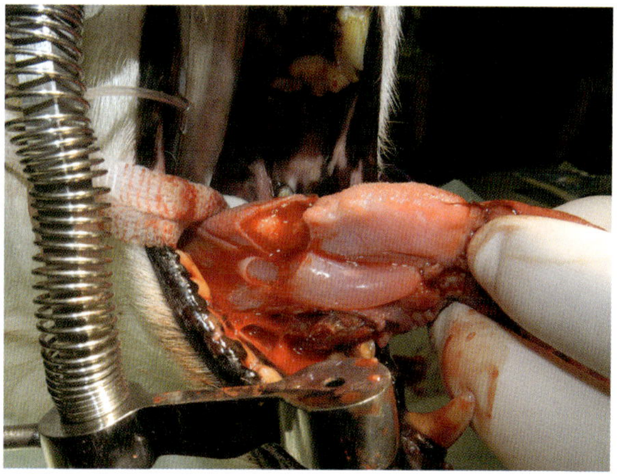

D-vii)
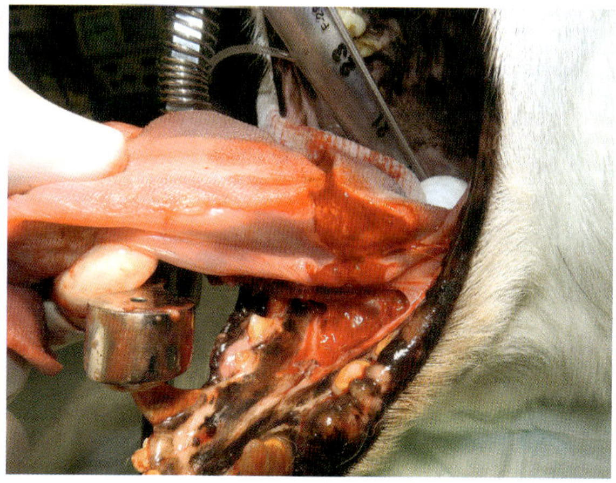

D-viii)
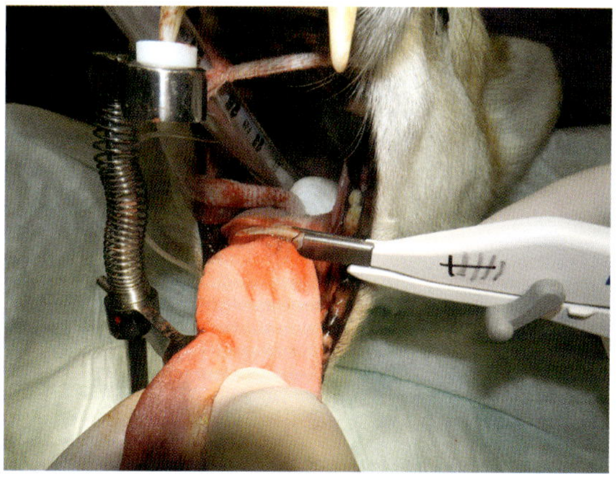

D-ix)
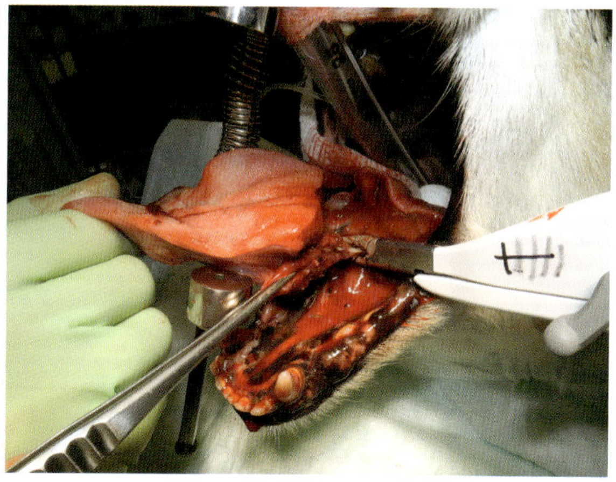

D-x)
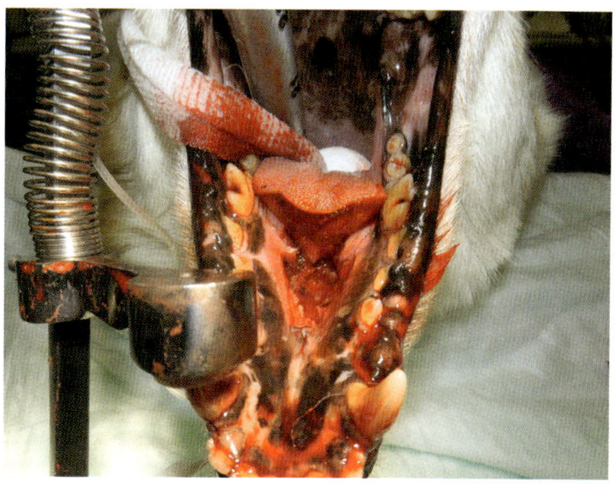

Surgical Technique (See Plate 7A–E) *continued*

E) The tongue defect is closed in one to three layers. For lateral (i) and transverse (ii) partial glossectomies, the ventral mucosa is sutured to the dorsal mucosa in a simple interrupted or continuous suture pattern using 3-0 to 4-0 absorbable suture material. For wedge partial glossectomies, the dorsal (iii) and ventral mucosa (iv) are closed separately in a two-layer closure in a simple interrupted or continuous suture pattern using 3-0 to 4-0 absorbable suture material. For partial-thickness glossectomies, the mucosa is sutured in a simple interrupted (v) or continuous suture pattern using 3-0 to 4-0 absorbable suture material. For lateral, transverse, and wedge partial glossectomies and partial-thickness glossectomies, the muscle can also be closed with a simple continuous suture pattern using 3-0 to 4-0 absorbable suture material. For near-total and total glossectomies, the tongue remnant is sutured to the floor of the intermandibular space using 3-0 to 4-0 absorbable suture material in a simple interrupted pattern (vi).

Postoperative Management

1) Multimodal analgesia
2) Elizabethan collar
3) ± Esophagostomy feeding tube and supplemental feeding (following subtotal or total glossectomy) [1, 2]

Complications – Dogs

Intraoperative Complications

- Blood loss [1]

Plate 7

Partial and Total Glossectomy *continued*

E-i)

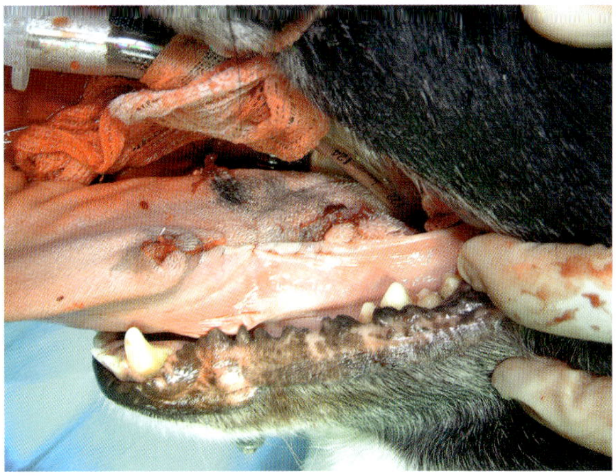

E-ii)

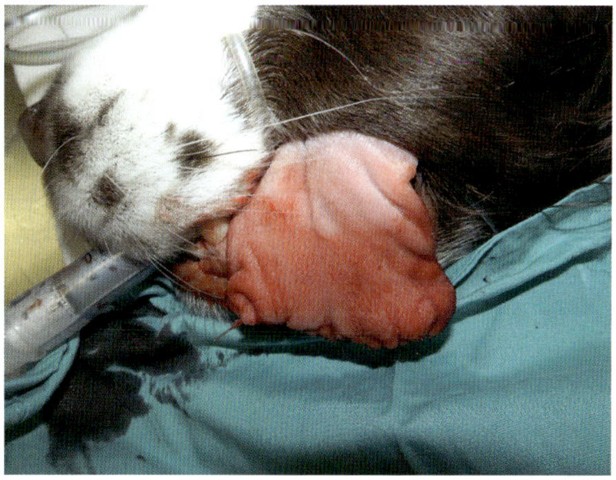

E-iii)

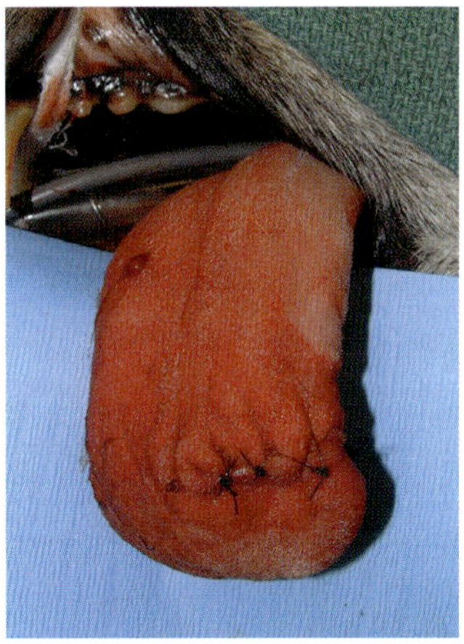

E-iv)

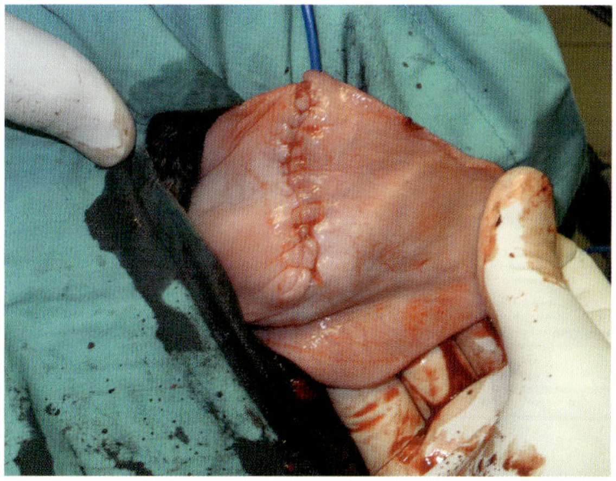

E-v)

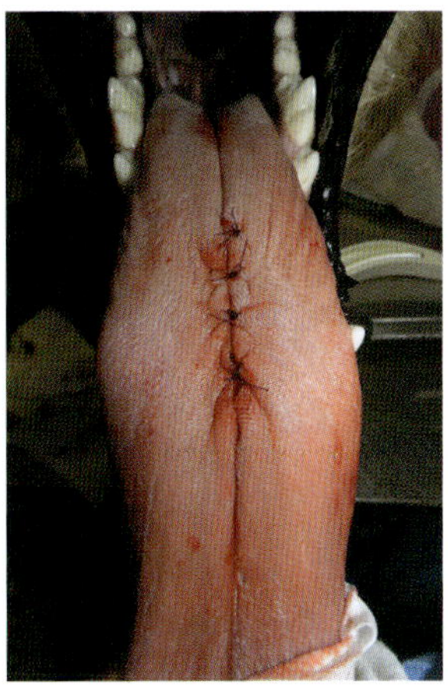

E-vi)

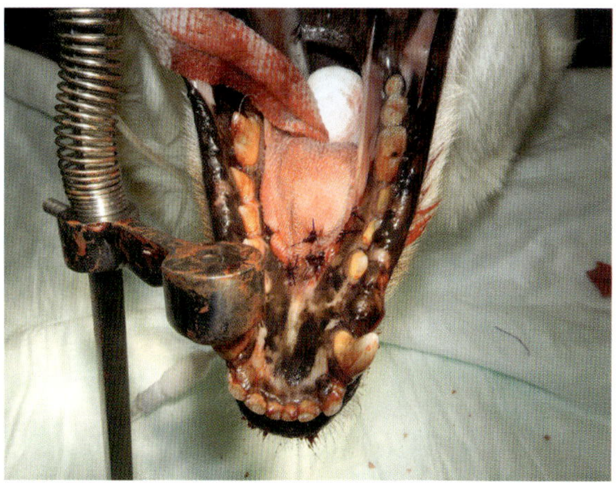

Postoperative Complications (See Plate 7F)

- Overall: 54% [2]
- Excessive drooling (38%) [2]
- Incisional dehiscence (2%–23%; F – i, ii, incisional dehiscence after second intention healing) [2, 4]
- Dysphagia/inappetence (0%–15% overall, common after near-total and total glossectomy) [1, 2, 4]
- Bleeding (10%) [4]
- Partial tongue paralysis (2%) [4]

Suggested Adjuvant Treatments

- ± Chemotherapy
- ± Radiation therapy, depending on tumor type and completeness of excision

Plate 7

Partial and Total Glossectomy *continued*

F-i)

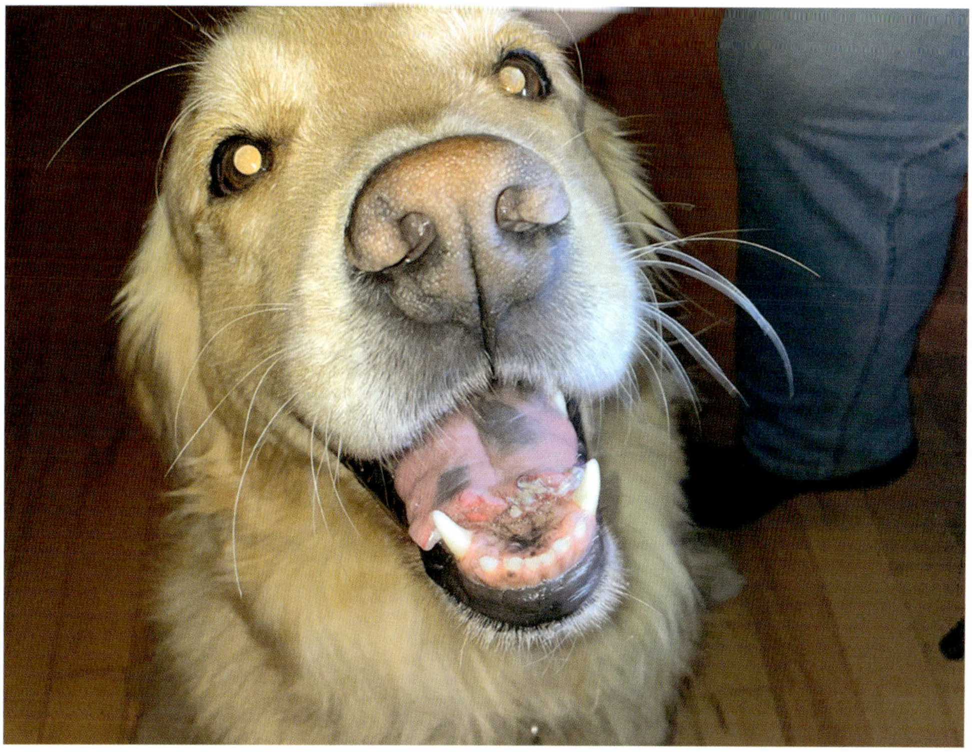

F-ii)

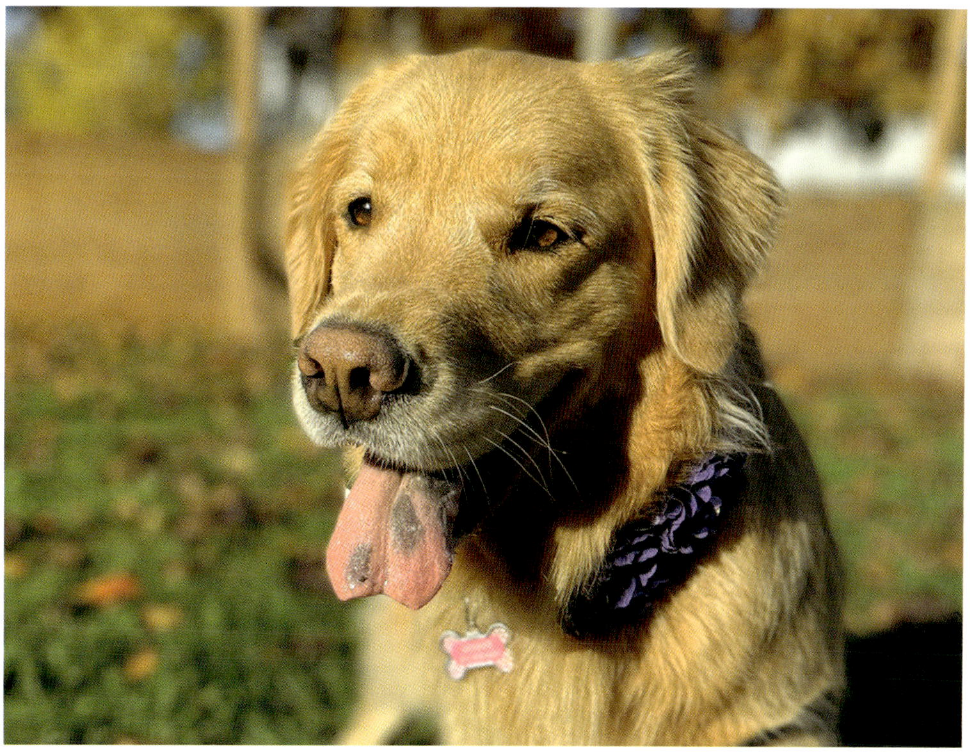

Prognosis and Oncologic Outcome – Dogs [2]

	Local Recurrence Rate	Metastatic Rate	Disease-Free Interval (d)	Median Survival Time (d)	1-Year Survival Rate	2-Year Survival Rate
Overall [2, 4]						
Overall	26%–27%	14%–19%	51–205	286	–	–
Tumor ≥ 2 cm [4]						
No	–	–	–	818	–	–
Yes	–	–	–	207	–	–
Metastasis [4]						
No	–	–	–	661	–	–
Yes	–	–	–	241	–	–
Feeding tube [4]						
No	–	–	–	532	–	–
Yes	–	–	–	207	–	–
Melanoma [2, 4]						
Overall	9%–31%	38%–45%	168	222	–	–
Squamous Cell Carcinoma [2, 4, 5]						
Overall	0%–32%	14%–19%	–	301	–	–
Histologic grade [5]						
I	–	–	–	487	–	–
II	–	–	–	116	–	–
III	–	–	–	91	–	–
Hemangiosarcoma [6]						
Overall	41%	45%	297	500	–	–
Clinical signs						
No	–	–	–	633	–	–
Yes	–	–	–	105	–	–
Tumor ≥ 2 cm [4]						
No	–	–	–	633	–	–
Yes	–	–	–	105	–	–
Extramedullary Plasmacytoma [2]						
Overall	20%	0%	–	>1607	–	–

References

1 Dvorak, L.D., Beaver, D.P., Ellison, G.W. et al. (2004). Major glossectomy in dogs: a case series and proposed classification system. *J. Am. Anim. Hosp. Assoc.* 40 (4): 331–337.

2 Syrcle, J.A., Bonczynski, J.J., Monette, S. et al. (2008). Retrospective evaluation of lingual tumors in 42 dogs: 1999–2005. *J. Am. Anim. Hosp. Assoc.* 44: 308–319.

3 Stiles, J., Weil, A.B., Packer, R.A., and Lantz, G.C. (2012). Post-anesthetic cortical blindness in cats: twenty cases. *Vet. J.* 193 (2): 367–373.

4 Culp, W.T.N., Ehrhart, N., Withrow, S.J. et al. (2013). Results of surgical excision and evaluation of factors associated with survival time in dogs with lingual neoplasia: 97 cases (1995-2008). *J. Am. Vet. Med. Assoc.* 242 (10): 1392–1397.

5 Carpenter, L.G., Withrow, S.J., Powers, B.E. et al. (1993). Squamous cell carcinoma of the tongue in 10 dogs. *J. Am. Anim. Hosp. Assoc.* 29: 17–24.

6 Burton, J.H., Powers, B.E., and Biller, B.J. (2014). Clinical outcome in 20 cases of lingual hemangiosarcoma in dogs: 1996–2011. *Vet. Comp. Oncol.* 12 (3): 198–204.

Chapter 8: Thyroidectomy

Indications

1) Resection of nonmetastatic mobile thyroid tumors
2) ± Resection of nonmetastatic fixed thyroid tumors
3) ± Resection of hyperplastic thyroid lobes
4) ± Palliative resection of metastatic mobile thyroid tumors if the tumor is symptomatic

Suggested Diagnostic Workup and Clinical Staging

- Complete blood count, serum biochemistry, and urinalysis
- Thyroid hormone testing
- Fine-needle aspirate cytology
- Precontrast and postcontrast CT scan of the head and neck for surgical planning
- Three-view thoracic radiographs or thoracic CT scan for assessment of lung metastasis

Patient Positioning

The patient is positioned in dorsal recumbency. A towel or sandbag can be placed under the neck to elevate the neck.

Surgical Technique (See Plate 8A–F)

A) A ventral midline skin incision is made extending from just caudal to the larynx and extending caudally to a few centimeters cranial to the thoracic inlet. Dissection is continued through the subcutaneous tissue using a combination of sharp and blunt dissection until the paired sternohyoideus muscles are exposed. Both the sternohyoideus and sternocephalicus muscles arise from the manubrium; the sternohyoideus muscles continue along the midline cranially while the four separate parts of the sternocephalicus muscles diverge laterally (paired on each of the left and right sides). Because of this divergence, it is unusual to need to separate the sternocephalicus muscles to expose the trachea and thyroid glands; however, this can be performed if necessary. The left and right sternohyoideus muscles are separated laterally using sharp dissection (i). Small blood vessels may be encountered during this dissection and can be managed with bipolar electrocautery. Gelpi (or other self-retraining) retractors are placed cranially and caudally in the incision to lateralize the sternohyoideus muscles and expose a deep fascial layer and the underlying trachea (ii).

B) Although the thyroid glands can have an isthmus connecting the left and right sides (i), most dogs have clearly delineated left and right thyroid glands (also referred to as lobes). The thyroid glands are generally attached to the trachea in a lateral position; however, neoplastic thyroid glands tend to be much larger than normal and are more easily visualized (ii, TH). To fully expose the thyroid gland, dissection through the deep fascial layer overlying the affected lobe needs to be performed. After exposing the ventral aspect of the thyroid tumor, self-retaining retractors should be repositioned to improve the visualization of the affected side and lateralize the trachea to the contralateral side of the tumor (iii). A sponge, or other protective device, should be placed on the trachea during lateralization to prevent iatrogenic trauma.

Color Atlas of Canine and Feline Surgical Oncology, First Edition. Julius M. Liptak, Paolo Buracco, William T. N. Culp, and Nicholas J. Bacon.

Plate 8

Thyroidectomy

A-I)

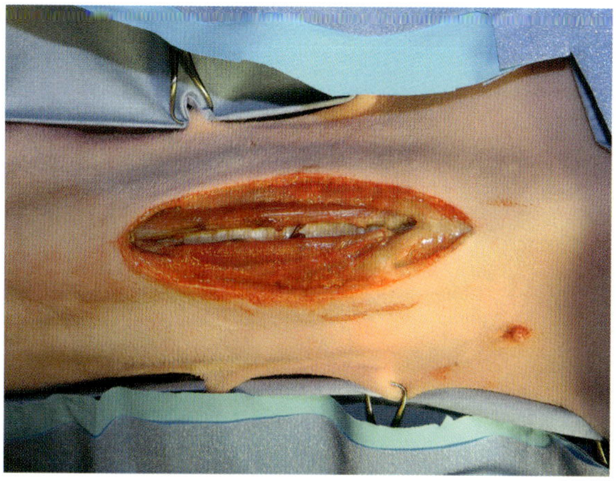

A-ii)

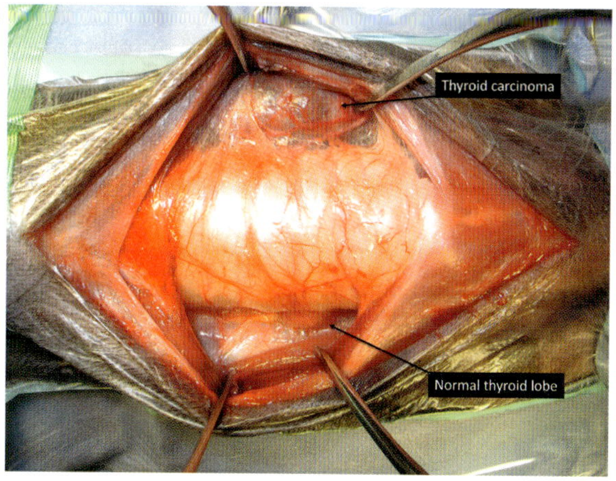

B-i)

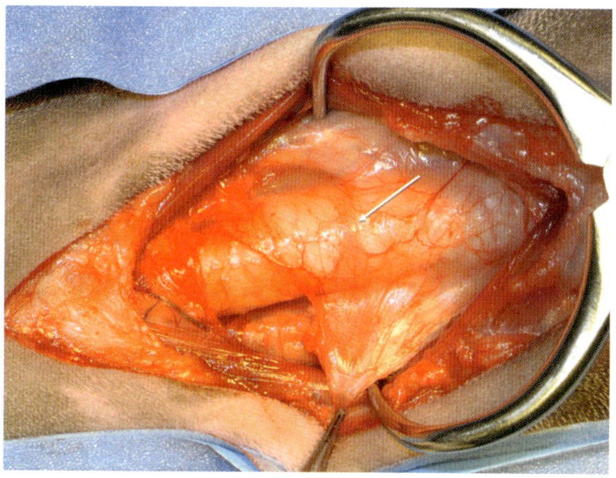

B-ii)

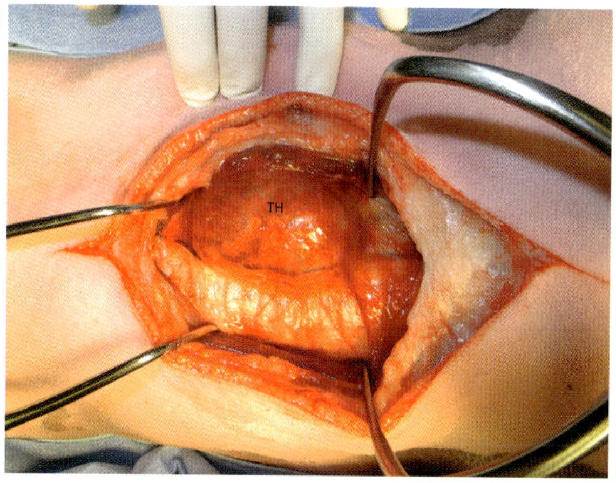

B-iii)

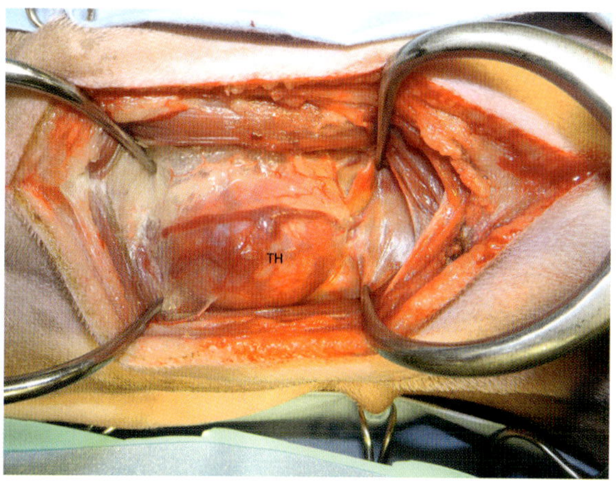

Surgical Technique (See Plate 8A–F) *continued*

C) In normal thyroid glands, the blood supply is quite small and arises from the cranial and caudal thyroid arteries (i), which may arise from the common carotid artery and/or the brachiocephalic trunk; however, cats do not have caudal thyroid arteries [1]. Thyroid tumors tend to be vascular (ii), and bleeding during dissection can be robust. A combination of monopolar electrosurgery, bipolar electrocautery, and vessel sealing devices (iii–vi) can be used to

Plate 8

Thyroidectomy *continued*

C-i)

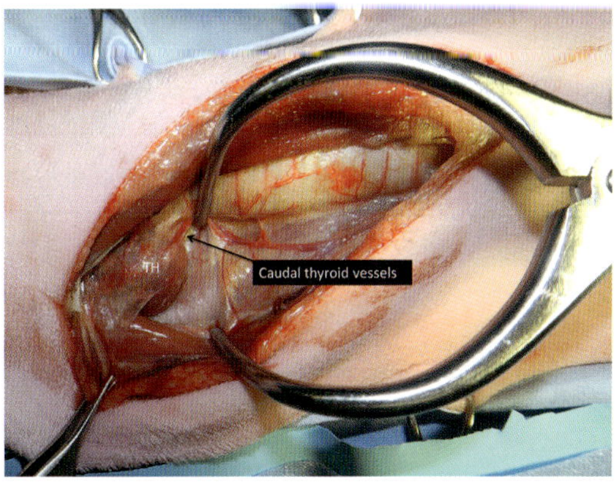

C-ii)

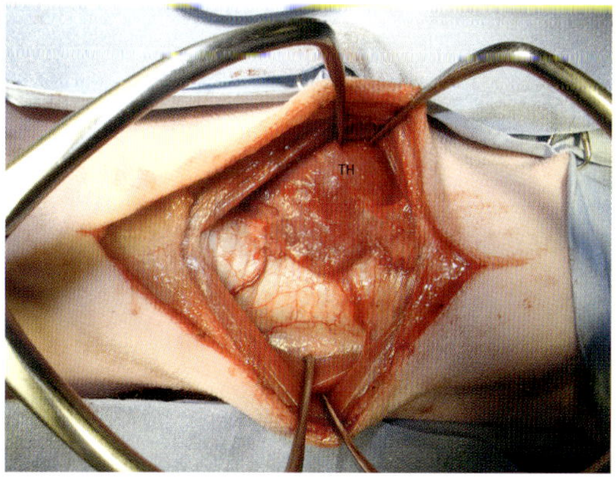

C-ii)

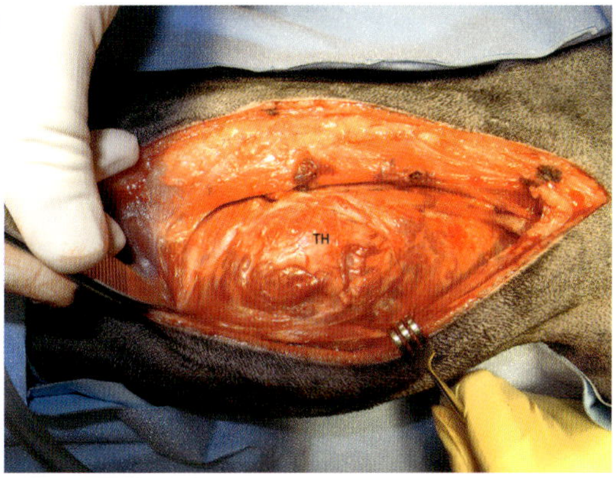

C-iii)

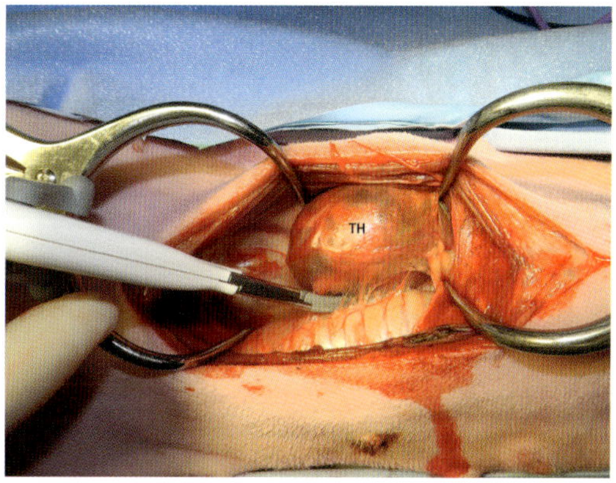

C-iv)

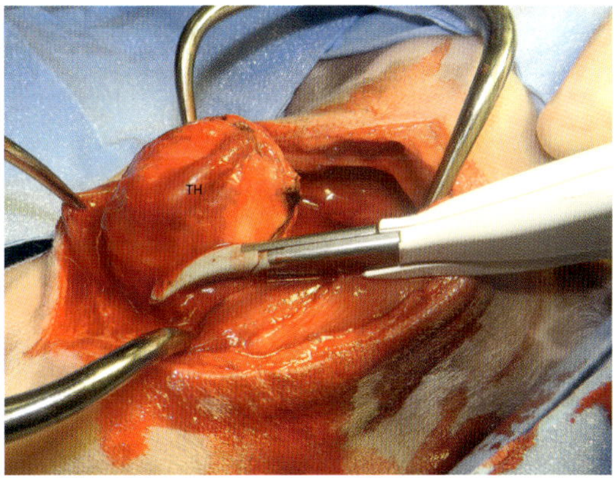

C-v)

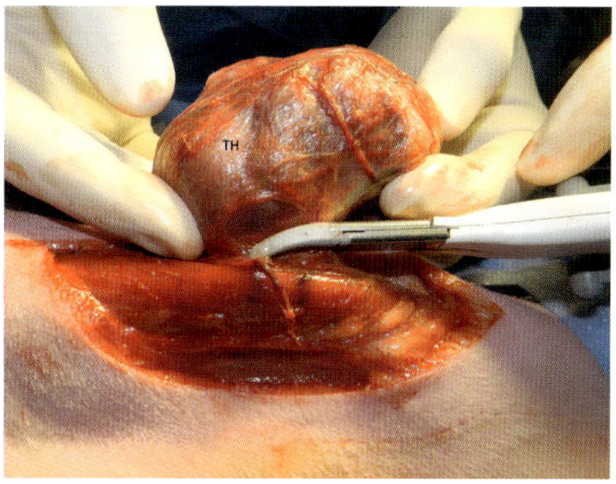

C-vi)

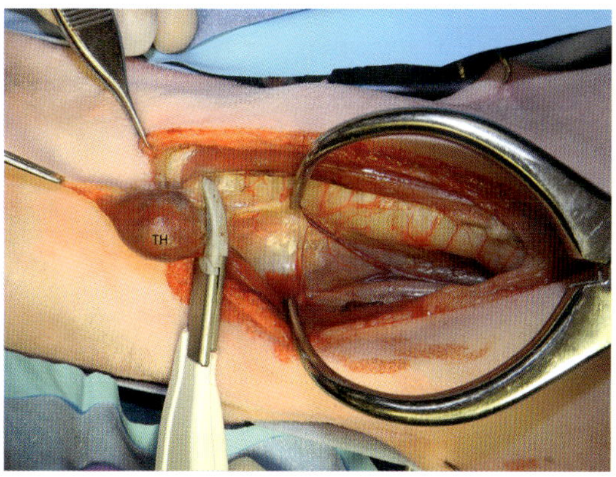

Surgical Technique (See Plate 8A–F) *continued*

begin to dissect the abnormal thyroid gland (TH) from the surrounding tissue. The surgeon should be cautious to avoid important adjacent structures, including the trachea (TR), esophagus (ES), carotid artery (CA), jugular vein (JV), vagosympathetic trunk, and recurrent laryngeal nerve (vii–x). In general, removal of an abnormal thyroid gland is most effectively performed by isolating either the cranial or caudal aspect of the mass first. This allows the mass (or attached fascial tissue) to be grasped and elevated to expose the blood supply to the mass and attachments to surrounding normal structures. Once the mass is freed from attachments, it is removed.

D) Macroscopic vascular invasion, which is seen in up to 35% of dogs with thyroid carcinomas, is frequently evident as a tumor thrombus (i–iii, arrow) extending caudally into the caudal thyroid vein and jugular vein, and occasionally the cranial thyroid vein. If possible, the affected veins should be isolated, and the tumor thrombus should be resected in its entirety en bloc with the thyroid tumor.

Plate 8

Thyroidectomy *continued*

C-vii)

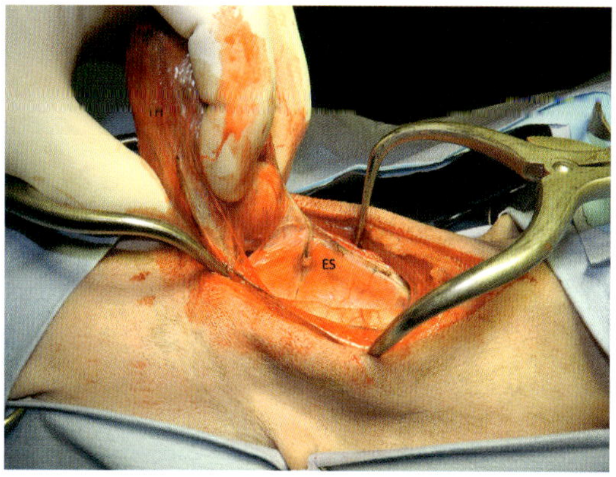

C-viii)

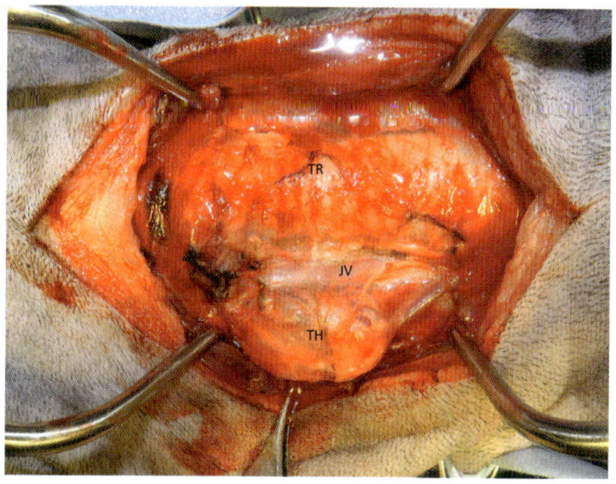

C-ix)

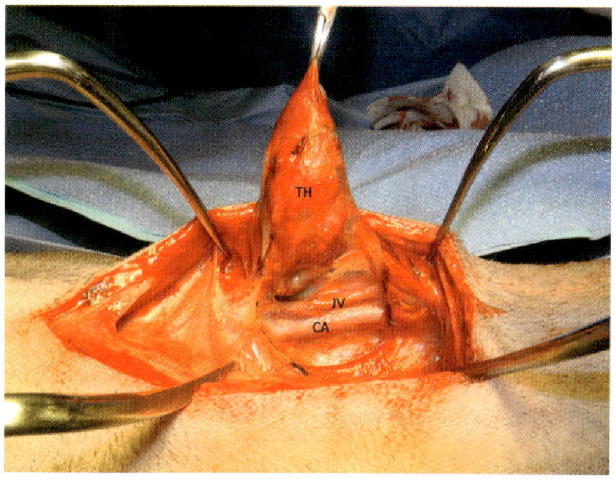

C-x)

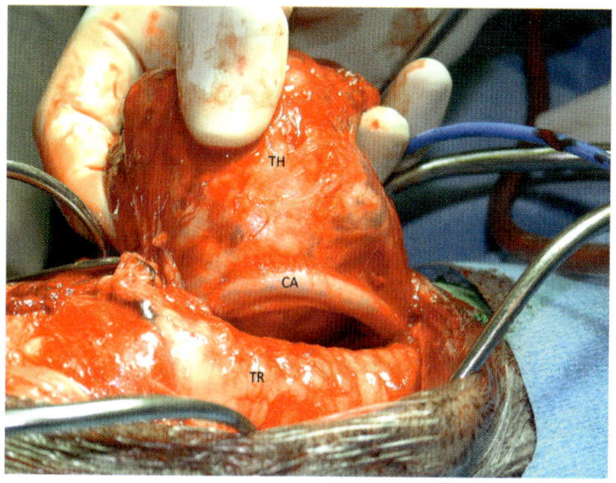

D-i)

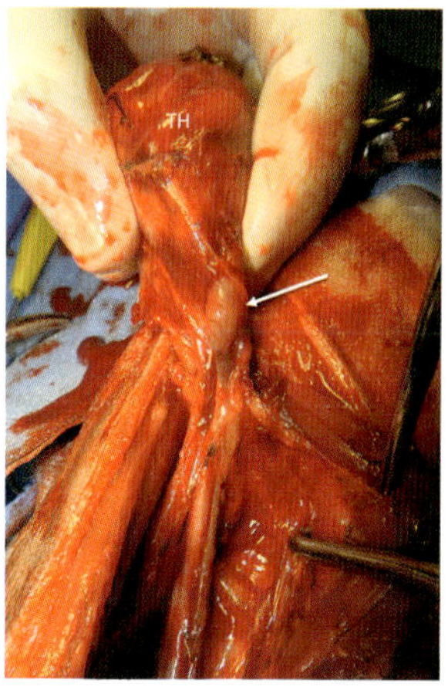

D-ii)

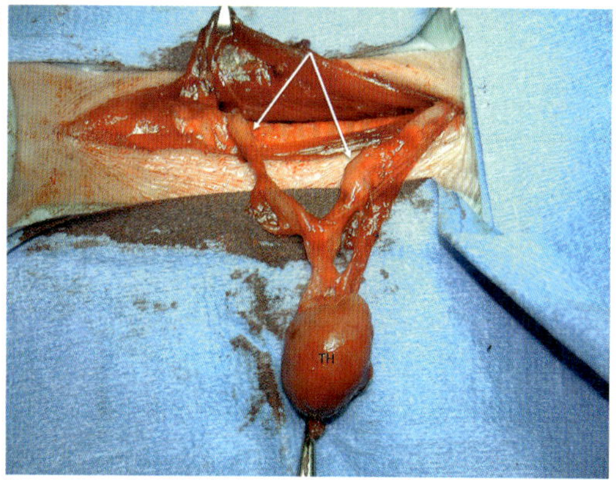

D-iii)

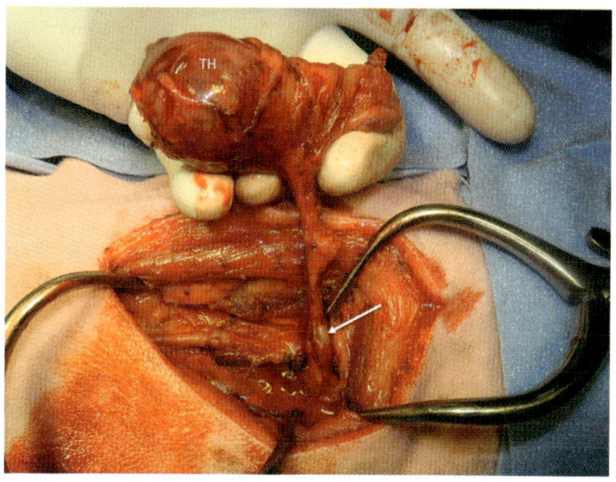

Surgical Technique (See Plate 8A–F) *continued*

E) The contralateral thyroid gland should be visually examined and palpated to determine whether there is any evidence of bilateral disease. The normal thyroid gland (N-TH) is salmon colored and soft (i), whereas thyroid tumors are often firm and rounded (ii). If a contralateral thyroid mass is noted (TH), then bilateral thyroidectomy (as described in C) is recommended. The owners should be counseled on the need for long-term vitamin D $\pm$ calcium and thyroid hormone supplementation. Reimplantation of one or more external parathyroid glands (PTG) into a muscle pocket created in the sternohyoideus muscle (SH) may result in revascularization of the parathyroid gland and return to normal calcium homeostasis (iii, iv).

F) The sternohyoideus muscles are reapposed with 3-0 or 4-0 monofilament absorbable suture in a simple continuous suture pattern (i). The subcutaneous tissue is reapposed with 3-0 or 4-0 monofilament absorbable suture in a simple continuous suture pattern (ii). An intradermal layer of 3-0 or 4-0 monofilament absorbable suture is placed followed by skin sutures if necessary (iii).

Plate 8

Thyroidectomy *continued*

E-i)

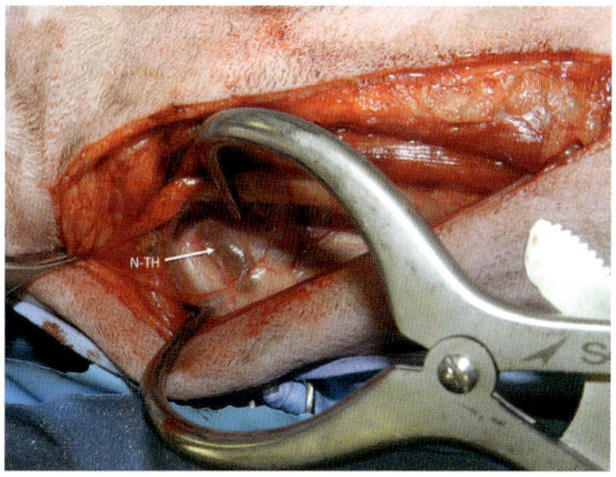

E-ii)

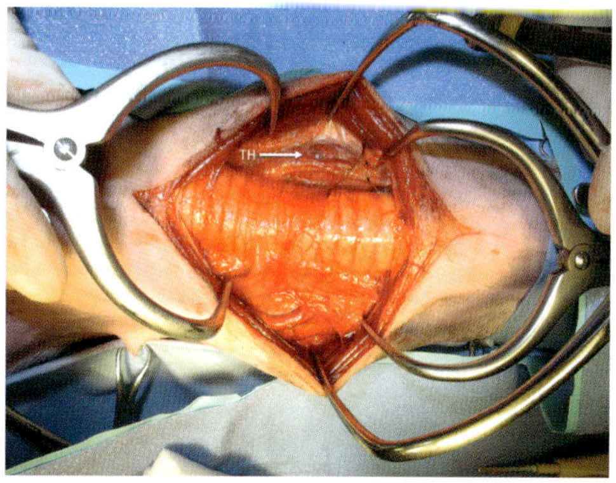

E-iii)

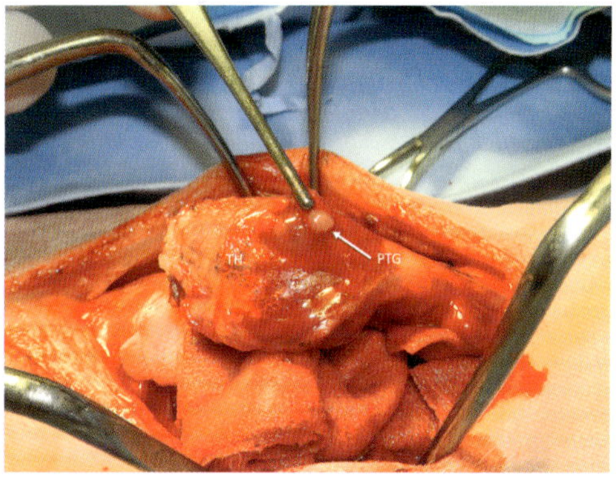

E-iv)

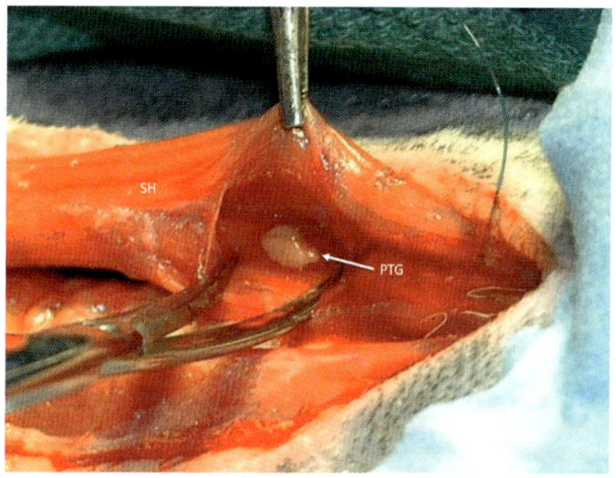

F-i)

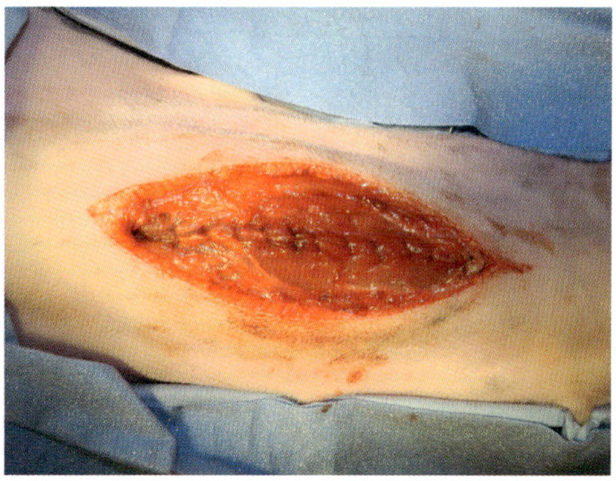

F-ii)

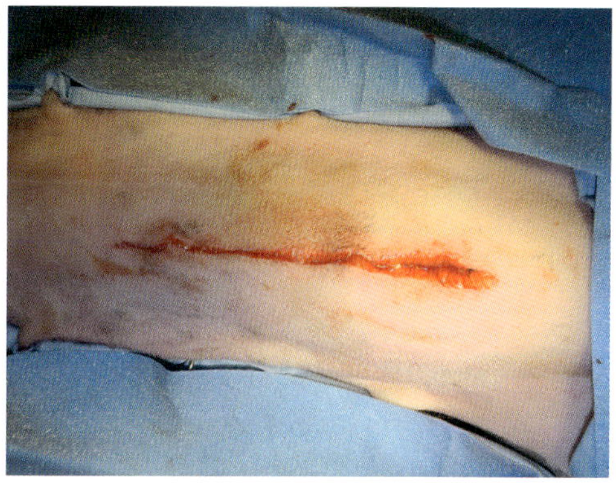

F-iii)

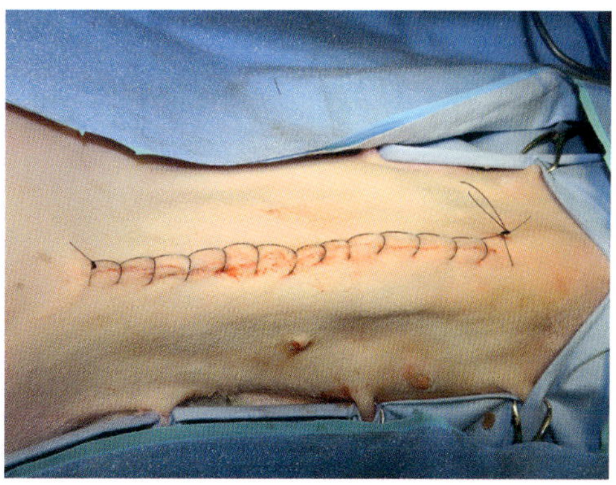

Postoperative Management

1) Multimodal analgesia
2) Elizabethan collar
3) Calcitriol ± calcium supplementation if bilateral thyroidectomy has been performed
4) Thyroid hormone supplementation after unilateral thyroidectomy for dogs presenting with functional thyroid carcinoma or if bilateral thyroidectomy has been performed

Complications – Dogs

Intraoperative Complications

- 2%–15% overall [2–4]
- Blood loss (3%–27%) [2, 4, 5]
- Vascular invasion (35%) [2]
- Esophageal trauma (1%) [3, 4]
- Tracheal trauma (rare) [4]
- Recurrent laryngeal nerve trauma resulting in laryngeal paresis or paralysis (0%–2%) [2, 4–6]
- Vagosympathetic trunk trauma resulting in Horner's syndrome (rare)

Postoperative Complications

- 6%–16% overall [2, 4, 6]
- Blood loss and hematoma formation (5%) [3]
- Incisional complications (seroma, infection, dehiscence; rare)
- Hypothyroidism (27% after bilateral thyroidectomy [5] and 64% in dogs with functional thyroid carcinomas [6])
- Hypocalcemia (2% after unilateral thyroidectomy [3, 6] and 43%–73% after bilateral thyroidectomy [4, 6])
- Laryngeal paralysis (rare)
- Aspiration pneumonia secondary to laryngeal paralysis (3%–5%) [2–4, 6]
- Horner's syndrome (1%) [4]

Complications – Cats

Postoperative Complications

- Incisional complications (seroma, infection, dehiscence; rare)
- Recurrence of hyperthyroidism (6%–44%) [7, 8]
- Hypothyroidism (49%) [7]
- Hypocalcemia (6% after unilateral thyroidectomy [8] and 82% after bilateral extracapsular thyroidectomy, 36% after bilateral intracapsular thyroidectomy, and 11% when bilateral thyroidectomies were staged by 3–4 weeks [9])

Suggested Adjuvant Treatments

- ± Chemotherapy
- ± Radiation therapy, depending on degree of fixation and completeness of excision

Prognosis and Oncologic Outcome – Dogs [2, 4–6, 10, 11]

Tumor Type	Local Recurrence Rate	Metastatic Rate	Disease-Free Interval (d)	Median Survival Time (d)	1-Year Survival Rate	2-Year Survival Rate
Carcinoma	0%–10%	0%–10%	238–375 [4]	911 to 2208 to >1095	89%	81%

Prognosis and Oncologic Outcome – Cats [8]

Tumor Type	Local Recurrence Rate	Metastatic Rate	Disease-Free Interval (d)	Mean Survival Time (d)	1-Year Survival Rate	2-Year Survival Rate
Overall	5%	–	–	694	–	–

References

1 Birchard, S.J. (2006). Thyroidectomy in the cat. *Clin. Tech. Small Anim. Pract.* 21 (1): 29–33.

2 Reagan, J.K., Selmic, L.E., Fallon, C. et al. (2019). Complications and outcomes associated with unilateral thyroidectomy in dogs with naturally occurring thyroid tumors: 156 cases (2003-2015). *J. Am. Vet. Med. Assoc.* 255 (8): 926–932.

3 Lorange, M., De Arburn, P.R., Huneault, L. et al. (2019). Use of a vessel-sealing device versus conventional hemostatic techniques in dogs undergoing thyroidectomy because of suspected thyroid carcinoma. *J. Am. Vet. Med. Assoc.* 254 (10): 1186–1191.

4 Latifi, M., Skinner, O.T., Spoldi, E. et al. (2021). Outcome and postoperative complications in 73 dogs with thyroid carcinoma with gross vascular invasion managed with thyroidectomy. *Vet. Comp. Oncol.* 19 (4): 685–696.

5 Tuohy, J.L., Worley, D.R., and Withrow, S.J. (2012). Outcome following simultaneous bilateral thyroid lobectomy for treatment of thyroid gland carcinoma in dogs: 15 cases (1994-2010). *J. Am. Vet. Med. Assoc.* 241 (1): 95–103.

6 Scharf, V.F., Oblak, M.L., Hoffman, K. et al. (2020). Clinical features and outcome of functional thyroid tumours in 70 dogs. *J. Small Anim. Pract.* 61: 504–511.

7 Covey, H.L., Chang, Y.M., Elliott, J. et al. (2019). Changes in thyroid and renal function after bilateral thyroidectomy in cats. *J. Vet. Intern. Med.* 33 (2): 508–515.

8 Naan, E.C., Kirpensteijn, J., Kooistra, H.S. et al. (2006). Results of thyroidectomy in 101 cats with hyperthyroidism. *Vet. Surg.* 35 (3): 287–293.

9 Flanders, J.A., Harvey, H.J., and Erb, H.N. (1987). Feline thyroidectomy: a comparison of postoperative hypocalcemia associated with three different surgical techniques. *Vet. Surg.* 16 (5): 362–366.

10 Klein, M.K., Powers, B.E., Withrow, S.J. et al. (1995). Treatment of thyroid carcinoma in dogs by surgical resection alone: 20 cases (1981-1989). *J. Am. Vet. Med. Assoc.* 206: 1007–1009.

11 Frederick, A.N., Pardo, A.D., Schmiedt, C.W. et al. (2020). Outcomes for dogs with functional thyroid tumors treated by surgical excision alone. *J. Am. Vet. Med. Assoc.* 256 (4): 444–448.

Chapter 9: Parathyroidectomy

Indications

1) Resection of hyperplastic tissue or benign adenomas causing functional hyperparathyroidism
2) Resection of malignant parathyroid adenocarcinomas

Suggested Diagnostic Workup and Clinical Staging

- Complete blood count, serum biochemistry, and urinalysis
- Parathyroid hormone panel
- Cervical ultrasound or computed tomography (CT) scan
- Thoracic radiographs or thoracic CT scan

Patient Positioning

The patient is positioned in dorsal recumbency. A towel or sandbag can be placed under the neck to elevate the neck.

Surgical Technique (See Plate 9A–G)

A) A ventral midline skin incision is made extending from just caudal to the larynx and extending caudally to a few centimeters cranial to the thoracic inlet.
B) Dissection is continued through the subcutaneous tissue using a combination of sharp and blunt dissection (i) until the paired sternohyoideus muscles (SHMs) are exposed (ii). Both the sternohyoideus and sternocephalicus muscles arise from the manubrium; the SHMs continue along the midline cranially, whereas the four separate parts of the sternocephalicus muscles diverge laterally (paired on each of the left and right sides). Because of this divergence, it is unusual to need to separate the sternocephalicus muscles to expose the trachea and thyroid glands; however, this can be performed if necessary.
C) The left and right SHMs are separated laterally using sharp dissection. Small blood vessels may be encountered during this dissection and can be managed with bipolar electrocautery.
D) Gelpi (or other self-retaining) retractors are placed cranially and caudally in the incision to lateralize the SHMs and expose a deep fascial layer and the underlying trachea.

Color Atlas of Canine and Feline Surgical Oncology, First Edition. Julius M. Liptak, Paolo Buracco, William T. N. Culp, and Nicholas J. Bacon.

Plate 9

Parathyroidectomy

A)

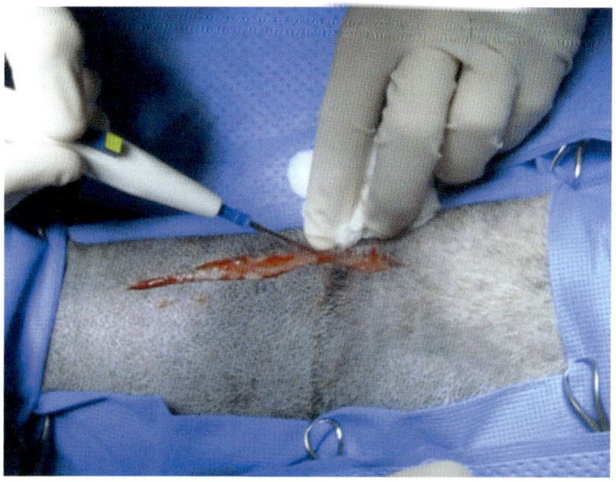

B-i)

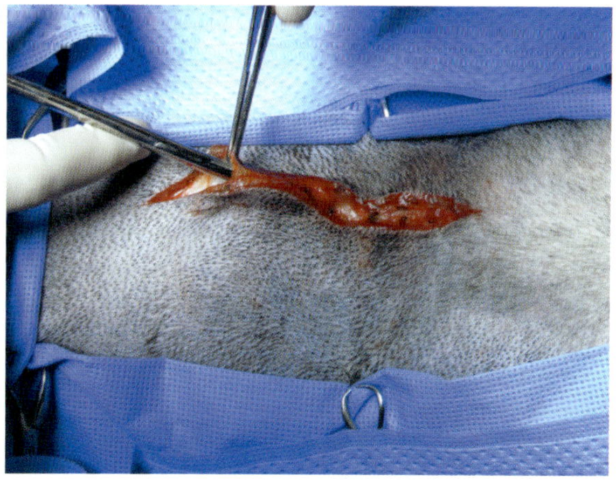

B-ii)

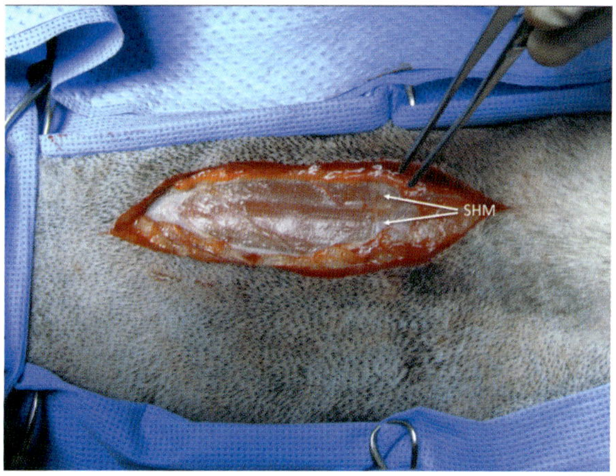

C)

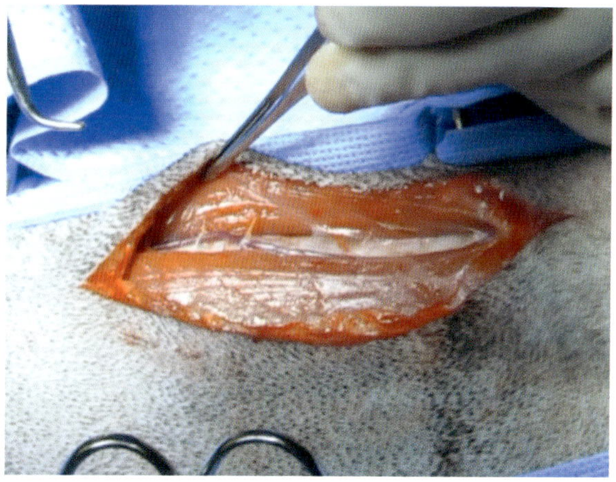

D)

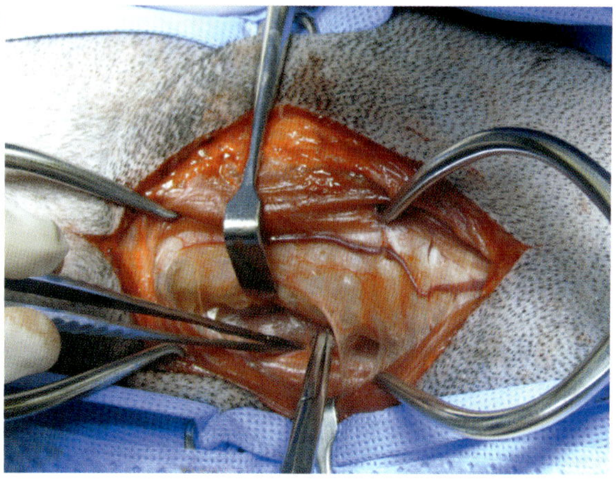

Surgical Technique (See Plate 9A–G) *continued*

E) There are two external parathyroid glands (PT) and two internal parathyroid glands in dogs and cats. The external parathyroid gland is located extracapsular to the thyroid gland, whereas the internal parathyroid gland is located within the parenchyma of the thyroid gland. The thyroid glands are generally attached to the trachea in a lateral position, and the parathyroid glands can be found closely associated with the thyroid glands (TH). After exposing the ventral aspect of the parathyroid gland that is to be removed, self-retaining retractors should be repositioned to improve the visualization of the affected side and lateralize the trachea to the contralateral side of the tumor. A sponge, or other protective device, should be placed on the trachea during lateralization to prevent trauma. In normal parathyroid glands, the blood supply is quite small and arises from the cranial and caudal thyroid arteries in dogs and the cranial thyroid artery in cats. Neoplastic parathyroid glands are relatively small (i–v), and a combination of monopolar electrosurgery and bipolar electrocautery can be used to control bleeding.

F) Neoplastic parathyroid glands (PT) can be removed with or without the thyroid gland (TH). For noninvasive parathyroid tumors, a surgical plane can be established by dissecting between the parathyroid gland and the capsule of the thyroid gland, leaving the entire thyroid gland intact. Small bleeding vessels can be controlled with bipolar electrocautery.

Plate 9

Parathyroidectomy *continued*

E-i)

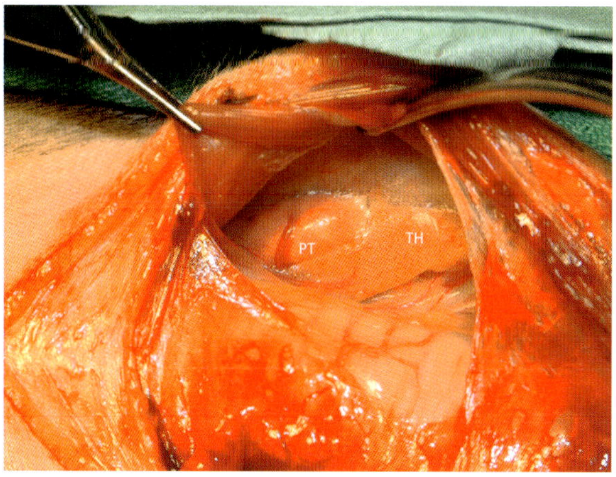

E-ii)

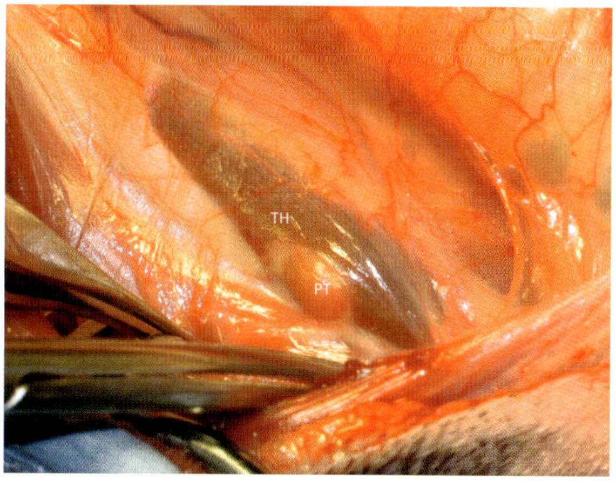

E-iii)

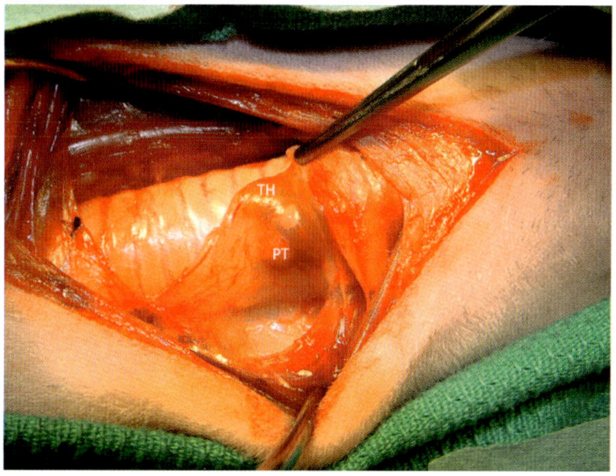

E-iv)

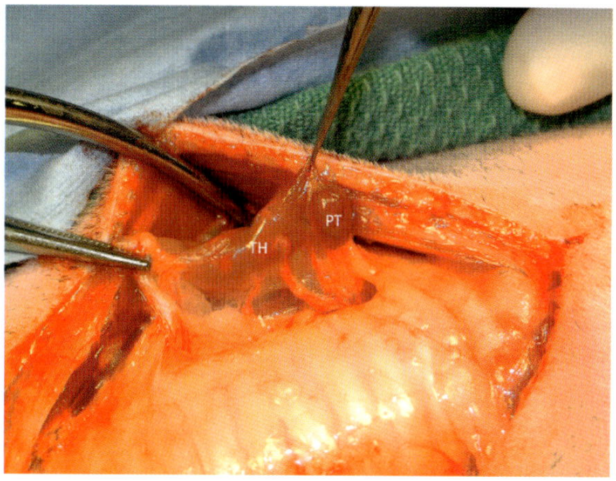

E-v)

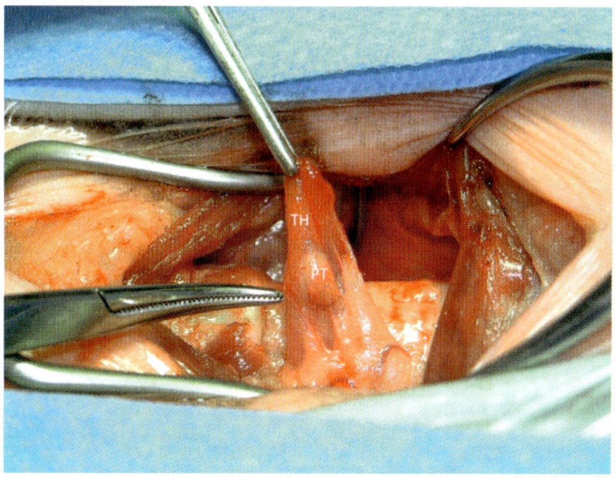

F)

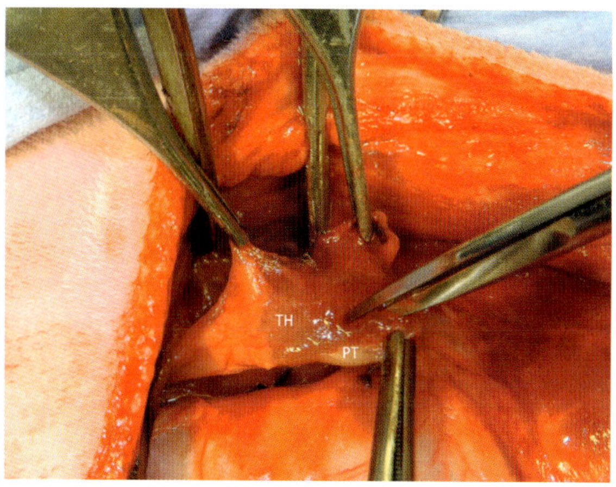

Surgical Technique (See Plate 9A–G) *continued*

G) For invasive parathyroid tumors, part or all of the thyroid gland can be removed in combination with the parathyroid gland tumor (see *8. Thyroidectomy*). A partial thyroidectomy with the associated parathyroid tumor can be performed with a vessel sealing device.

Closure (See Plate 9H, I)

H) The SHMs are reapposed with 3-0 or 4-0 monofilament absorbable suture in a simple continuous suture pattern.
I) The subcutaneous tissue is reapposed with 3-0 or 4-0 monofilament absorbable suture in a simple continuous suture pattern. An intradermal layer of 3-0 or 4-0 monofilament absorbable suture is placed followed by skin sutures if necessary.

Postoperative Management

1) Multimodal analgesia
2) Monitoring ionized calcium levels ± calcitriol supplementation if hypocalcemic
3) Elizabethan collar

Complications – Dogs

- Incisional complications (seroma, infection, dehiscence; rare)
- Persistent or recurrent hypercalcemia (5%–7%) [1, 2]
- Hypocalcemia (31%–58%) [2, 3]
- Chronic renal failure (24%) [1]

Complications – Cats [4]

- Respiratory distress secondary to presumed recurrent laryngeal nerve damage and laryngeal paralysis (9%)
- Persistent hypercalcemia (19%)
- Hypocalcemia (34%)

Suggested Adjuvant Treatments

- ± Calcitriol if hypocalcemic after surgery

Plate 9

Parathyroidectomy *continued*

G)

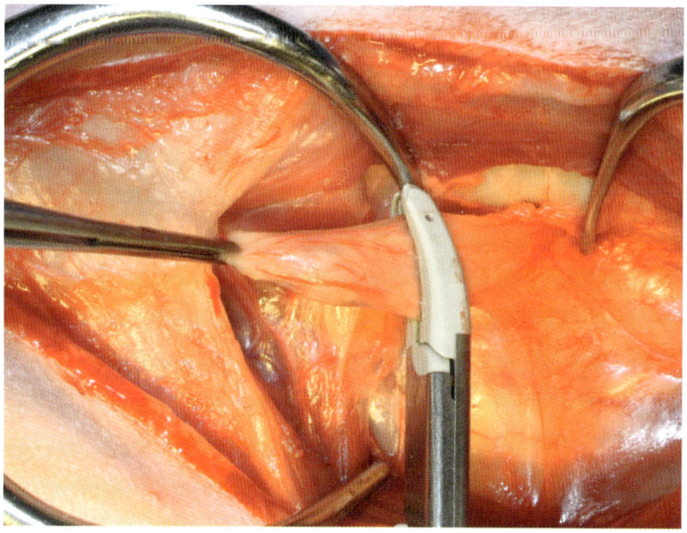

H)

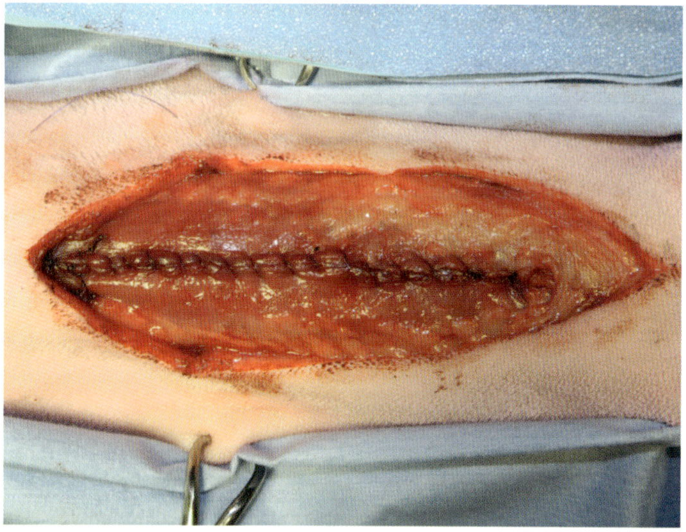

I)

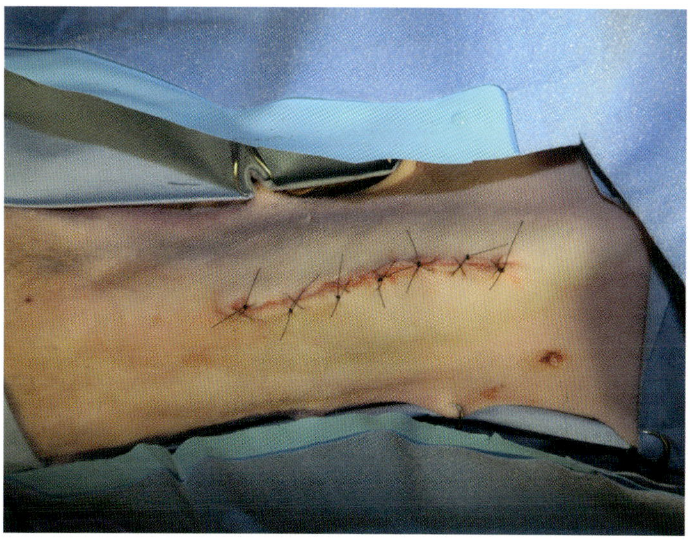

Prognosis and Oncologic Outcome – Dogs [1, 2]

Tumor Type	Local Recurrence Rate	Metastatic Rate	Disease-Free Interval (d)	Median Survival Time (d)	1-Year Survival Rate	2-Year Survival Rate
Carcinoma	0%–7%	0%	–	>547 to 1009	83%–100%	59%–100%

Prognosis and Oncologic Outcome – Cats [4]

Tumor Type	Local Recurrence Rate	Metastatic Rate	Disease-Free Interval (d)	Mean Survival Time (d)	1-Year Survival Rate	2-Year Survival Rate
Overall	3%	–	–	1109	–	–

References

1 Gear, R.N.A., Neiger, R., Skelly, B.J.S. et al. (2005). Primary hyperparathyroidism in 29 dogs: diagnosis, treatment, outcome and associated renal failure. *J. Small Anim. Pract.* 46: 10–16.

2 Sawyer, E.S., Northrup, N.C., Schmiedt, C.W. et al. (2012). Outcome of 19 dogs with parathyroid carcinoma after surgical excision. *Vet. Comp. Oncol.* 10 (1): 57–64.

3 Berger, B. and Feldman, E.C. (1987). Primary hyperparathyroidism in dogs: 21 cases (1976–1986). *J. Am. Vet. Med. Assoc.* 191 (3): 350–356.

4 Singh, A., Giuffrida, M.A., Thomson, C.B. et al. (2019). Perioperative characteristics, histologic diagnosis, and outcome in cats undergoing surgical treatment of primary hyperparathyroidism. *Vet. Surg.* 48: 367–374.

Section 3

Thoracic

Chapter 10: Surgical Approaches to the Thorax

10.1 Intercostal Thoracotomy

Indications

The surgical approach for resection of tumors is confined to either the left or right hemithorax, including lung tumors, small cranial mediastinal tumors, right atrial tumors, and tracheal and esophageal tumors, as well as subtotal pericardectomy for the palliative management of heart base tumors.

Patient Positioning

The patient is positioned in lateral recumbency with the affected side uppermost.

Surgical Technique (See Plate 10.1A–G)

A) The intended intercostal space for the lateral thoracotomy depends on the disease being treated. A fourth or fifth intercostal thoracotomy is recommended for resection of lung tumors, heart base tumors, and subtotal pericardectomy. Mediastinal masses can be approached through either a first or second intercostal thoracotomy. Esophageal and tracheal tumors are approached through the intercostal space that allows the best visualization based on the location of the tumor. An incision is made through the skin and subcutaneous tissue at the desired intercostal space extending from the costovertebral junction to a few centimeters dorsal to the sternum.

B) The cutaneous trunci muscle is incised, and the latissimus dorsi (LD) muscle is visualized.

C) The LD and pectoralis muscles can either be incised (i) or retracted with a retractor, such as an Army-Navy or Senn-Miller retractor, to expose the scalenus (SC) muscle inserting on the fifth rib and the external abdominal oblique (EAO) originating on the fifth rib (ii).

D) Depending on the chosen intercostal space, either the scalenus (pictured) or EAO muscle is incised off the fifth rib. The serratus ventralis (SV) muscle is also separated, revealing the external intercostal (IC) muscles. At this point, it is prudent to recount the intercostal spaces cranial to caudal to verify the correct location.

E) The external and internal intercostal muscles are identified, grasped with tissue forceps, and incised to expose the pleura (P). The incision is made in the middle of the intercostal muscles in the desired intercostal space. Care should be taken to not incise the internal thoracic artery.

Color Atlas of Canine and Feline Surgical Oncology, First Edition. Julius M. Liptak, Paolo Buracco, William T. N. Culp, and Nicholas J. Bacon.

Plate 10.1

Intercostal Thoracotomy

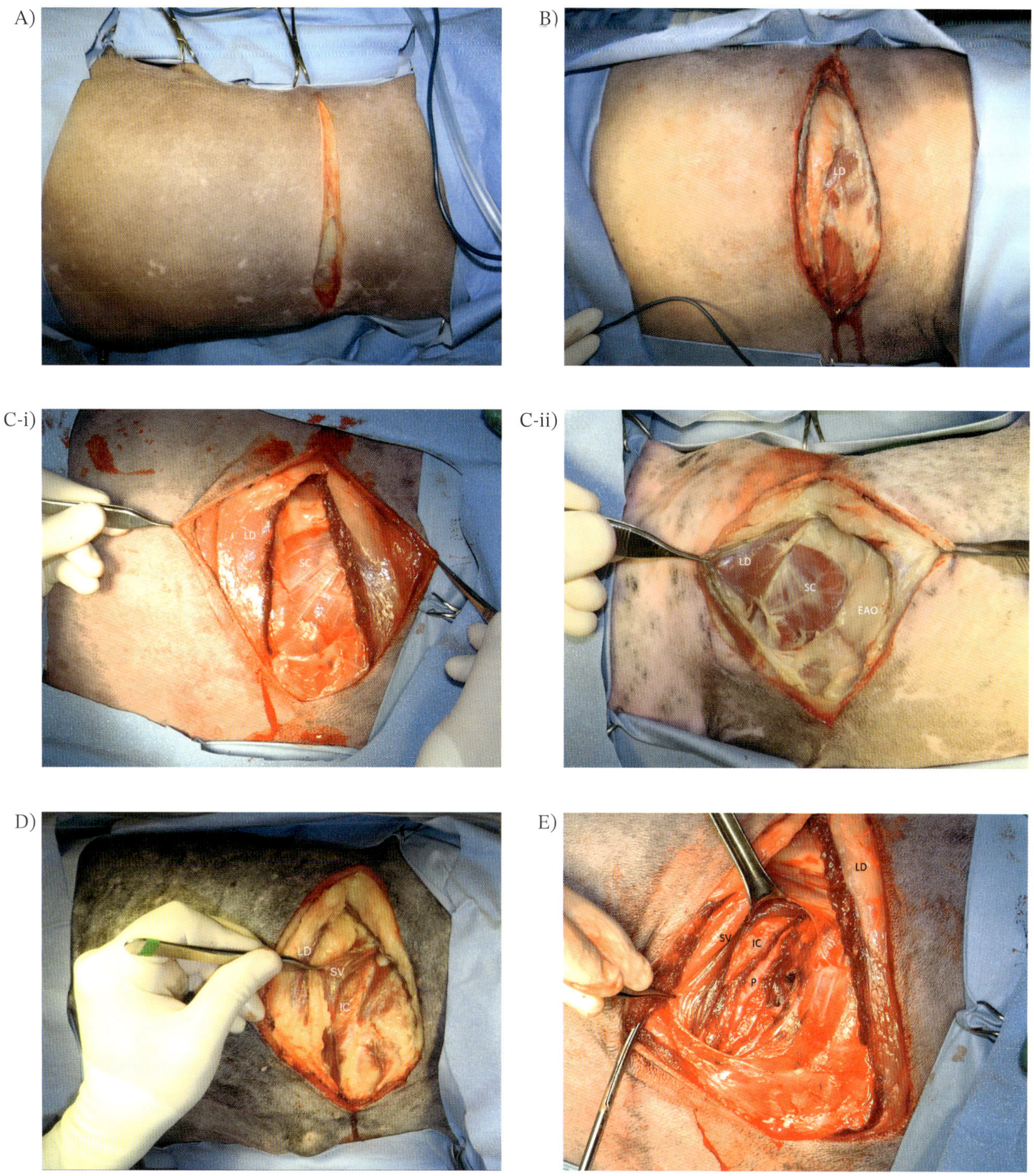

Surgical Technique (See Plate 10.1A–G) *continued*

F) Often the parietal pleura will be visualized, and this is elevated with tissue forceps, punctured gently with Metzenbaum scissors (i) and incised to create a pneumothorax (ii). Any remaining pleura within the intercostal space is incised, generally with sharp scissors.

G) Once the thorax is open, moistened laparotomy sponges are placed on the exposed edges of the incision, and a Finochietto retractor is placed to spread the ribs.

Closure (See Plate 10.1H–L)

H) A thoracostomy tube is placed before closure of the thorax and secured to the skin.

I) Large-gauge monofilament absorbable or nonabsorbable suture (1-0 to 2) is preplaced in a simple interrupted pattern around the rib cranial and caudal to the intercostal incision in either a simple interrupted or cruciate suture pattern. When the needle is inserted from a lateral-to-intrathoracic direction, the needle is reversed to avoid iatrogenic puncture of the lungs (i, arrow). After placement, the needle is cut off of the suture, and the two suture ends are secured with a hemostat. These sutures are generally placed 1–3 cm apart (ii).

J) After all sutures have been preplaced, an assistant approximates the ribs to decrease tension while tying each knot.

Plate 10.1

Intercostal Thoracotomy *continued*

F-i)

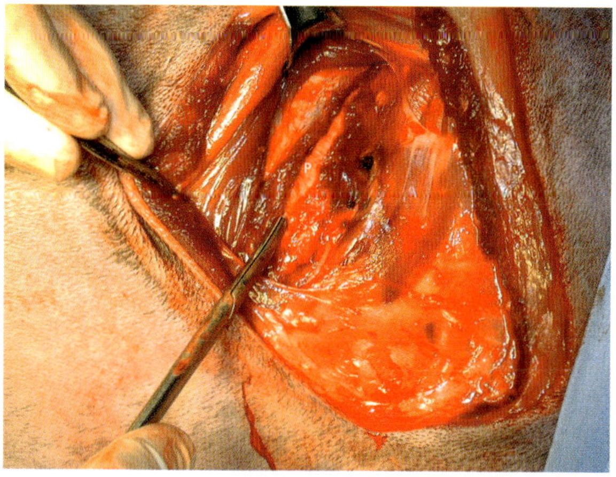

F-ii)

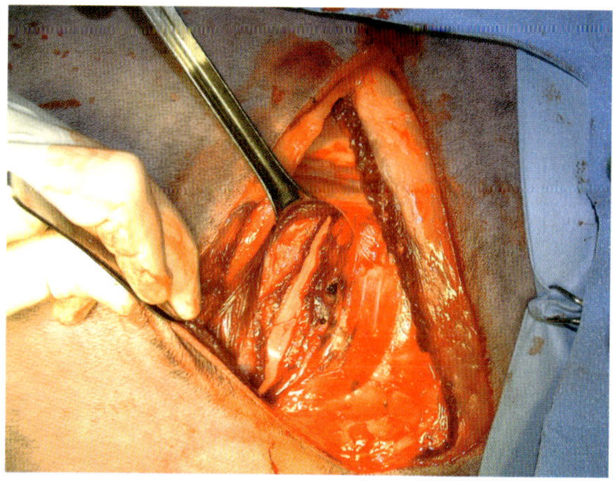

G)

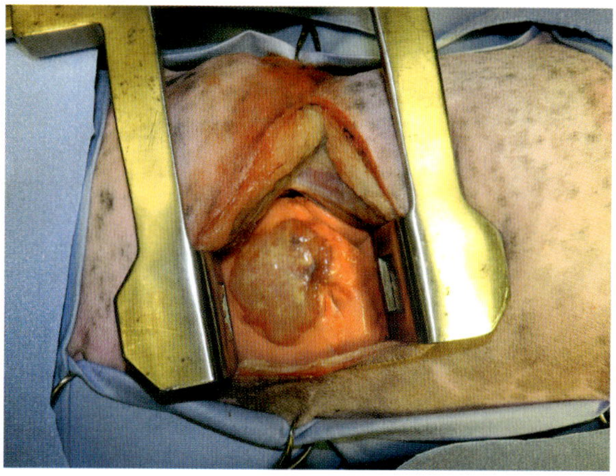

H)

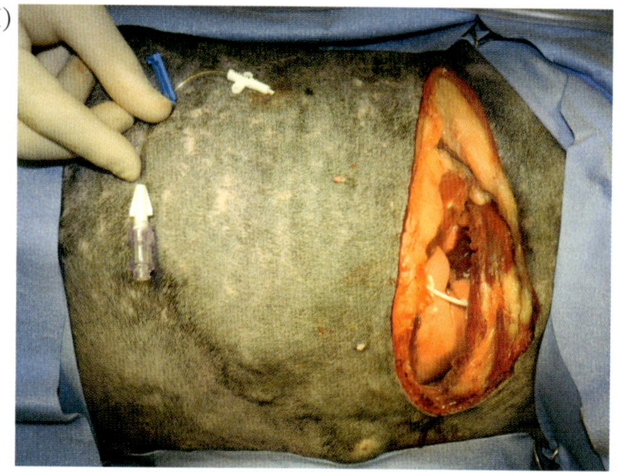

I-i)

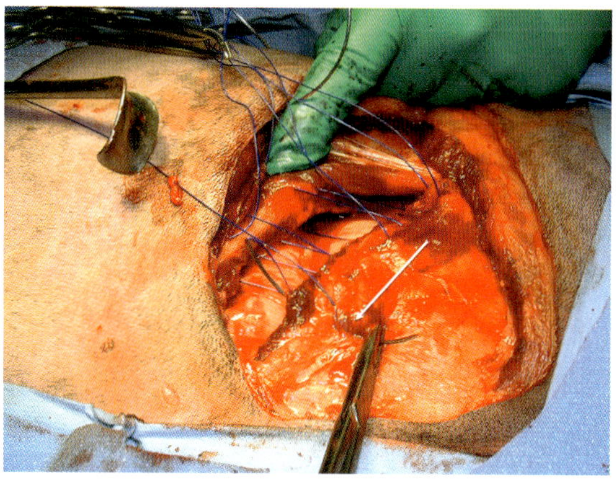

I-ii)

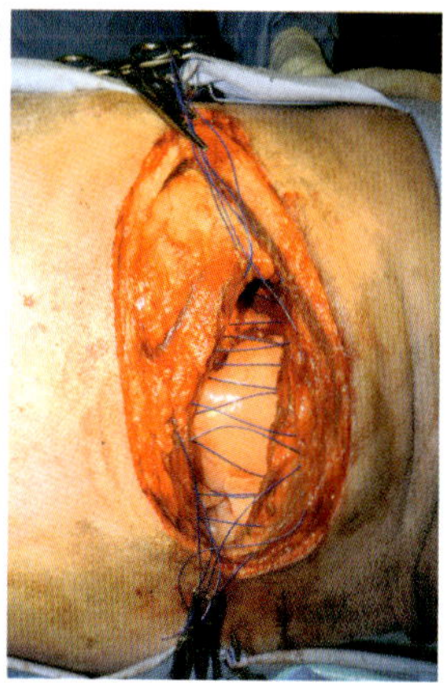

J)

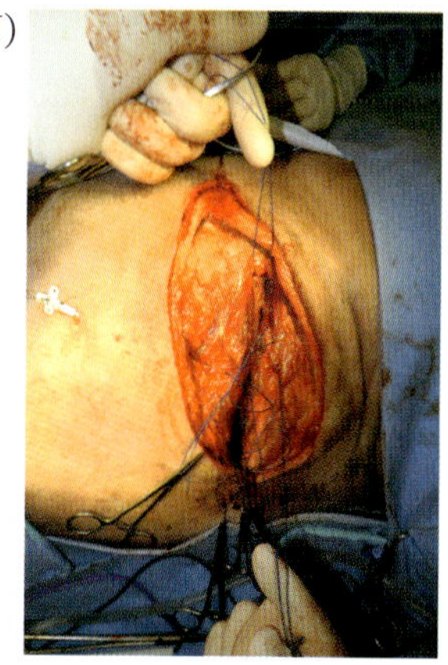

Closure (See Plate 10.1H–L) *continued*

K) As an alternative, small holes can be drilled into the caudal rib with a pin and hand chuck (i). The suture material is passed through these transcostal holes (ii) to avoid compression of the intercostal neurovascular bundles coursing along the caudal aspect of the rib and reduce postoperative pain [1].

L) The serratus ventralis and scalenus or EAO muscles are closed in an interrupted or continuous pattern with 2-0 to 3-0 monofilament absorbable suture (i). If the LD muscle has been transected, a simple continuous pattern of 3-0 monofilament absorbable suture in a simple continuous pattern is used to appose the cut edges of this muscle (ii). Removal of residual air from the thoracic cavity is performed using the preplaced chest tube once the thoracic cavity is closed. A wound diffuser catheter can be placed in the subcutaneous space to provide additional analgesia (iii). The subcutaneous tissue is closed with a simple continuous pattern of 3-0 to 4-0 absorbable suture (iv). An intradermal layer of 3-0 or 4-0 absorbable suture is placed followed by skin sutures if necessary (v).

Postoperative Management

1) Multimodal analgesia, including perioperative continuous rate infusion of an opioid ± ketamine, intercostal nerve blocks, local anesthesia instilled through the thoracostomy tube ± wound diffuser catheter, and oral analgesic drugs
2) Supplemental oxygen therapy, if required
3) Thoracostomy tube management
4) Elizabethan collar or body suit

Complications [2, 3]

Intraoperative Complications

- Bleeding (3%)
- Cardiac arrhythmias (10%)

Postoperative Complications

- Hypoxia (13%)
- Bleeding (4%)
- Pneumothorax (2%)
- Seroma and ventral edema (22%)
- Ipsilateral thoracic limb lameness (4%)

References

1 Rooney, M.B., Mehl, M., and Monnet, E. (2004). Intercostal thoracotomy closure: transcostal sutures as a less painful alternative to circumcostal suture placement. *Vet. Surg.* 33 (3): 209–213.

2 Moores, A.L., Halfacree, Z.J., Baines, S.J. et al. (2007). Indications, outcomes and complications following lateral thoracotomy in dogs and cats. *J. Small Anim. Pract.* 48 (12): 695–698.

3 Bleakley, S., Phipps, K., Petrovsky, B. et al. (2018). Median sternotomy versus intercostal thoracotomy for lung lobectomy: A comparison of short-term outcome in 134 dogs. *Vet. Surg.* 47 (1): 104–113.

Plate 10.1

Intercostal Thoracotomy *continued*

K-i)

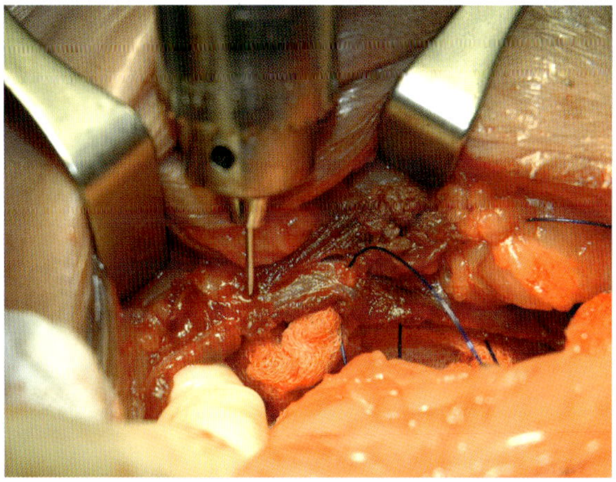

K-ii)

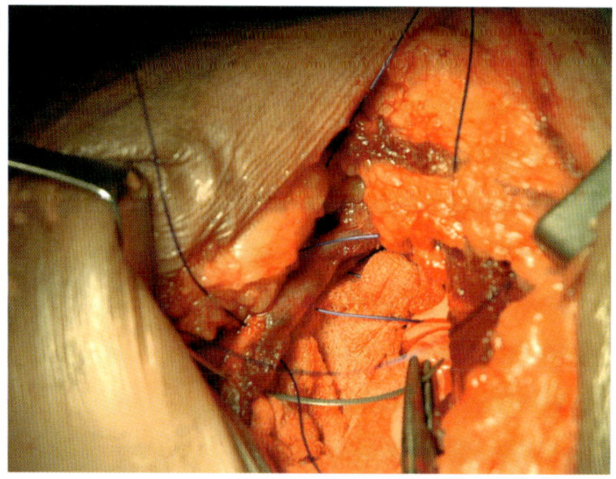

L-i)

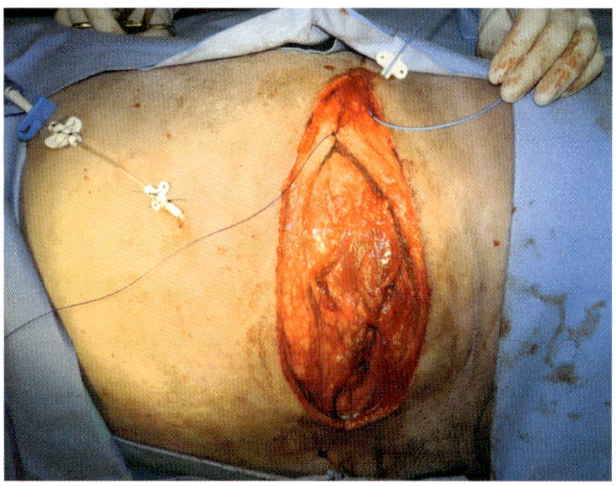

L-ii)

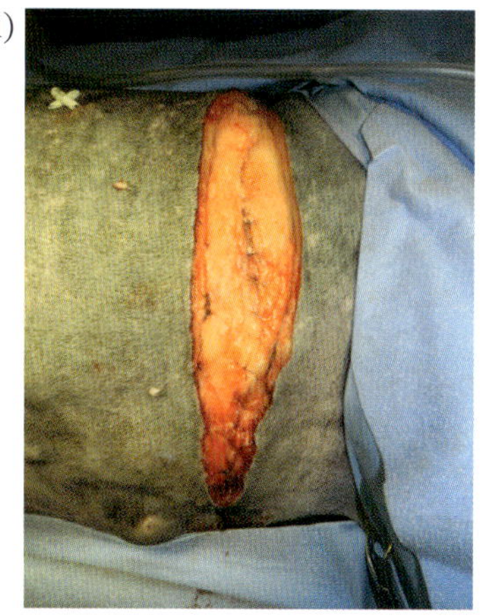

L-iii)

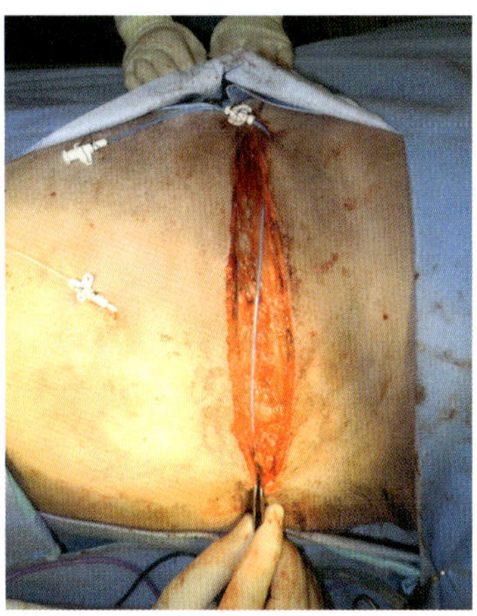

L-iv)

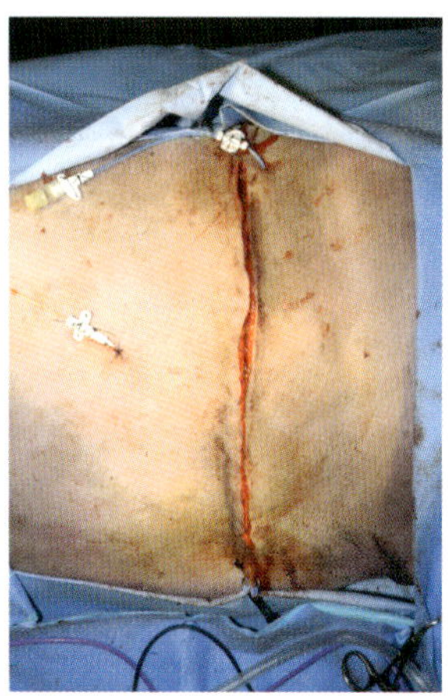

L-v)

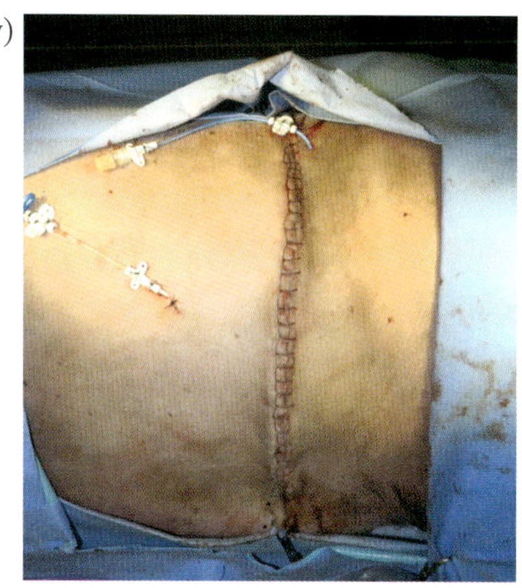

10.2 Median Sternotomy

Indications

This surgical approach is preferred for resection of tumors involving both hemithoraces, such as cranial mediastinal and heart base tumors. Subtotal pericardectomy for palliative management of heart base tumors is also possible through this approach, although an open intercostal (see *12.1. Open Subtotal Pericardectomy*) or thoracoscopic open intercostal (see *12.2. Thoracoscopic Pericardectomy*) approach is generally preferred for pericardectomy.

Patient Positioning

The patient is positioned in dorsal recumbency.

Surgical Technique (See Plate 10.2A–E)

A) A skin incision is made on the ventral midline of the sternum extending from the manubrium to the xiphoid process. The incision is extended through the subcutaneous tissue until the pectoral muscles are visualized.
B) Electrosurgery is preferred when available to separate the pectoral muscles from the sternum, although blunt elevation of the muscles off of the sternum is also acceptable. Effort should be made not to dissect the muscles too far laterally because perforating blood vessels can be encountered and these can bleed vigorously.
C) Once the ventral midline of the sternebrae is exposed, an oscillating or sagittal saw is used to osteotomize the sternum on the midline (i–iii). Care should be taken to avoid transecting the rib heads off of the sternum because this complicates closure.
D) Once a full-thickness cut has been made through a portion of the sternum, an elevator or other flat instrument can be introduced into the sternotomy and used to open the sternotomy laterally to allow better visualization of the dorsal-ventral depth of the sternum during the remainder of the osteotomy. In most cases, either the manubrium or xiphoid process can be left intact to facilitate easier closure of the sternum; however, this is not necessary for postoperative sternal stability. The choice as to which of these structures not to cut is based on the location of the lesion that is being treated. Once the sternotomy is complete, Gelpi retractors are initially used to expose and transect ventral pleural and mediastinal tissue with a vessel sealing device (pictured).
E) Once the thorax is open, a Finochietto retractor is inserted to spread the sternal components laterally.

Color Atlas of Canine and Feline Surgical Oncology, First Edition. Julius M. Liptak, Paolo Buracco, William T. N. Culp, and Nicholas J. Bacon.

Plate 10.2

Median Sternotomy

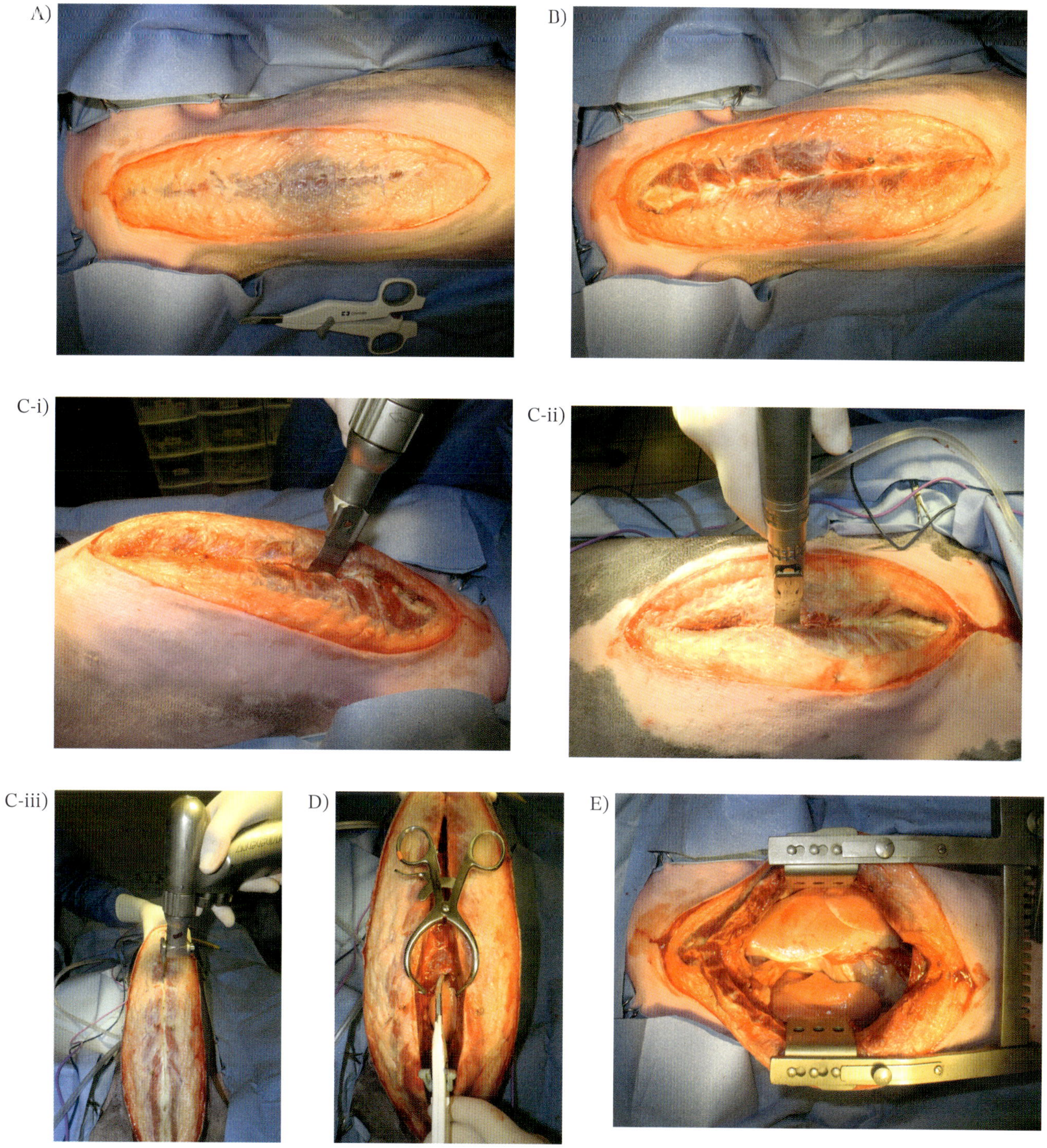

Closure (See Plate 10.2F–I)

F) A thoracostomy tube is placed before closure of the thorax and secured to the skin.

G) In medium to large breed dogs, the use of stainless steel wire is preferred for sternotomy closure (i, ii). The wire (generally 18–22 gauge) is placed in a figure-of-eight pattern centered on the sternal synchondroses. Alternatively, 80-lb nylon leader can be used in similar fashion to stainless steel wire [1], and a monofilament absorbable suture has been used in smaller patients (iii) [2].

H) After preplacement of all the wires, each wire is twisted while pulling up ventrally to allow for close apposition of the left and right segments of sternum; ideally, three unbent twists are left on the wire (i). In small animals or animals with poor soft tissue coverage, the knot can be bent, although this is less desirable because the security of the closure is weakened. Similarly, if using suture material to close the sternotomy, the preplaced sutures are tightened and knotted (ii). The pectoral muscles are closed in a simple continuous pattern with 2-0 or 3-0 monofilament absorbable suture. Removal of residual air from the thoracic cavity is performed using the preplaced chest tube once the thoracic cavity is closed.

Plate 10.2

Median Sternotomy *continued*

F)

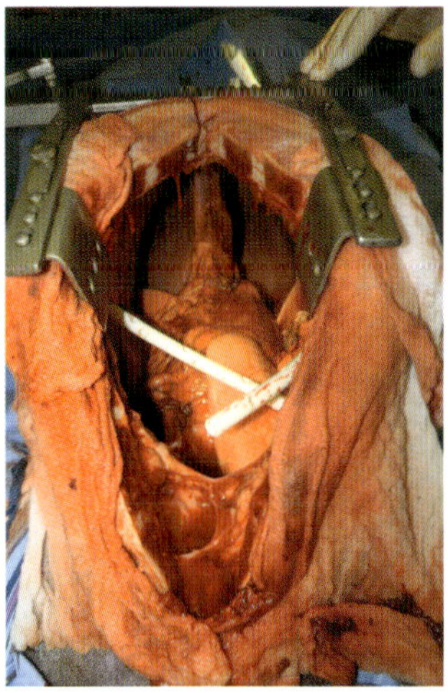

G-i)

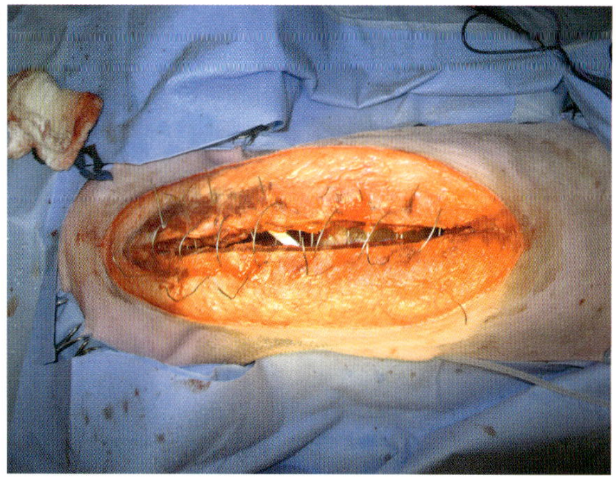

G-ii)

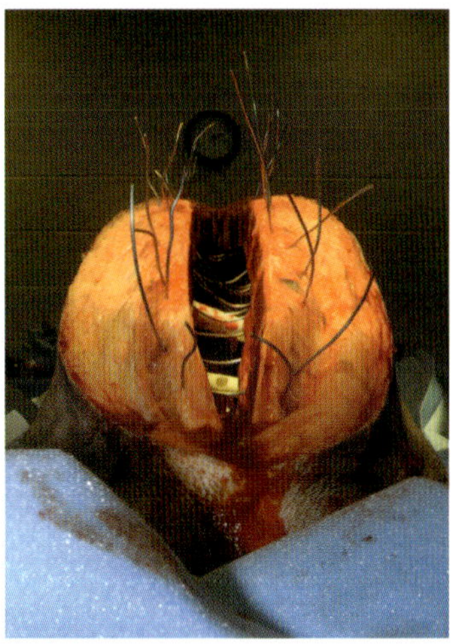

G-iii)

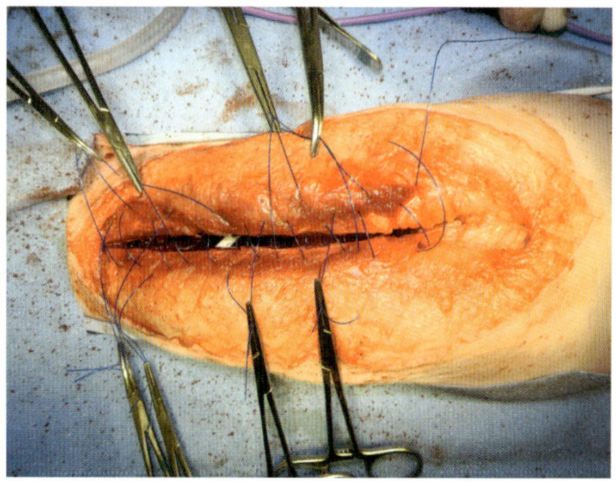

H-i)

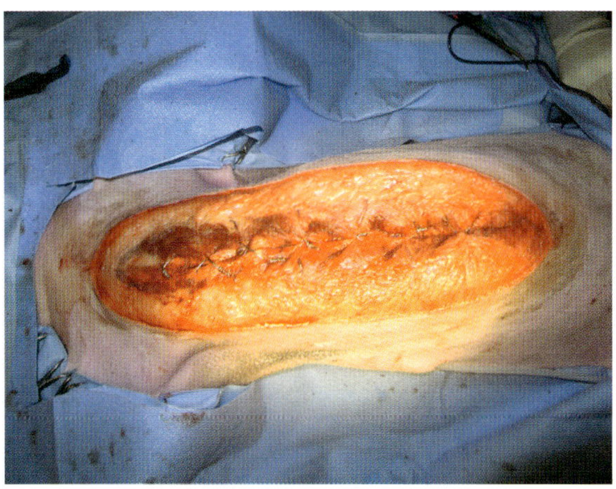

H-ii)

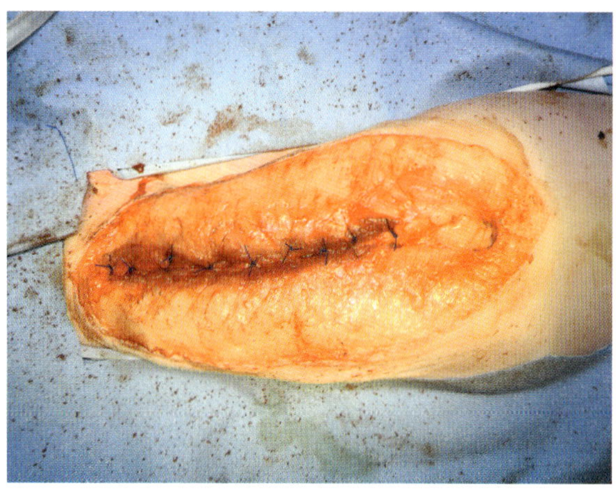

Closure (See Plate 10.2F–I) *continued*

I) The subcutaneous tissue is closed with a simple continuous pattern of 3-0 or 4-0 absorbable suture (i). An intradermal layer of 3-0 or 4-0 absorbable suture is placed followed by skin sutures if necessary (ii).

Postoperative Management

1) Multimodal analgesia, including perioperative continuous rate infusion of an opioid ± ketamine, intercostal nerve blocks, local anesthesia instilled through the thoracostomy tube ± wound diffuser catheter, and oral analgesic drugs
2) Supplemental oxygen therapy, if required
3) Thoracostomy tube management
4) Elizabethan collar or body suit

Complications [3, 4]

Intraoperative Complications

- Bleeding (2%)
- Cardiac arrhythmias (7%)
- Transection of costosternal junction

Postoperative Complications (0–14 days)

- Overall: 19%
- Hypoxia (34%)
- Bleeding (5%)
- Pneumothorax (5%)
- Pulmonary thromboembolism (2%)
- Surgical-site infection (5%) (J).
- Ipsilateral thoracic limb lameness (3%)

Postoperative Complications (>14 days) (See Plate 10.2J)

- Overall: 22%
- Surgical-site infection (5%)
- Sternal osteomyelitis (11%–14%) (J, 10 days postoperatively)

References

1 McCready, D.J., Bell, J.C., Ness, M.G. et al. (2015). Mechanical comparison of monofilament nylon leader and orthopaedic wire for median sternotomy closure. *J. Small Anim. Pract.* 56 (8): 510–515.
2 Gines, J.A., Friend, E.J., Vives, M.A. et al. (2011). Mechanical comparison of median sternotomy closure in dogs using polydioxanone and wire sutures. *J. Small Anim. Pract.* 52 (11): 582–586.
3 Burton, C.A. and White, R.N. (1996). Review of the technique and complications of median sternotomy in the dog and cat. *J. Small Anim. Pract.* 37 (11): 516–522.
4 Bleakley, S., Phipps, K., Petrovsky, B. et al. (2018). Median sternotomy versus intercostal thoracotomy for lung lobectomy: A comparison of short-term outcome in 134 dogs. *Vet. Surg.* 47 (1): 104–113.

Plate 10.2

Median Sternotomy *continued*

I-i)

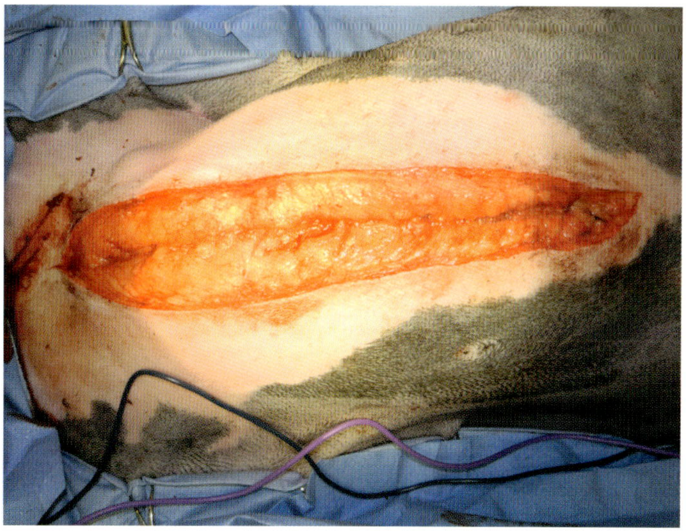

I-ii)

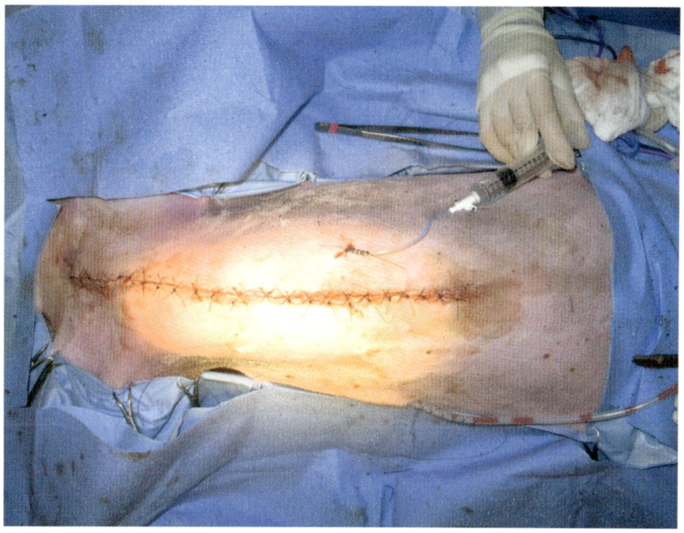

J)

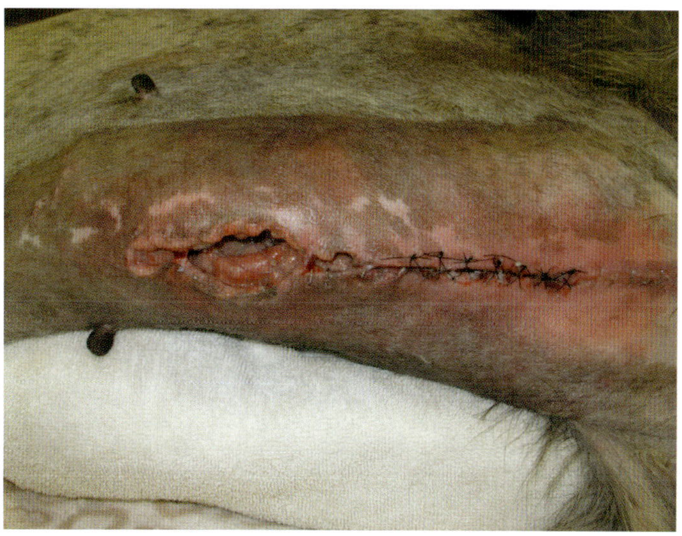

10.3 Thoracoscopy

Indications

Although the indications are still being defined, resection of pulmonary masses, mediastinal masses, and tracheobronchial lymph nodes have been described, as has subtotal pericardectomy and pericardial window formation [1–4].

Patient Positioning

The patient is positioned in lateral recumbency. An oblique positioning to the thorax with the dorsal aspect higher than the ventral aspect improves visualization of the thoracic cavity with fluoroscopy. The surgeon is positioned on the ventral side of the patient, and the monitor is across the table on the dorsum of the patient.

Surgical Technique – Access to Thoracic Cavity (See Plate 10.3C)

A) Initial access to the thoracic cavity is performed primarily using two primary techniques: open technique and optical entry technique (not pictured). A Veress needle technique is also an option; however, this is rarely employed in companion animals.
B) For the more traditional open technique, a skin incision is made that is slightly larger than the cannula that is going to be placed. A combination of blunt and sharp dissection, as well as electrosurgery, can then be used to penetrate the tissue from the level of the subcutaneous space to the level of the pleura. Once the pleura is visualized, the pleura can be incised to induce pneumothorax. A cannula with a blunt trocar can then be inserted through the hole that has been created (not pictured).
C) With the optical entry technique, a skin incision is made similar to the open technique, and the subcutaneous tissue is bluntly and sharply dissected open. A cannula is then inserted into the incision. The telescope is placed into the cannula, and the two instruments are used in unison to direct the placement of the cannula; the cannula is twisted until penetration is noted through the pleura.
D) Insufflation is rarely needed for video-assisted thoracoscopic surgery procedures (as opposed to laparoscopic procedures), which allows for the use of very simple cannulae (not pictured).

Color Atlas of Canine and Feline Surgical Oncology, First Edition. Julius M. Liptak, Paolo Buracco, William T. N. Culp, and Nicholas J. Bacon.

Plate 10.3

Thoracoscopy

C)

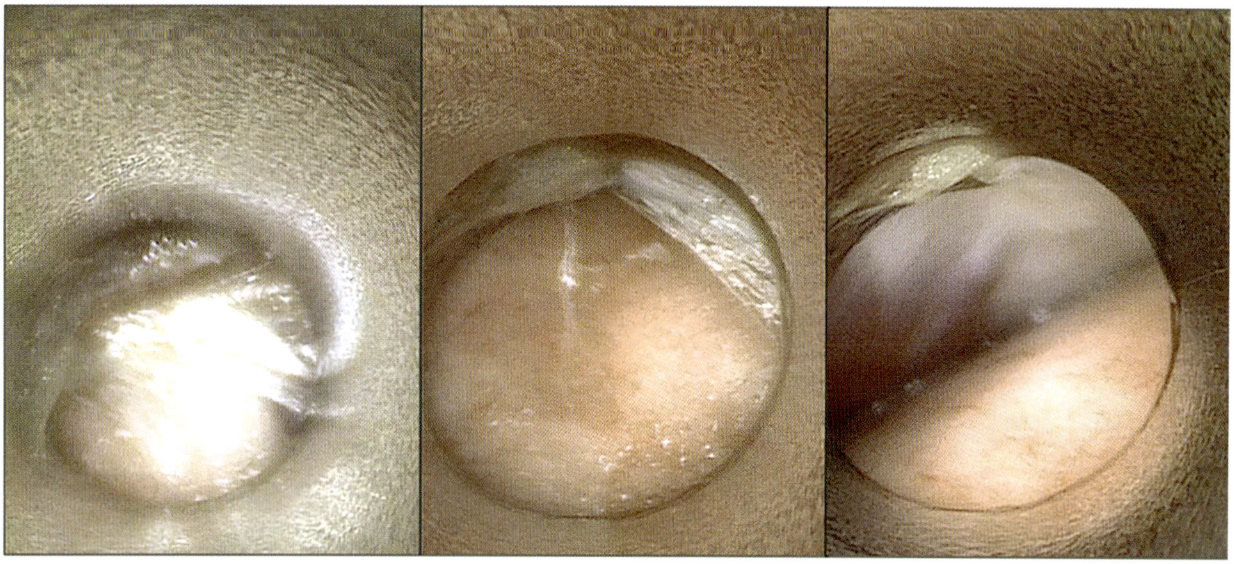

Surgical Technique – Dorsal Recumbency: Paraxiphoid Transdiaphragmatic Approach (See Plate 10.3E–G)

E) For procedures performed in dorsal recumbency, the endoscopic tower and monitor are generally placed at the head of the patient.

F) Initial access into the thorax is obtained through a paraxiphoid (or subxiphoid) transdiaphgramatic approach, and the telescope will be placed into this cannula. The skin incision (approximately 1–1.5 cm long) is made just lateral to the xiphoid; the incision will be positioned in a triangle formed by the angle of the 13th rib and xiphoid process. In addition, the skin incision is positioned on the side of the hemithorax that the surgeon would like to place the telescope.

G) The cannula is driven into the chest in a cranial direction with an angle of 45 degrees to the sagittal and perpendicular planes, as well as 45 degrees to the ventral midline. A significant amount of force may be necessary to introduce the cannula into the thorax. The goal is to pass the cannula through the ventral aspect of the diaphragm and into the hemithorax of choice.

Surgical Technique – Lateral Recumbency: Intercostal Approach (See Plate 10.3H, I)

H) For procedures performed in lateral recumbency, the endoscopic tower and monitor are generally placed on the contralateral side of the patient. For pulmonary tumors, the cranial-caudal position of the monitor may be altered depending on the location of the tumor that is being removed.

I) A 1.0- to 1.5-cm skin incision is created in the caudal aspect of the intercostal space. The intercostal space and the dorsal-ventral position are dependent on the procedure being performed. Blunt and sharp dissection and electrosurgery are used to dissect through the subcutaneous tissue. Dissection through the underlying muscle can be performed sharply or with electrosurgery; alternatively, the cannula with blunt trocar can be driven through these muscles until the thoracic cavity is penetrated (i). Once the cannulae are in position in the thoracic cavity (ii), the depth of the cannulae should be checked to avoid iatrogenic trauma to intrathoracic structures.

Closure

A thoracostomy tube is placed before closure, and the position is visualized by the telescope. Any equipment, as well as the cannulae and telescope, is removed. The muscle and subcutaneous tissue can be closed with 2-0 to 3-0 monofilament absorbable suture in a simple interrupted or cruciate pattern. The dermal layer is closed with 3-0 monofilament absorbable suture. The chest tube is secured to the skin.

Postoperative Management

1) Multimodal analgesia
2) Supplemental oxygen therapy, if required
3) Thoracostomy tube management
4) Elizabethan collar or body suit

Complications in Dogs

Intraoperative Complications

- When introducing cannulae into the thorax, it is possible for the cannulae not to be passed deep enough into the thorax. This results in visualization of subcutaneous tissue and muscle, or in the case of the paraxiphoid approach, a cannulae that may be intraabdominal.
- Similarly, cannulae can be placed into the mediastinum, which also impairs visualization.

Plate 10.3

Thoracoscopy *continued*

E-G)

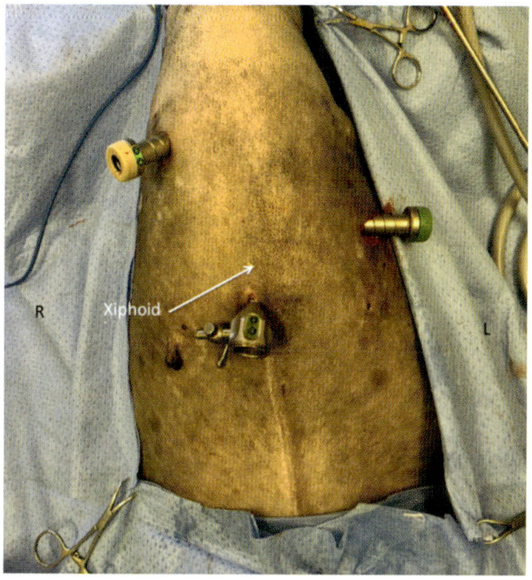

H)

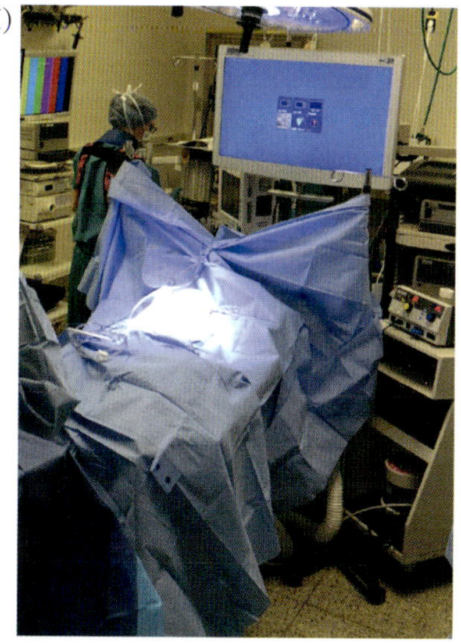

I-i)

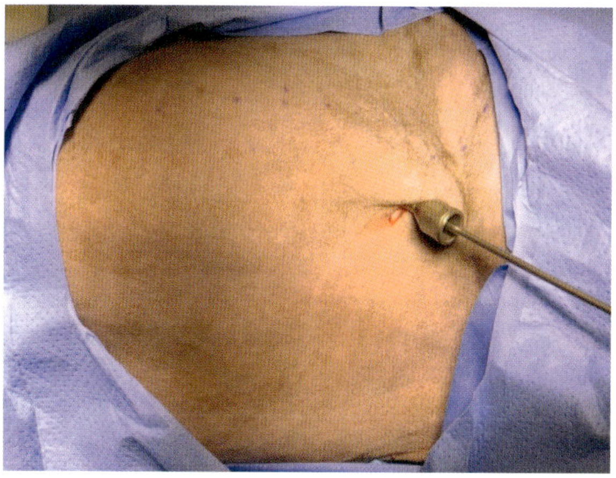

I-ii)

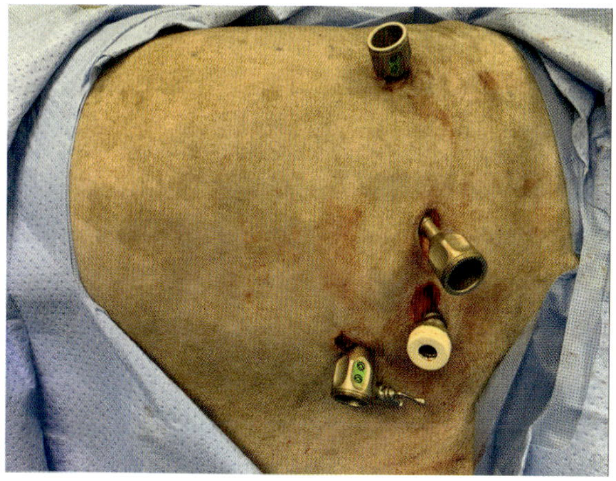

- Trauma to intrathoracic structures may also occur during cannula/trocar placement or equipment manipulation within the thorax.
- In some dogs (particularly brachycephalic breeds), the thoracic height may be too limited to allow for procedures such as pericardectomy. In these cases, the heart is often positioned just dorsal to the sternum, preventing the placement or manipulation of equipment in the space ventral to the heart.
- Conversion to an open procedure may be necessary as a result of an inability to complete the procedure because of patient size or conformation, or if a complication, such as excessive bleeding, occurs.

Postoperative Complications (0–14 Days)

- Surgical-site infections (rare) [5]

Postoperative Complications (>14 Days)

- Portal-site metastases (rare) [6, 7]

References

1 Lansdowne, J.L., Monnet, E., Twedt, D.C. et al. (2005). Thoracoscopic lung lobectomy for treatment of lung tumors in dogs. *Vet. Surg.* 34 (5): 530–535.

2 Mayhew, K.N., Mayhew, P.D., Sorrell-Raschi, L. et al. (2009). Thoracoscopic subphrenic pericardectomy using double-lumen endobronchial intubation for alternating one-lung ventilation. *Vet. Surg.* 38 (8): 961–966.

3 Mayhew, P.D. and Friedberg, J.S. (2008). Video-assisted thoracoscopic resection of noninvasive thymomas using one-lung ventilation in two dogs. *Vet. Surg.* 37 (8): 756–762.

4 Mayhew, P.D., Hunt, G.B., Steffey, M.A. et al. (2013). Evaluation of short-term outcome after lung lobectomy for resection of primary lung tumors via video-assisted thoracoscopic surgery or open thoracotomy in medium- to large-breed dogs. *J. Am. Vet. Med. Assoc.* 243 (5): 681–688.

5 Mayhew, P.D., Freeman, L., Kwan, T. et al. (2012). Comparison of surgical site infection rates in clean and clean-contaminated wounds in dogs and cats after minimally invasive versus open surgery: 179 cases (2007-2008). *J. Am. Vet. Med. Assoc.* 240 (2): 193–198.

6 Alwen, S.G., Culp, W.T., Szivek, A. et al. (2015). Portal site metastasis after thoracoscopic resection of a cranial mediastinal mass in a dog. *J. Am. Vet. Med. Assoc.* 247 (7): 793–800.

7 Brisson, B.A., Reggeti, F., and Bienzle, D. (2006). Portal site metastasis of invasive mesothelioma after diagnostic thoracoscopy in a dog. *J. Am. Vet. Med. Assoc.* 229 (6): 980–983.

Chapter 11: Lung Lobectomy

11.1 Open Lung Lobectomy

Indications

1) Resection of nonmetastatic primary lung tumors
2) Resection of metastatic lung tumors for either palliative purposes (such as management of hypertrophic osteopathy) or treatment (if the criteria for metastasectomy have been satisfied)

Suggested Diagnostic Workup and Clinical Staging

- Complete blood count, serum biochemistry, and urinalysis
- ± Preoperative ultrasound-guided fine-needle aspirate cytology
- Thoracic computed tomography (CT) scan for assessment of nodal and lung metastasis

Patient Positioning

Patient positioning is dependent on the surgical approach with lateral recumbency for an intercostal thoracotomy approach (see *10.1. Intercostal Thoracotomy*) and dorsal recumbency for a median sternotomy approach (see *10.2. Median Sternotomy*).

Surgical Technique – General Principles (See Plate 11.1A–D)

A) See *10.1. Intercostal Thoracotomy* or *10.2. Median Sternotomy* for details on the surgical approach for open lung lobectomy. A fourth or fifth intercostal thoracotomy is preferred for lung lobectomy (i). Rarely, a rib may require resection to allow adequate exposure of very large lung tumors for lung lobectomy. In these cases, the intercostal muscles are incised on either side of the rib intended for resection (usually the fifth rib). A circumcostal ligature is placed around the proximal aspect of the isolated rib (ii). The rib is then osteotomized with rib cutters distal to this circumcostal ligature (iii) and proximal to the costosternal articulation (iv), taking care to preserve the internal thoracic artery. The rib is then discarded (v) and Finochietto retractors are inserted to spread the ribs.
B) Following identification of the tumor (pictured, primary bronchogenic carcinoma), adjacent lung lobes should be gently moved away from the tumor and packed out of the surgical field with moistened laparotomy sponges (arrow).
C) If a caudal lung lobectomy is planned, then the ligamentous attachments (pulmonary ligaments, arrow) should be transected with scissors, electrosurgery, or a vessel sealing device before lung lobectomy.

Color Atlas of Canine and Feline Surgical Oncology, First Edition. Julius M. Liptak, Paolo Buracco, William T. N. Culp, and Nicholas J. Bacon.

Plate 11.1

Open Lung Lobectomy

A-i)

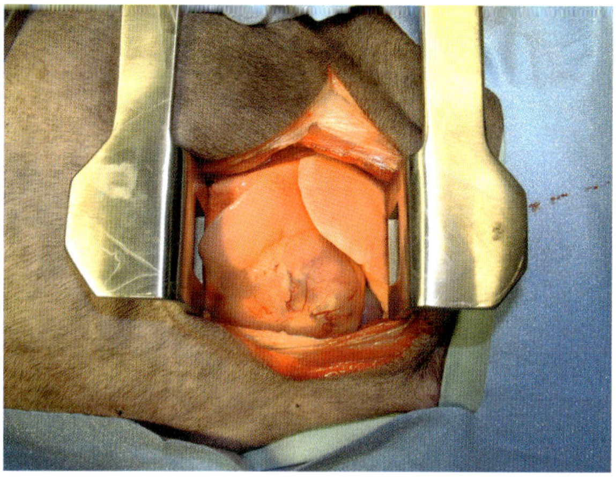

A-ii)

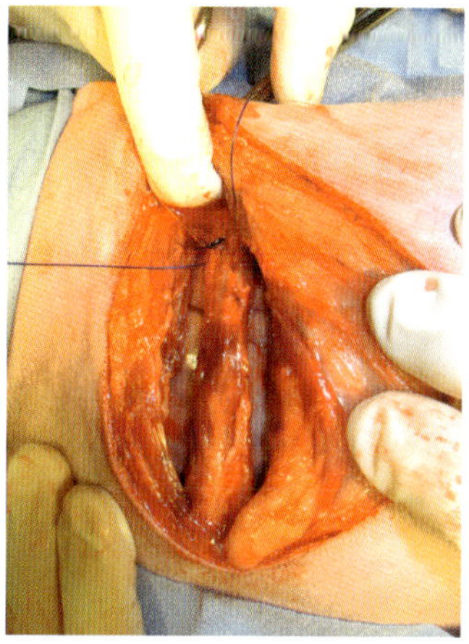

A-iii)

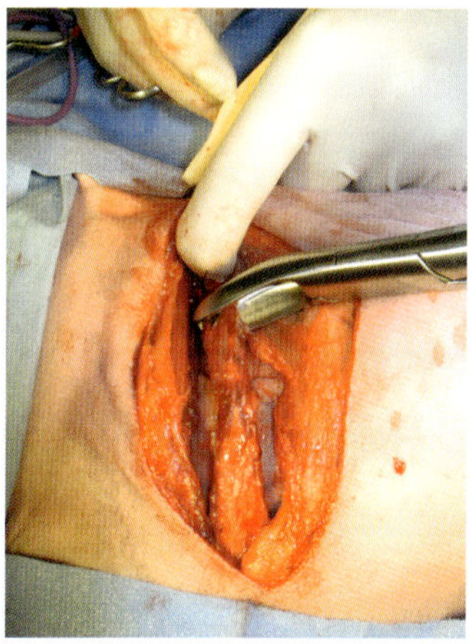

A-iv)

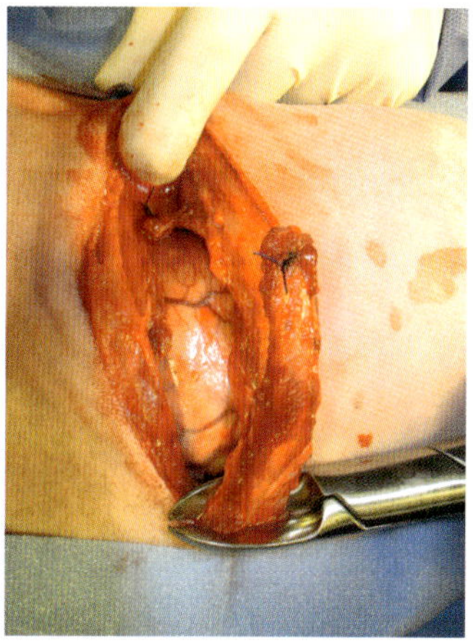

A-v)

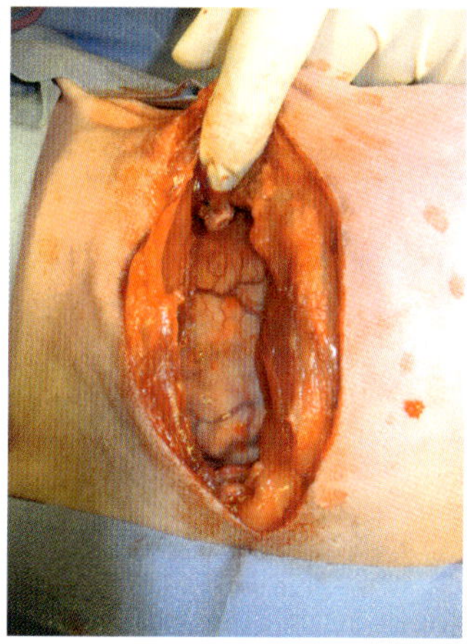

B)

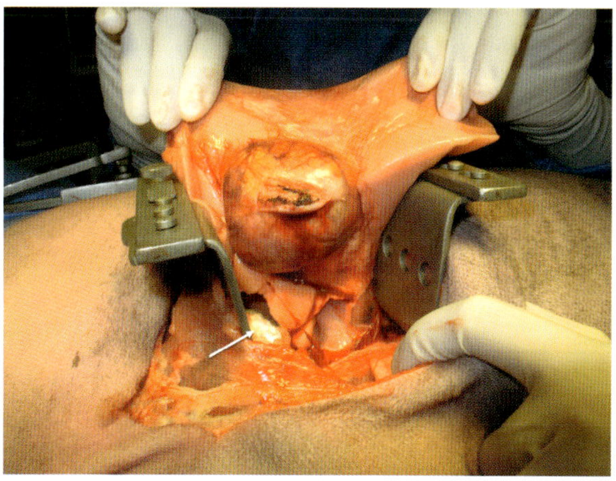

C)

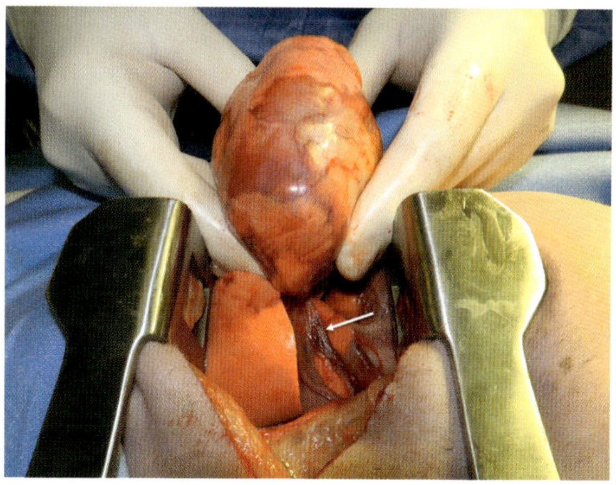

Surgical Technique – General Principles (See Plate 11.1A–D) *continued*

D) If there are adhesions between the lung lobe and other thoracic structures (e.g. adjacent lung lobes, ribs, pericardium), then these should be resected en bloc with the lung tumor if possible (i, primary bronchogenic carcinoma [PBC] with adhesions [with histologic evidence of invasion] to an adjacent lung lobe [LL]; ii, partial lung lobectomy of the adhesed normal lung lobe; iii, en bloc rib resection [R] in a dog with a primary bronchogenic carcinoma invasive into the ribs). If this is not possible, then these adhesions should be gently broken down with blunt dissection using cotton tip applicators, the tip of the inner stylet of a Poole suction instrument, or the tip of a cautery blade.

Surgical Technique – Stapled Lung Lobectomy (See Plate 11.1E–I)

E) The hilus of the lung lobe is visualized and isolated by dissecting any attached tissues (see step B). The thoracoabdominal (TA) stapler is passed around the hilus of the lung lobe. A vascular 30-mm TA stapler is preferred for lung lobectomies because the three rows of staples and 1.0-mm closing height of the staples provide a better seal than other available types of stapler cartridge. The retaining pin (arrow) is engaged, which allows for the tissues to be isolated within the opening of the stapler cartridge.

F) The handle of the stapler is compressed, which results in the staples engaging the tissue within the cartridge.

G) Large forceps should be applied across the lung lobe distal to the stapler cartridge to prevent tumor spillage after completion of the lung lobectomy.

Plate 11.1

Open Lung Lobectomy *continued*

D i)

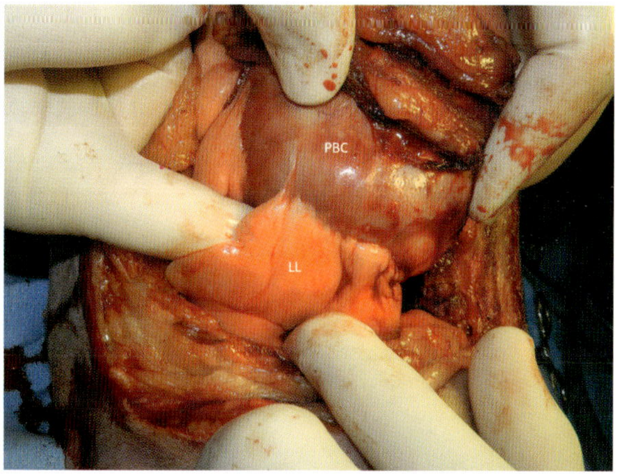

D-ii)

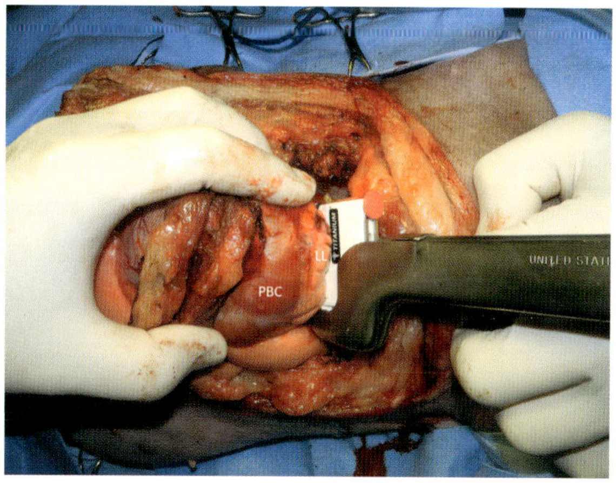

D-iii)

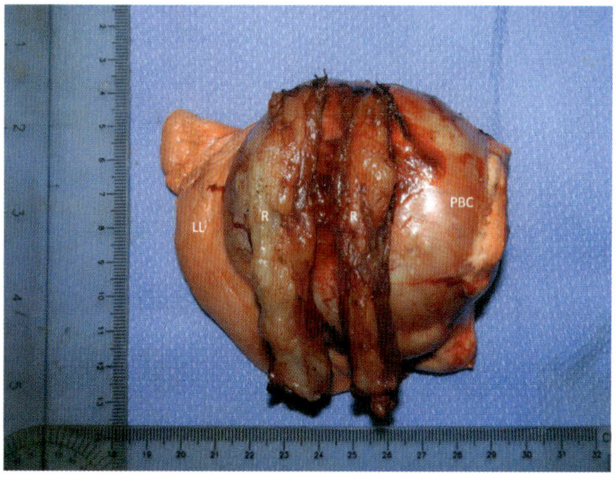

E)

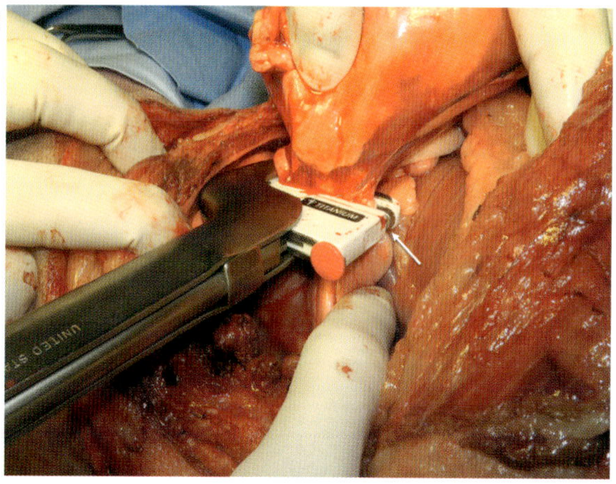

F)

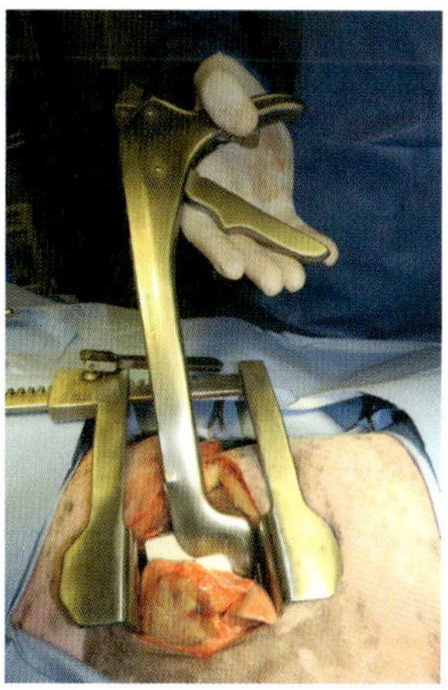

G)

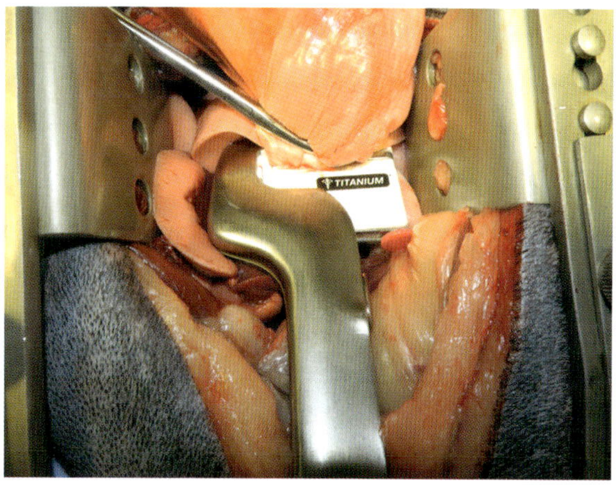

Surgical Technique – Stapled Lung Lobectomy (See Plate 11.1E–I) *continued*

H) The tissue is then transected distal to the staple cartridge. The staple cartridge will often have a small shelf that will allow for guidance of the scalpel blade during transection (pictured).

I) The stapler handle is then released (i) and the stapler is removed (ii). The staple line is assessed for bleeding or air leakage (ii, arrow). If any is noted, then the affected region can be sutured with 3-0 or 4-0 absorbable monofilament suture.

Surgical Technique – Sutured Lung Lobectomy (See Plate 11.1J–L)

J) The hilus of the lung lobe is visualized and isolated by dissecting any attached tissues.

Plate 11.1

Open Lung Lobectomy *continued*

H)

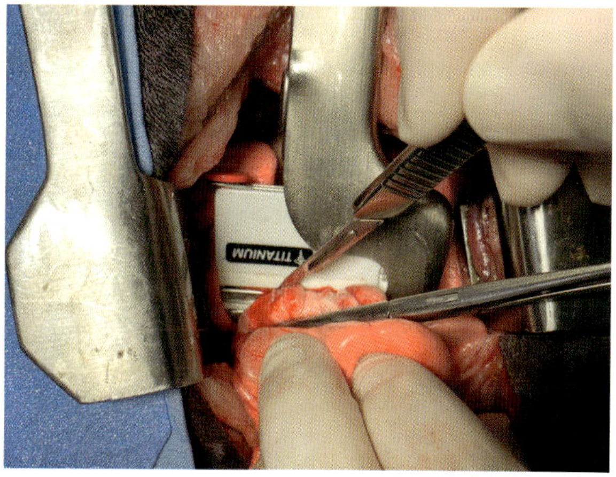

I-i)

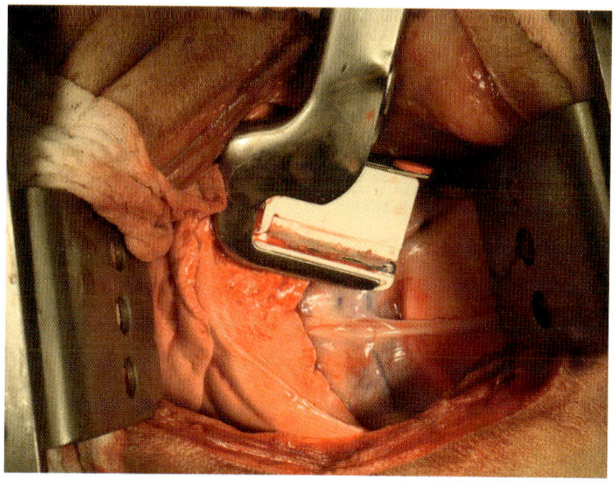

I-ii)

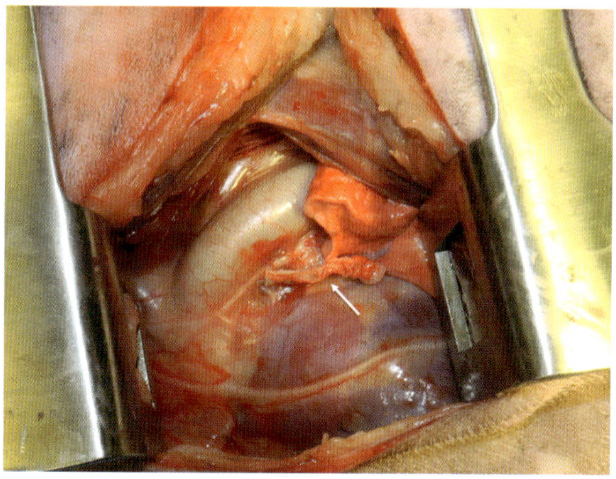

J)

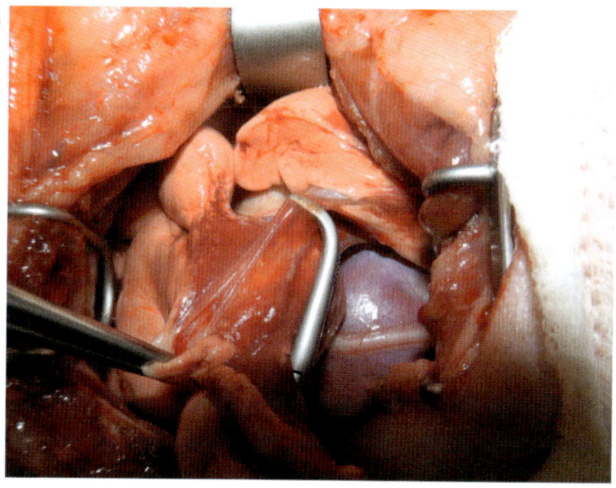

Surgical Technique – Sutured Lung Lobectomy (See Plate 11.1J–L) *continued*

K) The artery is skeletonized free from any attachments by a combination of blunt and sharp dissection. Right angle forceps are passed around the artery and an open section of 1–2 cm is established (i). A strand of 2-0 to 3-0 silk suture is passed around the artery (ii), and the artery is ligated at the most proximal location. A second strand of silk is then passed around the artery and ligated approximately 1 cm distal to the proximal ligature. Lastly, a transfixion suture (4-0 to 3-0 monofilament absorbable suture) is placed between the previously placed silk strands. The artery is transected between the transfixion ligature and the distal silk ligature (iii). A similar dissection and suturing technique to what is described earlier for the artery is used for the pulmonary vein (iv, ligation of the pulmonary vein; v, transection of the pulmonary vein between the proximal and distal ligatures).

Plate 11.1

Open Lung Lobectomy *continued*

K-i)

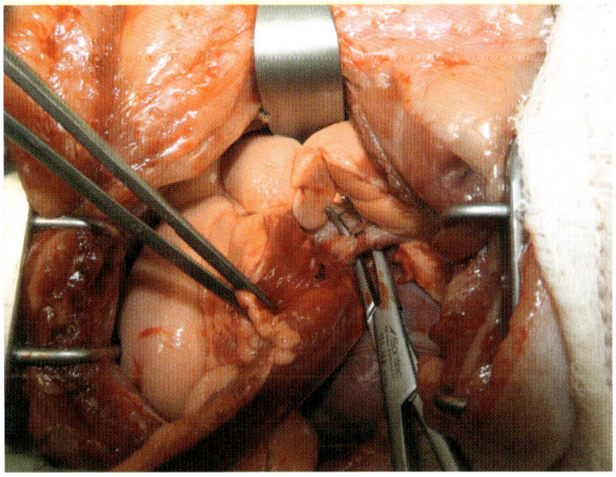

K-ii)

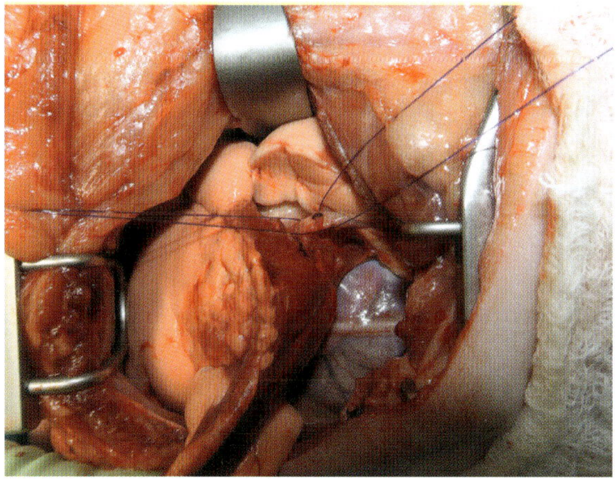

K-iii)

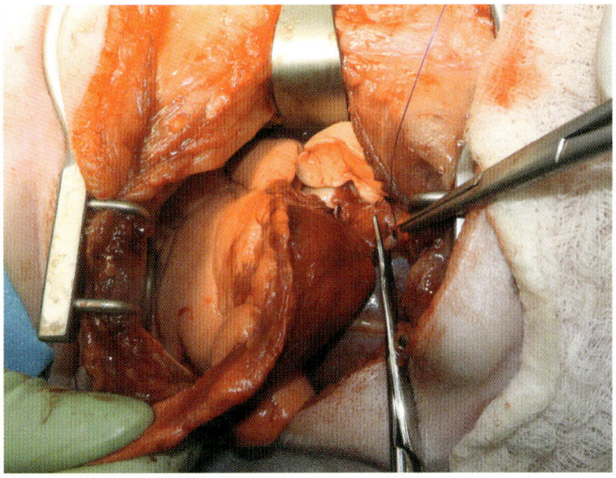

K-iv)

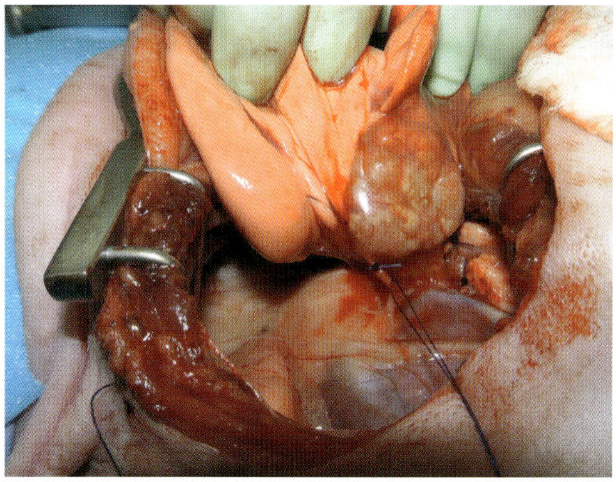

K-v)

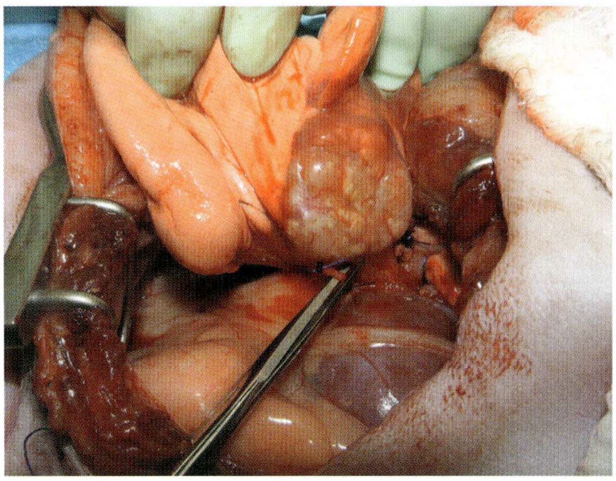

Surgical Technique – Sutured Lung Lobectomy (See Plate 11.1J–L) *continued*

L) The bronchus is dissected last (i, arrow). Similar to the artery and vein, the bronchus is dissected free from any surrounding tissue. Two noncrushing forceps are placed across the bronchus while maintaining a space between the forceps to allow for transection of the bronchus (ii, Satinsky forceps). After transection, the lung lobe (LL) is removed (iii). The bronchus is collapsed by placing a continuous or overlapping horizontal mattress suture pattern proximal to the remaining noncrushing forceps using 2-0 or 3-0 monofilament absorbable or nonabsorbable suture (iv). The end of the bronchus is sealed by placing a continuous oversew pattern using 3-0 or 4-0 monofilament absorbable suture. The suture line is assessed for bleeding or air leakage (v; see M – iv).

Plate 11.1

Open Lung Lobectomy *continued*

L-i)

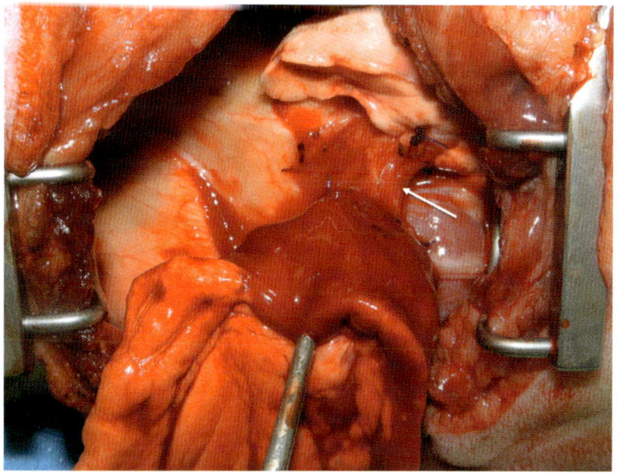

L ii)

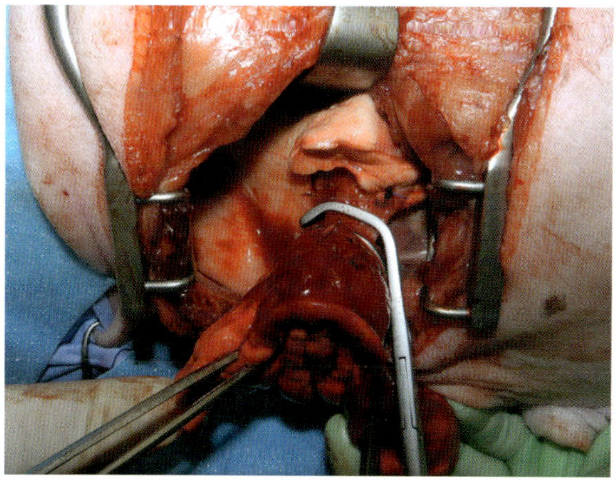

L-iii)

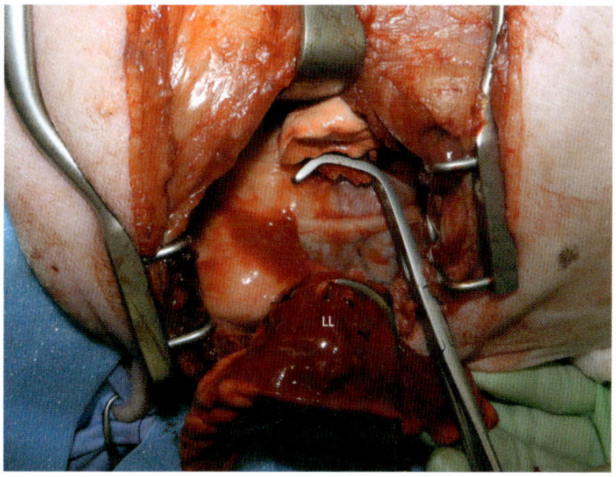

L-iv)

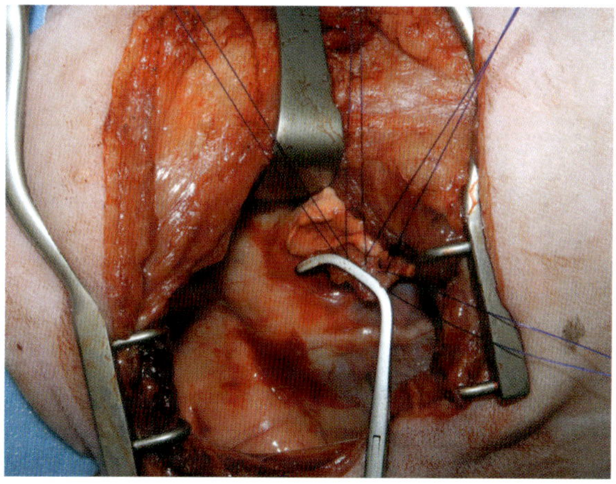

L-v)

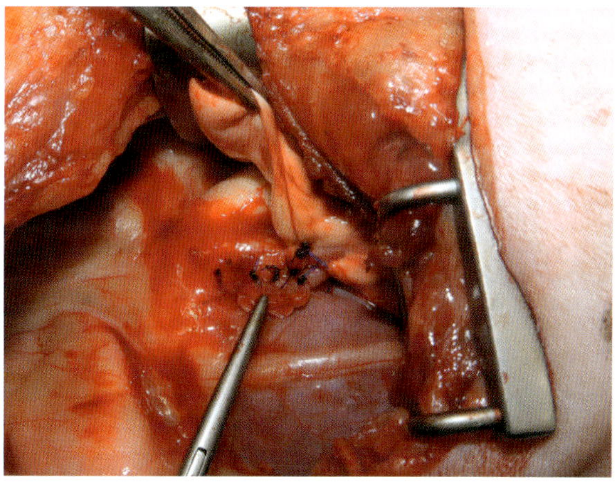

Closure (See Plate 11.1M)

Prior to closure, the tracheobronchial lymph nodes (i, arrows indicate metastatic tracheobronchial lymph nodes; SL, staple line) and sternal lymph node (ii, metastatic) are assessed and excised if necessary (iii, metastatic), and the thoracic cavity is lavaged with warmed sterile saline to assess for air leakage from the lung lobectomy site (iv, arrow). If air leakage is noted, additional sutures or staples over the site of leakage can be placed. A thoracostomy tube is placed in the ipsilateral hemithorax. Closure of the surgical approach is described in the appropriate chapter (see *10.1. Intercostal Thoracotomy* or *10.2. Median Sternotomy*).

Postoperative Management

1) Multimodal analgesia, including perioperative continuous rate infusion of an opioid ± ketamine, intercostal nerve blocks, local anesthesia instilled through the thoracostomy tube ± wound diffuser catheter, and oral analgesic drugs
2) Supplemental oxygen therapy, if required
3) Thoracostomy tube management
4) Elizabethan collar or body suit

Complications [1–3]

Intraoperative Complications

- Bleeding (2%–3%)
- Cardiac arrhythmias (10%)

Postoperative Complications

- Seroma and ventral edema (8%–22%)
- Hypoxia (2%–13%)
- Subcutaneous emphysema (10%)
- Ipsilateral thoracic limb lameness (4%)
- Hemorrhage requiring revision surgery (2%–4%)
- Pneumothorax (2%)
- Aspiration pneumonia (2%)
- Lung lobe torsion

Suggested Adjuvant Treatments

- ± Adjuvant chemotherapy, depending on histologic grade, lymph node metastasis, and other negative prognostic criteria

Plate 11.1

Open Lung Lobectomy *continued*

M-i)

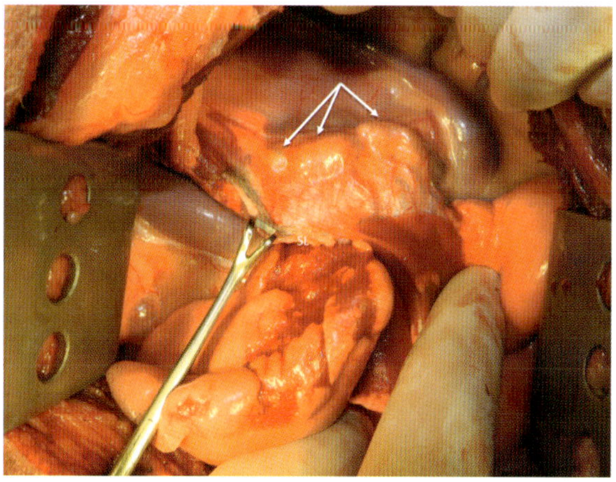

M-ii)

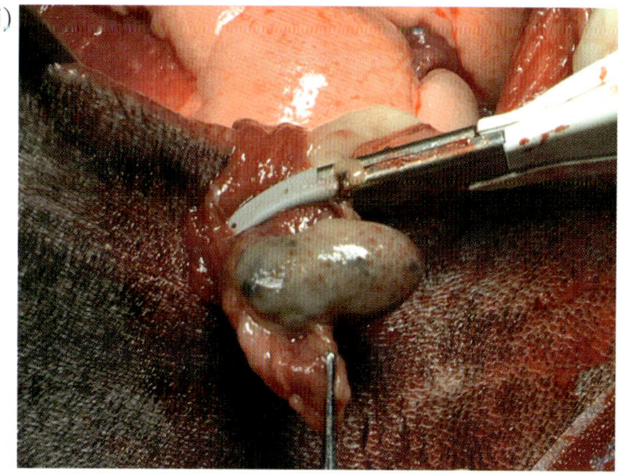

M-iii)

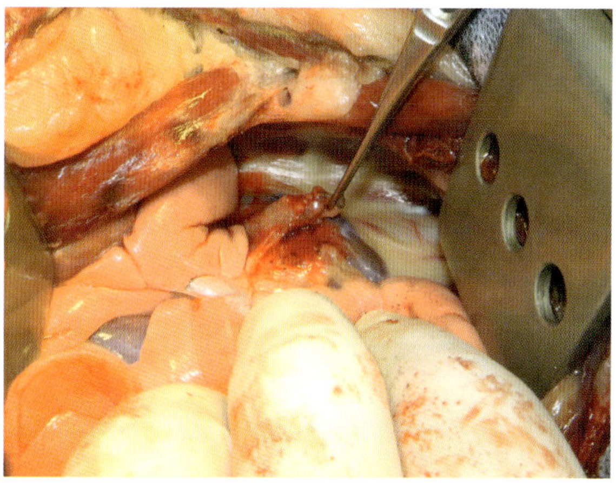

M-iv)

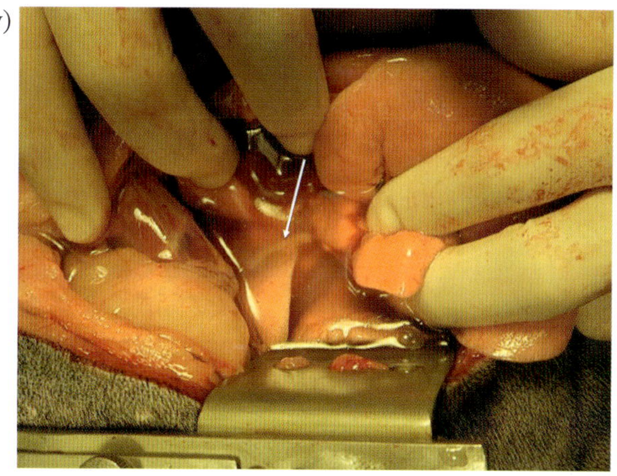

Prognosis and Oncologic Outcome – Dogs

	Local Recurrence Rate	Metastatic Rate	Disease-Free Interval (d)	Median Survival Time (d)	1-Year Survival Rate	2-Year Survival Rate
			Primary Lung Carcinoma			
Overall [3–7]	5%	24%–28%	223–754	361–716	–	–
Clinical signs [4]						
No	–	–	461	545	–	–
Yes	–	–	177	240	–	–
Tumor size [5, 7]						
<100 cm [2]	–	–	–	644	–	–
≥100 cm [2]	–	–	–	198	–	–
Tumor size [5, 7]						
≤3 cm	–	–	NR	597–1064	–	–
>3 to ≤5 cm	–	–	754	704–721	–	–
>5 to ≤7 cm	–	–	366	493–574	–	–
>7 cm	–	–	95	110–157	–	–
Lymph node metastasis [4, 6, 7]						
No	–	–	351	452 to NR	–	–
Yes	–	–	6	26–167	–	–
Distant metastasis [7]						
Yes	–	–	–	459	–	–
No	–	–	–	52	–	–
Clinical stage [7]						
I: Nonmetastatic, tumor <3 cm	–	–	–	952	–	–
II: Nonmetastatic, tumor 3–7 cm; or tracheobronchial lymph node metastasis, tumor ≤5 cm	–	–	–	658	–	–
III: Nonmetastatic, tumor >7 cm; or tracheobronchial lymph node metastasis, tumor >5 cm	–	–	–	158	–	–
IV: Distant metastasis or malignant pleural effusion	–	–	–	52	–	–
Histologic margins [7]						
Complete	–	–	–	467	–	–
Narrow	–	–	–	731		
Incomplete	–	–	–	211	–	–
Histologic grade [7]						
I	–	–	493	658 to NR	–	–
II	–	–	191	208–251	–	–
III	–	–	0	5–43	–	–
			Histiocytic Sarcoma			
Overall[a] [8]	–	–	276	374	–	–

[a] The majority of these dogs were treated with lung lobectomy and chemotherapy (CCNU).
NR, not reached.

Prognosis and Oncologic Outcome – Cats

	Local Recurrence Rate	Metastatic Rate	Disease-Free Interval (d)	Median Survival Time (d)	1-Year Survival Rate	2-Year Survival Rate
			Primary Lung Carcinoma			
Overall	–	74%–86%	–	64–156	–	–
Clinical signs [9]						
No	–	–	–	578	–	–
Yes	–	–	–	4	–	–
Pleural effusion [9, 10]						
No	–	–	–	31–467	–	–
Yes	–	–	–	03–Feb	–	–
Lymph node size [10, 11]						
No	–	–	–	412–498	–	–
Yes	–	–	–	65–73	–	–
Clinical stage [9]						
I: Solitary lung tumor with no invasion	–	–	–	190	–	–
Other: ≥T2, N1, M1	–	–	–	3	–	–
Degree of differentiation [9, 11]						
Well	–	–	–	68	–	–
Moderate	–	–	–	3–698		
Poor	–	–	–	6–75	–	–
Histologic grade [10]						
I/II	–	–	–	730	–	–
III	–	–	–	105	–	–

References

1 Moores, A.L., Halfacree, Z.J., Baines, S.J. et al. (2007). Indications, outcomes and complications following lateral thoracotomy in dogs and cats. *J. Small Anim. Pract.* 48 (12): 695–698.

2 Bleakley, S., Phipps, K., Petrovsky, B. et al. (2018). Median sternotomy versus intercostal thoracotomy for lung lobectomy: a comparison of short-term outcome in 134 dogs. *Vet. Surg.* 47 (1): 104–113.

3 Ichimata, M., Kagawa, Y., Namiki, K. et al. (2023). Prognosis of primary pulmonary adenocarcinoma after surgiczl resection in small-breed dogs: 52 cases (2005-2021). *J. Vet. Intern. Med.* 37 (4): 1466–1474.

4 McNiel, E.A., Ogilvie, G.K., Powers, B.E. et al. (1997). Evaluation of prognostic factors for dogs with primary lung tumors: 67 cases (1985-1992). *J. Am. Vet. Med. Assoc.* 211 (11): 1422–1427.

5 Rose, R.J. and Worley, D.R. (2020). A contemporary retrospective study of survival in dogs with primary lung tumors: 40 cases (2005-2017). *Front. Vet. Sci.* 7: 519703.

6 Paoloni, M.C., Adams, W.M., Dubielzig, R.R. et al. (2006). Comparison of results of computed tomography and radiography with histopathologic findings in tracheobronchial lymph nodes in dogs with primary lung tumors: 14 cases (1999-2002). *J. Am. Vet. Med. Assoc.* 228 (11): 1718–1722.

7 Lee, B.M., Clarke, D., Watson, M. et al. (2020). Retrospective evaluation of a modified human lung cancer stage classification in dogs with surgically excised primary pulmonary carcinomas. *Vet. Comp. Oncol.* 18 (4): 590–598.

8 Marlowe, K.W., Robat, C.S., Clarke, D. et al. (2018). Primary pulmonary histiocytic sarcoma in dogs: a retrospective analysis of 37 cases (2000-2015). *Vet. Comp. Oncol.* 16 (4): 658–663.

9 Maritato, K.C., Schertel, E.R., Kennedy, S.C. et al. (2014). Outcome and prognostic indicators in 20 cats with surgically treated primary lung tumors. *J. Feline Med. Surg.* 16 (12): 979–984.

10 Nunley, J., Sutton, J., Culp, W. et al. (2015). Primary pulmonary neoplasia in cats: assessment of computed tomography findings and survival. *J. Small Anim. Pract.* 56 (11): 651–656.

11 Hahn, K.A. and McEntee, M.F. (1998). Prognosis factors for survival in cats after removal of a primary lung tumor: 21 cases (1979-1994). *Vet. Surg.* 27 (4): 307–311.

11.2 Thoracoscopic and Thoracoscopic-Assisted Lung Lobectomy

Indications

1) Resection of nonmetastatic primary lung tumors
2) Resection of metastatic lung tumors for either palliative purposes (such as management of hypertrophic osteopathy) or treatment (if the criteria for metastatectomy have been satisfied)

Suggested Diagnostic Workup and Clinical Staging

- Complete blood count, serum biochemistry, and urinalysis
- ± Preoperative ultrasound-guided fine-needle aspirate cytology
- Thoracic computed tomography scan for assessment of nodal and lung metastasis

Patient Positioning

The patient is placed in lateral recumbency with the affected side uppermost. An oblique positioning to the thorax with the dorsal aspect higher than the ventral aspect improves visualization of the hilus of the lung lobe during dissection and stapling.

Surgical Technique – Thoracoscopic Lung Lobectomy (See Plate 11.2A–E)

A) One-lung ventilation is recommended whenever possible because this greatly improves visualization and movement of instrumentation during the procedure. A three- to four-port technique is used. The ports can be placed in the same intercostal space or can be staggered in a triangular pattern (pictured). Ports are placed in the ventral third of the thorax to allow for increased working space within the thoracic cavity. For cranial lung lobe tumors, ports are placed caudally, generally in the seventh to ninth intercostal space, and the monitor is positioned close to the head of the patient. For right middle or caudal lung lobe tumors, ports are placed cranially in the third or fourth intercostal space with the monitor positioned close to the tail of the patient. Cannulae diameter sizes are generally between 6 and 12 mm, and smooth or threaded versions can be used. Insufflation is generally not needed for thoracoscopic lung lobectomy.
B) Once all cannulae have been placed, the lung lobe (LL) is mobilized by placing a blunt probe (P) on the ventral surface and lifting the lung lobe (pictured). This allows the surgeon to determine the location of the tumor in relation to the hilus and whether adhesions are present that need to be broken down. If adhesions exist, these can be gently broken down with a blunt probe or dissected free using J-hook electrocautery or a vessel sealing device.

Color Atlas of Canine and Feline Surgical Oncology, First Edition. Julius M. Liptak, Paolo Buracco, William T. N. Culp, and Nicholas J. Bacon.

Plate 11.2

Thoracoscopic and Thoracoscopic-Assisted Lung Lobectomy

A)

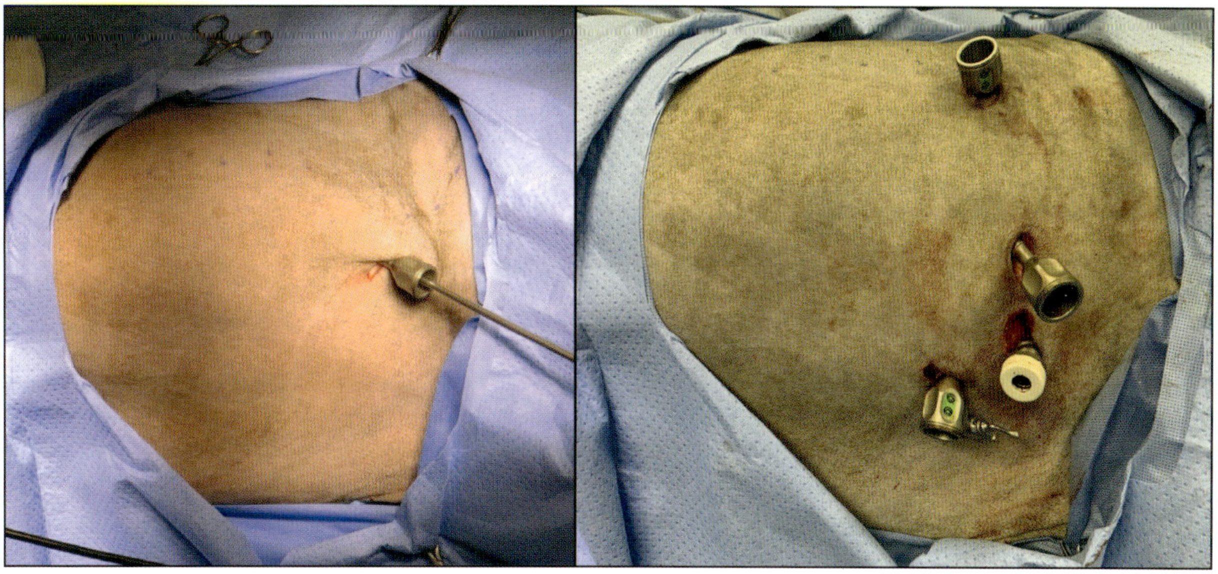

B)

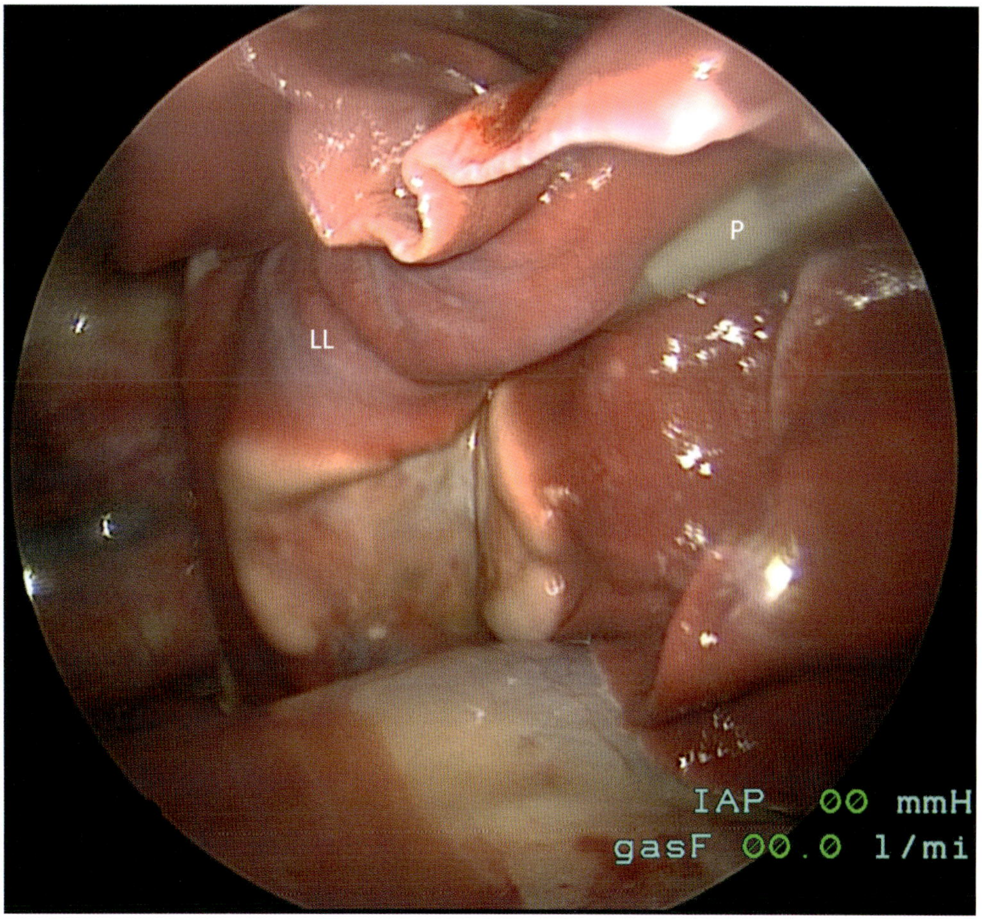

Surgical Technique – Thoracoscopic Lung Lobectomy (See Plate 11.2A–E) *continued*

C) If a caudal or accessory lung lobe is being removed, then pulmonary ligamentous attachments are transected using J-hook electrocautery or a vessel sealing device.

D) The lung lobe is then elevated by placing the blunt probe (P) across the major region of parenchyma, and this is then used to position the lobe dorsolaterally to allow visualization of the hilus. The lung lobectomy is performed by the use of a thoracoscopic stapling device (Endo GIA). The Endo GIA device is capable of articulating to allow for easier placement across the hilus. The device is placed across the hilus, ensuring the staple line extends across the entire base of the hilus before deploying the stapler. The stapler is engaged and the lung lobe is simultaneously transected free from the hilus.

E) The lung lobe is placed into a retrieval bag after transection (arrow). Because many of these tumors are quite large, the port incision through which the retrieval bag has been introduced may need to be extended to allow for extraction.

Plate 11.2

Thoracoscopic and Thoracoscopic-Assisted Lung Lobectomy *continued*

C)

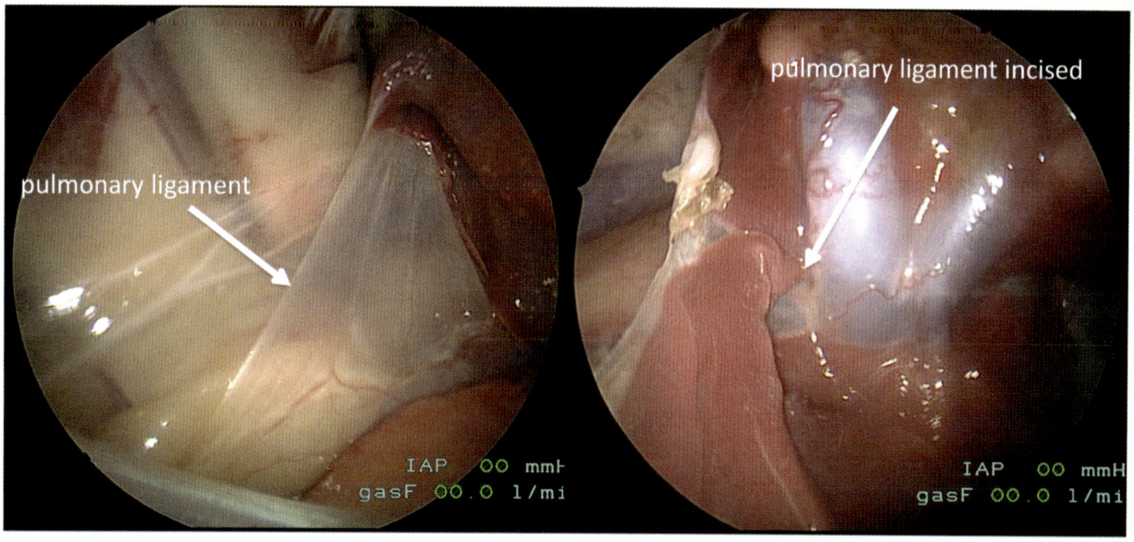

D)

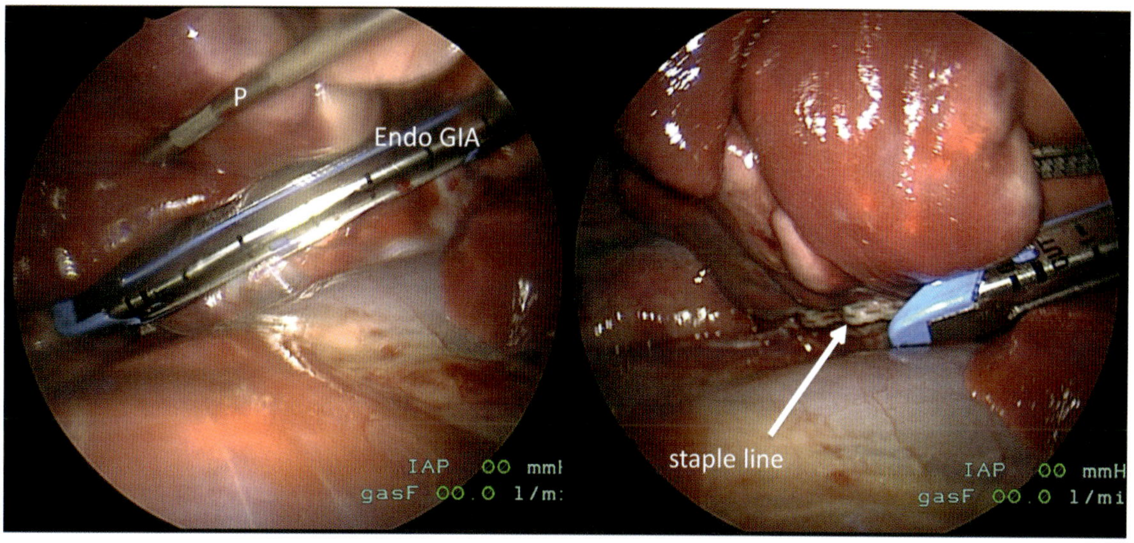

E)

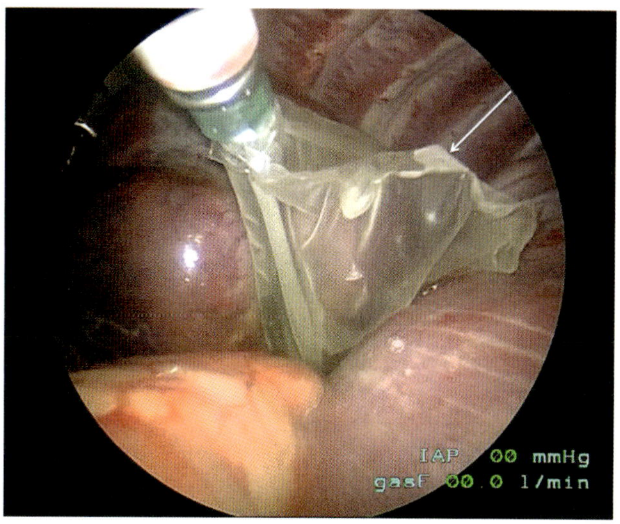

Surgical Technique – Thoracoscopic-Assisted Lung Lobectomy (See Plate 11.2F–H)

F) Two techniques have been described for thoracoscopic-assisted lung lobectomy: stapling within the thorax or stapling outside of the thorax. In both situations, a telescope cannula is placed at a site distant to the lung tumor and a small thoracotomy is created over the hilus of the lung lobe that is going to be removed. Thoracoscopy is used to guide dissection.

G) For the intrathoracic stapling technique, a 30-mm vascular thoracoabdominal (TA) stapler is placed across the hilus of the lung lobe, secured, and deployed (see *11.1. Open Lung Lobectomy*, steps E and F). A scalpel blade is then used to complete the lung lobectomy by incising the lung tissue distal to the cartridge. The stapler is then released and removed from the surgical field (see *11.1. Open Lung Lobectomy*, steps H and I).

H) For the extrathoracic stapling technique, the lung lobe is grasped and pulled outside of the thorax through the small thoracotomy (i). The TA stapler is then used to staple the hilus as is done via the traditional intercostal thoracotomy approach (ii, see *11.1. Open Lung Lobectomy*, steps E–I).

Closure

A thoracostomy tube is placed before closure, and the position is visualized by the telescope. All equipment, including the cannulae and telescope, are removed. The muscle and subcutaneous tissue can be closed with 2-0 to 3-0 monofilament absorbable suture in a simple interrupted or cruciate pattern. The dermal layer is closed with 3-0 monofilament absorbable suture. The thoracostomy tube is secured to the skin.

Postoperative Management

1) Multimodal analgesia
2) Supplemental oxygen therapy, if required
3) Thoracostomy tube management
4) Elizabethan collar or body suit

Complications – Dogs

Intraoperative Complications

- Iatrogenic lung lobe trauma (10%) [1]
- Intercostal artery hemorrhage (10%) [1]

Postoperative Complications (0–14 Days)

- Surgical-site infections (rare) [2]
- Air leakage (uncommon and usually self-limiting)
- See *11.1. Open Lung Lobectomy* for complications associated with lung lobectomy

Postoperative Complications (>14 Days)

- Portal-site metastases (rare) [3, 4]

Plate 11.2

Thoracoscopic and Thoracoscopic-Assisted Lung Lobectomy *continued*

H-i)

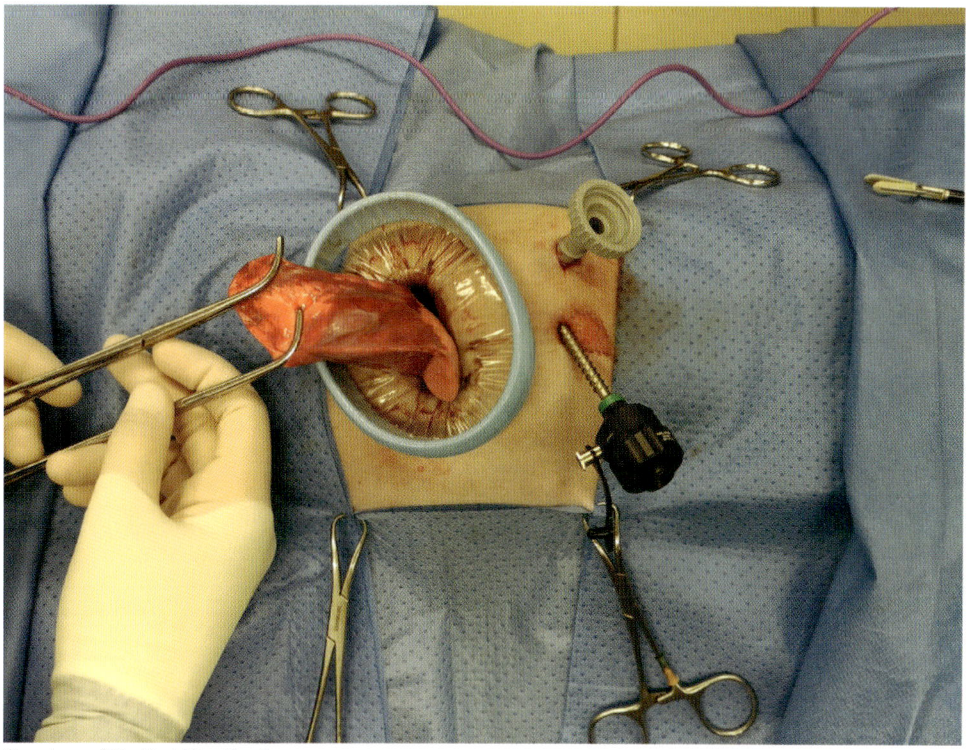

Courtesy of Dr. Bart Van Goethem

H-ii)

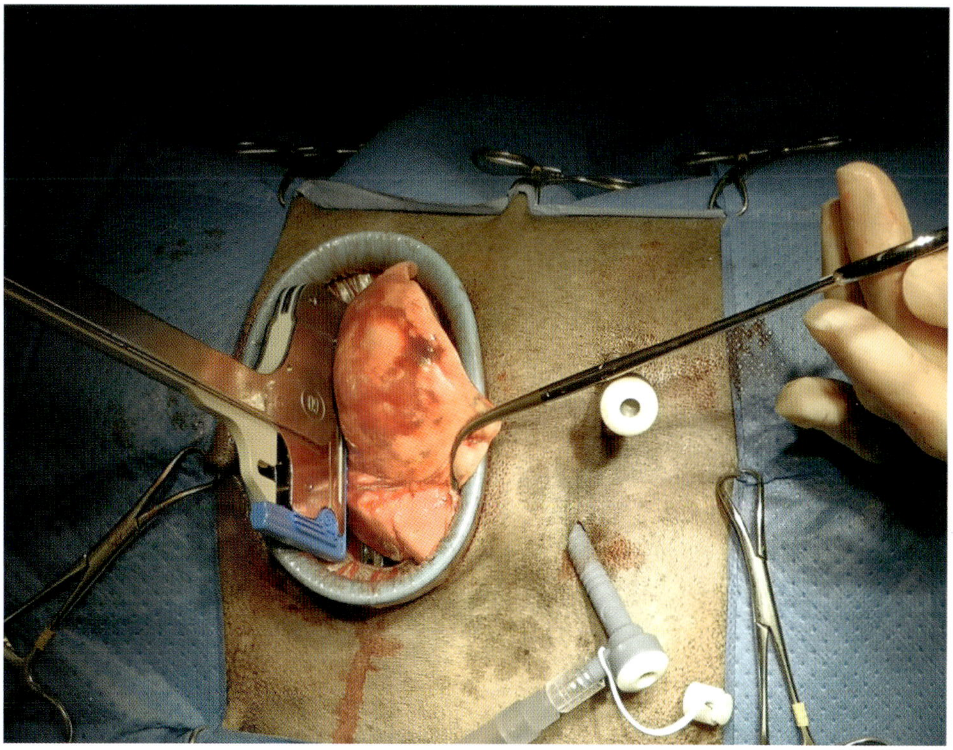

Courtesy of Dr. Bart Van Goethem

Suggested Adjuvant Treatments

- See *11.1. Open Lung Lobectomy*.

Prognosis and Oncologic Outcome

- See *11.1. Open Lung Lobectomy*.

References

1 Mayhew, P.D., Hunt, G.B., Steffey, M.A. et al. (2013). Evaluation of short-term outcome after lung lobectomy for resection of primary lung tumors via video-assisted thoracoscopic surgery or open thoracotomy in medium- to large-breed dogs.*J. Am. Vet. Med. Assoc.* 243 (5): 681–688.

2 Mayhew, P.D., Freeman, L., Kwan, T. et al. (2012). Comparison of surgical site infection rates in clean and clean-contaminated wounds in dogs and cats after minimally invasive versus open surgery: 179 cases (2007-2008). *J. Am. Vet. Med. Assoc.* 240 (2): 193–198.

3 Brisson, B.A., Reggeti, F., and Bienzle, D. (2006). Portal site metastasis of invasive mesothelioma after diagnostic thoracoscopy in a dog. *J. Am. Vet. Med. Assoc.* 229 (6): 980–983.

4 Alwen, S.G., Culp, W.T., Szivek, A. et al. (2015). Portal site metastasis after thoracoscopic resection of a cranial mediastinal mass in a dog. *J. Am. Vet. Med. Assoc.* 247 (7): 793–800.

Chapter 12: Subtotal Pericardectomy

12.1 Open Subtotal Pericardectomy

Indications

1) Palliation of heart base tumors, bleeding right atrial tumors, and mesotheliomas causing pericardial effusion

Suggested Diagnostic Workup and Clinical Staging

- Complete blood count, serum biochemistry, and urinalysis
- Pericardiocentesis
- Cytologic analysis of pericardial fluid
- Echocardiogram
- Three-view thoracic radiographs or thoracic computed tomography scan

Patient Positioning

Patient positioning is dependent on the surgical approach with lateral recumbency for an intercostal thoracotomy approach (see *10.1. Intercostal Thoracotomy*) and dorsal recumbency for a median sternotomy approach (see *10.2. Median Sternotomy*). A median sternotomy allows for easier access to the entire pericardium; however, an intercostal thoracotomy allows for clearer delineation of the phrenic nerve on the ipsilateral side and is a less invasive approach.

Surgical Technique (See Plate 12.1A–F)

A) See *10.1. Intercostal Thoracotomy* or *10.2. Median Sternotomy* for details on the surgical approach for open subtotal pericardectomy. A right fifth intercostal thoracotomy is recommended for open subtotal pericardectomy (pictured) (i, pericardial effusion [PE] secondary to right atrial hemangiosarcoma; phrenic nerve, arrow) (ii; HBT, heart base tumor; PN, phrenic nerve).
B) The ventral surface of the pericardium is grasped with forceps (toothed forceps are often required), lifted away from the heart, and then a stab incision is made with either sharp scissors or a scalpel blade with the blade facing away from the heart (i). Once a hole is created in the pericardium, the edge of the hole is elevated to allow for extension of the incision (ii; PN, phrenic nerve). A tongue depressor can be inserted into the hole to elevate the pericardium and act as a barrier to protect the heart during incision of the pericardium (iii).

Color Atlas of Canine and Feline Surgical Oncology, First Edition. Julius M. Liptak, Paolo Buracco, William T. N. Culp, and Nicholas J. Bacon.

Plate 12.1

Open Subtotal Pericardectomy

A-i)

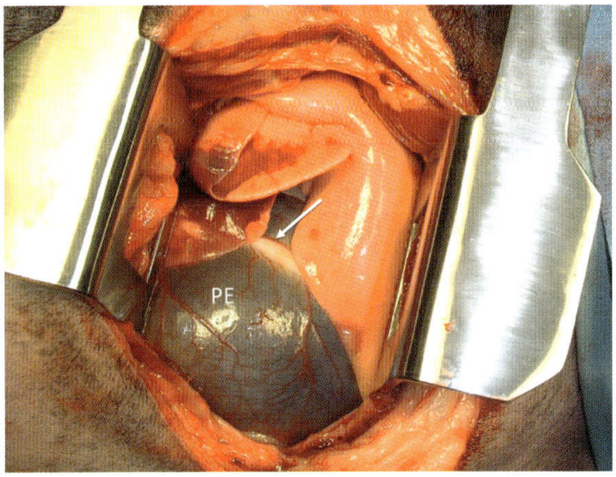

A-ii)

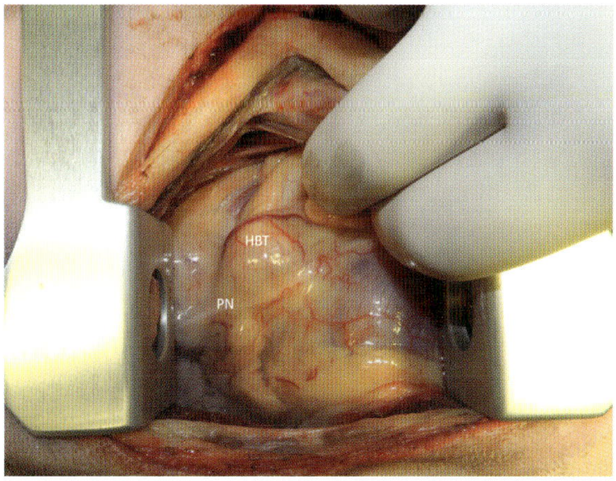

B-i)

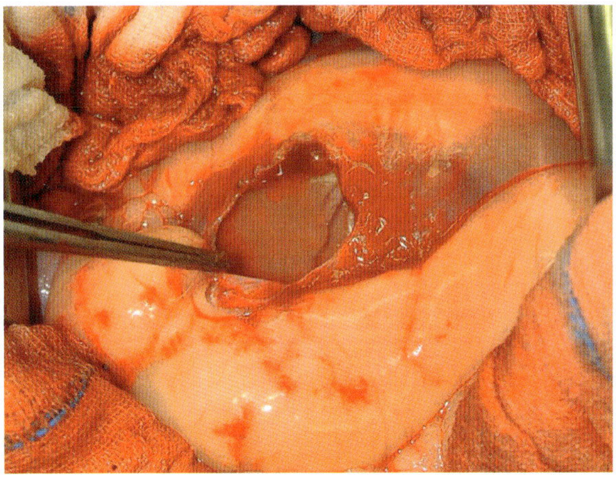

B-ii)

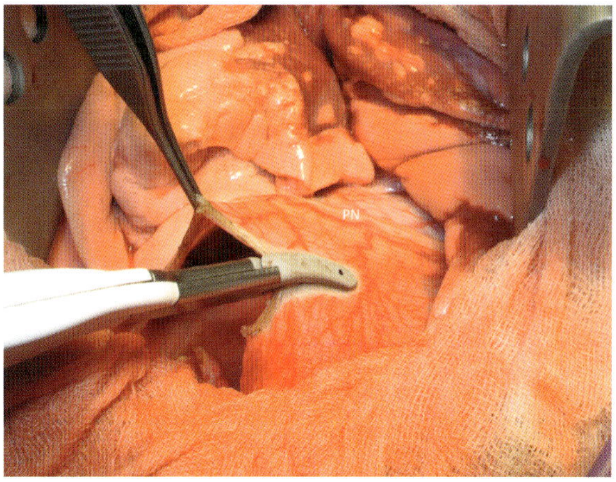

B-iii)

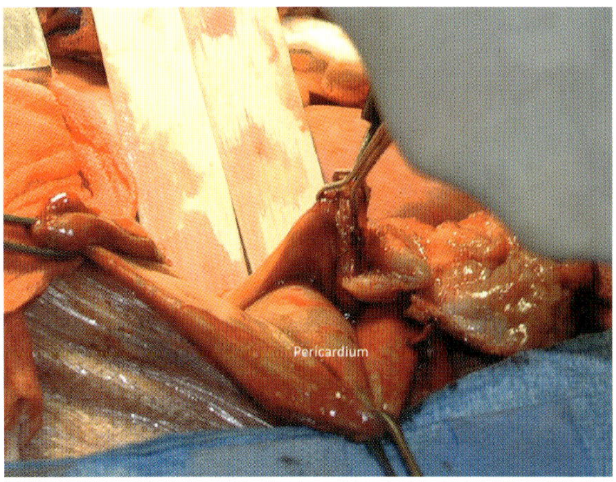

Surgical Technique (See Plate 12.1A–F) *continued*

C) Several techniques can be used to complete the pericardectomy. Sharp dissection can be done with scissors, although the pericardium is vascular and bleeding can be robust (see B – i). Alternatively, electrosurgery or a vessel sealing device (pictured) can be used to incise the pericardial tissue ventral to the phrenic nerve. These instruments should not contact the heart because cardiac arrhythmias are possible.

D) The majority of pericardium ventral to the phrenic nerve can be excised from a median sternotomy approach (i, ii), although it can be difficult to visualize the phrenic nerves in deep-chested dogs.

E) For a subtotal pericardectomy from an intercostal thoracotomy approach, the ipsilateral pericardium is incised ventral to the phrenic nerve initially as the phrenic nerve is easily visualized (see B – i, ii). The heart often needs to be elevated to allow for removal of the pericardium on the contralateral side (i). Depending on the size of the patient and mobility of the heart, it may be challenging to incise the pericardium as far dorsally on the contralateral side as compared with the ipsilateral side (ii).

F) A biopsy can be taken from the tumor causing the pericardial effusion, although the risks of the biopsy should be considered, especially because pericardectomy is a palliative procedure and the biopsy results are unlikely to change postoperative management recommendations (i, right auricular hemangiosarcoma; ii, right atrial appendage mesothelioma; iii, suspected aortic body tumor [ABT]).

Closure

The thoracic cavity is lavaged with warmed sterile saline. A thoracostomy tube is placed in the ipsilateral hemithorax. Closure of the surgical approach is described in the appropriate chapter (see *10.1. Intercostal Thoracotomy* or *10.2. Median Sternotomy*).

Postoperative Management

1) Multimodal analgesia, including perioperative continuous rate infusion of an opioid ± ketamine, intercostal nerve blocks, local anesthesia instilled through the thoracostomy tube ± wound diffuser catheter, and oral analgesic drugs
2) Supplemental oxygen therapy, if required
3) Thoracostomy tube management
4) Elizabethan collar

Complications

- There are anecdotal reports of arrhythmias after use of electrocautery and vessel sealing devices to perform pericardectomy
- Pleural effusion
- Other intraoperative and postoperative complications are dependent on the surgical approach; see *10.1. Intercostal Thoracotomy* or *10.2. Median Sternotomy*

Suggested Alternative or Adjuvant Treatments

- Chemotherapy is recommended for dogs with cardiac hemangiosarcomas [1, 2]
- ± Stereotactic radiation therapy for dogs with heart base tumors such as chemodectomas or ectopic thyroid carcinomas [3, 4]
- ± Toceranib phosphate for dogs with heart base tumors [5]

Plate 12.1

Open Subtotal Pericardectomy *continued*

C)

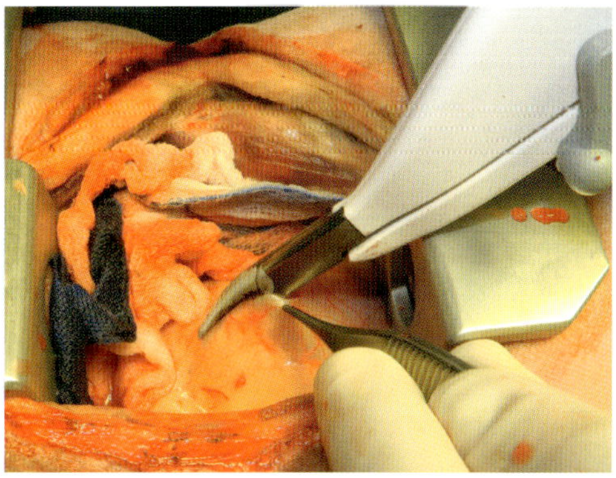

D-i)

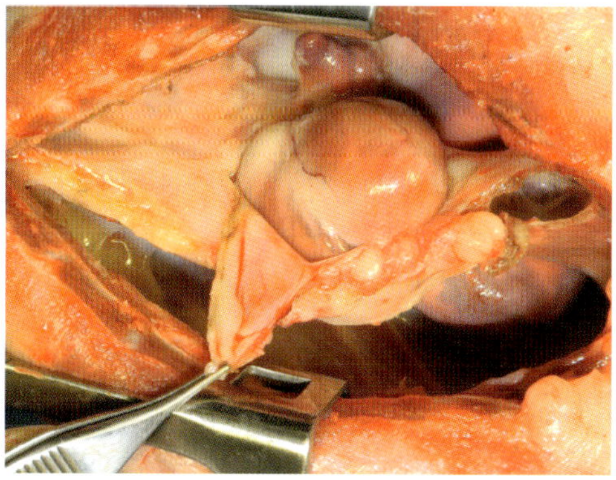

D-ii)

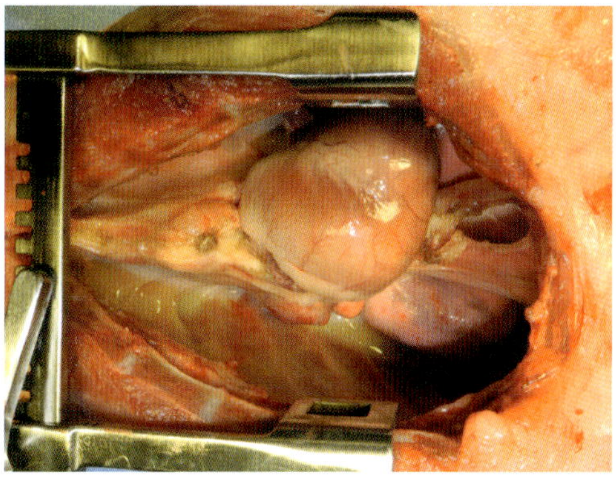

E-i)

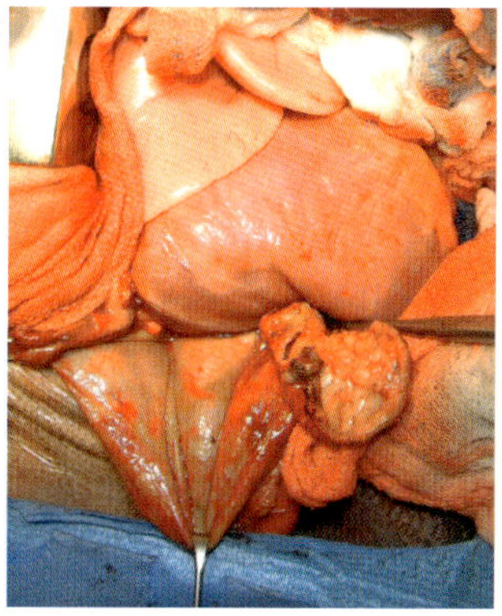

E-ii)

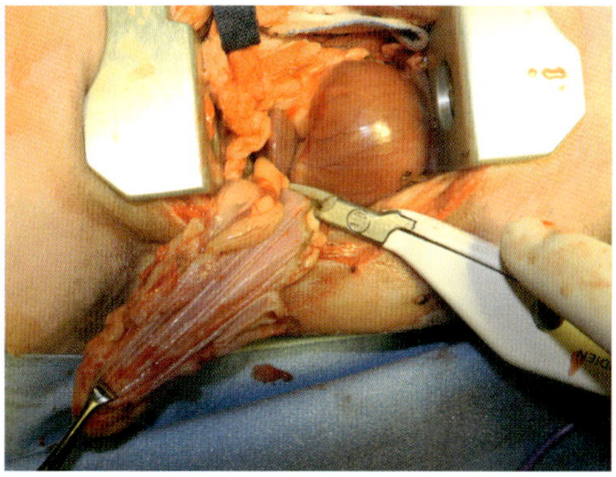

F-i)

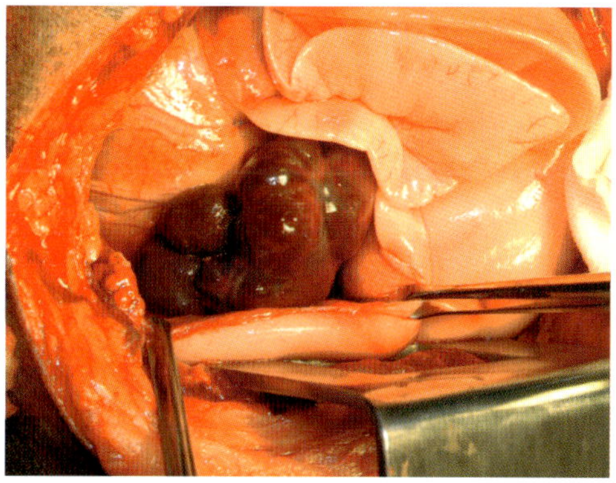

F-ii)

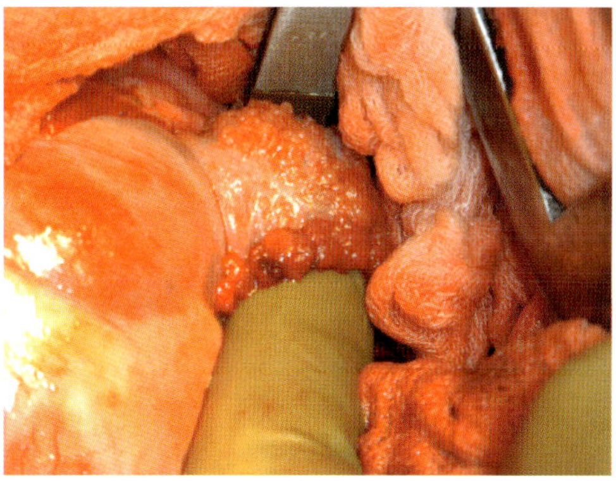

F-iii)

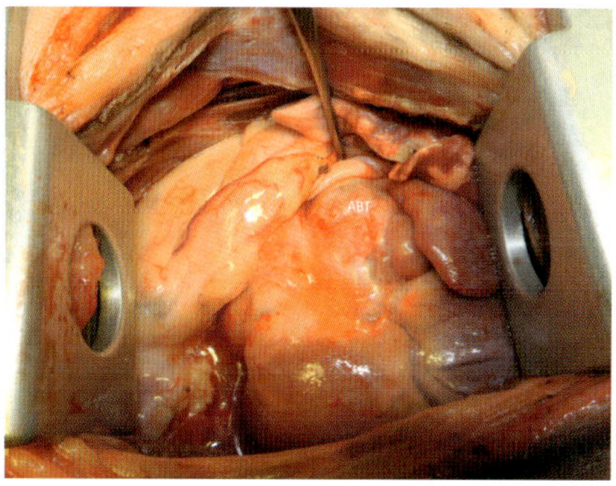

Prognosis and Oncologic Outcome – Dogs

Tumor Type	Local Recurrence Rate	Metastatic Rate	Disease-Free Interval (d)	Median Survival Time (d)	1-Year Survival Rate	2-Year Survival Rate
Hemangiosarcoma [6]	–	–	–	16	0%	0%
Adjuvant chemotherapy [2]						
• Chemotherapy	–	–	–	175	–	–
• No chemotherapy	–	–	–	42	–	–
Mesothelioma [6]	–	–	–	414	80%	40%
Aortic body tumor [7, 8]	–	–	–	661[a]–720	–	–

[a] Mean survival time.

References

1. Ghaffari, S., Pelio, D.C., Lange, A.J. et al. (2014). A retrospective evaluation of doxorubicin-based chemotherapy for dogs with right atrial masses and pericardial effusion. *J. Small Anim. Pract.* 55 (5): 254–257.
2. Weisse, C., Soares, N., Beal, M.W. et al. (2005). Survival times in dogs with right atrial hemangiosarcoma treated by means of surgical resection with or without adjuvant chemotherapy: 23 cases (1986-2000). *J. Am. Vet. Med. Assoc.* 226: 575–579.
3. Magestro, L.M., Gieger, T.L., and Nolan, M.W. (2018). Stereotactic body radiation therapy for heart-base tumors in six dogs. *J. Vet. Cardiol.* 20 (3): 186–197.
4. Kruckman-Gatesy, C.R., Ames, M.K., Griffin, L.R. et al. (2020). A retrospective analysis of stereotactic body radiation therapy for canine heart base tumors: 26 cases. *J. Vet. Cardiol.* 27: 62–77.
5. Lew, F.H., McQuown, B., Borrego, J. et al. (2019). Retrospective evaluation of canine heart base tumours treated with toceranib phosphate (Palladia): 2011-2018. *Vet. Comp. Oncol.* 17 (4): 465–471.
6. Dunning, D., Monnet, E., Orton, E.C. et al. (1998). Analysis of prognostic indicators for dogs with pericardial effusion: 46 cases (1985-1996). *J. Am. Vet. Med. Assoc.* 212 (8): 1276–1280.
7. Vicari, E.D., Brown, D.C., Holt, D.E. et al. (2001). Survival times of and prognostic indicators for dogs with heart base masses: 25 cases (1986-1999). *J. Am. Vet. Med. Assoc.* 219 (4): 485–487.
8. Ehrhart, N., Ehrhart, E.J., Willis, J. et al. (2002). Analysis of factors affecting survival in dogs with aortic body tumors. *Vet. Surg.* 31 (1): 44–48.

12.2 Thoracoscopic Pericardectomy – Pericardial Window and Subtotal Pericardectomy

Indications

1) Palliation of heart base tumors, bleeding right atrial tumors, and mesotheliomas causing pericardial effusion.
2) Thoracoscopic pericardial window formation and subtotal pericardectomy can be performed in most dogs, but dogs with less dorsal-ventral height, such as brachycephalic breeds, present a challenge because of limited space to manipulate equipment between the sternum and heart.

Suggested Diagnostic Workup and Clinical Staging

- Complete blood count, serum biochemistry, and urinalysis
- Pericardiocentesis
- Cytologic analysis of pericardial fluid
- Echocardiogram
- Three-view thoracic radiographs or thoracic computed tomography scan

Patient Positioning

The patient is positioned in dorsal recumbency.

Surgical Technique (See Plate 12.2A–D)

A) One-lung ventilation is recommended whenever possible because this greatly improves visualization and movement of instrumentation during the procedure [1]. A paraxiphoid transdiaphragmatic port is established (pictured), and the telescope is inserted intrathoracically; a 6-mm cannula is generally selected to allow for placement of a 5-mm diameter telescope. The intercostal port can either be placed bilaterally [1, 2] or with two unilateral ports [3]. Intercostal ports are generally placed in the ventral third of the fourth to sixth intercostal spaces when a bilateral port technique is used. For dogs undergoing unilateral placement of two ports, the caudal port is placed between the eighth to tenth intercostal spaces, and the cranial port is placed between the second to fourth intercostal spaces. The intercostal cannula size is generally between 6 and 10 mm in diameter.
B) A thoracoscopic grasper is introduced into an intercostal cannula, and the ventral aspect of the pericardium is grasped. Thoracoscopic scissors are placed into the contralateral intercostal cannula, and a small incision is made into the pericardium (pictured). Once a hole can be clearly visualized in the pericardium, the pericardium on the edge of the hole is grasped and elevated.

Plate 12.2

Thoracoscopic Pericardectomy – Pericardial Window and Subtotal Pericardectomy

A)

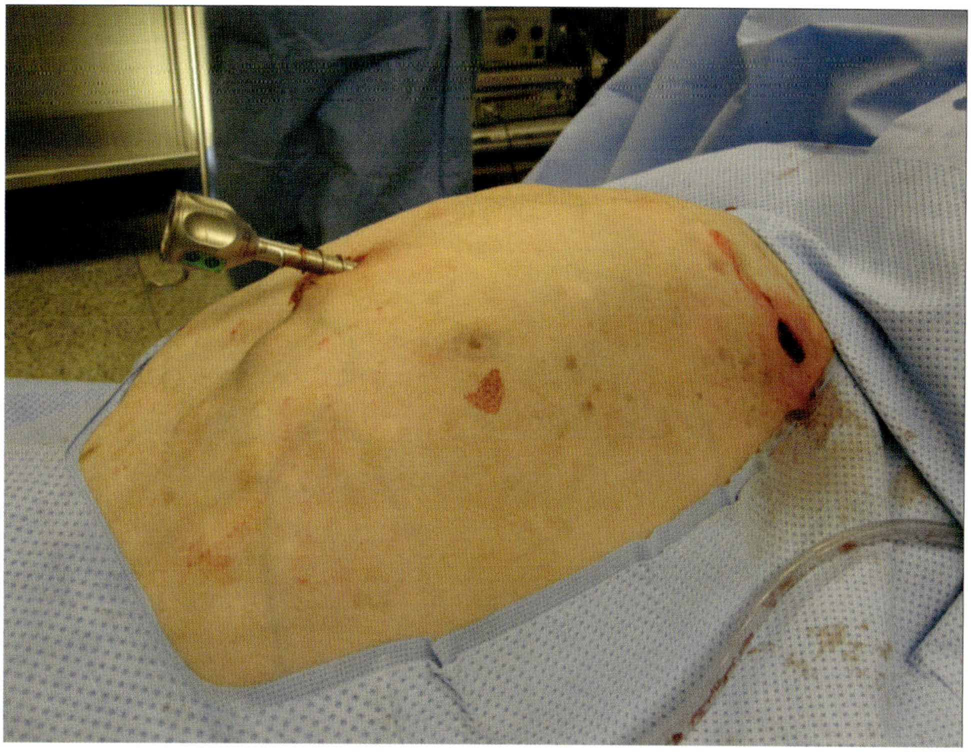

B)

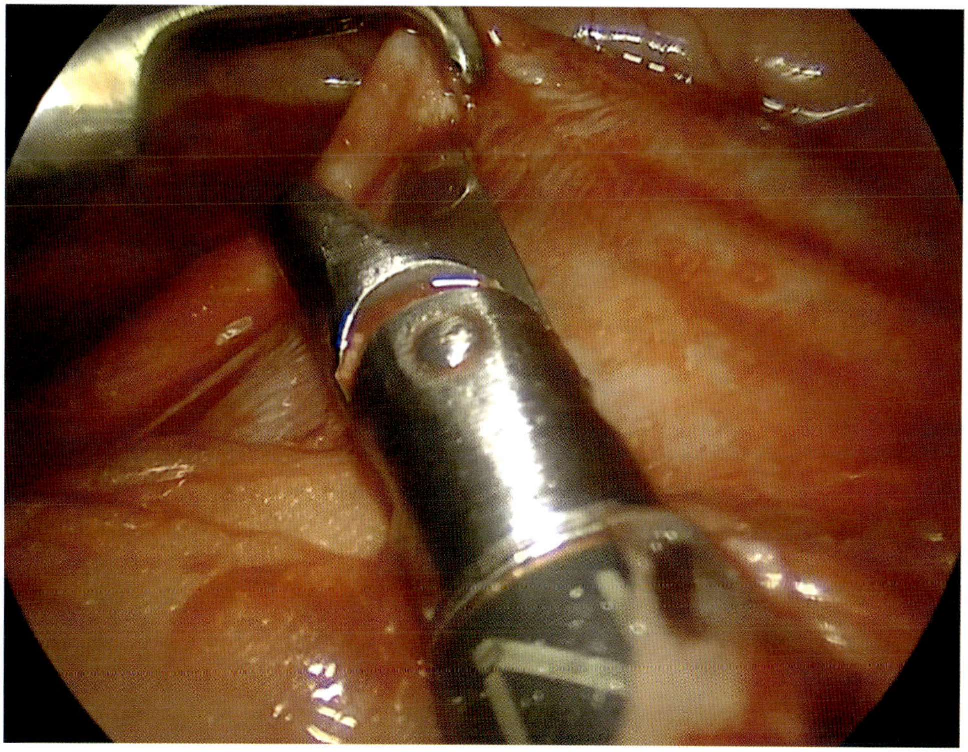

Suggested Adjuvant Treatments

- See *12.1. Open Subtotal Pericardectomy.*

Prognosis and Oncologic Outcome

- See *12.1. Open Subtotal Pericardectomy.*

References

1 Mayhew, K.N., Mayhew, P.D., Sorrell-Raschi, L. et al. (2009). Thoracoscopic subphrenic pericardectomy using double-lumen endobronchial intubation for alternating one-lung ventilation. *Vet. Surg.* 38 (8): 961–966.
2 Dupre, G.P., Corlouer, J.P., and Bouvy, B. (2001). Thoracoscopic pericardectomy performed without pulmonary exclusion in 9 dogs. *Vet. Surg.* 30 (1): 21–27.
3 Michelotti, K.P., Youk, A., Payne, J.T. et al. (2019). Outcomes of dogs with recurrent idiopathic pericardial effusion treated with a 3-port right-sided thoracoscopic subtotal pericardiectomy. *Vet. Surg.* 48 (6): 1032–1041.
4 Mayhew, P.D., Freeman, L., Kwan, T. et al. (2012). Comparison of surgical site infection rates in clean and clean-contaminated wounds in dogs and cats after minimally invasive versus open surgery: 179 cases (2007-2008). *J. Am. Vet. Med. Assoc.* 240 (2): 193–198.
5 Brisson, B.A., Reggeti, F., and Bienzle, D. (2006). Portal site metastasis of invasive mesothelioma after diagnostic thoracoscopy in a dog. *J. Am. Vet. Med. Assoc.* 229 (6): 980–983.
6 Alwen, S.G., Culp, W.T., Szivek, A. et al. (2015). Portal site metastasis after thoracoscopic resection of a cranial mediastinal mass in a dog. *J. Am. Vet. Med. Assoc.* 247 (7): 793–800.

Chapter 13: Atrial Appendage Amputation

13.1 Open Right Atrial Appendage Amputation

Indications

1) Resection of tumors involving the right atrial appendage (RAA)
2) Case selection is important because RAA amputation is not recommended for dogs with tumor invasion into the right atrium

Suggested Diagnostic Workup and Clinical Staging

- Complete blood count, serum biochemistry, and urinalysis
- Pericardiocentesis
- Cytologic analysis of pericardial fluid
- Echocardiogram
- Three-view thoracic radiographs or thoracic computed tomography scan
- Blood typing ± cross matching

Patient Positioning

The patient is positioned in lateral recumbency for an intercostal thoracotomy approach.

Surgical Technique (See Plate 13.1A–D)

A) See *10.1. Intercostal Thoracotomy* for details on the surgical approach for open RAA amputation. A right fifth intercostal thoracotomy is recommended for the best exposure to perform an open RAA amputation. A subtotal pericardectomy (PC) is performed to expose the RAA mass (i, ii) (see *12.1. Open Subtotal Pericardectomy*).
B) The RAA mass is assessed to determine its extent and resectability. If not resectable (i), then RAA amputation should not be attempted unless bypass facilities are available. If resectable (ii), then there are two techniques for amputation of the RAA: suture or stapler.
C) For the suture technique, a noncrushing vascular clamp is placed proximal to the base of the tumor (i). The tumor is resected by incising the RAA distal to the vascular clamp, leaving adequate tissue for closure of the RAA stump distal to the clamp (ii). The stump of the RAA is closed with one to two rows of 3-0 to 5-0 polypropylene in a simple continuous suture pattern (iii). Alternatively, a Parker-Kerr suture pattern can be used with a continuous suture pattern performed loosely over the vascular clamp; the vascular clamp is then removed and the suture material tightened and secured. After removal of the vascular clamp, the stump of the RAA is inspected for bleeding (iv).

Color Atlas of Canine and Feline Surgical Oncology, First Edition. Julius M. Liptak, Paolo Buracco, William T. N. Culp, and Nicholas J. Bacon.

Plate 13.1

Open Right Atrial Appendage Amputation

A-i)

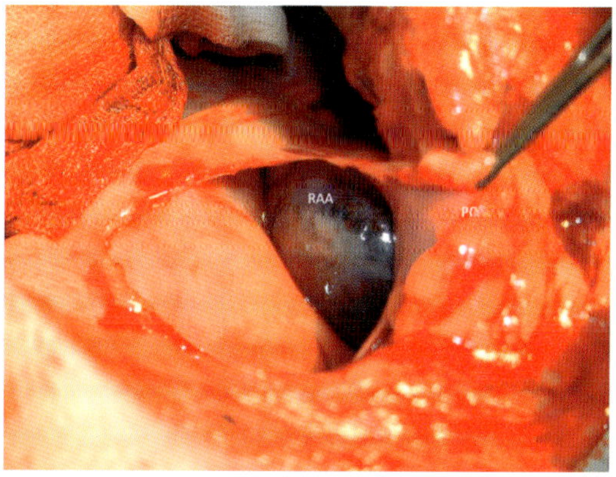

A-ii)

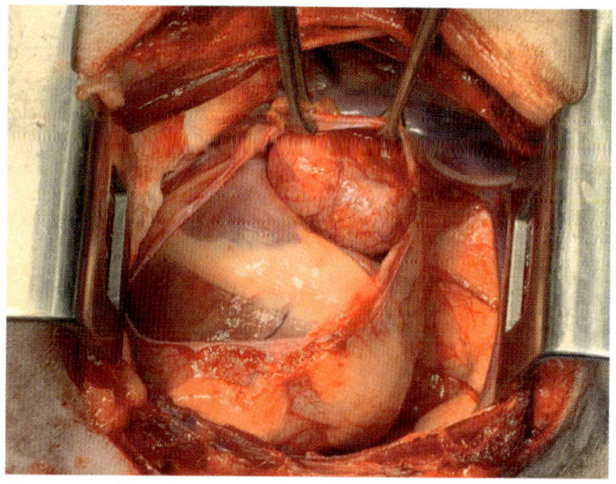

Courtesy of Dr. Roberto Bussadori

B-i)

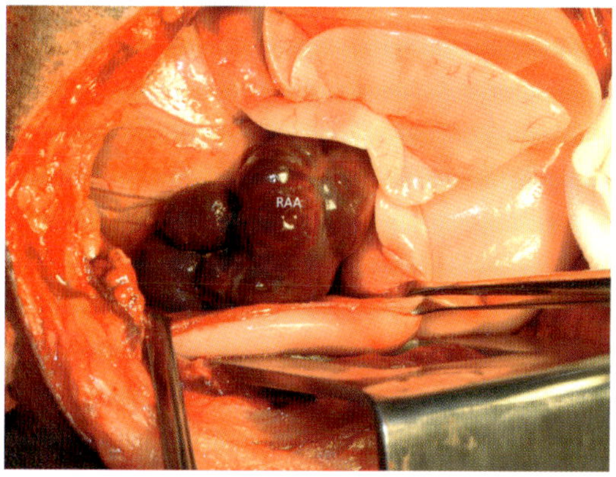

B-ii)

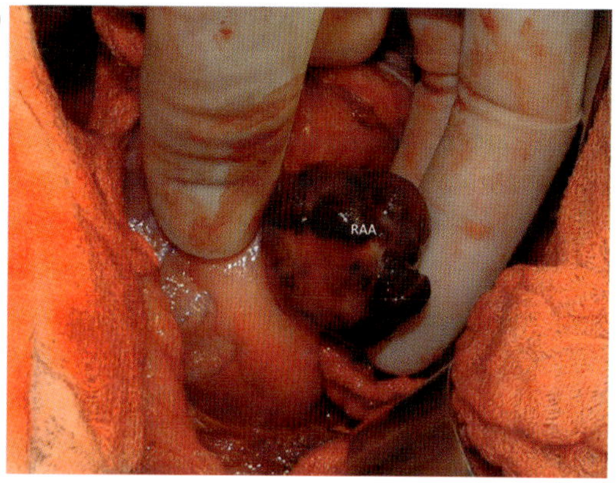

C-i)

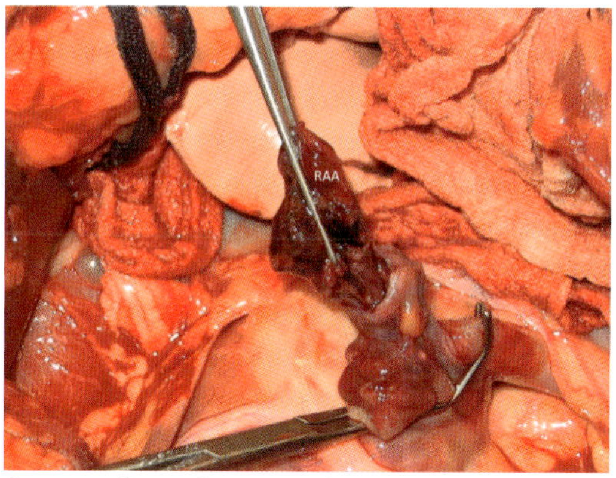

Courtesy of Dr. Roberto Bussadori

C-ii)

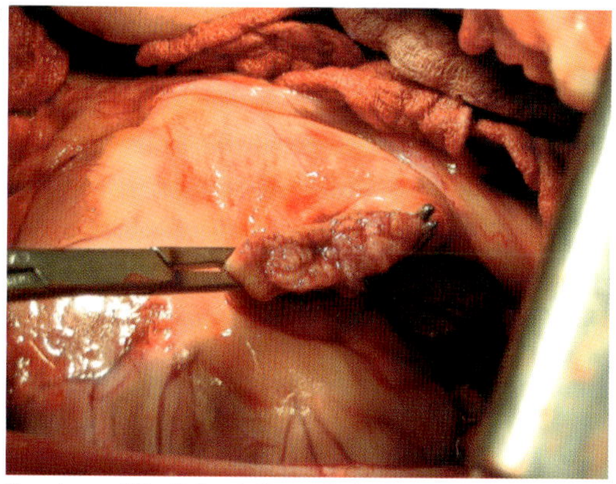

Courtesy of Dr. Roberto Bussadori

C-iii)

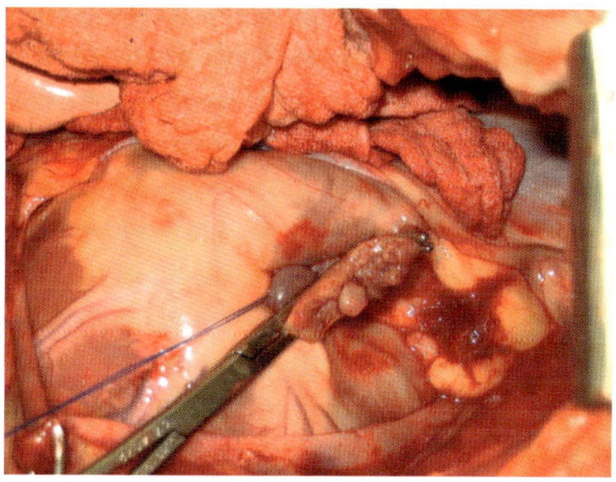

Courtesy of Dr. Roberto Bussadori

C-iv)

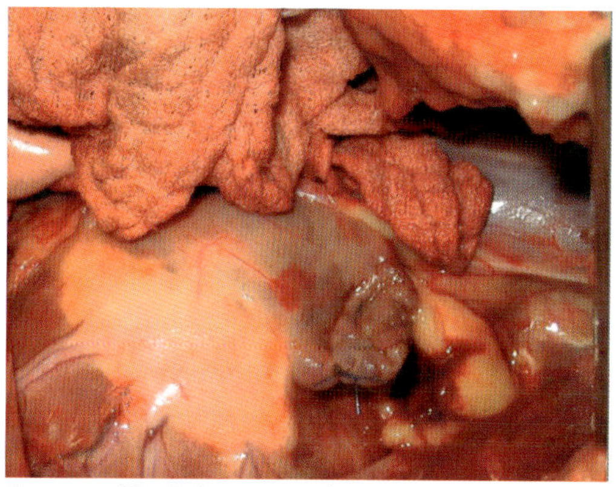

Courtesy of Dr. Roberto Bussadori

Surgical Technique (See Plate 13.1A–D) *continued*

D) For the stapler technique, a vascular 30-mm thoracoabdominal (TA) stapler is preferred because the three rows of staples and 1.0-mm closing height of the staples provide a better seal than other available stapler cartridges. The TA stapler is passed around the base of the mass, ideally with a cuff of normal tissue for surgical margins (i). The retaining pin (arrow) is engaged, which allows for the tissues to be isolated within the opening of the stapler cartridge (ii). The handle of the stapler is compressed, which results in the staples engaging the tissue within the cartridge. The tissue is then transected distal to the staple cartridge. The staple cartridge will often have a small shelf that will allow for guidance of the scalpel blade during transection (iii; note that this image is of a lung lobectomy). The stapler handle is then released and the stapler is removed, and the amputated RAA is removed from the surgical field (iv). The staple line is assessed for bleeding (v). If any is noted, then the staple line can be reinforced with a continuous suture pattern using 3-0 to 5-0 polypropylene over the staple line. Alternatively, a curved endo gastrointestinal anastomosis stapler can be used (vi).

Closure

The thoracic cavity is lavaged with warmed sterile saline. A thoracostomy tube is placed in the ipsilateral hemithorax. Closure of the surgical approach is described in *10.1. Intercostal Thoracotomy*.

Postoperative Management

1) Multimodal analgesia, including perioperative continuous rate infusion of an opioid ± ketamine, intercostal nerve blocks, local anesthesia instilled through the thoracostomy tube ± wound diffuser catheter, and oral analgesic drugs
2) Supplemental oxygen therapy, if required
3) Thoracostomy tube management
4) Elizabethan collar or body suit

Complications

Intraoperative Complications

- Hemorrhage (whole blood transfusion should be available)

Postoperative Complications [1]

- Cardiac arrhythmias (13%)
- Surgical-site infection or incisional dehiscence (9%)
- Anemia (4%)
- Pneumonia (4%)

Suggested Adjuvant Treatments

- Chemotherapy is recommended for dogs with cardiac hemangiosarcomas [1–3].

Plate 13.1

Open Right Atrial Appendage Amputation *continued*

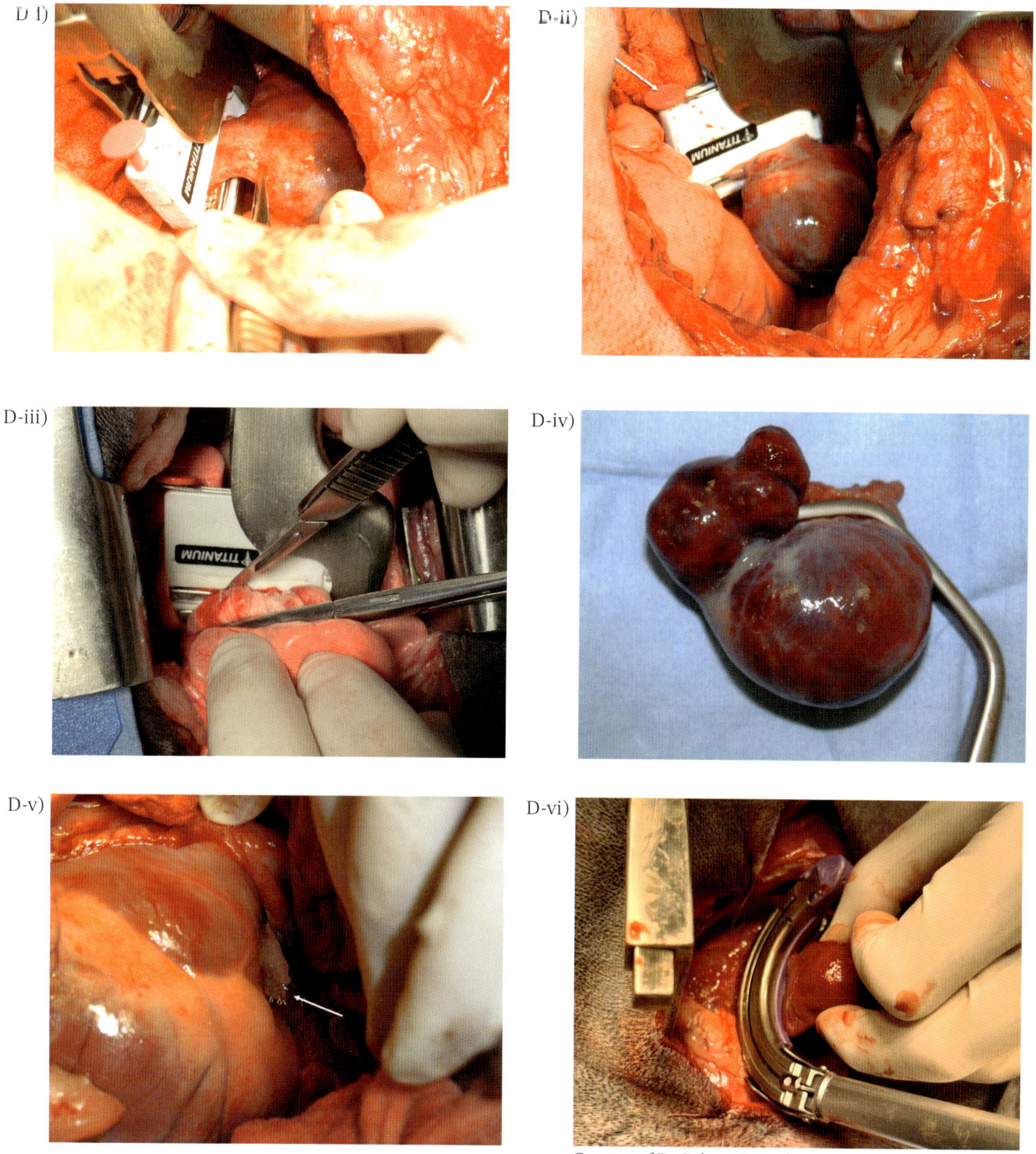

Courtesy of Dr. Roberto Bussadori

Prognosis and Oncologic Outcome – Dogs

Tumor Type	Local Recurrence Rate	Metastatic Rate	Disease-Free Interval (d)	Median Survival Time (d)	1-Year Survival Rate	2-Year Survival Rate
Hemangiosarcoma [1, 3, 4]	–	75%	–	56–90	0%	0%
Adjuvant chemotherapy [1, 3]						
• Chemotherapy	–	–	–	175–189	0%	0%
• No chemotherapy	–	–	–	42–86	0%	0%

References

1. Weisse, C., Soares, N., Beal, M.W. et al. (2005). Survival times in dogs with right atrial hemangiosarcoma treated by means of surgical resection with or without adjuvant chemotherapy: 23 cases (1986-2000). *J. Am. Vet. Med. Assoc.* 226: 575–579.
2. Ghaffari, S., Pelio, D.C., Lange, A.J. et al. (2014). A retrospective evaluation of doxorubicin-based chemotherapy for dogs with right atrial masses and pericardial effusion. *J. Small Anim. Pract.* 55 (5): 254–257.
3. Yamamoto, S., Hoshi, K., Hirakawa, A. et al. (2013). Epidemiological, clinical and pathological features of primary cardiac hemangiosarcoma in dogs: a review of 51 cases. *J. Vet. Med. Sci.* 75 (11): 1433–1441.
4. Ployart, S., Libermann, S., Doran, I. et al. (2013). Thoracoscopic resection of right auricular masses in dogs: 9 cases (2003-2011). *J. Am. Vet. Med. Assoc.* 242 (2): 237–241.

13.2 Thoracoscopic Right Atrial Appendage Amputation

Indications

1) Resection of tumors confined to the apex of the right atrial appendage
2) Case selection is important because right atrial appendage amputation is not recommended for dogs with tumor invasion into the right atrium

Suggested Diagnostic Workup and Clinical Staging

- Complete blood count, serum biochemistry, and urinalysis
- Pericardiocentesis
- Cytologic analysis of pericardial fluid
- Echocardiogram
- Three-view thoracic radiographs or thoracic computed tomography scan
- Blood typing ± cross matching

Patient Positioning

The patient is positioned in dorsal recumbency.

Surgical Technique (See Plate 13.2A–C)

A) A paraxiphoid transdiaphragmatic port is established and the telescope is inserted intrathoracically; a 6-mm cannula is generally selected to allow for placement of a 5-mm diameter telescope. Two to three intercostal ports are placed with one intercostal port at the right fifth or sixth intercostal space and one to two intercostal ports at the left sixth and ninth intercostal spaces. The intercostal cannula size is generally between 6 and 10 mm in diameter.
B) A large pericardial window is created (see *12.2. Thoracoscopic Pericardectomy – Pericardial Window and Subtotal Pericardectomy*) to allow for visualization of the right atrial appendage and the right atrium. The extent of the tumor is assessed by grasping the incised pericardium and inserting the telescope into the pericardial sac.
C) The right atrial appendage is grasped and elevated through one of the intercostal ports. An Endo GIA stapler is introduced from a contralateral intercostal port and placed across the base of the atrial appendage, leaving a cuff of normal tissue for surgical margins. It is essential that the staple line extends along the entire base of the appendage before deployment of the stapler (i). The stapler is engaged and the right atrial appendage is simultaneously transected free from stump of the right atrial appendage (ii).

Color Atlas of Canine and Feline Surgical Oncology, First Edition. Julius M. Liptak, Paolo Buracco, William T. N. Culp, and Nicholas J. Bacon.

Plate 13.2

Thoracoscopic Right Atrial Appendage Amputation

A)

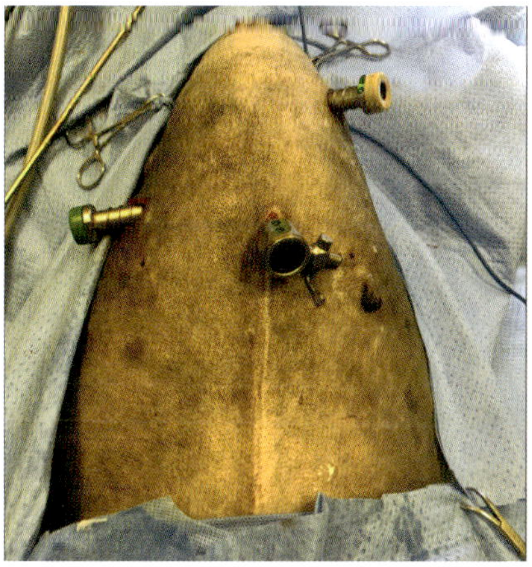

Courtesy of Dr. Brad Case

B)

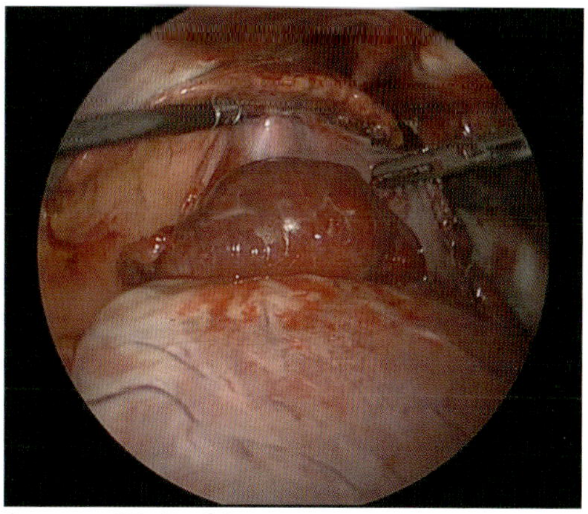

Courtesy of Dr. Brad Case

C-i)

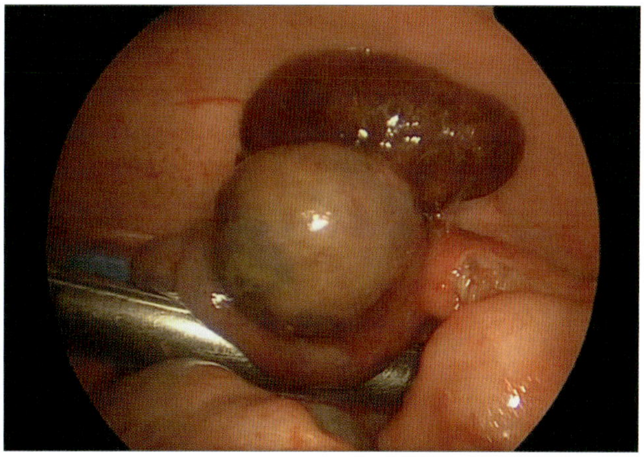

Courtesy of Dr. Brad Case

C-ii)

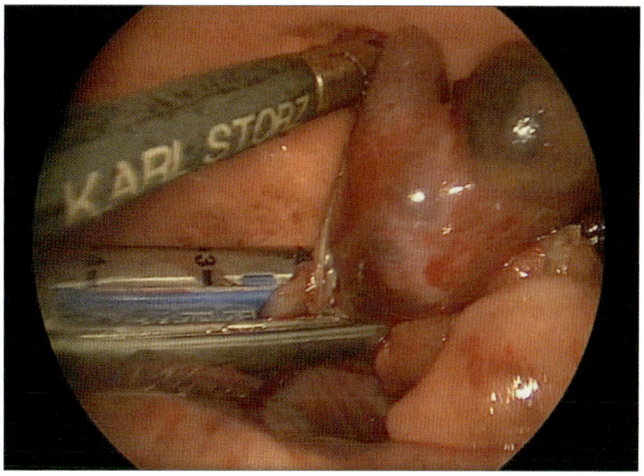

Courtesy of Dr. Brad Case

Surgical Technique (See Plate 13.2A–C) *continued*

D) Limited contact of the atrial appendage mass with the port sites is important. A retrieval device should be introduced into one of the ports. Grasping forceps are used to grasp the amputated right atrial appendage and insert this into the retrieval device. The retrieval device is closed and removed from the thorax.

Closure

A thoracostomy tube is placed before closure and the position is visualized by the telescope. All equipment, including the cannulae and telescope, are removed. The muscle and subcutaneous tissue can be closed with 2-0 to 3-0 monofilament absorbable suture in a simple interrupted or cruciate pattern. The dermal layer is closed with 3-0 monofilament absorbable suture. The thoracostomy tube is secured to the skin.

Postoperative Management

1) Multimodal analgesia
2) Supplemental oxygen therapy, if required
3) Thoracostomy tube management
4) Elizabethan collar or body suit

Complications

Intraoperative Complications

- Hemorrhage (whole blood transfusion should be available) [1]

Postoperative Complications (0–14 Days)

- Premature ventricular complexes (33%) [1]
- Surgical-site infections (rare) [2]

Postoperative Complications (>14 Days)

- Portal-site metastases (rare) [3, 4]

Suggested Adjuvant Treatments

- Chemotherapy is recommended for dogs with cardiac hemangiosarcomas [5–7]

Prognosis and Oncologic Outcome

- See *13.1. Open Right Atrial Appendage Amputation.*

References

1 Ployart, S., Libermann, S., Doran, I. et al. (2013). Thoracoscopic resection of right auricular masses in dogs: 9 cases (2003-2011). *J. Am. Vet. Med. Assoc.* 242 (2): 237–241.

2 Mayhew, P.D., Freeman, L., Kwan, T. et al. (2012). Comparison of surgical site infection rates in clean and clean-contaminated wounds in dogs and cats after minimally invasive versus open surgery: 179 cases (2007-2008). *J. Am. Vet. Med. Assoc.* 240 (2): 193–198.

3 Brisson, B.A., Reggeti, F., and Bienzle, D. (2006). Portal site metastasis of invasive mesothelioma after diagnostic thoracoscopy in a dog. *J. Am. Vet. Med. Assoc.* 229 (6): 980–983.

4 Alwen, S.G., Culp, W.T., Szivek, A. et al. (2015). Portal site metastasis after thoracoscopic resection of a cranial mediastinal mass in a dog. *J. Am. Vet. Med. Assoc.* 247 (7): 793–800.

5 Weisse, C., Soares, N., Beal, M.W. et al. (2005). Survival times in dogs with right atrial hemangiosarcoma treated by means of surgical resection with or without adjuvant chemotherapy: 23 cases (1986-2000). *J. Am. Vet. Med. Assoc.* 226: 575–579.

6 Ghaffari, S., Pelio, D.C., Lange, A.J. et al. (2014). A retrospective evaluation of doxorubicin-based chemotherapy for dogs with right atrial masses and pericardial effusion. *J. Small Anim. Pract.* 55 (5): 254–257.

7 Yamamoto, S., Hoshi, K., Hirakawa, A. et al. (2013). Epidemiological, clinical and pathological features of primary cardiac hemangiosarcoma in dogs: a review of 51 cases. *J. Vet. Med. Sci.* 75 (11): 1433–1441.

Chapter 14: Chest Wall Resection and Reconstruction

Indications

1) Resection of tumors involving the rib or ribs, including primary rib sarcomas, tumors invading into the ribs, or where resection of the chest wall is required for deep margins.
2) The maximum number of ribs that can be resected is unknown. Six ribs can be safely resected without the need for rigid reconstruction of the chest wall [1].
3) Primary rib tumors can be adherent to lung lobes or the pericardium. In these cases, chest wall resection can be combined with en bloc lung lobectomy (see *11.1. Open Lung Lobectomy*) or subtotal pericardectomy (see *12.1. Open Subtotal Pericardectomy*).

Suggested Diagnostic Workup and Clinical Staging (See Plate 14 – 1, 2)

- Complete blood count, serum biochemistry, and urinalysis
- Preoperative biopsy
- Thoracic computed tomography (CT) scan (primary rib osteosarcoma; 1, axial CT image; 2, reconstructed CT image)

Patient Positioning

The patient is positioned in lateral recumbency with the affected side uppermost.

Surgical Technique – Chest Wall Resection (See Plate 14A–J)

A) A vertical skin incision is performed over the rib mass from the costovertebral junction to the sternocostal junction. If a preoperative biopsy has been done (B), then the skin incision should be modified with an elliptical incision around the biopsy site so this and the biopsy tract can be resected en bloc with the chest wall resection. The skin incision is continued deeply through subcutaneous tissue and the cutaneous trunci muscle.
B) If the latissimus dorsi (LD) muscle is not adhered to or invaded by the rib tumor, then this muscle can be used for later reconstruction of the chest wall defect. The ventral border of the LD muscle (i) is dissected free from its fascial attachments using blunt dissection or a vessel sealing device (ii). The caudal border of the muscle inserts on the 13th rib; this insertion should be released with sharp dissection or a vessel sealing device (ii). The dorsal border of the LD muscle, extending from the caudal border of the triceps muscle to the head of the 13th rib, is dissected free from its fascial attachments using blunt dissection or a vessel sealing device. Once freed of its ventral, caudal, and dorsal attachments, the LD muscle is raised (iii), progressively ligating and dividing perforating intercostal vessels, reflected craniodorsally (iv), and protected with moistened laparotomy sponges (v).

Color Atlas of Canine and Feline Surgical Oncology, First Edition. Julius M. Liptak, Paolo Buracco, William T. N. Culp, and Nicholas J. Bacon.

Plate 14

Chest Wall Resection and Reconstruction

1)

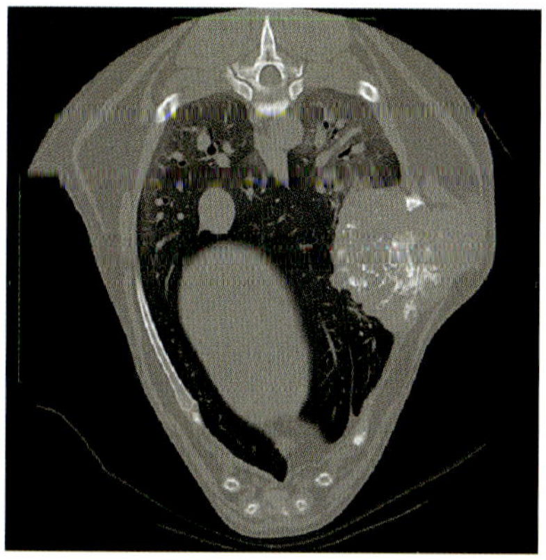

2)

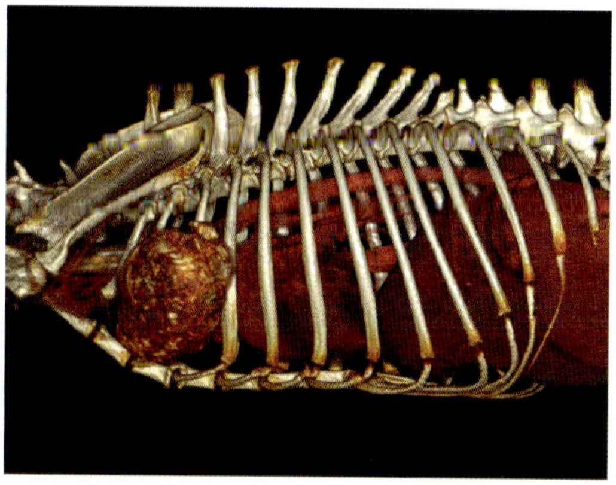

A)

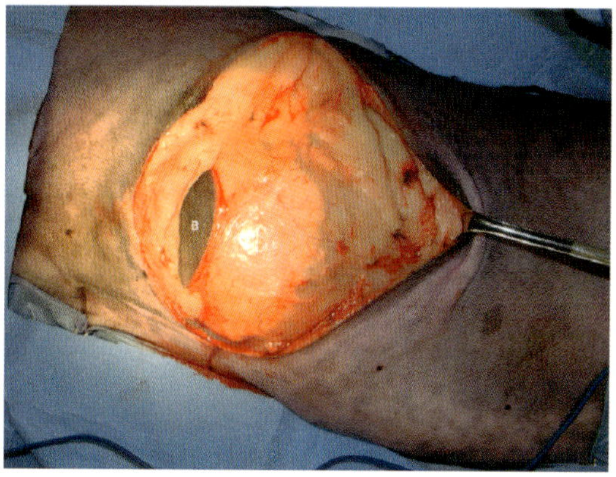

B-i)

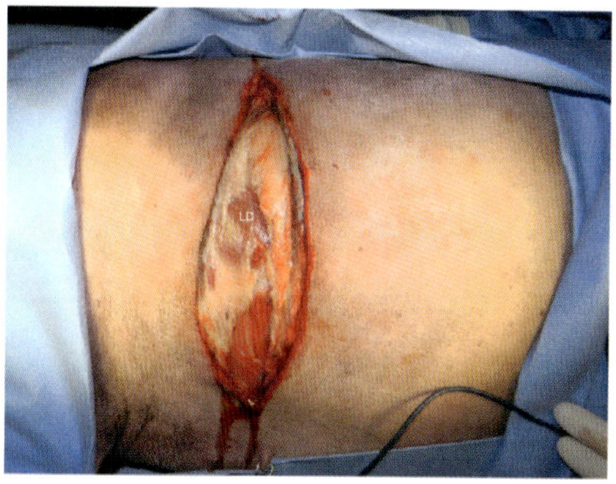

B-ii)

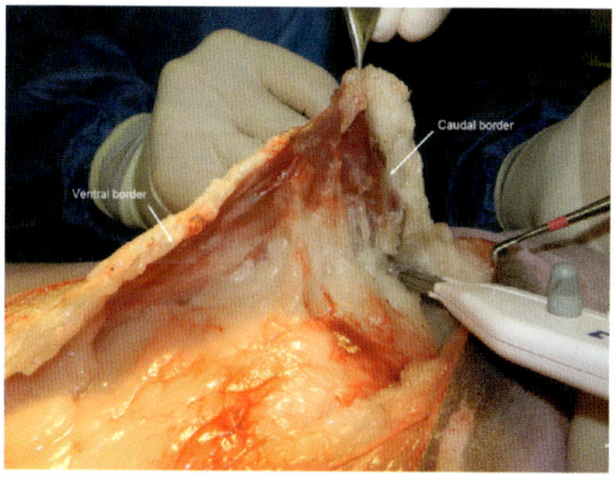

B-iii)

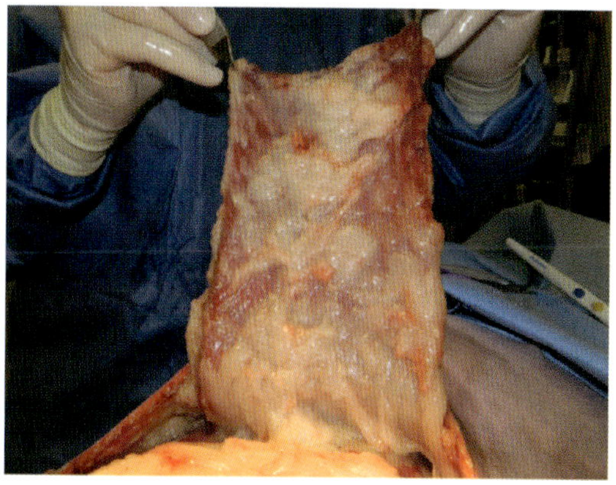

B-iv)

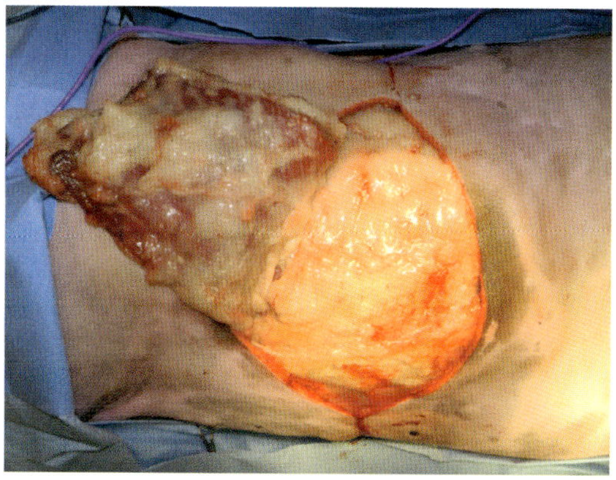

B-v)

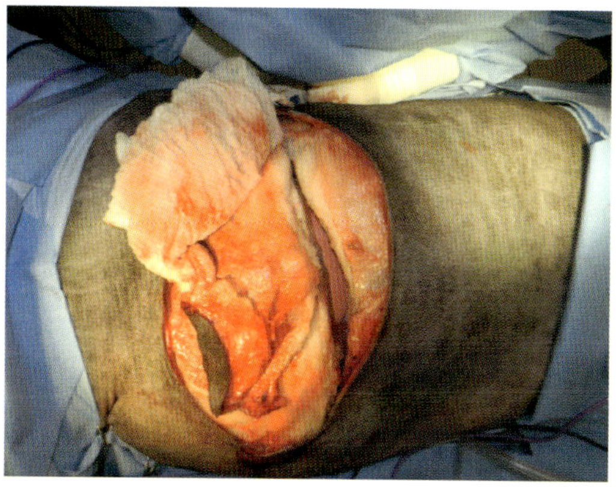

Surgical Technique – Chest Wall Resection (See Plate 14A–J) *continued*

C) A normal rib cranial and caudal to the rib tumor is resected for cranial and caudal margins, respectively. The caudal intercostal thoracotomy is performed first. Depending on the location of the rib tumor, muscles bellies are either incised or separated to expose the appropriate intercostal space (see *10.1. Intercostal Thoracotomy*). The external and internal intercostal muscles (i) and pleura (ii) are incised from the rib head to the sternocostal junction. Once the caudal intercostal thoracotomy is completed, the rib cranial to the thoracotomy is elevated to expose the rib tumor and verify the resection margins (iii, iv).

D) The dorsal margin should be a minimum of 3 cm proximal to the rib tumor; however, resection of the entire rib has also been recommended because rib tumors can extend beyond their palpable and visible limits along the intramedullary canal of the rib [1]. Circumcostal ligatures, using 0 or 2-0 monofilament absorbable suture material, are placed around the dorsal aspect of each of the ribs to be resected at a minimum of 4 cm proximal to the rib tumor (i, ii). These ligatures minimize the risk of bleeding from the intercostal vessels coursing along the caudal aspect of the ribs during osteotomy of the ribs. Alternatively, these vessels can be individually identified, ligated, and divided.

E) Osteotomies of the dorsal aspect of the ribs are performed with either bone cutters (i) or an oscillating or sagittal saw (ii). These osteotomies are performed ventral to the circumcostal ligatures and a minimum of 3 cm proximal to the rib tumor (iii).

Plate 14

Chest Wall Resection and Reconstruction *continued*

C-i)

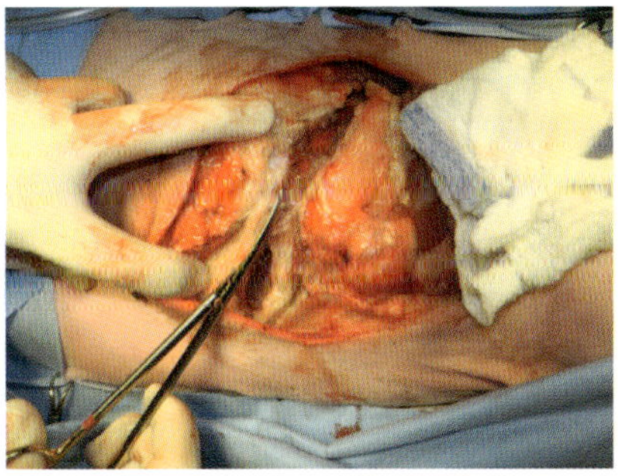

C-ii)

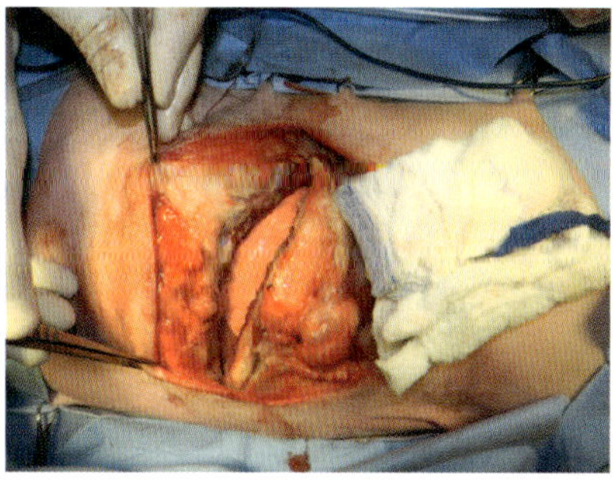

C-iii)

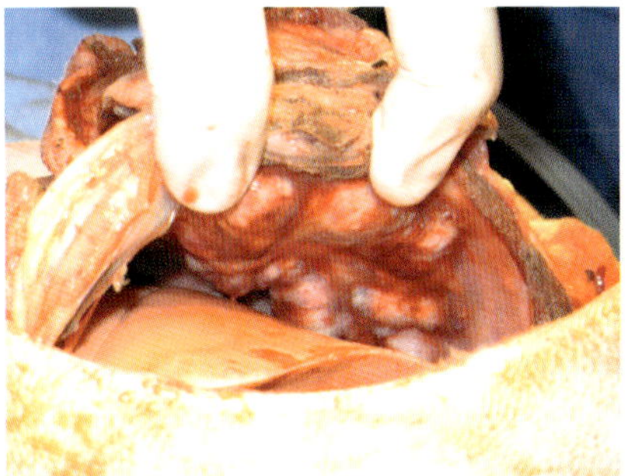

C-iv)

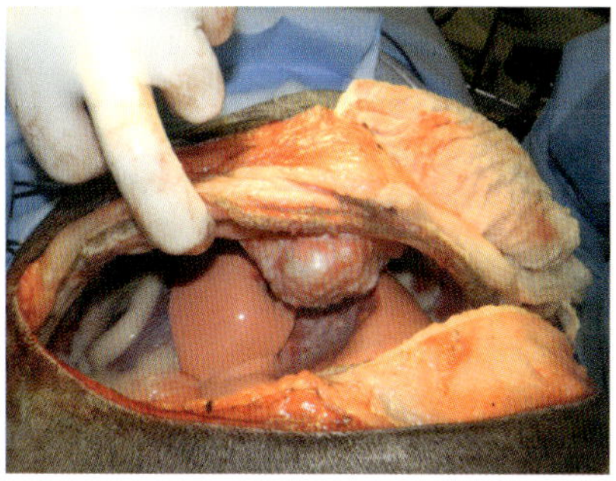

D-i)

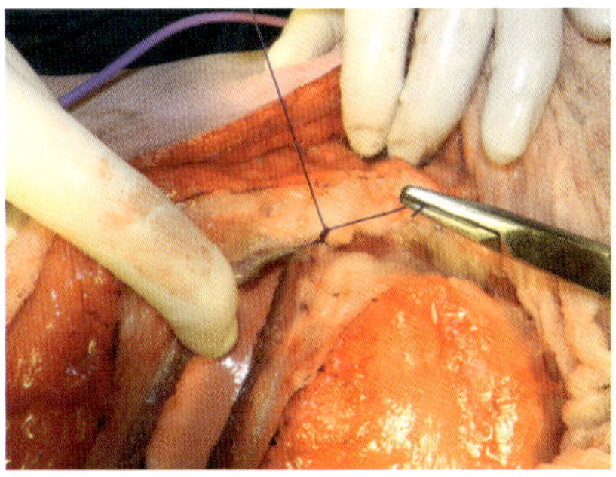

D-ii)

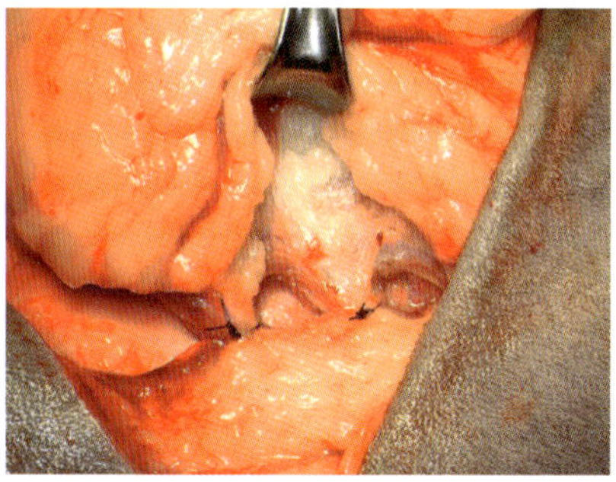

E-i)

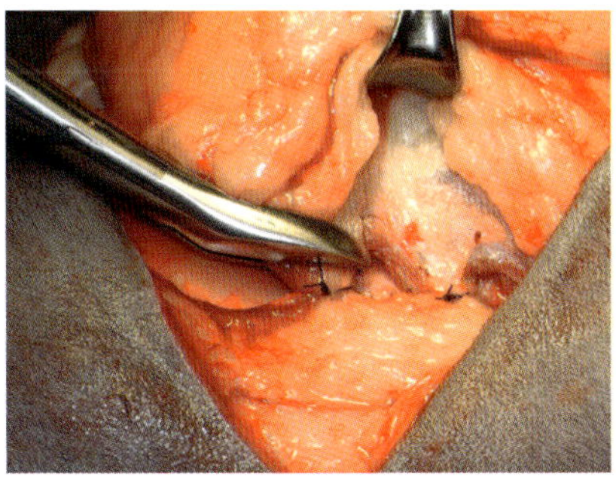

E-ii)

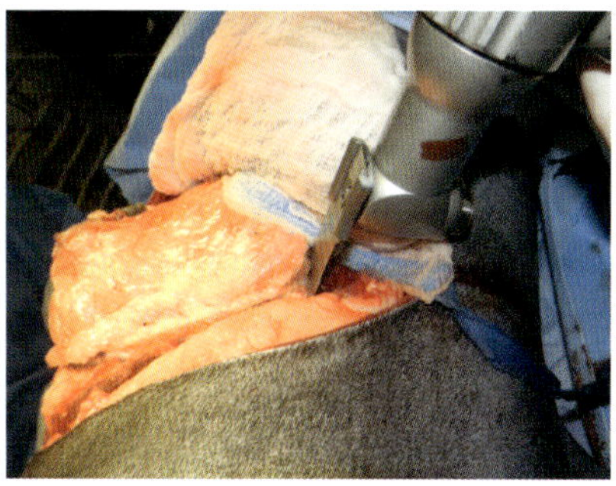

E-iii)

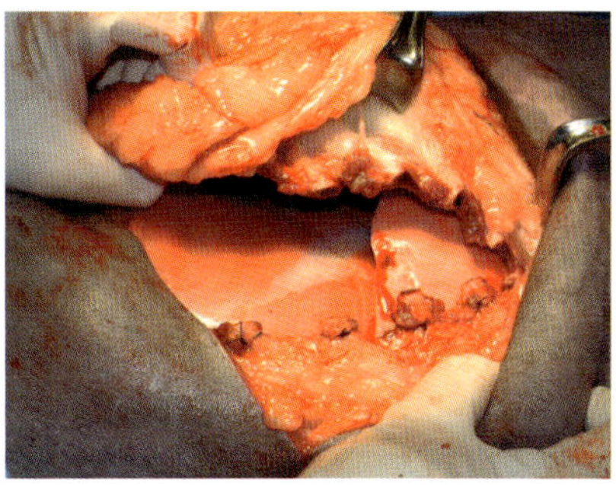

Surgical Technique – Chest Wall Resection (See Plate 14A–J) *continued*

F) Osteotomies of the ventral aspect of the ribs is then performed with a minimum of 3-cm margins distal to the rib tumor (i–iii). If 3-cm margins cannot be obtained with osteotomies of the ventral aspect of the ribs, then an en bloc partial sternebrectomy should be performed with an oscillating or sagittal saw (iv, arrow).

G) The chest wall resection is completed with an intercostal thoracotomy cranial to the normal rib being used for cranial margins (i–iv; see *10.1. Intercostal Thoracotomy*). Depending on the location of the rib tumor, muscle bellies are either incised or separated to expose the appropriate intercostal space. The external and internal intercostal muscles and the pleura are incised from the rib head to the sternocostal junction (iii).

H) The internal thoracic artery and vein course along the ventrolateral aspect of the thoracic cavity at the level of the sternocostal junction. These vessels should be identified and protected or ligated and divided (pictured, arrow) if the chest wall resection is planned to extend further ventrally than the internal thoracic artery and vein.

Plate 14

Chest Wall Resection and Reconstruction *continued*

F-i)

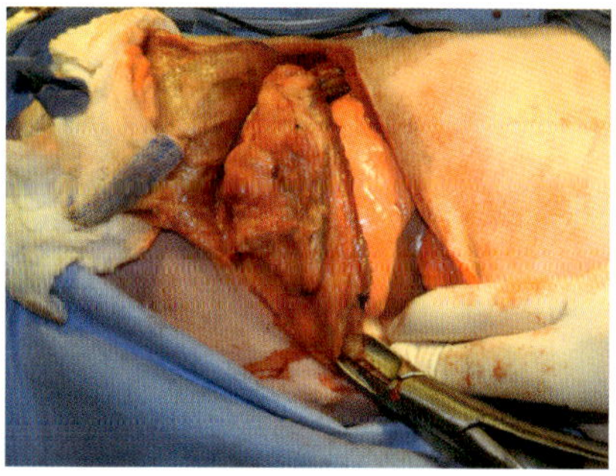

F-ii)

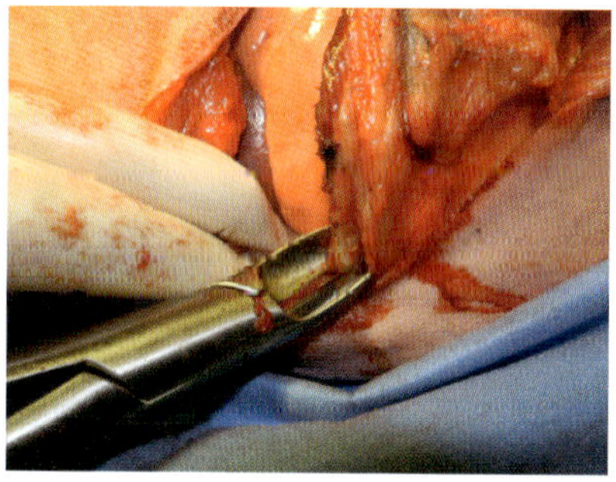

F-iii)

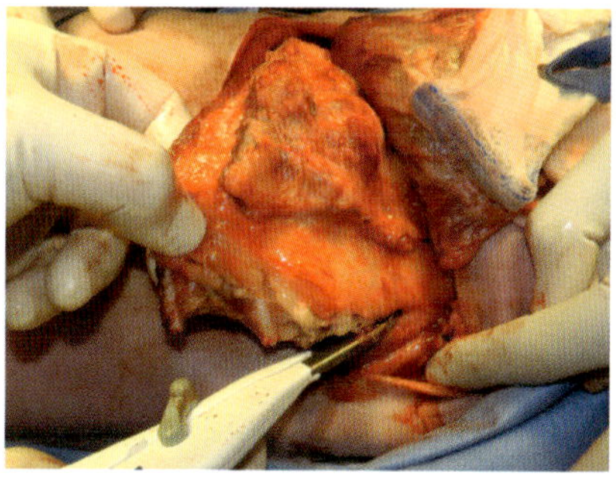

F-iv)

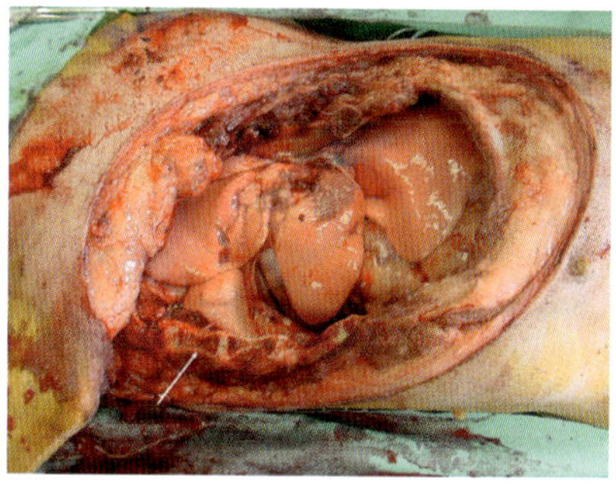

G-i)

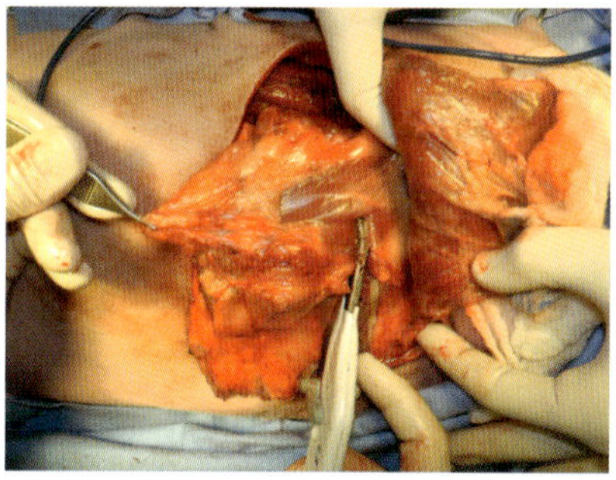

G-ii)

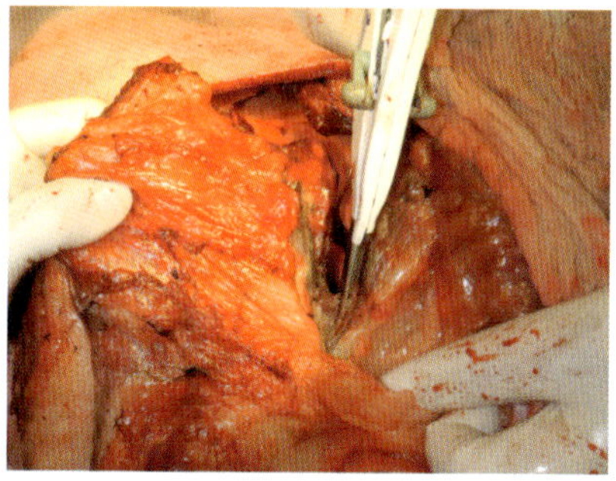

G-iii)

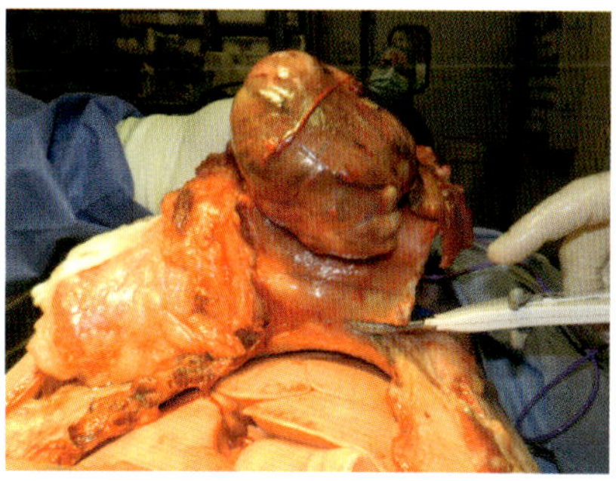

G-iv)

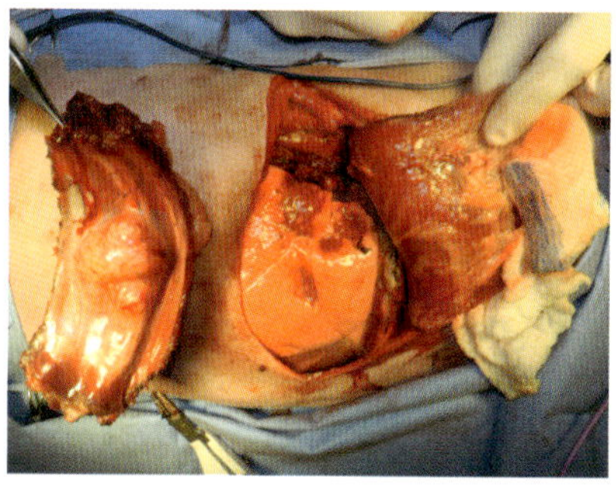

H)

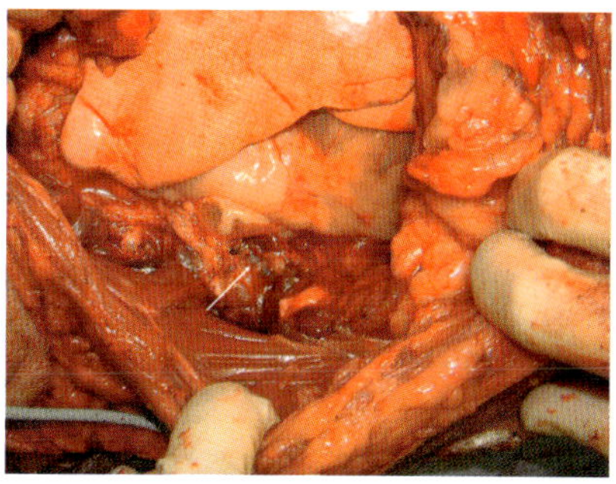

Surgical Technique – Chest Wall Resection (See Plate 14A–J) *continued*

I) If there are adhesions to either lung lobes or the pericardium, which are reported in 26% and 8% of dogs, respectively [1], then en bloc lung lobectomy (i, adhesion; ii, lung lobectomy with a thoracoabdominal stapler; iii, completed lung lobectomy) (see *11.1. Open Lung Lobectomy*) or subtotal pericardectomy (see *12.1. Open Subtotal Pericardectomy*) should be performed. For caudal primary rib tumors, a portion of the diaphragm may need to be resected (iv, adhesion; v, vi, partial diaphragmatic resection).

Plate 14

Chest Wall Resection and Reconstruction *continued*

I-i)

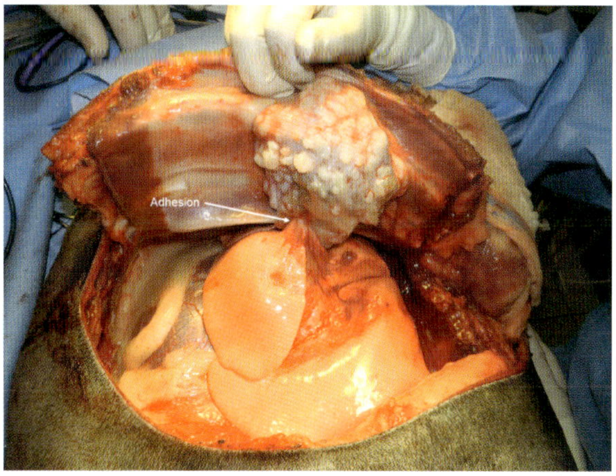

I-ii)

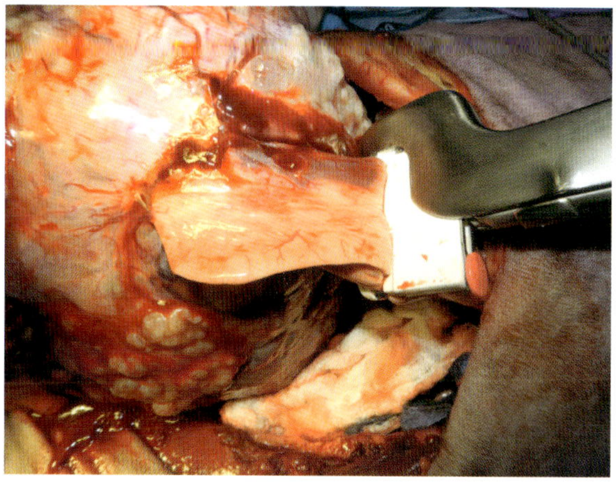

I-iii)

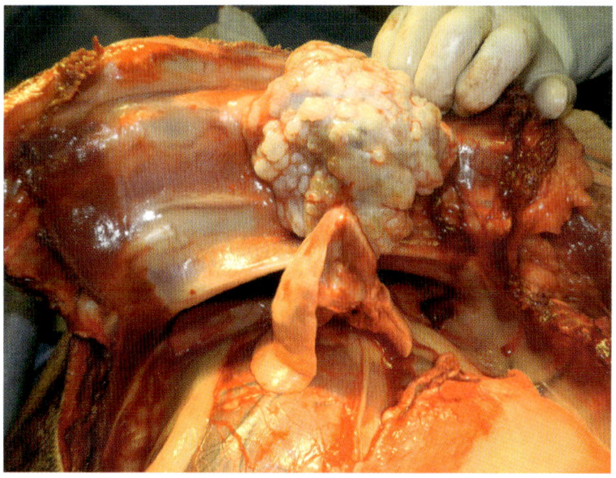

I-iv)

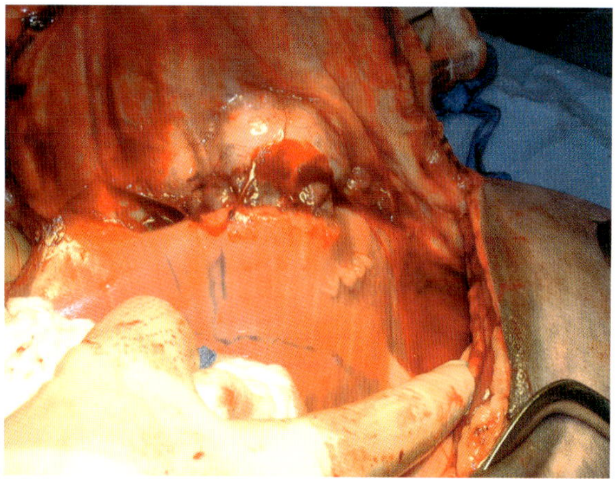

I-v)

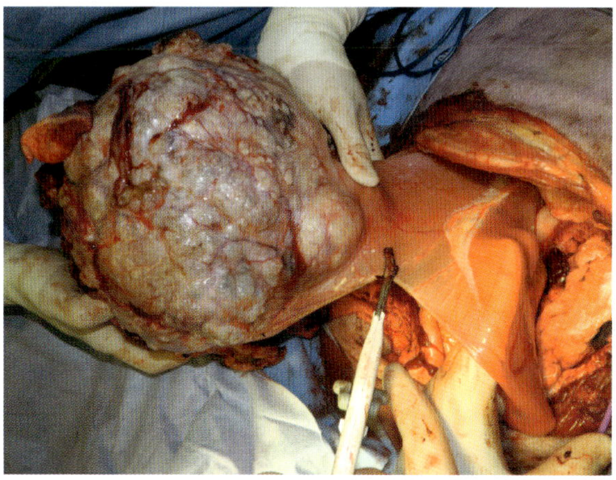

I-vi)

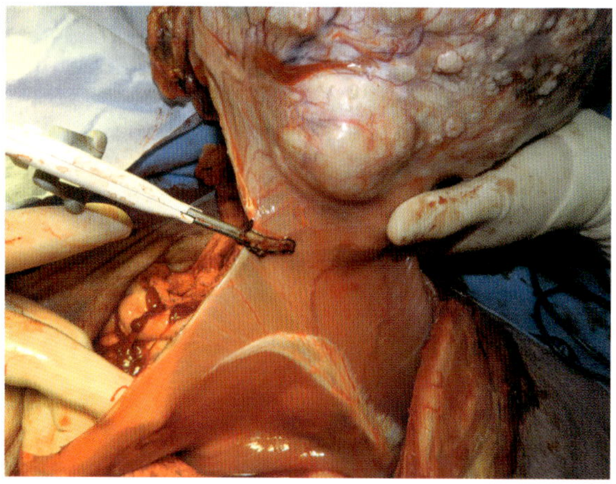

Surgical Technique – Chest Wall Resection (See Plate 14A–J) *continued*

J) An appropriately sized thoracostomy tube is inserted into the ipsilateral hemithorax.

Closure (See Plate 14K–N)

K–N) There are a number of different techniques to reconstruct chest wall defects after chest wall resections. The choice of reconstruction technique depends on the location of the chest wall defect and personal preference. Cranial to mid-chest wall defects can be reconstructed with a LD muscle flap, LD myocutaneous flap, or prosthetic mesh. These can be used as sole methods of reconstruction or they can be combined. If they are combined, then the prosthetic mesh should be sutured into the chest wall defect first and then the LD muscle flap should be sutured over the lateral aspect of the prosthetic mesh. An omental pedicle graft can be used as a supplemental autogenous technique, especially for coverage of the pleural surface of prosthetic mesh, but this should not be used as the sole method of chest wall reconstruction. The pectoral muscle flap (K) can also be used to reconstruct the ventral portion of large chest wall defects. If greater than six ribs are resected, consideration should be given for more rigid chest wall reconstruction using plastic spinal or other plates (L), autogenous split rib grafts, or allogeneic free rib grafts. Segmental sternal defects can be reconstructed with prosthetic mesh (M), mesh-methylmethacrylate-mesh sandwiches, or patient-specific 3D-printed implants (N – i, ii). Caudal chest wall defects are reconstructed with diaphragmatic advancement and reconstruction of the subsequent abdominal wall defect.

Plate 14

Chest Wall Resection and Reconstruction *continued*

J)

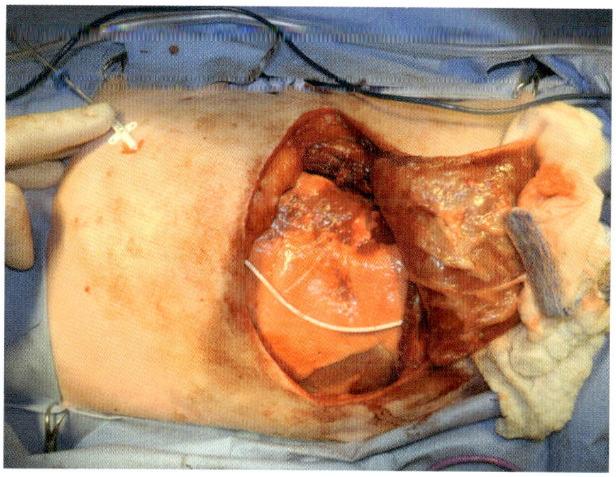

K)

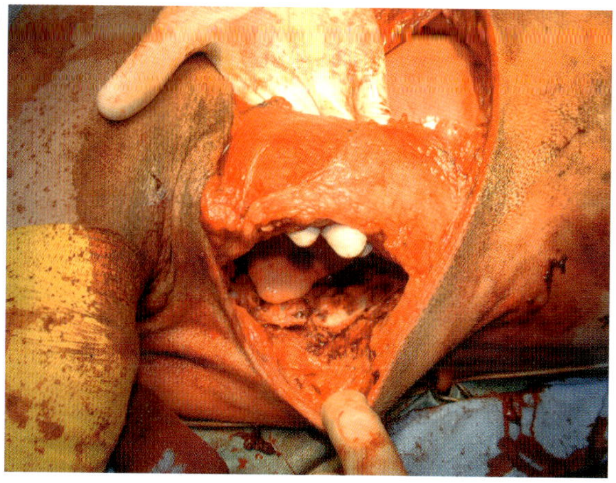

L)

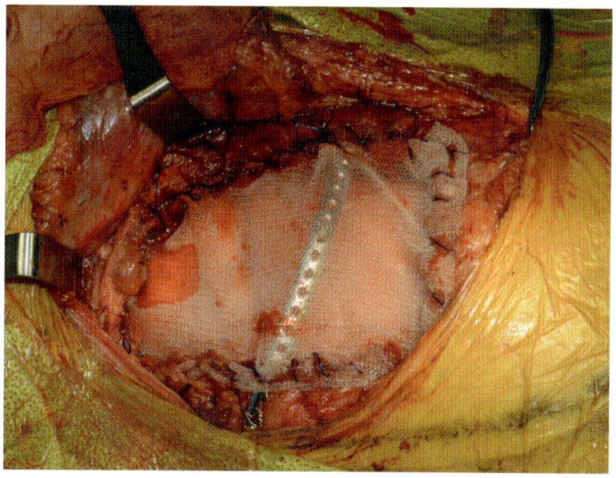

Courtesy of Dr. Takeshi Aikawa

M)

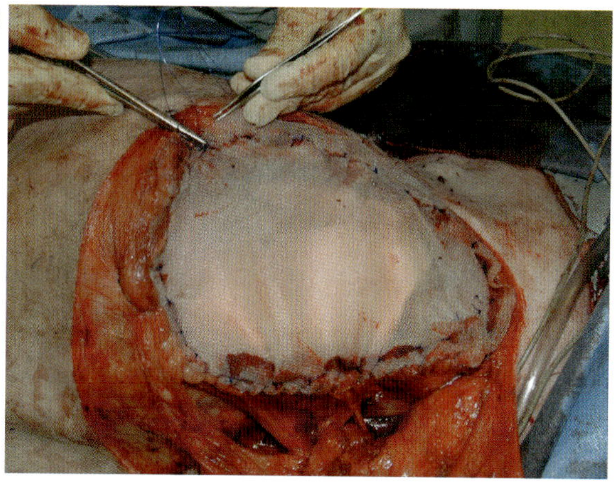

N-i)

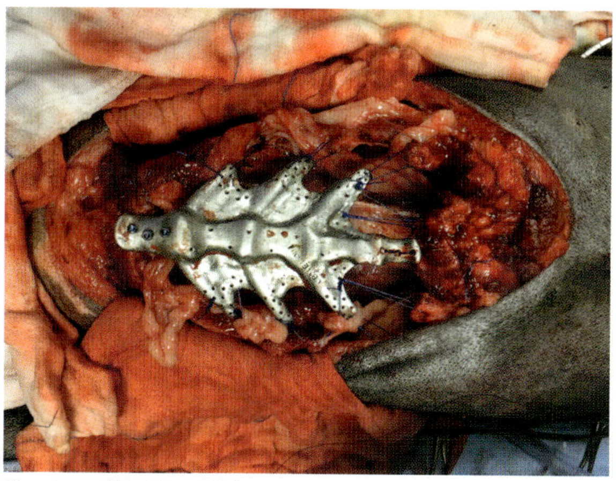

Courtesy of Dr. Hervé Brissot

N-ii)

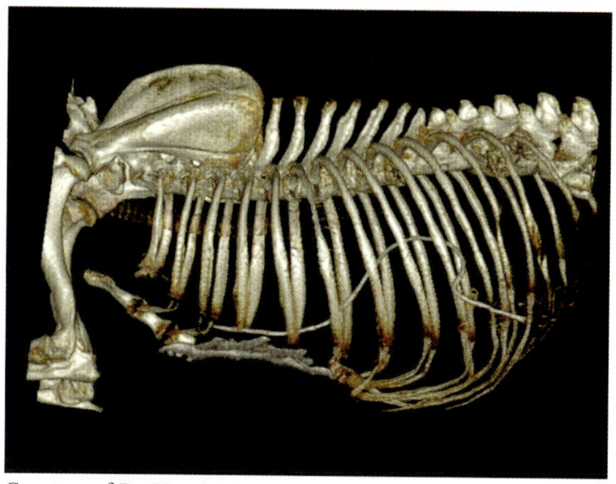

Courtesy of Dr. Hervé Brissot

Surgical Technique – Chest Wall Reconstruction with a Supplemental Omental Pedicle Graft [2] (See Plate 140–U)

O) The cranial abdominal cavity is exposed through either the chest wall resection site (pictured) or a separate paracostal abdominal approach (see *15.2. Paracostal Approach*).

P) The omentum and spleen are exteriorized and the visceral leaf of the greater omentum is retracted cranially to identify and transect its pancreatic attachments to the level of the spleen.

Q) The omental vessels originating from the splenic artery are ligated and transected (arrows) to allow caudal retraction of the visceral leaf of the omentum.

R) An inverted L-shaped incision is then made in the bursal portion of the greater omentum, based on either the left (LGEA) or right gastroepiploic arteries.

S) The omental vessels are ligated along the left border of the greater omentum caudal to the gastrosplenic ligament, and the omental incision is then continued caudally parallel to the remaining omental vessels for two thirds of its length (arrows).

T) The epiploic branches to the greater curvature of the stomach and the opposite gastroepiploic artery are ligated and divided.

Plate 14

Chest Wall Resection and Reconstruction *continued*

O)

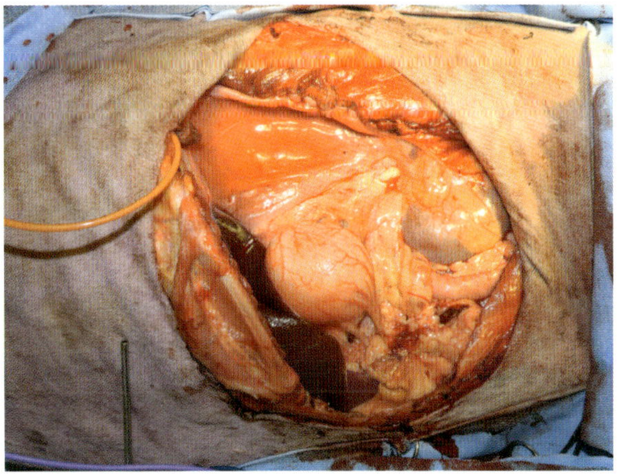

P)

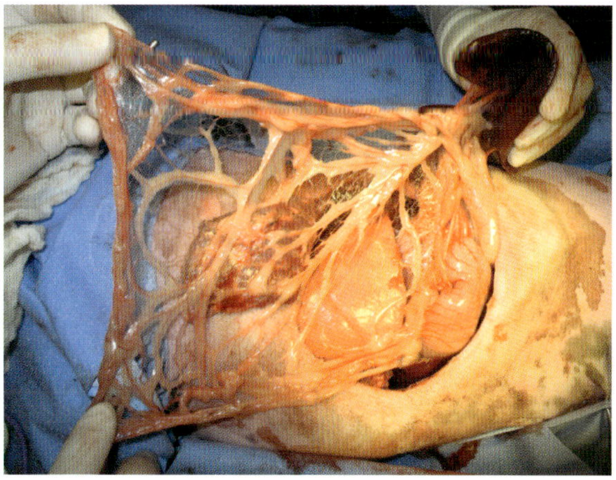

Q)

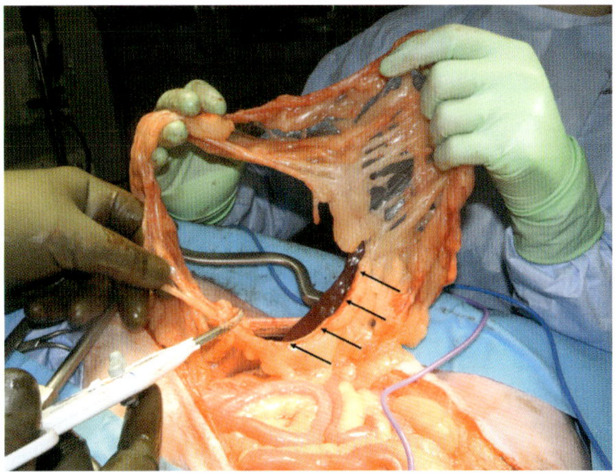

R)

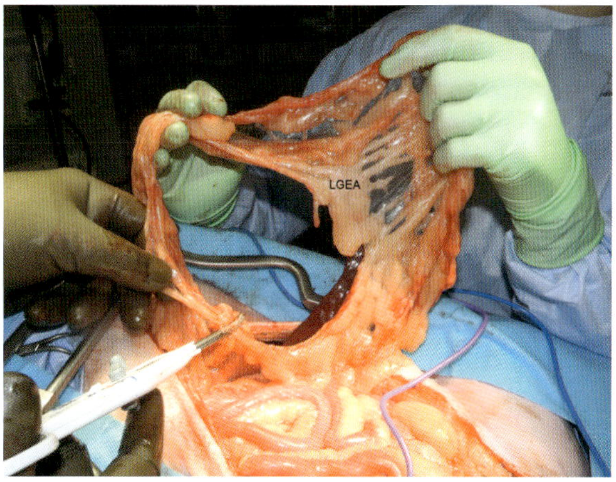

S)

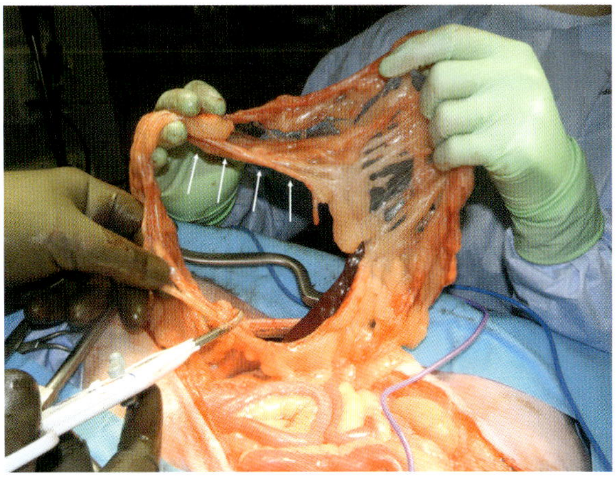

T)

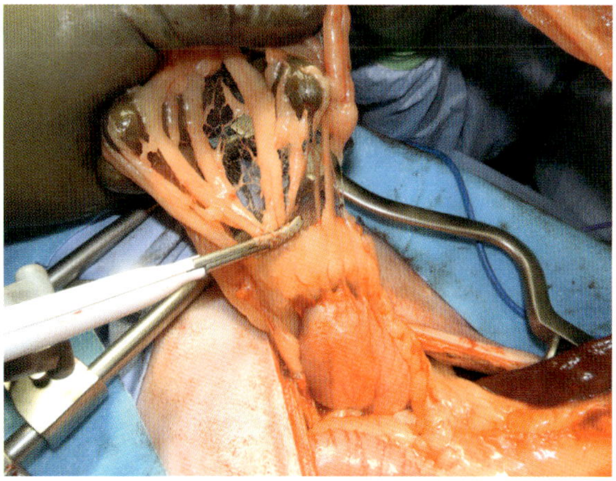

Surgical Technique – Chest Wall Reconstruction with a Supplemental Omental Pedicle Graft [2] (See Plate 140–U) *continued*

U) The omental pedicle graft (i) is extended into the thoracic cavity to the chest wall defect through either the diaphragm (ii, arrow) or a subcutaneous tunnel between the paracostal approach and chest wall resection site (iii), and then sutured to the edges of the chest wall defect (iv).

Surgical Technique – Chest Wall Reconstruction with Prosthetic Mesh (See Plate 14V, W)

V) Nonabsorbable mesh (polypropylene or polytetrafluoroethylene) is tailored to the size of the chest wall defect so that the edges of the mesh are either doubled over or a double thickness of mesh is used. The mesh is sutured under mild tension to either the pleural or lateral surface of the defect using either absorbable or nonabsorbable monofilament suture material (i). If a composite reconstruction is planned, then omental pedicle grafts should cover the pleural surface of the mesh (see step U) and autogenous muscle flaps should be sutured over the lateral surface of the mesh (ii, see step W).

Plate 14

Chest Wall Resection and Reconstruction *continued*

U-i)

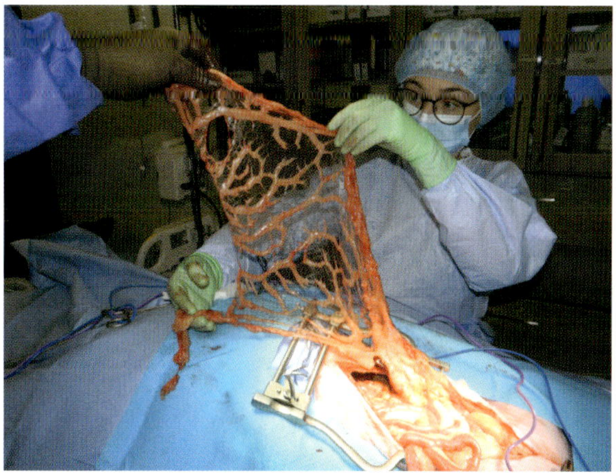

U-ii)

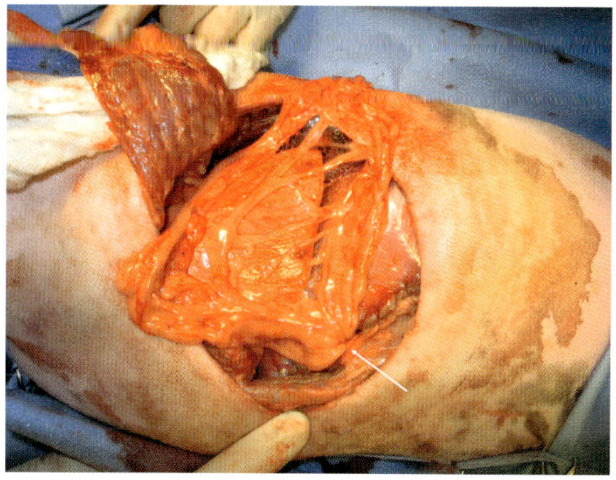

U-iii)

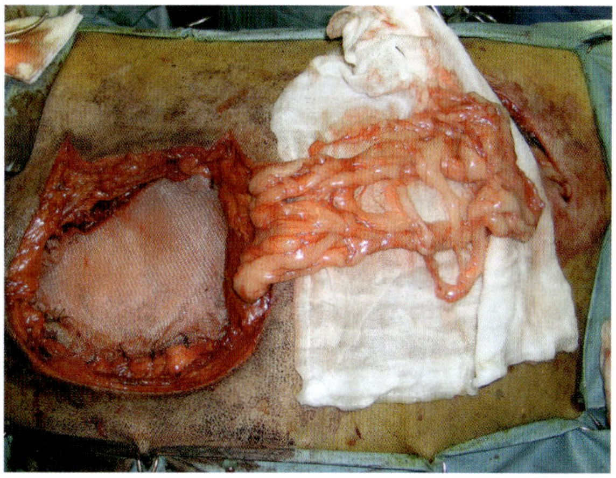

U-iv)

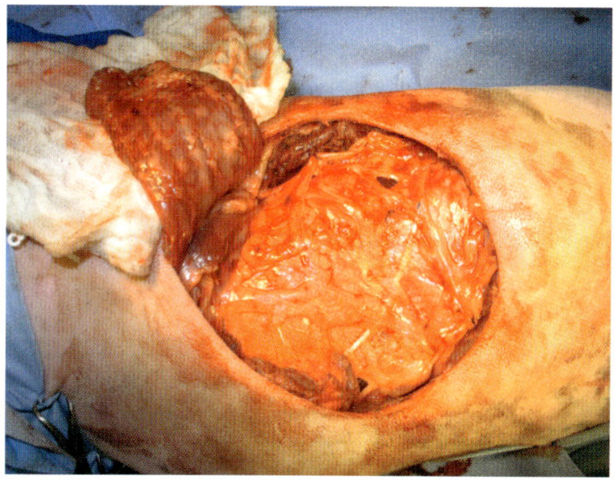

V-i)

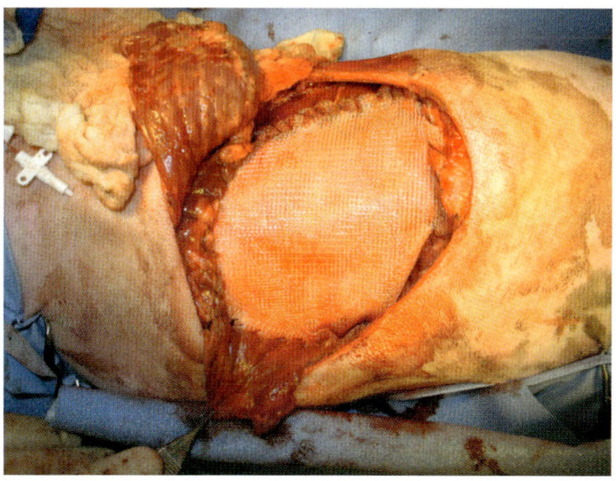

V-ii)

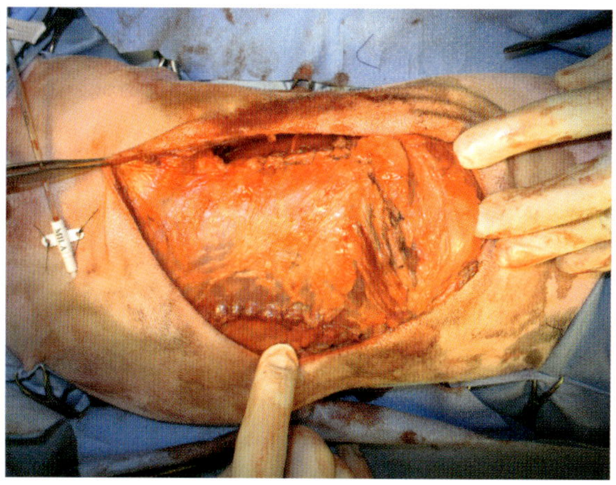

Surgical Technique – Chest Wall Reconstruction with a Latissimus Dorsi Muscle Flap (See Plate 14W)

W) The LD muscle flap is elevated as described earlier (i, see B). The LD muscle is rotated into the defect and sutured ventrally to the pectoral muscles (ii), cranially to either the rib or musculature along the cranial border of the chest wall defect (iii), and caudally to either the rib or musculature along the caudal border of the chest wall defect (iii). Monofilament absorbable suture material is used in either an interrupted or simple continuous suture pattern. The LD myocutaneous flap has been reported as an alternative to the LD muscle flap to improve vascularization of the LD muscle and reduce the risk of distal flap necrosis [3].

Surgical Technique – Diaphragmatic Advancement (See Plate 14X–Z)

X) If diaphragmatic advancement will result in a significant reduction in the ability of the ipsilateral caudal lung lobe to expand during inspiration (i), then a lung lobectomy should be performed (ii) to provide adequate pleural volume to allow expansion of the remaining lungs and avoid respiratory complications (iii) (see *11.1. Open Lung Lobectomy*).

Plate 14

Chest Wall Resection and Reconstruction *continued*

W-i)

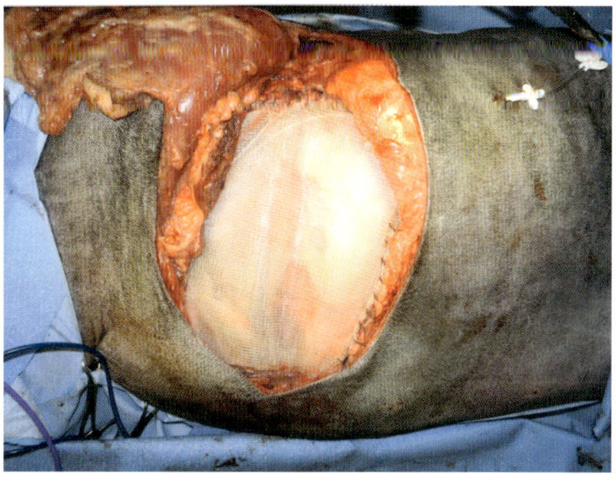

W-ii)

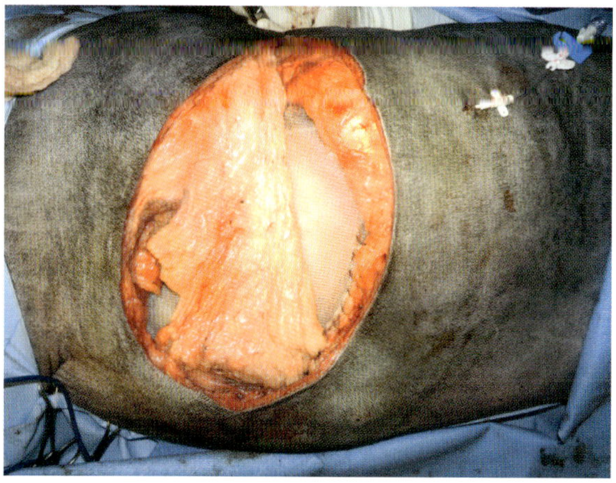

W-iii)

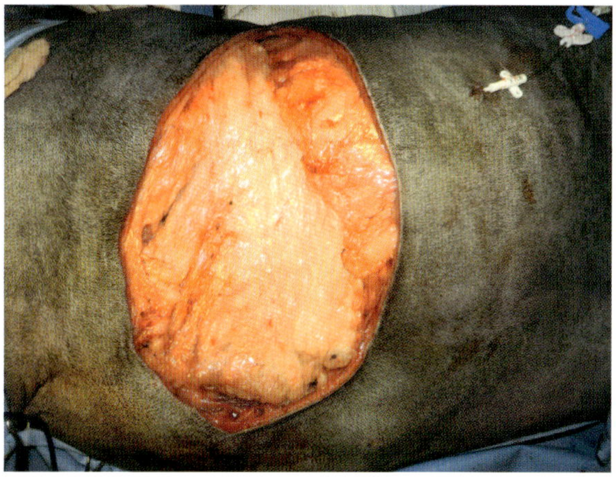

X-i)

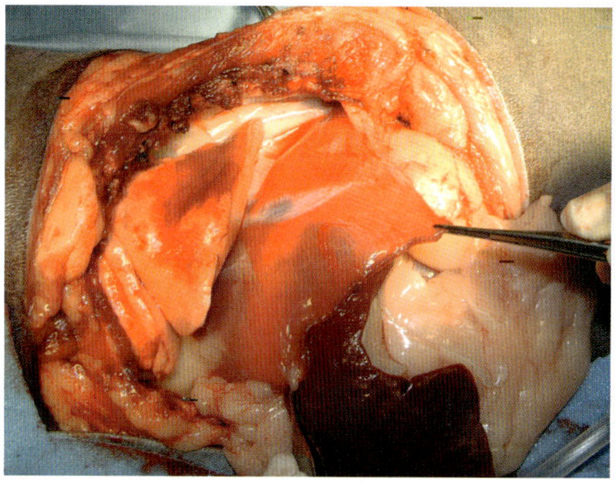

X-ii)

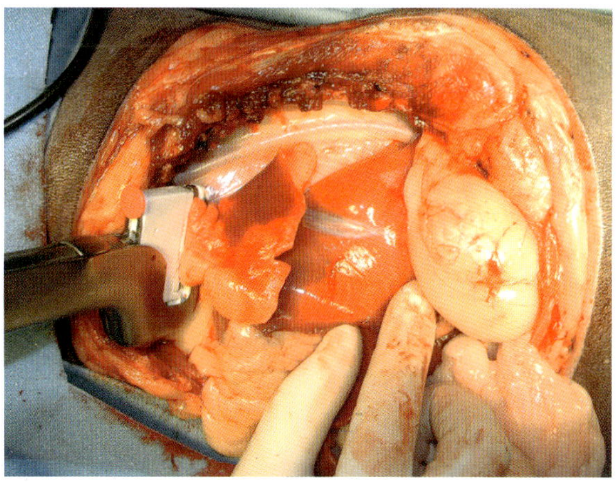

X-iii)

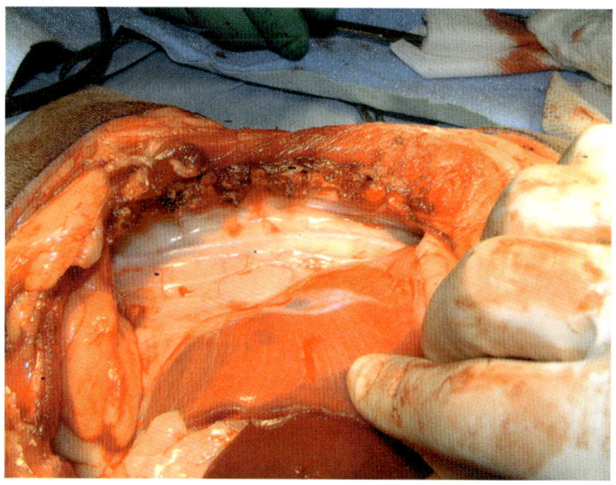

Surgical Technique – Diaphragmatic Advancement (See Plate 14X–Z) *continued*

Y) The diaphragm is sutured to the caudal-most rib in a simple continuous suture pattern using 0 to 3-0 monofilament absorbable suture material (i). A temporary thoracostomy should be placed before completion of the closure, and the pleural space aspirated until negative pleural pressure is reestablished (ii). The thoracostomy tube can be removed either at this stage or after closing the abdomen.

Z) The resultant abdominal wall defect (i) is reconstructed with an omental flap; however, the omental leaves can be sutured directly into the abdominal defect without requiring the creation of an omental pedicle graft (ii). Nonabsorbable mesh is tailored to the size of the abdominal wall defect; rigidity is not as important for abdominal wall reconstruction as for chest wall reconstruction and hence a single thickness of mesh is adequate. The mesh is sutured under mild tension to either the mesothelial or lateral surface of the defect using either absorbable or nonabsorbable monofilament suture material (iii).

Surgical Technique – Closure (See Plate 14AA)

After chest wall reconstruction, the wound is closed routinely in three layers. A simple continuous suture pattern using monofilament absorbable suture material is used to close the cutaneous trunci muscle and subcutis. An interrupted or continuous suture pattern using monofilament nonabsorbable suture material is used to close the skin.

Postoperative Management

1) Multimodal analgesia, including perioperative continuous rate infusion of an opioid ± ketamine, intercostal nerve blocks, local anesthesia instilled through the thoracostomy tube ± wound diffuser catheter, and oral analgesic drugs
2) Supplemental oxygen therapy, if required
3) Thoracostomy tube management
4) Elizabethan collar or body suit

Complications in Dogs [1]

Intraoperative Complications

- Intraoperative blood loss (30%) with 23% of these dogs requiring a blood transfusion

Plate 14

Chest Wall Resection and Reconstruction *continued*

Y-i)

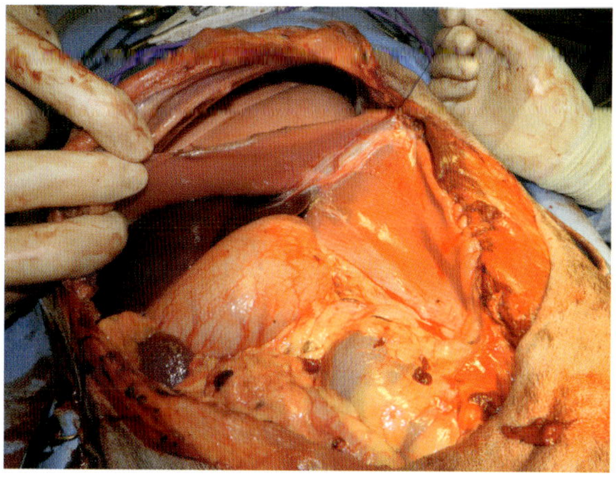

Y-ii)

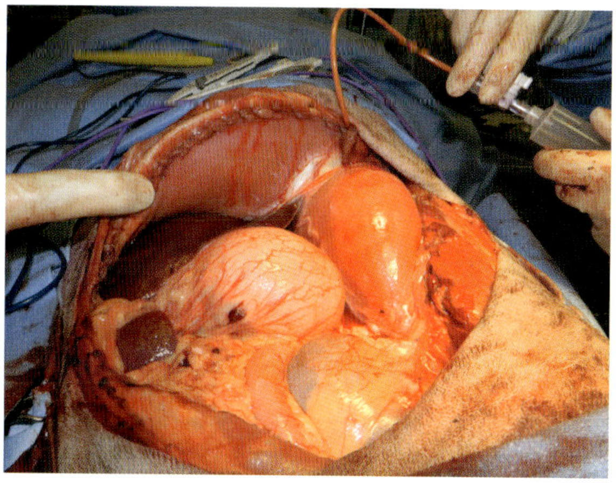

Z-i)

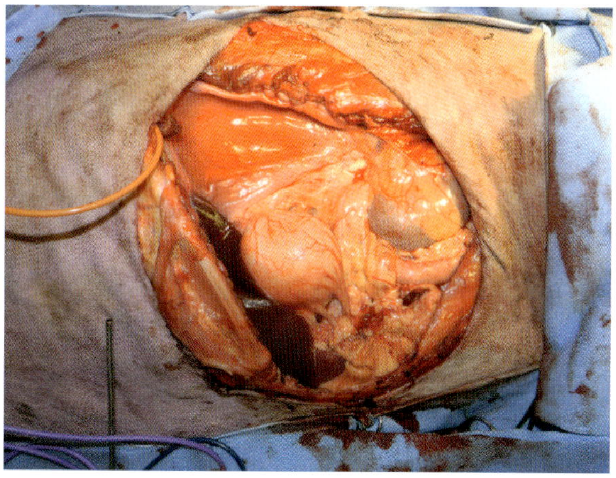

Z-ii)

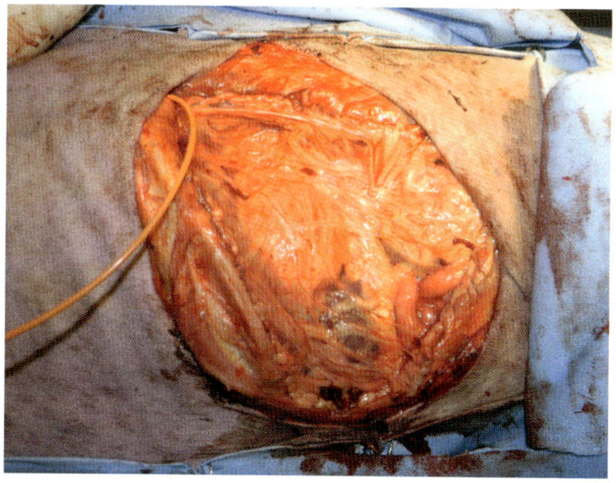

Z-iii)

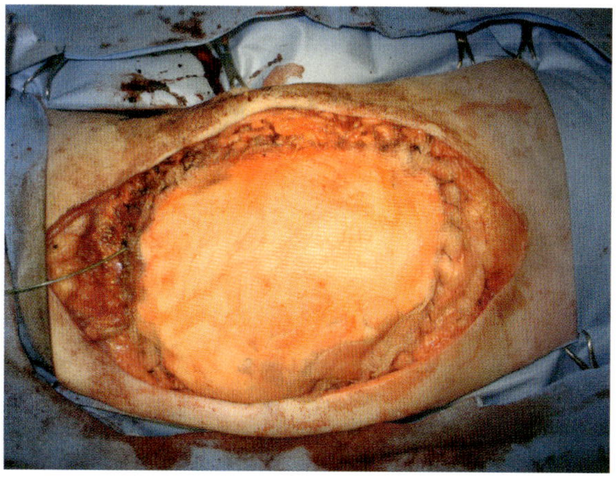

AA)

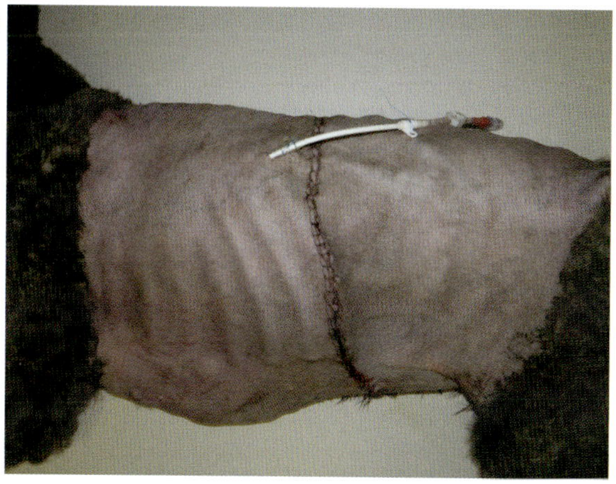

Postoperative Complications (0–14 Days) (See Plate 14BB)

- Incisional seroma (11%) (BB)
- Pleural effusion and peripheral edema (5%)

Postoperative Complications (>14 Days) (See Plate 14CC)

- Infection (2%)
- LD muscle necrosis (CC)

Suggested Adjuvant Treatments

- Chemotherapy for dogs with primary rib osteosarcoma and hemangiosarcoma [4, 5]

Prognosis and Oncologic Outcome

Tumor Type	Local Recurrence Rate	Metastatic Rate	Disease-Free Interval (d)	Median Survival Time (d)	1-Year Survival Rate	2-Year Survival Rate
			Osteosarcoma			
Overall [4, 5]	7%–12%	75%	149	290	32%	0%
Preoperative ALP [5]						
• Normal	–	–	–	675	–	–
• Increased	–	–	–	210	–	–
Chemotherapy [4]						
• No chemotherapy	–	–	60	90	–	–
• Chemotherapy	–	–	225	240	–	–
			Chondrosarcoma [4, 5]			
Overall	13%–17%	17%–53%	316–1080	1080 to >3820	75%	50%

ALP, alkaline phosphatase.

References

1 Liptak, J.M., Dernell, W.S., Rizzo, S.A. et al. (2008). Reconstruction of chest wall defects after rib tumor resection: a comparison of autogenous, prosthetic, and composite techniques in 44 dogs. *Vet. Surg.* 37 (5): 479–487.
2 Ross, W.E. and Pardo, A.D. (1993). Evaluation of an omental pedicle extension technique in the dog. *Vet. Surg.* 22 (1): 37–43.
3 Halfacree, Z.J., Baines, S.J., Lipscomb, V.J. et al. (2007). Use of a latissimus dorsi myocutaneous flap for one-stage reconstruction of the thoracic wall after en bloc resection of primary rib chondrosarcoma in five dogs. *Vet. Surg.* 36 (6): 587–592.
4 Pirkey-Ehrhart, N., Withrow, S.J., Straw, R.C. et al. (1995). Primary rib tumors in 54 dogs. *J. Am. Anim. Hosp. Assoc.* 31 (1): 65–69.
5 Liptak, J.M., Kamstock, D.A., Dernell, W.S. et al. (2008). Oncologic outcome after curative-intent treatment in 39 dogs with primary chest wall tumors (1992-2005). *Vet. Surg.* 37 (5): 488–496.

Plate 14

Chest Wall Resection and Reconstruction *continued*

BB)

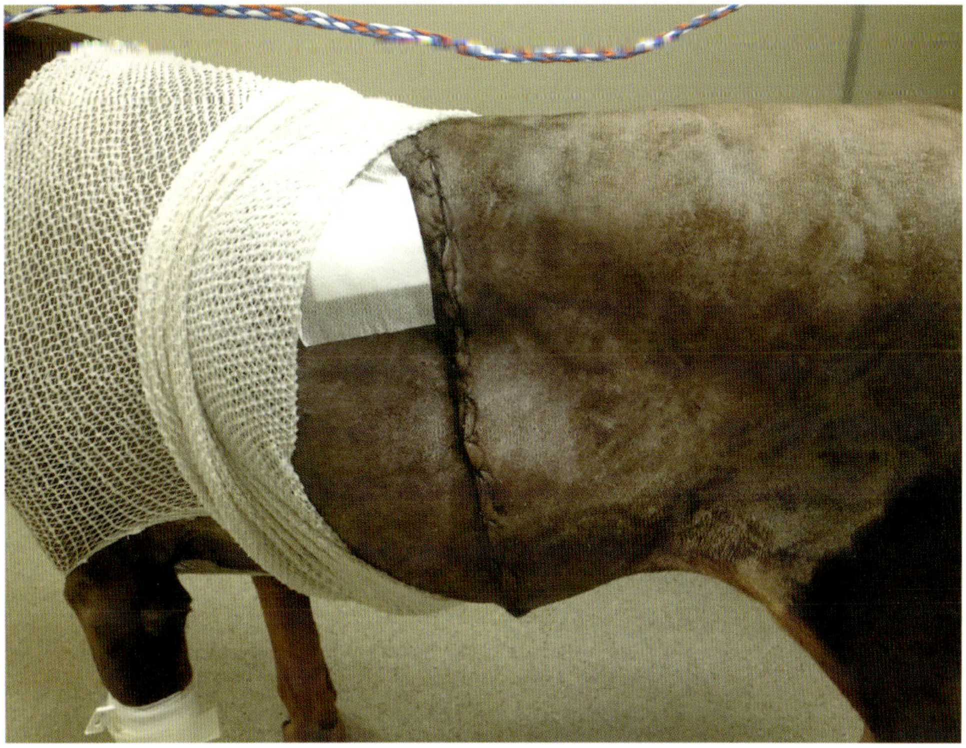

CC)

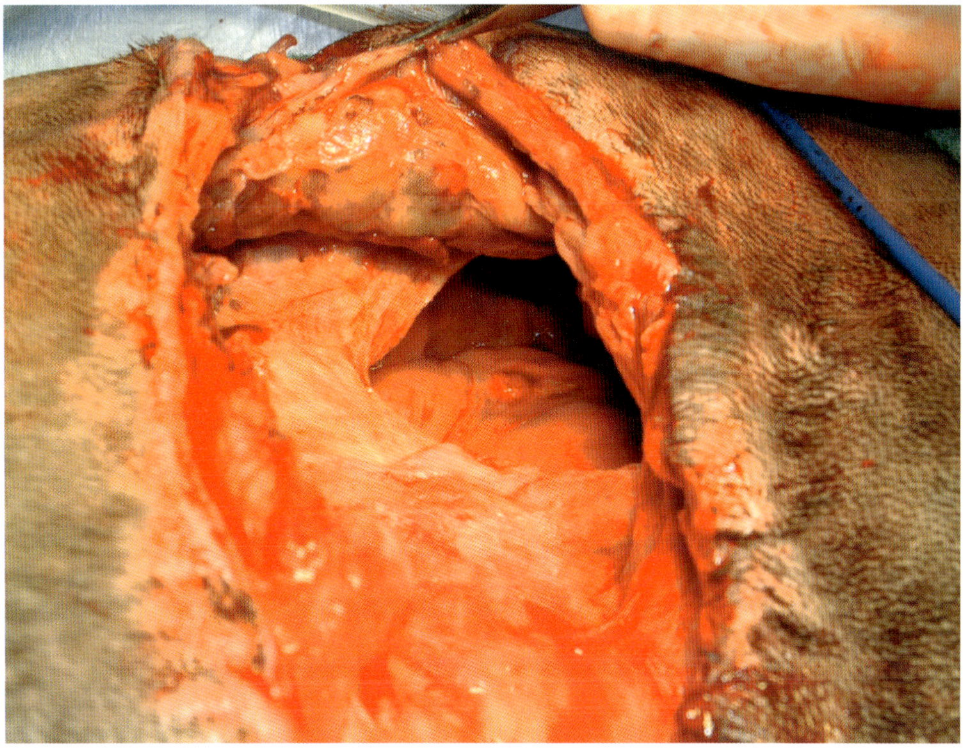

Section 4

Abdominal

Chapter 15: Surgical Approaches to the Abdomen

15.1 Ventral Midline Celiotomy

Indications

1) A ventral midline celiotomy provides access to the peritoneal and retroperitoneal spaces and is the preferred approach for the treatment of most intra-abdominal cancers.
2) A ventral midline celiotomy can be combined with a paracostal approach (see *15.2. Paracostal Approach*) for resection of large adrenal and hepatic tumors.

Patient Positioning

The patient is positioned in dorsal recumbency.

Surgical Technique (See Plate 15.1A–F)

A) The landmarks for skin incision location are the xiphoid process cranially and the pelvis caudally. A skin incision of this length does not need to be made in every case, and the length should be determined by the type of procedure that is being conducted. Incision lengths are usually made longer in patients with diseases of the retroperitoneal space (e.g. adrenal or renal tumors) or when very large masses (often liver and spleen) are being resected. In cats and female dogs, the skin incision is made in a straight line (i). In male dogs, the skin incision needs to be continued caudally in a paramedian direction around the prepuce if the incision is to be extended caudally (ii). A scalpel blade or electrosurgery can be used to make the skin incision.
B) The subcutaneous tissue is bluntly and sharply dissected using a scalpel blade, Metzenbaum scissors (i), or electrosurgery. In male dogs, the subcutaneous dissection lateral to the prepuce is continued in a paramedian direction through the subcutaneous tissue and preputialis muscle (ii). The preputialis muscle should be transected in the middle of the muscle with electrosurgery to allow for future closure. After the subcutaneous dissection has continued to the abdominal wall (iii), the prepuce and penis are mobilized laterally away from the incision to expose the linea alba on midline (iv, female dog; v, male dog).
C) The linea alba is formed by the aponeurosis of the external and internal abdominal obliques and the aponeurosis of the transversus abdominus muscles. The junction of all of these muscles forms a dorsal sheath and a ventral sheath. The linea alba can be incised with one of the following techniques:
    a. A toothed forcep is used to grasp the linea alba. A #15 scalpel blade is introduced into the linea alba with the blade turned upward.
    b. The scalpel blade can be used to create a hole in the linea alba through a series of painted strokes (not pictured).

Color Atlas of Canine and Feline Surgical Oncology, First Edition. Julius M. Liptak, Paolo Buracco, William T. N. Culp, and Nicholas J. Bacon.

Plate 15.1

Ventral Midline Celiotomy

A-i)
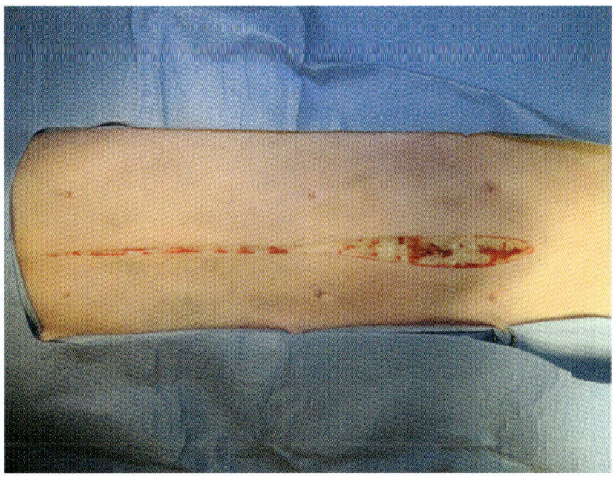

A-ii)
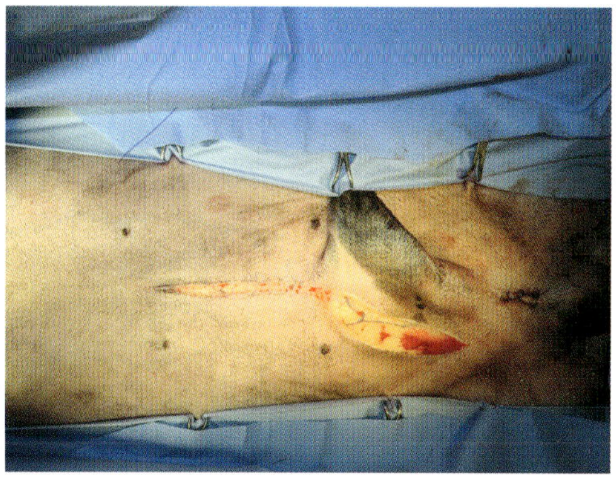

B-i)
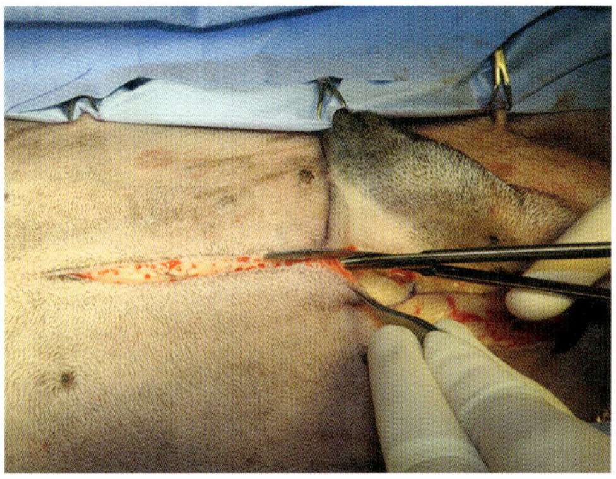

B-ii)
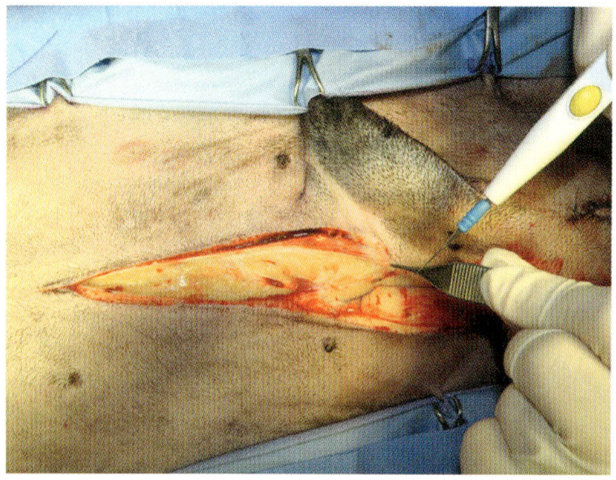

B-iii)
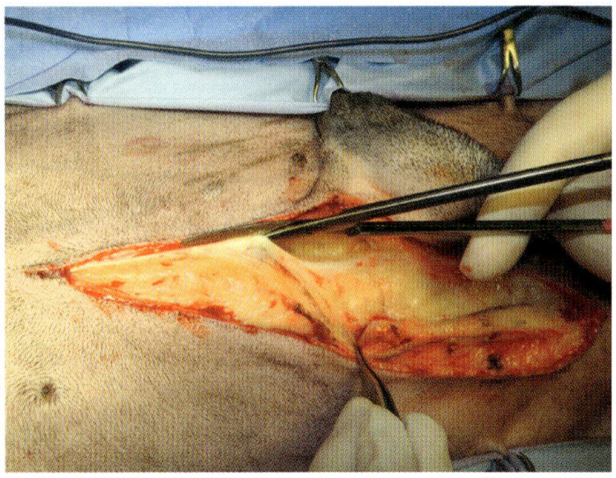

B-iv)
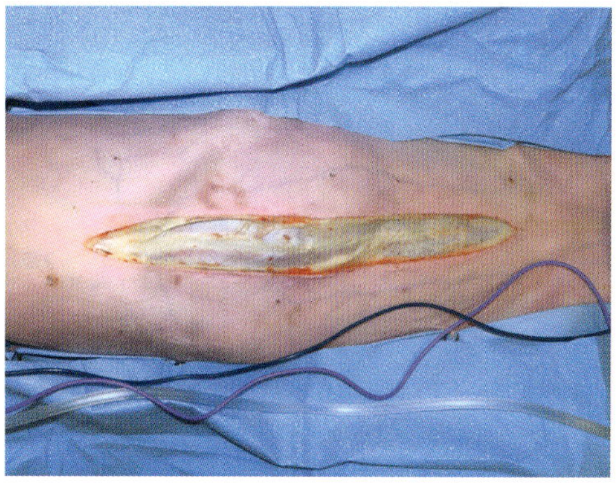

B-v)
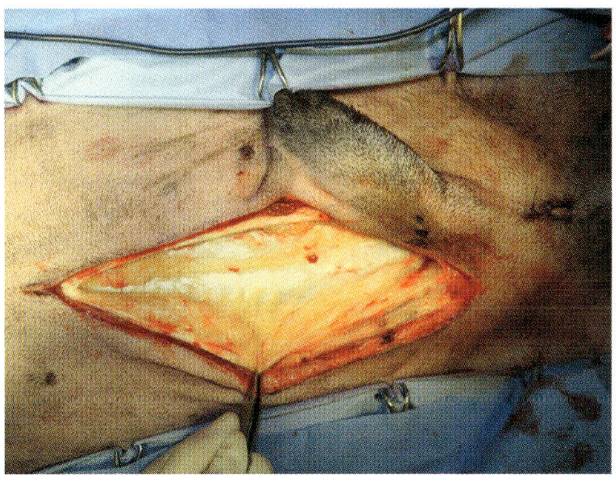

C)
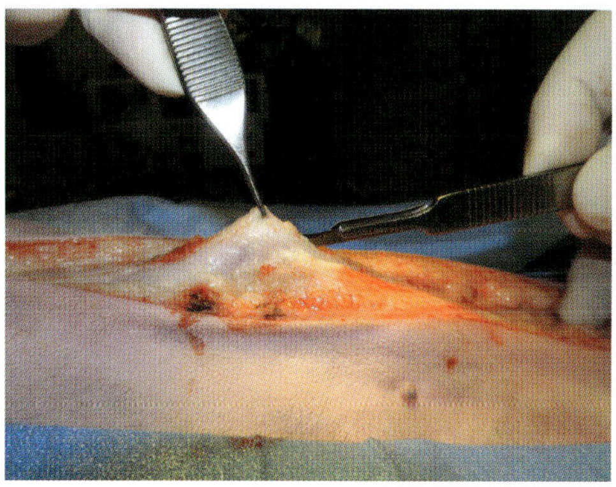

Surgical Technique (See Plate 15.1A–F) *continued*

D) After the creation of a hole in the linea alba, a finger should be introduced into the abdomen to free any underlying tissues from the linea alba to prevent iatrogenic trauma during entrance into the abdomen. When the linea alba has been sufficiently freed from underlying tissues, the linea alba is incised for the desired length. This can be done using Mayo scissors with the scissors being used to lift the linea alba away from the abdominal contents (pictured). Alternatively, nontoothed forceps can be introduced into the hole and used to elevate the linea alba, and the linea alba can be incised to the desired length using a scalpel blade or Mayo scissors.

E) Once the linea alba has been incised, the falciform ligament is visualized. The falciform ligament can be grasped and retracted with moist laparotomy sponges or, preferably, incised and removed from its attachment to the body wall at the level of the xyphoid cartilage (i). Paired vessels entering the cranial aspect of the falciform ligament should be either cauterized or sealed (ii). If removed, the falciform ligament can be discarded. The bladder may contain a ligament with attachment to the ventral aspect of the body wall. This may need to be separated during the approach to the abdomen.

F) Balfour (pictured) or Gosset retractors are placed to allow for visualization of the abdominal cavity. This retractor is self-retaining and will allow for exposure of the abdominal cavity throughout the entire abdominal procedure. Moistened laparotomy sponges can be placed along the edges of the abdominal incision to protect soft tissues. Additional retractors (e.g. Army-Navy retractors or malleable ribbon retractors) may be used to provide additional retraction if necessary.

Plate 15.1

Ventral Midline Celiotomy *continued*

D)

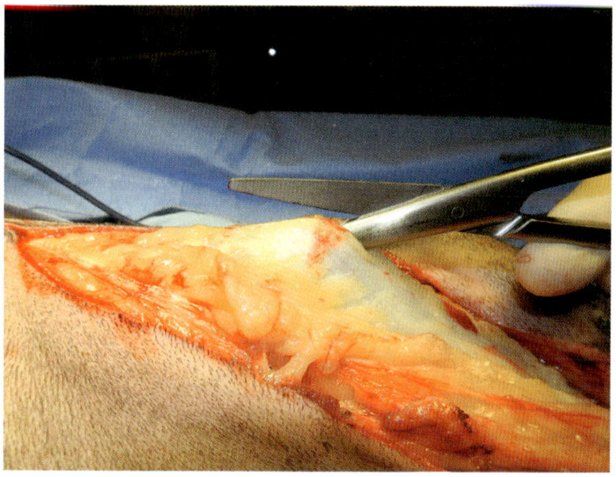

E-i)

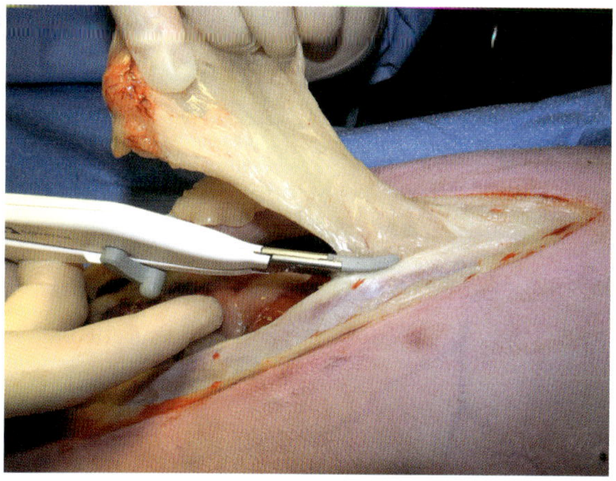

E-ii)

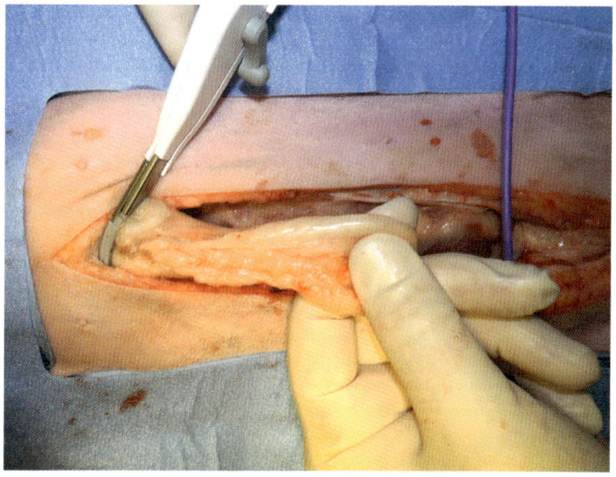

F)

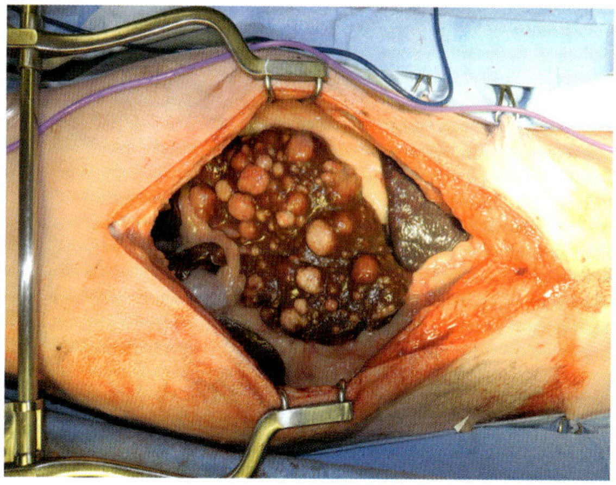

Closure (See Plate 15.1G, H)

G) Before closure, the abdomen may require irrigation with warm, sterile saline (pictured); this saline should be gently suctioned afterward. Surgeons should be careful not to traumatize the intra-abdominal contents during the process. In addition, all sponges should be accounted for before closure, and all instrumentation that had been placed within the abdomen (including retractors) should be removed.

H) The linea alba can be closed in either a simple interrupted or simple continuous pattern (i, ii), preferably in a caudal-to-cranial direction so that the sutures that are being placed last are less likely to cause iatrogenic damage to abdominal organs because of their distance away from the linea alba at the level of the xyphoid cartilage (arrow, iii). The ventral sheath of the rectus abdominis should be included in the closure because this is the holding layer of the linea alba. Both absorbable and nonabsorbable sutures can be used for closure, but generally a monofilament absorbable suture is used. The size of the suture will vary depending on the size of the animal, but, in general, sutures sizes are between 4-0 and 0. Sutures should be placed between 5 and 10 mm from the incised edge of the linea alba, and sutures can be placed 3–12 mm apart depending on the size of the patient. Depending on the depth of subcutaneous tissue, this layer can be closed in one to two layers using monofilament absorbable suture material (iv). The skin is closed using either a continuous intradermal technique with 4-0 to 2-0 monofilament absorbable suture material, or 4-0 to 2-0 nonabsorbable suture material in a simple interrupted or cruciate suture pattern (v) or with skin staples.

Postoperative Management

1) Multimodal analgesia
2) Elizabethan collar or body suit

Complications

- Incisional complications (4%) [1]
- Surgical-site infections (3%–5%) [2, 3]

References

1 Boothe, H.W., Slater, M.R., Hobson, H.P. et al. (1992). Exploratory celiotomy in 200 nontraumatized dogs and cats. *Vet. Surg.* 21 (6): 452–457.

2 Brown, D.C., Conzemius, M.G., Shofer, F. et al. (1997). Epidemiologic evaluation of postoperative wound infections in dogs and cats. *J. Am. Vet. Med. Assoc.* 210 (9): 1302–1306.

3 Vasseur, P.B., Levy, J., Dowd, E. et al. (1988). Surgical wound infection rates in dogs and cats. Data from a teaching hospital. *Vet. Surg.* 17 (2): 60–64.

Plate 15.1

Ventral Midline Celiotomy *continued*

G)

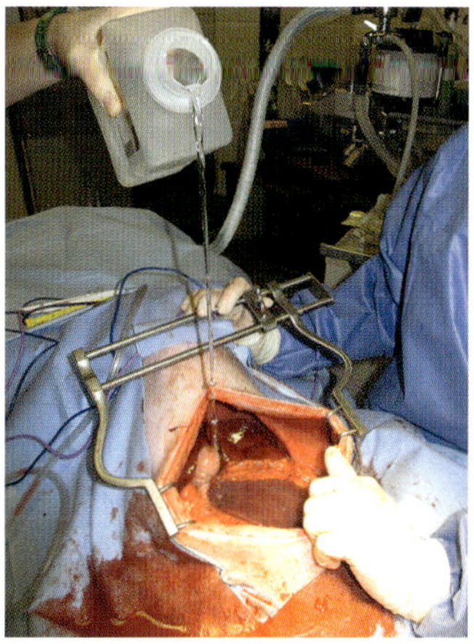

H-i)

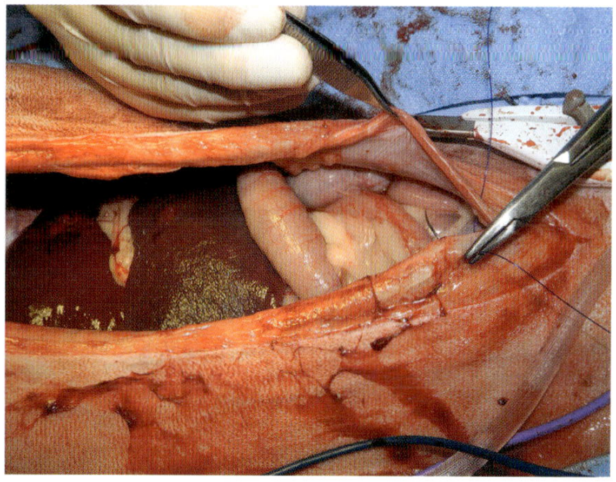

H-ii)

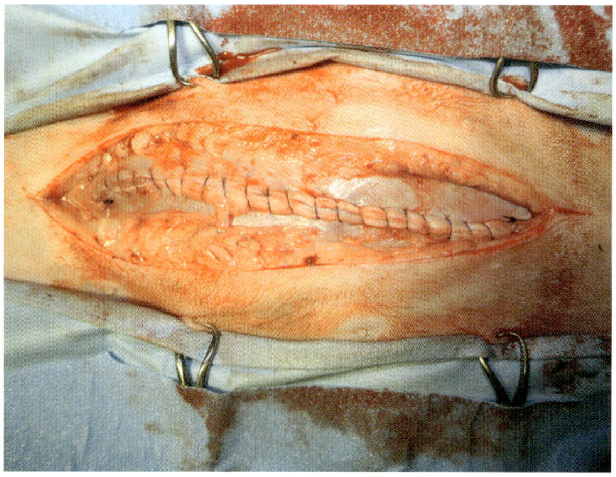

H-iii)

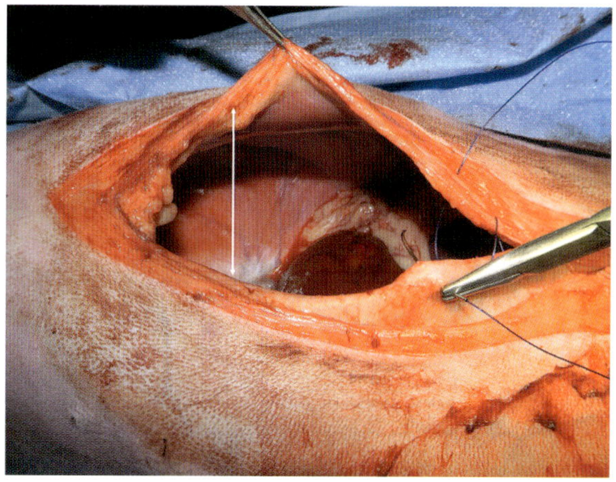

H-iv)

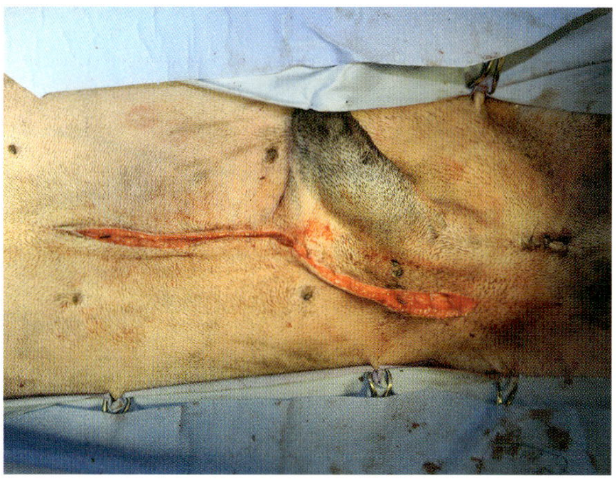

H-v)

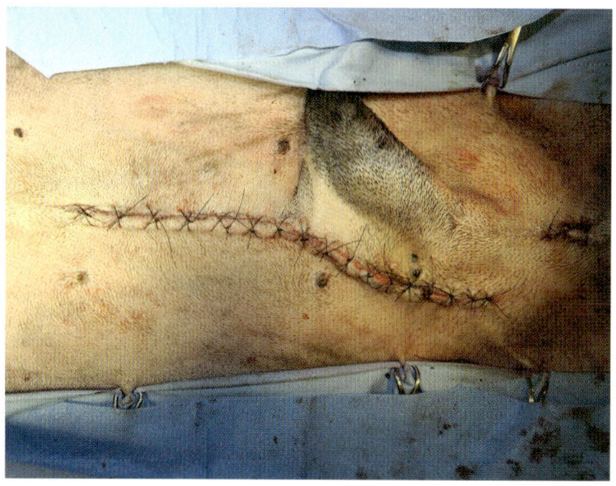

15.2 Paracostal Approach

Indications

1) Sole approach for resection of noninvasive adrenal tumors [1, 2]
2) A paracostal approach can be combined with a ventral midline celiotomy (see *15.1. Ventral Midline Celiotomy*) for resection of large adrenal and hepatic tumors

Patient Positioning

The patient is positioned in lateral recumbency with the side to be approached uppermost, or dorsal recumbency if the paracostal approach is being combined with a ventral midline celiotomy.

Surgical Technique – Isolated Paracostal Approach (See Plate 15.2A, B)

A) A skin incision is made just caudal to the last rib (dashed line) extending proximally to the epaxial muscles and distally to the costochondral junction (pictured, paracostal incision for placement of a low-profile gastrostomy tube).
B) The incision is continued through the rectus abdominis, the aponeurosis of the internal and external abdominal obliques (i), and the deeper transversus abdominis to expose the dorsal abdominal structures (ii). To access the caudal thorax, the muscular attachment of the diaphragm to the last rib is transected, leaving a small cuff of muscle attached to the rib to help reattachment.

Surgical Technique – Combined Approach (See Plate 15.2C–F)

C) A ventral midline celiotomy is performed (see *15.1. Ventral Midline Celiotomy*) to the level of the xiphoid cartilage and the diaphragmatic attachment. A full-thickness mattress stay suture (3-0 or 2-0 monofilament suture material) is then placed in the body wall at the cranial end of the incision (arrow).
D) The skin is then incised in a dorsal direction directly over the outline of the last rib to the level of the right kidney.
E) The incision is continued through the rectus abdominis (i), the aponeurosis of the internal and external abdominal obliques (ii), and the deeper transversus abdominis (iii). These incisions are made with scissors (iv), electrosurgery, or a vessel sealing device as traction is applied caudally on the preplaced stay suture. The muscles are incised approximately 5–10 mm caudal to the last rib to allow adequate tissue for closure of the paracostal approach.

Color Atlas of Canine and Feline Surgical Oncology, First Edition. Julius M. Liptak, Paolo Buracco, William T. N. Culp, and Nicholas J. Bacon.

Plate 15.2

Paracostal Approach

A)

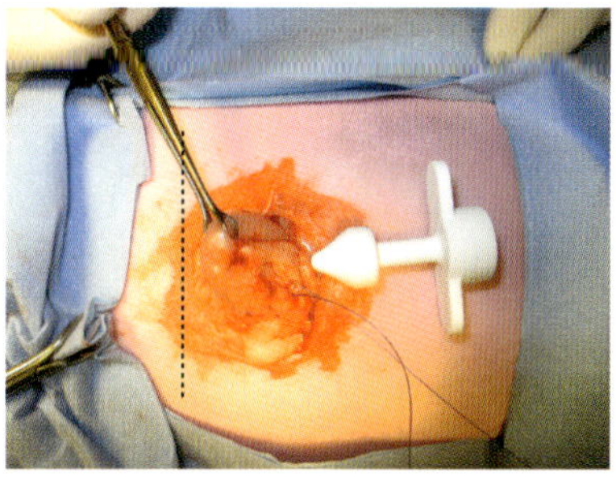

B-i)

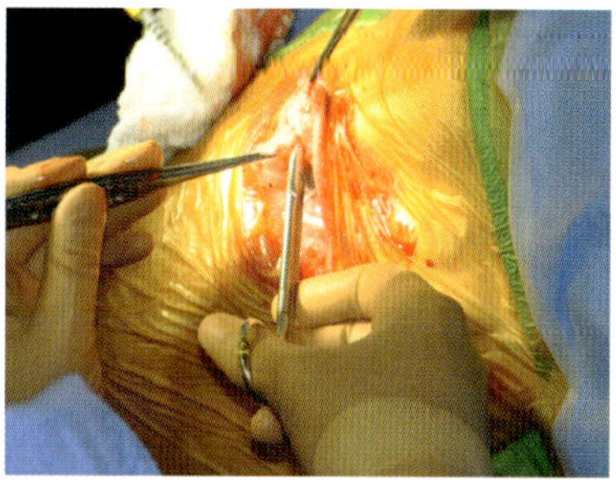

B-ii)

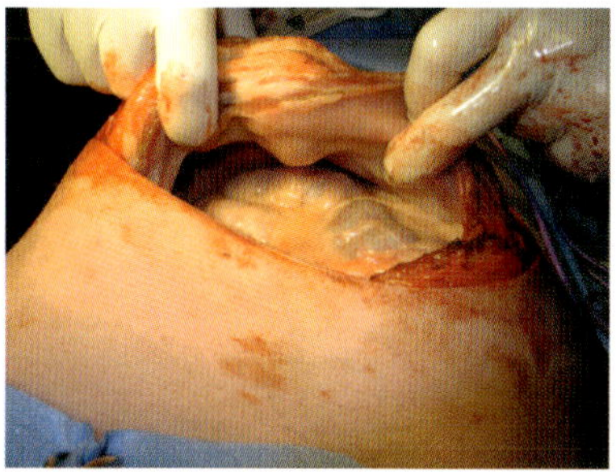

C)

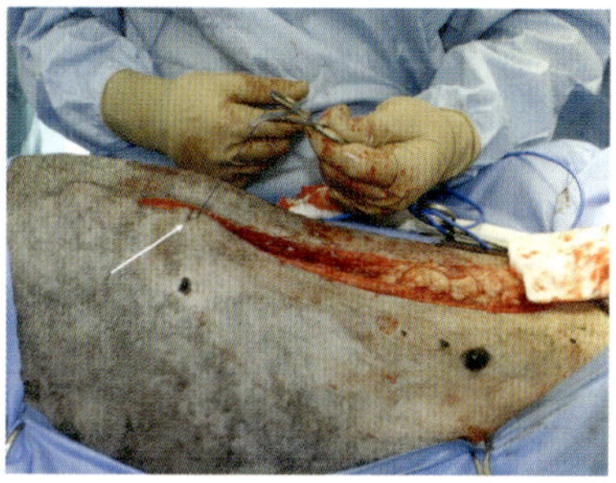

D)

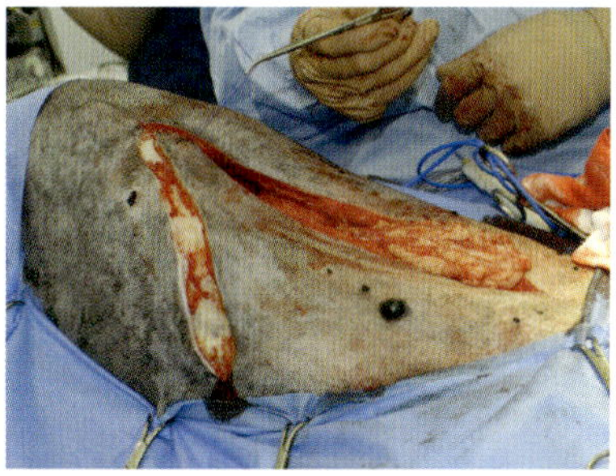

E-i)

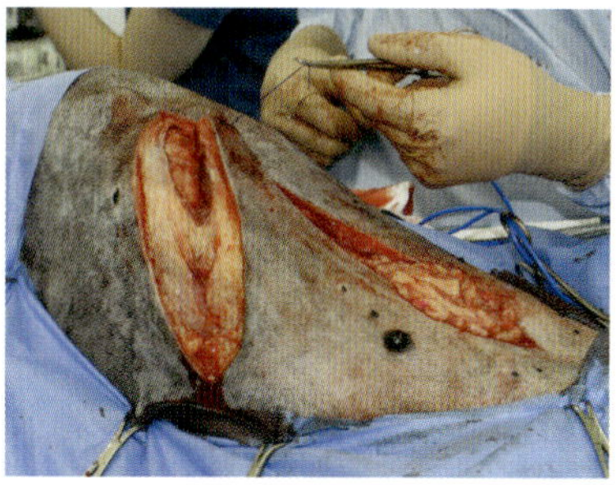

E-ii)

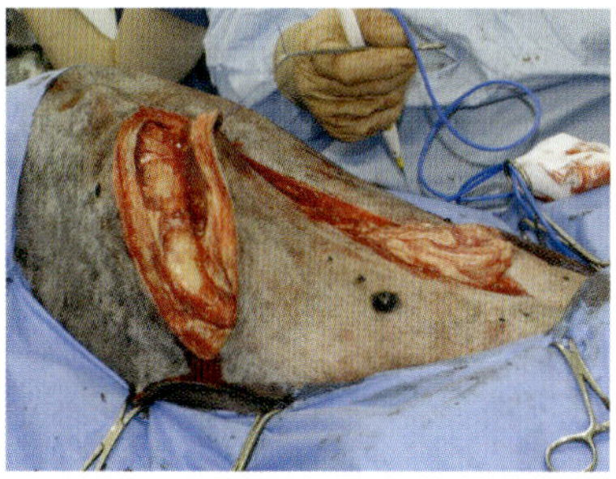

E-iii)

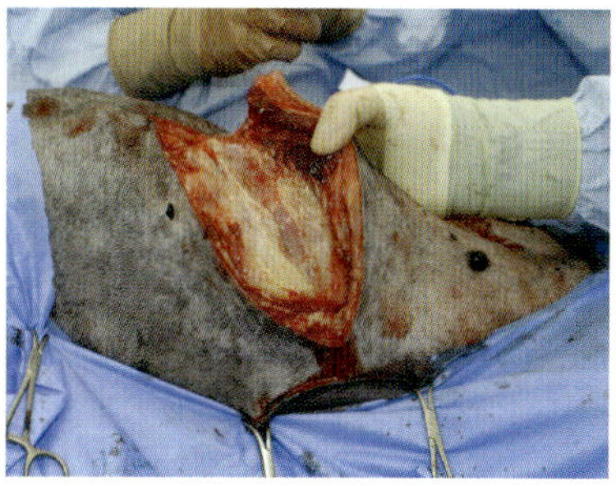

E-iv)

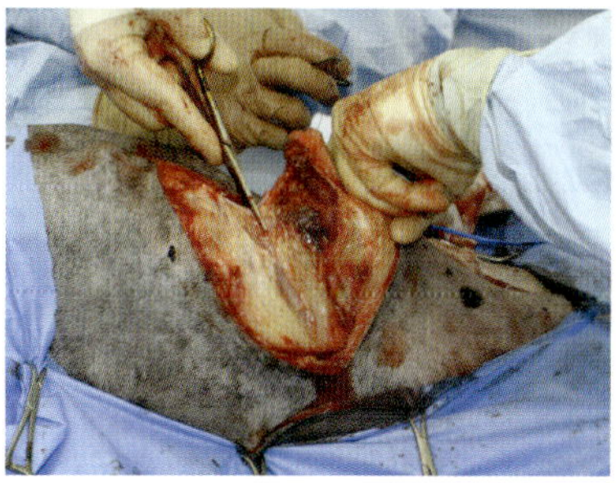

Surgical Technique – Combined Approach (See Plate 15.2C–F) *continued*

F) The peritoneum is incised and the triangular myocutaneous flap (i) wrapped in moist laparotomy swabs and folded caudally to allow full exposure of the dorsal abdominal cavity (ii, iii, hepatocellular carcinoma in the right lateral liver lobe).

Closure – Isolated Paracostal Approach (See Plate 15.2G, H)

The diaphragm is attached to the costal arch with a continuous suture of monofilament material. The muscles of the abdominal wall are closed in two to three layers with absorbable suture material in a continuous pattern (G). The subcutaneous tissue is closed in one to two layers using monofilament absorbable suture material. The skin is closed using either a continuous intradermal technique with 4-0 to 2-0 monofilament absorbable suture material, or 4-0 to 2-0 nonabsorbable suture material in a simple interrupted, cruciate, or continuous (H) suture pattern or with skin staples.

Plate 15.2

Paracostal Approach *continued*

F-i)

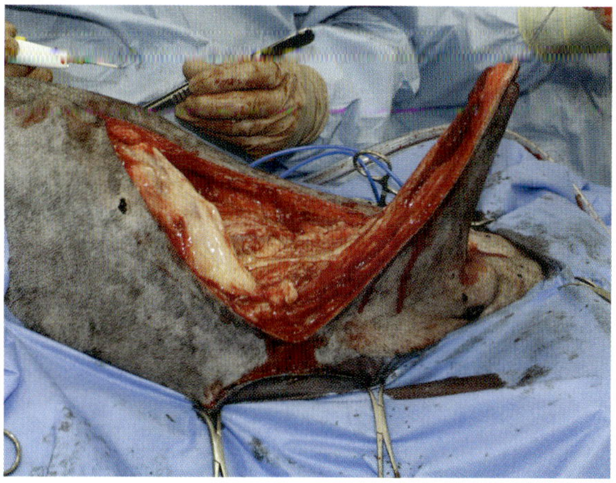

F-ii)

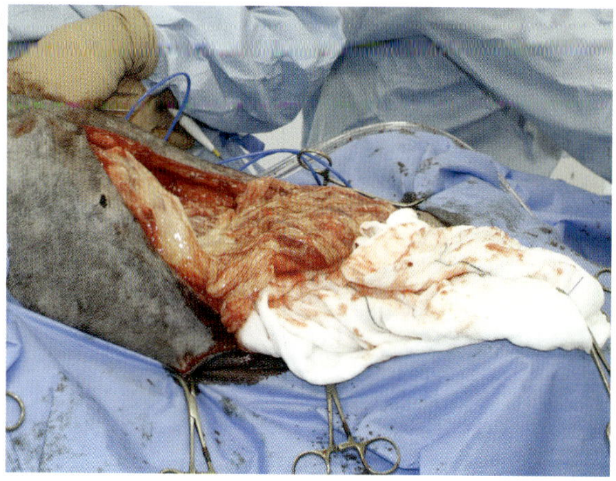

F-iii)

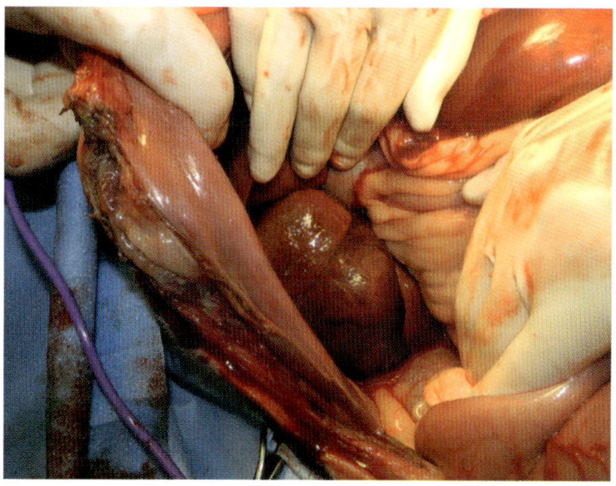

G)

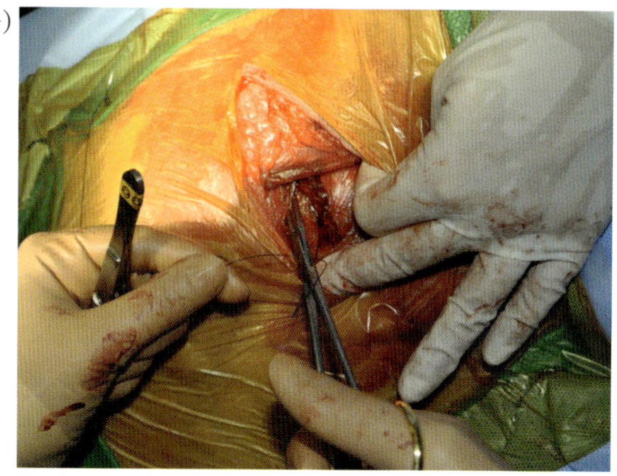

H)

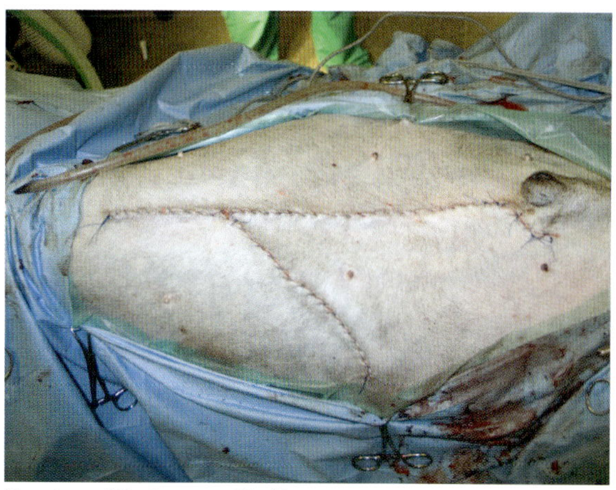

Courtesy of Dr. Laurent Findji

Closure – Combined Approach (See Plate 15.2I–M)

The stay suture is used to realign the tip of the muscular flap to the cranial midline (I), and the muscle layer is closed in a single mattress suture at the level of the xiphoid cartilage (J). The muscles of the abdominal wall are closed in two to three layers with absorbable suture material in a continuous pattern (K – i, ii). The subcutaneous tissue is closed in one to two layers using monofilament absorbable suture material (L). The skin is closed using either a continuous intradermal technique with 4-0 to 2-0 monofilament absorbable suture material, or 4-0 to 2-0 nonabsorbable suture material in a simple interrupted, cruciate, or continuous pattern (M) or with skin staples.

Postoperative Management

1) Multimodal analgesia
2) Elizabethan collar or body suit

Complications

- Incisional complications
- Tissue necrosis at the tip of the paracostal skin flap

References

1 Andrade, N., Rivas, L.R., Milovancev, M. et al. (2014). Intercostal approach for right adrenalectomy in dogs. *Vet. Surg.* 43: 99–104.

2 Van Sluijs, F., Sjollema, B.E., Voorhout, G. et al. (1995). Results of adrenalectomy in 36 dogs with hyperadrenocorticism caused by adreno-cortical tumour. *Vet. Q.* 3: 113–116.

Plate 15.2

Paracostal Approach *continued*

I)

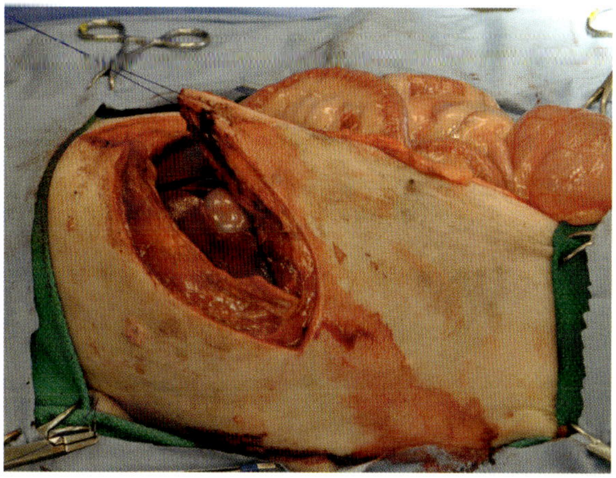

J)

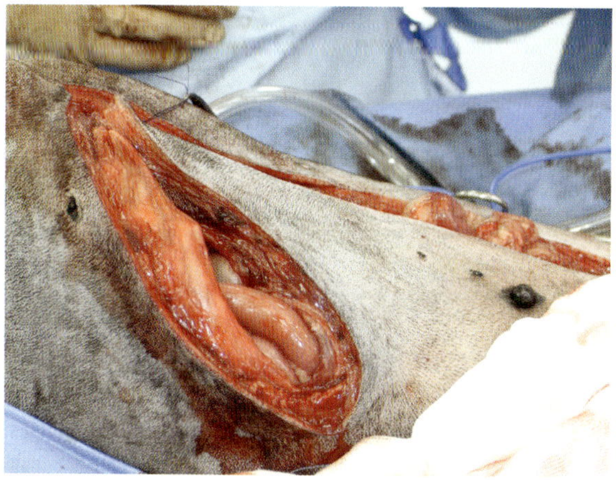

K-i)

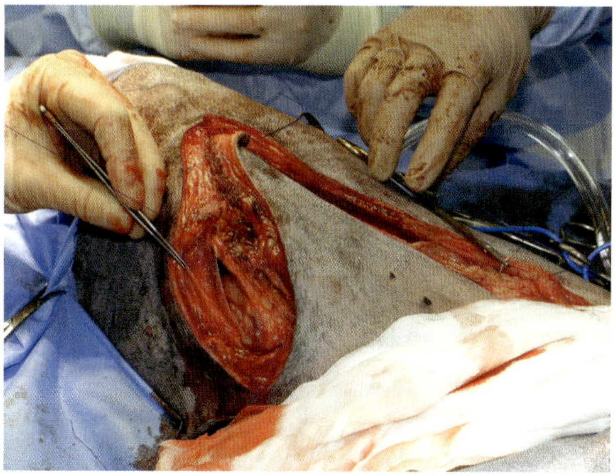

K-ii)

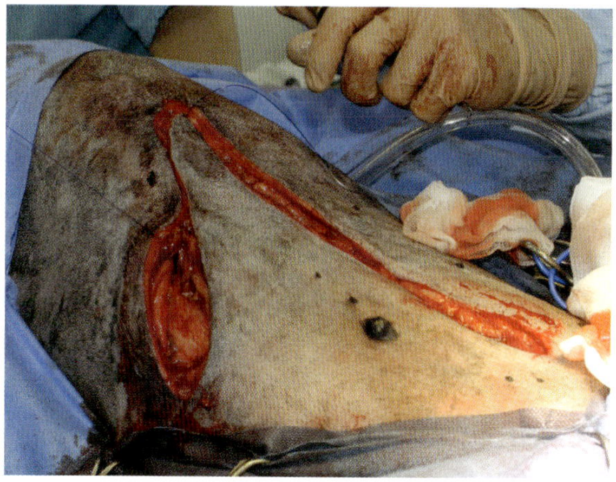

L)

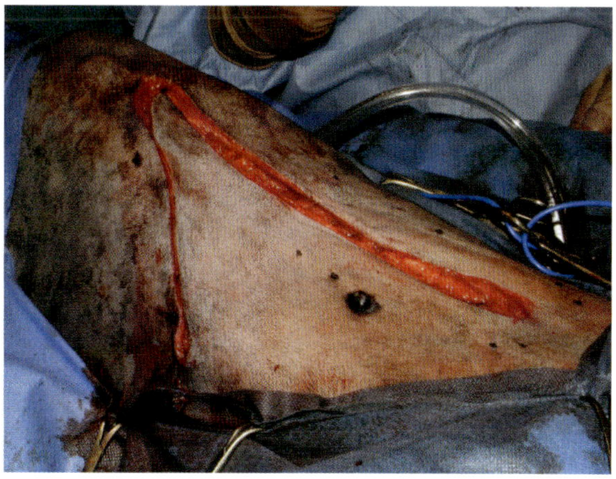

M)

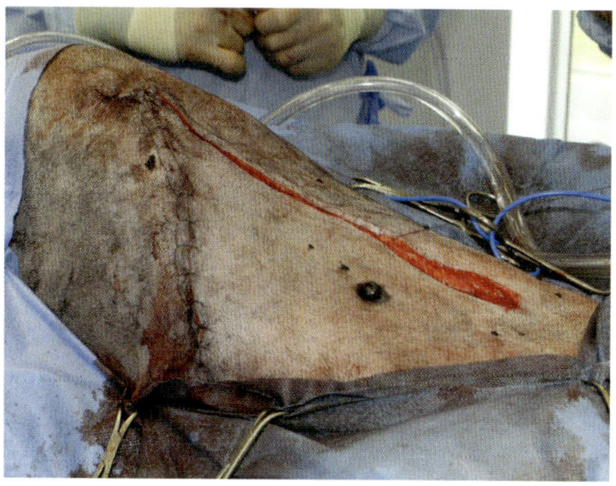

15.3 Laparoscopic Approach

Indications

1) Laparoscopy is routinely used in veterinary patients for prophylactic procedures such as ovariectomy, ovariohysterectomy, and gastropexy, but it is also increasingly being used for the diagnosis and treatment of intra-abdominal cancer.
2) The major laparoscopic procedures currently being performed in veterinary cancer care are adrenalectomy, nephrectomy, splenectomy, ovariohysterectomy or orchiectomy for reproductive tract tumors, and sublumbar lymph node extirpation. Laparoscopic partial pancreatectomy, liver lobectomy, and prostatectomy are currently being investigated. In addition, laparoscopic-assisted procedures, such as intestinal biopsy procurement and intestinal resection and anastomosis, have also been described.

Patient Positioning

The patient is positioned in dorsal recumbency for laparoscopic splenectomy, intestinal procedures, and lymph node extirpation. The patient is positioned in lateral recumbency with the affected side uppermost for laparoscopic ureteronephrectomy and adrenalectomy.

Surgical Technique (See Plate 15.3B–E)

A) Several descriptions of laparoscopic access have been described with techniques categorized as open, closed, blind, and visual. Most commonly in companion animals, the Veress needle (closed or blind) or modified Hasson (open) techniques are used. After access to the abdominal cavity has been achieved, the abdomen is insufflated with CO_2 to cause a pneumoperitoneum. Veress needles are specifically designed for gaining access into the body cavity and allowing for creation of a pneumoperitoneum before insertion of camera or instrument cannulae. The location of Veress needle placement is clinician dependent, but common locations are caudal/caudolateral to the umbilicus or through the last palpable intercostal space. For Veress needle insertion, a small stab incision is made in the skin. A towel clamp can be used to lift the abdominal wall and provide tension against which the needle will be pushing. The needle should be inserted in a caudal direction with the intent of avoiding intra-abdominal organs. Once the needle is inserted, saline can be injected into the needle to be certain that it is positioned within the abdominal cavity. If the needle is in an appropriate position, no saline should be able to be aspirated from the needle after injection. The insufflation tubing can then be connected to the needle and insufflation can begin. This allows for the creation of a pneumoperitoneum, before cannulae insertion, to protect the intra-abdominal organs.
B) For the modified Hasson technique, a small skin incision large enough for a cannula to be introduced without incorporating the skin is created (arrow). The incision is continued deep to the skin with blunt and sharp dissection of the subcutaneous tissues until the abdominal wall is visualized. The abdominal wall is grasped with toothed forceps, and a stab incision is made into the abdomen.

Color Atlas of Canine and Feline Surgical Oncology, First Edition. Julius M. Liptak, Paolo Buracco, William T. N. Culp, and Nicholas J. Bacon.

Plate 15.3

Laparoscopic Approach

B)

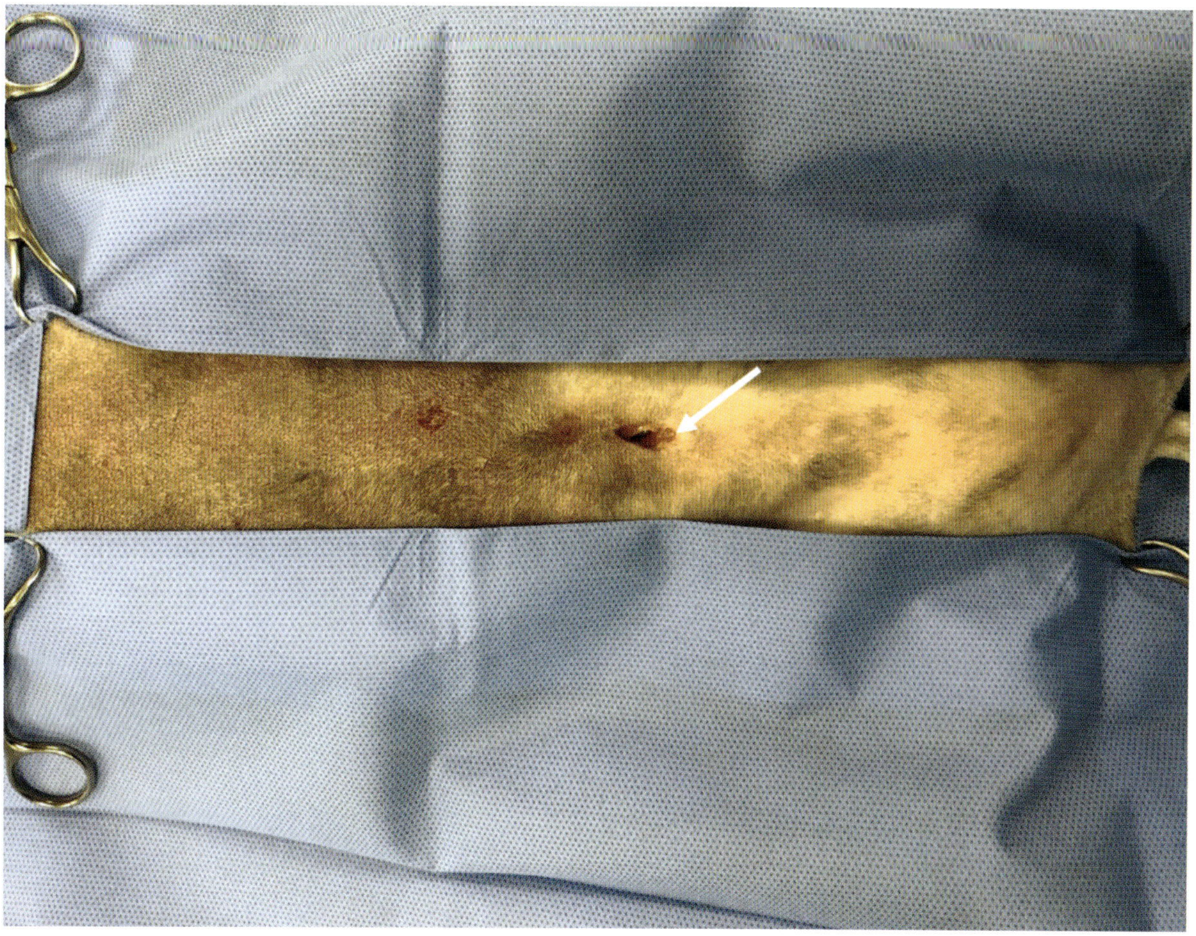

Surgical Technique (See Plate 15.3B–E) *continued*

C) If a cannula with a tip (generally threaded version) is used, the tip of the cannula can be inserted into the stab incision and twisted until it has been placed within the abdominal cavity (i). Alternatively, a blunt tip trocar can be inserted into the cannula and used to guide the cannula into the abdomen. The cannula is directed toward the right side of the patient in an attempt to avoid the spleen during introduction. If the Hasson technique is used, a cannula with an attachment for CO_2 should be used initially so that a pneumoperitoneum can be achieved before placement of instrument cannulae (ii). For procedures performed in dorsal recumbency, the first cannula is most often placed into a subumbilical position on ventral midline. For procedures performed in lateral recumbency, the first cannula is often placed a 1–3 cm lateral of midline.

D) Additional cannulae are placed as needed. Because a pneumoperitoneum has been created, placement of these cannulae is generally safer than the initial telescope cannula. Whenever possible, the telescope should be placed within the initial cannula to allow for visualization of the placement of the instrument cannulae. Before introduction of the instrument cannulae, it is helpful for the surgeon to digitally compress the abdominal wall in the region of the proposed port placement so that it can be predetermined whether the position is safe while watching intra-abdominally with the telescope.

Plate 15.3

Laparoscopic Approach *continued*

C-i)

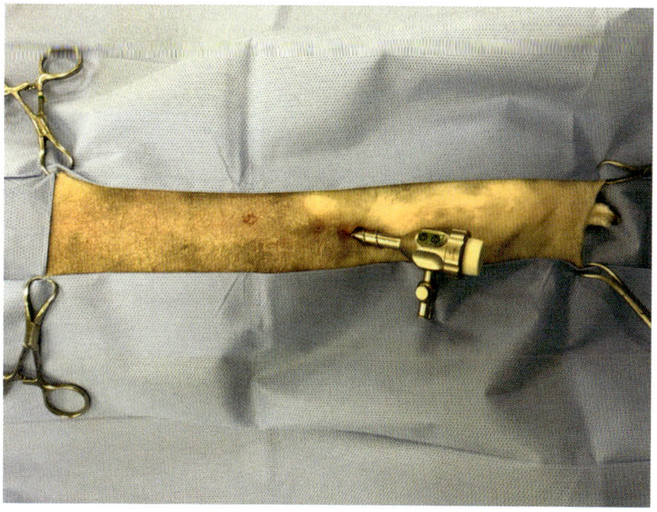

C-ii)

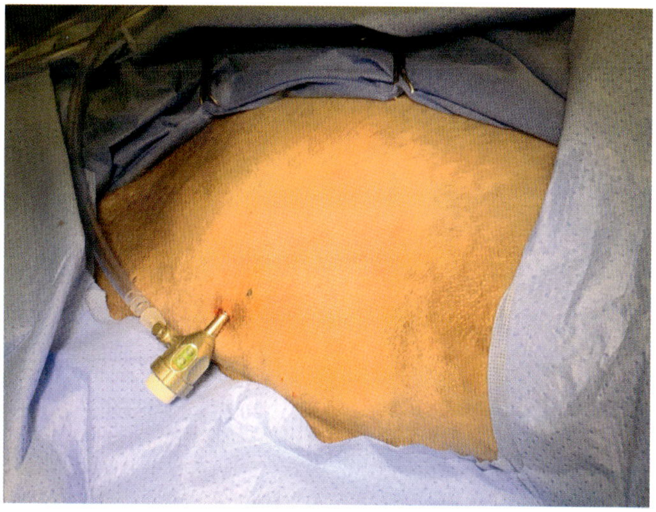

D)

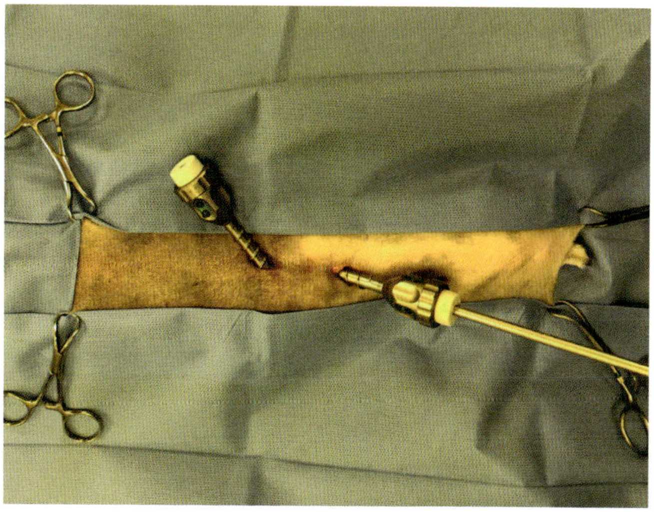

Surgical Technique (See Plate 15.3B–E) *continued*

E) To create the instrument ports (i), a modified Hasson technique can also be used as described earlier, although when performed lateral to the ventral midline, dissection occurs through multiple muscle layers. Alternatively, a closed/blind technique can be used in which a sharp-tipped trocar is loaded into a cannula and used to penetrate the abdominal wall. Because the tip of the trocar is quite sharp, the introduction of these devices needs to be very controlled and monitored via the telescope intra-abdominally (ii–iv).

Closure

Once the procedure is completed, CO_2 is released from the abdomen before closure by removing the caps of the cannula and allowing the gas to passively flow out or compressing the abdominal wall to forcibly cause removal. The muscular layers are closed with 2-0 to 3-0 monofilament absorbable suture in a simple interrupted or cruciate pattern. The subcutaneous tissue is closed with 3-0 monofilament absorbable suture if needed. The dermal layer is apposed with 3-0 to 4-0 monofilament nonabsorbable suture in a simple interrupted or simple continuous pattern.

Postoperative Management

1) Multimodal analgesia
2) Elizabethan collar or body suit

Complications

Intraoperative Complications

- Trauma to intra-abdominal organs while obtaining access to the abdomen. Splenic laceration was the most common complication (38%) [1].
- Conversion to an open procedure (31%) [1].
- Lack of visualization after introducing the initial telescope cannula into the abdomen may happen because of the cannula being inserted into the falciform ligament. To correct this, the cannula can be driven farther into the abdomen slowly and, if no resistance is met, it is possible to puncture through the falciform ligament. Alternatively, a blunt probe can be introduced into the cannula to try to move the falciform ligament off the end of the cannula. If these techniques are not successful, the cannula can be pulled out and replaced using a different entry angle.
- Lack of visualization can happen as a result of the cannulae being inserted into the mediastinum.

Postoperative Complications

- Surgical-site infection (1.7%) [2]

References

1 Maurin, M.P., Mullins, R.A., Singh, A. et al. (2020). A systematic review of complications related to laparoscopic and laparoscopic-assisted procedures in dogs. *Vet. Surg.* 49 (suppl 1): O5–O14.

2 Mayhew, P.D., Freeman, L., Kwan, T. et al. (2012). Comparison of surgical site infection rates in clean and clean-contaminated wounds in dogs and cats after minimally invasive versus open surgery: 179 cases (2007-2008). *J. Am. Vet. Med. Assoc.* 240 (2): 193–198.

Plate 15.3

Laparoscopic Approach *continued*

E-i)

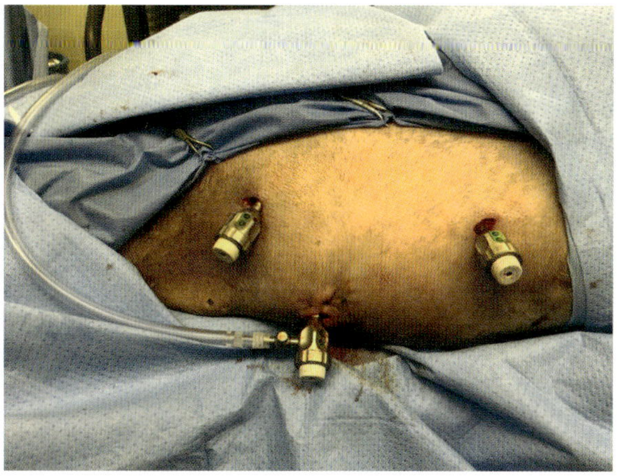

E-ii)

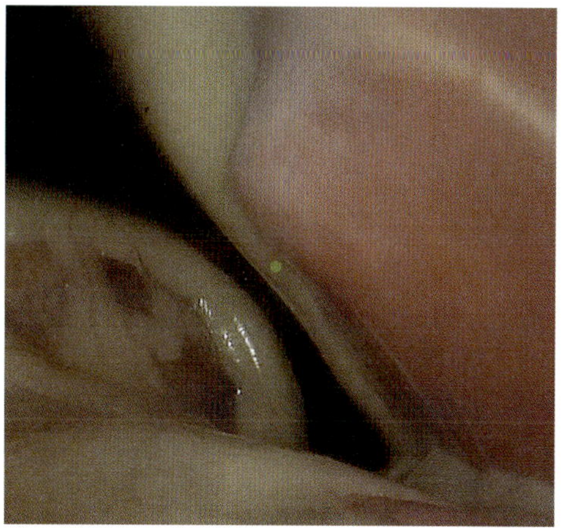

E-iii)

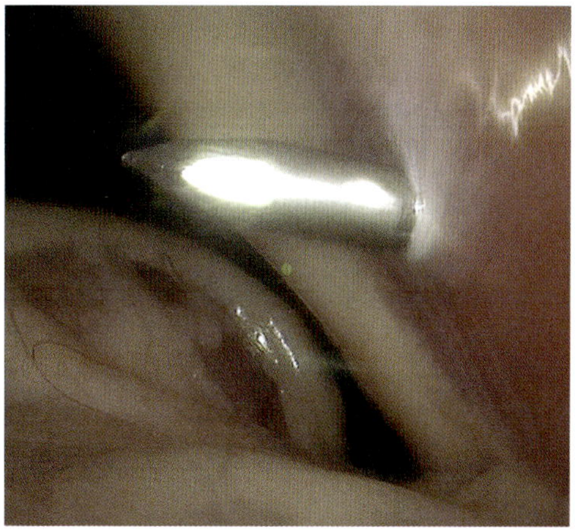

E-iv)

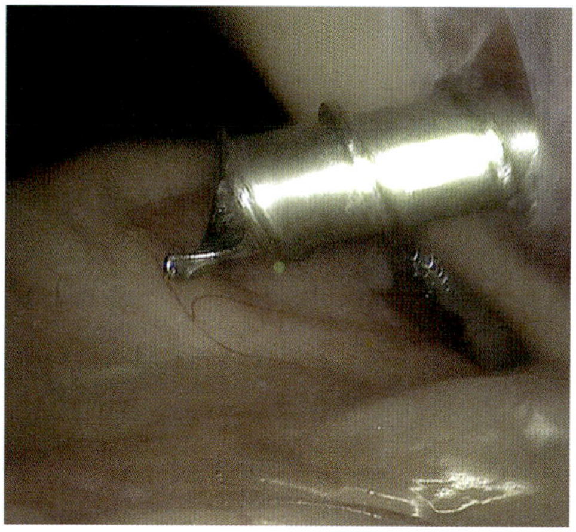

15.4 Abdominal Wall Resection and Reconstruction

Indications

1) Resection of primary malignant tumors of the abdominal wall, or for deep margins for the wide resection of invasive cutaneous and subcutaneous malignant tumors
2) Abdominal wall resection and reconstruction can be combined with chest wall resection (see *14. Chest Wall Resection and Reconstruction*)

Suggested Diagnostic Workup and Clinical Staging

- Complete blood count, serum biochemistry, and urinalysis
- Preoperative biopsy
- Precontrast and postcontrast computed tomography (CT) scan of the abdomen for surgical planning
- Abdominal and thoracic CT scan for assessment of intra-abdominal and lung metastasis

Patient Positioning

The patient is positioned in lateral recumbency with the affected side uppermost.

Surgical Technique (See Plate 15.4A–C)

A) An incision is performed either over a primary abdominal wall tumor (i, primary abdominal wall soft tissue sarcoma) or around a cutaneous or subcutaneous tumor with appropriate lateral margins for the tumor type (ii, incompletely excised subcutaneous soft tissue sarcoma surgical scar).
B) The skin incision is continued through the subcutaneous tissue with appropriate margins to the level of the abdominal wall (i, primary abdominal wall soft tissue sarcoma; ii, fixed cutaneous mast cell tumor).
C) The abdominal wall is resected with appropriate margins for the tumor type (i). Although scissors or electrosurgery can be used for full-thickness abdominal wall resection, a vessel sealing device is preferred (ii).

Color Atlas of Canine and Feline Surgical Oncology, First Edition. Julius M. Liptak, Paolo Buracco, William T. N. Culp, and Nicholas J. Bacon.

Plate 15.4

Abdominal Wall Resection and Reconstruction

A-i)

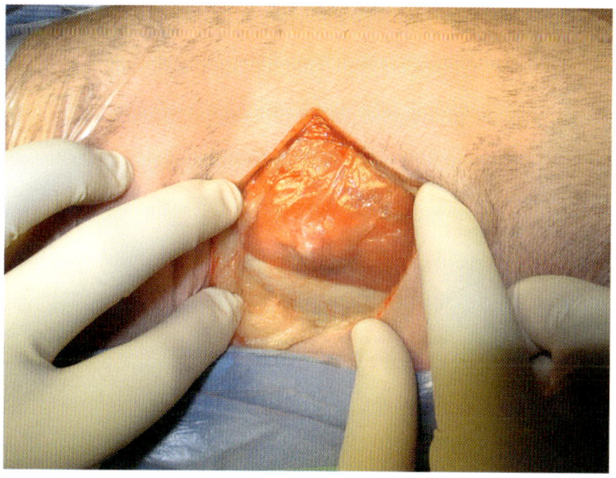

A-ii)

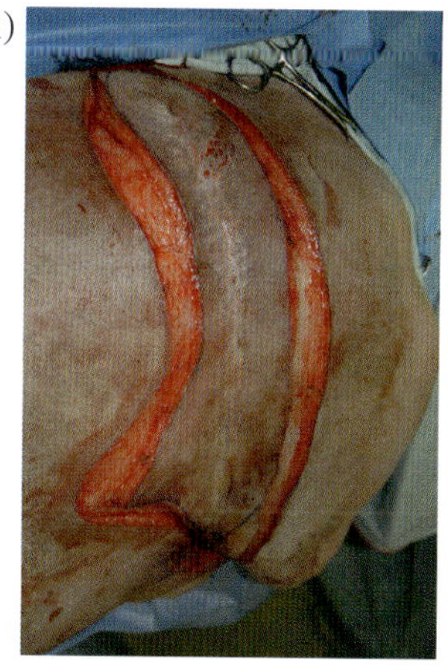

B-i)

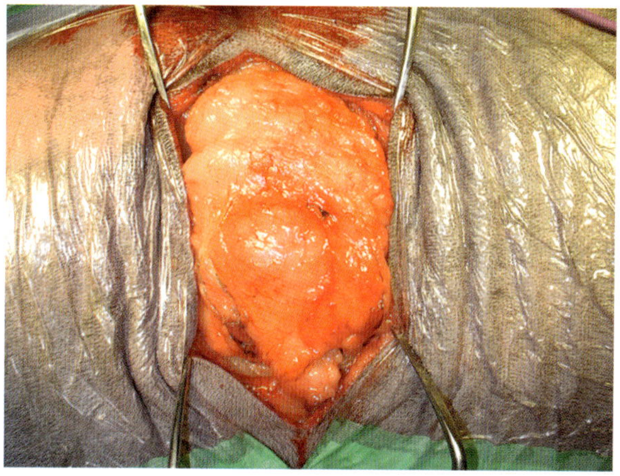

B-ii)

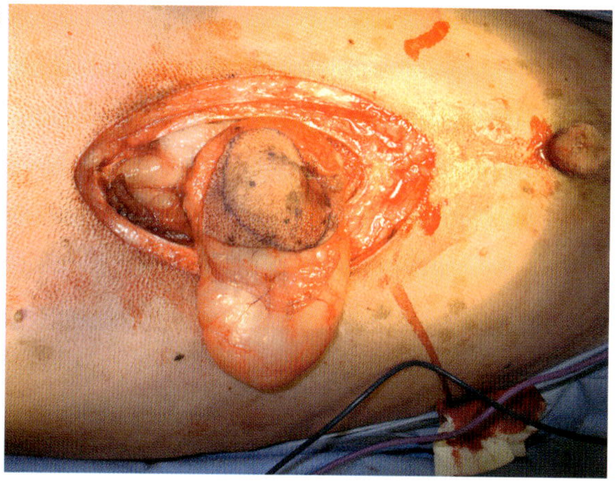

C-i)

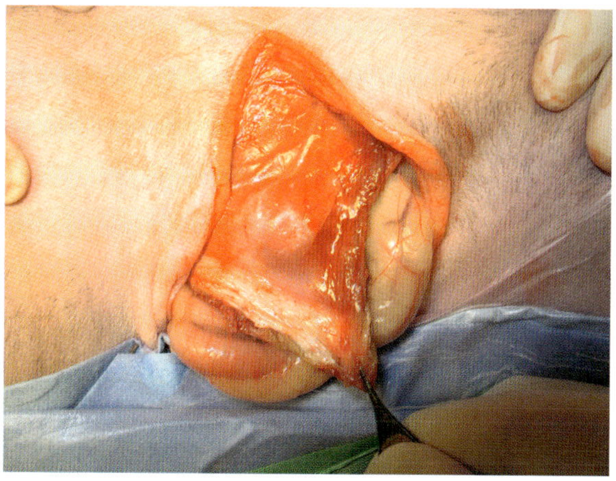

C-ii)

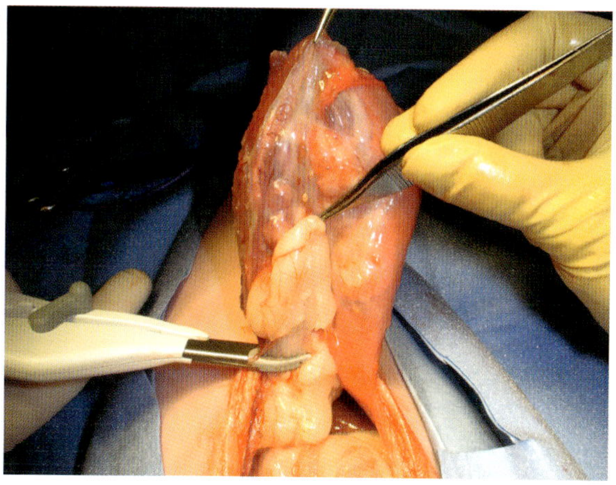

Closure (See Plate 15.4D–H)

Abdominal wall defects should be closed primarily if possible or reconstructed if primary closure is not possible. An interrupted technique using absorbable suture material is recommended for primary closure of abdominal wall defects (D). If reconstruction is required (E), then a number of autogenous and prosthetic techniques have been described for closure of abdominal wall defects. Autogenous techniques, which are not described in this section, include the cranial sartorius muscle flap (see *37. Hemipelvectomy*) [1], complete sartorius muscle flap [2], external abdominal oblique muscle flap [3], internal abdominal oblique muscle flap [4], rectus abdominal muscle flap [5], and transversus abdominis muscle flap [6].

When reconstructing with prosthetic mesh, omentum is sutured to the medial or mesothelial aspect of the abdominal wall defect, either with a simple continuous or interrupted tacking suture pattern using absorbable monofilament suture material (F). An omental pedicle technique is rarely required because of the mobility and proximity of the omental leaves to the abdominal wall defect. The omentum serves as a barrier between the abdominal organs and mesh, and to potentially improve fibrovascular tissue formation into the interstices of the mesh and thus decrease the risk of implant-associated infection. Nonabsorbable mesh (polypropylene or polytetrafluoroethylene) is tailored to the size of the abdominal wall defect so that the edges of the mesh are either doubled over (preferred) or a double thickness of mesh is used. The mesh is sutured under mild tension to either the lateral or medial/mesothelial aspect of the defect using either absorbable or nonabsorbable monofilament suture material (G). After abdominal wall reconstruction, the wound is closed routinely in two to three layers. A simple continuous suture pattern using monofilament absorbable suture material is used to close the cutaneous trunci muscle and subcutis. An interrupted or continuous suture pattern using monofilament nonabsorbable suture material is used to close the skin (H).

Postoperative Management

1) Multimodal analgesia, including perioperative continuous rate infusion of an opioid ± ketamine, local anesthesia instilled through a wound diffuser catheter, and oral analgesic drugs
2) ± Bandage
3) Elizabethan collar or body suit

Complications

- Incisional complications (seroma, dehiscence, infection)
- Implant-associated infection (0%–7%) [7, 8]

References

1 Weinstein, M.J., Pavletic, M.M., Boudrieau, R.J. et al. (1989). Cranial sartorius muscle flap in the dog. *Vet. Surg.* 18 (4): 286–291.

2 Mejia, S., Boston, S.E., and Skinner, O.T. (2018). Sartorius muscle flap for body wall reconstruction: Surgical technique description and retrospective case series. *Can. Vet. J.* 59 (11): 1187–1194.

3 Alexander, L.G., Pavletic, M.M., and Engler, S.J. (1991). Abdominal wall reconstruction with a vascular external abdominal oblique myofascial flap. *Vet. Surg.* 20 (6): 379–384.

4 Cronin, A. and Hall, J.L. (2021). A novel internal abdominal oblique muscle flap to close a major abdominal wall defect. *J. Small Anim. Pract.* 62 (1): 55–58.

5 Archipow, W. and Lanz, O.I. (2011). Rectus abdominis muscle flap for repair of prepubic tendon rupture in 8 dogs. *Can. Vet. J.* 52 (11): 1215–1218.

6 Liptak, J.M. and Brebner, N.S. (2006). Hemidiaphragmatic reconstruction with a transversus abdominis muscle flap after resection of a solitary diaphragmatic mesothelioma in a dog. *J. Am. Vet. Med. Assoc.* 228 (8): 1204–1208.

7 Bowman, K.L.T., Birchard, S.J., and Bright, R.M. (1998). Complications associated with the implantation of polypropylene mesh in dogs and cats: a retrospective study of 21 cases (1984–1996). *J. Am. Anim. Hosp. Assoc.* 34: 225–233.

8 Liptak, J.M., Dernell, W.S., Rizzo, S.A. et al. (2008). Reconstruction of chest wall defects after rib tumor resection: a comparison of autogenous, prosthetic, and composite techniques in 44 dogs. *Vet. Surg.* 37 (5): 479–487.

Plate 15.4

Abdominal Wall Resection and Reconstruction *continued*

D)

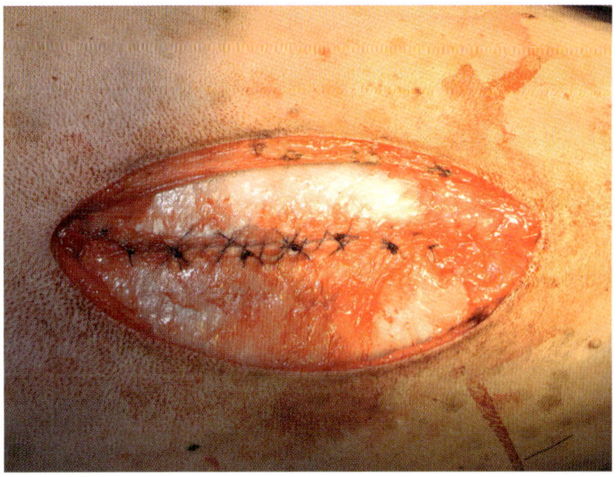

E)

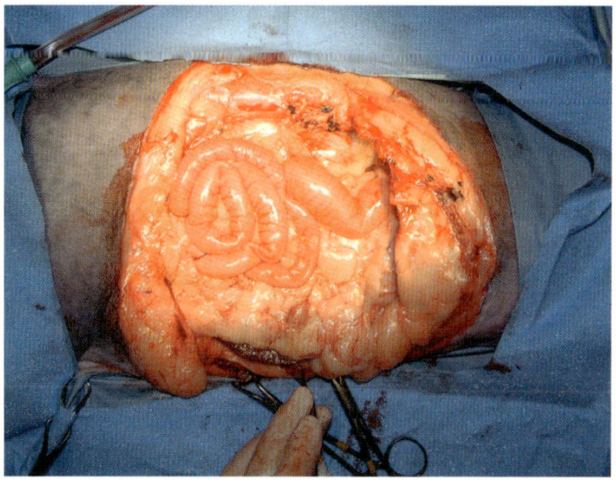

F)

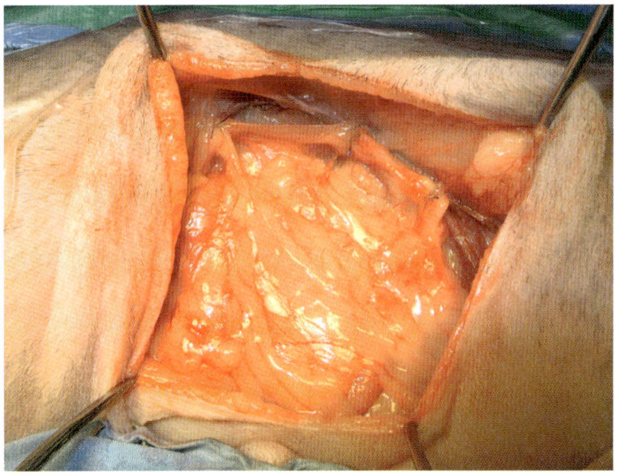

G)

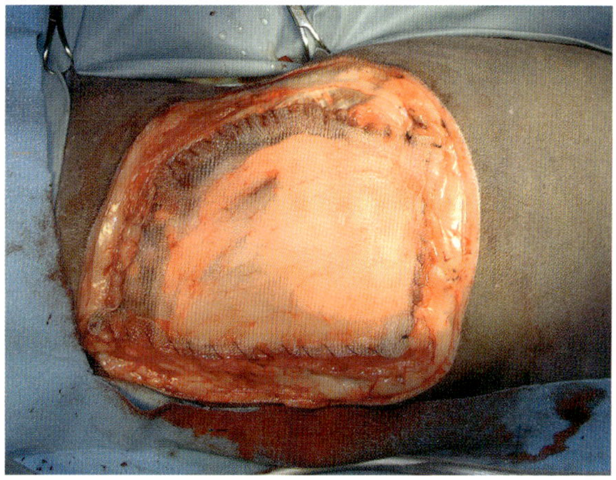

H)

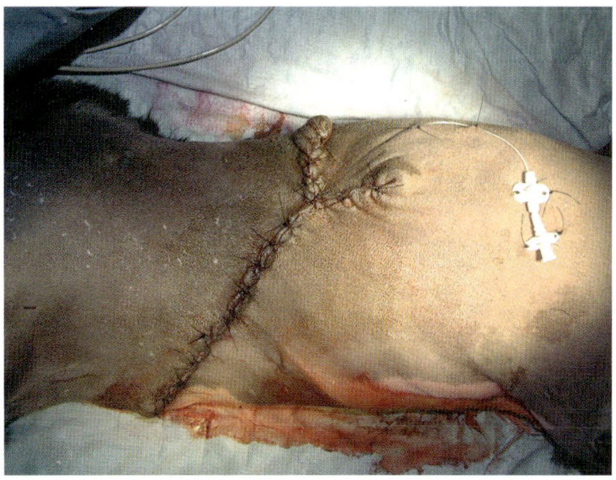

15.5 Pubic Symphysiotomy

Indications

1) To increase exposure for resection of malignant intrapelvic tumors, such as colic, rectal, or prostatic tumors
2) Pubic symphysiotomy is often combined with a ventral midline celiotomy (see *15.1. Ventral Midline Celiotomy*)

Patient Positioning

The patient is positioned in dorsal recumbency. The urethra should be catheterized to allow intraoperative identification and to minimize the risk of iatrogenic trauma.

Surgical Technique [1] (See Plate 15.5A–D)

A) A ventral midline celiotomy is performed (see *15.1. Ventral Midline Celiotomy*) and extended caudally to the level of the scrotum or vulva. The subcutaneous tissues are incised caudally to expose the adductor muscles (AM) over the ventral aspect of the pubis. The aponeurosis of the adductor muscles is divided in the midline (i) and exposes the fibrocartilaginous pubic symphysis (ii, arrows).
B) The adductor muscles are elevated with periosteal elevators bilaterally in a medial-to-lateral direction to expose the medial pubis and medial one third of the obturator foramina (i). Two to three holes (arrows) are drilled (ii) either side of the pubic symphysis for later fixation of the pubic symphysiotomy (iii, arrows), if desired. The intrapelvic contents are protected with a retractor, such as a malleable (MR; see C – i) or ribbon retractor, positioned along the dorsal aspect of the pubis while drilling and performing the osteotomies.
C) A symphysiotomy is performed along the fibrocartilaginous pubic symphysis with an oscillating (i, pictured) or sagittal saw or osteotome and mallet. The soft tissue dorsal to the completed symphysiotomy (ii, arrow) needs to be incised with either Metzenbaum scissors, electrosurgery, or a vessel sealing device to expose the pelvic cavity.
D) A Finochietto self-retaining rib retractor (FR) is used to retract the pubic bones and pelvis to expose the contents of the pelvic canal (asterisk, rectal leiomyoma).

Color Atlas of Canine and Feline Surgical Oncology, First Edition. Julius M. Liptak, Paolo Buracco, William T. N. Culp, and Nicholas J. Bacon.

Plate 15.5

Pubic Symphysiotomy

A-i)

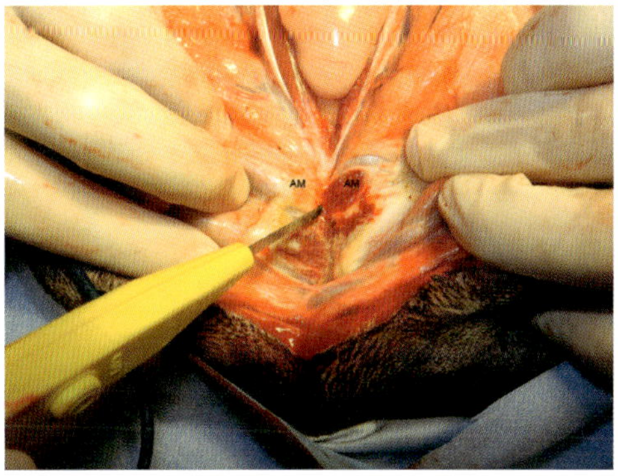

A-ii)

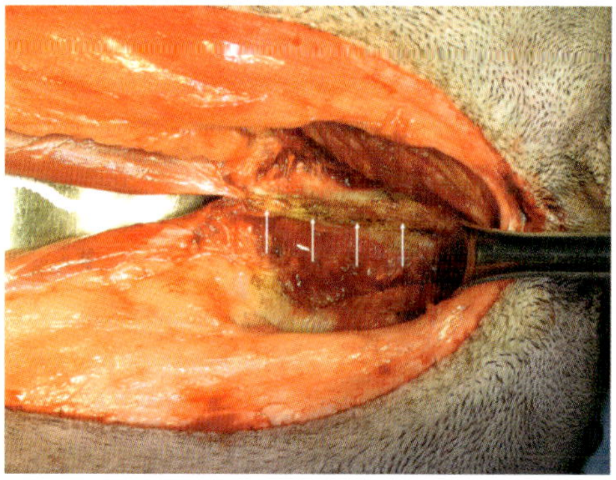

B-i)

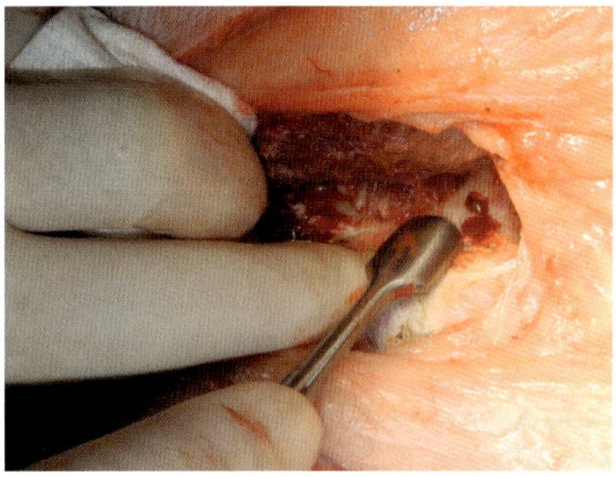

B-ii)

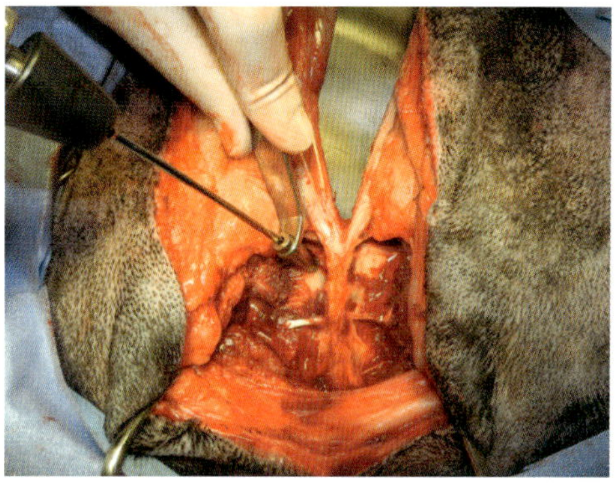

B-iii)

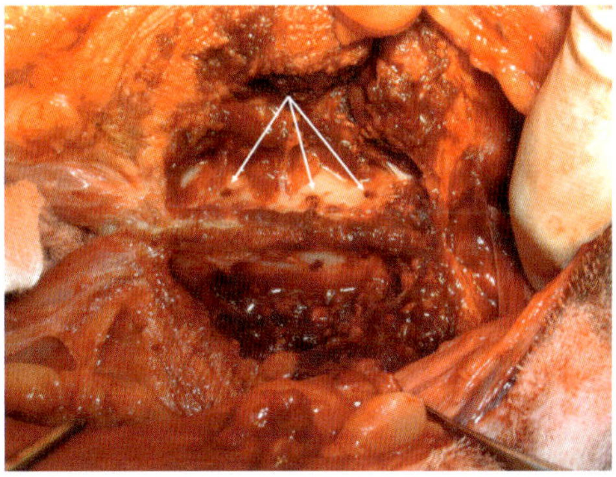

C-i)

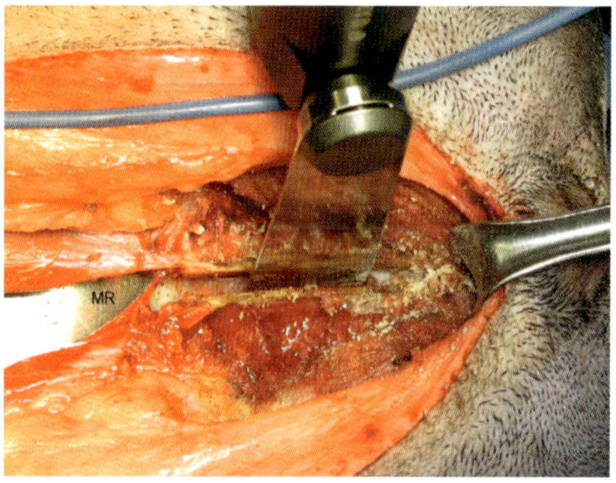

C-ii)

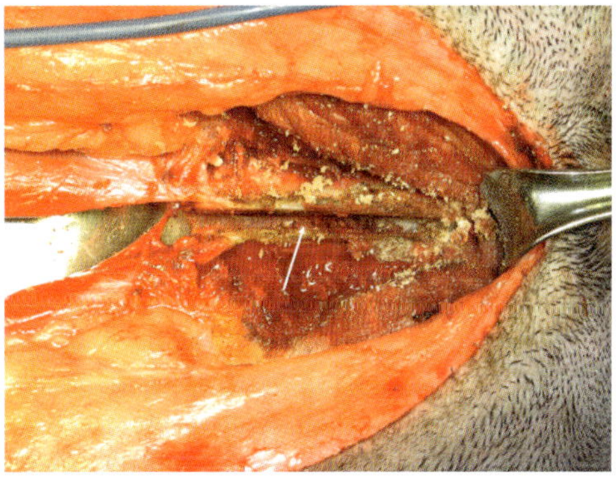

D)

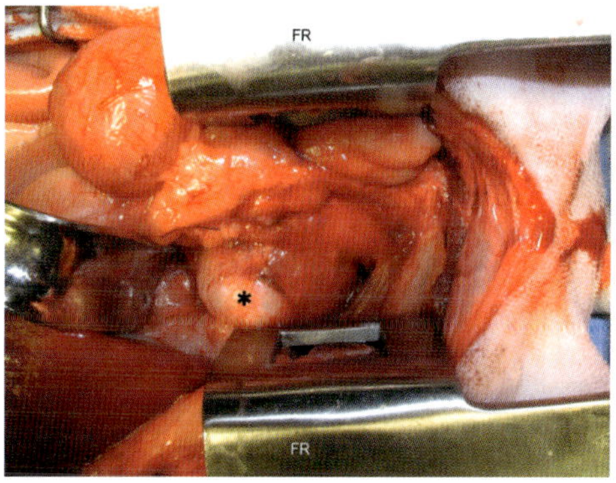

Closure (See Plate 15.5E–H)

The pubic symphysis can be stabilized with either stainless steel wire or heavy gauge absorbable material, depending on the size of the animal. These can be passed through the medial borders of obturator foraminae (E) or through predrilled holes (F, see step C). Because of the short distance between the symphysiotomy and the predrilled holes, collapse of this bone is possible during tightening of the orthopedic wire. Care is taken not to incorporate any vessels or nerves in the wire suture loop. The wire is then tightened while being bent, and then the ends are cut with wire cutters (G). The adductor muscles are closed with 2-0 to 0 absorbable monofilament suture material using a cruciate or horizontal mattress technique (H). The subcutaneous tissue and skin are closed routinely as described in *15.1. Ventral Midline Celiotomy*.

Postoperative Management

1) Multimodal analgesia
2) Elizabethan collar
3) ± Hobbles at the level of the hocks for the first 5 days may help to avoid an excessive abduction of the pelvic limbs
4) ± Exercise restriction for 4 weeks

Complications

- Incisional complications
- Sacroiliac subluxation/luxation [2]
- Nonunion of the osteotomy site
- Implant-associated infection [1]

References

1 Davies, J.V. and Read, H.M. (1990). Sagittal pubic osteotomy in the investigation and treatment of intrapelvic neoplasia in the dog. *J. Sm. Anim. Pract.* 31: 123–130.

2 Schlicksup, M.D., Holt, D.E., Mai, W. et al. (2013). The effect of abaxial retraction on pelvic geometry after pelvic symphysiotomy. *Vet. Surg.* 42 (8): 958–962.

Plate 15.5

Pubic Symphysiotomy *continued*

E)

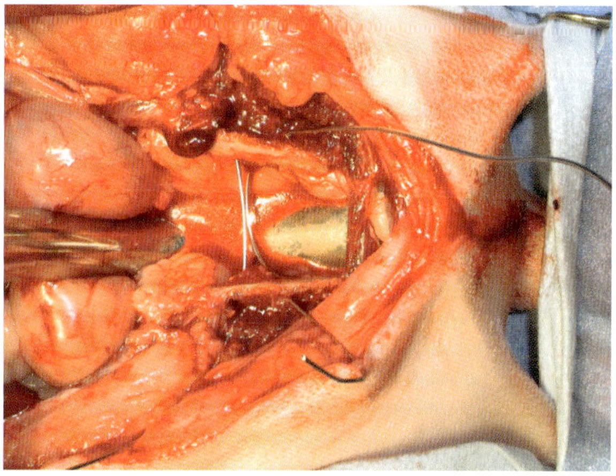

F)

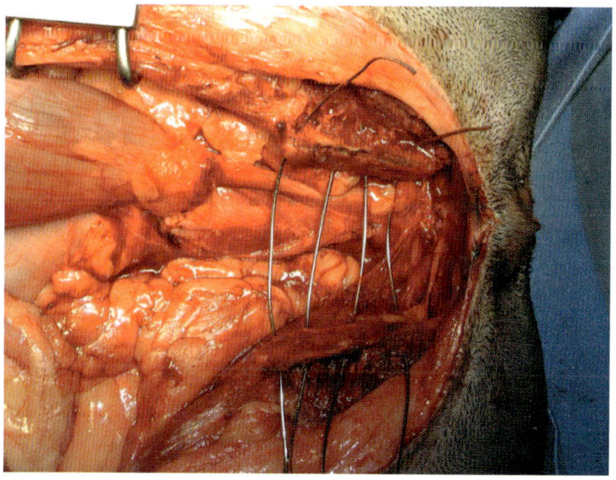

G)

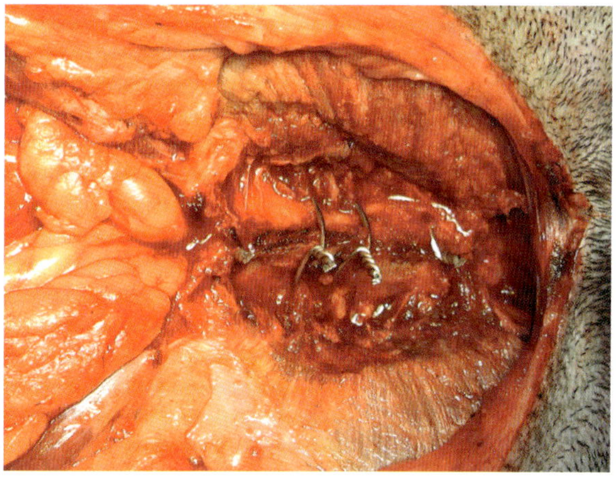

H)

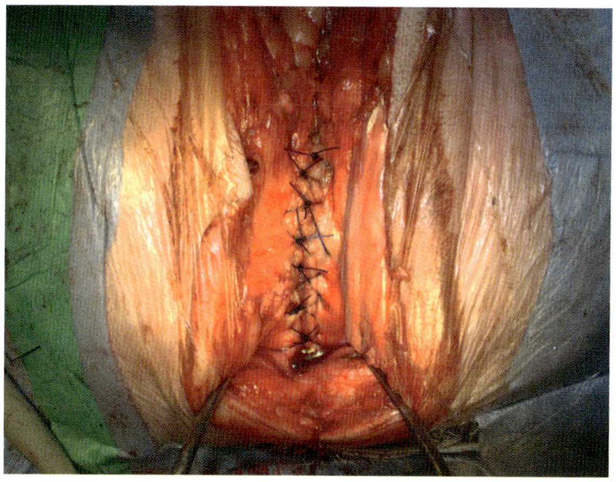

15.6 Pubic Flap

Indications

1) To increase exposure for resection of malignant intrapelvic tumors, such as colic, rectal, or prostatic tumors
2) Pubic flap is often combined with a ventral midline celiotomy (see *15.1. Ventral Midline Celiotomy*)

Patient Positioning

The patient is positioned in dorsal recumbency. The urethra should be catheterized to allow intraoperative identification and to minimize the risk of iatrogenic trauma.

Surgical Technique [1] (See Plate 15.6A–G)

A) A ventral midline celiotomy is performed (see *15.1. Ventral Midline Celiotomy*) and extended caudally to the level of the scrotum or vulva. The subcutaneous tissues are incised caudally to expose the aponeurosis of the adductor muscles (AMs).
B) The aponeurosis of the AMs is divided in the midline to expose the ventral pubis. The AMs are elevated with periosteal elevators bilaterally in a medial-to-lateral direction to expose up to two thirds of the obturator foramina (double arrows). The prepubic tendon is transected bilaterally along the cranial pubic margin (single arrow).
C) Two to three holes (arrows) are drilled (i) bilaterally along the cranial pubis for later reattachment of the prepubic tendon (ii, arrows). The intrapelvic contents are protected with a retractor, such as a malleable (MR) or ribbon retractor, positioned along the dorsal aspect of the pubis while drilling and performing the osteotomies.
D) One to two holes are drilled on either side of the intended osteotomies for later fixation of the elevated pubic flap back into its normal position (pictured, cranial holes have been drilled and caudal hole is being drilled).
E) The cranial pubic osteotomies (arrows) are performed with an oscillating or sagittal saw (i) lateral to the pubic symphysis (PS) cranially to medial to the craniolateral aspect of the obturator foramen (OF) caudally (ii).

Color Atlas of Canine and Feline Surgical Oncology, First Edition. Julius M. Liptak, Paolo Buracco, William T. N. Culp, and Nicholas J. Bacon.

Plate 15.6

Pubic Flap

A)

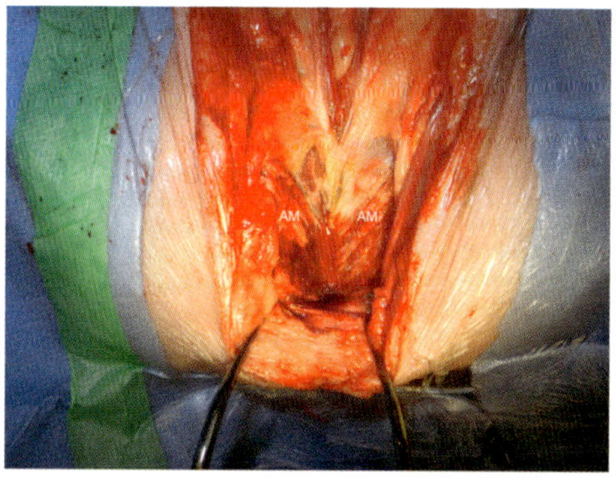

B)

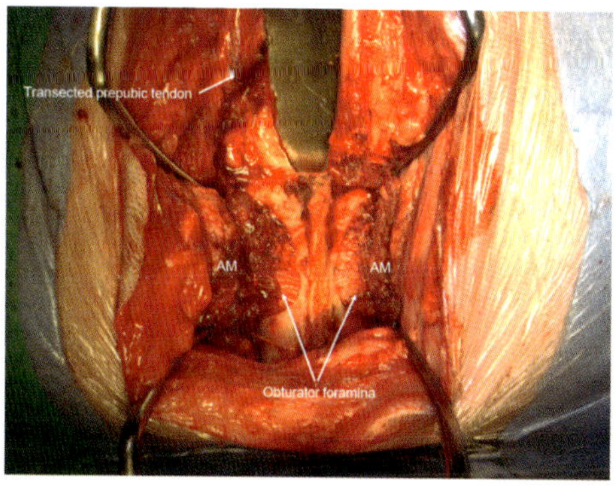

C-i)

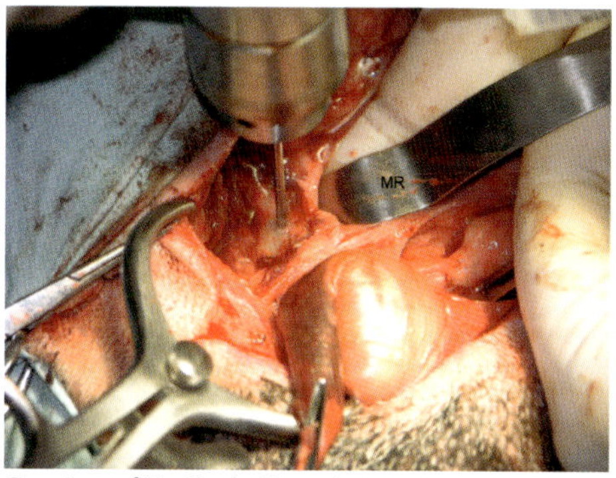

Courtesy of Dr. Paolo Bogoni

C-ii)

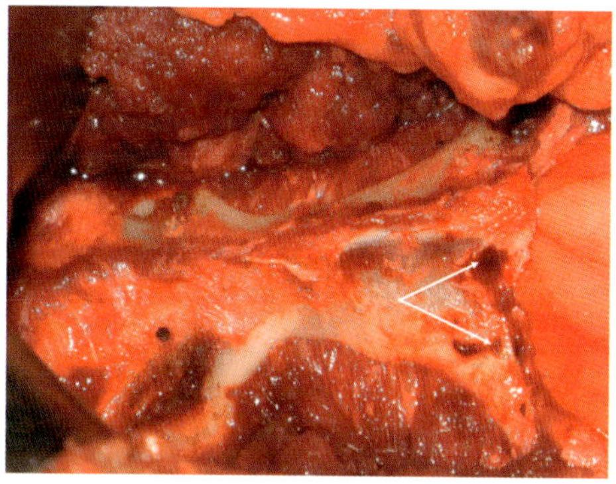

D)

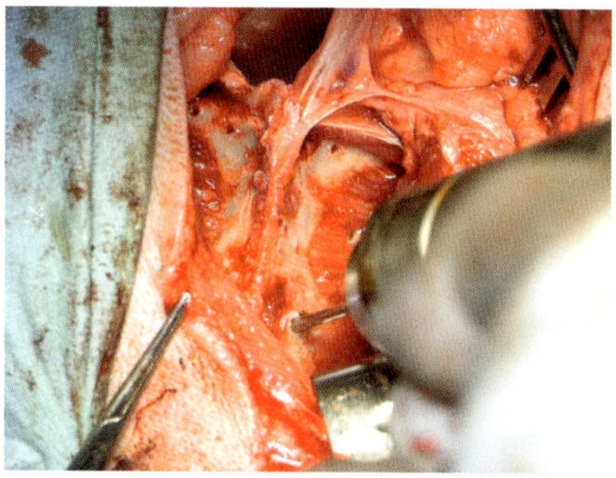

Courtesy of Dr. Paolo Bogoni

E-i)

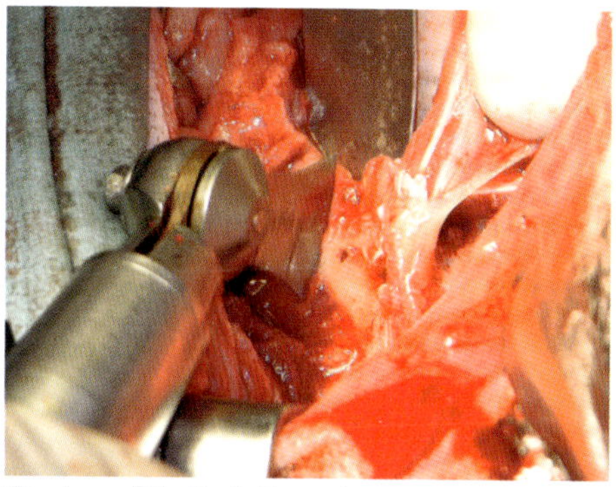

Courtesy of Dr. Paolo Bogoni

E-ii)

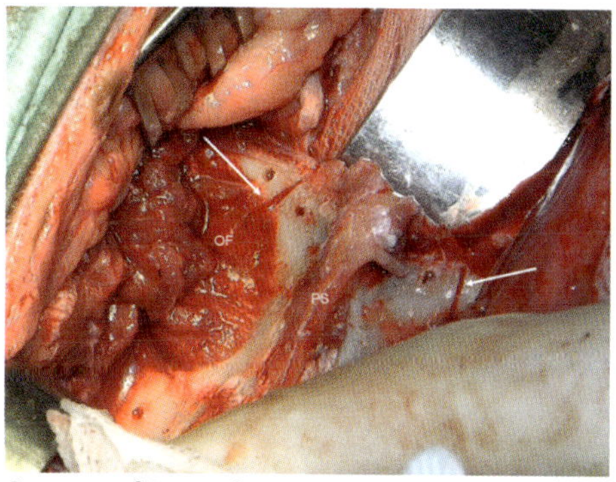

Courtesy of Dr. Paolo Bogoni

Surgical Technique (See Plate 15.6A–G) *continued*

F) The caudal osteotomies are performed with an oscillating or sagittal saw (i) medial to the caudolateral aspect of the obturator foramen (OF) cranially to the lateral third of the ischiatic arch caudally (ii, arrow).

G) The pubic bone flap (i, ii) is then reflected caudally (iii) or laterally (iii) to expose the contents of the pelvic canal.

Plate 15.6

Pubic Flap *continued*

F-i)

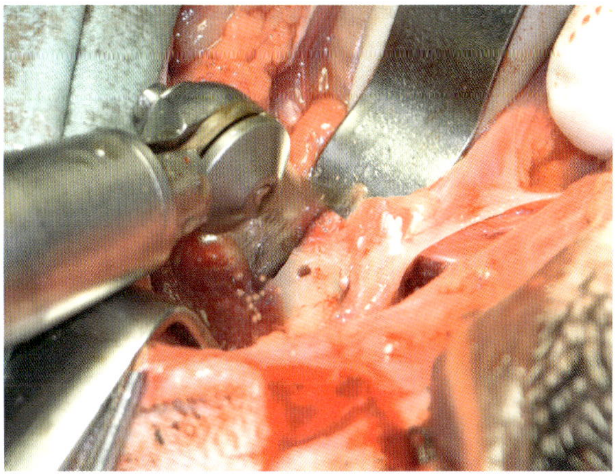

Courtesy of Dr. Paolo Bogoni

F-ii)

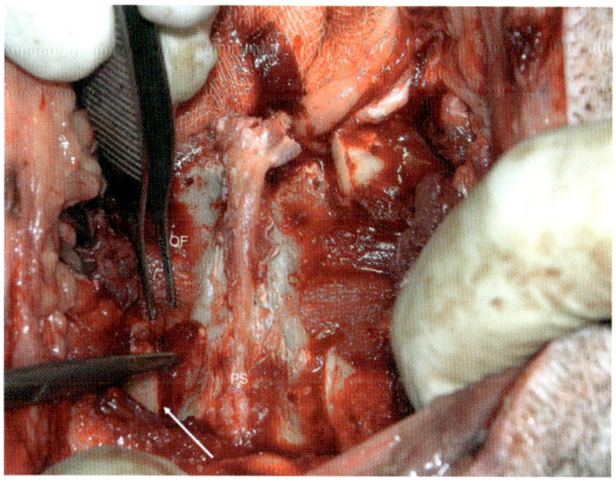

Courtesy of Dr. Paolo Bogoni

G-i)

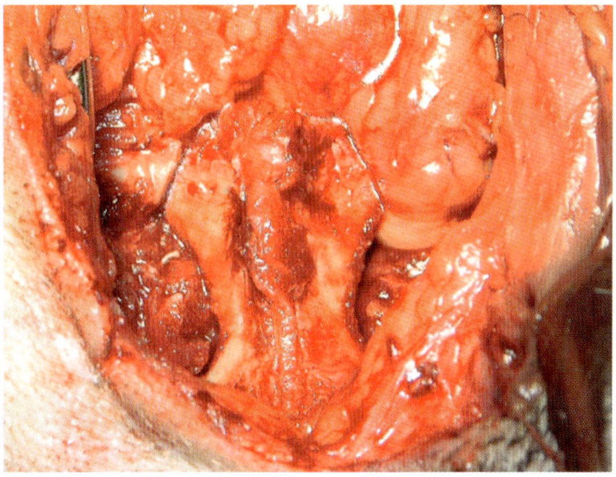

Courtesy of Dr. Paolo Bogoni

G-ii)

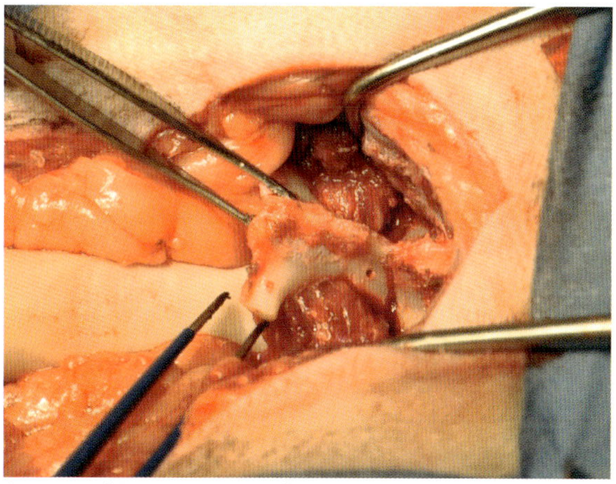

Courtesy of Dr. Bart Van Goethem

G-iii)

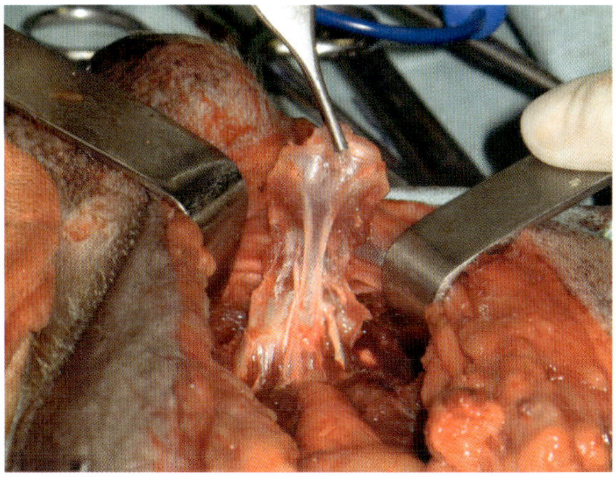

G-iv)

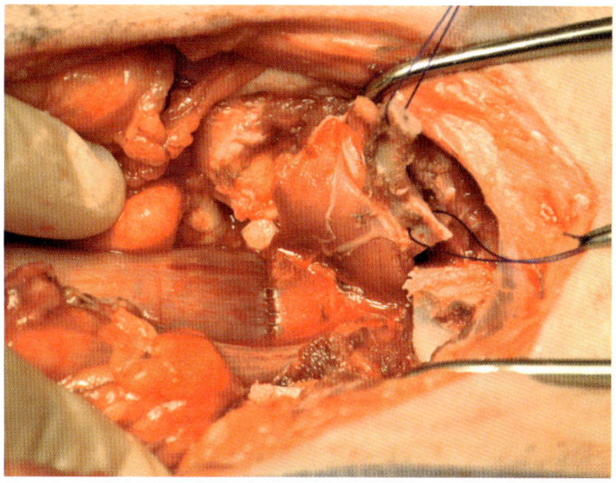

Courtesy of Dr. Bart Van Goethem

Closure (See Plate 15.6H–K)

The pubic bone flap is returned to its normal location and fixed by passing either orthopedic wire (H) or heavy (2-0 to 1) absorbable suture material (I – i, ii), depending on the size of the animal, through the predrilled holes. The prepubic tendon is reattached to the cranial pubis with four to six sutures using heavy (2-0 to 1) absorbable suture material (J – i, ii). The AMs are closed with 2-0 to 0 absorbable monofilament suture material using a cruciate or horizontal mattress technique (K). The subcutaneous tissue and skin are closed routinely as described in *15.1. Ventral Midline Celiotomy*.

Postoperative Management

1) Multimodal analgesia
2) Elizabethan collar
3) ± Hobbles at the level of the hocks for the first 5 days may help to avoid excessive abduction of the pelvic limbs
4) ± Exercise restriction for 4 weeks [2]

Complications

- Prepubic herniation [3]
- Nonunion of the osteotomy site(s)
- Avascular necrosis of the pubic bone flap [1]

References

1 Yoon, H.Y. and Mann, F.A. (2008). Bilateral pubic and ischial osteotomy for surgical management of caudal colonic and rectal masses in six dogs and a cat. *J. Am. Vet. Med. Assoc.* 232 (7): 1016–1020.

2 Allen, S.W. and Crowell, S.W. (1991). Ventral approach to the pelvic canal in the female dog. *Vet. Surg.* 20 (2): 118–121.

3 Bennett, T.C., Matz, B.M., Henderson, R.A. et al. (2018). Total prostatectomy as a treatment for prostatic carcinoma in 25 dogs. *Vet. Surg.* 47 (3): 367–377.

Plate 15.6

Pubic Flap *continued*

H)

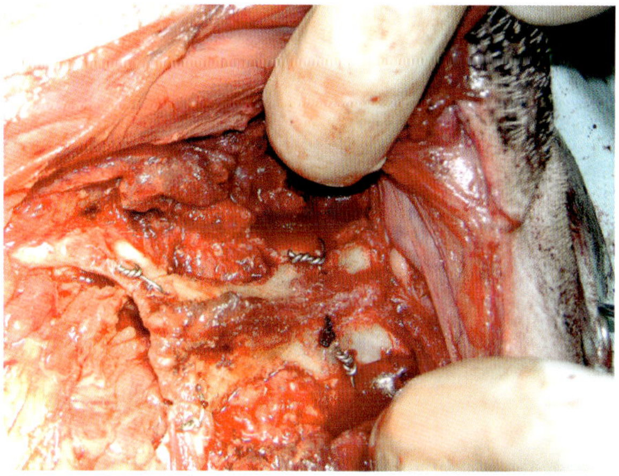

Courtesy of Dr. Paolo Bogoni

I-i)

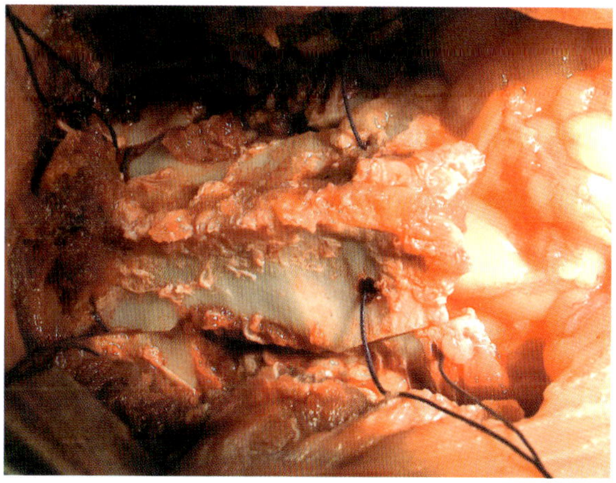

I-ii)

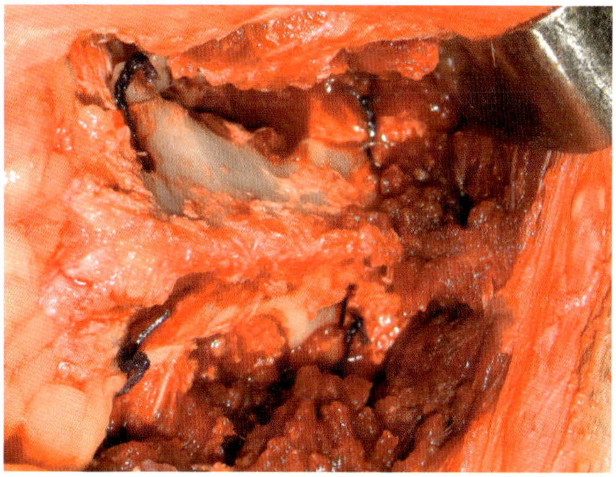

J-i)

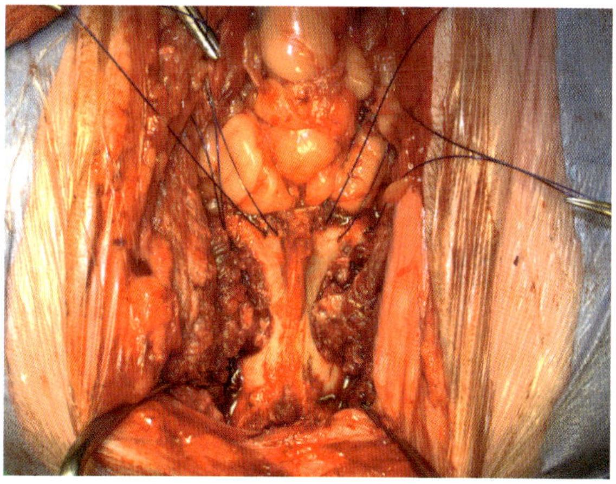

J-ii)

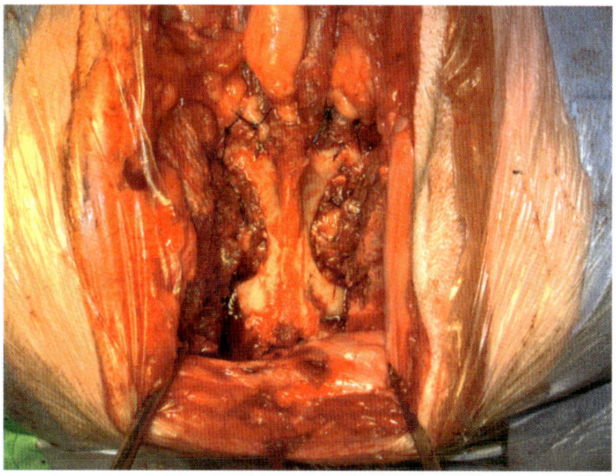

K)

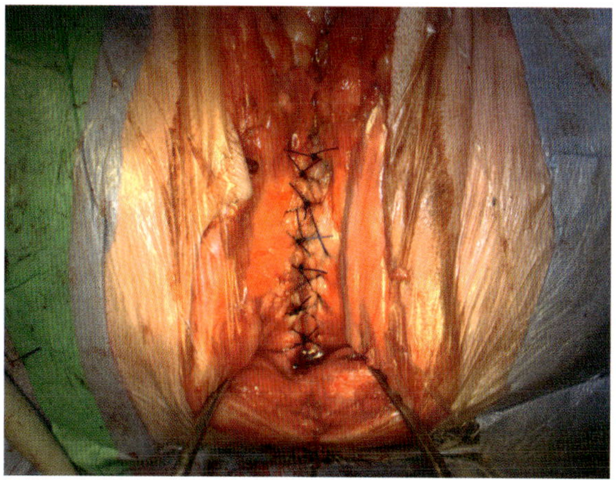

Chapter 16: Liver Lobectomy

Indications

1) Resection of benign and malignant massive morphology liver masses
2) Management of nonneoplastic conditions, such as liver lobe torsion, hepatic abscess, and hepatic trauma

Suggested Diagnostic Workup and Clinical Staging

- Complete blood count, serum biochemistry, and urinalysis
- ± Coagulation profile
- ± Cross matching or blood typing
- Abdominal ultrasound or precontrast and postcontrast computed tomography (CT) scan of the abdomen for characterization of the liver mass and assessment of intra-abdominal metastasis
- ± Ultrasound- or CT-guided fine-needle aspirate cytology
- Three-view thoracic radiographs or thoracic CT scan for assessment of lung metastasis

Patient Positioning

The patient is positioned in dorsal recumbency.

Surgical Technique – Approach (See Plate 16A–F)

A) A ventral midline celiotomy is performed (i; see *15.1. Ventral Midline Celiotomy*). The falciform ligament should be resected to improve exposure (ii).

B) A ventral midline celiotomy can be combined with a paracostal approach (see *15.2. Paracostal Approach*) for improved visualization and exposure (i, paracostal approach; ii, right-sided hepatocellular carcinoma (HCC) and caudal vena cava [CaVC]; iii, CaVC).

C) A diaphragmatic incision (arrow), with either a sharp incision in the pars sternalis using an inverted scalpel blade or continuing the linea alba incision through into the diaphragm, releases the tethering effect of the diaphragm and improves caudal mobilization of the liver and exposure of the hilus of the liver, if required. Care should be taken to avoid the diaphragmatic insertions of the phrenic nerves laterally, intrathoracic structures cranially, and the CaVC, esophagus, and aorta as they pass through the caval foramen, esophageal hiatus, and aortic hiatus, respectively [1].

D) In some cases, there will be omentum adhered to the liver mass (i, arrow). The omentum should not be detached because this may represent tumor invasion into the omentum rather than adhesions. The adhesed omentum should be isolated by blunt dissection (ii) and then either ligated with 2-0 or 3-0 absorbable monofilament suture material, transected with a vessel sealing device, or cauterized using electrosurgery (iii), leaving a cuff of approximately 5 cm of omentum attached to the liver mass.

Color Atlas of Canine and Feline Surgical Oncology, First Edition. Julius M. Liptak, Paolo Buracco, William T. N. Culp, and Nicholas J. Bacon.

Plate 16

Liver Lobectomy

A-i)

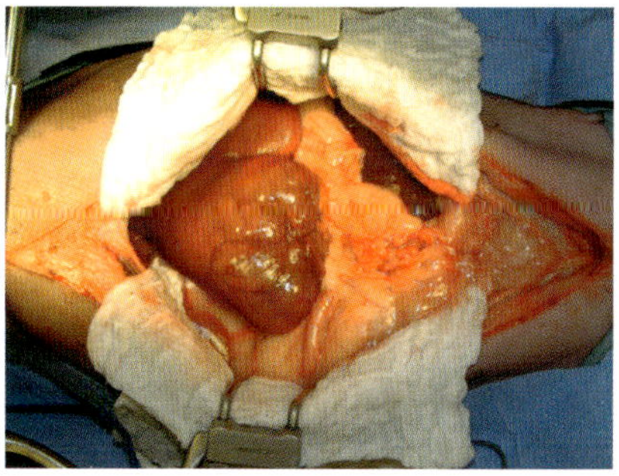

A-ii)

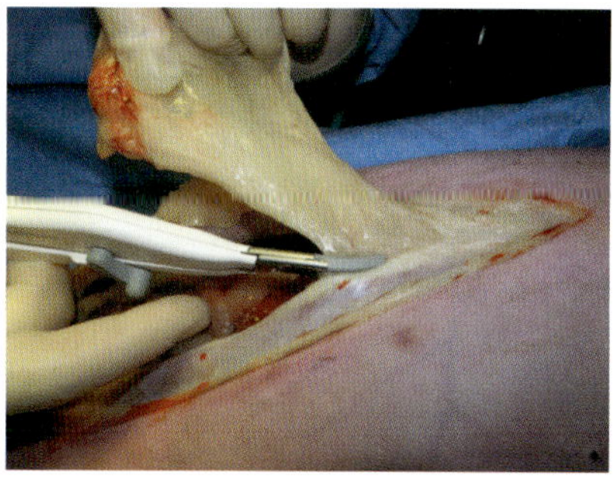

B-i)

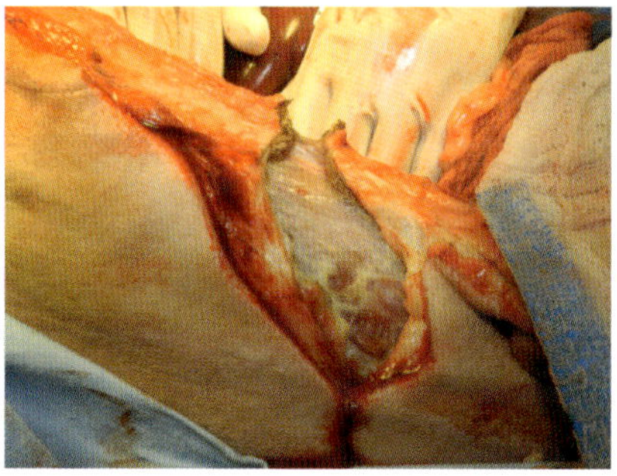

B-ii)

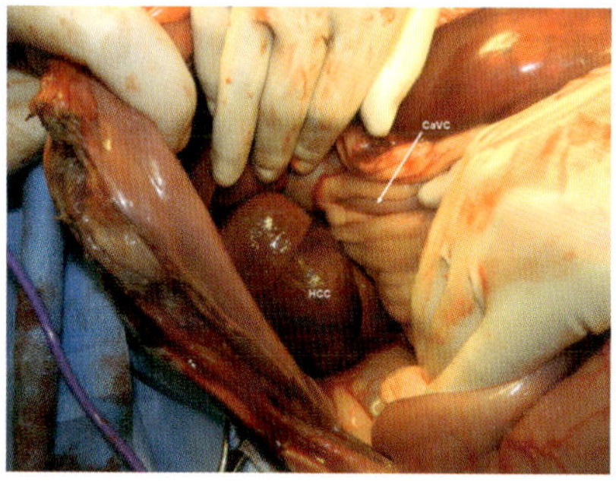

B-iii)

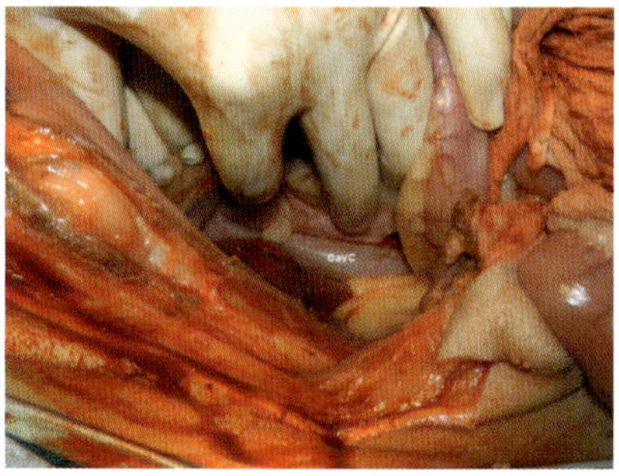

C)

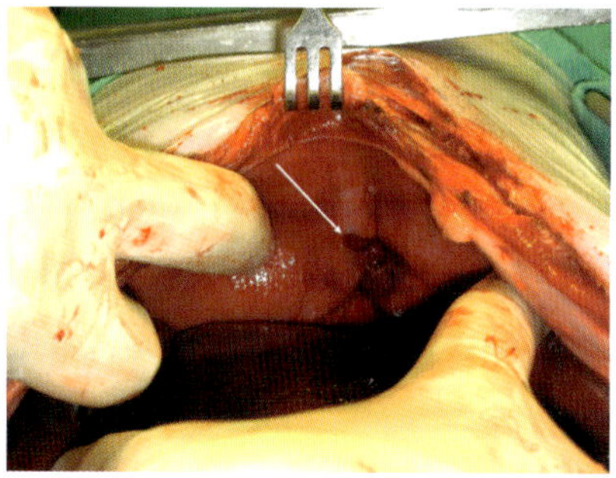

D-i)

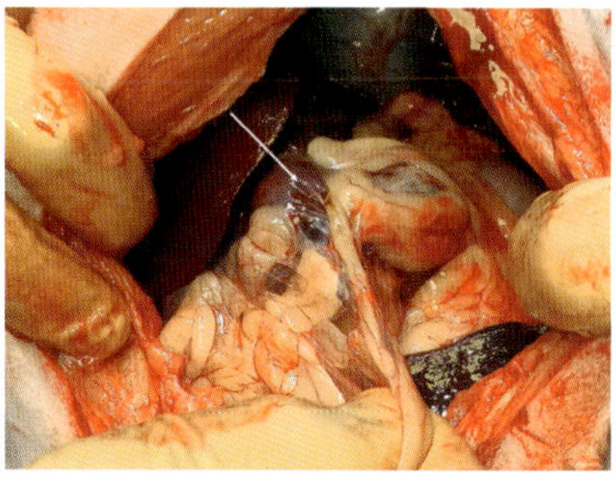

D-ii)

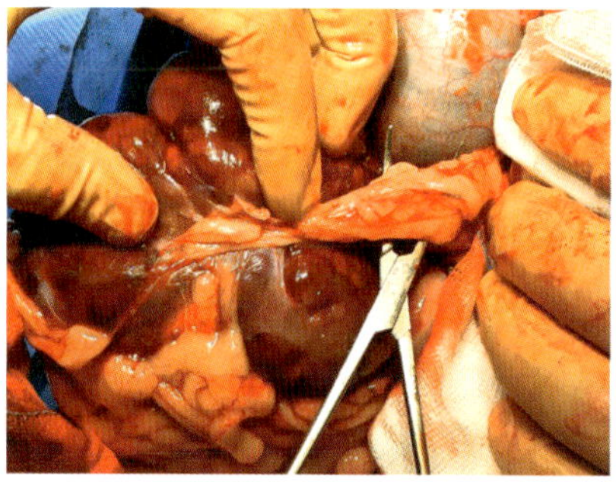

D-iii)

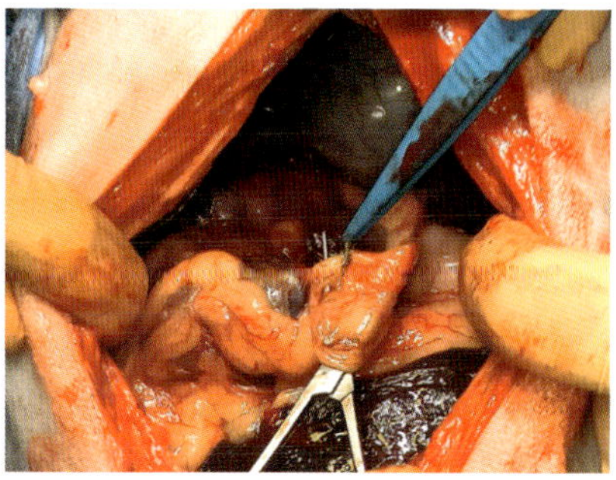

Surgical Technique – Approach (See Plate 16A–F) *continued*

E) The abdominal cavity should be explored to determine which liver lobe(s) the mass is originating. If right sided, then the proximity of the mass (HCC) to the CaVC should be assessed to determine whether liver lobectomy is possible (i). If not, then an appropriately sized punch biopsy should be used to collect a biopsy from the liver mass (ii).

F) For tumors involving the central division of the liver (quadrate [i] or right medial liver lobes), the gallbladder (GB) may need to be dissected free from the hepatic fossa (HF) to provide adequate exposure of the affected liver lobe (ii).

Surgical Technique – Stapling [2] (See Plate 16G–J)

G) An appropriately sized thoracoabdominal (TA) stapler is passed around the affected liver lobe, either at the hilus of the liver lobe or within the parenchyma of the liver lobe, with a minimum of 1-cm surgical margins cranial to the liver mass. A vascular 30-mm TA stapler is preferred for liver lobectomies because the three rows of staples and 1.0 mm closing height of the staples provide a better seal than other available stapler cartridges (i); however, larger TA staplers (ii; i.e. 55–60 mm) may be required, especially for partial liver lobectomies, because of the width of the liver lobe at the lobectomy site.

H) The retaining pin is engaged, which allows for the tissues to be isolated within the opening of the stapler cartridge (arrow). The handle of the stapler is compressed, which results in the staples engaging the tissue within the cartridge.

I) The tissue is then transected distal to the staple cartridge using either sharp dissection (i) or a vessel sealing device (ii). The staple cartridge will often have a small shelf that will allow for guidance of the scalpel blade during transection.

Plate 16

Liver Lobectomy *continued*

E-i)

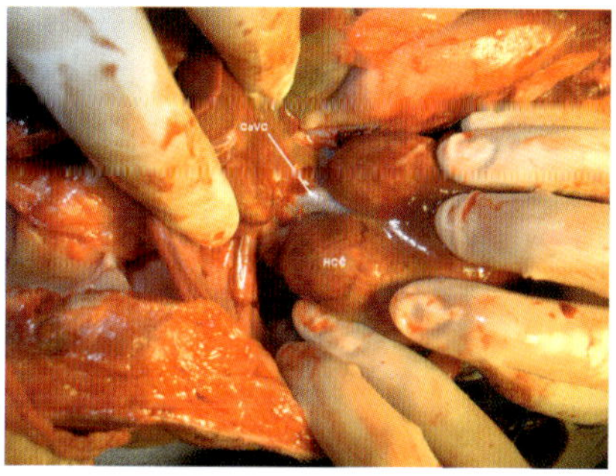

E-ii)

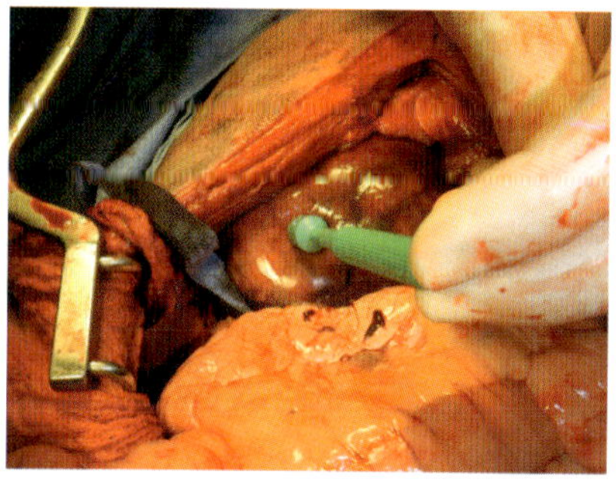

F-i)

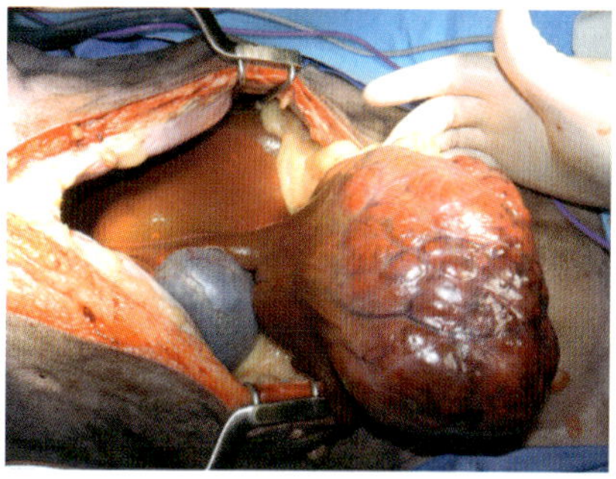

F-ii)

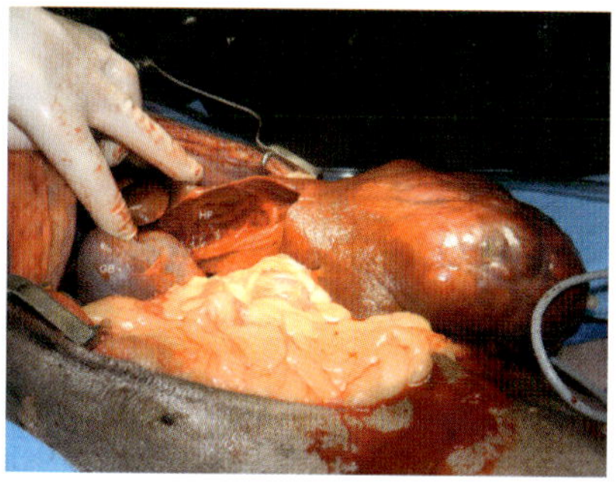

G-i)

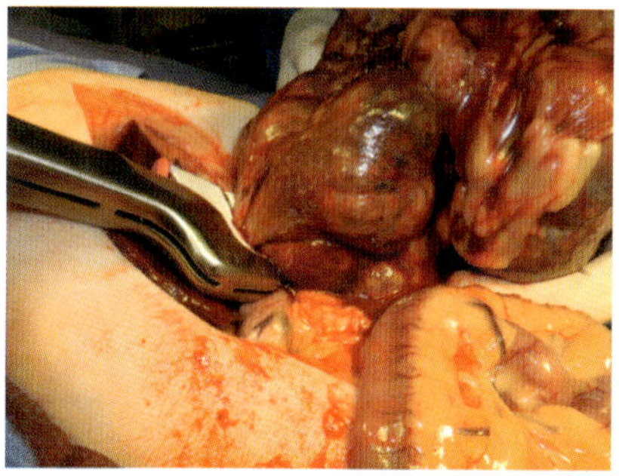

G-ii)

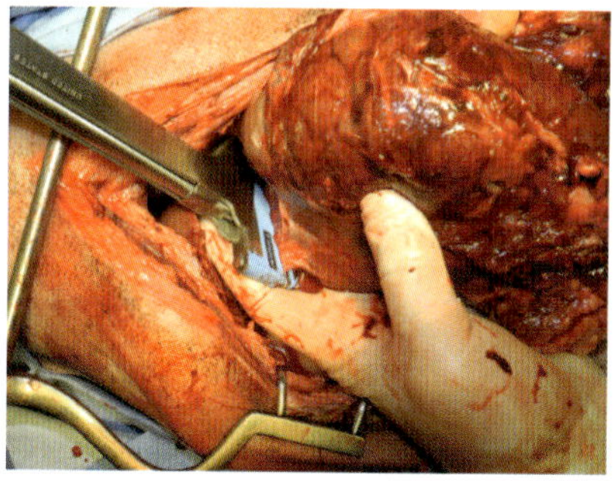

H)

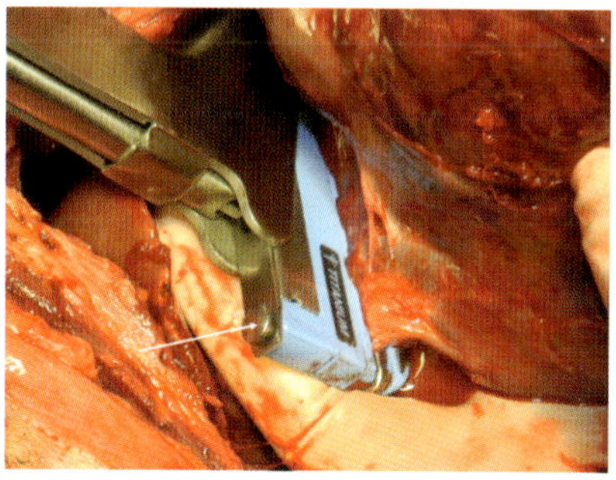

I-i)

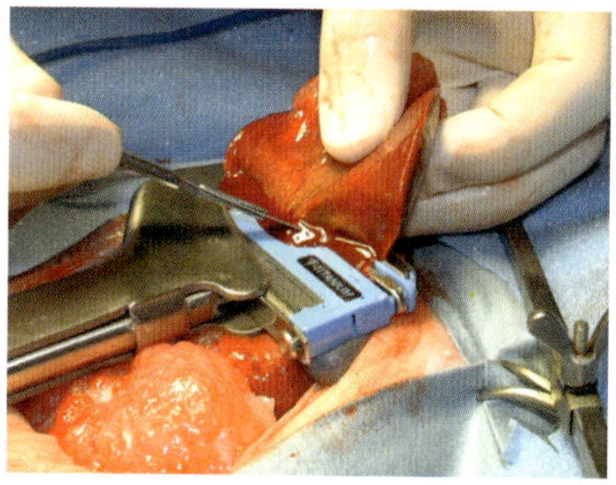

I-ii)

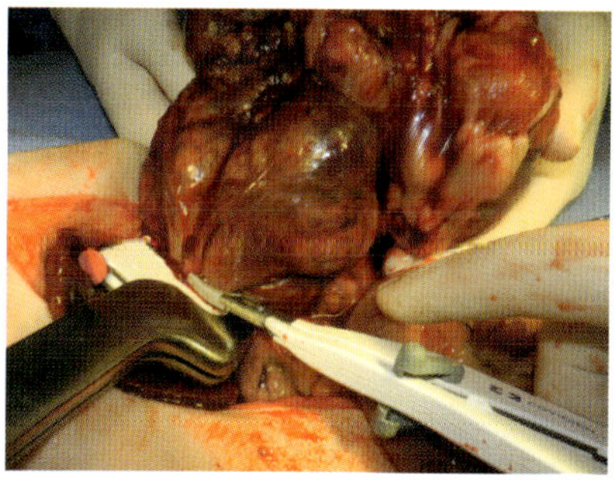

Surgical Technique – Stapling [2] (See Plate 16G–J) *continued*

J) The stapler handle is then released and the stapler is removed. The staple line is assessed for bleeding. If any is noted, then the affected region can be sutured with 3-0 or 4-0 absorbable monofilament suture.

Surgical Technique – Vessel Sealing Device [2] (See Plate 16K)

K) A vessel sealing device can be used to sequentially seal and divide hepatic parenchyma with a minimum of 1-cm surgical margins cranial to the liver mass (i, ii).

Surgical Technique – Pretied Suture Loop [2, 3] (See Plate 16L, M)

L) A prefabricated lasso-like suture loop on a single-use applicator (i) is slid over the isolated liver lobe (ii).
M) The applicator tip is broken off and the suture loop pulled closed over the liver lobe with a minimum of 1-cm surgical margins cranial to the liver mass (pictured). The tissue is then transected distal to the suture loop using either sharp dissection or a vessel sealing device.

Plate 16

Liver Lobectomy *continued*

J)

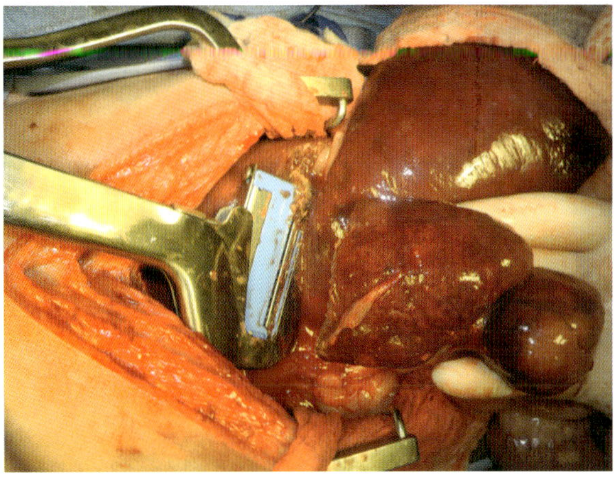

K-i)

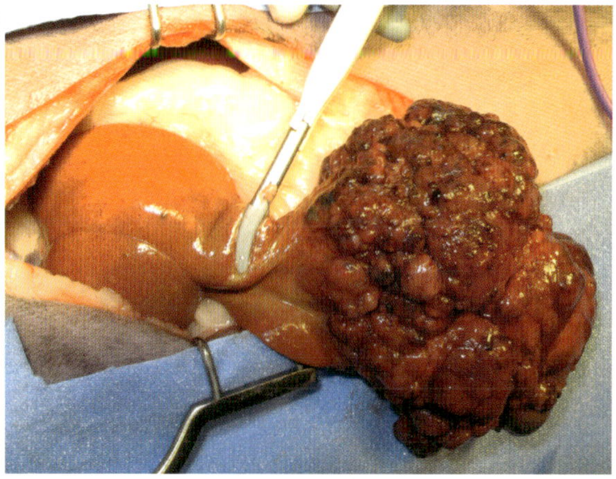

K-ii)

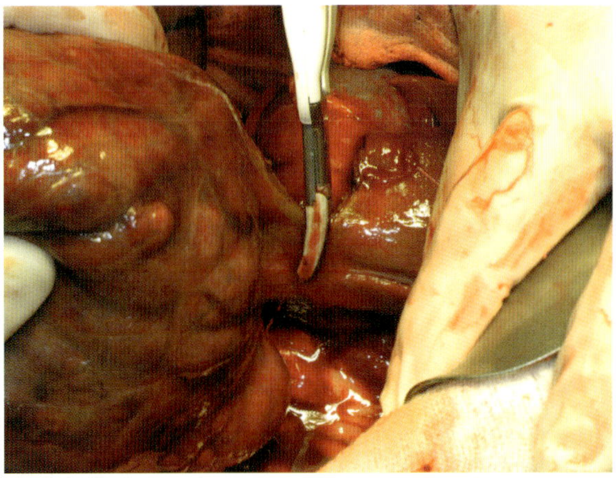

L-i)

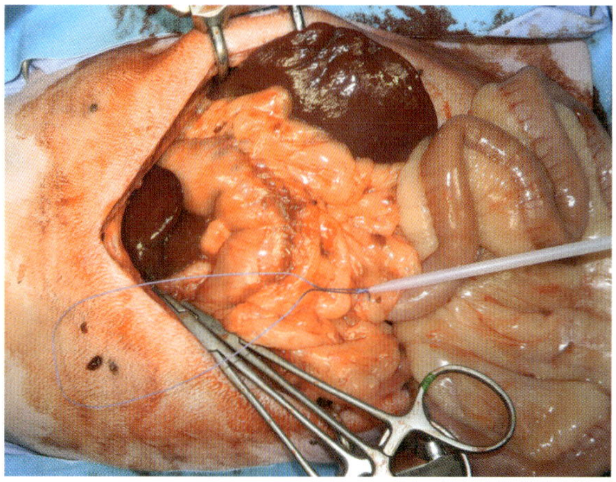

L-ii)

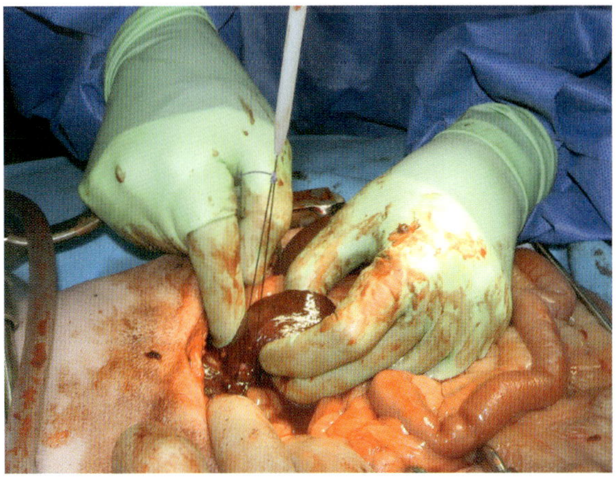

M)

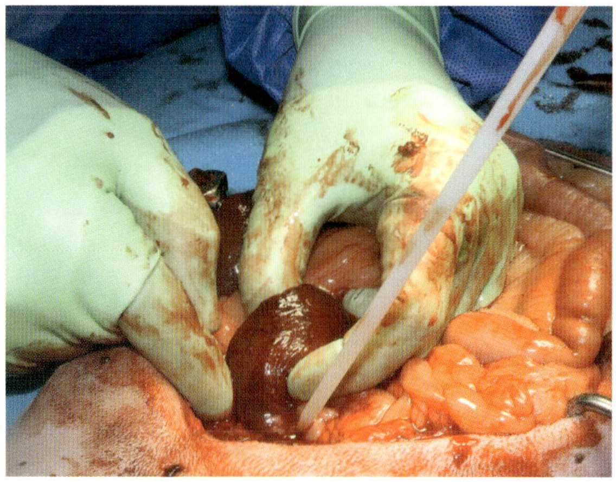

Surgical Technique – Hilar Suturing

Hilar ligation for liver lobectomy differs based on the affected liver lobe. A description for hilar ligation of each liver lobe is included later; however, these are not accompanied with step-by-step images.

Hilar Suturing of the Caudate Liver Lobe [4]

1) The hepatorenal ligament between the caudate lobe and right kidney is incised at the level of the vena cava, allowing the right kidney to be retracted caudally and the caudate lobe to be retracted to the right side.
2) Stay sutures are placed in the gastric pylorus and the stomach is retracted caudally.
3) Vital local anatomic structures are identified, including the CaVC, celiac artery, portal vein, and common bile duct.
4) The right medial and quadrate liver lobes and GB are gently retracted to the left and cranially to expose the right hilar region.
5) The right triangular ligament is transected to improve mobility of the right lateral lobe.
6) At the level of the right hilus, additional structures are identified, such as the cystic duct, hepatic ducts (especially from the left liver division, which will be vital), branching of the right portal vein into the caudate lobar portal vein, and the right lateral lobar portal vein.
7) For caudate liver lobectomy, the peritoneum over the hilus is bluntly dissected. The superficially located lobar bile duct is isolated using right angled forceps and double ligated with monofilament absorbable suture material and divided.
8) The adjacent lobar hepatic artery is likewise isolated, double ligated, and divided; alternatively, a vessel sealing device can be used.
9) The deeper caudate lobar portal vein is then isolated, ligated or sealed with a vessel sealing device, and divided, as described earlier. This will result in a more mobile liver lobe and mass.
10) The insert of a Poole suction tip is then used to bluntly dissect deeper through hepatic parenchyma in a cranioventral direction to the lobar hepatic vein. This is facilitated by gentle caudal traction on the caudate liver lobe.
11) The lobar hepatic vein is then ligated or sealed with a vessel sealing device and divided, thus completing the caudate liver lobectomy. The lobar hepatic vein can be very short in length, almost a venous window into the CaVC in some dogs. A Satinsky vascular clamp should be available to partially clamp the caval wall to oversew this window if required, using 4-0 or 5-0 polypropylene in a simple continuous suture pattern.

Surgical Technique – Hilar Suturing of the Right Lateral Liver Lobe [4]

1) For right lateral liver lobectomy, a similar approach to earlier is made as described earlier with blunt dissection of the peritoneum over the hilus and the more superficial biliary duct and hepatic artery being isolated, ligated or sealed with a vessel sealing device, and divided.
2) The lobar portal vein can then be circumferentially isolated, ligated or sealed with a vessel sealing device, and divided.
3) The insert of a Poole suction tip is used to bluntly dissect the hilar parenchyma toward the CaVC. The right lateral lobar hepatic vein is deep within parenchyma and is separate to the quadrate lobar hepatic vein. This vein is then ligated or sealed with a vessel sealing device and divided, thus completing the right lateral liver lobectomy.

Surgical Technique – Hilar Suturing of the Caudate and Right Lateral Liver Lobes [4]

For combined right divisional liver lobectomy, a similar approach to earlier is made as described earlier. The hepatic bile ducts and arterial branches are isolated, ligated or sealed with a vessel sealing device, and divided at the conjoined hilus. The right portal vein is ligated before it divides into the quadrate and right lateral branches. The separate lobar hepatic veins are then identified, isolated, and ligated or sealed with a vessel sealing device, as described earlier, thus completing the right divisional liver lobectomy.

Surgical Technique – Hilar Suturing of the Papillary Process of the Caudate Lobe [4]

1) For liver lobectomy of the papillary process of the caudate liver lobe, the omental bursa is entered by opening the lesser omentum. Stay sutures are placed in the gastric pylorus, and the stomach is retracted caudally.
2) The lobar hepatic artery lies superficial to the hilus and is isolated, ligated or sealed, and transected. This allows the deeper lobar portal vein to be dissected with right angled forceps; this vein is then double ligated or sealed with a vessel sealing device and divided. The left divisional portal vein, which often courses from right to left across the hilus, should be preserved.
3) The deeper bile duct is then identified, ligated, and divided, which results in mobilization and better exposure of the lobar hilus.
4) The insert of a Poole suction tip is used to bluntly dissect through the hepatic parenchyma a cranial and dorsal direction toward the hepatic vein, which is located slightly to the left in most cases. The hepatic vein is ligated or sealed with a vessel sealing device and divided. Residual parenchymal attachments to the caudate process are then bluntly dissected or sealed and divided with a vessel sealing device to complete lobectomy of the papillary process of the caudal liver lobe.

Surgical Technique – Hilar Suturing of the Central Divisional Liver Lobes [4]

1) The right medial and quadrate lobes have separate draining hepatic veins that merge into a single central hepatic vein. The common central hepatic vein then drains into the left hepatic vein, all within the hepatic parenchyma. For simplicity, combined lobectomy of the right medial and quadrate liver lobes is preferred. Note that the right medial lobe also has an accessory hepatic vein that enters the vena cava separately to the right of midline at the diaphragm.
2) The right triangular ligament attachment to the right medial liver lobe is divided to improve mobility of the right medial liver lobe.
3) Stay sutures are placed in the gastric pylorus and the stomach is retracted caudally.
4) The right medial and quadrate liver lobes and GB are retracted cranially to expose the central hilar region.
5) The GB is freed from the hepatic fossa to the level of the cystic duct with blunt dissection. Alternatively, if the mass is adhered to the GB, then an en bloc cholecystectomy can be performed by isolating the cystic duct with right-angled forceps, and then double ligating and dividing the cystic duct.
6) The lobar bile ducts and hepatic arteries to each lobe lie superficial to the lobar portal veins in the hilus, to the right and left of the right medial and quadrate lobar portal veins, respectively. Each is dissected using right-angled forceps and double ligated or sealed with a vessel sealing device and divided.
7) The lobar portal veins to each lobe are then identified, isolated, and individually ligated or sealed with a vessel sealing device and divided.
8) The insert of a Poole suction tip is used to bluntly dissect between the quadrate and left medial lobe toward the CaVC, allowing for the central division liver lobes to be retracted farther to the right and caudally to expose the central vein.
9) The insert of a Poole suction tip is used to skeletalize the central vein, which is double ligated or sealed with a vessel sealing device and divided before it joins the left hepatic vein.
10) This further mobilizes the central division. The insert of a suction tip is then used to bluntly dissect the parenchyma between the right medial and right lateral liver lobes.
11) The last attachment is the accessory right hepatic vein entering the CaVC to the right of midline at the level of the diaphragm. If this vein is long enough, then it should be ligated or sealed with a vessel sealing device and divided. If the vein is short, then a Satinsky vascular clamp should be used to partially clamp the caval wall, and then the CaVC is oversewn using 4-0 or 5-0 polypropylene in a simple continuous suture pattern.
12) If the GB has been preserved, then it can be pexied to the exposed left medial liver parenchyma.

Surgical Technique – Hilar Suturing of the Left Lateral Liver Lobe [4]

1) The left triangular ligament attachment to the left lateral liver lobe is divided to improve mobility of the left lateral liver lobe.
2) Stay sutures are placed in the gastric pylorus, and the stomach is retracted caudally and to the right.

3) The left lateral liver lobe is reflected craniolaterally to expose the hepatoduodenal ligament. The hepatoduodenal ligament includes the bile ducts and arteries that can be ligated en masse at the base of the lobe, or individually identified and ligated depending on their size. Large liver masses recruit additional blood flow, and the hepatic artery in this location is often prominent.
4) The peritoneum over the left lateral lobar portal vein is opened and right-angled forceps are used to dissect around the vein. Once isolated, the vein is double ligated or sealed with a vessel sealing device and divided.
5) This allows the liver lobe to be retracted farther laterally. The insert of a Poole suction tip is used to bluntly dissect the parenchyma between the left lateral and left medial liver lobes until the left lateral lobar vein, coursing in a craniomedial direction, is isolated, ligated or sealed with a vessel sealing device, and divided, thus completing the left lateral liver lobectomy.

Surgical Technique – Hilar Suturing of the Left Medial Liver Lobe [4]

1) The left medial liver lobe is retracted cranially and the left medial lobar portal vein identified entering the lobe. The peritoneum overlying the vein is divided, and the vein is ligated or sealed with a vessel sealing device and divided.
2) The lobar bile duct and artery lie deep to the lobar portal vein. These are individually isolated, double ligated, and divided.
3) The insert of a Poole suction tip is used to bluntly dissect the parenchyma between the quadrate and left medial liver lobes, and between the left medial and left lateral lobes.
4) Gentle caudal traction on the left medial liver lobe exposes the left medial hepatic vein, which can be isolated and skeletalized before it enters the common left hepatic vein with the insert of a Poole suction tip. Note that some dogs have two or three left medial hepatic veins; if this is the case, these veins should be individually ligated or sealed with a vessel sealing device and divided. The left lateral hepatic vein should be preserved.

Closure (See Plate 16N)

N) If a diaphragmotomy has been performed, a temporary tracheostomy tube is inserted through the diaphragmatic incision and into the pleural space (i). The diaphragmotomy is then closed with a simple continuous suture pattern using 2-0 to 3-0 monofilament absorbable suture material (ii). The pleural space is evacuated of air, and the temporary thoracostomy tube is then removed (iii). The linea alba, subcutaneous tissue, and skin are closed as described in *15.1. Ventral Midline Celiotomy*.
If a paracostal approach has been used, then the muscle, subcutaneous tissue, and skin are closed as described in *15.2. Paracostal Approach*.

Complications

Dogs

Intraoperative Complications

- Overall: 7%–38% [5–7]
- Blood loss (12%–33%), with 79%–95% of these dogs requiring a blood transfusion [3, 5–7] or 17%–31% of dogs treated with liver lobectomy requiring blood transfusions [7, 8]
- Iatrogenic injury to the extrahepatic biliary system (5%) [7]
- Iatrogenic vascular compromise to the left lateral liver lobe during left medial liver lobectomy (5%) [5]
- Iatrogenic occlusion of the CaVC (1%) [6]
- Hypotension
- Unresectable tumor
- Dogs treated with hilar resections were significantly more likely to have intraoperative complications for central division liver lobectomies [7]
- Dogs treated with right medial liver lobectomies were significantly more likely to have intraoperative complications than dogs treated with quadrate liver lobectomies [7]

Plate 16

Liver Lobectomy *continued*

N-i)

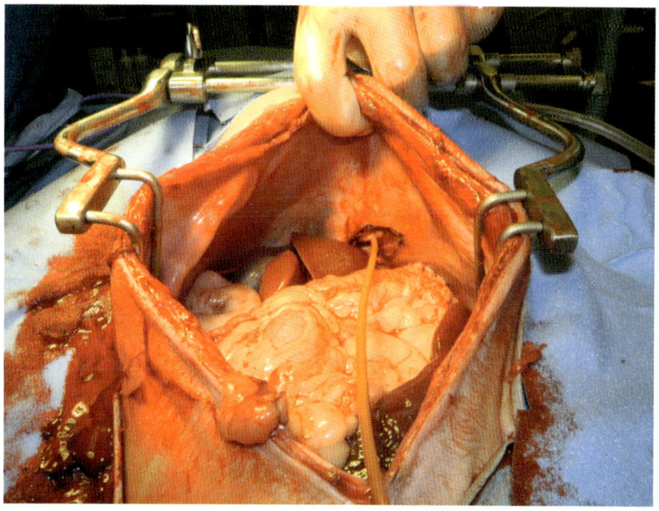

N-ii)

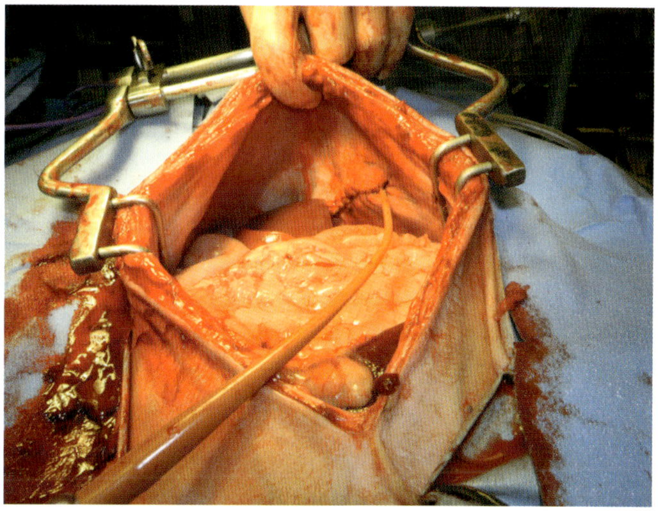

N-iii)

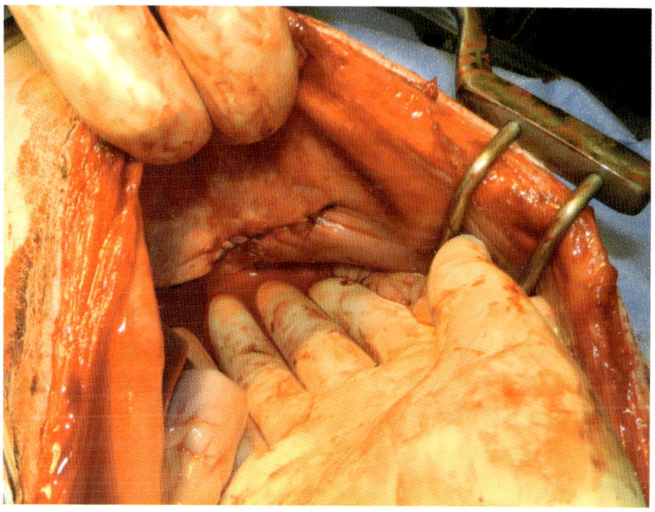

Perioperative Mortality

- Overall: 5%–12% [5, 7–9]

Immediate Postoperative Complications (0–48 Hours)

- Overall: 33% [7]
- Anemia (17%) [7]
- Cardiac arrhythmia (10%) [7]
- Coagulation abnormalities (10%) [7]
- Hypotension (6%), with these dogs having a 100 times greater risk of mortality than dogs with an uncomplicated anesthetic recovery [6]
- Hemoabdomen (3%) [3]
- Hypoglycemia (2%) [7]

Short-Term Postoperative Complications (2–14 Days) [7]

- Overall: 20%
- Aspiration pneumonia (5%)
- Surgical-site infection (5%)
- Bleeding (5%)
- Incisional dehiscence (2%)
- Seroma (2%)
- Hyperglycemia (2%)
- Perforated duodenal ulcer and septic peritonitis (2%)
- Multiorgan dysfunction syndrome (2%)
- Dogs treated with hilar resections were significantly more likely to have short-term complications

Long-Term Postoperative Complications (>14 Days) [7]

- Overall: 2%
- Pancreatitis (2%)

Cats [10]

Intraoperative Complications

- Overall: 41%
- Unresectable tumors (29%)
- Blood loss (12%), with 25% of these cats requiring a blood transfusion

Short-Term Postoperative Complications (During Hospitalization)

- Overall: 54%
- Mild (23% overall)
  - Hyporexia (8%)
  - Esophagitis (4%)
  - Pancreatitis (4%)
- Moderate (15%)
  - Blood transfusion (15%)
- Death (15%)

Suggested Adjuvant Treatment

- ± Chemotherapy for primary hepatic sarcomas
- ± Chemotherapy for primary hepatic neuroendocrine carcinomas

Prognosis and Oncologic Outcome – Dogs

	Local Recurrence Rate	Metastatic Rate	Disease-Free Interval (d)	Median Survival Time (d)	1-Year Survival Rate	2-Year Survival Rate
Hepatocellular Carcinoma [5–7, 9, 11, 12]						
Overall	0%–3%	5%–9%	36 712	707 to >1460	82%	82%
Treatment [5]						
Liver lobectomy	–	–	–	>1460	–	–
No surgery	–	–	–	270	–	–
Tumor location 1 [5]						
Left division liver lobectomies	–	–	–	>1460	–	–
Right division liver lobectomies	–	–	–	365	–	–
Tumor location 2 [11]						
Liver lobe other than quadrate lobe	–	–	–	834	–	–
Quadrate liver lobe	–	–	–	489	–	–
ASA score [11]						
2 or 3	–	–	–	775	–	–
4 or 5	–	–	–	393	–	–
Histologic margins[a] [9]						
Complete histologic margins	12%	–	1000	>1836	–	–
Incomplete histologic margins	58%	–	521	765	–	–

[a] Note that histologic margins were not prognostic for local tumor recurrence, disease-free interval, or median survival in four studies [5, 7, 11, 12].
ASA, American Society of Anesthesiologists.

Prognosis and Oncologic Outcome – Cats

	Local Recurrence Rate	Metastatic Rate	Disease-Free Interval (d)	Median Survival Time (d)	1-Year Survival Rate	2-Year Survival Rate
			Overall [10, 13]			
Overall	0%–29%	0%–21%	151 (local recurrence) 186 (metastasis)	375–877	–	–
			Hepatocellular Carcinoma [10]			
Overall	6%	0%	–	868	–	–
			Bile Duct Carcinoma [10]			
Overall	7%	15%	–	270	–	–
			Neuroendocrine Carcinoma [10]			
Overall	50%	0%	–	246 (n = 1)	–	–
			Primary Sarcoma [10]			
Overall	17%	0%	–	16	–	–

References

1 Dean, B., Anderson, T., Garcia-Pertierra, S. et al. (2020). Diaphragmotomy to aid exposure during hepatobiliary surgery: a multi-centre retrospective review of 31 dogs. *J. Small Anim. Pract.* 61 (5): 278–284.

2 Risselada, M., Ellison, G.W., Bacon, N.J. et al. (2010). Comparison of 5 surgical techniques for partial liver lobectomy in the dog for intraoperative blood loss and surgical time. *Vet. Surg.* 39 (7): 856–862.

3 Goodman, A.R. and Casale, S.A. (2014). Short-term outcome following partial or complete liver lobectomy with a commercially prepared self-ligating loop in companion animals: 29 cases (2009-2012). *J. Am. Vet. Med. Assoc.* 244 (6): 693–698.

4 Covey, J.L., Degner, D.A., Jackson, A.H. et al. (2009). Hilar liver resection in dogs. *Vet. Surg.* 38 (1): 104–111.

5 Liptak, J.M., Dernell, W.S., Monnet, E. et al. (2004). Massive hepatocellular carcinoma in dogs: 48 cases (1992-2002). *J. Am. Vet. Med. Assoc.* 225 (8): 1225–1230.

6 Kinsey, J.R., Gilson, S.D., Hauptman, J. et al. (2015). Factors associated with long-term survival in dogs undergoing liver lobectomy as treatment for liver tumors. *Can. Vet. J.* 56 (6): 598–604.

7 Linden, D.S., Liptak, J.M., Vinayak, A. et al. (2019). Outcomes and prognostic variables associated with central division hepatic lobectomies: 61 dogs. *Vet. Surg.* 48 (3): 309–314.

8 Hanson, K.R., Pigott, A.M., and Linklater, A.K. (2017). Incidence of blood transfusion requirements and factors associated with transfusion following liver lobectomy in dogs and cats: 72 cases (2007-2015). *J. Am. Vet. Med. Assoc.* 251 (8): 929–934.

9 Matsuyama, A., Takagi, S., Hosoya, K. et al. (2017). Impact of surgical margins on survival of 37 dogs with massive hepatocellular carcinoma. *N Z Vet. J.* 65 (5): 227–231.

10 Brandstetter, V., Schmidt, J.M., Findji, L. et al. (2023). Feline primary nonhematopoietic malignant liver tumours: a multicenter retrospective study (2000-2021). *Vet. Comp. Oncol.* 21 (2): 191–199.

11 Moyer, J., Lopez, D.J., Balkman, C.E. et al. (2021). Factors associated with survival in dogs with a histopathological diagnosis of hepatocellular carcinoma: 94 cases (2007-2018). *Open Vet. J.* 11 (1): 144–153.

12 Lapsley, J.M., Wavreille, V., Barry, S. et al. (2022). Risk factors and outcome in dogs with recurrent massive hepatocellular carcinoma: a veterinary society of surgical oncology case-control study. *Vet. Comp. Oncol.* 20 (3): 697–709.

13 Goussev, S.A., Center, S.A., Randolph, J.F. et al. (2016). Clinical characteristics of hepatocellular carcinoma in 19 cats from a single institution (1980-2013). *J. Am. Anim. Hosp. Assoc.* 52 (1): 36–41.

Chapter 17: Splenectomy

17.1 Open Splenectomy

Indications

1) Resection of benign and malignant splenic masses
2) Management of nonneoplastic conditions, such as splenic torsion, splenic rupture, splenic necrosis associated with gastric dilatation-volvulus, generalized infiltrative disease, and immune-mediated disease

Suggested Diagnostic Workup and Clinical Staging

- Complete blood count, serum biochemistry, and urinalysis
- ± Coagulation profile
- ± Cross matching or blood typing
- Abdominal ultrasound or precontrast and postcontrast computed tomography (CT) scan of the abdomen for characterization of the splenic mass and assessment of intra-abdominal metastasis
- ± Ultrasound- or CT-guided fine-needle aspirate cytology
- Three-view thoracic radiographs or thoracic CT scan for assessment of lung metastasis
- ± Echocardiography for assessment of cardiac masses

Patient Positioning

The patient is positioned in dorsal recumbency.

Surgical Technique (See Plate 17.1A–H)

A) A ventral midline celiotomy is performed (see *15.1. Ventral Midline Celiotomy*). If there is a hemoabdomen, then the blood should either be removed by suction (i, ii) or collected for autotransfusion.
B) The splenic mass should be exteriorized (i). For large splenic masses, the abdominal incision may need to be extended to avoid rupture of the splenic mass during exteriorization (ii, arrow).
C) In some cases, there will be omentum adhered to the splenic capsule, usually if there has been a recent bleed. The omentum should not be detached because this may represent tumor invasion into the omentum rather than adhesions. The omentum should be ligated with 2-0 or 3-0 absorbable monofilament suture material or transected with a vessel sealing device (pictured), leaving a cuff of approximately 5 cm of omentum attached to the spleen.

Color Atlas of Canine and Feline Surgical Oncology, First Edition. Julius M. Liptak, Paolo Buracco, William T. N. Culp, and Nicholas J. Bacon.

Plate 17.1

Open Splenectomy

A-i)

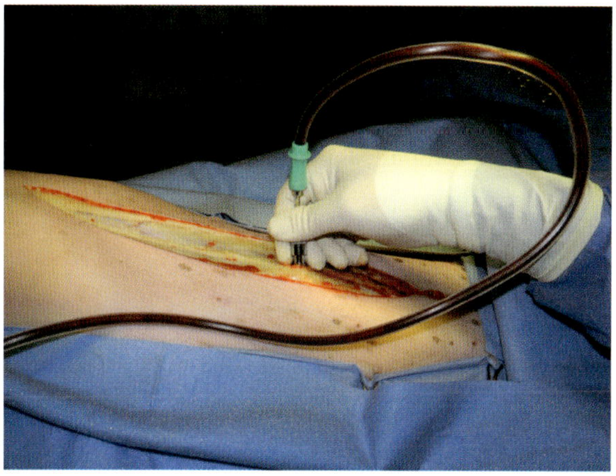

A-ii)

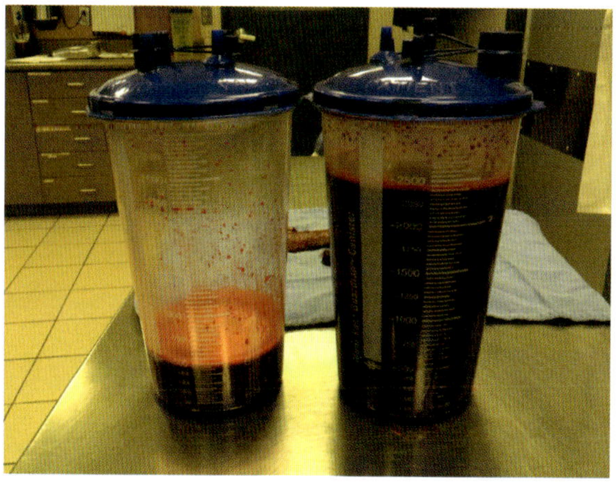

B-i)

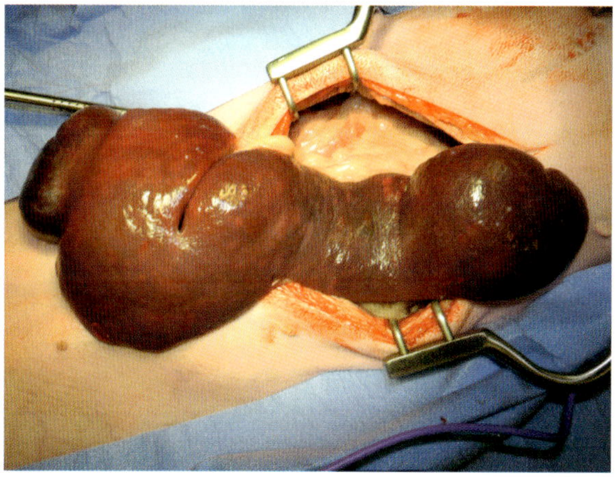

B-ii)

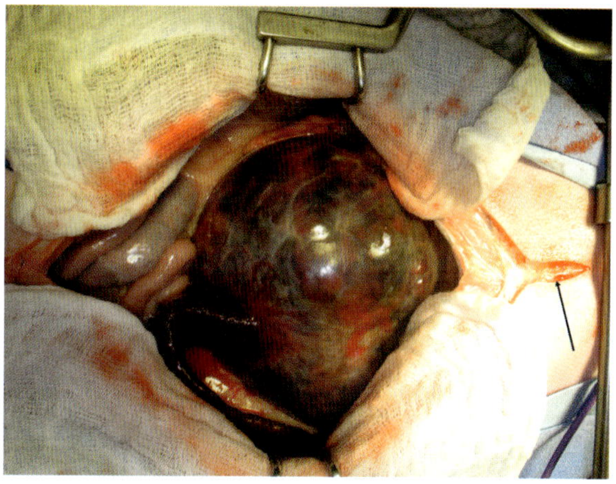

C)

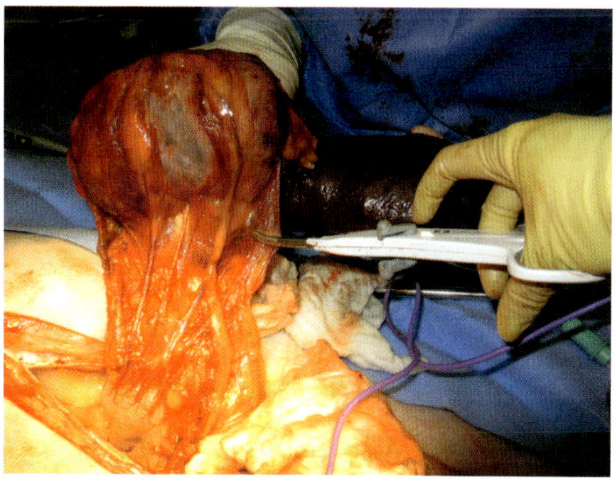

Surgical Technique (See Plate 17.1A–H) *continued*

D) **Suture technique 1:** The splenic hilar vessels are sequentially clamped with hemostats approximately 2 cm from the hilus of the spleen (i). The hilar vessels are then ligated using a simple circumferential ligature of 3-0 absorbable suture material from the tail to the head of the spleen (ii). After ligation, these vessels are transected with Metzenbaum scissors between the hemostats and ligatures (iii). The ends of the ligated and transected vessels should be checked for bleeding (iv). The splenic artery (v) should be ligated with a simple and a transfixion ligature of 2-0 to 3-0 absorbable suture material, and the splenic vein (v) with a single simple ligature of 3-0 absorbable suture material. After ligation, these vessels are transected with Metzenbaum scissors between the hemostats and ligatures (vi). The ends of the ligated and transected vessels should be checked for bleeding.

Plate 17.1

Open Splenectomy *continued*

D-i)

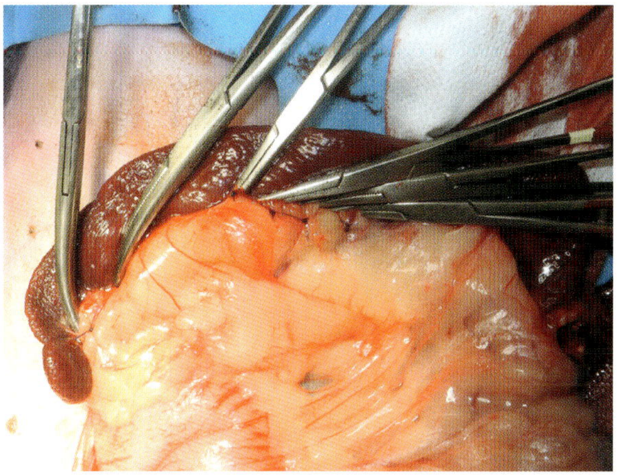

D-ii)

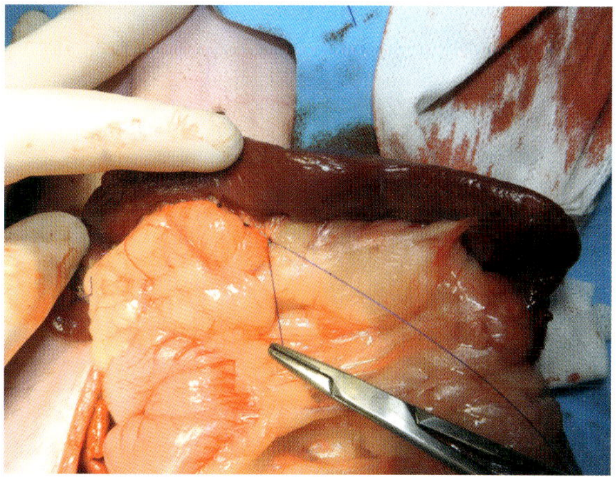

D-iii)

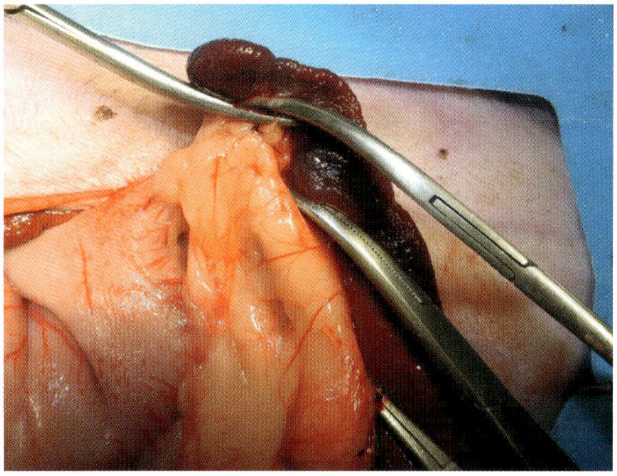

D-iv)

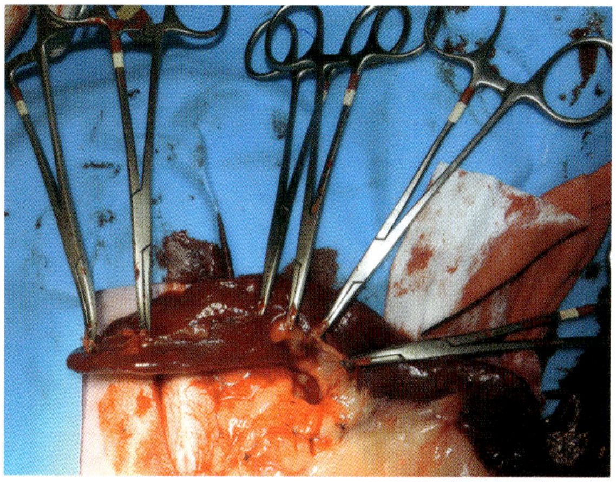

D-v)

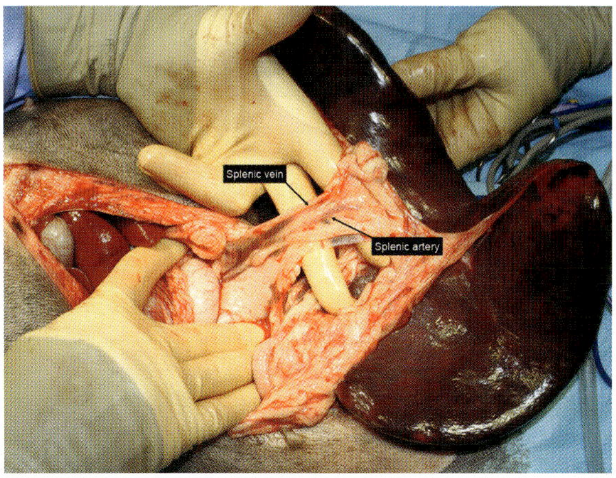

Courtesy of Dr. Laurent Findji

D-vi)

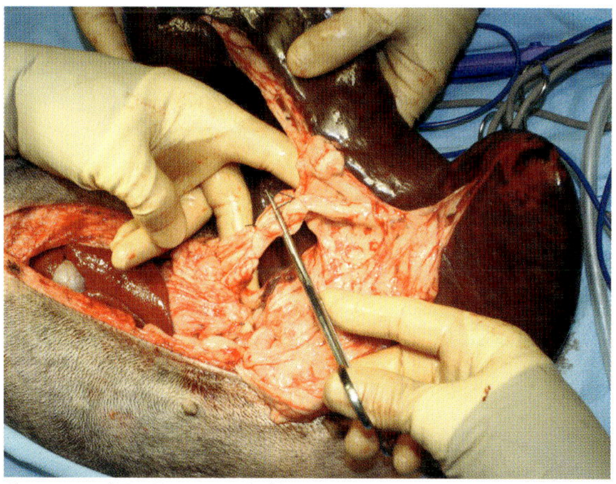

Courtesy of Dr. Laurent Findji

Surgical Technique (See Plate 17.1A–H) *continued*

E) **Suture technique 2 [1]:** The splenic artery is ligated immediately lateral to the tip of the left limb of the pancreas and proximal to the branching of the left gastroepiploic artery with 2-0 or 3-0 absorbable suture material. A second transfixion ligature, distal to the first ligature, is recommended on the splenic artery. The splenic vein is similarly ligated with a single circumferential ligature using 3-0 absorbable suture material (dashed line). The gastroepiploic artery and vein feeding the greater curvature are then ligated, followed by ligation of the short gastric arteries and veins. After ligation, these vessels are transected with Metzenbaum scissors between the hemostats and ligatures. The ends of the ligated and transected vessels should be checked for bleeding.

F) **Stapler technique [2, 3]:** The hilar suture technique can be performed with staples rather than suture material. Two different types of stapler can be used for this purpose: hemostatic clips (i, Autosuture Premium Surgiclip, Covidien) or a ligating and dividing stapler (LDS; ii, iii, ligating and dividing stapler; Covidien). These staplers are not as secure as ligatures, and this technique is less commonly performed with the increasing popularity of vessel sealing devices. The splenic artery should be ligated with a simple and a transfixion ligature of 2-0 to 3-0 absorbable suture material, and the splenic vein with a single simple ligature of 3-0 absorbable suture material. After ligation, these vessels are transected with Metzenbaum scissors between the hemostats and ligatures. The ends of the ligated and transected vessels should be checked for bleeding.

Plate 17.1

Open Splenectomy *continued*

E)

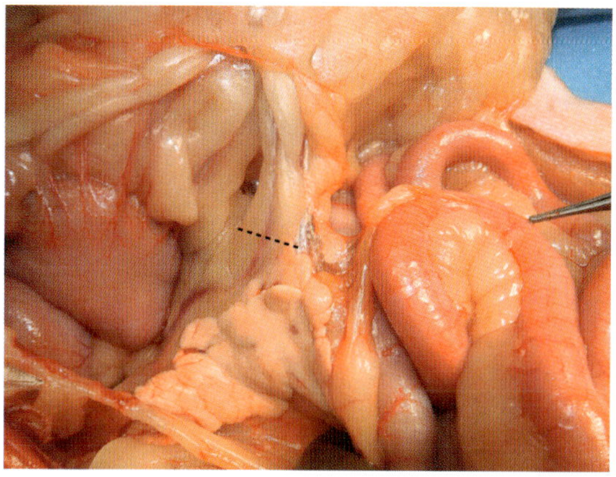

F-i)

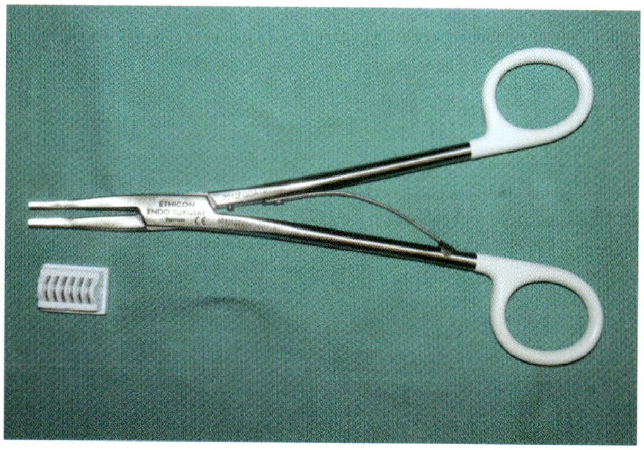

F-ii)

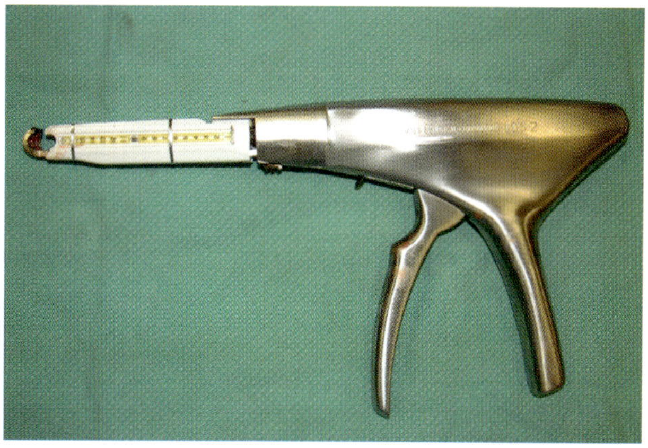

F-iii)

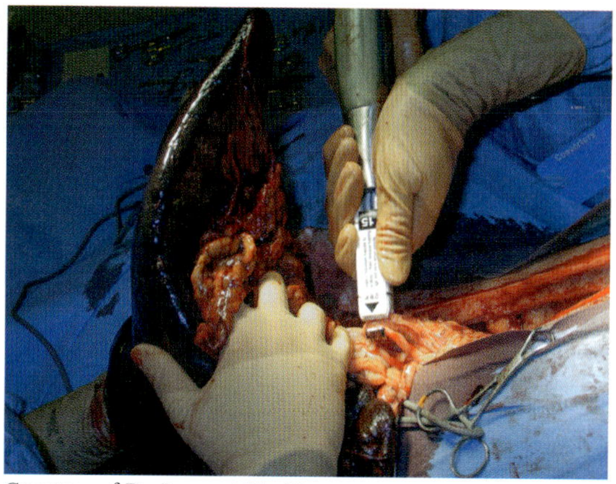

Courtesy of Dr. Laurent Findji

Surgical Technique (See Plate 17.1A–H) *continued*

G) **Vessel sealing device technique [3, 4]:** The hilar suture technique can be performed with a vessel sealing device (i–vi) rather than suture material, such as a LigaSure (Covidien, pictured), EnSeal (Ethicon Endo-Surgery, Johnson & Johnson), and harmonic handpieces (Ethicon Endo-Surgery, Johnson & Johnson). LigaSure and EnSeal can seal blood vessels up to 7 mm in diameter. For medium to large breed dogs, it is prudent to ligate the splenic artery with a simple and a transfixion ligature of 2-0 to 3-0 absorbable suture material, and the splenic vein with a single simple ligature of 3-0 absorbable suture material (vii, viii). After these vessels have been ligated, then they are sealed and transected with the vessel sealing device (ix).

Plate 17.1

Open Splenectomy *continued*

G-i)

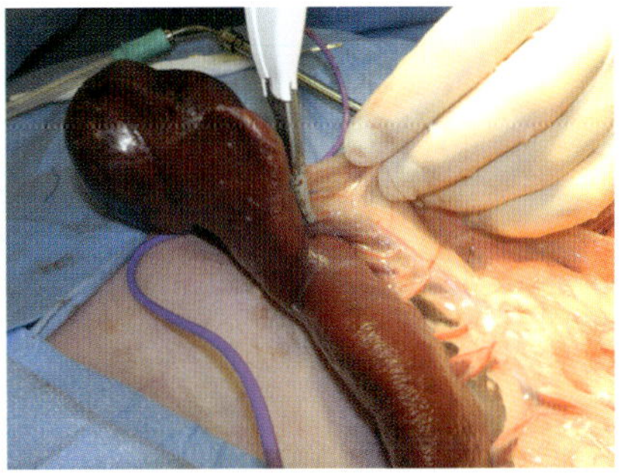

G-ii)

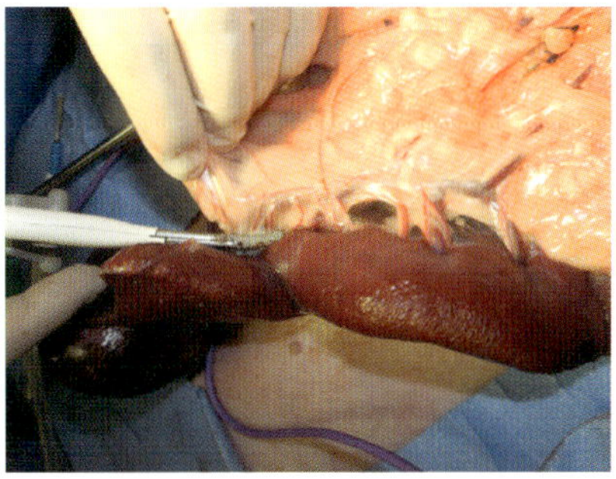

G-iii)

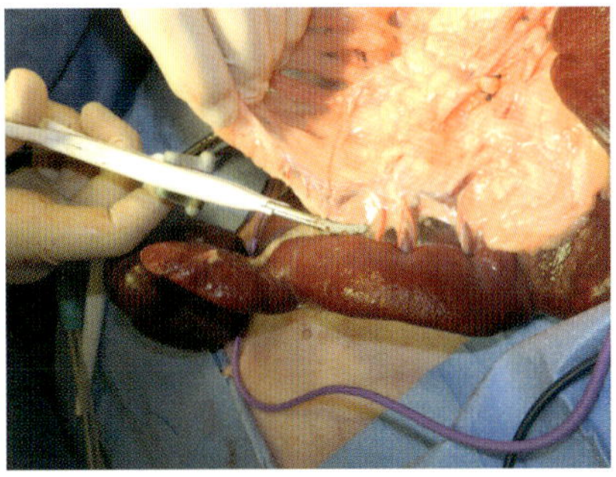

G-iv)

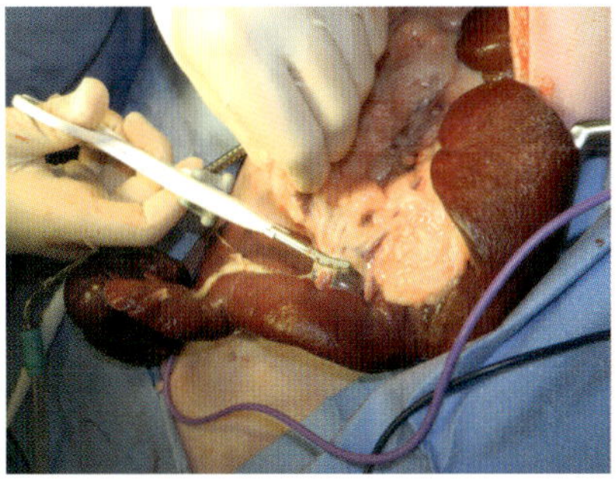

G-v)

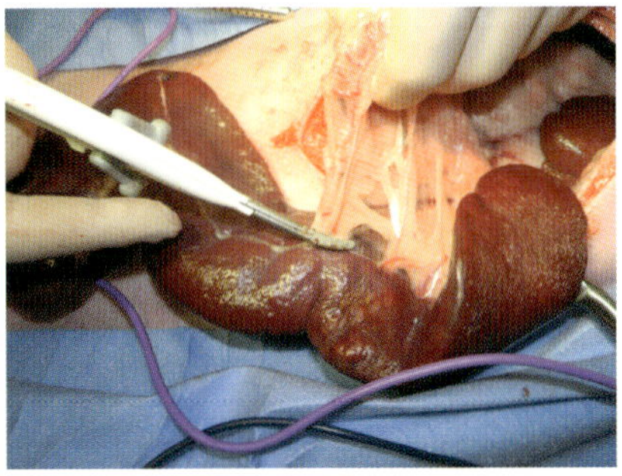

G-vi)

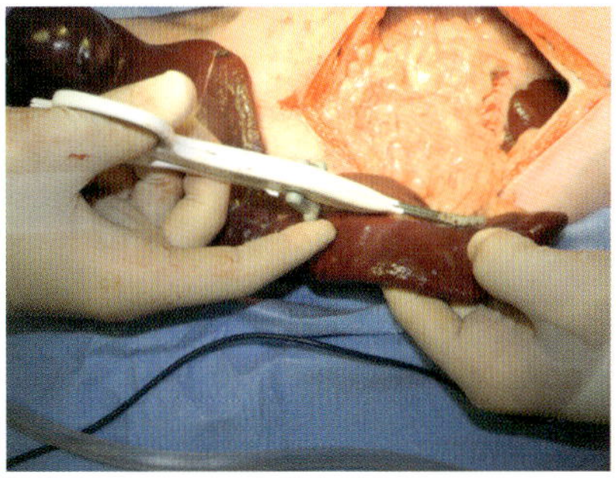

G-vii)

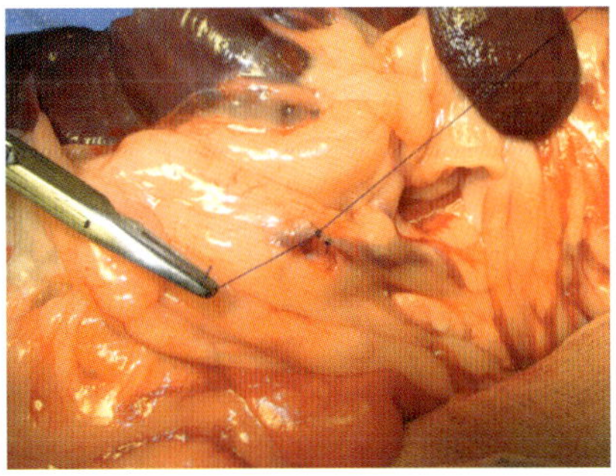

G-viii)

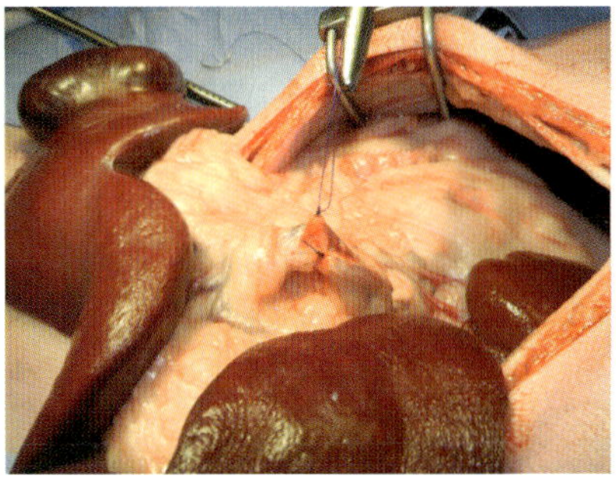

G-ix)

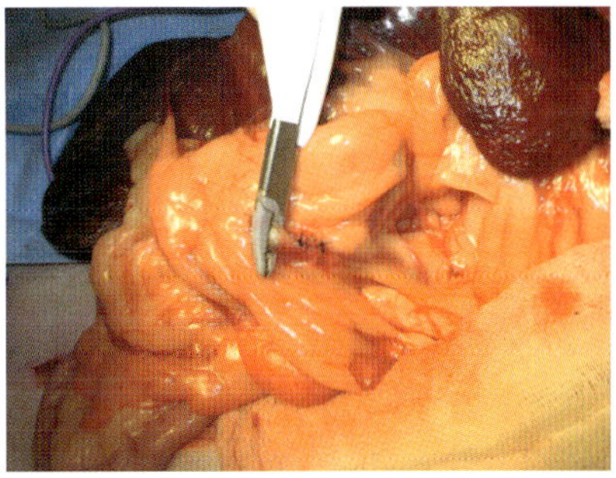

Surgical Technique (See Plate 17.1A–H) *continued*

H) The abdominal cavity should be systematically explored for metastatic disease. The most common metastatic sites for splenic hemangiosarcoma include the liver (i–iii), omentum (iv), kidneys (v, arrow), adrenal gland, and abdominal wall (vi, vii). After completion of the splenectomy and abdominal exploration, the abdominal cavity should be lavaged with warmed, sterile isotonic saline.

Plate 17.1

Open Splenectomy *continued*

H-i)
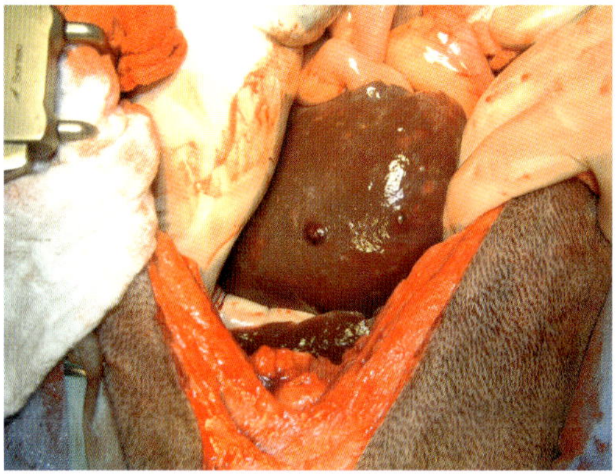

H-ii)
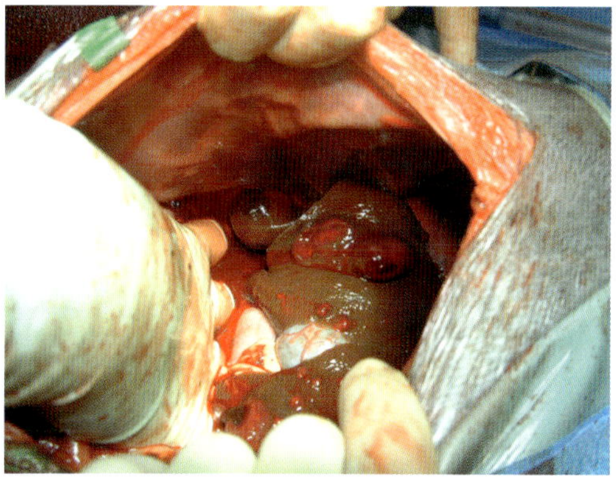

H-iii)
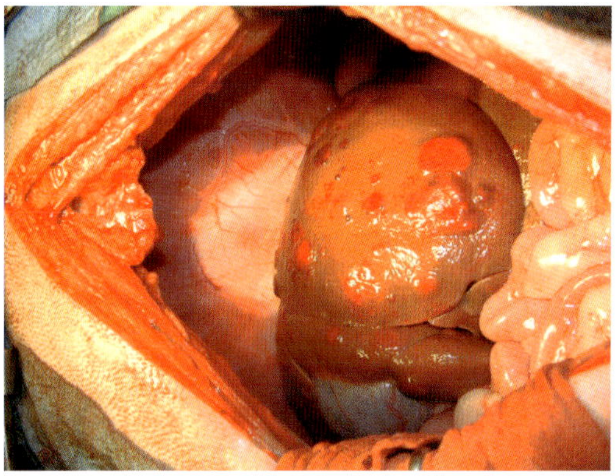

H-iv)
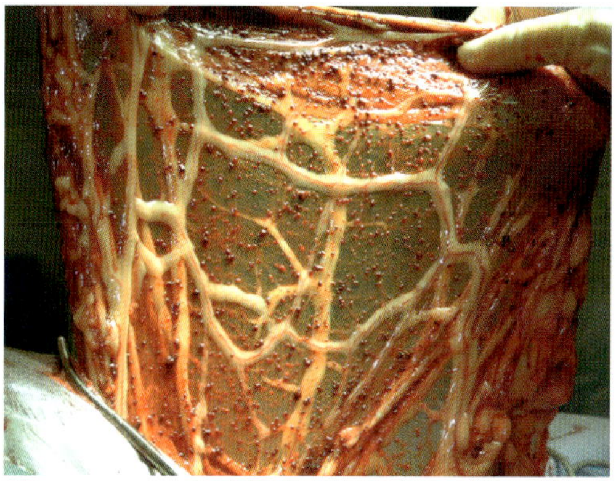

H-v)
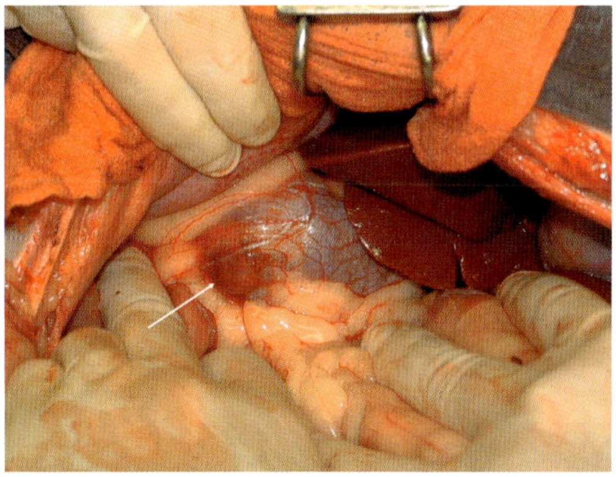

H-vi)
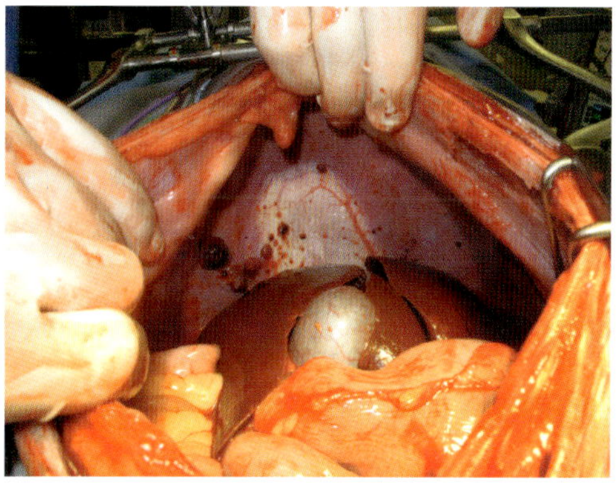

H-vii)
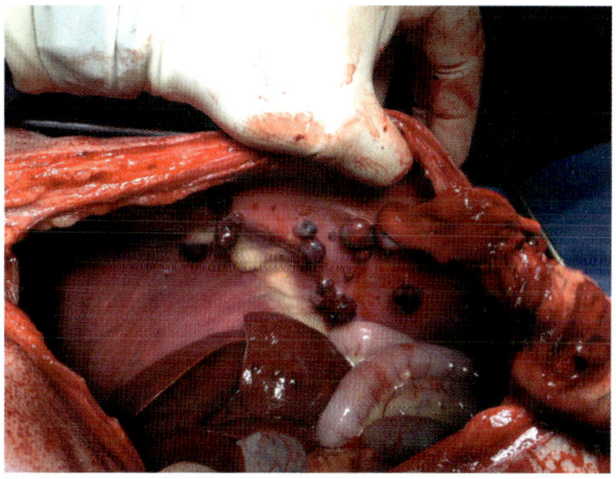

Closure

The linea alba, subcutaneous tissue, and skin are closed as described in *15.1. Ventral Midline Celiotomy*.

Postoperative Management

1) Multimodal analgesia
2) Elizabethan collar or body suit
3) Electrocardiogram monitoring
4) ± Blood transfusion (autotransfusion or allotransfusion)

Complications

Intraoperative Complications

- Splenic rupture and bleeding
- Ventricular arrhythmias
- Hypovolemia

Postoperative Complications

- Perioperative mortality (7.6%–10.8%), associated with preoperative thrombocytopenia and anemia, intraoperative ventricular arrhythmias, increased anesthetic duration, and intraoperative or postoperative administration of blood products [5, 6]
- Incisional complications
- Cardiac arrhythmias (especially ventricular premature complexes)
- Ischemic necrosis of the left limb of the pancreas (suture technique 2)
- Transfusion reactions
- Hemoabdomen
- Portal vein thrombosis
- Disseminated intravascular coagulation

Suggested Adjuvant Treatments

- Chemotherapy for dogs with splenic hemangiosarcomas, splenic histiocytic sarcomas, and high-grade nonangiomatous/nonlymphomatous splenic sarcomas

Prognosis and Oncologic Outcome

Tumor Type	Local Recurrence Rate	Metastatic Rate	Disease-Free Interval (d)	Median Survival Time (d)	1-Year Survival Rate	2-Year Survival Rate
Hemangiosarcoma						
Overall [7–13]	0%	62%–96%	125–185	50–200	9%–29%	9%
Treatment [7–18]						
• Surgery	–	–	–	19–86	11%	4%
– I	–	–	–	167–238	35%	12%
– II	–	–	–	61–82	13%	5%
– III	–	–	–	27–65	0%	0%
• Surgery and chemotherapy	–	–	126–178	103–274	12%–23%	3%
– I	–	–	259–338	196–983	–	–
– II	–	–	125–151	96–303	0–23%	–
– III	–	–	62	23–195	8%	–
Thrombocytopenia [19]						
• Stage I/II						
– No	–	–	203	259	–	–
– Yes	–	–	138	159	–	–
• Stage III						
– No	–	–	77	154	–	–
– Yes	–	–	60	60	–	–
Sternal lymphadenopathy [20]						
• No	–	–	–	68	–	–
• Yes	–	–	–	33	–	–
Nonangiomatous/Nonlymphomatous Sarcoma [21–24]						
Overall	–	40%–70%	147	76–599	0%–20%	–
Metastasis at diagnosis [21, 23]						
• No	–	–	–	274–590	–	–
• Yes	–	–	–	30–65	–	–
Mitotic count [22, 23]						
• ≤9/10 hpf	–	–	–	NR	40%	–
• >9/10 hpf	–	–	–	30–269	0%–20%	–
Histologic grade [23]						
• I	–	20%	–	NR	–	–
• II	–	27%	–	589	–	–
• III	–	60%	–	158	–	–
Histiocytic Sarcoma						
Surgery [22, 25]	–	66%	–	29–30	–	–
Surgery and chemotherapy [26]	–	36%	205	427	–	–

(Continued)

Tumor Type	Local Recurrence Rate	Metastatic Rate	Disease-Free Interval (d)	Median Survival Time (d)	1-Year Survival Rate	2-Year Survival Rate
			Liposarcoma [27]			
Overall	–	42%	–	623	–	–
Metastasis at diagnosis						
• No	–	–	–	767	–	–
• Yes	–	–	–	45	–	–
Histologic grade						
• I	–	–	–	1009	–	–
• II	–	–	–	206	–	–
• III	–	–	–	74	–	–
			Lymphoma			
Overall [28, 29]	–	37%	377	377–383	60%	–
Clinical signs [29]						
• Asymptomatic	–	–	–	1153	–	–
• Symptomatic	–	–	–	309	–	–
Hemoabdomen [28]						
• No	–	–	–	NR	–	–
• Yes	–	–	–	120	–	–
Lymphoma type [29]						
• Marginal zone	–	–	NR	NR	64%	–
• Mantle cell	–	–	NR	NR	89%	–
• Other B cell	–	–	561	561	50%	–
• NU/NK cell	–	–	0	8	0%	–
• Peripheral T cell	–	–	0	4	0%	–
			Benign Splenic Masses [30, 31]			
Overall	–	11%	–	436 to NR	64%	–

hpf, high-power fields; NR, not reached.

References

1 Hosgood, G., Bone, D.L., Vorhees, W.D. et al. (1989). Splenectomy in the dog by ligation of the splenic and short gastric arteries. *Vet. Surg.* 18 (2): 110–113.

2 Tobias, K.M. (2007). Surgical stapling devices in veterinary medicine: a review. *Vet. Surg.* 36 (4): 341–349.

3 Monarski, C.J., Jaffe, M.H., and Kass, P.H. (2014). Decreased surgical time with a vessel sealing device versus a surgical stapler in performance of canine splenectomy. *J. Am. Anim. Hosp. Assoc.* 50 (1): 42–45.

4 Rivier, P. and Monnet, E. (2011). Use of a vessel sealant device for splenectomy in dogs. *Vet. Surg.* 40 (1): 102–105.

5 Wendelburg, K.M., O'Toole, T.E., McCobb, E. et al. (2014). Risk factors for perioperative death in dogs undergoing splenectomy for splenic masses: 539 cases (2001-2012). *J. Am. Vet. Med. Assoc.* 245 (12): 1382–1390.

6 Sirochman, A.L., Milovancev, M., Townsend, K. et al. (2020). Influence of a bipolar vessel sealing device on short-term postoperative mortality after splenectomy: 203 dogs (2005-2018). *Vet. Surg.* 49 (2): 291–303.

7 Lana, S., U'ren, L., Plaza, S. et al. (2007). Continuous low-dose oral chemotherapy for adjuvant therapy of splenic hemangiosarcoma in dogs. *J. Vet. Intern. Med.* 21 (4): 764–769.

8 Kahn, S.A., Mullin, C.M., de Lorimier, L.P. et al. (2013). Doxorubicin and deracoxib adjuvant therapy for canine splenic hemangiosarcoma: a pilot study. *Can. Vet. J.* 54 (3): 237–242.

9 Göritz, M., Müller, K., Krastel, D. et al. (2013). Canine splenic haemangiosarcoma: influence of metastases, chemotherapy and growth pattern on post-splenectomy survival and expression of angiogenic factors. *J. Comp. Pathol.* 149 (1): 30–39.

10 Matsuyama, A., Poirier, V.J., Mantovani, F. et al. (2017). Adjuvant doxorubicin with or without metronomic cyclophosphamide for canine splenic hemangiosarcoma. *J. Am. Anim. Hosp. Assoc.* 53 (6): 304–312.
11 Batchinski, K., Nobre, A., Vargas-Mendez, E. et al. (2018). Canine visceral hemangiosarcoma treated with surgery alone or surgery and doxorubicin: 37 cases (2005-2014). *Can. Vet. J.* 59 (9): 967–972.
12 Bray, J.P., Orbell, G., Cave, N. et al. (2018). Does thalidomide prolong survival in dogs with splenic haemangiosarcoma? *J. Small Anim. Pract.* 59 (2): 85–91.
13 Treggiari, E., Borrego, J.F., Gramer, I. et al. (2020). Retrospective comparison of first-line adjuvant anthracycline vs metronomic-based chemotherapy protocols in the treatment of stage I and II canine splenic haemangiosarcoma. *Vet. Comp. Oncol.* 18 (1): 43–51.
14 Kim, S.E., Liptak, J.M., Gall, T.T. et al. (2007). Epirubicin in the adjuvant treatment of splenic hemangiosarcoma in dogs: 59 cases (1997–2004). *J. Am. Vet. Med. Assoc.* 231 (10): 1550–1557.
15 Teske, E., Rutteman, G.R., Kirpenstein, J. et al. (2011). A randomized controlled study into the efficacy and toxicity of pegylated liposome encapsulated doxorubicin as an adjuvant therapy in dogs with splenic haemangiosarcoma. *Vet. Comp. Oncol.* 9 (4): 283–289.
16 Alvarez, F.J., Hosoya, K., Lara-Garcia, A. et al. (2013). VAC protocol for treatment of dogs with stage III hemangiosarcoma. *J. Am. Anim. Hosp. Assoc.* 49 (6): 370–377.
17 Wendelburg, K.M., Price, L.L., Burgess, K.E. et al. (2015). Survival time of dogs with splenic hemangiosarcoma treated by splenectomy with or without adjuvant chemotherapy: 208 cases (2001-2012). *J. Am. Vet. Med. Assoc.* 247 (4): 393–403.
18 Moore, A.S., Rassnick, K.M., and Frimberger, A.E. (2017). Evaluation of clinical and histologic factors associated with survival time in dogs with stage II splenic hemangiosarcoma treated by splenectomy and adjuvant chemotherapy: 30 cases (2011-2014). *J. Am. Vet. Med. Assoc.* 251 (5): 559–565.
19 Masyr, A.R., Rendahl, A.K., Winter, A.L. et al. (2021). Retrospective evaluation of thrombocytopenia and tumor stage as prognostic indicators in dogs with splenic hemangiosarcoma. *J. Am. Vet. Med. Assoc.* 258 (6): 630–637.
20 Kelsey, J., Balfour, R., Szabo, D. et al. (2022). Prognostic value of sternal lymphadenopathy on malignancy and outcome in dogs undergoing splenectomy. *Vet. Comp. Oncol.* 20 (1): 1–7.
21 Weinstein, M.J., Carpenter, J.L., and Schunk, C.J. (1989). Nonangiogenic and nonlymphomatous sarcomas of the canine spleen: 57 cases (1975-1987). *J. Am. Vet. Med. Assoc.* 195 (6): 784–788.
22 Sprangler, W.L., Culbertson, M.R., and Kass, P.H. (1994). Primary mesenchymal (nonangiomatous/nonlymphomatous) neoplasms occurring in the canine spleen: Anatomic classification, immunohistochemistry, and mitotic activity correlated with patient survival. *Vet. Pathol.* 31 (1): 37–47.
23 Linden, D., Liptak, J.M., Vinayak, A. et al. (2019). Outcomes and prognostic variables associated with primary abdominal visceral soft tissue sarcomas in dogs: a veterinary society of surgical oncology retrospective study. *Vet. Comp. Oncol.* 17 (3): 265–270.
24 Ferarri, R., Marconato, L., Boracchi, P. et al. (2024). Splenic stromal factors in dogs: Outcome and clinicopathological prognostic factors in 32 cases. *Vet. Comp. Oncol.* 22 (1): 12–21.
25 Constantino-Casas, F., Mayhew, D., Hoather, T.M. et al. (2011). The clinical presentation and histopathologic-immunohistochemical classification of histiocytic sarcomas in the flat-coated retriever. *Vet. Pathol.* 48 (3): 764–771.
26 Latifi, M., Tuohy, J.L., Coutermarsh-Ott, S.L. et al. (2020). Clinical outcomes in dogs with localized splenic histiocytic sarcoma treated with splenectomy with or without chemotherapy. *J. Vet. Intern. Med.* 34 (6): 2645–2650.
27 Gower, K.L.A., Liptak, J.M., WTN, C. et al. (2015). Splenic liposarcoma in dogs: 13 cases (2002-2012). *J. Am. Vet. Med. Assoc.* 247 (12): 1404–1407.
28 O'Brien, D., Moore, P.F., Vernau, W. et al. (2013). Clinical characteristics and outcome in dogs with splenic marginal zone lymphoma. *J. Vet. Intern. Med.* 27 (4): 949–954.
29 van Stee, L.L., Boston, S.E., Singh, A. et al. (2015). Outcome and prognostic factors for canine splenic lymphoma treated by splenectomy (1995-2011). *Vet. Surg.* 44 (8): 976–982.
30 Cleveland, M.J. and Casale, S. (2016). Incidence of malignancy and outcomes for dogs undergoing splenectomy for incidentally detected nonruptured splenic nodules or masses: 105 cases (2009-2013). *J. Am. Vet. Med. Assoc.* 248 (11): 1267–1273.
31 Patten, S.G., Boston, S.E., and Monteith, G.J. (2016). Outcome and prognostic factors for dogs with a histologic diagnosis of splenic hematoma following splenectomy: 35 cases (2001-2013). *Can. Vet. J.* 57 (8): 842–846.

17.2 Laparoscopic and Laparoscopic-Assisted Splenectomy

Indications

1) Laparoscopic and laparoscopic-assisted splenectomy are generally indicated for diffuse splenic disease or splenic masses that are relatively small.
2) Note that a laparoscopic approach for splenectomy does not allow for a full abdominal exploration, and this needs to be considered when choosing a laparoscopic approach for resection of a potentially malignant splenic tumor.

Suggested Diagnostic Workup and Clinical Staging

- Complete blood count, serum biochemistry, and urinalysis
- ± Coagulation profile
- ± Cross matching or blood typing
- Abdominal ultrasound or precontrast and postcontrast computed tomography (CT) scan of the abdomen for characterization of the splenic mass and assessment of intra-abdominal metastasis
- ± Ultrasound- or CT-guided fine-needle aspirate cytology
- Three-view thoracic radiographs or thoracic CT scan for assessment of lung metastasis
- ± Echocardiography for assessment of cardiac masses

Patient Positioning

The patient is positioned in dorsal recumbency.

Surgical Technique – Multiport Laparoscopic Splenectomy (See Plate 17.2B–H)

A) For multiport laparoscopic splenectomy, three or four separate ports are established to perform the procedure. A skin incision is made in a subumbilical location, and a 6-mm cannula is placed as described in *15.3. Laparoscopic Approach*. After placement of this initial cannula, a pneumoperitoneum is created.
B) Two to three additional cannulae are introduced to allow for placement of instrumentation. At least one of the instrument ports should be a 10-mm-diameter cannula to allow for placement of a retrieval bag. Although multiple port placement positions have been described, placement of all the ports on midline appears to be successful in the majority of cases. When this is performed, one port is placed cranial and one port is placed caudal to the subumbilical telescope port.
C) Through the cranial instrument port, a blunt probe or fan retractor is inserted (i), and this is used to elevate the tail of the spleen ventrally to expose the hilar blood vessels (ii).

Color Atlas of Canine and Feline Surgical Oncology, First Edition. Julius M. Liptak, Paolo Buracco, William T. N. Culp, and Nicholas J. Bacon.

Plate 17.2

Laparoscopic and Laparoscopic-Assisted Splenectomy

B)

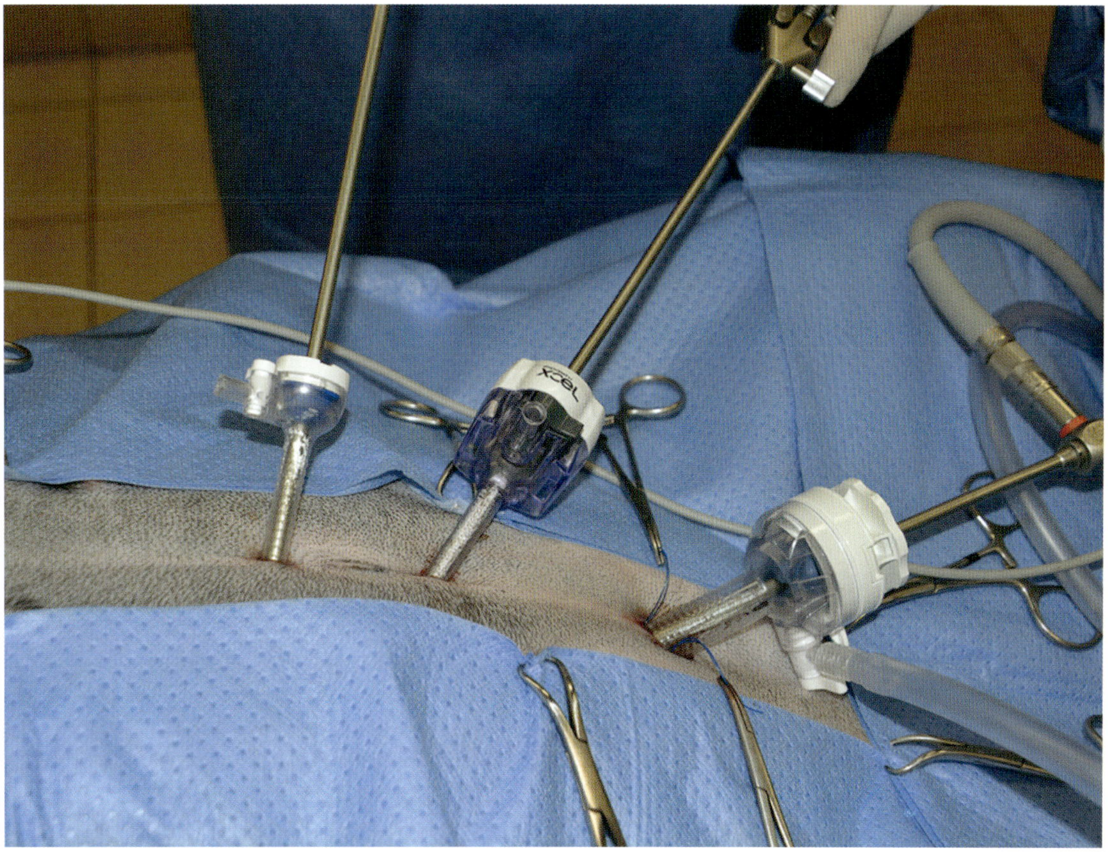

Courtesy of Dr. Bart Van Goethem

C-i)

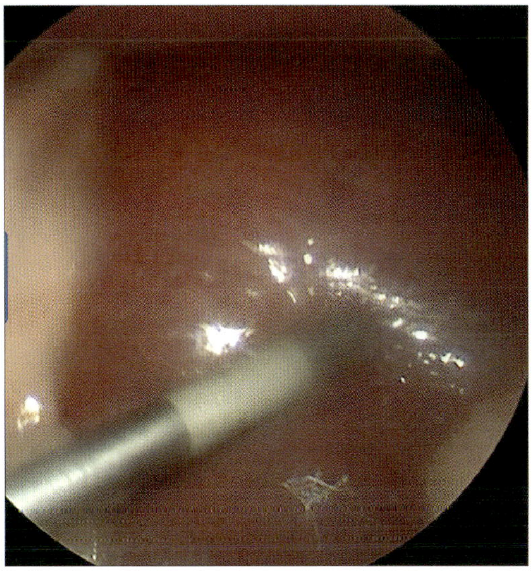

C-ii)

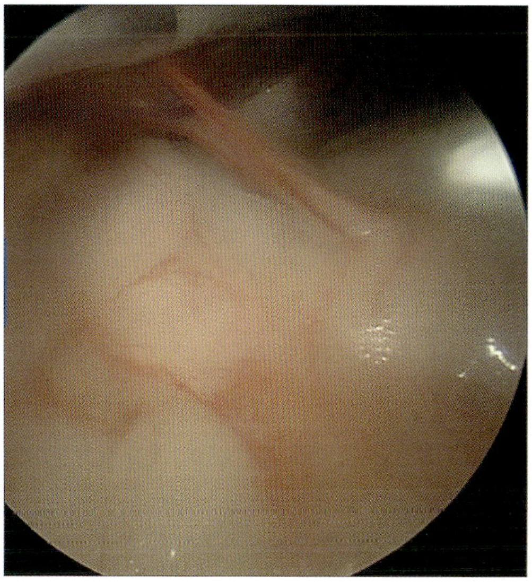

Surgical Technique – Multiport Laparoscopic Splenectomy (See Plate 17.2B–H) *continued*

D) A vessel sealing device is then inserted into the caudal instrument port, and the hilar blood vessels are sealed from the tail to the head of the spleen (i). As the location of the blunt probe or retractor holding the spleen is reached with the vessel sealing device, the instrument can be moved toward the head of the spleen to allow for further visualization of the hilar blood vessels (ii).

E) When the spleen has been completely separated from the blood supply, the vessel sealing device is removed and a retrieval bag is introduced into the abdomen (i). One of the midline incisions will need to be enlarged to allow for removal of the spleen in dogs (ii). In some cats with small spleens, the spleen can be removed via one of the midline portals after removal of the cannula.

Surgical Technique – Single-Port Laparoscopic Splenectomy

F) Single-port laparoscopic splenectomy is performed by placement of a single-port device into a small celiotomy. The most common devices currently used in veterinary patients are the single-incision laparoscopic surgery (SILS) port and the GelPOINT access system. A skin incision is made at the level of the umbilicus or just caudal to the umbilicus. The skin incision length is dependent on the length of the single-port device that is going to be used to perform the procedure. The SILS port is smaller, and an approximately 3-cm-long incision is usually sufficient to introduce this port. The GelPOINT access system requires an approximately 6-cm-long incision.

G) After continuation of the skin incision through the linea alba (see *15.1. Ventral Midline Celiotomy*), the single-port device is inserted through the celiotomy into the abdomen. The falciform ligament is retracted to allow for introduction of the device; alternatively, if the incision is large enough to visualize the falciform ligament, then this can be transected.

H) The cannulae that are designed for these devices are then inserted into the single-port device and the patient is insufflated with CO_2. Three ports are needed to perform the procedure.

I) A 5-mm-diameter telescope is inserted into the port and the spleen is visualized (not pictured). Through an instrument port, a blunt probe or fan retractor is inserted, and this is used to elevate the tail of the spleen ventrally to exposure the hilar blood vessels.

J) A vessel sealing device is then inserted into another instrument port, and the hilar blood vessels are sealed in a direction from the tail to the head of the spleen (not pictured). As the location of the instrument holding the spleen is reached, the instrument can be moved more toward the head of the spleen to allow for further visualization of the hilar blood vessels.

K) When the spleen has been completely separated from the blood supply, the vessel sealing device is removed from the abdomen and the spleen is removed via the celiotomy (after removal of the single-port device) or by placement in a retrieval bag (not pictured).

Plate 17.2

Laparoscopic and Laparoscopic-Assisted Splenectomy *continued*

D-i)
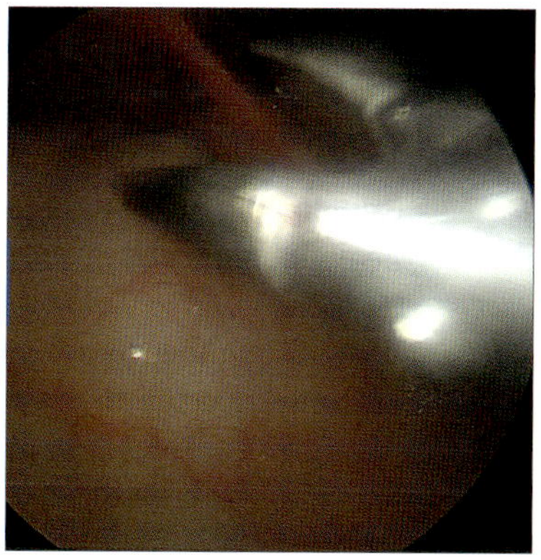

D-ii)
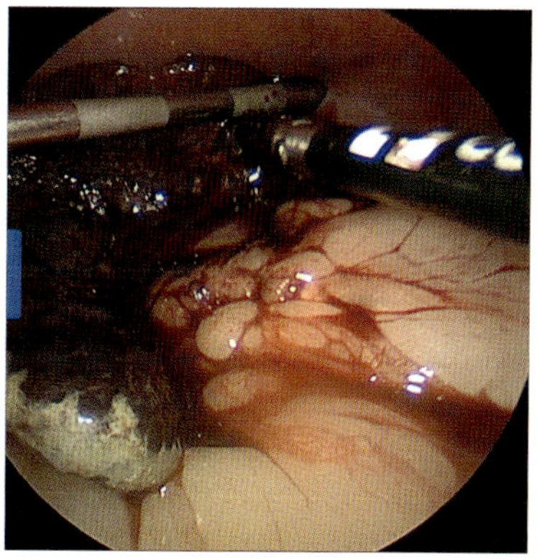

E-i)
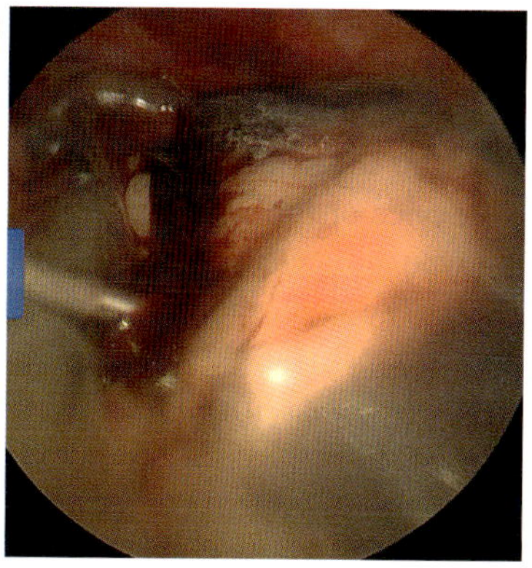

E-ii)
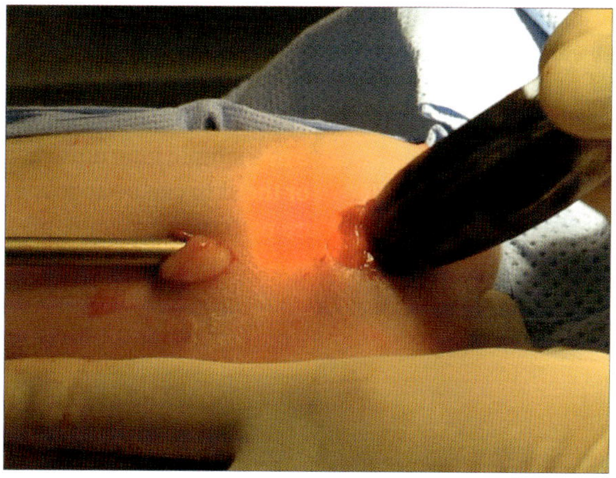

F)
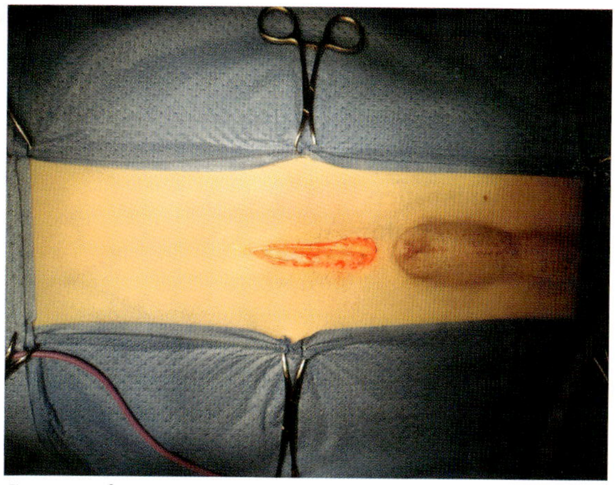

Courtesy of Dr. Bart Van Goethem

G)
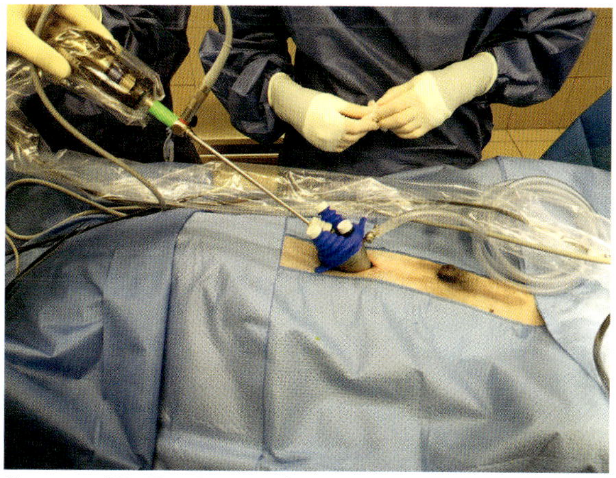

Courtesy of Dr. Bart Van Goethem

H)
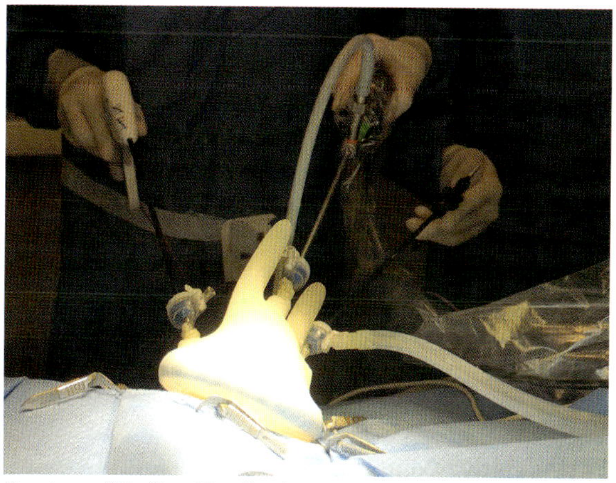

Courtesy of Dr. Bart Van Goethem

Chapter 18: Partial Pancreatectomy

Indications

1) Resection of localized malignant pancreatic tumors: Up to 90% of the pancreas can be resected provided the pancreatic ducts are preserved.
2) Partial pancreatectomy can be combined with a Billroth I if required (see *21.2. Billroth I*).

Suggested Diagnostic Workup and Clinical Staging

- Paired serum glucose-insulin assay (for dogs with suspected pancreatic insulinomas)
- Abdominal ultrasound or computed tomography (CT) scan for assessment of primary tumor location and assessment of intra-abdominal metastasis ± guided fine-needle aspirate cytology
- Double- or triple-phase CT angiography (for dogs with suspected pancreatic insulinomas)
- Three-view thoracic radiographs or thoracic CT scan for assessment of lung metastasis

Patient Positioning

The patient is positioned in dorsal recumbency.

Surgical Technique (See Plate 18A–H)

A) A ventral midline celiotomy is performed (see *15.1. Ventral Midline Celiotomy*). The deep leaf of the greater omentum (GO) is incised to expose the left limb of the pancreas (LLP) (insulinoma, arrow). Branches of the gastroepiploic artery are ligated and divided if necessary; alternatively, a vessel sealing device can be used. The splenic branches should be preserved.

B) The mesoduodenum and duodenum (DD) are reflected ventrally and toward the midline to expose the right limb of the pancreas (RLP) (insulinoma, arrow). The cranial and caudal pancreaticoduodenal arteries should be preserved.

C) Localized pancreatic masses (star) should be resected with 1-cm margins if possible; however, this may not be possible for pancreatic tumors located in the head of the pancreas. In these cases, the pancreatic tumor should be enucleated with minimal margins to preserve the pancreatic ducts and exocrine pancreatic function.

D) **Partial pancreatectomy technique 1 – Dissection and ligation [1]**: The pancreatic lobules are gently separated from adjacent pancreatic lobules by blunt dissection using either mosquito forceps (i, ii) or cotton swabs. Once the ducts, ductules, and vessels are completely exposed (iii), these structures are ligated and divided (iv). After division of these ducts and vessels, the tissue distal to the ligatures is resected and the partial pancreatectomy is completed.

Color Atlas of Canine and Feline Surgical Oncology, First Edition. Julius M. Liptak, Paolo Buracco, William T. N. Culp, and Nicholas J. Bacon.

Plate 18

Partial Pancreatectomy

A)
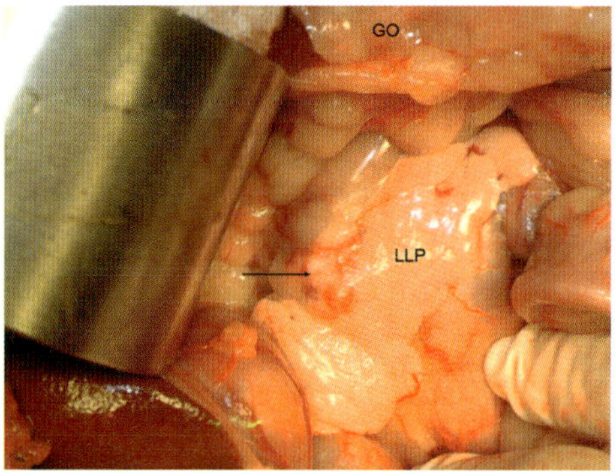

B)
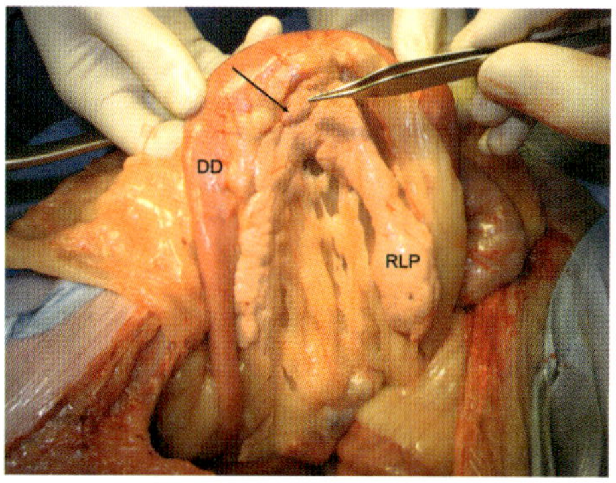

C)
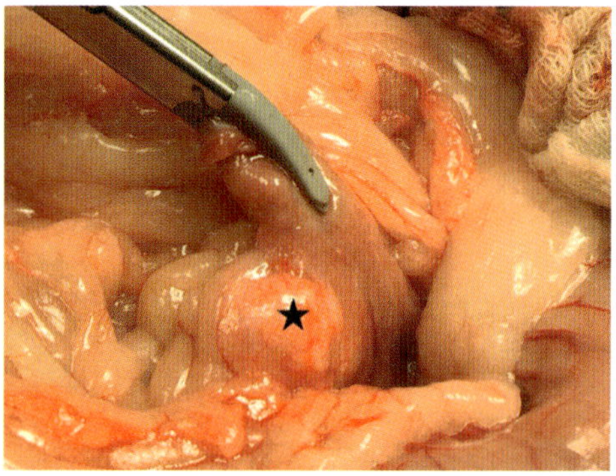

D-i)
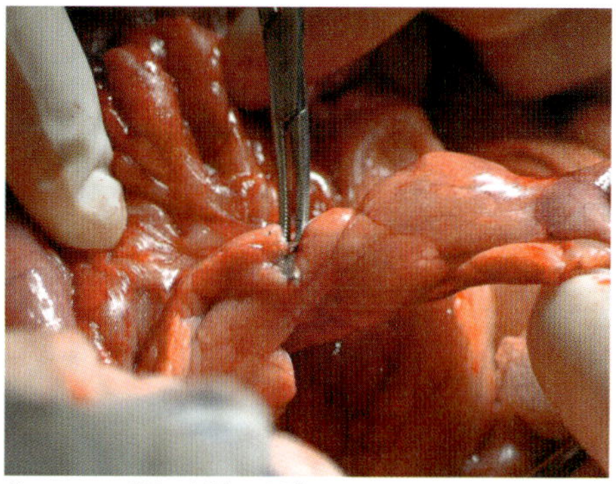
Courtesy of Dr. Milan Milovancev

D-ii)
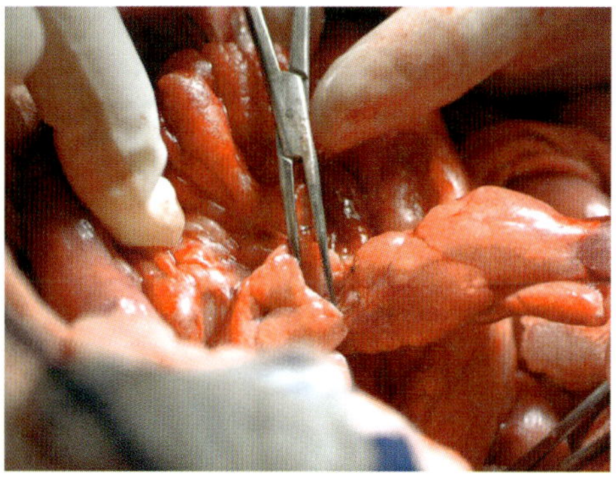
Courtesy of Dr. Milan Milovancev

D-iii)
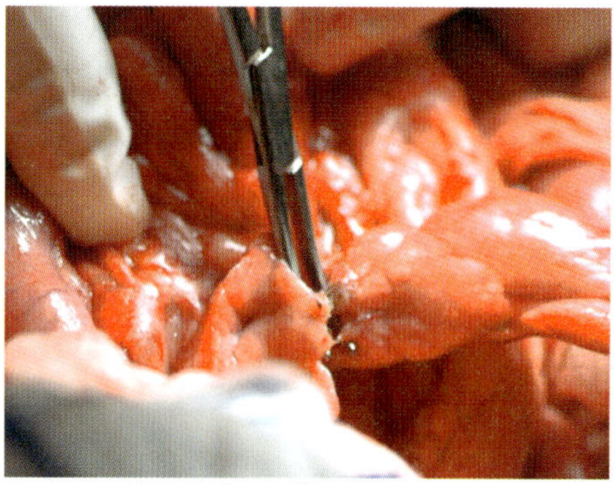
Courtesy of Dr. Milan Milovancev

D-iv)
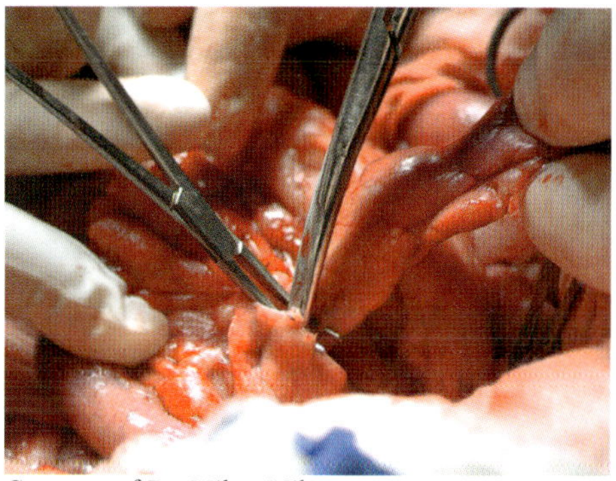
Courtesy of Dr. Milan Milovancev

Surgical Technique (See Plate 18A–H) *continued*

E) **Partial pancreatectomy technique 1 – Suture fracture [1]**: An incision is made into the mesoduodenum (for tumors of the right limb of the pancreas) or greater omentum (for tumors of the left limb of the pancreas) either side of the pancreas to be resected. Absorbable monofilament suture material is passed through these incisions proximal to the planned partial pancreatectomy site, and the ligature is tightened to crush the pancreatic parenchyma, ducts, ductules, and vessels (i). The pancreatic tissue distal to the ligature is resected to complete the partial pancreatectomy (ii).

F) **Partial pancreatectomy technique 3 – Vessel sealing device [2]**: An incision is made into the mesoduodenum (for tumors of the right limb of the pancreas) or greater omentum (for tumors of the left limb of the pancreas) either side of the pancreas to be resected. A vessel sealing device is used to complete the partial pancreatectomy either between or through the pancreatic lobules with appropriate margins (i–iv).

Plate 18

Partial Pancreatectomy *continued*

E-i)
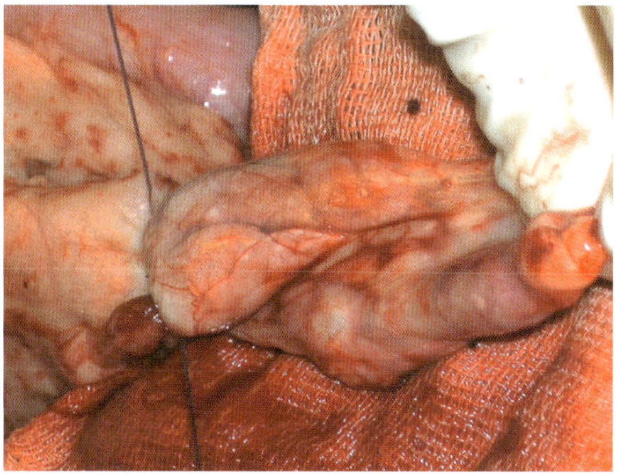

E-ii)
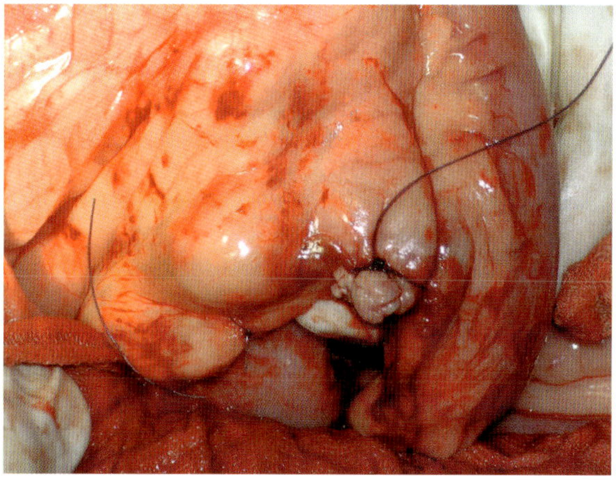

F-i)
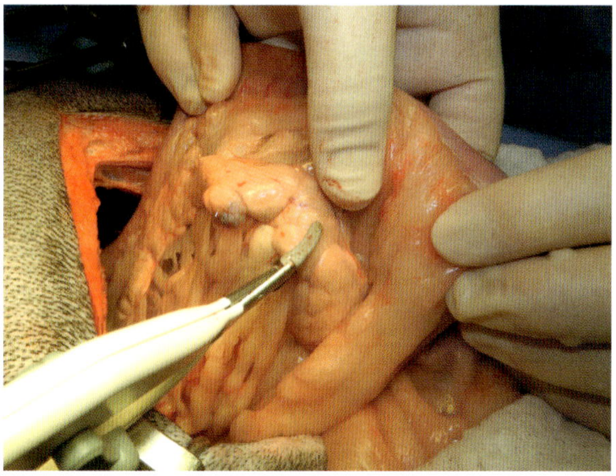

F-ii)
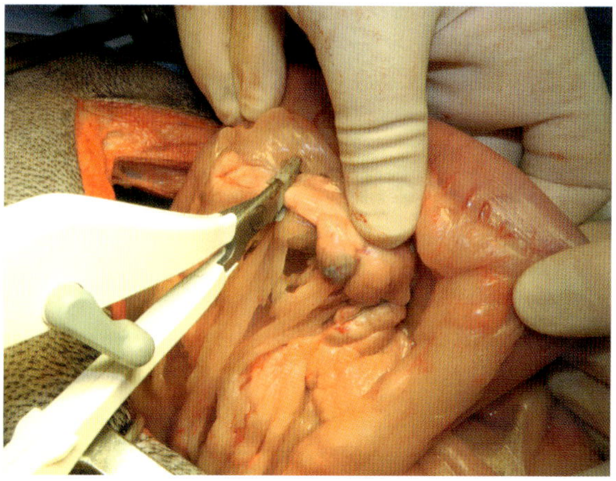

F-iii)
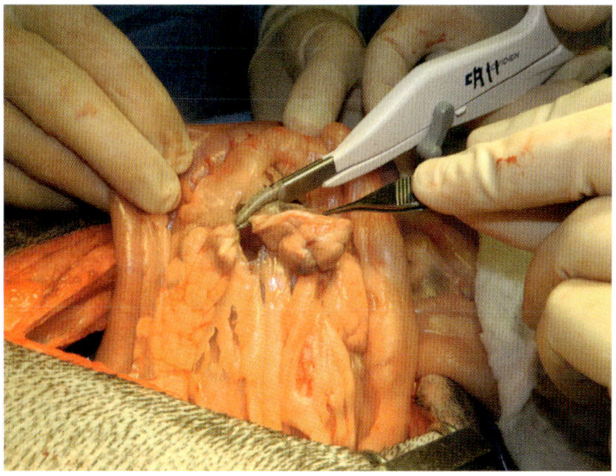

F-iv)
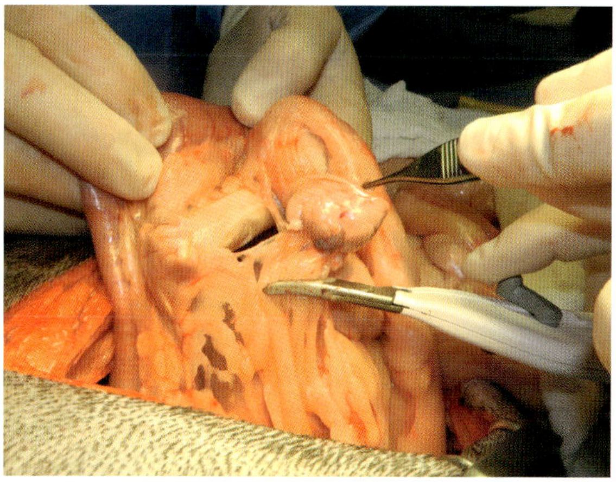

Surgical Technique (See Plate 18A–H) *continued*

G) The abdominal cavity should be systematically explored for metastatic disease. The most common metastatic sites for pancreatic insulinomas are the regional lymph nodes (i, arrow) and liver (ii, iii). Metastasis to the regional lymph nodes and liver and carcinomatosis (iv) are common in animals with pancreatic carcinomas.

H) Either a biopsy should be performed of the enlarged lymph nodes (i, arrow) and suspected metastatic lesions (ii, partial liver lobectomy with a vessel sealing device to perform a biopsy on a metastatic lesion from a pancreatic insulinoma) or they should be resected. Blood glucose should be measured after resection of the insulinoma and after each suspected metastatic lesion. Blood glucose should increase to within the normal reference range if all disease has been resected [3]. The abdominal cavity should be lavaged with warmed sterile isotonic saline.

Closure

The linea alba, subcutaneous tissue, and skin are closed as described in *15.1. Ventral Midline Celiotomy*.

Postoperative Management

1) Multimodal analgesia
2) Elizabethan collar or body suit
3) Glucose monitoring for dogs with pancreatic insulinoma

Complications

Complications in Dogs with Pancreatic Insulinomas [3–9]

- Unresectable tumors because of location or diffuse disease (17%–21%)
- Intraoperative blood loss (6%)
- Hyperglycemia (8%–36%); transient (15%–26%) or permanent (10%–19%)
- Persistent hypoglycemia (15%–27%)
- Delayed wound healing (13%)
- Pancreatitis (8%–43%)
- Ventricular arrhythmias (6%)
- Seizures (unrelated to hypoglycemia, 3%–6%)
- Diabetic ketoacidosis (4%)
- Pancreatic cyst (4%)

Complications in Cats with Exocrine Pancreatic Carcinomas [10, 11]

- Unresectable tumors because of location or diffuse disease (25%)
- Hyporexia (11%)

Complications in Cats with Insulinomas [12]

- Overall: 25%
- Pancreatitis (10%)
- Seizures (10%)
- Hyperglycemia (5%)
- Perioperative mortality (10%)

Plate 18

Partial Pancreatectomy *continued*

G-i)

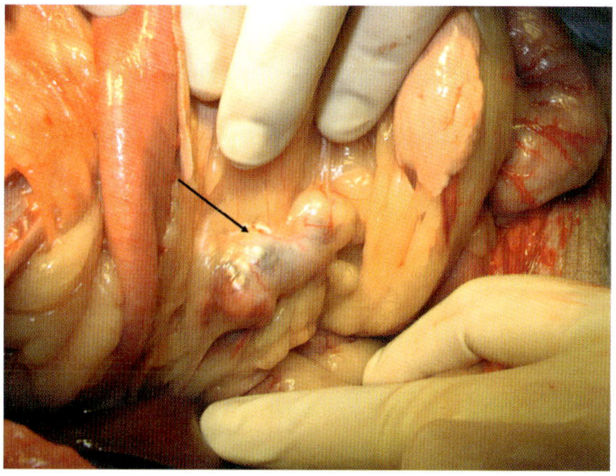

G-ii)

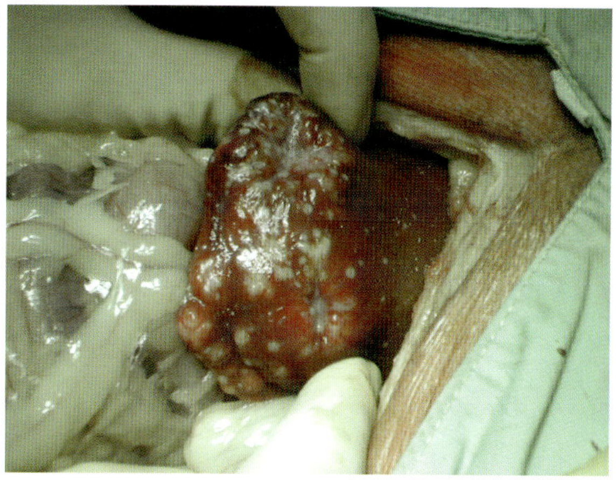

G-iii)

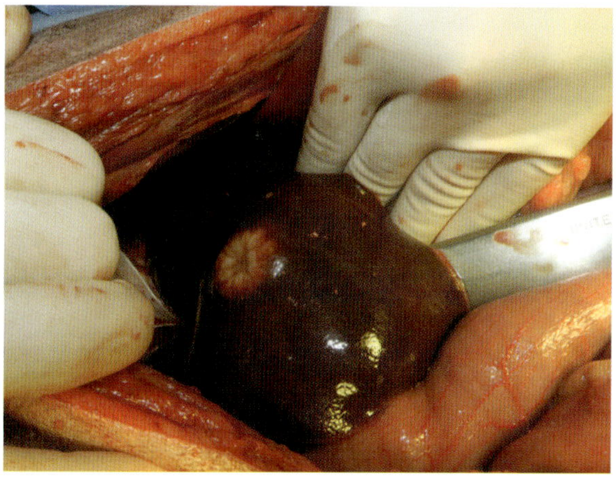

G-iv)

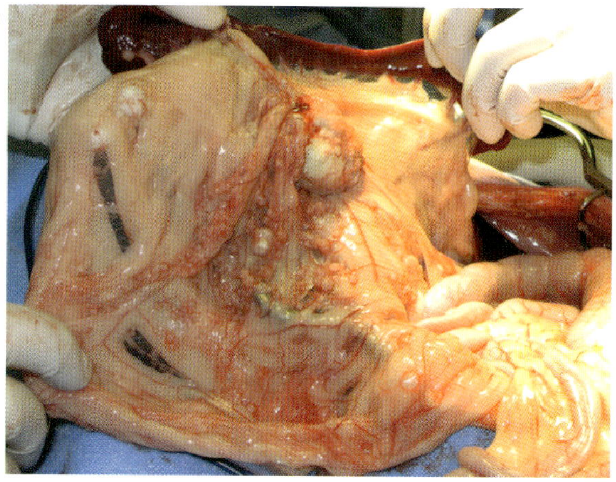

H-i)

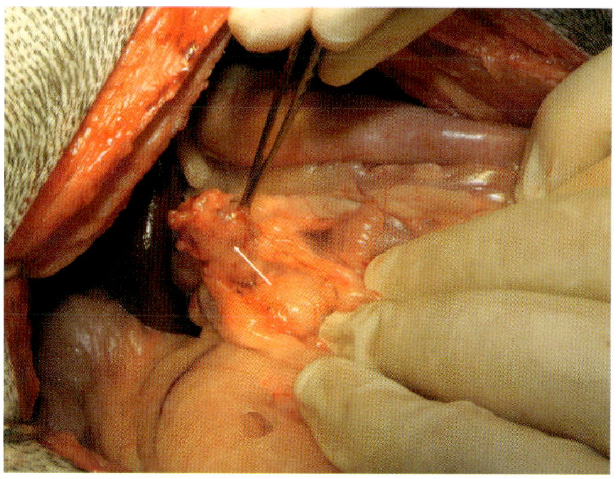

H-ii)

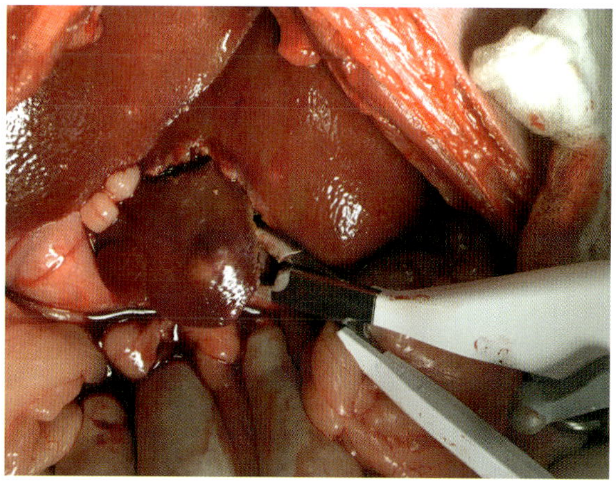

Suggested Adjuvant Treatments

- Chemotherapy for dogs and cats with pancreatic adenocarcinomas
- Prednisone or chemotherapy for dogs with stage II or stage III pancreatic insulinomas

Prognosis and Oncologic Outcome

Prognosis and Oncologic Outcome – Dogs

	Local Recurrence Rate	Metastatic Rate	Disease-Free Interval (d)	Median Survival Time (d)	1-Year Survival Rate	2-Year Survival Rate
		Insulinoma				
Overall [3–5, 7, 9]	–	42%–73%	244–496	258–762	–	–
Treatment [7]						
• Surgery	–	–	–	381	–	–
• Medical	–	–	–	74	–	–
Clinical stage [5, 8, 9]						
• Stage I	–	–	–	549–785	–	–
• Stage II	–	–	–	547–549	–	–
• Stage III	–	–	–	183–217	–	–
Surgical technique [6]						
• Partial pancreatectomy	–	–	–	546	–	–
• Enucleation	–	–	–	351	–	–
Postoperative glycemia [4]						
• Normoglycemia or hyperglycemia	–	–	–	680	–	–
• Hypoglycemia	–	–	–	90	–	–

Prognosis and Oncologic Outcome – Cats

	Local Recurrence Rate	Metastatic Rate	Disease-Free Interval (d)	Median Survival Time (d)	1-Year Survival Rate	2-Year Survival Rate
		Exocrine Pancreatic Carcinoma				
Overall [10, 11]						
Preoperative ascites [10]						
• No ascites						
• Ascites						
		Insulinoma [12]				
Overall	0%	39%	214	863	75%	51%

References

1 Allen, S.W., Cornelius, L.M., and Mahaffey, E.A. (1989). A comparison of two methods of partial pancreatectomy in the dog. *Vet. Surg.* 18 (4): 274–278.

2 Wouters, E.G.H., Buishand, F.O., Kik, M., and Kirpensteijn, J. (2011). Use of a bipolar vessel-sealing device in resection of canine insulinoma. *J. Small Anim. Pract.* 52 (3): 139–145.

3 Collgros, N.C. and Bray, J.P. (2023). Blood glucose monitoring during surgery in dogs to assess completeness of surgical resection of insulinoma: 11 cases. *J. Am. Vet. Med. Assoc.* 261 (2): 229–236.

4 Trifonidou, M.A., Kirpensteijn, J., and Robben, J.H. (1998). A retrospective evaluation of 51 dogs with insulinoma. *Vet. Q.* 20 (Suppl 1): S114–S115.

5 Polton, G.A., White, R.N., Brearley, M.J., and Eastwood, J.M. (2007). Improved survival in a retrospective cohort of 28 dogs with insulinoma. *J. Small Anim. Pract.* 48 (3): 151–156.

6 Mehlhaff, C.J., Peterson, M.E., Patnaik, A.K. et al. (1984). Insulin producing islet cell neoplasms: Surgical considerations and general management in 35 dogs. *J. Am. Anim. Hosp. Assoc.* 21: 607–612.

7 Tobin, R.L., Nelson, R.W., Lucroy, M.D. et al. (1999). Outcome of surgical versus medical treatment of dogs with beta cell neoplasia: 39 cases (1990-1997). *J. Am. Vet. Med. Assoc.* 215 (2): 226–230.

8 Caywood, D.D., Klausner, J.S., O'Leary, T.P. et al. (1988). Pancreatic insulin-secreting neoplasms: clinical, diagnostic and prognostic features in 73 dogs. *J. Am. Anim. Hosp. Assoc.* 24: 577–584.

9 Del Busto, I., German, A.J., Treggiari, E. et al. (2020). Incidence of postoperative complications and outcome of 48 dogs undergoing surgical management of insulinoma. *J. Vet. Intern. Med.* 34 (3): 1135–1143.

10 Linderman, M.J., Brodsky, E.M., de Lorimier, L.P. et al. (2013). Feline exocrine pancreatic carcinoma: a retrospective study of 34 cases. *Vet. Comp. Oncol.* 11 (3): 208–218.

11 Nicoletti, R., Chun, R., Curran, K.M. et al. (2018). Postsurgical outcome in cats with exocrine pancreatic carcinoma: nine cases (2007-2016). *J. Am. Anim. Hosp. Assoc.* 54 (5): 291–295.

12 Veytsman, S., Amsellem, P., Husbands, B.D. et al. (2023). Retrospective study of 20 cats surgically treated for insulinoma. *Vet. Surg.* 52 (1): 42–50.

Chapter 19: Adrenalectomy

19.1 Open Adrenalectomy

Indications

1) Resection of functional adrenal tumors (adrenocortical tumors and pheochromocytomas) ± nonfunctional adrenal tumors, especially if >2 cm at presentation or growing to >2 cm over a 3-month period [1, 2]
2) Resection of functional or nonfunctional adrenal tumors with tumor thrombus formation in the phrenicoabdominal vein, caudal vena cava, or renal veins
3) Adrenalectomy can be combined with nephrectomy (see *27.1. Open Ureteronephrectomy*) if the adrenal tumor is invasive into the kidney

Suggested Diagnostic Workup and Clinical Staging

- Complete blood count, serum biochemistry, and urinalysis
- Blood pressure measurements
- ± Cross matching or blood typing
- Coagulation panel
- Adrenal function testing for suspected hyperadrenocorticism with combinations of urine protein-to-creatinine ratio, adrenocorticotropic hormone (ACTH) stimulation test, endogenous ACTH assay, low-dose dexamethasone suppression test, and high-dose dexamethasone suppression test
- Adrenal function testing for suspected pheochromocytoma with combinations of plasma-free normetanephrine and metanephrine [3, 4], urinary metanephrine-to-creatinine ratio [4, 5], and urinary normetanephrine [4]
- Abdominal ultrasound or precontrast and postcontrast computed tomography (CT) scan of the abdomen for assessment of adrenal mass(es), vascular invasion, and intra-abdominal metastasis
- Three-view thoracic radiographs or thoracic CT scan for assessment of lung metastasis
- ± Echocardiography for assessment of extension of caval tumor thrombus beyond the hepatic hilus

Patient Positioning

The patient is positioned in dorsal recumbency for a ventral midline celiotomy approach or lateral recumbency with the affected side uppermost for either a paracostal or intercostal thoracotomy approach [6].

Color Atlas of Canine and Feline Surgical Oncology, First Edition. Julius M. Liptak, Paolo Buracco, William T. N. Culp, and Nicholas J. Bacon.

Surgical Technique – Approach

A) A ventral midline celiotomy is performed (see *15.1. Ventral Midline Celiotomy*). The falciform ligament should be resected to improve exposure.
B) A paracostal approach (see *15.2. Paracostal Approach*) can be done for small nonmetastatic and noninvasive adrenal tumors, or a paracostal approach can be combined with a ventral midline celiotomy for improved visualization and exposure.

Surgical Technique – Noninvasive Adrenalectomy (See Plate 19.1C–H)

C) For left-sided adrenal tumors (AT), the descending colon (DC) is retracted to the right lateral abdominal wall to act as a mesocolic basket (MC) to expose the left adrenal gland immediately cranial to the left kidney (K). Moist laparotomy sponges and malleable retractors are used to retract the mesentery and intestines toward the midline, and the left lateral and left medial lobes of the liver toward the cranial abdomen.

D) For right-sided adrenal tumors (AT), the duodenum is retracted to the left lateral abdominal wall to act as a mesoduodenal basket (MD) to expose the right adrenal gland cranial to the right kidney (K) and dorsal to the caudal vena cava (CaVC). The hepatorenal ligament is transected, and a narrow malleable retractor is placed between the cranial pole of the right adrenal gland and caudate process of the caudate liver lobe.

E) Dissection starts by entering the retroperitoneum lateral to the adrenal mass and dissecting through fat a few millimeters from the mass. A vessel sealing device is beneficial with this dissection (pictured), and Q-tips or Debakey forceps can help to gently manipulate the adrenal mass and aid in dissection. The cranial pole of the adrenal mass is dissected free, and this dissection is continued dorsally.

F) The lateral dissection is continued caudally (i), gently separating the adrenal mass (AT) from the kidney (K) (ii). A cleavage plane usually exists between the adrenal gland and kidney (ii, arrow). For right-sided adrenal tumors, additional care is taken when dissecting the caudal pole of the adrenal gland free because the right renal vein (RV) is in close proximity to the adrenal gland (AT) (iii; PAV, phrenicoabdominal vein; CaVC, caudal vena cava). In some cases, the adrenal mass invades into the kidney; in these cases, an ipsilateral nephroureterectomy is performed en bloc with the adrenalectomy (see *27.1. Open Ureteronephrectomy*).

G) The loose fascial and adventitial attachments between the aortic wall (for left adrenal masses, arrow) or the wall of the caudal vena cava (for right adrenal masses) and the medial wall of the adrenal mass should be divided with blunt dissection. There are multiple small penetrating vessels entering the adrenal gland dorsally, and these should be sealed and transected with a vessel sealing device.

H) The phrenicoabdominal vein is isolated and ligated with two simple ligatures of 3-0 or 4-0 monofilament absorbable suture material (i) or hemoclips lateral to the gland, and then divided. Alternatively, a vessel sealing device can be used to seal and transect the phrenicoabdominal vein (ii). The adrenal gland is removed from the retroperitoneal fossa to complete the adrenalectomy. The retroperitoneal fossa should be inspected for evidence of residual bleeding.

Plate 19.1

Open Adrenalectomy

C)

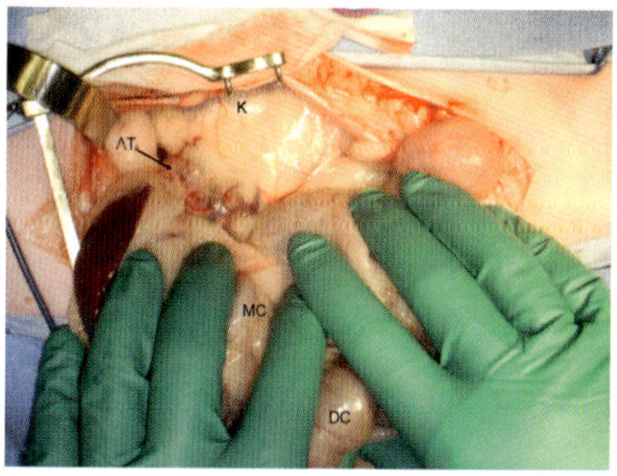

D)

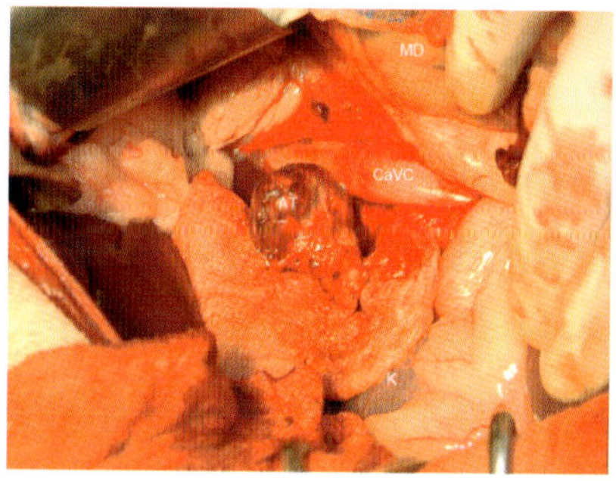

E)

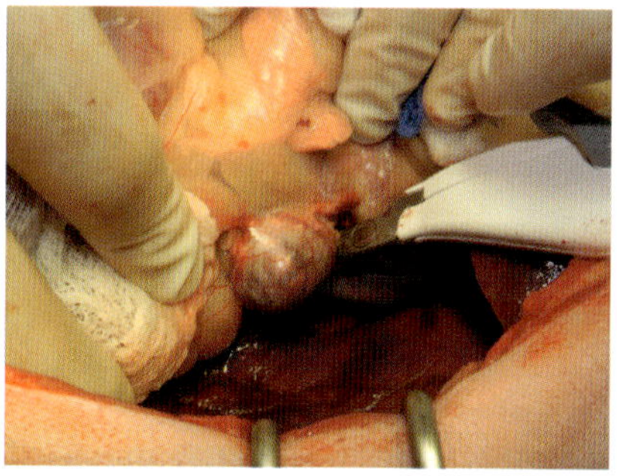

F-i)

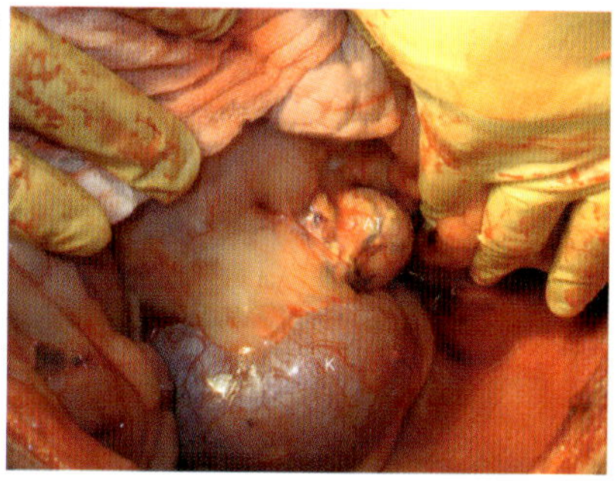

F-ii)

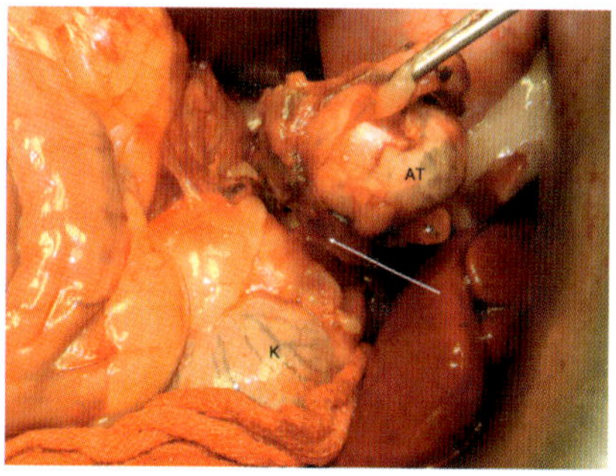

F-iii)

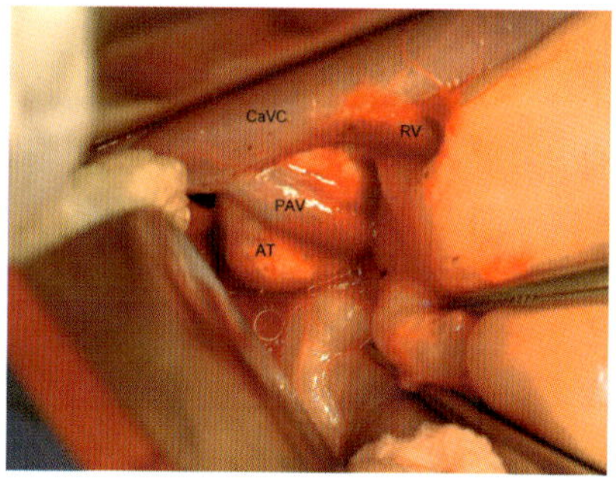

G)

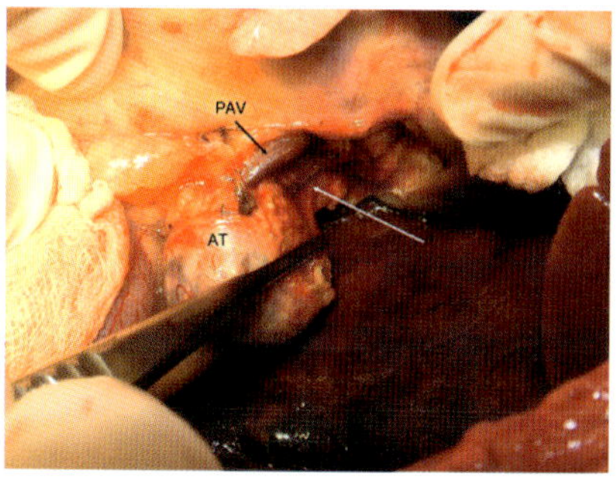

H-i)

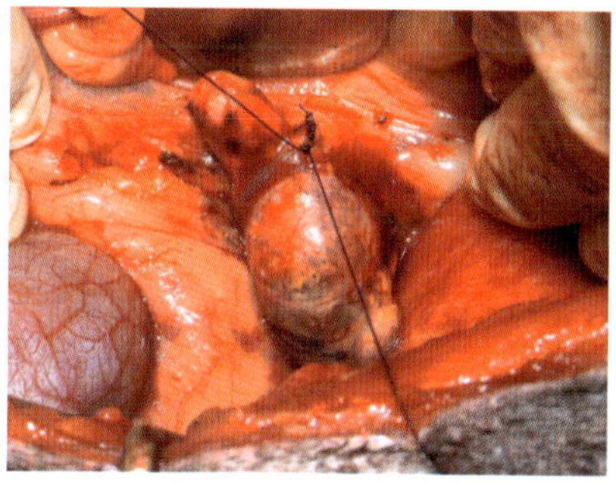

H-ii)

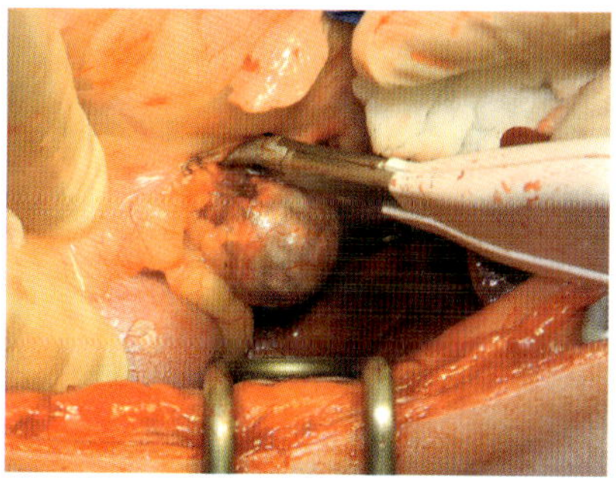

Surgical Technique – Tumor Thrombus in Phrenicoabdominal Vein (See Plate 19.1I)

I) There are two options for when a tumor thrombus extends into the phrenicoabdominal vein but not into the caudal vena cava, or when a small thrombus extends into the caudal vena cava but does not occlude the lumen of the caudal vena cava. Gently apply lateral traction on the adrenal mass (AT) to stretch the phrenicoabdominal vein (PAV) (i) and create a small window of grossly normal phrenicoabdominal vein at the junction with the caudal vena cava (CaVC) (dashed arrow). The first option for management of the tumor thrombus is ligation of the small window of the phrenicoabdominal vein with two simple ligatures of 3-0 or 4-0 monofilament absorbable suture material and then divide the vein between the two ligatures (not pictured). The second option is to apply a curved Satinsky clamp across the small window of the phrenicoabdominal vein, parallel to the caudal vena cava (ii). The phrenicoabdominal vein is then transected under traction, and the resulting defect in the phrenicoabdominal vein or caudal vena caval wall is closed with a simple interrupted or continuous suture pattern of 5-0 polypropylene (iii). The Satinsky clamp is then gently removed, and the venotomy site is inspected for bleeding (iv).

Surgical Technique – Tumor Thrombus Occluding the Caudal Vena Cava (See Plate 19.1J–M)

J) Rumel tourniquets are preplaced around the caudal vena cava, and occasionally the renal veins, cranial and caudal to the proposed venotomy site. The most cranial Rumel tourniquet is usually placed just caudal to the liver margin. A small hole is made in the peritoneum to the left of the caudal vena cava, and then a curved Satinsky clamp or right-angled forceps are used to pass 2-0 or 3-0 polypropylene or umbilical tape from right to left and dorsal to the caudal vena cava, exiting through the soft tissue hole. The loose ends of the suture material or umbilical tape are passed through a semirigid 8 or 10 Fr polyurethane tube, and then these are loosely clamped with mosquito forceps as they exit the polyurethane tube.

K) The more caudal Rumel tourniquets are placed around the caudal vena cava (CaVC) and possibly the renal veins, depending on whether the mass is left- or right-sided and the caudal extent of the adrenal mass. For a left-sided adrenal tumor, a Rumel tourniquet is placed caudal to the left adrenal gland and cranial to the left renal vein (LRV), and often a second Rumel tourniquet is required around the right renal vein (RRV) (pictured). A single Rumel tourniquet placed immediately caudal to the right adrenal gland and cranial to the right renal vein is the minimum recommended for a right-sided adrenal tumor (see step J). For larger adrenal tumors or those invading the renal veins or kidneys, Rumel tourniquets on individual renal veins are required, in addition to those on the caudal vena cava cranial and caudal to the adrenal mass. The Rumel tourniquets are tightened so that the suture within the tube snares and occludes the vessel with minimal trauma, and these are then held closed by clamping the suture with the mosquito forceps. An appropriate tightness is identified by a gentle bend appearing in the tubing.

Plate 19.1

Open Adrenalectomy *continued*

I-i)

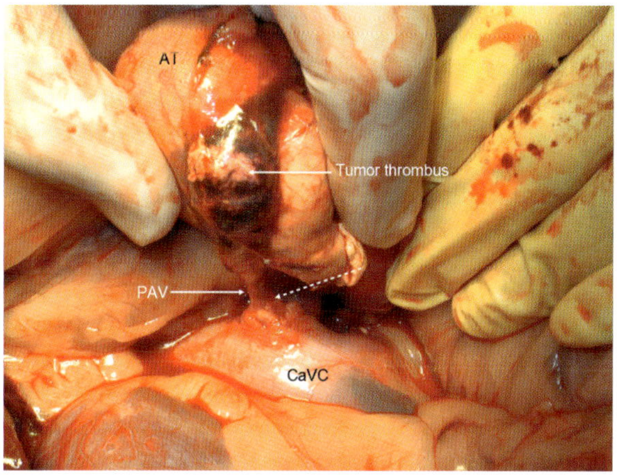

I-ii)

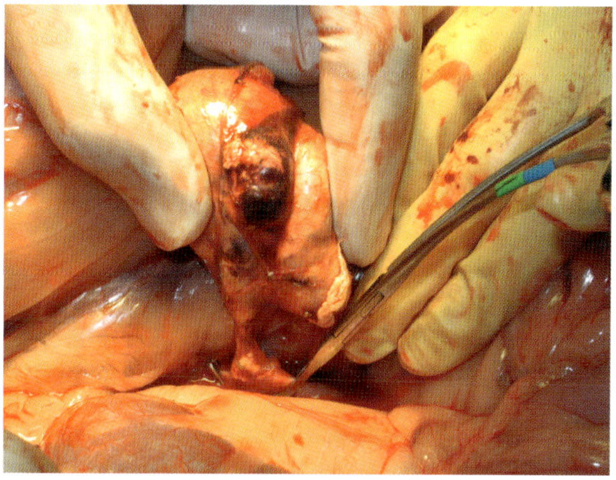

I-iii)

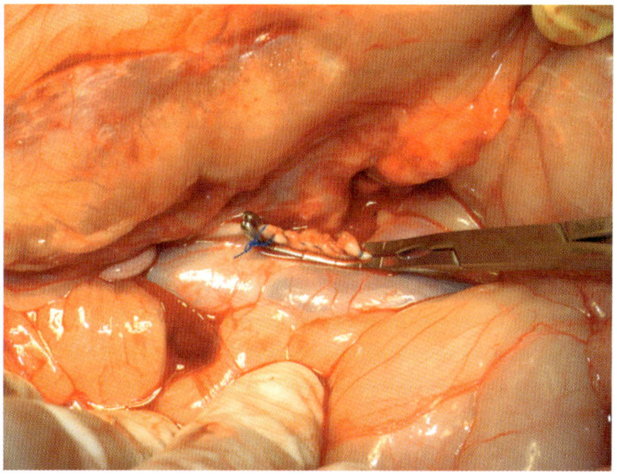

I-iv)

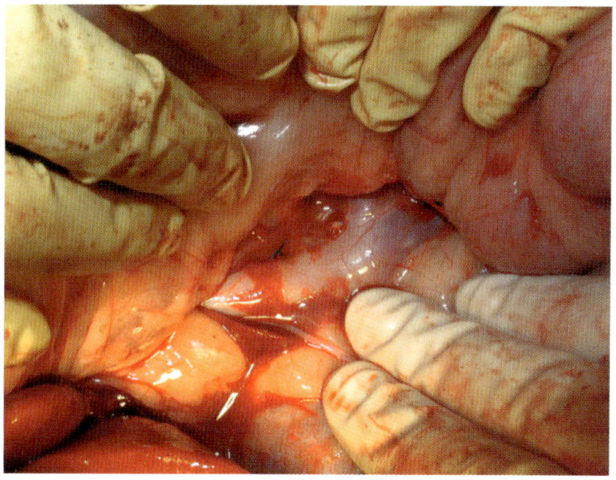

J)

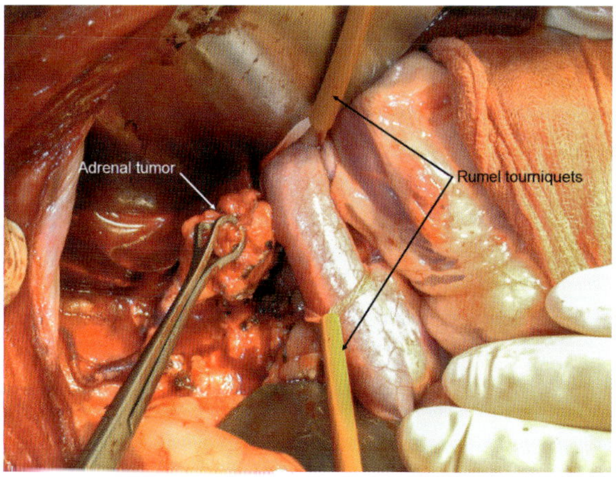

K)

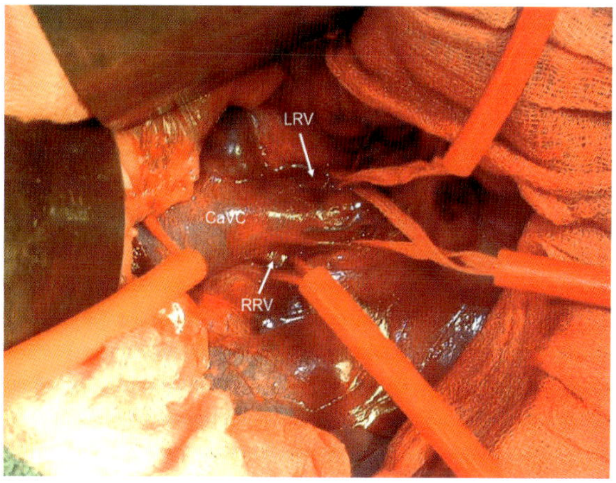

Surgical Technique – Tumor Thrombus Occluding the Caudal Vena Cava (See Plate 19.1J–M) *continued*

L) For a caval thrombus that occludes the lumen of the caudal vena cava (CaVC) but does not extend beyond the hilus of the liver, the adrenal gland (AT) is dissected free (i) and the Rumel tourniquets are placed as described in steps C–G and steps J and K, respectively. A time check should start when the caudal vena cava is occluded. A venotomy (ii, arrows) is made with a No. 11 scalpel blade in the wall of the cava circumferentially around the dilated phrenicoabdominal vein. Sharp, curved iris scissors are sometimes helpful to minimize a jagged venotomy edge. Gentle caudal traction on the adrenal tumor usually results in extraction of the tumor thrombus (TT) from within the lumen of the caudal vena cava en bloc with the adrenal tumor (iii). Once the thrombus is removed, the venotomy (arrow) is closed with a simple continuous pattern of 5-0 polypropylene. The needle is passed 2–3 mm from each wound edge, at intervals of approximately 2–3 mm (iv). Operating loupes are recommended to ensure the best possible tissue apposition. After completion of the venotomy closure, the Rumel tourniquets are released, starting with the cranial Rumel tourniquet first, to restore blood flow through the caudal vena cava (v). The period of caudal vena cava occlusion should not exceed 8 minutes, but longer occlusion times may be tolerated without irreversible hemodynamic effects. Mild hemorrhage from the suture holes can be managed with gentle pressure. Defects in the venotomy closure require the Rumel tourniquets to be reapplied and the defect repaired.

M) For a caval thrombus (TT) that occludes the lumen of the caudal vena cava (CaVC) and extends beyond the hilus of the liver (L) (i), the same technique is used as described in step L, but tightening of the cranial Rumel tourniquet is delayed until the tumor thrombus has been extracted caudal to the level of the hilus of the liver (AT, adrenal tumor). In these cases, although rare, the tumor thrombus can also extend into the hepatic veins. Extraction of the tumor thrombus is more challenging and sometimes impossible in these cases, thus necessitating intraoperative euthanasia (ii, dog with adrenocortical adenocarcinoma with a tumor thrombus [TT] extending into the heart [H]; D, diaphragm).

Closure

The method of closure depends on the surgical approach. For ventral midline celiotomy approaches, the linea alba, subcutaneous tissue, and skin are closed as described in *15.1. Ventral Midline Celiotomy*. For paracostal approaches, the muscle, subcutaneous tissue, and skin are closed as described in *15.2. Paracostal Approach*. For an intercostal approach, the ribs, muscle, subcutaneous tissue, and skin are closed as described in *10.1. Intercostal Thoracotomy*.

Postoperative Management

1) Multimodal analgesia: Nonsteroidal anti-inflammatory drugs should be avoided in dogs with suspected adrenocortical tumors.
2) Elizabethan collar or body suit.
3) For dogs with suspected hyperadrenocorticism, a continuous rate infusion of dexamethasone is started intraoperatively and extended for 6 hours postoperatively, and is then followed by two doses every 8–12 hours. Oral prednisolone can be used postoperatively either in all cases (tapered over a 9- to 12-week period) [7] or guided by ACTH stimulation test 24–48 hours postsurgery. Oral prednisolone is not administered in dogs with a normal ACTH stimulation test but is administered in dogs with an abnormal ACTH stimulation test [8].
4) Consider perioperative heparin continuous rate infusion to achieve a prothrombin time (PTT) of 1.5× baseline PTT to reduce the risk of pulmonary thromboembolism [8].
5) Electrolytes and blood glucose are checked every 6–8 hours.

Plate 19.1

Open Adrenalectomy *continued*

L-i)

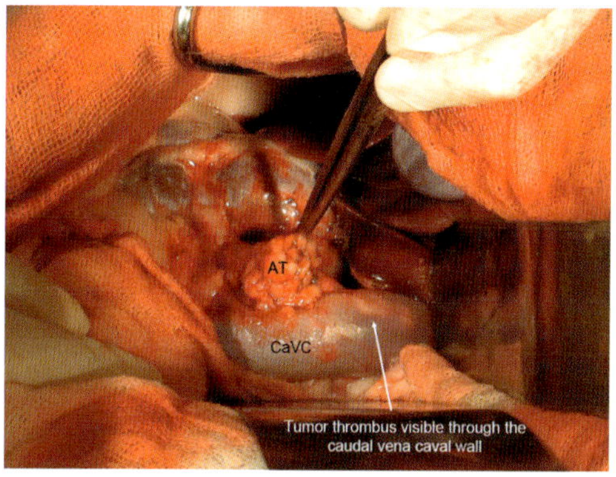

L-ii)

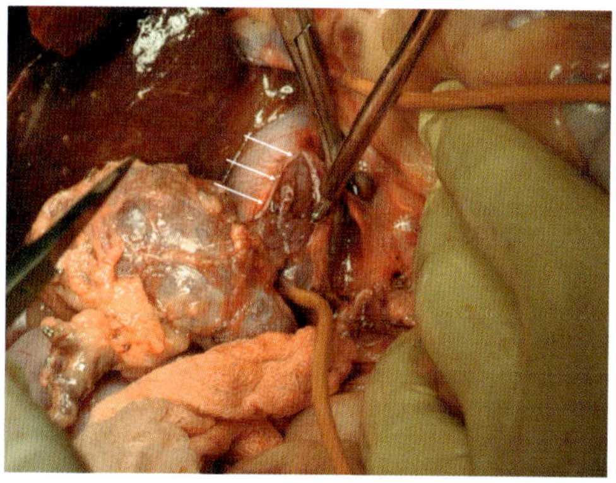

L-iii)

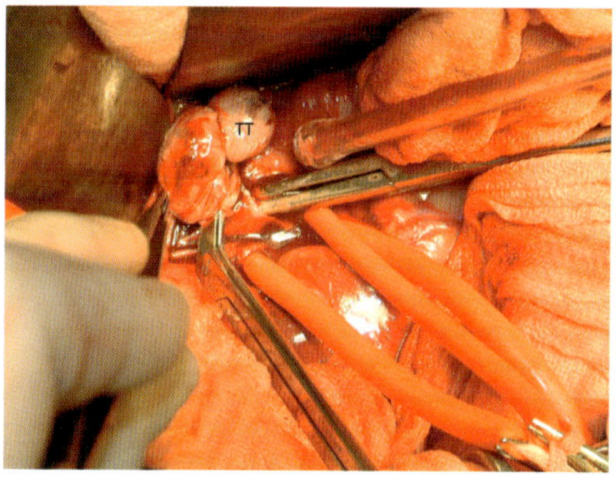

L-iv)

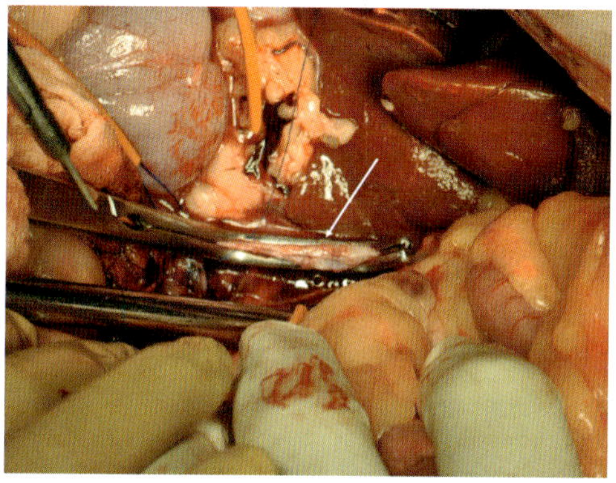

L-v)

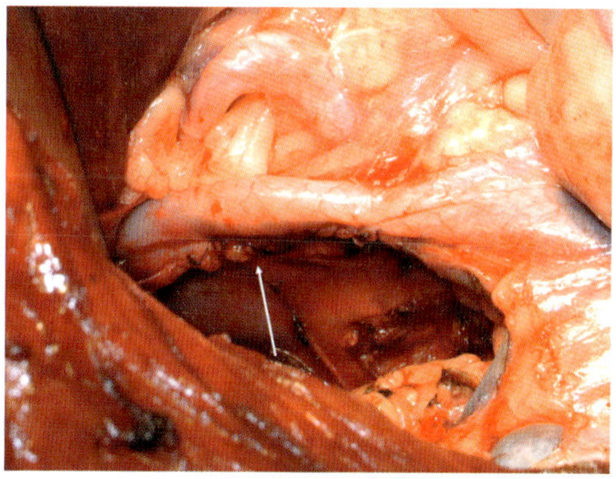

M-i)

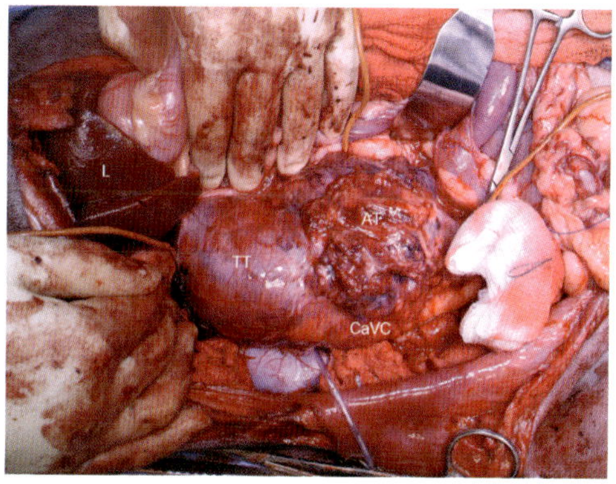

M-ii)

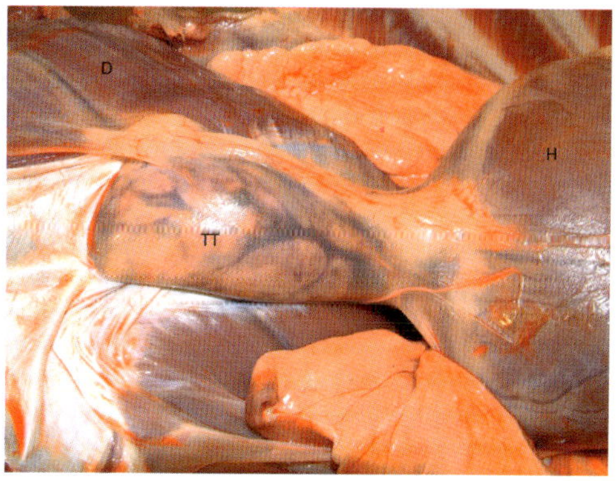

Complications

Intraoperative Complications

- Overall (4%–83%) [7, 9–15]
- Hypotension (2%–63%) [7–10, 12, 14–16]
- Hypertension (2%–15%) [7–9, 12, 14–16]
- Blood loss requiring a blood transfusion (2%–32%) [7–14, 16]
- Cardiac arrhythmias (7%–20%) [7–9, 12]
- Ventricular tachycardia (6%–40%) [7, 14, 15]
- Bradycardia (20%–23%) [14, 15]
- Hypoxemia or hypoxia (8%–12%) [8, 9]
- Hypercapnia (15%) [8]
- Tumor capsule rupture (4%–13%) [14, 17, 18]
- Unresectable tumor (5%) [16]

Postoperative Complications (0–14 Days)

- Overall (23%–72%) [9, 11–14, 19]
- Perioperative mortality
  - Overall (2%–60%) [7–11, 13, 15–22]: Perioperative mortality is associated with dogs with pheochromocytoma not pretreated with phenoxybenzamine (48% vs. 13%; note this is not a consistent finding and there is evidence that pretreatment with phenoxybenzamine is either contraindicated [15] or ineffective), older age, preoperative thrombocytopenia, emergency adrenalectomy, intraoperative arrhythmias, intraoperative blood loss and treatment with a blood transfusion, tumor size, invasion and extensive invasion into the caudal vena cava, concurrent nephrectomy, surgery time, tumor type (pheochromocytoma in one study [9] and adenocarcinoma in another study [10]), postoperative hypotension, postoperative hypoxemia, disseminated intravascular coagulation, pancreatitis, and renal failure [9, 16, 20]
  - Adrenalectomy alone (13%–47%) versus adrenalectomy and cavotomy (0%–71%) [7, 9, 11–13]
  - Elective (6%) versus emergency adrenalectomy (50%) [7]
- Ventricular tachycardia (13%) [7, 11]
- Vomiting ± diarrhea (4%–23%) [7, 9, 11, 14, 15]
- Hypotension (2%–16%) [7, 9, 12, 14]
- Hypertension (2%–6%) [11, 12, 14]
- Hypoxemia (10%) [9]
- Hypoadrenocorticism (6%–24%) [14, 16, 19]
- Unclassified respiratory disease (12%–13%) [7, 11]
- Pulmonary thromboembolism (0%–11%) [8, 12, 16, 17, 19]
- Aspiration pneumonia (2%–11%) [11, 12, 14, 17, 19]
- Pancreatitis (2%–8%) [8, 9, 11, 14, 16, 17, 19]
- Acute renal failure/renal insufficiency (3%–14%) [8, 9, 11, 12, 14, 16, 19]
- Disseminated intravascular coagulation (5%–10%) [8, 9, 11]
- Septic peritonitis (3%–5%) [9, 16]
- Abdominal wall dehiscence (8%) [11]

Postoperative Complications (>14 Days)

- Recurrent clinical signs in dogs with adrenal-dependent hyperadrenocorticsm because of postoperative local tumor recurrence, contralateral adrenal-dependent hyperadrenocorticism, or pituitary-dependent hyperadrenocorticsm [18]

Suggested Adjuvant Treatments

- None for dogs with adrenocortical adenoma or adenocarcinoma
- None for dogs with pheochromocytoma

Prognosis and Oncologic Outcome

Tumor Type	Local Recurrence Rate	Metastatic Rate	Disease-Free Interval (d)	Median Survival Time (d)	1-Year Survival Rate	2-Year Survival Rate
			Adrenocortical Adenoma and Adenocarcinoma Combined [23]			
Overall	–	–	–	1664	–	–
Utrecht score						
• <6	–	–	–	NR	–	–
• 6–10	–	–	–	1566	–	–
• >10	–	–	–	438	–	–
			Adrenocortical Adenoma [9, 16, 21]			
Overall	–	–	–	688 to NR	–	–
			Adrenocortical Adenocarcinoma [9, 10, 13, 16, 18, 19, 21]			
Overall	4%–14%	14%–50%	–	230–1460	88%	88%
			Pheochromocytoma [9, 10, 13, 16, 21, 24]			
Overall	9%	13%–22%	–	374 to NR	83%	60%
			Invasion into the Caudal Vena Cava [9]			
No invasion	–	–	–	NR	–	–
Invasion	–	–	–	1460	–	–

NR, not reached.

References

1 Pagani, E., Tursi, M., Lorenzi, C. et al. (2016). Ultrasonographic features of adrenal gland lesions in dogs can aid in diagnosis. *BMC Vet. Res.* 12 (1): 267.

2 Cook, A.K., Spaulding, K.A., and Edwards, J.F. (2014). Clinical findings in dogs with incidental adrenal gland lesions determined by ultrasonography: 151 cases (2007-2010). *J. Am. Vet. Med. Assoc.* 244 (10): 1181–1185.

3 Gostelow, R., Bridger, N., and Syme, H.M. (2013). Plasma-free metanephrine and free normetanephrine measurement for the diagnosis of pheochromocytoma in dogs. *J. Vet. Intern. Med.* 27 (1): 83–90.

4 Salesov, E., Boretti, F.S., Sieber-Ruckstuhl, N.S. et al. (2015). Urinary and plasma catecholamines and metanephrines in dogs with pheochromocytoma, hypercortisolism, nonadrenal disease and in healthy dogs. *J. Vet. Intern. Med.* 29 (2): 597–602.

5 Quante, S., Boretti, F.S., Kook, P.H. et al. (2010). Urinary catecholamine and metanephrine to creatinine ratios in dogs with hyperadrenocorticism or pheochromocytoma, and in healthy dogs. *J. Vet. Intern. Med.* 24 (5): 1093–1097.

6 Andrade, N., Rivas, L.R., Milovancev, M. et al. (2014). Intercostal approach for right adrenalectomy in dogs. *Vet. Surg.* 43 (2): 99–104.

7 Lang, J.M., Schertel, E., Kennedy, S. et al. (2011). Elective and emergency surgical management of adrenal gland tumors: 60 cases (1999-2006). *J. Am. Anim. Hosp. Assoc.* 47 (6): 428–435.

8 Taylor, C.J. and Monnet, E. (2021). A comparison of outcomes between laparoscopic and open adrenalectomies in dogs. *Vet. Surg.* 50 (Suppl 1): O99–O107.

9 Barrera, J.S., Bernard, F., Ehrhart, E.J. et al. (2013). Evaluation of risk factors for outcome associated with adrenal gland tumors with or without invasion of the caudal vena cava and treated via adrenalectomy in dogs: 86 cases (1993-2009). *J. Am. Vet. Med. Assoc.* 242 (12): 1715–1721.

10 Massari, F., Nicoli, S., Romanelli, G. et al. (2011). Adrenalectomy in dogs with adrenal gland tumors: 52 cases (2002-2008). *J. Am. Vet. Med. Assoc.* 239 (2): 216–221.

11 Kyles, A.E., Feldman, E.C., de Cock, H.E.V. et al. (2003). Surgical management of adrenal gland tumors with and without associated tumor thrombi in dogs: 40 cases (1994-2001). *J. Am. Vet. Med. Assoc.* 223 (5): 654–662.

12 Knight, R.C., Lamb, C.R., Brockman, D.J. et al. (2019). Variations in surgical technique for adrenalectomy with caudal vena cava venotomy in 19 dogs. *Vet. Surg.* 48 (5): 751–759.

13 Mayhew, P.D., Boston, S.E., Zwingenberger, A.L. et al. (2019). Perioperative morbidity and mortality in dogs with invasive adrenal neoplasms treated by adrenalectomy and cavotomy. *Vet. Surg.* 48 (5): 742–750.

14 Cavalcanti, J.V.J., Skinner, O.T., Mayhew, P.D. et al. (2020). Outcome in dogs undergoing adrenalectomy for small adrenal gland tumours without vascular invasion. *Vet. Comp. Oncol.* 18 (4): 599–606.

15 Appelgrein, C., Hosgood, G., Drynan, E. et al. (2020). Short-term outcome of adrenalectomy in dogs with adrenal gland tumours that did not receive pre-operative medical management. *Aust. Vet. J.* 98 (9): 449–454.

16 Schwartz, P., Kovak, J.R., Koprowski, A. et al. (2008). Evaluation of prognostic factors in the surgical treatment of adrenal gland tumors in dogs: 41 cases (1999-2005). *J. Am. Vet. Med. Assoc.* 232 (1): 77–84.

17 Mayhew, P.D., Culp, W.T.N., Hunt, G.B. et al. (2014). Comparison of perioperative morbidity and mortality rates in dogs with noninvasive adrenocortical masses undergoing laparoscopic versus open adrenalectomy. *J. Am. Vet. Med. Assoc.* 245 (9): 1028–1035.

18 van Sluijs, F.J., Sjollema, B.E., Voorhout, G. et al. (1995). Results of adrenalectomy in 36 dogs with hyperadrenocorticism caused by adrenocortical tumour. *Vet. Q.* 17 (3): 113–116.

19 Scavelli, T.D., Peterson, M.E., and Matthiesen, D.T. (1986). Results of surgical treatment for hyperadrenocorticism caused by adrenocortical neoplasia in the dog: 25 cases (1980-1984). *J. Am. Vet. Med. Assoc.* 189 (10): 1360–1364.

20 Herrera, M.A., Mehl, M.L., Kass, P.H. et al. (2008). Predictive factors and the effect of phenoxybenzamine on outcome in dogs undergoing adrenalectomy for pheochromocytoma. *J. Vet. Intern. Med.* 22 (6): 1333–1339.

21 Anderson, C.R., Birchard, S.J., Powers, B.E. et al. (2001). Surgical treatment of adrenocortical tumors: 21 cases (1990-1996). *J. Am. Anim. Hosp. Assoc.* 37 (1): 93–97.

22 Piegols, H.J., Abrams, B.E., Lapsley, J.M. et al. (2023). Risk factors influencing death prior to discharge in 302 dogs undergoing unilateral adrenalectomy for treatment of primary adrenal gland tumours. *Vet. Comp. Oncol.* 21 (4): 673–684.

23 Sanders, K., Cirkel, K., Grinwis, G.C.M. et al. (2019). The Utrecht Score: a novel histopathological scoring system to assess the prognosis of dogs with cortisol-secreting adrenocortical tumours. *Vet. Comp. Oncol.* 17 (3): 329–337.

24 Barthez, P.Y., Marks, S.L., Woo, J. et al. (1997). Pheochromocytoma in dogs: 61 cases (1984-1995). *J. Vet. Intern. Med.* 11 (5): 272–278.

19.2 Laparoscopic Adrenalectomy

Indications

1) Dogs and cats with adrenal masses <5 cm with no evidence of vascular invasion beyond the phrenicoabdominal vein (i.e., not caudal vena cava or renal vein)

Suggested Diagnostic Workup and Clinical Staging

- See *19.1. Open Adrenalectomy*.

Patient Positioning

The patient is positioned in lateral recumbency with the affected side uppermost. An oblique positioning to the abdomen with the dorsal aspect higher than the ventral aspect improves visualization of the retroperitoneal region during dissection. The surgeon is positioned on the ventral side of the patient, and the monitor is across the table on the dorsal aspect of the patient.

Surgical Technique (See Plate 19.2A–F)

A) For laparoscopic adrenalectomy, three to four separate ports are established to perform the procedure. Variations of the technique described later have also been described using single-port device access or placing dogs in sternal recumbency. A skin incision is made in a subumbilical location or just lateral to the umbilicus on the affected side. Placement of the telescope cannula commences as is described in *15.3. Laparoscopic Approach*. A 5-mm 30-degree telescope (T) is commonly used, and this is introduced into the initial cannula after a pneumoperitoneum is established. Two to three additional cannulae (C) are introduced to allow for placement of instrumentation. The first two instrument cannulae are triangulated with the telescope cannula by placing one cannula caudodorsal and one cannula craniodorsal as compared with the telescope cannula. If an additional cannula is needed for retraction, this is generally placed over the affected adrenal gland.

B) Organs covering the adrenal tumor (AT) need to be mobilized out of the way to allow for adrenalectomy. This is usually most easily accomplished by using a blunt probe to drag the organs off the kidney and adrenal gland and toward the abdominal midline or the opposite side of the abdomen.

Color Atlas of Canine and Feline Surgical Oncology, First Edition. Julius M. Liptak, Paolo Buracco, William T. N. Culp, and Nicholas J. Bacon.

Plate 19.2

Laparoscopic Adrenalectomy

A)

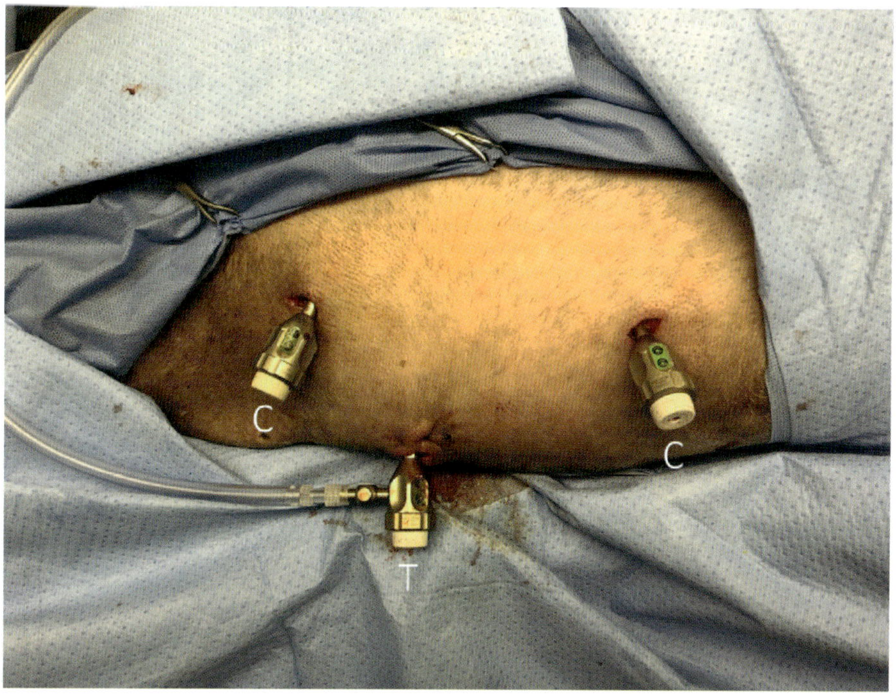

B)

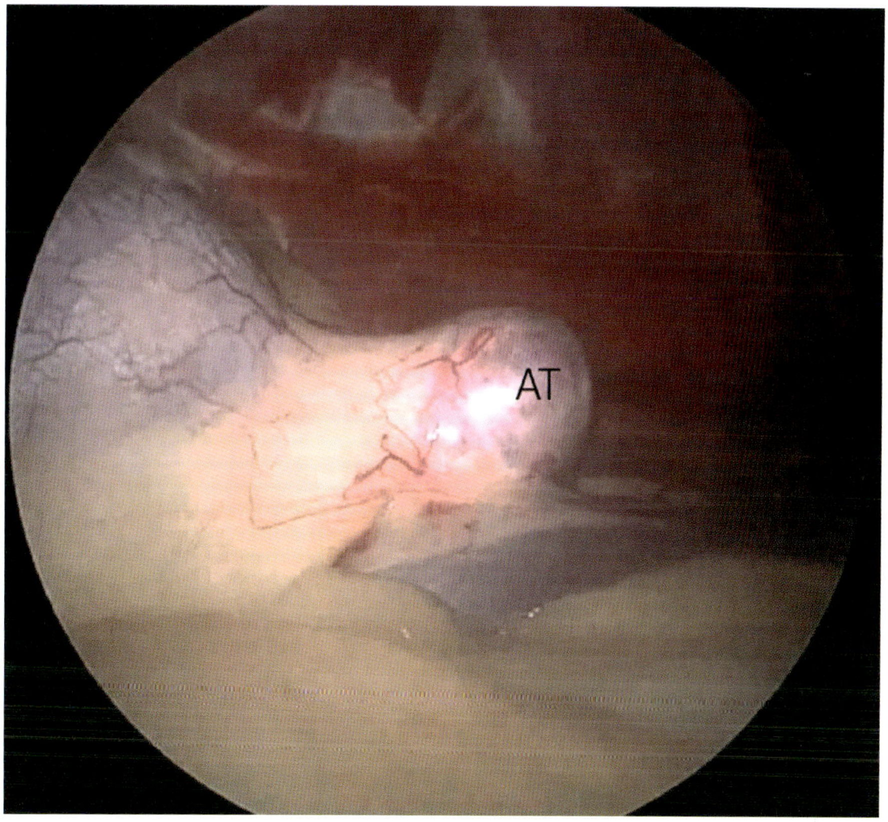

Surgical Technique (See Plate 19.2A–F) *continued*

C) Dissection is usually initiated by gently retracting the kidney or adrenal gland caudally (from the caudal instrument port) using a blunt probe or fan retractor, depending on the region of the adrenal gland that is going to be dissected first; the kidney is retracted caudally to allow visualization of the caudal adrenal gland or the adrenal gland is retracted caudally to open up the space between the cranial aspect of the adrenal gland and the vena cava. The dissection of the adrenal gland usually commences along the margin most closely associated with the caudal vena cava (CaVC). Many surgeons prefer starting cranially for right-sided tumors and caudally for left-sided tumors; however, each case should be assessed individually. A laparoscopic right-angle forceps can be used initially to create a plane between the adrenal gland and the vena cava. Depending on the amount of space created by blunt dissection, a J-hook electrocautery instrument or vessel sealing device can then be used to further dissect open the tissue connecting the adrenal gland to the vena cava.

D) Dissection laterally and dorsally to the adrenal gland is performed almost exclusively with a vessel sealing device. The adrenal gland is mobilized by using a blunt probe to hold it in different positions or by grasping fatty or connective tissue attached to the adrenal gland; it is preferable not to grasp the adrenal gland itself to prevent capsular rupture. The dorsolateral aspect of the phrenicoabdominal vessels is encountered during this dissection, and the vessel sealing device can be used for sealing this aspect of the vessels.

E) If possible, it is advantageous to dissect the medial aspect of the phrenicoabdominal vein free of surrounding tissues to allow for safe placement of the vessel sealing device completely around the vein. This location should be several millimeters away from the vena cava to allow room for thermal spread from the vessel sealing device. If caudal dissection has not been performed to this point, this can commence after transection of the phrenicoabdominal vessels by continuing the dissection along the caudal vena cava in a caudal direction. If the tumor is associated with the renal vein, a right-angle forceps can be used to dissect between the renal vein and the tumor.

F) When the adrenal gland has been completely separated from the surrounding tissues, the vessel sealing device is removed and a retrieval bag is introduced into the abdomen. With small adrenal gland tumors, the thumb of a sterile glove can also be used as a retrieval device (i, ii).

Closure

The muscular layers are closed with 2-0 to 3-0 monofilament absorbable suture in a simple interrupted or cruciate pattern. The subcutaneous tissue is closed with 3-0 monofilament absorbable suture if needed. The dermal layer is apposed with 3-0 to 4-0 monofilament nonabsorbable suture in a simple interrupted or simple continuous pattern.

Postoperative Management

1) Multimodal analgesia
2) Elizabethan collar or body suit
3) Adrenal function testing

Complications

Intraoperative Complications

- Hypotension (14%) [1]
- Hypertension (14%–80%) [1, 2]
- Cardiac arrhythmias (7%–20%) [1, 2]
- Hypercapnia (29%) [1]
- Minor capsular rupture/impingement (0%–32%) [1–6]

Plate 19.2

Laparoscopic Adrenalectomy *continued*

C)

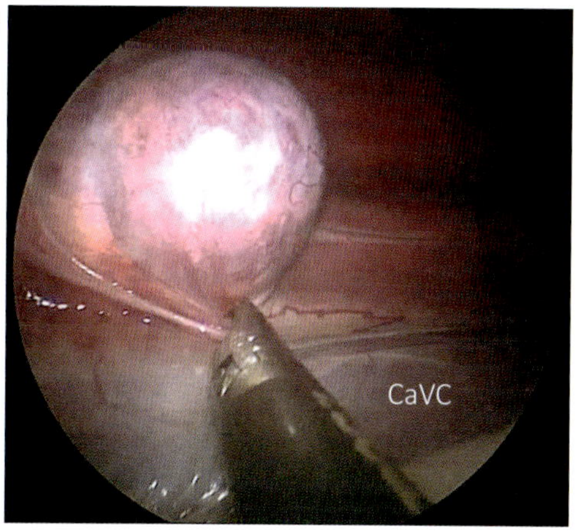

D)

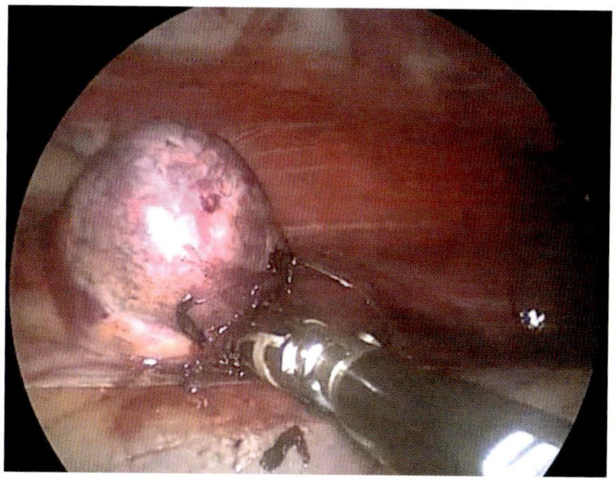

E)

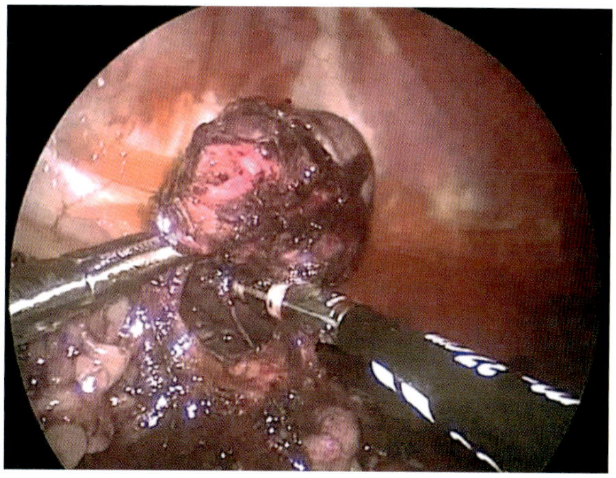

F-i)

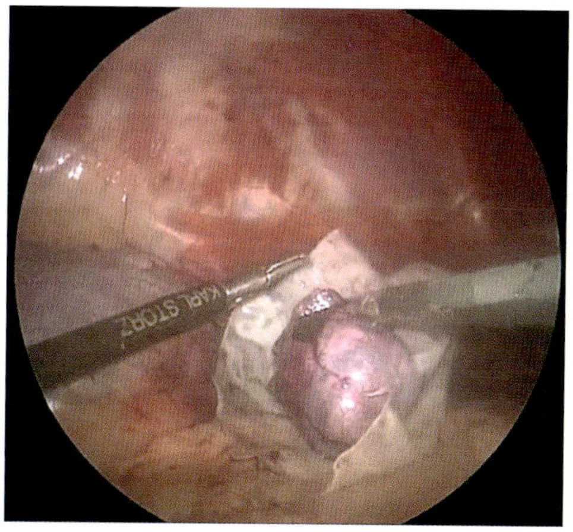

F-ii)

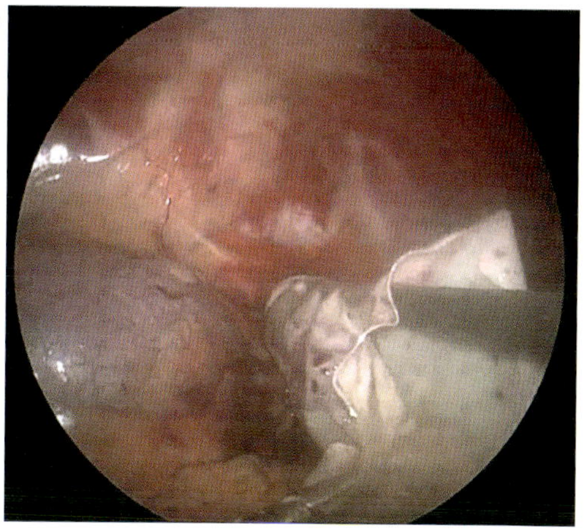

- Minor hemorrhage (14%) [1, 5]
- Splenic laceration during port placement (10%) [2]
- Pneumothorax (11%) [5]
- Conversion to an open adrenalectomy (0%–10% in dogs [2–6] and 36% in cats [7])
- For complications specific to all laparoscopic procedures, see *15.3. Laparoscopic Approach*

Postoperative Complications

- Perioperative mortality (0%–29%) [1–6]
- Subcutaneous cellulitis around portals (43%) [4]
- Surgical-site infection (5%) [6]
- Pulmonary thromboembolism or pneumonia (0%–29%) [1, 4, 5]
- Acute renal failure/renal insufficiency (8%) [1]
- Hypoadrenocorticism (11%) [5]

Suggested Adjuvant Treatments

- See *19.1. Open Adrenalectomy*.

Prognosis and Oncologic Outcome

- See *19.1. Open Adrenalectomy*.

References

1 Taylor, C.J. and Monnet, E. (2021). A comparison of outcomes between laparoscopic and open adrenalectomies in dogs. *Vet. Surg.* suppl 1: O99–O107.

2 Pitt, K.A., Mayhew, P.D., Steffey, M.A. et al. (2016). Laparoscopic adrenalectomy for removal of unilateral noninvasive pheochromocytomas in 10 dogs. *Vet. Surg.* 45 (S1): O70–O76.

3 Mayhew, P.D. (2009). Advanced laparoscopic procedures (hepatobiliary, endocrine) in dogs and cats. *Vet. Clin. North Am. Small Anim. Pract.* 39 (5): 925–939.

4 Jiménez Peláez, M., Bouvy, B.M., and Dupré, G.P. (2008). Laparoscopic adrenalectomy for treatment of unilateral adrenocortical carcinomas: technique, complications, and results in seven dogs. *Vet. Surg.* 37 (5): 444–453.

5 Naan, E.C., Kirpensteijn, J., Dupré, G.P. et al. (2013). Innovative approach to laparoscopic adrenalectomy for treatment of unilateral adrenal gland tumors in dogs. *Vet. Surg.* 42 (6): 710–715.

6 Mayhew, P.D., Culp, W.T., Hunt, G.B. et al. (2014). Comparison of perioperative morbidity and mortality rates in dogs with noninvasive adrenocortical masses undergoing laparoscopic versus open adrenalectomy. *J. Am. Vet. Med. Assoc.* 245 (9): 1028–1035.

7 Mitchell, J.W., Mayhew, P.D., Culp, W.T.N. et al. (2017). Outcome of laparoscopic adrenalectomy for resection of unilateral noninvasive adrenocortical tumors in 11 cats. *Vet. Surg.* 46 (5): 714–721.

Chapter 20: Sublumbar Lymph Node Resection

20.1 Open Sublumbar Lymph Node Resection

Indications

1) Resection of enlarged or metastatic sublumbar lymph nodes (medial iliac, hypogastric, and sacral): This is most common in dogs with apocrine gland anal sac adenocarcinoma but can also be observed in dogs and cats with urogenital, mammary, and pelvic limb malignancies.
2) Resection of normal-sized sublumbar lymph nodes for clinical staging purposes.
3) Open sublumbar lymph node resection can be combined with a closed anal sacculectomy (see *26. Anal Sacculectomy*) in dogs with apocrine gland anal sac adenocarcinoma.

Suggested Diagnostic Workup and Clinical Staging

- Complete blood count, serum biochemistry, and urinalysis
- Ionized calcium blood test
- ± Fine-needle aspirate cytology of the anal sac mass ± enlarged sublumbar lymph nodes
- Abdominal ultrasound or precontrast and postcontrast computed tomography (CT) scan of the abdomen and pelvis for assessment of sublumbar lymph nodes and other intra-abdominal metastasis; abdominal CT scan is preferred because of better imaging of the sacral lymph nodes within the pelvic canal [1, 2]
- Three-view thoracic radiographs or thoracic CT scan for assessment of lung metastasis

Patient Positioning

The patient is positioned in dorsal recumbency.

Surgical Technique (See Plate 20.1A–E, G)

A) A ventral midline celiotomy is performed (see *15.1. Ventral Midline Celiotomy*). The length of the incision is typically from the umbilicus to the pubic brim. The ventral ligament of the bladder is incised to allow the bladder to be mobilized to one side or the other. Large abdominal retractors (e.g. Balfour retractors) are inserted to aid surgical exposure and visualization. These can be inserted as a single retractor for lateral-to-lateral abdominal wall retraction (i) or two retractors perpendicular to each other for lateral-to-lateral and cranial-to-caudal abdominal wall retraction (ii). For both retraction techniques, moistened laparotomy sponges are inserted into the abdominal cavity between the blades of the retractor and intra-abdominal structures to aid in maintaining their retraction from the surgical field and exposure of the sublumbar lymph node (SLLN).

Color Atlas of Canine and Feline Surgical Oncology, First Edition. Julius M. Liptak, Paolo Buracco, William T. N. Culp, and Nicholas J. Bacon.

Plate 20.1

Open Sublumbar Lymph Node Resection

A-i)

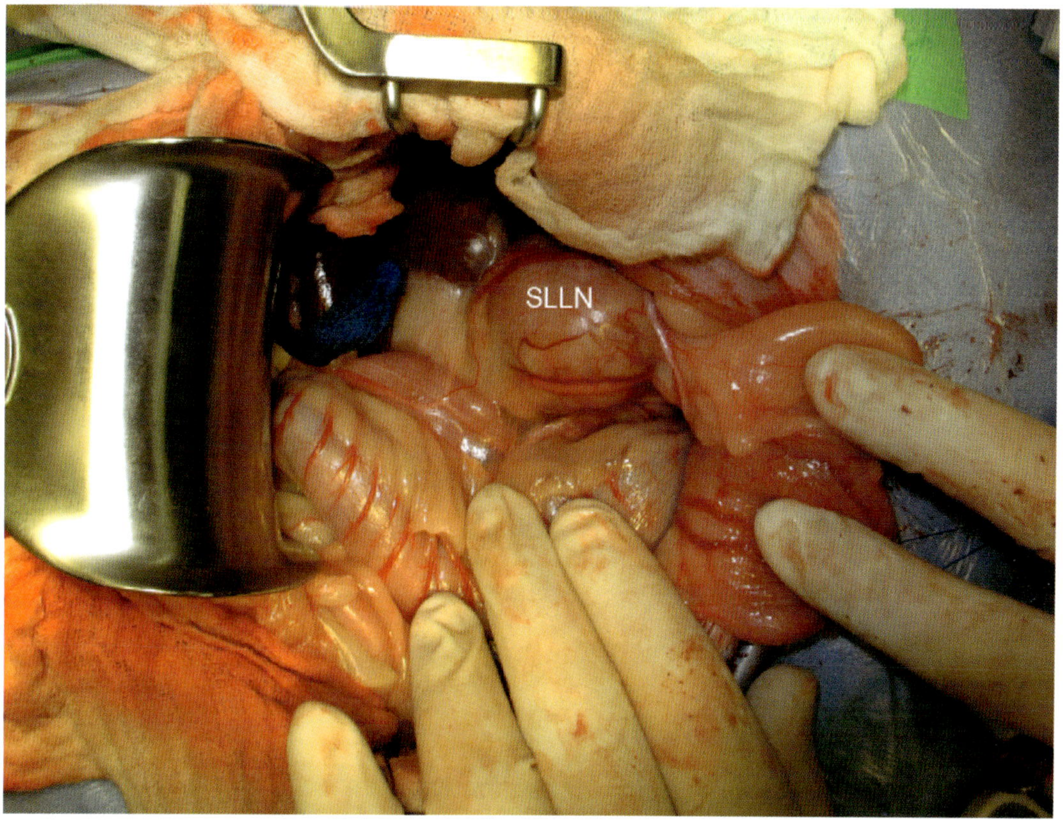

A-ii)

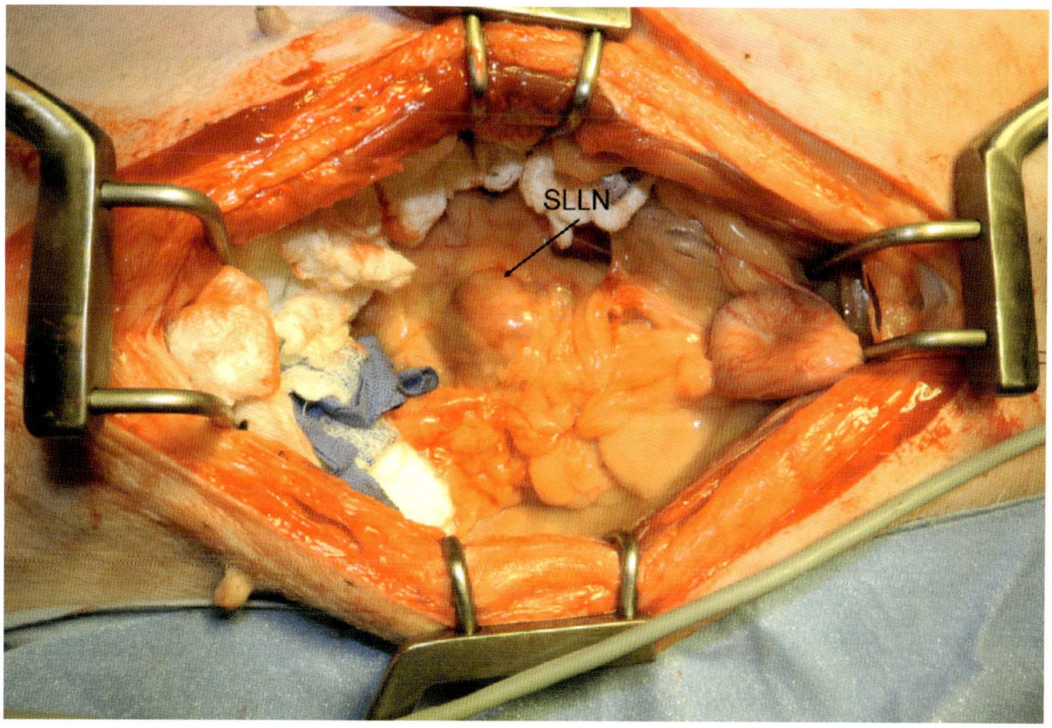

Surgical Technique (See Plate 20.1A–E, G) *continued*

B) The ureters should be identified (arrow) before extirpation of the sublumbar lymph nodes (SLLN) to minimize the risk of iatrogenic ureteral trauma.

C) A longitudinal paramedian defect is created in the retroperitoneum overlying the enlarged lymph node (SLLN), medial to the ipsilateral ureter and cranial to the palpable iliac arteries (i). If there are several enlarged lymph nodes, then the medial iliac lymph node (MILN) should be excised first because this is the most accessible of the sublumbar lymph nodes (ii) and, once extirpated, will make subsequent excision of the hypogastric (iii, iv) and sacral nodes (SLN) easier.

D) Enlarged sublumbar lymph nodes are excised using a combination of blunt dissection to separate the lymph node from adjacent soft tissues, which can be done with Metzenbaum scissors or gentle digital dissection, and either electrosurgery or vessel sealing device (pictured) for sealing and transection of blood vessels and fascial attachments (A, aorta; EIA, external iliac artery; IIA, internal iliac artery).

Plate 20.1

Open Sublumbar Lymph Node Resection *continued*

B)

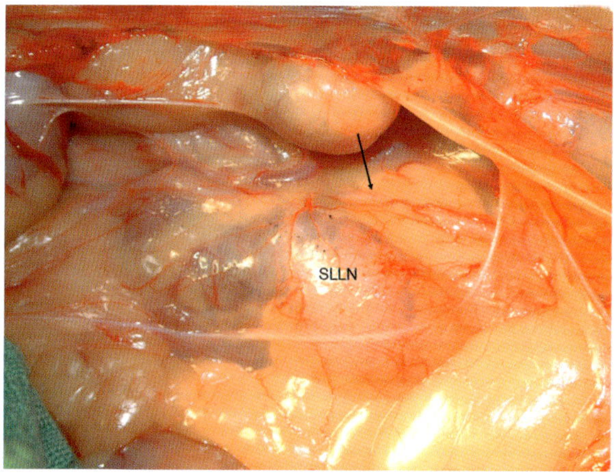

C-i)

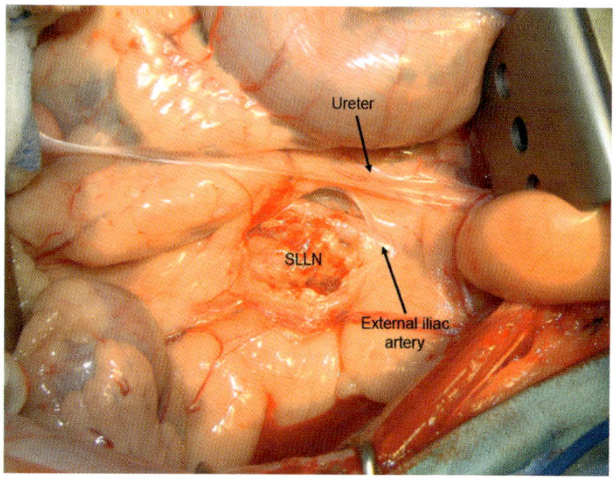

C-ii)

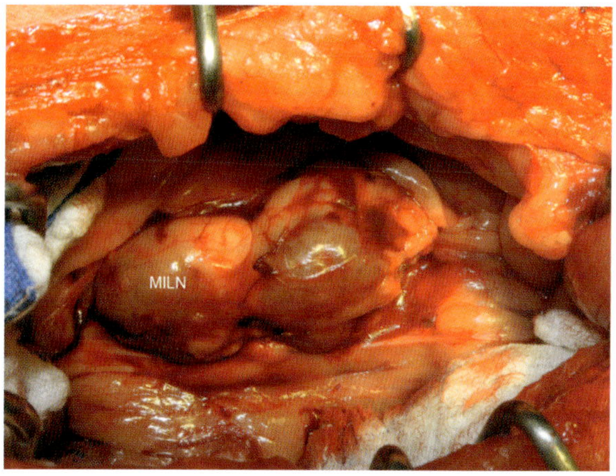

C-iii)

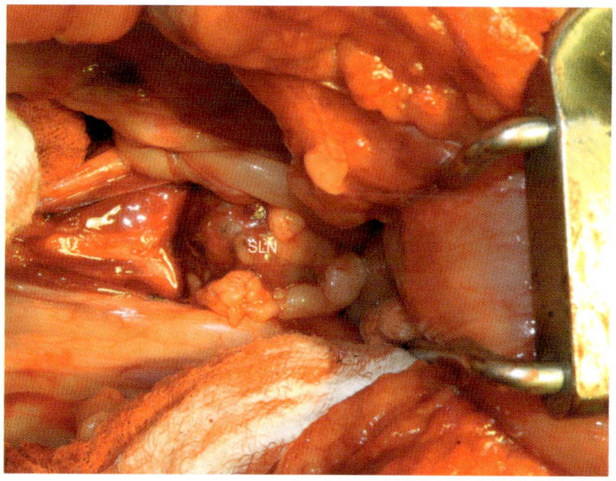

C-iv)

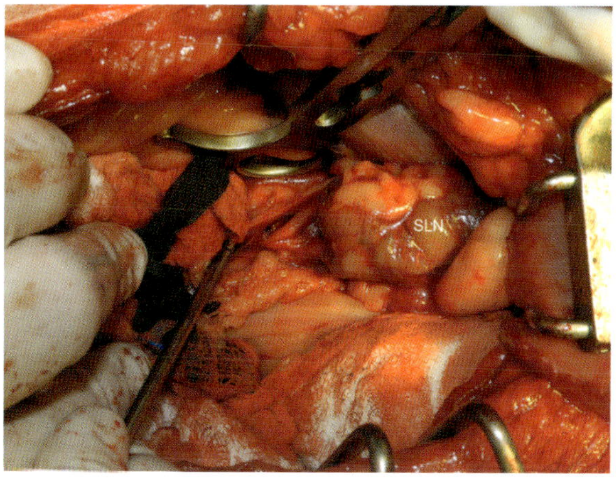

D)

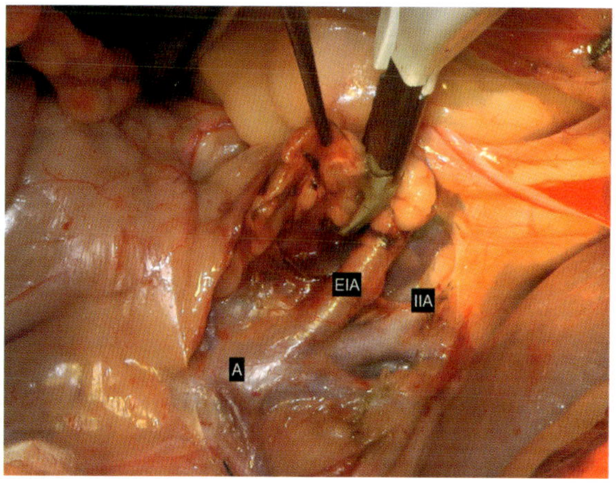

Surgical Technique (See Plate 20.1A–E, G) *continued*

E) The enlarged sublumbar lymph nodes (SLLN) may be intimately associated with the iliac arteries (A, aorta; EIA, external iliac artery; IIA, internal iliac artery) and veins (i–iv; EIV, external iliac vein). In these cases, the lymph node should be gently dissected away from these vessels. This can be done with the flat blade of an electrosurgery pen, the inner stylet of a Poole suction tip (v), or blunt dissection with Metzenbaum scissors. In rare cases, the external or internal iliac artery or vein, but not both, can be sacrificed unilaterally, but this should be avoided (vi, iliac artery entering metastatic lymph node, arrow; vii, internal iliac artery clipped with two hemoclips).

F) The enlarged sublumbar lymph nodes may be firmly fixed to the lumbar spine. In these cases, a periosteal elevator is used to elevate the dorsal aspect of the lymph nodes away from the periosteum and fascia along the ventral aspect of the lumbar vertebrae (not pictured).

Plate 20.1

Open Sublumbar Lymph Node Resection *continued*

E-i)

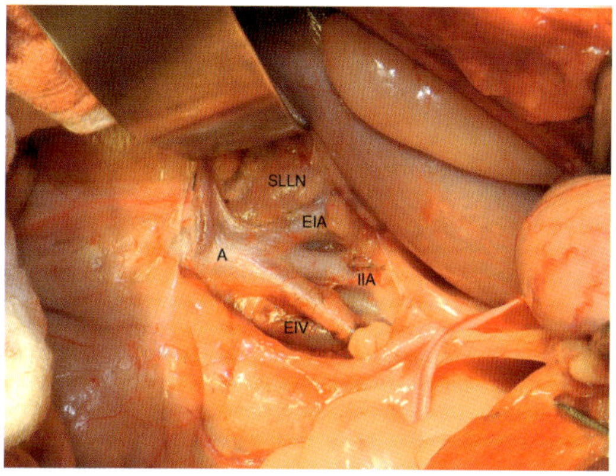

E-ii)

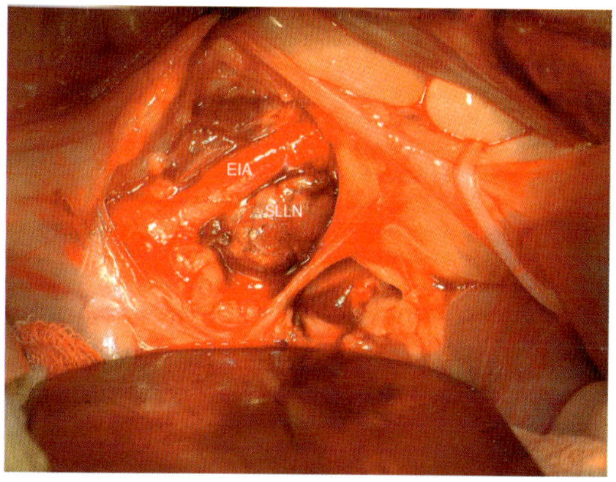

E-iii)

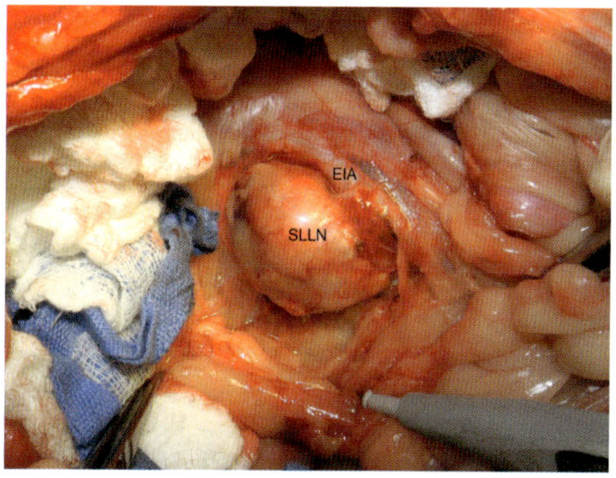

E-iv)

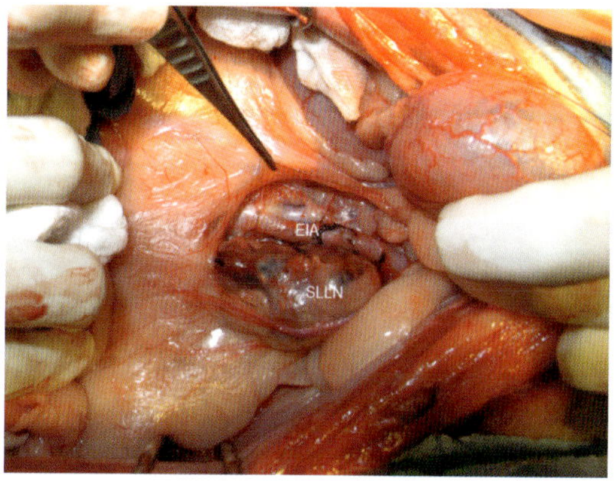

E-v)

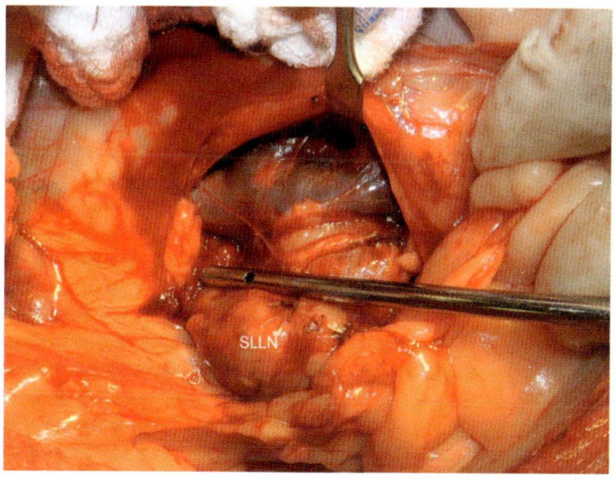

E-vi)

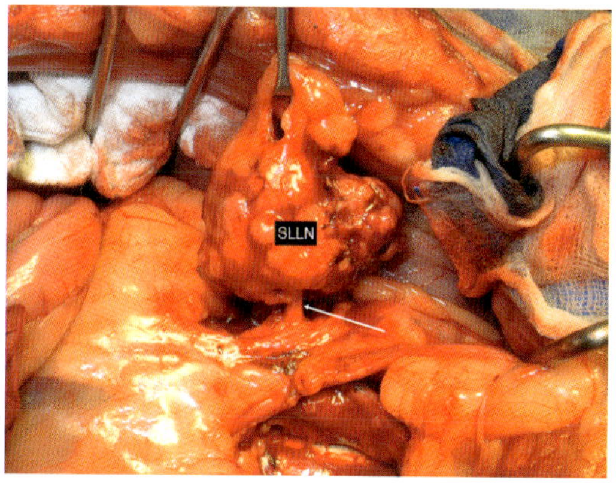

E-vii)

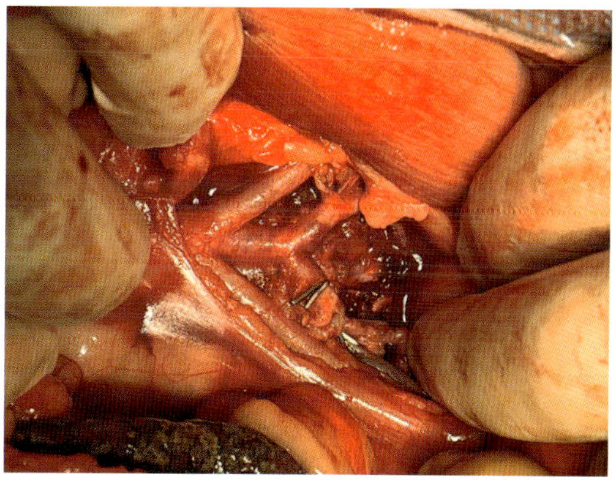

Surgical Technique (See Plate 20.1A–E, G) *continued*

G) The abdominal cavity should be systematically explored for metastatic disease. The most common metastatic sites for apocrine gland anal sac adenocarcinoma after the sublumbar lymph nodes are the spleen (i) and liver (ii), but the colonic (iii) and superficial inguinal lymph nodes should also be examined because metastasis can occur to these lymph nodes. After completion of the lymph node excision and abdominal exploration, the abdominal cavity should be lavaged with warmed, sterile isotonic saline.

Closure

The linea alba, subcutaneous tissue, and skin are closed as described in *15.1. Ventral Midline Celiotomy*.

Postoperative Management

1) Multimodal analgesia
2) Elizabethan collar or body suit
3) ± Monitor ionized calcium levels if hypercalcemic before surgery

Complications [3–6]

- Overall: 26% [5]

Intraoperative Complications

- Overall: 18% [5]
- Bleeding from the retroperitoneal space or iatrogenic trauma to the aorta or iliac arteries or caudal vena cava or iliac veins (5%–18%)
- Unresectable or residual disease because of adhesion to the vertebrae or involvement of the iliac arteries ± veins (5%)
- Lymph node rupture (3%)
- Iatrogenic ureteral trauma (rare)

Postoperative Complications

- Overall: 10% [5]
- Transient neuropraxia to the pelvic limbs (obturator nerve) (3%)
- Abdominal wall dehiscence (1%–2%)
- Pelvic limb lymphedema (0%–3%)
- Urinary incontinence (2%)
- Surgical-site infection (1%)
- Hypocalcemia

Suggested Adjuvant Treatments

- See *26. Anal Sacculectomy*.

Prognosis and Oncologic Outcome

- See *26. Anal Sacculectomy*.

Plate 20.1

Open Sublumbar Lymph Node Resection *continued*

G-i)

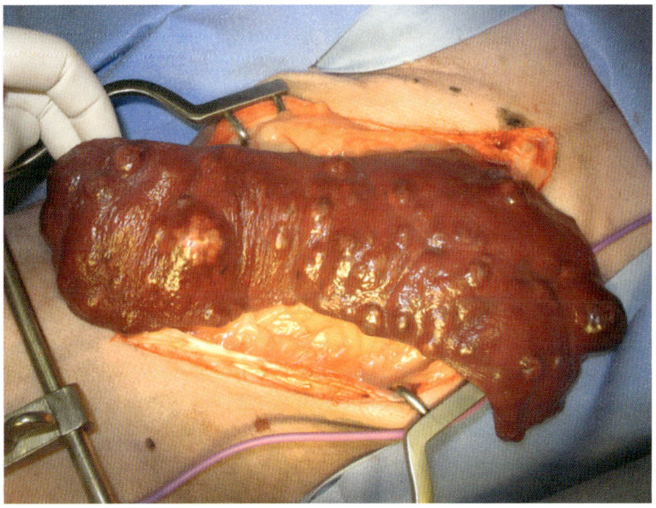

G-ii)

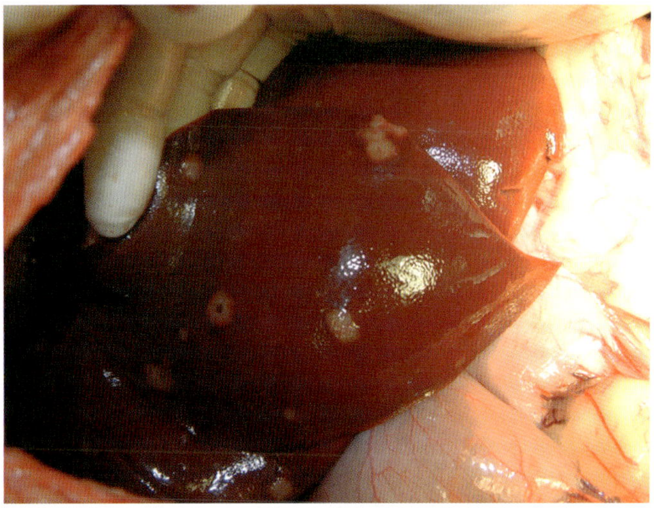

G-iii)

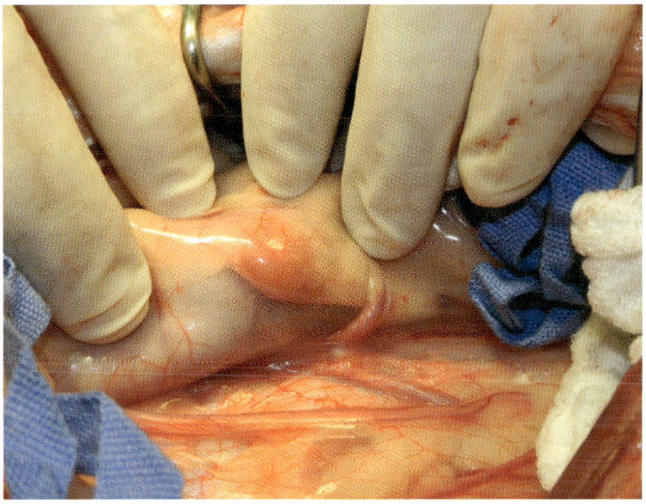

References

1 Palladino, S., Keyerleber, M.A., King, R.G. et al. (2016). Utility of computed tomography versus abdominal ultrasound examination to identify iliosacral lymphadenomegaly in dogs with apocrine gland adenocarcinoma of the anal sac. *J. Vet. Intern. Med.* 30 (6): 1858–1863.

2 Pollard, R.E., Fuller, M.C., and Steffey, M.A. (2017). Ultrasound and computed tomography of the iliosacral lymphatic centre in dogs with anal sac gland carcinoma. *Vet. Comp. Oncol.* 15 (2): 299–306.

3 Barnes, D.C. and Demetriou, J.L. (2017). Surgical management of primary, metastatic and recurrent anal sac adenocarcinoma in the dog: 52 cases. *J. Small Anim. Pract.* 58 (5): 263–268.

4 Liptak, J.M., Selmic, L., Amsellem, P. et al. (2015). Apocrine gland anal sac adenocarcinoma and sublumbar lymph node metastasis: a VSSO retrospective study. *Am. Coll. Vet. Surg. Annu. Meet.* .

5 Huerta, Y., De Mello Souza, C.H., Selmic, L.E. et al. (2022). Complications associated with iliosacral lymphadenectomy in dogs with metastatic apocrine gland anal sac adenocarcinoma. *Can. Vet. J.* 63: 929–934.

6 Tanis, J.B., Simlett-Moss, A.B., Ossowksa, M. et al. (2022). Canine anal sac gland carcinoma with regional lymph node metastases treated with sacculectomy and lymphadenectomy: outcome and possible prognostic factors. *Vet. Comp. Oncol.* 20: 276–292.

20.2 Laparoscopic Sublumbar Lymph Node Resection

Indications

1) Resection of enlarged or metastatic sublumbar lymph nodes (medial iliac, hypogastric, and sacral): This is most common in dogs with apocrine gland anal sac adenocarcinoma but can also be observed in dogs and cats with urogenital, mammary, and pelvic limb malignancies.
2) Resection of normal-sized sublumbar lymph nodes for clinical staging purposes.
3) Laparoscopic sublumbar lymph node resection can be combined with a closed anal sacculectomy (see *26. Anal Sacculectomy*) in dogs with apocrine gland anal sac adenocarcinoma.

Suggested Diagnostic Workup and Clinical Staging

- Complete blood count, serum biochemistry, and urinalysis
- Ionized calcium blood test
- ± Fine-needle aspirate cytology of the anal sac mass ± enlarged sublumbar lymph nodes
- Abdominal ultrasound or precontrast and postcontrast computed tomography (CT) scan of the abdomen and pelvis for assessment of sublumbar lymph nodes and other intra-abdominal metastasis; abdominal CT scan is preferred because of better imaging of the sacral lymph nodes within the pelvic canal [1, 2]
- Three-view thoracic radiographs or thoracic CT scan for assessment of lung metastasis

Patient Positioning

Techniques for performing lymphadenectomy with patients in both dorsal and lateral recumbency have been described [3, 4]. With the approach in dorsal recumbency, the patient is rotated 30 degrees away from the affected side during identification and dissection to allow for organs to fall away from the region of interest. With the approach in lateral recumbency, the side of the lymph node resection is positioned uppermost. If bilateral lymph node resections are to be performed, then the patient will need to be rotated to the opposite side to allow for contralateral lymphadenectomy.

Surgical Technique – Dorsal Recumbency: Instrumentation and Access

A) A three-port technique is used (not pictured). A skin incision is made craniolateral to the umbilicus in the right upper abdomen. Placement of the telescope cannula commences as is described in *15.3. Laparoscopic Approach*. A 5-mm 30-degree telescope is most commonly used, and this is introduced into the initial cannula after a pneumoperitoneum is established.
B) Two additional cannulae are introduced to allow for placement of instrumentation (not pictured). The first is placed in the left upper quadrant in a position equal to the telescope cannula on the left side. A third cannula is placed in the caudal abdomen about one third of the distance from the pubic brim to the cranially placed port on the ipsilateral side. One of the instrument cannulae should be 10 mm to allow for eventual placement of a specimen retrieval bag.

Color Atlas of Canine and Feline Surgical Oncology, First Edition. Julius M. Liptak, Paolo Buracco, William T. N. Culp, and Nicholas J. Bacon.

Surgical Technique – Lateral Recumbency: Instrumentation and Access (See Plate 20.2C/D)

C) A three-port technique is used. A skin incision is made in a subumbilical location or just lateral to the umbilicus on the affected side. The skin incision is located directly ventral to the most cranial margin of the ilial wing. Placement of the telescope cannula (T) commences as is described in *15.3. Laparoscopic Approach*. A 5-mm 30-degree telescope is most commonly used, and this is introduced into the initial cannula after a pneumoperitoneum is established.

D) Two additional cannulae are introduced to allow for placement of instrumentation (C). The two-instrument cannulae are triangulated with the telescope cannula by placing one cannula caudodorsal and one cannula craniodorsal as compared with the telescope cannula. The cranial cannula should be 10 mm to allow for eventual placement of a specimen retrieval bag.

Surgical Technique – Lymphadenectomy (See Plate 20.2E–H)

E) A dissection plane is created cranial to the affected lymph node(s) by using laparoscopic right-angle forceps to create a window in the retroperitoneum. This dissection often starts immediately caudal to the deep circumflex blood vessels, although variations exist. Once a defect in the retroperitoneal lining has been created, a J-hook electrocautery device or vessel sealing device can be used to dissect the tissue around the lymph node.

F) Lateral and dorsal dissection of the lymph node (SLLN) is performed almost exclusively with a vessel sealing device. The lymph node is mobilized by grasping fatty or connective tissue attached to the node; it is preferable not to grasp the capsule of the lymph node itself to prevent capsular rupture.

G) These lymph nodes (SLLN) are often closely associated with major blood vessels, including the iliac arteries and veins (arrow). Dissection between the lymph node and these major blood vessels should be performed with right-angle forceps. Instrumentation that may be useful in the other instrument cannula includes a blunt probe for gentle retraction, laparoscopic hemostat, or Babcock forceps to gently elevate the lymph node away from adjacent blood vessels.

H) When the lymph node (SLLN) has been completely separated from the surrounding tissues, the lymph node is grasped and placed in a retrieval bag. For small lymph nodes, the thumb of a sterile glove can also be used as a retrieval device.

Plate 20.2

Laparoscopic Sublumbar Lymph Node Resection

C/D)

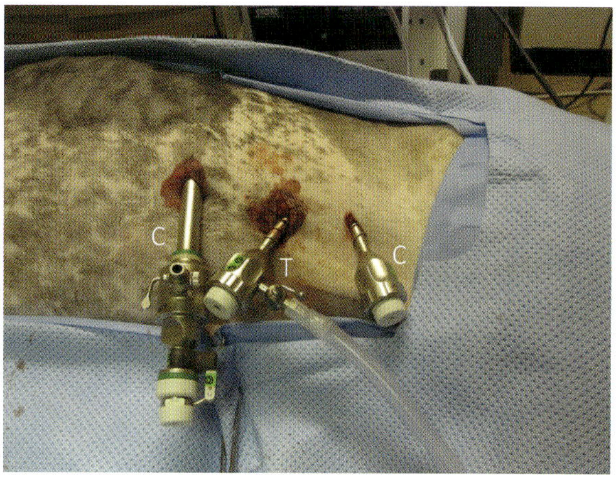

Courtesy of Dr. Phillip Mayhew

E)

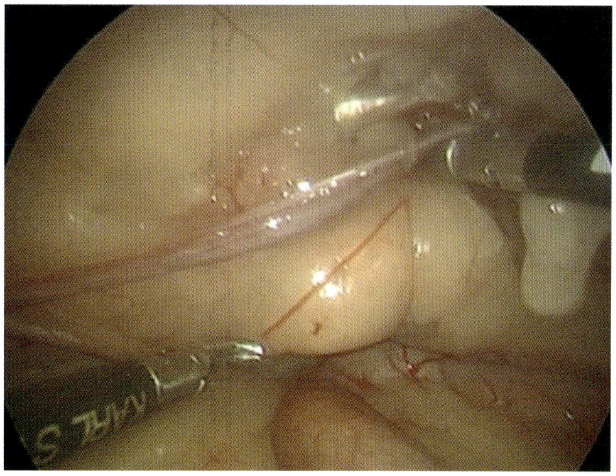

Courtesy of Dr. Phillip Mayhew

F)

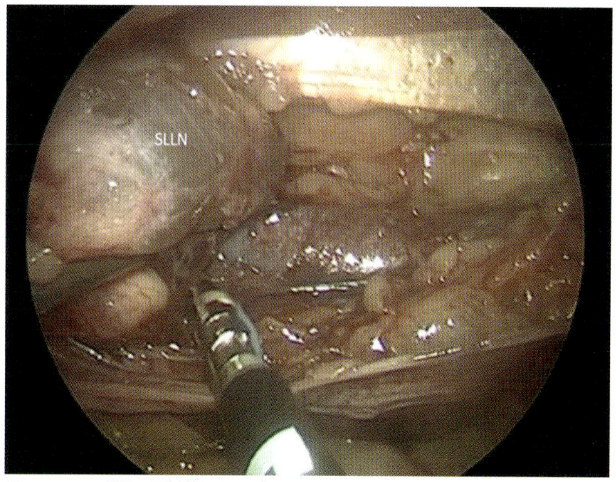

Courtesy of Dr. Phillip Mayhew

G)

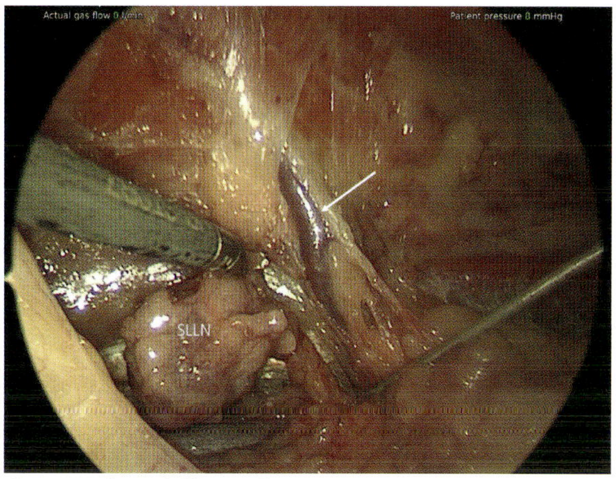

Courtesy of Dr. Phillip Mayhew

H)

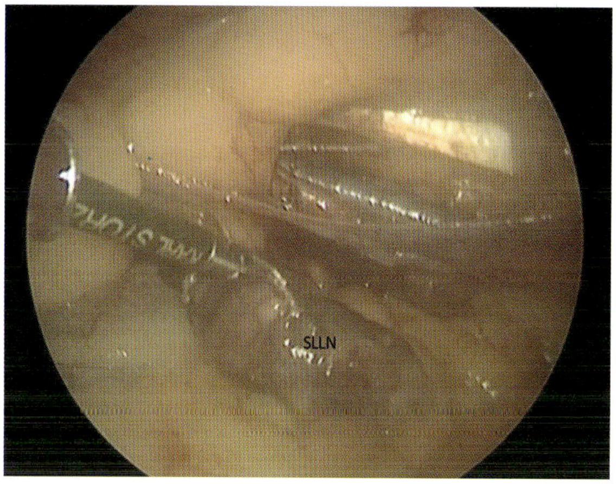

Courtesy of Dr. Phillip Mayhew

Closure

The muscular layers are closed with 2-0 to 3-0 monofilament absorbable suture in a simple interrupted or cruciate pattern. The subcutaneous tissue is closed with 3-0 monofilament absorbable suture if needed. The dermal layer is apposed with 3-0 to 4-0 monofilament absorbable suture in a simple interrupted or simple continuous pattern.

Postoperative Management

1) Multimodal analgesia
2) Elizabethan collar or body suit
3) ± Monitor ionized calcium levels if hypercalcemic before surgery

Complications

Intraoperative Complications

- Mild to moderate hemorrhage (controlled laparoscopically) (50%) [4]
- Lymph node capsule rupture (38%) [4]
- For complications specific to all laparoscopic procedures, see *15.3. Laparoscopic Approach*.

Postoperative Complications

- For complications specific to all laparoscopic procedures, see *15.3. Laparoscopic Approach*.

Suggested Adjuvant Treatments

- See *26. Anal Sacculectomy*.

Prognosis and Oncologic Outcome

- See *26. Anal Sacculectomy*.

References

1 Palladino, S., Keyerleber, M.A., King, R.G. et al. (2016). Utility of computed tomography versus abdominal ultrasound examination to identify iliosacral lymphadenomegaly in dogs with apocrine gland adenocarcinoma of the anal sac. *J. Vet. Intern. Med.* 30 (6): 1858–1863.

2 Pollard, R.E., Fuller, M.C., and Steffey, M.A. (2017). Ultrasound and computed tomography of the iliosacral lymphatic centre in dogs with anal sac gland carcinoma. *Vet. Comp. Oncol.* 15 (2): 299–306.

3 Lim, H., Kim, J., Li, L. et al. (2017). Bilateral medial iliac lymph node excision by a ventral laparoscopic approach: technique description. *J. Vet. Med. Sci.* 79 (9): 1603–1610.

4 Steffey, M.A., Daniel, L., Mayhew, P.D. et al. (2015). Laparoscopic extirpation of the medial iliac lymph nodes in normal dogs. *Vet. Surg.* 44 (Suppl 1): 59–65.

Section 5
Gastrointestinal

Chapter 21: Gastrectomy

The two main surgical techniques for resection of gastric tumors are partial gastric resection and Billroth I (pylorectomy and gastroduodenostomy). A partial gastric resection is recommended for gastric body tumors, whereas a Billroth I is recommended for resection of tumors involving the pylorus and pyloric antrum. A Billroth II (pyloric and duodenal resection with gastrojejunostomy and cholecystojejunostomy) is not recommended in dogs and cats because of significant postoperative morbidity [1]. Although not detailed in this chapter, submucosal resection of benign tumors from the gastric cardiac region has been described in dogs with excellent outcomes [2].

Suggested Diagnostic Workup and Clinical Staging

- Complete blood count, serum biochemistry, and urinalysis
- Endoscopy with endoscopic biopsies
- Abdominal ultrasound or computed tomography (CT) scan with image-guided aspirates
- Three-view thoracic radiographs or thoracic CT scan for assessment of lung metastasis

Suggested Adjuvant Treatments

- Chemotherapy for dogs with gastric carcinomas
- Chemotherapy for cats with solitary gastric lymphomas

Prognosis and Oncologic Outcome

Prognosis and Oncologic Outcome – Dogs

	Local Recurrence Rate	Metastatic Rate	Disease-Free Interval (d)	Median Survival Time (d)	1-Year Survival Rate	2-Year Survival Rate
			Carcinoma [3]			
Overall	8%–30%	45%–70%	54	178	18%	–
			Leiomyosarcoma[a] [4, 5]			
Overall	10%	54%	–	238–650	75%	66%
			Gastrointestinal Stromal Tumor[a] [5]			
Overall	0%	7%	–	354	–	–

[a] Includes all gastrointestinal sites (stomach, small intestines, cecum, and colon).

Color Atlas of Canine and Feline Surgical Oncology, First Edition. Julius M. Liptak, Paolo Buracco, William T. N. Culp, and Nicholas J. Bacon.

Prognosis and Oncologic Outcome – Cats

	Local Recurrence Rate	Metastatic Rate	Disease-Free Interval (d)	Median Survival Time (d)	1-Year Survival Rate	2-Year Survival Rate
			Lymphoma[a] [6]			
Overall	50%		357	417	–	–

[a] Includes all gastrointestinal sites (stomach, small intestines, and colon), and all cats were treated with an adjuvant cyclophosphamide-doxorubicin-vincristine-prednisone (CHOP) protocol.

References

1 Ahmadu-Suka, F., Withrow, S.J., Nelson, A.W. et al. (1988). Billroth II gastrojejunostomy in dogs. Stapling technique and postoperative complications. *Vet. Surg.* 17 (4): 211–219.

2 Kerpsack, S.J. and Birchard, S.J. (1994). Removal of leiomyomas and other noninvasive masses from the cardiac region of the canine stomach. *J. Am. Anim. Hosp. Assoc.* 30: 500–504.

3 Abrams, B., Wavreille, V.A., Husbands, B.D. et al. (2019). Perioperative complications and outcome after surgery for treatment of gastric carcinoma in dogs: A Veterinary Society of Surgical Oncology retrospective study of 40 cases (2004-2018). *Vet. Surg.* 48 (6): 923–932.

4 Cohen, M., Post, G.S., and Wright, J.C. (2003). Gastrointestinal leiomyosarcoma in 14 dogs. *J. Vet. Intern. Med.* 17 (1): 107–110.

5 Russell, K.N., Mehler, S.J., Skorupski, K.A. et al. (2007). Clinical and immunohistochemical differentiation of gastrointestinal stromal tumors from leiomyosarcomas in dogs: 42 cases (1990-2003). *J. Am. Vet. Med. Assoc.* 230 (9): 1329–1333.

6 Gouldin, E.D., Mullin, C., Morges, M. et al. (2017). Feline discrete high-grade gastrointestinal lymphoma treated with surgical resection and adjuvant CHOP-based chemotherapy: retrospective study of 20 cases. *Vet. Comp. Oncol.* 15 (2): 328–335.

21.1 Partial Gastrectomy

Indications

1) Resection of localized benign and malignant tumors of the gastric body

Suggested Diagnostic Workup and Clinical Staging

- See *21. Gastrectomy*.

Patient Positioning

The patient is positioned in dorsal recumbency.

Surgical Technique (See Plate 21.1A–F)

A) A ventral midline celiotomy is performed (see *15.1. Ventral Midline Celiotomy*). The stomach is protected from the remainder of the abdominal cavity with moistened laparotomy sponges. Stay sutures (i, carcinoma, arrow) or Babcock forceps (ii, leiomyoma, arrow) are used to manipulate the stomach during surgery and minimize the risk of spillage of gastric contents into the abdominal cavity.
B) Branches of the left and right gastric and gastroepiploic arteries supplying the affected portion of the stomach are ligated and divided (not pictured). Alternatively, this can be done with a vessel sealing device. The principal gastric and gastroepiploic arteries must be preserved.
C) The greater and lesser omental attachments to the affected portion of the stomach are transected.
D) **Partial gastrectomy and closure technique 1 – Suture:** The localized gastric tumor is resected with 2- to 3-cm margins of grossly normal gastric wall (i, leiomyoma [L]; ii, carcinoma [C]; iii, leiomyosarcoma [LS]). The resected gastric tumor is removed from the surgical field. Gastric contents are suctioned to reduce the risk of spillage. The partial gastrectomy is closed in two layers using 2-0 to 4-0 monofilament absorbable suture material with a simple continuous pattern in the mucosal-submucosal layer and either a continuous inverting pattern (Cushing or Lembert) or simple continuous pattern in the seromuscular layer (iv).

Color Atlas of Canine and Feline Surgical Oncology, First Edition. Julius M. Liptak, Paolo Buracco, William T. N. Culp, and Nicholas J. Bacon.

Plate 21.1

Partial Gastrectomy

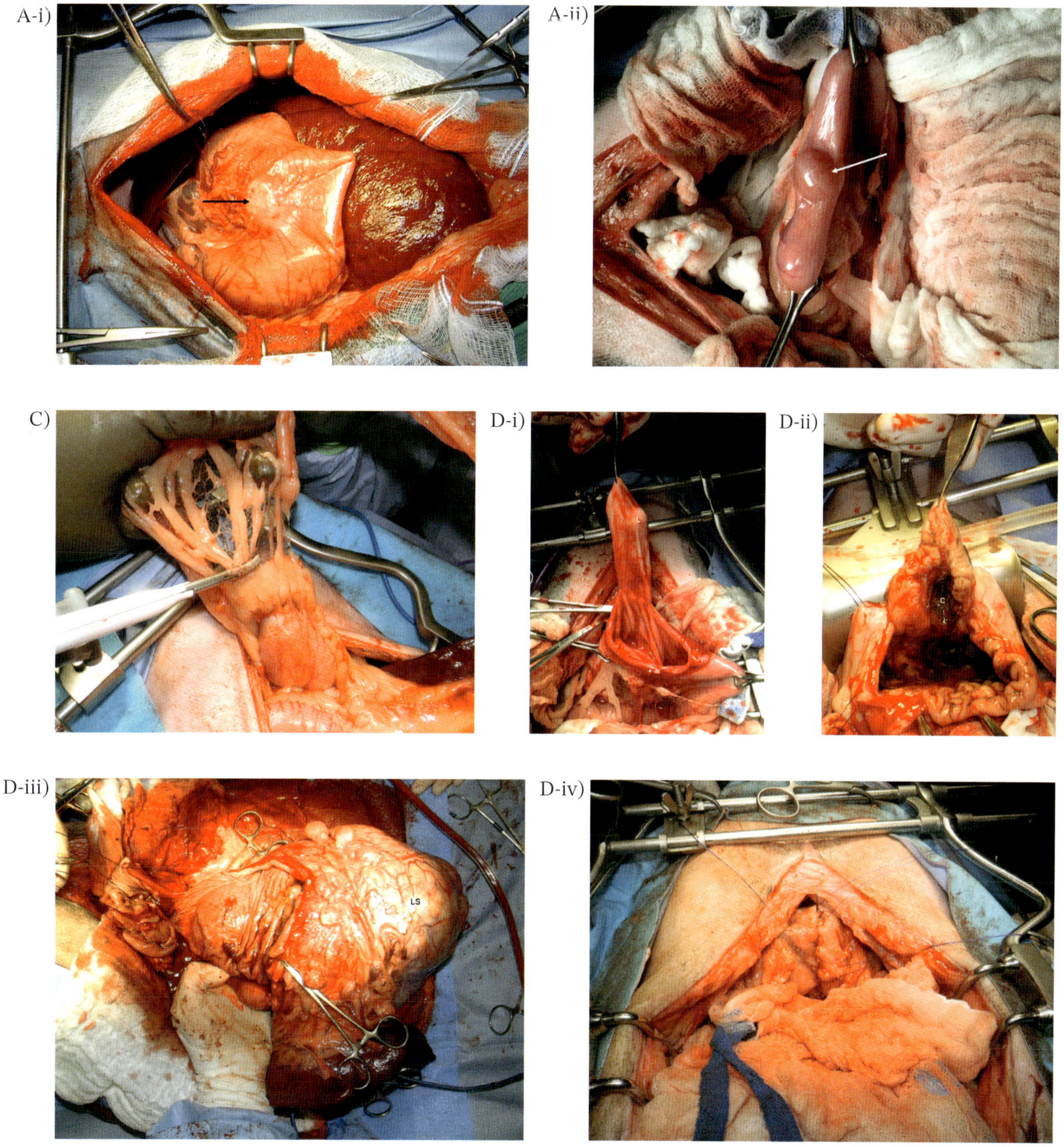

Surgical Technique (See Plate 21.1A–F) *continued*

E) **Partial gastrectomy and closure technique 2 – Stapler:** An appropriately sized gastrointestinal anastomosis (GIA) stapler is applied across the stomach with 2–3 cm of grossly normal gastric wall around the localized gastric tumor for margins (i, solitary lymphoma). The GIA stapler is locked and fired to both resect the gastric tumor and close the partial gastrectomy simultaneously (ii). More than one GIA stapler may be required depending on the length of the planned partial gastrectomy (iii, iv).

F) The abdominal cavity should be systematically explored for metastatic disease. The most common metastatic sites for gastric tumors include the regional lymph nodes and liver (pictured, leiomyosarcoma). After completion of the partial gastrectomy and abdominal exploration, the abdominal cavity should be lavaged with warmed, sterile isotonic saline.

Closure

The linea alba, subcutaneous tissue, and skin are closed as described in *15.1. Ventral Midline Celiotomy*.

Postoperative Management

1) Multimodal analgesia, but consider avoiding the use of steroids and nonsteroidal anti-inflammatory drugs because of their negative effects on intestinal healing
2) Elizabethan collar or body suit
3) Feed normal diet

Complications [1]

- Septic peritonitis (but for reasons unrelated to the partial gastrectomy site, 11%)
- Gastric stasis (4%)
- Pancreatitis (4%)

Suggested Adjuvant Treatments

- See *21. Gastrectomy*.

Prognosis and Oncologic Outcome

- See *21. Gastrectomy*.

Reference

1 Abrams, B., Wavreille, V.A., Husbands, B.D. et al. (2019). Perioperative complications and outcome after surgery for treatment of gastric carcinoma in dogs: A Veterinary Society of Surgical Oncology retrospective study of 40 cases (2004-2018). *Vet. Surg.* 48 (6): 923–932.

Plate 21.1

Partial Gastrectomy *continued*

E-i)

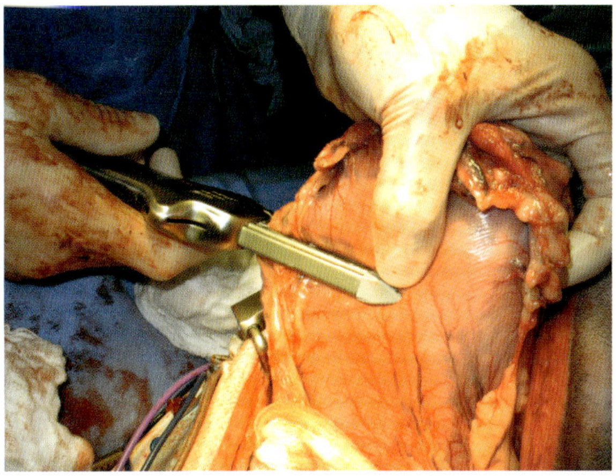

E-ii)

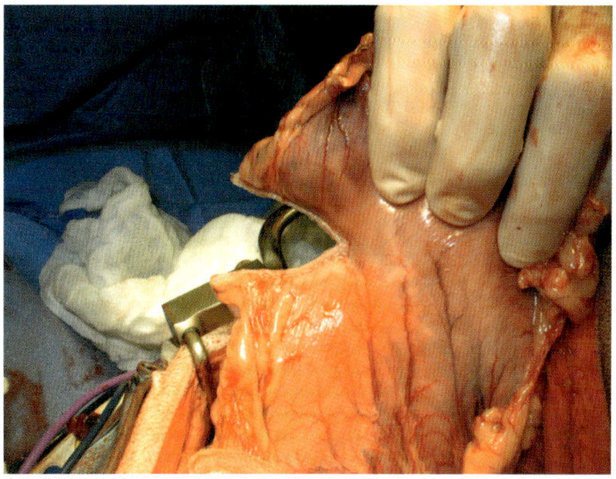

E-iii)

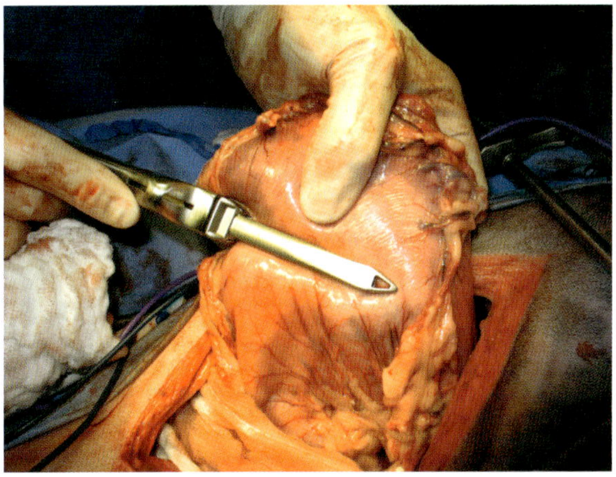

E-iv)

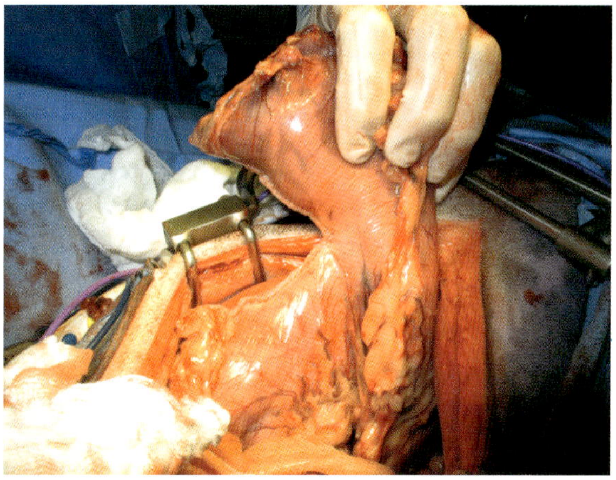

F)

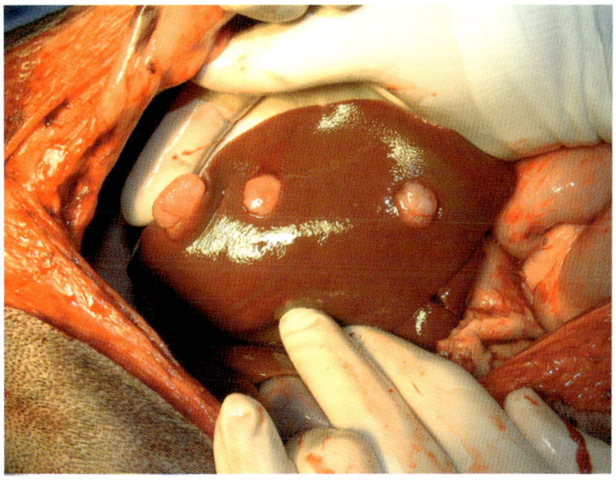

21.2 Billroth I

Indications

1) Resection of localized benign and malignant tumors of the pyloric region
2) Billroth I can be combined with a partial pancreatectomy if required (see *18. Partial Pancreatectomy*)

Suggested Diagnostic Workup and Clinical Staging

- See *21. Gastrectomy*.

Patient Positioning

The patient is positioned in dorsal recumbency.

Surgical Technique [1] (See Plate 21.2A–L)

A) A ventral midline celiotomy is performed (see *15.1. Ventral Midline Celiotomy*). The stomach is protected from the remainder of the abdominal cavity with moistened laparotomy sponges. Stay sutures (i, plasmacytoma, arrow) or Babcock forceps (ii, leiomyoma, arrow) are used to manipulate the stomach during surgery and minimize the risk of spillage of gastric contents into the abdominal cavity.
B) Branches of the left (L) and right (R) gastric (GA) and gastroepiploic arteries (GEA) supplying the pyloric region (i) are ligated and divided. Alternatively, this can be done with a vessel sealing device or bipolar cautery (ii). The principal gastric and gastroepiploic arteries must be preserved.
C) The greater and lesser omental attachments (arrows) to the pyloric region (P) are transected (also see B – ii).
D) Caudal retraction of the pylorus is facilitated by transection of the section of lesser omentum forming the gastrohepatic ligament (arrow). This should be done with care to avoid iatrogenic trauma to the portal vein, hepatic artery, and bile duct.

Color Atlas of Canine and Feline Surgical Oncology, First Edition. Julius M. Liptak, Paolo Buracco, William T. N. Culp, and Nicholas J. Bacon.

Plate 21.2

Billroth I

A-i)

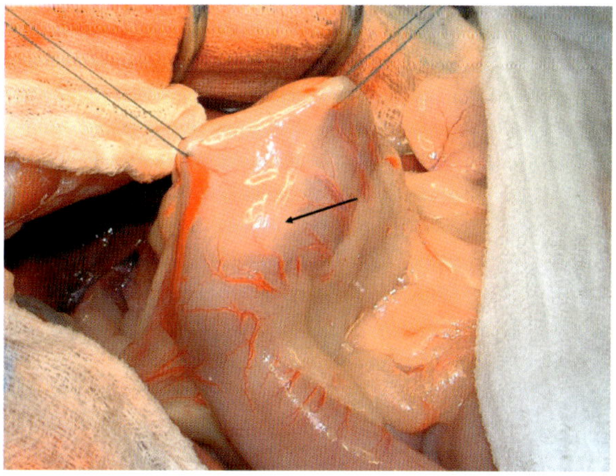

A-ii)

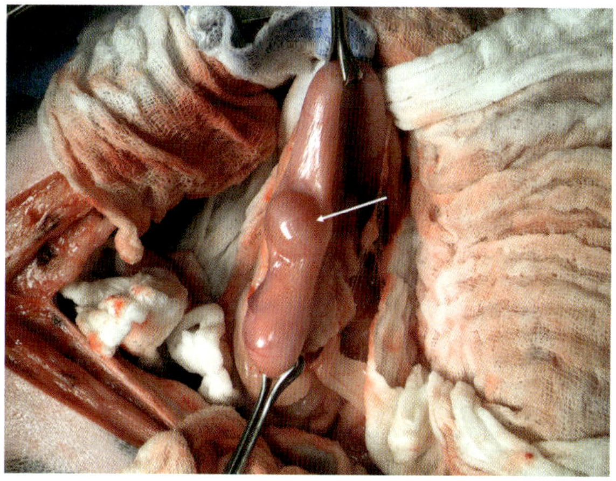

B-i)

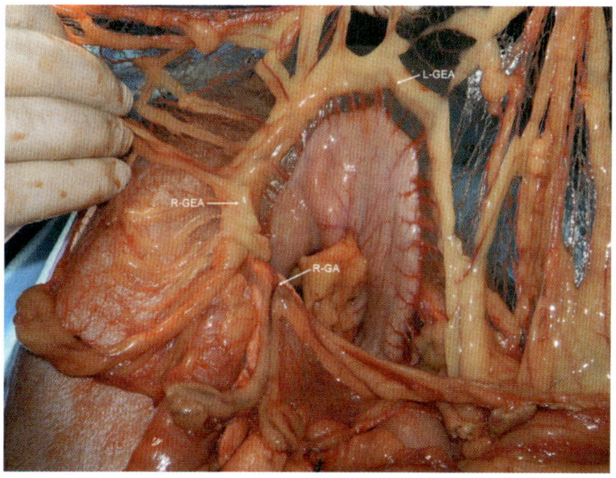

B-ii)

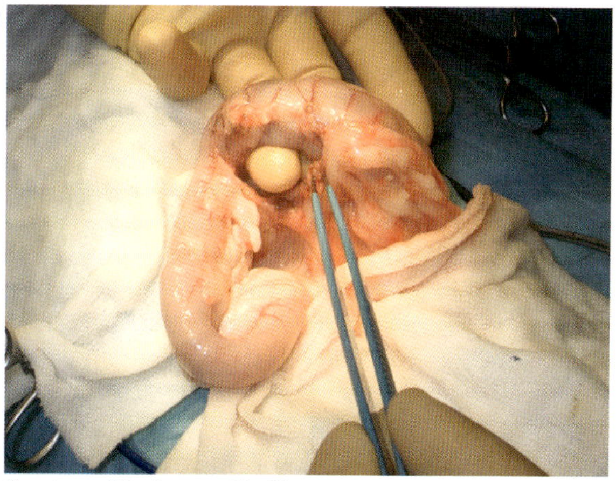

Courtesy of Dr. Laurent Findji

C)

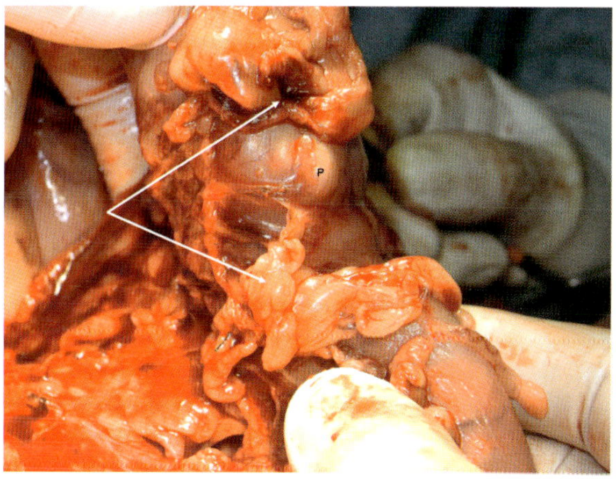

D)

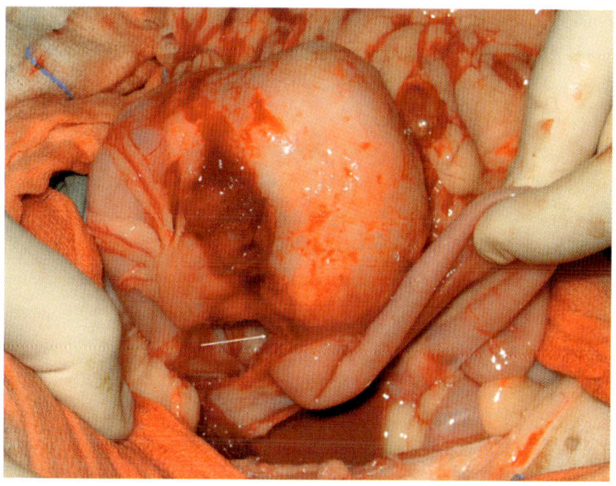

Surgical Technique [1] (See Plate 21.2A–L) *continued*

E) An assistant's fingers or atraumatic Doyen forceps are placed oral to the planned gastrectomy site and aboral to the planned duodenectomy site (i). The duodenectomy (ii) and gastrectomy (iii) sites should be positioned a minimum of 2 cm from the pyloric mass. The pyloric mass is resected with Metzenbaum scissors or scalpel blade (pictured) and removed from the surgical field. If possible, a minimum of 5-mm margins should be preserved oral to the insertion of the common bile duct and pancreatic ducts into the duodenal papilla (iv). If this is not possible, the common bile duct and pancreatic ducts should be ligated and divided, and a cholecystoduodenostomy performed for biliary diversion. If necessary, a partial pancreatectomy can be performed en bloc with resection of the pyloric mass (see *18. Partial Pancreatectomy*).

F) **Gastroduodenostomy technique 1 – Suture:** The transected gastric and duodenal ends can be anastomosed end to end using a simple interrupted (i), modified Gambee, or simple continuous suture pattern (ii, iii). For sutured anastomoses, 3-0 or 4-0 absorbable monofilament suture material is used with 2- to 3-mm bites every 3–4 mm. An end-to-end anastomosis with a simple continuous suture pattern should be done with two overlapping 180-degree continuous suture patterns (ii, first 180-degree simple continuous suture closure; iii, second 180-degree simple continuous suture closure) to minimize the risk of iatrogenic stricture of the gastroduodenostomy site. If there is a mismatch in luminal size between the duodenum and the stomach, then the additional gastric resection site should be closed with 3-0 or 4-0 absorbable monofilament suture material in a simple continuous suture pattern (iii, arrow).

Plate 21.2

Billroth I *continued*

E-i)

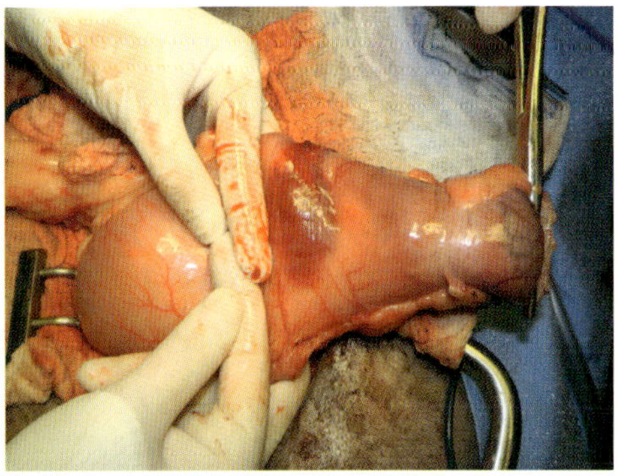

E-ii)

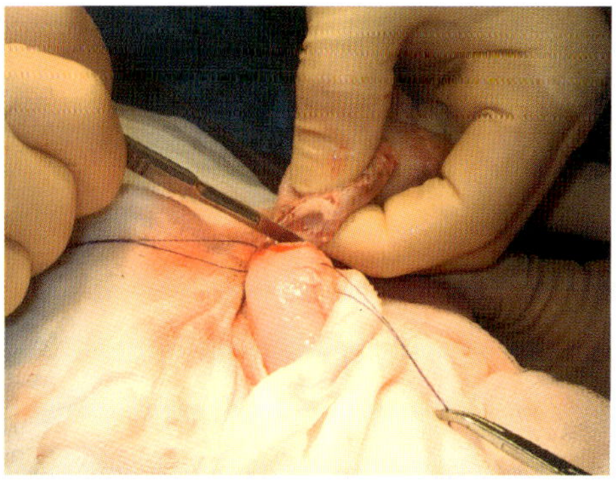

Courtesy of Dr. Laurent Findji

E-iii)

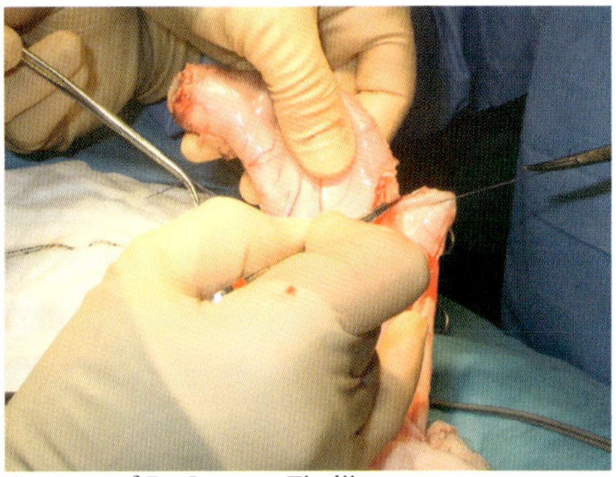

Courtesy of Dr. Laurent Findji

E-iv)

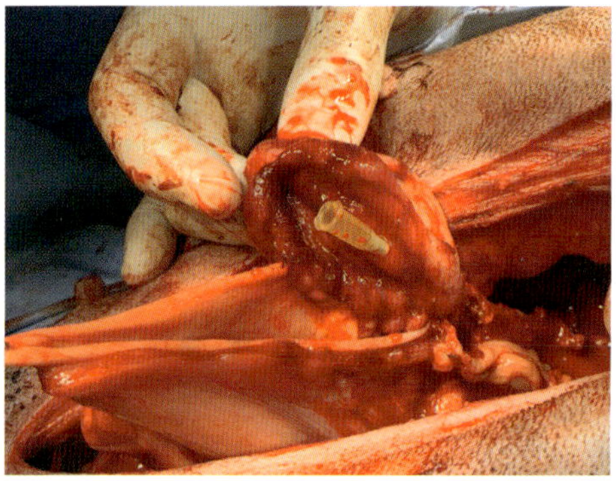

F-i)

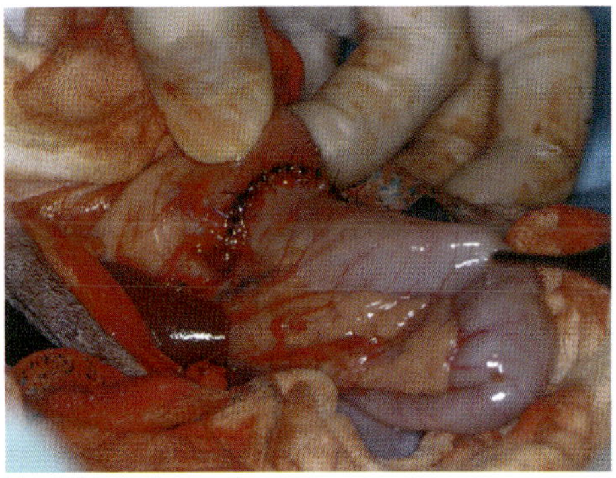

F-ii)

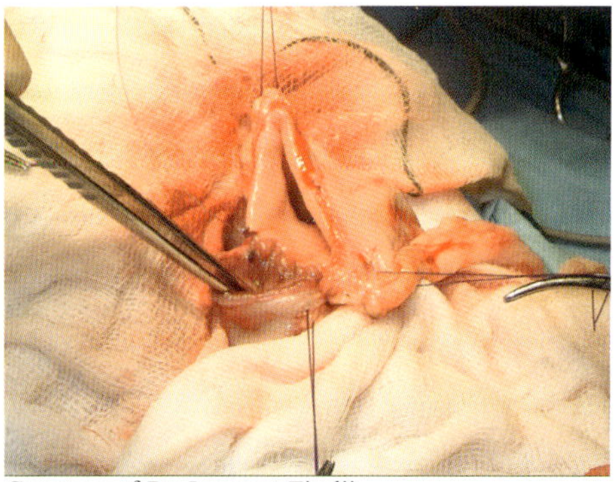

Courtesy of Dr. Laurent Findji

F-iii)

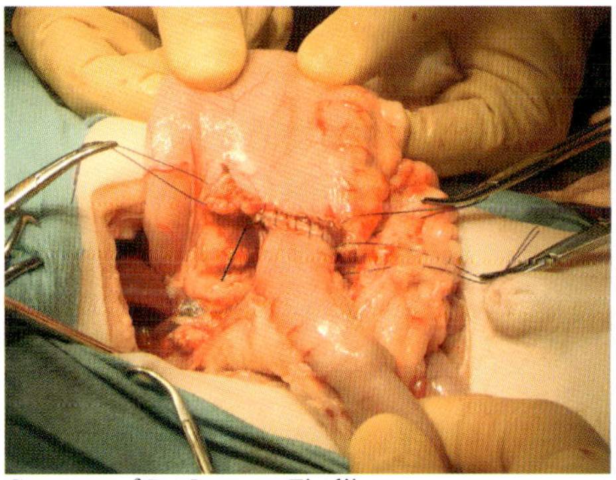

Courtesy of Dr. Laurent Findji

Surgical Technique [1] (See Plate 21.2A–L) *continued*

G) **Gastroduodenostomy technique 2 – Stapler:** The duodenectomy site is closed with an appropriately sized thoraco-abdominal (TA) stapler (usually a 30-mm or 55- to 60-mm TA stapler) (i) or Parker-Kerr continuous suture pattern; alternatively, the duodenectomy site can initially be left open. An incision is performed along the TA stapler cartridge with a scalpel blade to complete the duodenal transection (ii).

H) The gastrectomy is performed with one or more gastrointestinal anastomosis (GIA) staplers or the gastrectomy site (i) is closed with an appropriately sized TA stapler (usually a 55- to 60-mm or 90-mm TA stapler) or single- or double-layered continuous suture pattern (ii).

I) Stab incisions are made through the gastric and duodenal walls in close proximity to the gastrectomy and duodenectomy sites, respectively, with a scalpel blade (arrows); alternatively, if the duodenectomy site has not been closed, then the only stab incision is made adjacent to the gastrectomy site.

J) A GIA stapler is inserted through the stab incisions into the lumen of the stomach and duodenum; alternatively, if the duodenectomy site has not been closed, then one arm of the GIA stapler is inserted directly into the lumen of the duodenum.

K) The GIA stapler is locked and fired to create a side-to-side gastroduodenostomy (asterisk). The gastric and duodenal stab incisions (or, alternatively, the duodenectomy site) are closed using 3-0 or 4-0 absorbable monofilament suture material in a simple interrupted, modified Gambee or simple continuous suture pattern (arrows).

L) The abdominal cavity should be systematically explored for metastatic disease. The most common metastatic sites for gastric tumors include the regional lymph nodes and liver. After completion of the Billroth I and abdominal exploration, the abdominal cavity should be lavaged with warmed, sterile isotonic saline.

Plate 21.2

Billroth I *continued*

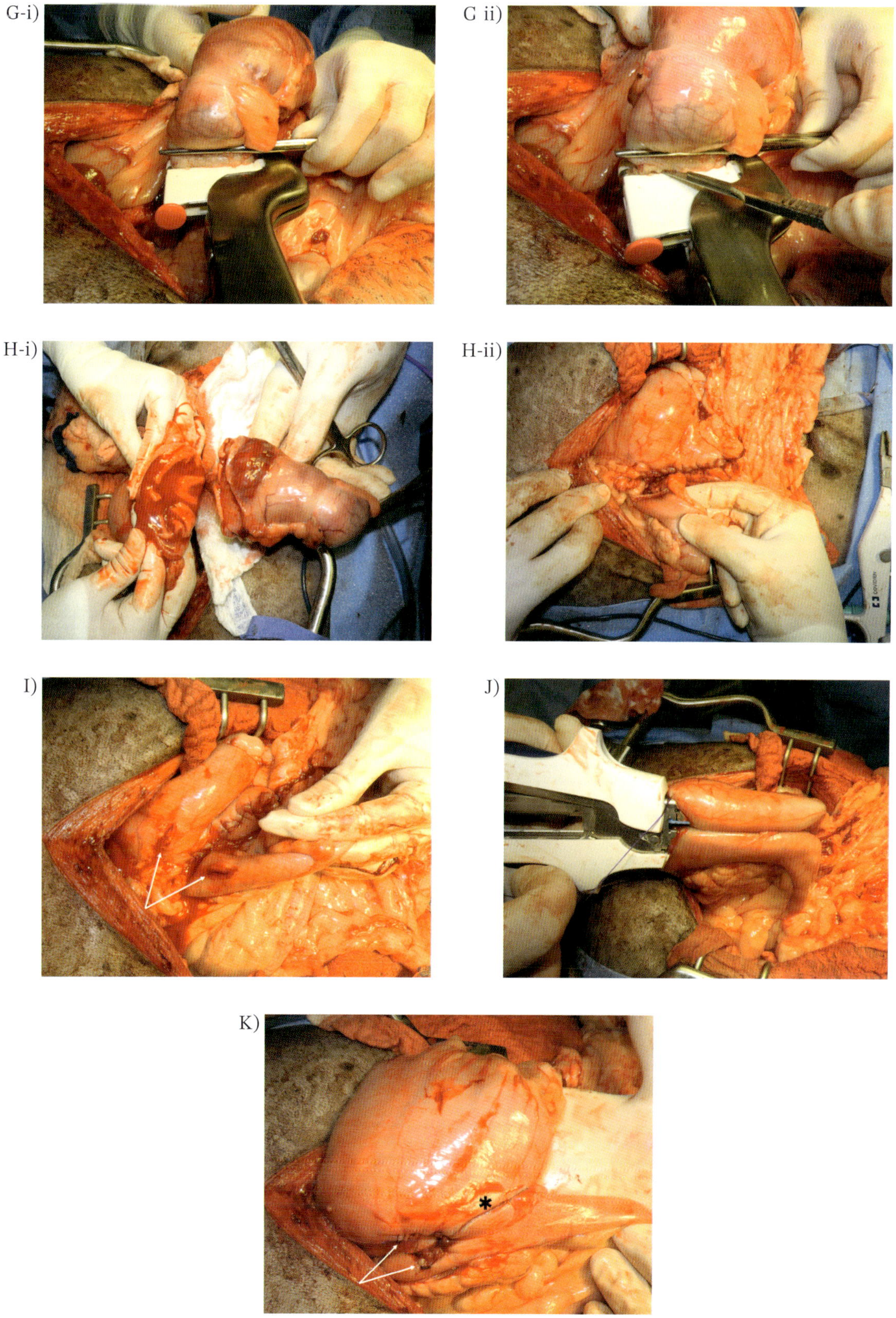

Closure

The linea alba, subcutaneous tissue, and skin are closed as described in *15.1. Ventral Midline Celiotomy*.

Postoperative Management

1) Multimodal analgesia, but consider avoiding the use of steroids and nonsteroidal anti-inflammatory drugs because of their negative effects on intestinal healing
2) Elizabethan collar or body suit
3) Feed normal diet

Complications [1, 2]

- Intraoperative blood loss requiring a blood transfusion (33%)
- Pancreatitis (13%–33%)
- Hypoglycemia (11%–17%)
- Aspiration pneumonia (0%–13%)
- Ascending cholangiohepatitis (0%–11%)
- Septic peritonitis (0%–8%)
- Exocrine pancreatic insufficiency if the pancreatic ducts are sacrificed

Suggested Adjuvant Treatments

- See *21. Gastrectomy*.

Prognosis and Oncologic Outcome

- See *21. Gastrectomy*.

References

1 Eisele, J., McClaran, J.K., Runge, J.J.S. et al. (2010). Evaluation of risk factors for morbidity and mortality after pylorectomy and gastroduodenostomy in dogs. *Vet. Surg.* 39 (2): 261–267.
2 Abrams, B., Wavreille, V.A., Husbands, B.D. et al. (2019). Perioperative complications and outcome after surgery for treatment of gastric carcinoma in dogs: a veterinary society of surgical oncology retrospective study of 40 cases (2004-2018). *Vet. Surg.* 48 (6): 923–932.

Chapter 22: Small Intestinal Resection and Anastomosis

Intestinal resection and anastomosis for resection of small intestinal tumors can be done through either open or laparoscopic-assisted approaches. The intestinal ends, particularly when performed through an open approach, can be anastomosed using a sutured end-to-end technique or a stapled functional end-to-end technique.

Suggested Diagnostic Workup and Clinical Staging

- Complete blood count, serum biochemistry, and urinalysis
- Abdominal ultrasound or CT scan with image-guided aspirates
- Three-view thoracic radiographs or thoracic CT scan for assessment of lung metastasis

Suggested Adjuvant Treatments

- Chemotherapy for dogs and cats with small intestinal lymphomas
- Chemotherapy for dogs and cats with intestinal mast cell tumors
- ± Chemotherapy for dogs and cats with small intestinal adenocarcinomas with evidence of lymphatic or vascular invasion, or metastatic to regional lymph nodes or distant sites
- ± Chemotherapy for dogs with high-grade intestinal leiomyosarcomas or undifferentiated sarcomas
- ± Tyrosine kinase inhibitors for gastrointestinal stromal tumors

Prognosis and Oncologic Outcome

Prognosis and Oncologic Outcome – Dogs

	Local Recurrence Rate	Metastatic Rate	Disease-Free Interval (d)	Median Survival Time (d)	1-Year Survival Rate	2-Year Survival Rate
			Adenocarcinoma [1]			
Overall	–	28%	–	544	60%	36%
Age						
• <8 years	–	–	–	1193	86%	69%
• ≥8 years	–	–	–	488	51%	26%
			Leiomyosarcoma[a] [2, 3]			
Overall	10%	54%	–	238–650	75%	66%

Color Atlas of Canine and Feline Surgical Oncology, First Edition. Julius M. Liptak, Paolo Buracco, William T. N. Culp, and Nicholas J. Bacon.

	Local Recurrence Rate	Metastatic Rate	Disease-Free Interval (d)	Median Survival Time (d)	1-Year Survival Rate	2-Year Survival Rate
			Gastrointestinal Stromal Tumor[a] [3]			
Overall	0%	7%	–	354	–	–
			Leiomyosarcoma and Gastrointestinal Stromal Tumor[b] [4]			
Overall	29%		–	–	63%	52%

[a] Includes all gastrointestinal sites (stomach, small intestines, cecum, and colon).
[b] Outcome for reclassified small intestinal leiomyosarcomas and gastrointestinal stromal tumors reported as a combined group.

Prognosis and Oncologic Outcome – Cats

	Local Recurrence Rate	Metastatic Rate	Disease-Free Interval (d)	Median Survival Time (d)	1-Year Survival Rate	2-Year Survival Rate
			Adenocarcinoma[a] [5]			
Overall	–	60%	–	365	–	–
Histologic excision						
• Complete	–	–	–	1320	–	–
• Incomplete	–	–	–	60	–	–
			Lymphoma[b] [6]			
Overall	50%		357	417	–	–
			Mast Cell Tumor[c] [7]			
Overall	–	–	–	531	–	–

[a] Includes all gastrointestinal sites (small intestines, cecum, and colon).
[b] Includes all gastrointestinal sites (stomach, small intestines, and colon) and all cats were treated with an adjuvant cyclophosphamide-doxorubicin-vincristine-prednisone (CHOP) protocol.
[c] Includes both small and large intestinal mast cell tumors. Note that there was no difference in outcome in cats treated with surgery and chemotherapy and cats treated with chemotherapy alone.

References

1 Smith, A.A., Frimberger, A.E., and Moore, A.S. (2019). Retrospective study of survival time and prognostic factors for dogs with small intestinal adenocarcinoma treated by tumor excision with or without adjuvant chemotherapy. *J. Am. Vet. Med. Assoc.* 254 (2): 243–250.

2 Cohen, M., Post, G.S., and Wright, J.C. (2003). Gastrointestinal leiomyosarcoma in 14 dogs. *J. Vet. Intern. Med.* 17 (1): 107–110.

3 Russell, K.N., Mehler, S.J., Skorupski, K.A. et al. (2007). Clinical and immunohistochemical differentiation of gastrointestinal stromal tumors from leiomyosarcomas in dogs: 42 cases (1990-2003). *J. Am. Vet. Med. Assoc.* 230 (9): 1329–1333.

4 Maas, C.P.H.J., ter Haar, G., van der Gaag, I. et al. (2007). Reclassification of small intestinal and cecal smooth muscle tumors in 72 dogs: clinical, histologic, and immunohistochemical evaluation. *Vet. Surg.* 36 (4): 302–313.

5 Green, M.L., Smith, J.D., and Kass, P.H. (2011). Surgical versus non-surgical treatment of feline small intestinal adenocarcinoma and the influence of metastasis on long-term survival in 18 cats (2000-2007). *Can. Vet. J.* 52 (10): 1101–1105.

6 Gouldin, E.D., Mullin, C., Morges, M. et al. (2017). Feline discrete high-grade gastrointestinal lymphoma treated with surgical resection and adjuvant CHOP-based chemotherapy: retrospective study of 20 cases. *Vet. Comp. Oncol.* 15 (2): 328–335.

7 Barrett, L.E., Skorupski, K., Brown, D.C. et al. (2018). Outcome following treatment of feline gastrointestinal mast cell tumours. *Vet. Comp. Oncol.* 16 (2): 188–193.

22.1 Open Small Intestinal Resection and Anastomosis

Indications

1) Resection of benign and malignant tumors involving the small intestine

Suggested Diagnostic Workup and Clinical Staging

- See *22. Small Intestinal Resection and Anastomosis.*

Patient Positioning

The patient is positioned in dorsal recumbency.

Surgical Technique (See Plate 22.1A–M)

A) A ventral midline celiotomy is performed (see *15.1. Ventral Midline Celiotomy*). The affected intestinal segment should be isolated from the abdominal cavity with moistened laparotomy sponges (pictured).

B) The terminal arcade of the jejunal branches of the cranial mesenteric artery supplying the affected intestinal segment is ligated with monofilament absorbable suture material (i) or metallic clips and divided (ii, iii). Alternatively, this can be done with a vessel sealing device (iv).

C) Crushing clamps are placed across the intestines orally and aborally at an appropriate distance from the intestinal tumor to prevent spillage of intestinal contents from the resected intestinal segment. The oral and aboral margins for resection of small intestinal tumors depends on the tumor type. In dogs, 3-cm margins in all directions are recommended for intestinal carcinomas, and 2-cm margins in all directions are recommended for intestinal sarcomas [1]. In cats, 4-cm margins in all directions are recommended for intestinal carcinomas, sarcomas, and mast cell tumors [2]. In both dogs and cats, discrete lymphomas tend to have extensive microscopic invasion extending beyond 4 cm [1, 2]. Mesenteric margins should also be considered when resecting small intestinal tumors with a minimum of 1-cm margins recommended (see B – iv, arrow).

Color Atlas of Canine and Feline Surgical Oncology, First Edition. Julius M. Liptak, Paolo Buracco, William T. N. Culp, and Nicholas J. Bacon.

Plate 22.1

Open Small Intestinal Resection and Anastomosis

A)

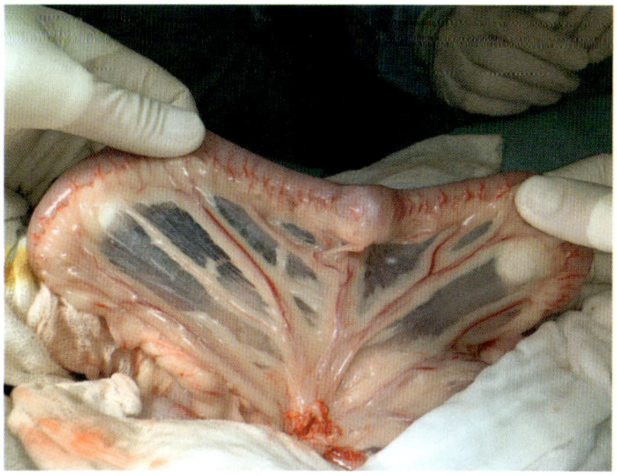

B-i)

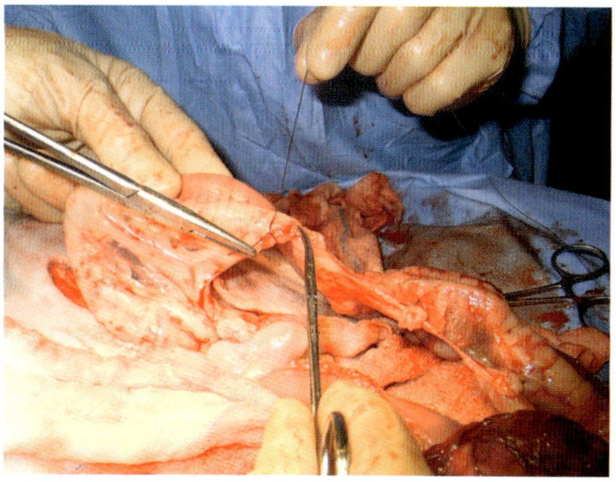

Courtesy of Dr. Laurent Findji

B-ii)

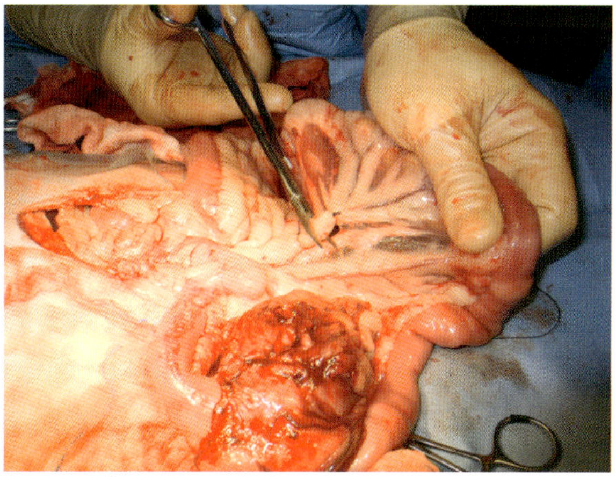

Courtesy of Dr. Laurent Findji

B-iii)

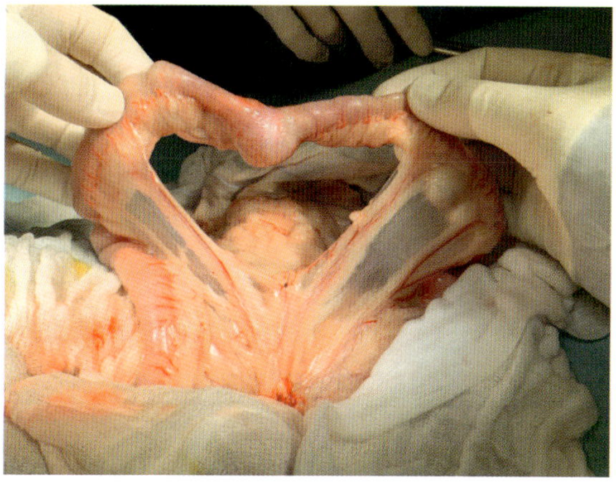

B-iv)

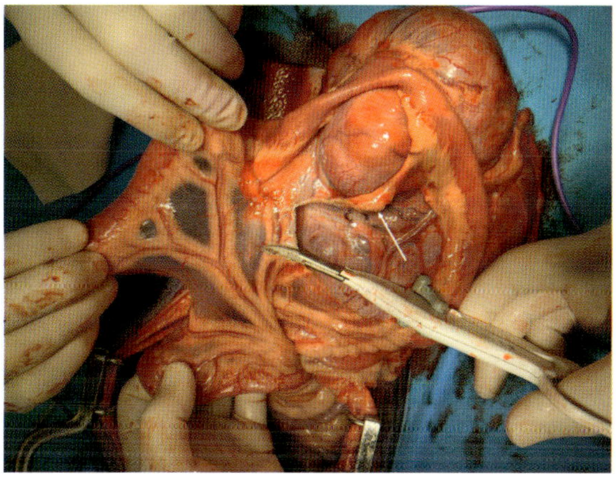

C)

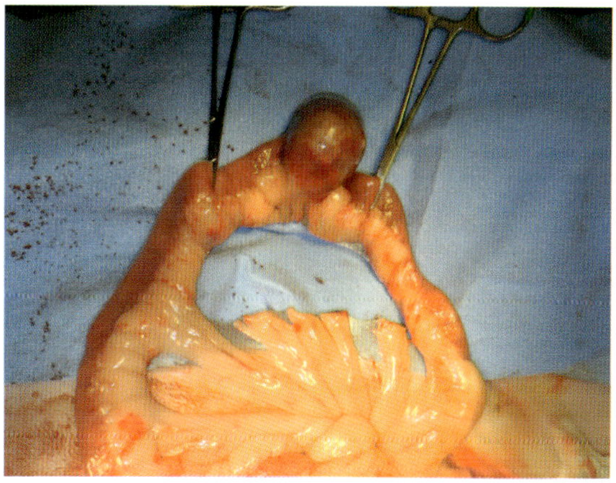

Surgical Technique (See Plate 22.1A–M) *continued*

D) The intestinal contents are milked away from the crushing clamps, and the intestines are occluded 4–6 cm orally and aborally to the crushing clamps with either an assistant's fingers (i) or atraumatic Doyen forceps (ii).

E) The intestines are transected along the crushing clamps, at the junction between the divided and nondivided terminal arcade of the jejunal branches of the cranial mesenteric artery, either perpendicular to the length of the intestines or angled such that the mesenteric border is longer than the antimesenteric border (pictured).

F) The resected intestinal segment is removed from the surgical field, and occlusion of the transected ends of the intestines is maintaining occlusion oral and aboral to the resection site. The transected intestinal ends are anastomosed using either a suture or a staple technique.

G) **End-to-end anastomosis technique 1 – Sutured anastomosis:** The transected intestinal ends can be anastomosed using a simple interrupted (i), modified Gambee, or simple continuous suture pattern, or with skin staples. For sutured anastomoses, 3-0 or 4-0 absorbable monofilament suture material is used with 2- to 3-mm bites every 3–4 mm. An end-to-end anastomosis with a simple continuous suture pattern should be done with two overlapping continuous suture patterns: one from the mesenteric border to the antimesenteric border in one direction (ii), and the other from the antimesenteric border to the mesenteric border in the opposite direction, to minimize the risk of iatrogenic stricture of the intestinal anastomosis. The mesenteric defect should be sutured with 3-0 or 4-0 absorbable monofilament suture material in a simple continuous pattern (iii).

H) **End-to-end anastomosis technique 2 – Functional end-to-end stapled anastomosis:** Stay sutures on the mesenteric side of the oral and aboral intestines are used to elevate the intestines in a vertical direction such that the antimesenteric borders of both intestines are opposed.

Plate 22.1

Open Small Intestinal Resection and Anastomosis *continued*

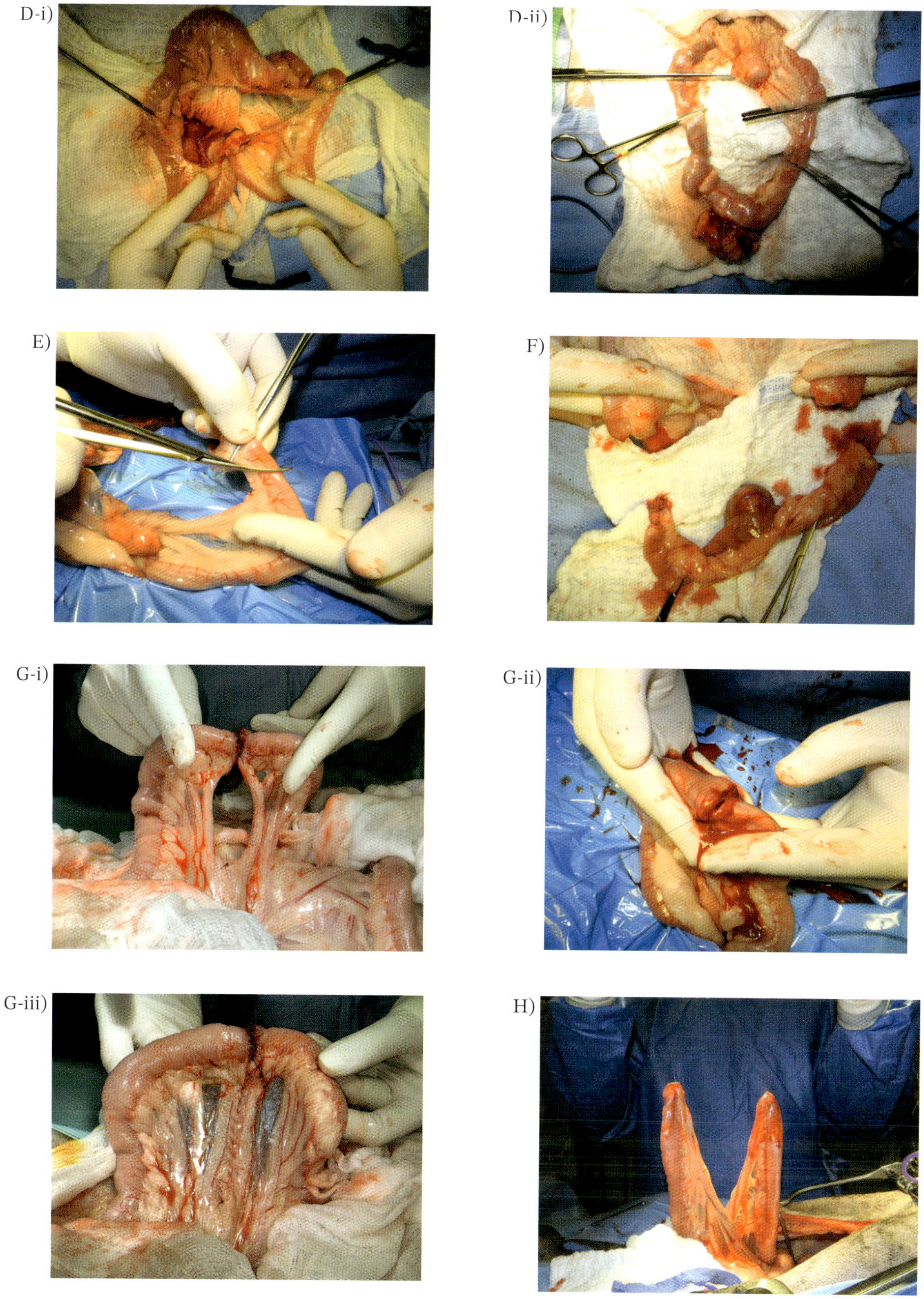

Surgical Technique (See Plate 22.1A–M) *continued*

I) A gastrointestinal anastomosis (GIA) stapler is inserted into the lumen of both intestinal segments (i, ii). The GIA stapler is locked and fired to create a side-to-side anastomosis along the antimesenteric border of the intestinal segments (iii, arrow; iv, intraluminal view).

J) With the intestines still elevated by the stay sutures, an appropriately sized thoracoabdominal (TA) stapler (usually a 55- to 60-mm TA stapler) is then placed across the transected intestinal ends, locked, and fired to complete the stapled anastomosis (i). The excessive intestinal tissue within the TA stapler (ii) is incised with a scalpel blade (iii) and either discarded or submitted for histopathologic assessment of surgical margins (iv, post-stapled anastomosis appearance of the intestines). Alternatively, a GIA stapler can be used for this step instead of a TA stapler.

Plate 22.1

Open Small Intestinal Resection and Anastomosis *continued*

I-i)

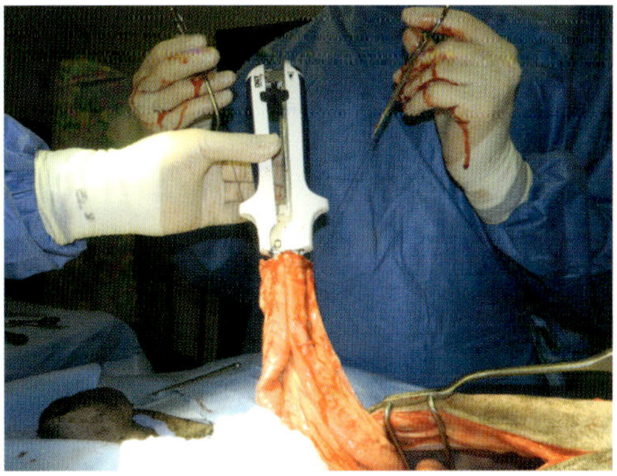

I-ii)

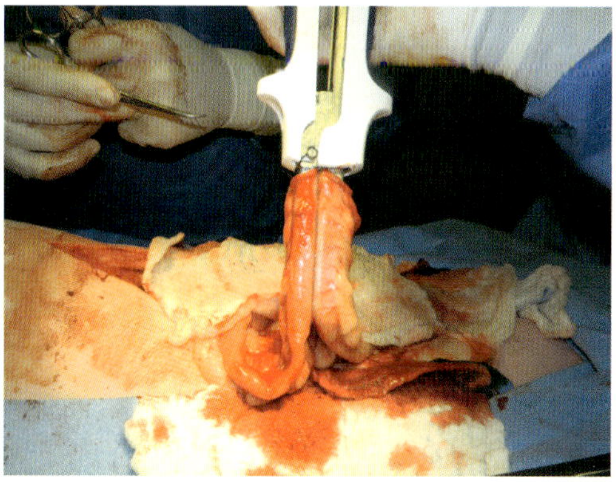

I-iii)

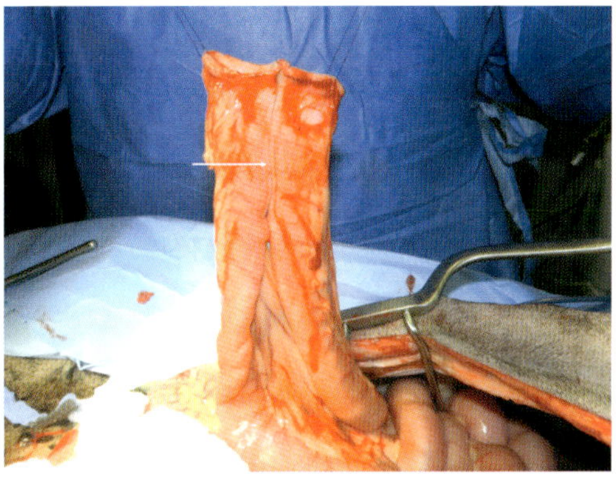

I-iv)

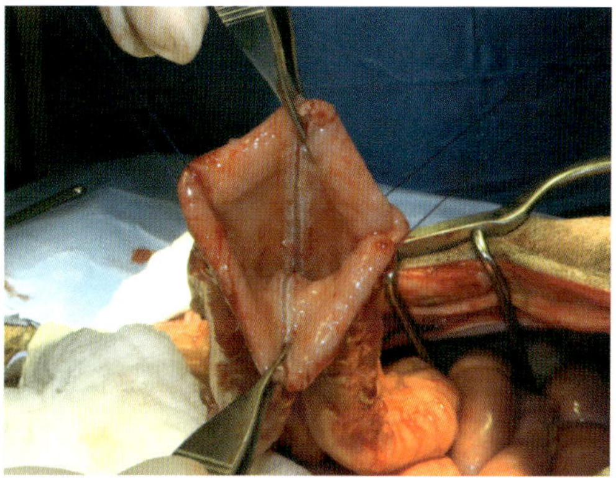

J-i)

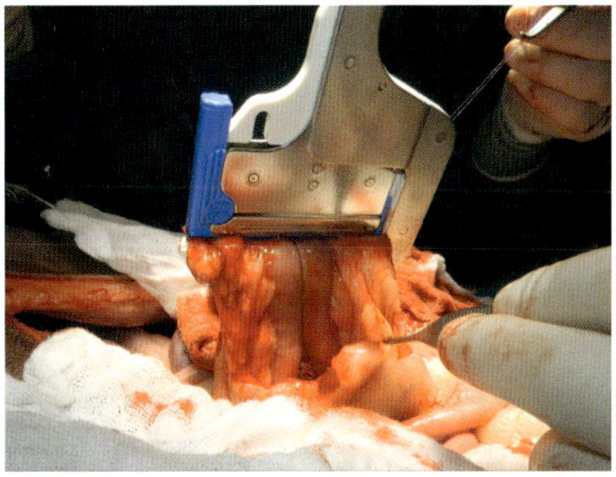

J-ii)

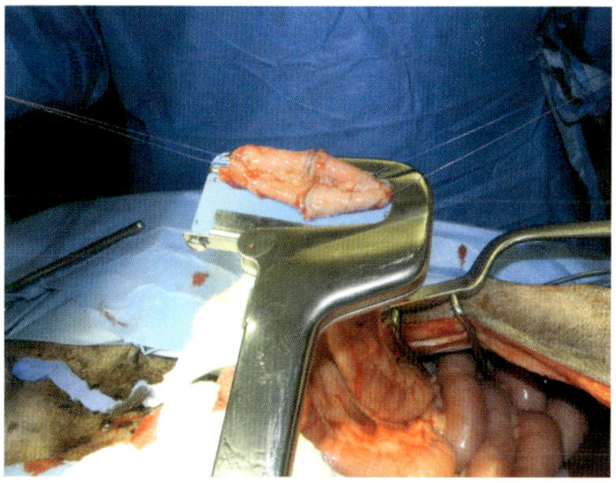

J-iii)

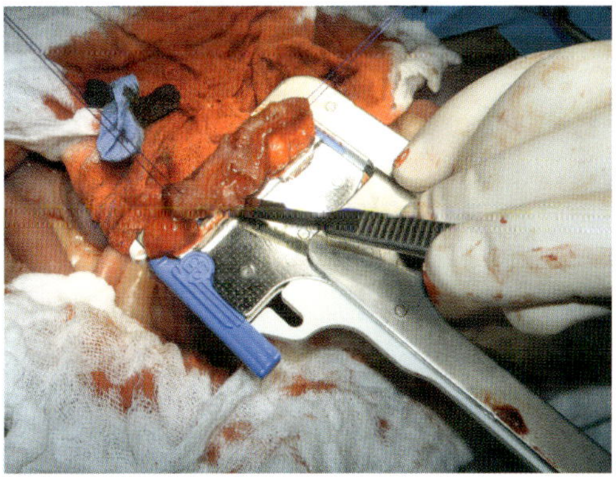

J-iv)

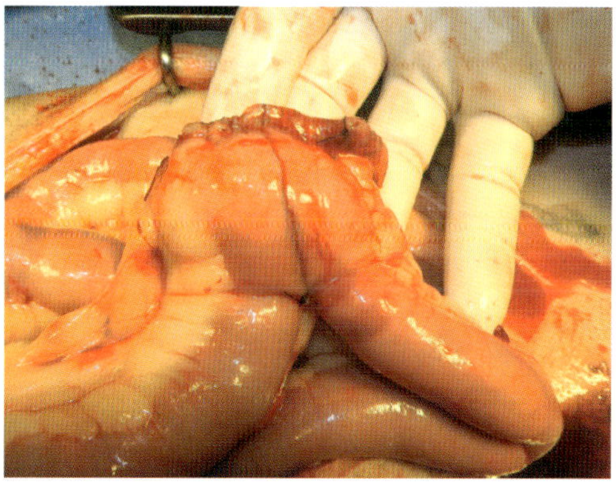

Surgical Technique (See Plate 22.1A–M) *continued*

K) The patency of the anastomosis should be tested by occluding the intestines oral and aboral to the anastomosis site with an assistant's fingers (i, ii) or atraumatic Doyen forceps, and then injecting sterile isotonic saline into the lumen of the anastomosed intestines. Any visible leaks should be sutured with 3-0 or 4-0 absorbable monofilament suture material in a simple interrupted pattern or, if along the TA staple line for a functional end-to-end stapled anastomosis, a simple continuous suture pattern to oversew the staple line.
L) The anastomosis should be wrapped in omentum (i, ii).
M) The abdominal cavity should be systematically explored for metastatic disease. The most common metastatic sites for small intestinal tumors include the regional lymph nodes and liver (i, ii), and carcinomatosis for small intestinal carcinomas (iii, iv). After completion of the intestinal resection and anastomosis and abdominal exploration, the abdominal cavity should be lavaged with warmed, sterile isotonic saline.

Closure

The linea alba, subcutaneous tissue, and skin are closed as described in *15.1. Ventral Midline Celiotomy*.

Postoperative Management

1) Multimodal analgesia, but consider avoiding the use of steroids and nonsteroidal anti-inflammatory drugs because of their negative effects on intestinal healing
2) Elizabethan collar or body suit
3) Feed normal diet

Complications

Intraoperative Complications

- Hypotension (33%) [3]

Postoperative Complications

- Anastomotic dehiscence and septic peritonitis (5%–14% overall; 13%–16% for sutured anastomoses, and 0%–15% for stapled anastomoses) [3–7]
- Incisional complications (10%) [4]
- Hyporexia (9%) [8]
- Impaction at the stapled anastomosis site (3%) [6]
- Abscess at the stapled anastomosis site (3%) [4]

Suggested Adjuvant Treatments

- See *22. Small Intestinal Resection and Anastomosis.*

Prognosis and Oncologic Outcome

- See *22. Small Intestinal Resection and Anastomosis.*

Plate 22.1

Open Small Intestinal Resection and Anastomosis *continued*

K i)

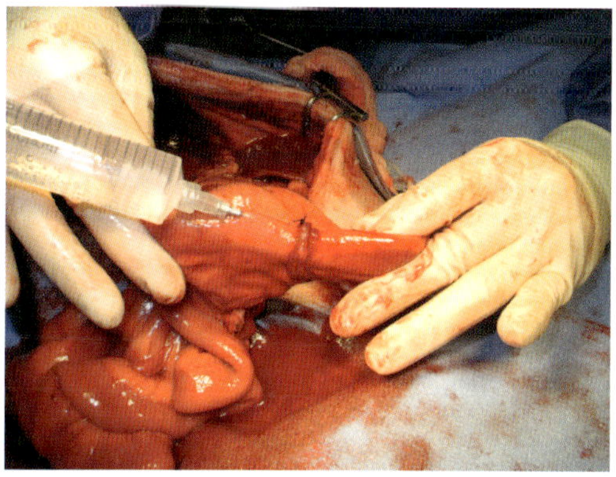

K-ii)

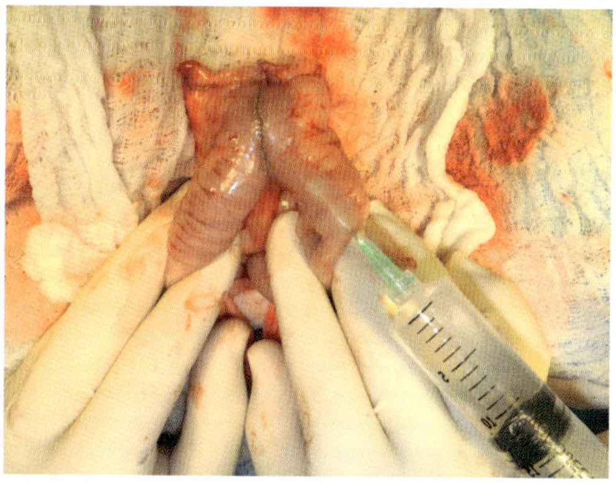

L-i)

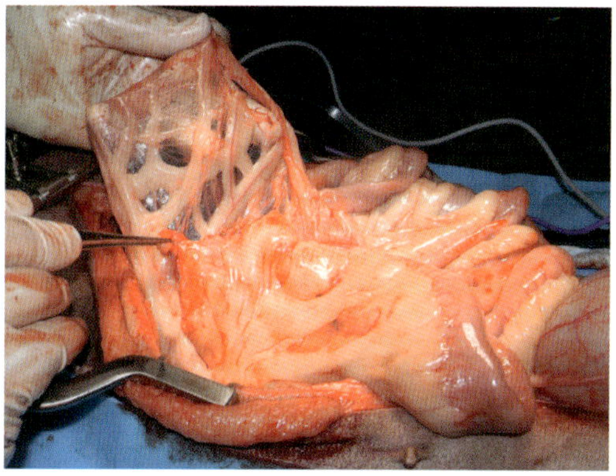

L-ii)

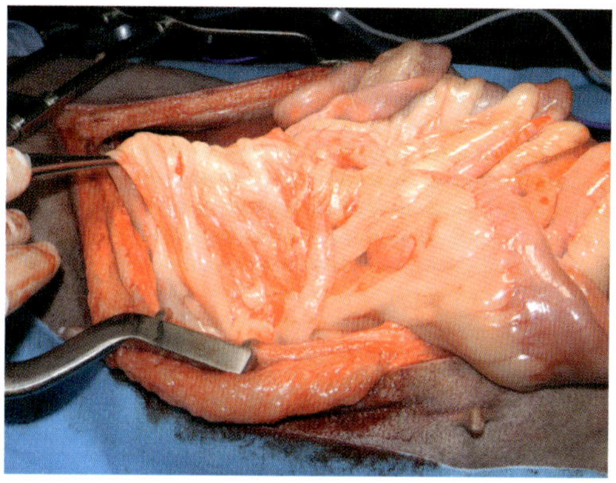

M-i)

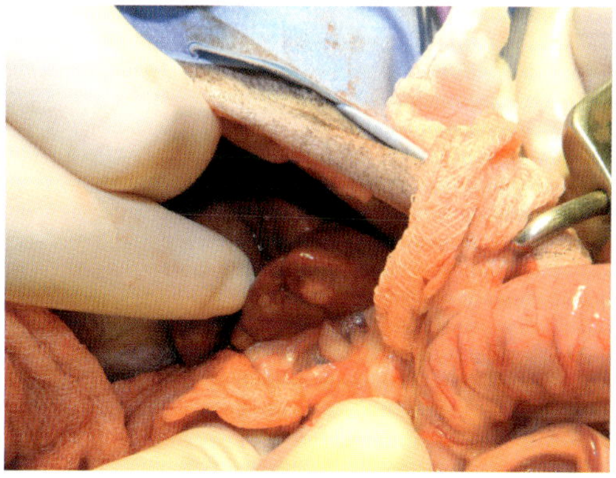

M-ii)

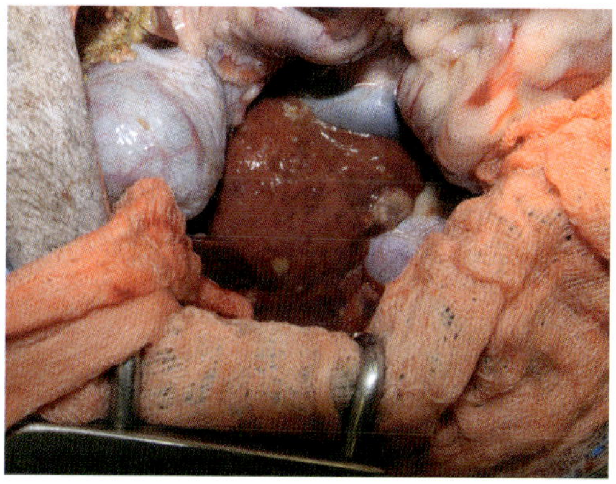

M-iii)

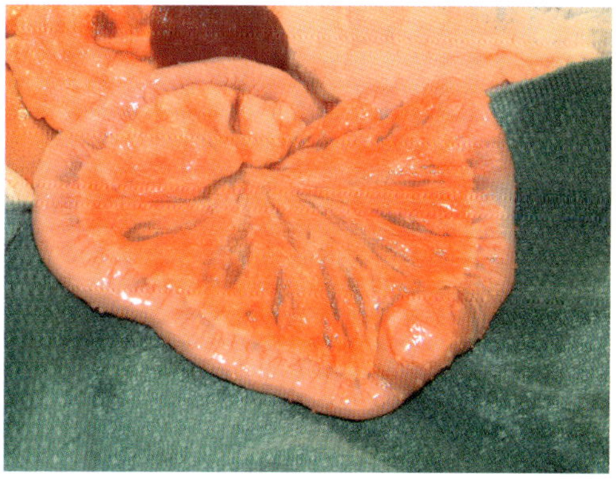

M-iv)

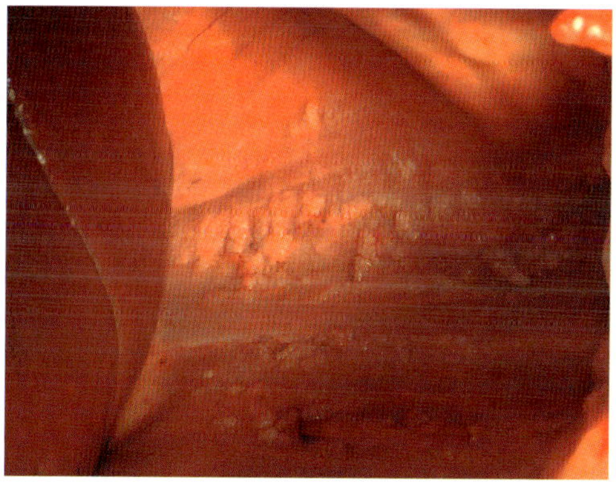

References

1 Morrice, M., Polton, G., and Beck, S. (2019). Evaluation of the extent of neoplastic infiltration in small intestinal tumours in dogs. *Vet. Med. Sci.* 5 (2): 189–198.

2 Morrice, M., Polton, G., and Beck, S. (2019). Evaluation of the histopathological extent of neoplastic infiltration in intestinal tumours in cats. *Vet. Med. Sci.* 5 (3): 307–316.

3 Snowdon, K.A., Smeak, D.D., and Chiang, S. (2016). Risk factors for dehiscence of stapled finctional end-to-end intestinal anastomoses in dogs: 53 dogs (2001-2012). *Vet. Surg.* 45 (1): 91–99.

4 Jardel, N., Hidalgo, A., Leperlier, D. et al. (2011). One stage functional end-to-end stapled anastomosis and resection performed by nonexpert surgeons for the treatment of small intestinal obstruction in 30 dogs. *Vet. Surg.* 40 (2): 216–222.

5 Duell, J.R., Thieman Mankin, K.M., Rochat, M.C. et al. (2016). Frequency of dehiscence in hand-sutured and stapled intestinal anastomoses in dogs. *Vet. Surg.* 45 (1): 100–103.

6 DePompeo, C.M., Bond, L., George, Y.E. et al. (2018). Intra-abdominal complications following intestinal anastomoses by suture and staple techniques in dogs. *J. Am. Vet. Med. Assoc.* 253 (4): 437–443.

7 Summer, S.M., Regier, P.J., Case, J.B. et al. (2019). Evaluation of suture reinforcement for stapled intestinal anastomoses: 77 dogs (2008-2018). *Vet. Surg.* 48 (7): 1188–1193.

8 White, R.N. (2008). Modified functional end-to-end stapled intestinal anastomosis: technique and clinical results in 15 dogs. *J. Small Anim. Pract.* 49 (6): 274–281.

22.2 Laparoscopic-Assisted Small Intestinal Resection and Anastomosis

Indications

1) Resection of small benign and malignant tumors involving the small intestine that can be readily exteriorized through a small opening in the abdomen

Suggested Diagnostic Workup and Clinical Staging

- See *22. Small Intestinal Resection and Anastomosis.*

Patient Positioning

The patient is positioned in dorsal recumbency.

Surgical Technique (See Plate 22.2A–E)

A) Laparoscopic-assisted intestinal resection and anastomosis can be performed either as a multiport or single-port procedure. For the multiport procedure, two ports are created to perform the procedure. A skin incision is made in a subumbilical location and a 6-mm cannula is placed as described in *15.3. Laparoscopic Approach*. After placement of this initial cannula, a pneumoperitoneum is created. An additional cannula is introduced to allow for placement of instrumentation; both cannulae are placed on the ventral midline. The second cannula is placed cranial or caudal to the telescope cannula depending on the suspected location of the mass.

B) For single-port laparoscopic intestinal resection and anastomosis, a single-port device is introduced into the abdomen via a small celiotomy. The most common devices currently used in veterinary patients are the single-incision laparoscopic surgery (SILS) port and the GelPOINT access system. A skin incision is made at the level of the umbilicus or just caudal to the umbilicus. The skin incision length is dependent on the length of the single-port device that is going to be used to perform the procedure. The SILS port is small and requires a 3-cm-long incision (pictured). The GelPOINT access system requires a 6-cm-long incision. After continuation of the skin incision through the linea alba (as per a typical celiotomy), the single-port device is inserted through the celiotomy into the abdomen. The falciform ligament is retracted to allow for introduction of the device; alternatively, if the incision is large enough to visualize the falciform ligament, this can be transected using an open technique. The cannulae that are designed for these devices are then inserted into the single-port device, and the patient is insufflated with CO_2.

C) For either the single-port device or multiport technique, a 5-mm-diameter telescope is inserted into the abdomen and the intestinal tract is visualized (not pictured). Through an instrument port, a blunt probe is inserted to allow for mobilization of the intestines and identification of the intestinal mass. In addition, a limited exploration of the abdomen is possible.

Color Atlas of Canine and Feline Surgical Oncology, First Edition. Julius M. Liptak, Paolo Buracco, William T. N. Culp, and Nicholas J. Bacon.

Plate 22.2

Laparoscopic-Assisted Small Intestinal Resection and Anastomosis

A)

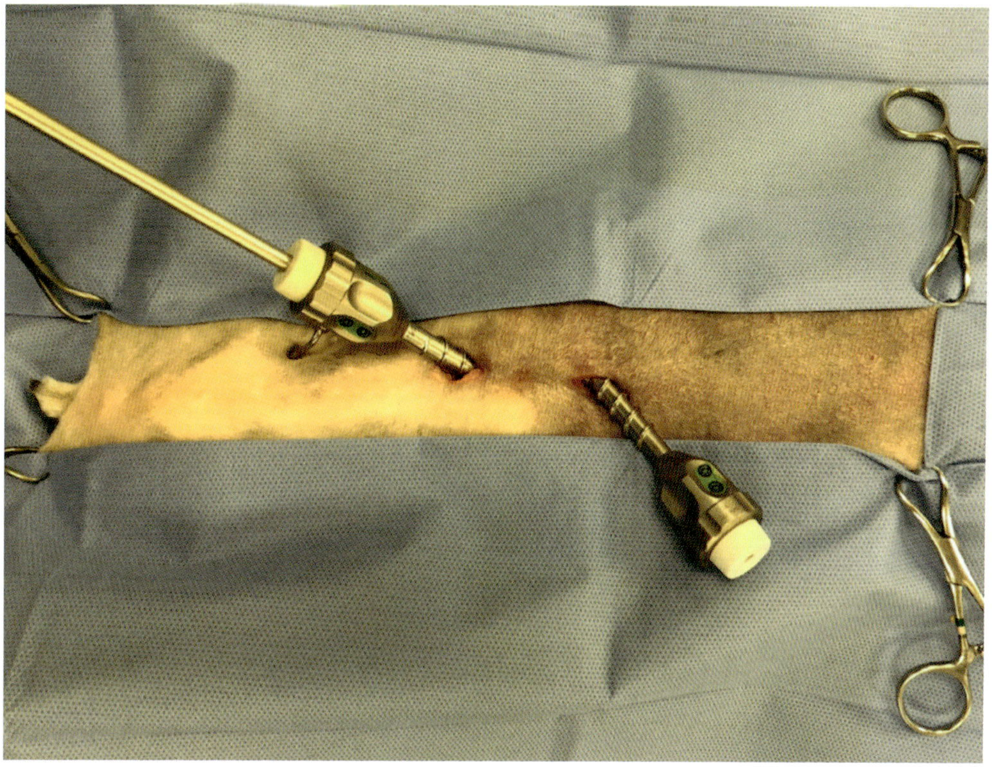

B)

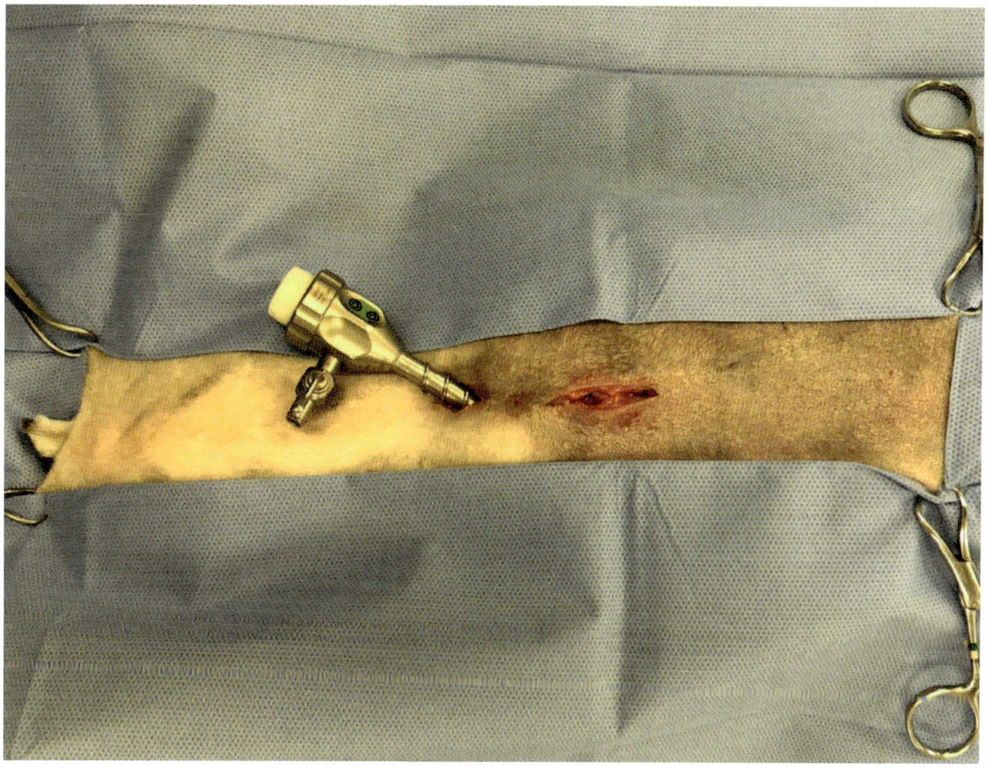

Surgical Technique (See Plate 22.2A–E) *continued*

D) After the mass has been located and evaluation of other abdominal structures has been performed, a wound retractor device can be inserted into the abdomen. If a single-port device was used, a wound retractor (pictured, inner ring of the Alexis wound retractor device) can likely be inserted directly into the abdomen through the previously created mini-celiotomy. If the multiport technique was used, the two ports can be connected for placement of the wound retractor device or one of the ports can be enlarged (i.e. more cranial port for a duodenal or jejunal lesion or more caudal port for an ileal, cecal, or colonic lesion).
E) Once the wound retraction device has been inserted into the abdomen (arrow), the mass and adjacent/associated intestine is exteriorized out of the abdomen through the wound retractor device. A traditional intestinal resection and anastomosis can then be performed as described in *22.1. Open Small Intestinal Resection and Anastomosis*.

Closure

The linea alba, subcutaneous tissue, and skin are closed as described in *15.1. Ventral Midline Celiotomy*.

Postoperative Management

1) Multimodal analgesia, but consider avoiding the use of steroids and nonsteroidal anti-inflammatory drugs because of their negative effects on intestinal healing
2) Elizabethan collar or body suit
3) Feed normal diet

Complications

Intraoperative Complications

- Inadequate exposure of the intestinal mass requiring conversion to an open intestinal resection and anastomosis (13%–25%) [1–3]
- Extension of celiotomy incision because of inability to exteriorize the intestinal mass (38%) [2]
- For complications specific to all laparoscopic procedures, see *15.3. Laparoscopic Approach*

Postoperative Complications

- Anastomotic dehiscence and septic peritonitis [4]
- Incisional complications
- Hyporexia

Suggested Adjuvant Treatments

- See *22. Small Intestinal Resection and Anastomosis*.

Prognosis and Oncologic Outcome

- See *22. Small Intestinal Resection and Anastomosis*.

Plate 22.2

Laparoscopic-Assisted Small Intestinal Resection and Anastomosis *continued*

D)

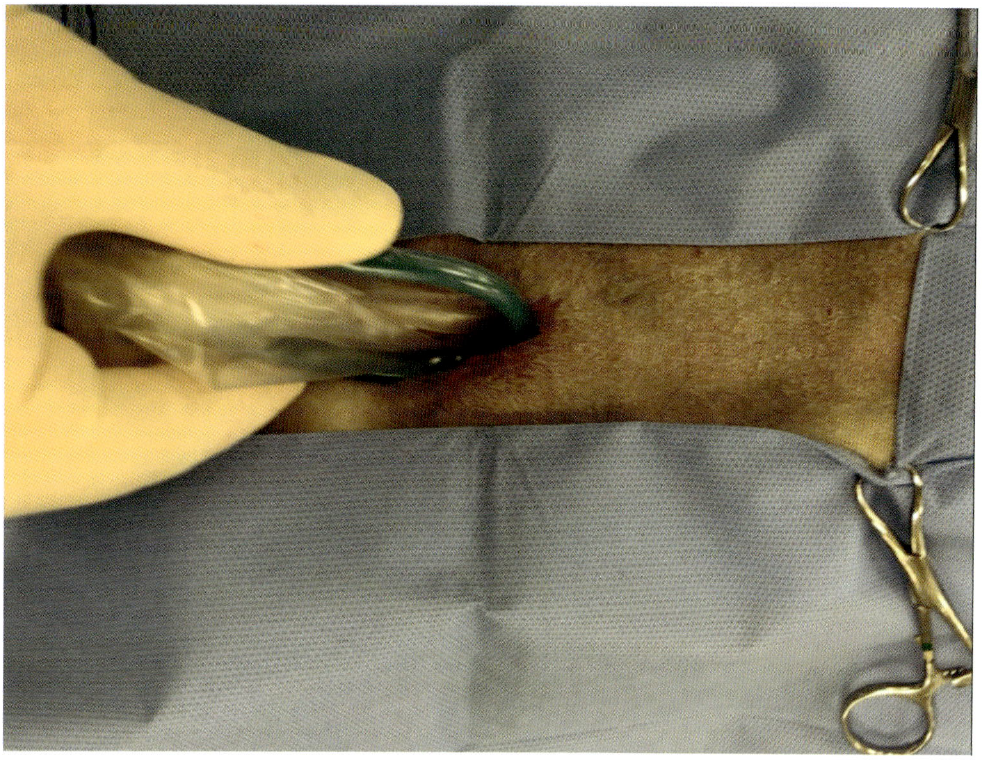

E)

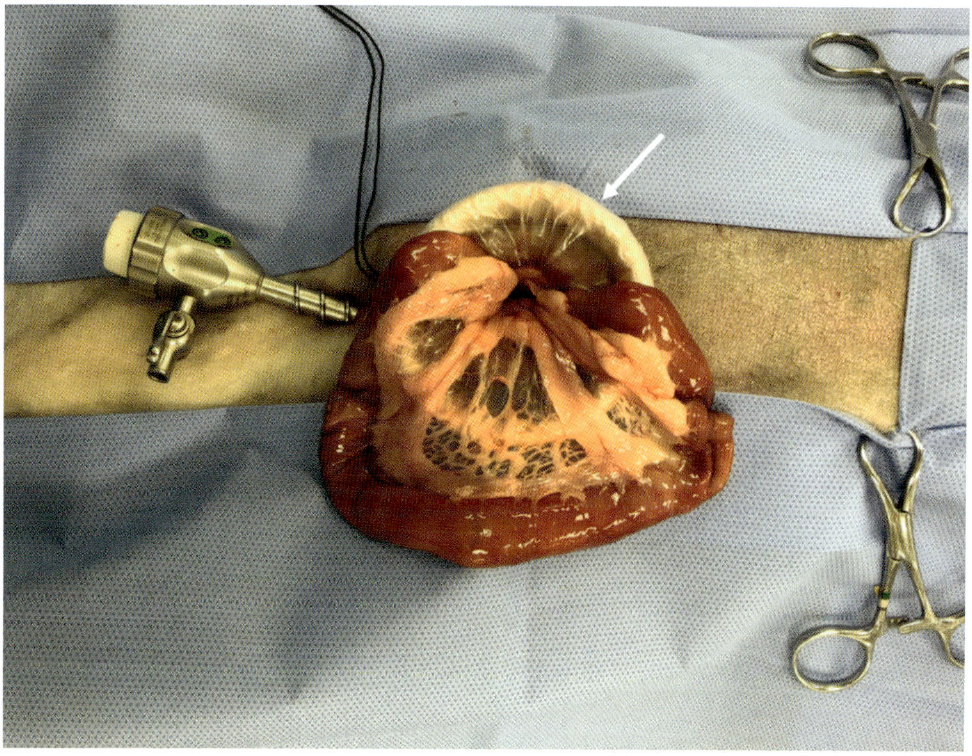

References

1 Gower, S.B. and Mayhew, P.D. (2011). A wound retraction device for laparoscopic-assisted intestinal surgery in dogs and cats. *Vet. Surg.* 40 (4): 485–488.
2 Case, B.J. and Ellison, G. (2013). Single incision laparoscopic-assisted intestinal surgery (SILAIS) in 7 dogs and 1 cat. *Vet. Surg.* 42 (5): 629–634.
3 Otomo, A., Singh, A., Valverde, A. et al. (2019). Comparison of outcome in dogs undergoing single-incision laparoscopic-assisted intestinal surgery and open laparotomy for simple small intestinal foreign body removal. *Vet. Surg.* 48 (S1): O83–O90.
4 Baron, J., Giuffrida, M., Mayhew, P.D. et al. (2017). Minimally invasive small intestinal exploration and targeted abdominal organ biopsy with a wound retraction device in 42 cats (2005-2015). *Vet. Surg.* 46 (7): 925–932.

Chapter 23: Typhlectomy

Indications

1) Resection of benign and malignant cecal tumors
2) For extensive cecal tumors, an end-to-end resection of the ileocecocolic junction should be performed rather than a typhlectomy (see *22.1. Open Small Intestinal Resection and Anastomosis*)

Suggested Diagnostic Workup and Clinical Staging

- Complete blood count, serum biochemistry, and urinalysis
- Abdominal ultrasound or computed tomography (CT) scan with image-guided aspirates
- Three-view thoracic radiographs or thoracic CT scan for assessment of lung metastasis

Patient Positioning

The patient is positioned in dorsal recumbency.

Surgical Technique (See Plate 23B–E)

A) A ventral midline celiotomy is performed (see *15.1. Ventral Midline Celiotomy*). The cecum and cecal mass are protected from the remainder of the abdominal cavity with moistened laparotomy sponges.
B) The ileocecal fold (i, dashed line) attaching the cecum to the ileum and the smaller accessory ileocecal fold attaching the cecum to the colon are incised. The ileocecal artery within the ileocecal fold should be ligated and divided; alternatively, a vessel sealing device can be used (ii). The antimesenteric artery should be preserved. Division of the ileocecal fold allows greater mobilization of the cecum and cecal mass (iii).
C) **Typhlectomy technique 1 – Suture:** Two atraumatic Doyen forceps are applied across the base of the cecum. The cecum is incised with a scalpel blade between the two Doyen forceps (i), and the cecum and cecal mass are removed from the surgical field. The typhlectomy site is closed with 3-0 to 4-0 monofilament absorbable suture material using a Parker-Kerr suture pattern over the Doyen forceps or a simple continuous suture (ii, iii) or interrupted sutures.

Color Atlas of Canine and Feline Surgical Oncology, First Edition. Julius M. Liptak, Paolo Buracco, William T. N. Culp, and Nicholas J. Bacon.

Plate 23

Typhlectomy

B-i)

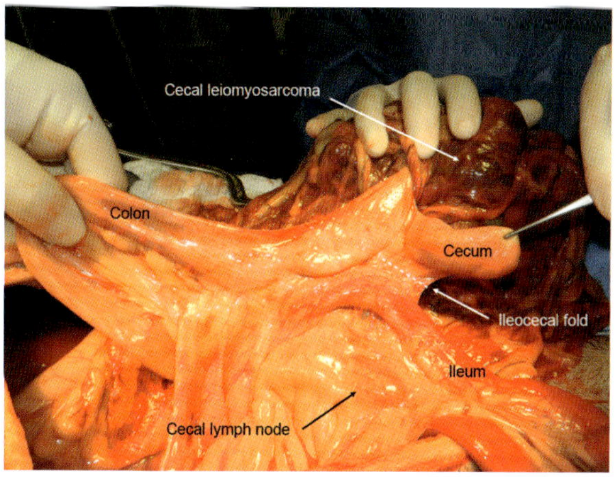

B-ii)

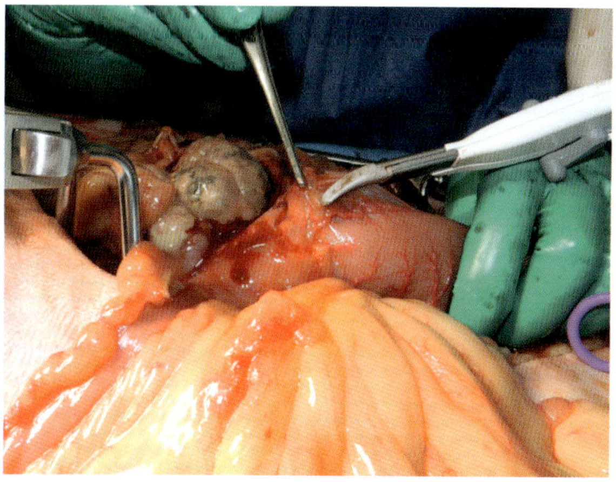

B-iii)

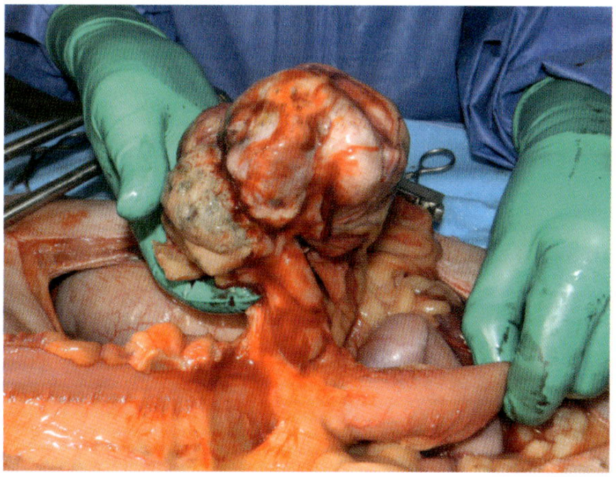

C-i)

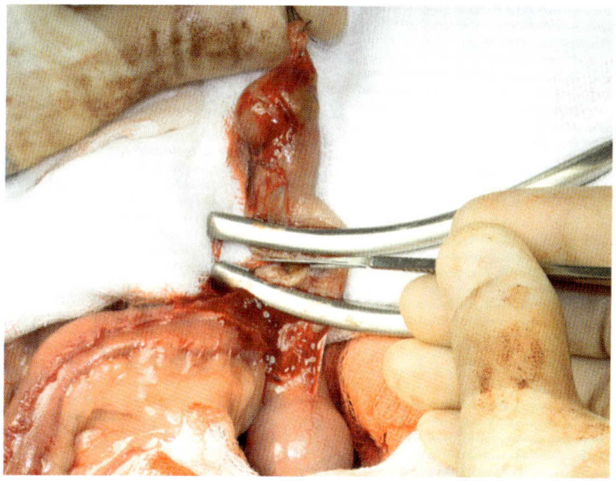

Courtesy of Dr. Laurent Findji

C-ii)

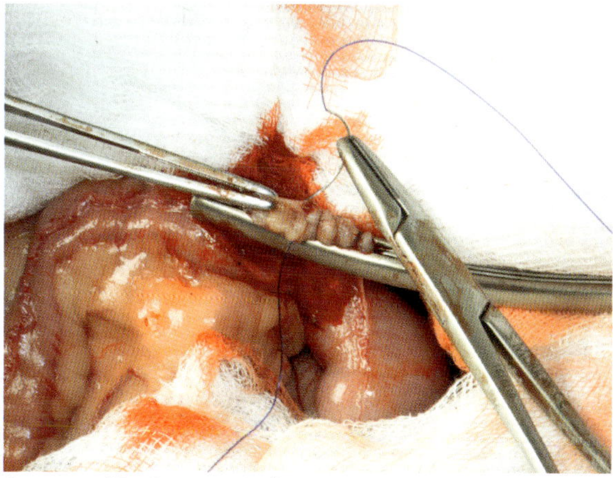

Courtesy of Dr. Laurent Findji

C-iii)

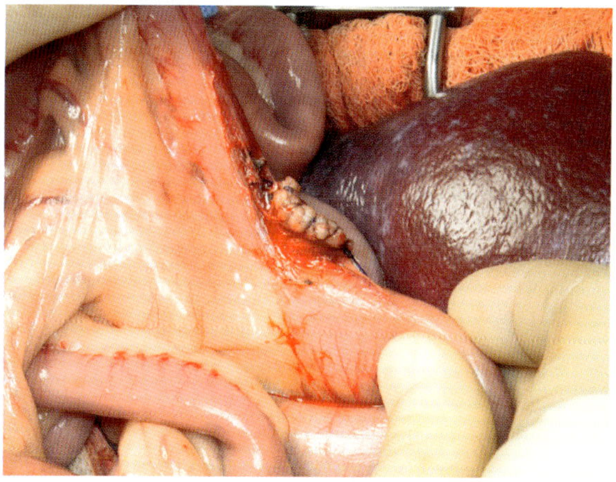

Courtesy of Dr. Laurent Findji

Surgical Technique (See Plate 23B–E) *continued*

D) **Typhlectomy technique 2 – Stapler:** An appropriately sized thoracoabdominal (TA) stapler (usually a 30-mm or 55- to 60-mm TA stapler) is placed across the base of the cecum (i), and crushing forceps are placed above the TA stapler (ii). The TA stapler is locked and fired. The cecum is incised with a scalpel blade between the TA stapler and forceps (iii), and the cecum and cecal mass are removed from the surgical field (iv). The staple line should be inspected and reinforced with a continuous suture pattern, using 3-0 to 4-0 monofilament absorbable material, if necessary. Alternatively, an appropriately sized gastrointestinal stapler can be used (v).

E) The abdominal cavity should be systematically explored for metastatic disease. The most common metastatic sites for cecal tumors include the regional lymph nodes (i and ii, LN) and liver (iii, arrow). After completion of the typhlectomy and abdominal exploration, the abdominal cavity should be lavaged with warmed, sterile isotonic saline.

Closure

The linea alba, subcutis, and skin are closed as described in *15.1. Ventral Midline Celiotomy*.

Postoperative Management

1) Multimodal analgesia, but consider avoiding the use of steroids and nonsteroidal anti-inflammatory drugs because of negative effects on intestinal healing
2) Elizabethan collar or body suit
3) Feed normal diet

Complications

- Anastomotic dehiscence and septic peritonitis (5%–16%)

Suggested Adjuvant Treatments

- Chemotherapy for cats and dogs with malignant intestinal tumors

Prognosis and Oncologic Outcome – Dogs

	Local Recurrence Rate	Metastatic Rate	Disease-Free Interval (d)	Median Survival Time (d)	1-Year Survival Rate	2-Year Survival Rate
			Leiomyosarcoma[a] [1, 2]			
Overall	10%	54%	–	238	75%	66%
			Gastrointestinal Stromal Tumor[a] [2]			
Overall	0%	7%	–	354	63%	52%
			Leiomyosarcoma and Gastrointestinal Stromal Tumor[b] [3]			
Overall	37%		–	–	84%	66%

[a] Includes all gastrointestinal sites (small intestines, cecum, and colon).
[b] Outcome for reclassified small intestinal leiomyosarcomas and gastrointestinal stromal tumors reported as a combined group.

Plate 23

Typhlectomy *continued*

D-i)

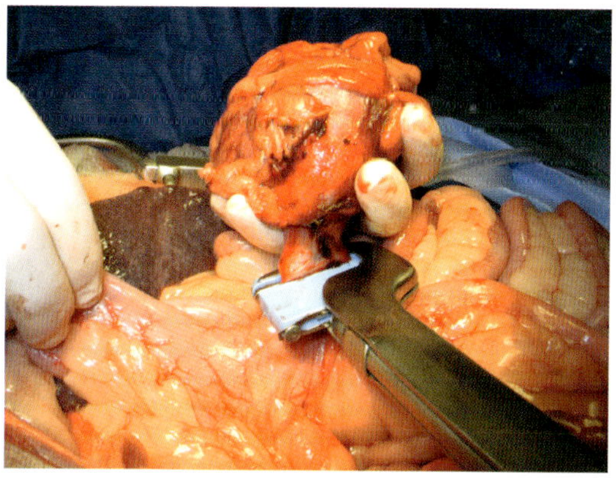

D-ii)

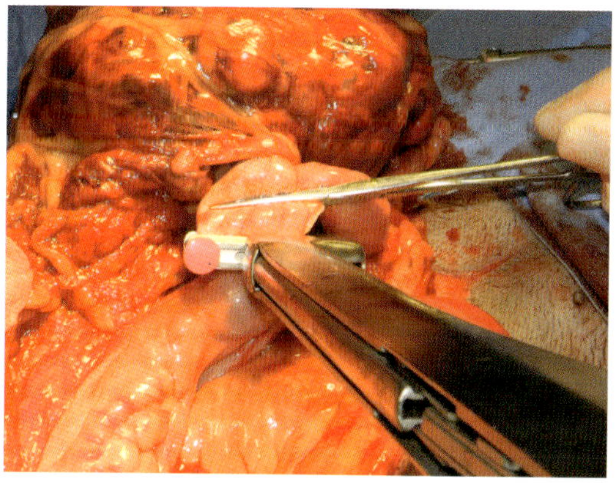

D-iii)

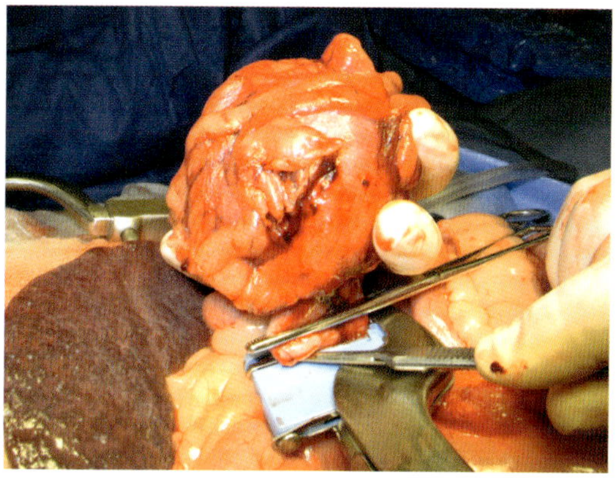

D-iv)

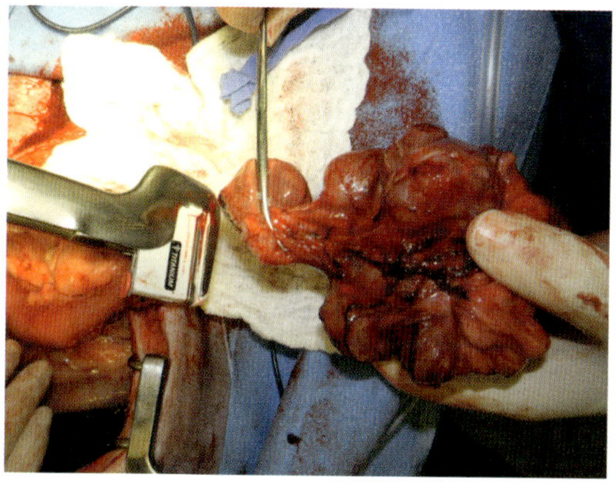

D-v)

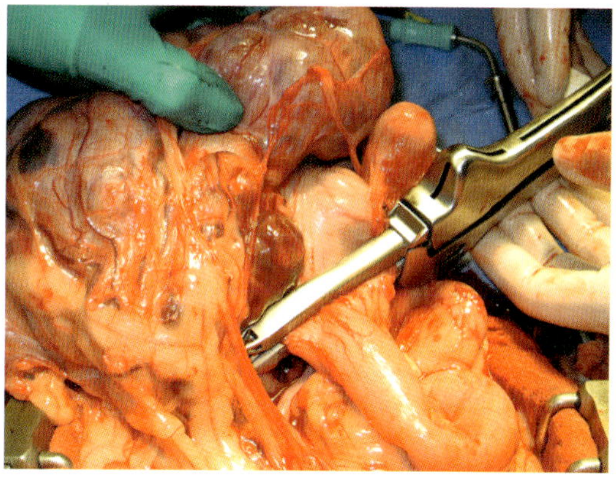

E-i)

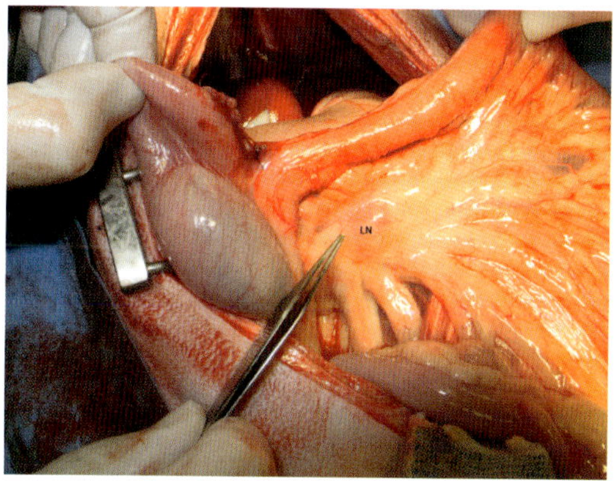

E-ii)

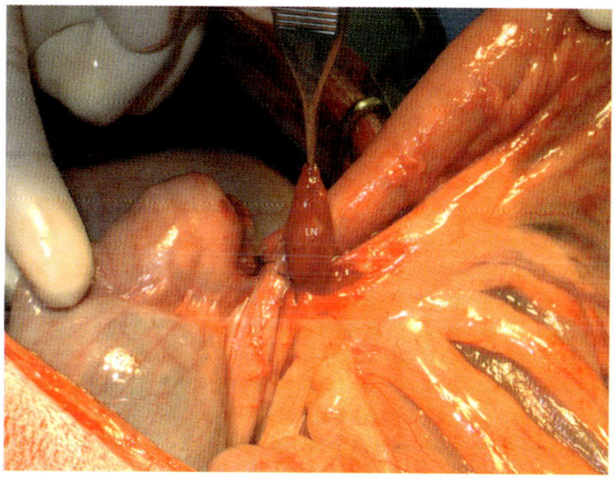

E-iii)

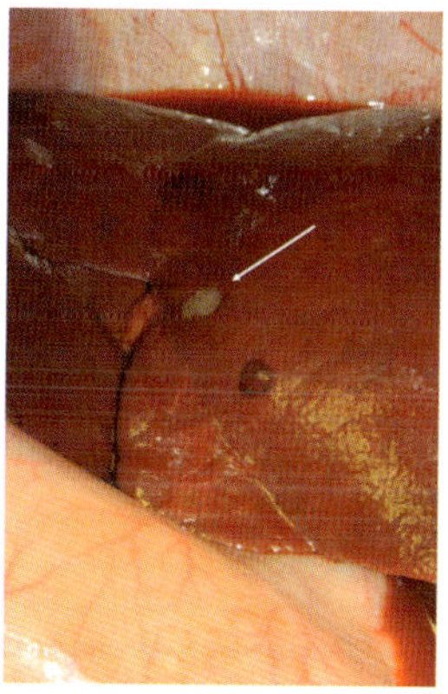

References

1 Cohen, M., Post, G.S., and Wright, J.C. (2003). Gastrointestinal leiomyosarcoma in 14 dogs. *J. Vet. Intern. Med.* 17 (1): 107–110.

2 Russell, K.N., Mehler, S.J., Skorupski, K.A. et al. (2007). Clinical and immunohistochemical differentiation of gastrointestinal stromal tumors from leiomyosarcomas in dogs: 42 cases (1990-2003). *J. Am. Vet. Med. Assoc.* 230 (9): 1329–1333.

3 Maas, C.P.H.J., ter Haar, G., van der Gaag, I. et al. (2007). Reclassification of small intestinal and cecal smooth muscle tumors in 72 dogs: clinical, histologic, and immunohistochemical evaluation. *Vet. Surg.* 36 (4): 302–313.

Chapter 24: Colorectal Resection and Anastomosis

Indications

1) Resection of benign and malignant tumors involving the large intestine
2) Large intestinal resection and end-to-end anastomosis (EEA) can be combined with either a pubic symphysiotomy (see *15.5. Pubic Symphysiotomy*) or pubic flap (see *15.6. Pubic Flap*) if additional caudal exposure is required.

Suggested Diagnostic Workup and Clinical Staging

- Complete blood count, serum biochemistry, and urinalysis
- Abdominal ultrasound or computed tomography (CT) scan with image-guided aspirates
- Three-view thoracic radiographs or thoracic CT scan for assessment of lung metastasis

Patient Positioning

The patient is positioned in dorsal recumbency.

Surgical Technique [1, 2] (See Plate 24A–E, G–L)

A) A ventral midline celiotomy is performed (see *15.1. Ventral Midline Celiotomy*). This can be combined with either a pubic symphysiotomy (see *15.5. Pubic Symphysiotomy*) or a pubic flap (see *15.6. Pubic Flap*) if additional caudal exposure is required. The affected intestinal segment should be isolated from the abdominal cavity with moistened laparotomy sponges.
B) The terminal branches of the ileocolic branch of the cranial mesenteric artery and the caudal mesenteric artery supplying the affected intestinal segment are ligated with monofilament absorbable suture material or metallic clips and divided. Alternatively, this can be done with a vessel sealing device (pictured).
C) Crushing clamps are placed across the intestines orally and aborally at an appropriate distance from the intestinal tumor to prevent spillage of intestinal contents from the resected intestinal segment. Oral, aboral, and mesenteric margins should be a minimum of 3–5 cm; however, lesser margins are likely sufficient for dogs with leiomyomas and low-grade leiomyosarcomas.
D) The intestinal contents are milked away from the crushing clamps, and the intestines are occluded 4–6 cm orally and aborally to the crushing clamps with either an assistant's fingers (see step C) or atraumatic Doyen forceps (DF, pictured).

Plate 24

Colorectal Resection and Anastomosis

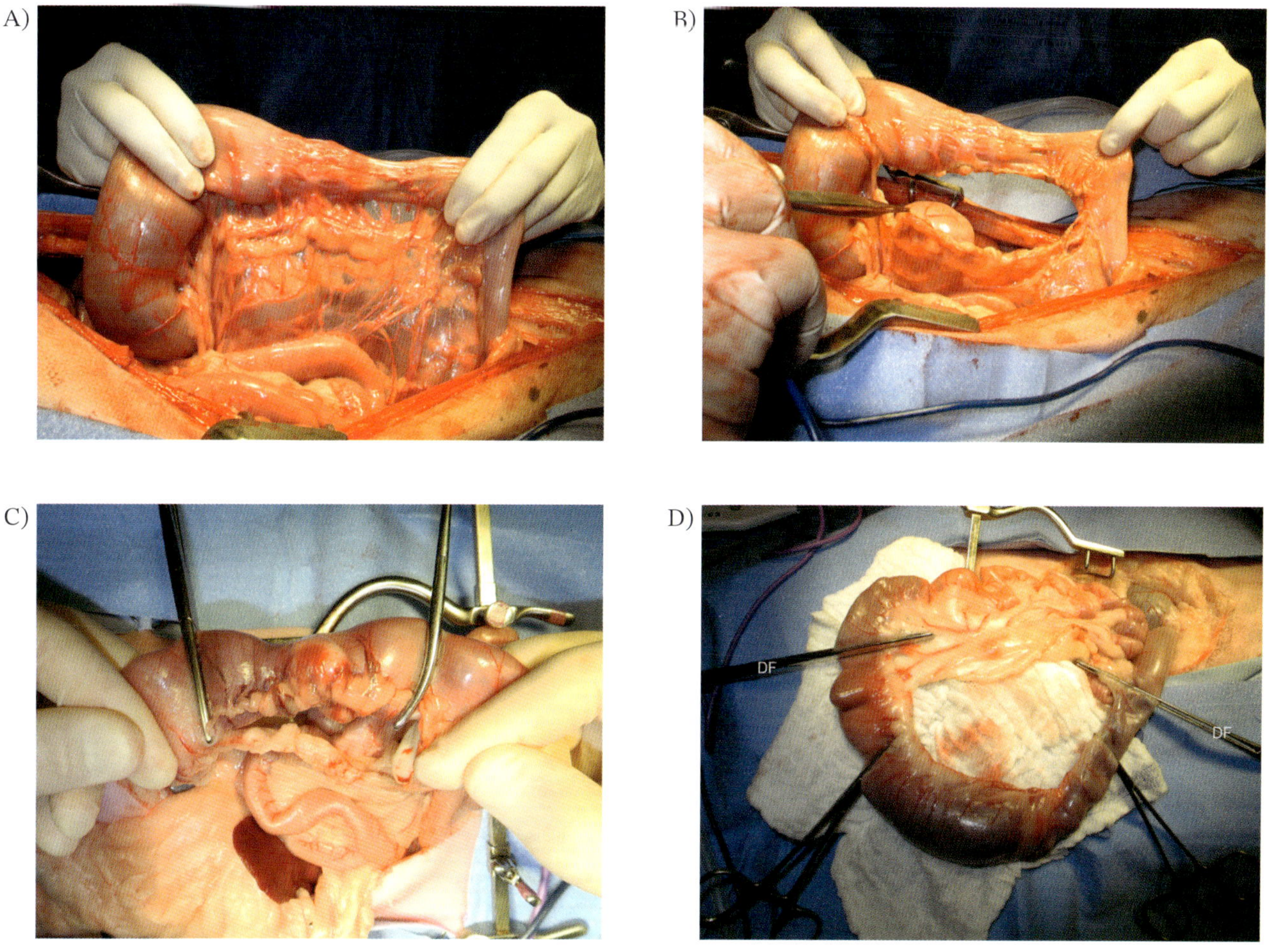

Surgical Technique [1, 2] (See Plate 24A–E, G–L) *continued*

E) The intestines are transected along the crushing clamps, at the junction between the divided and nondivided terminal branches of the ileocolic branch of the cranial mesenteric artery and the caudal mesenteric artery (i, orad colonic resection being performed with Metzenbaum scissors; ii, orad colonic resection completed; iii, aborad colonic resection being performed with Metzenbaum scissors; iv, aborad colonic resection completed).

F) The resected intestinal segment is removed from the surgical field (not pictured) and the transected ends of the intestines are opposed while maintaining occlusion of the intestines oral and aboral to the resection site. The opposed intestinal ends are anastomosed using either a suture or staple technique.

G) **EEA technique 1 – suture:** The transected intestinal ends can be anastomosed using a simple interrupted, modified Gambee, or simple continuous suture pattern, or with skin staples. For sutured anastomoses, 3-0 or 4-0 absorbable monofilament suture material is used with 2- to 3-mm bites every 3–4 mm. An EEA with a simple continuous suture pattern should be done with two overlapping 180-degree continuous suture patterns to minimize the risk of iatrogenic stricture of the colonic anastomosis (i, first 180-degree simple continuous suture pattern; ii, second overlapping 180-degree simple continuous suture pattern).

Plate 24

Colorectal Resection and Anastomosis *continued*

E-i)

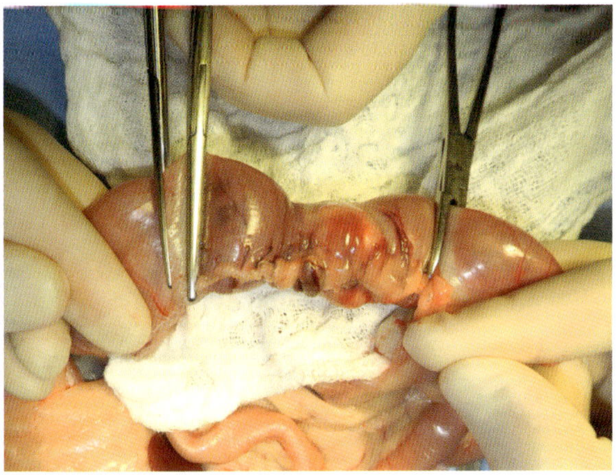

E-ii)

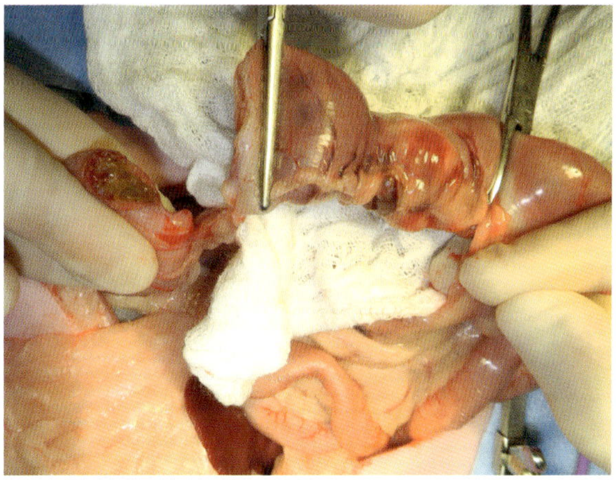

E-iii)

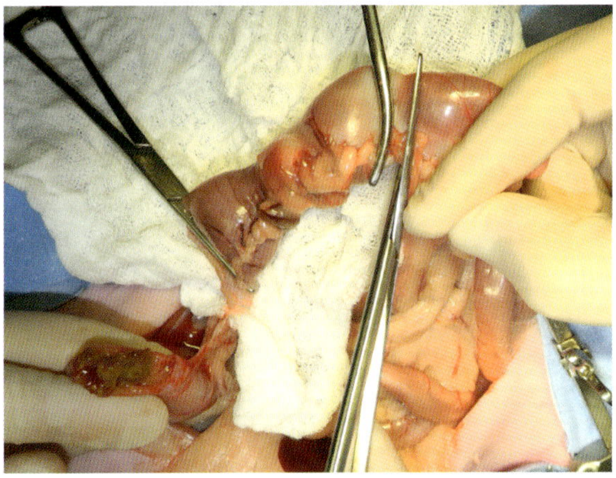

E-iv)

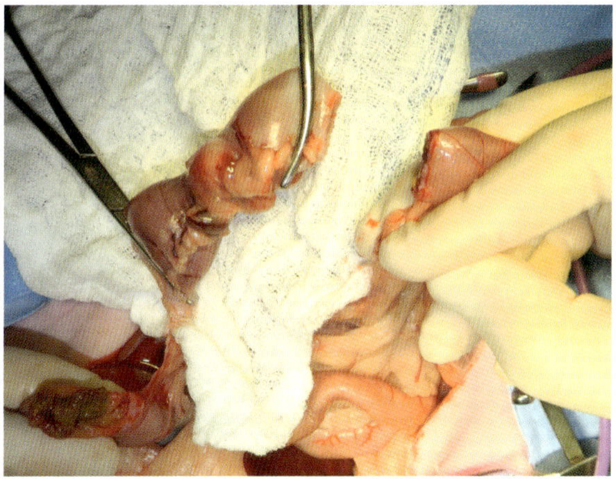

G-i)

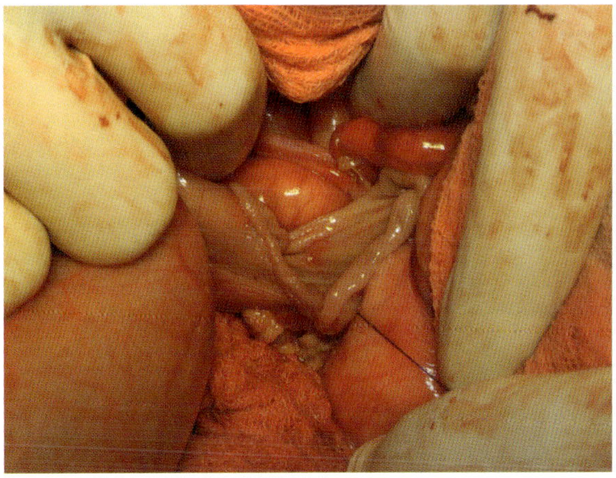

G-ii)

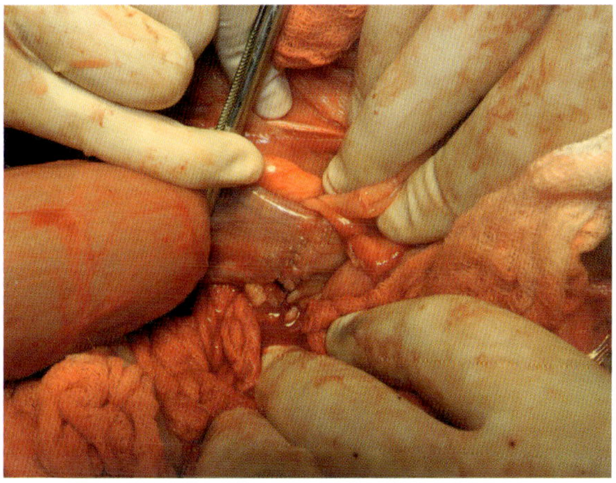

Surgical Technique [1, 2] (See Plate 24A–E, G–L) *continued*

H) **EEA technique 2 – functional end-to-end stapled anastomosis:** Stay sutures on the mesenteric side of the orad and aborad intestines are used to elevate the intestines in a vertical direction such that the antimesenteric borders of both intestines are opposed. A gastrointestinal anastomosis (GIA) stapler is inserted into the lumen of both intestinal segments (i). The GIA stapler is locked and fired to create a side-to-side anastomosis along the antimesenteric border of the intestinal segments (ii, intraluminal view). With the intestines still elevated by the stay sutures, an appropriately sized thoracoabdominal (TA) stapler is then placed across the transected intestinal ends, locked, and fired to complete the stapled anastomosis (iii). The excessive intestinal tissue within the TA stapler is incised with a scalpel blade and either discarded or submitted for histopathologic assessment of surgical margins.

I) **EEA technique 3 – end-to end anastomosis stapler:** A purse-string suture is placed in the orad and aborad ends of the colon with monofilament suture material on a straight needle passed through a Furniss clamp (i) or manually (ii). An appropriately sized EEA stapler (21, 25, 28, or 31 mm) is inserted through either the cecum (via a typhylotomy) or rectum [3] (pictured, iii). Insertion through the rectum is preferred in dogs, whereas either approach is feasible in cats [4].

Plate 24

Colorectal Resection and Anastomosis *continued*

H-i)

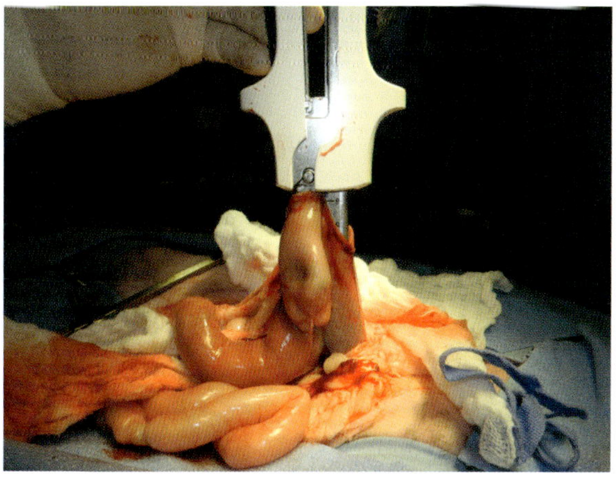

H-ii)

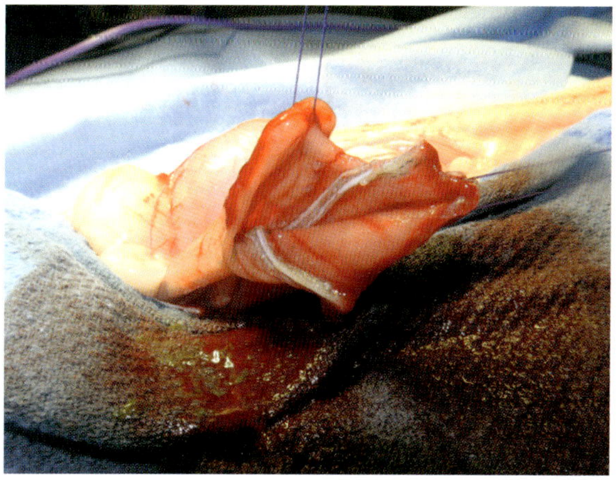

H-iii)

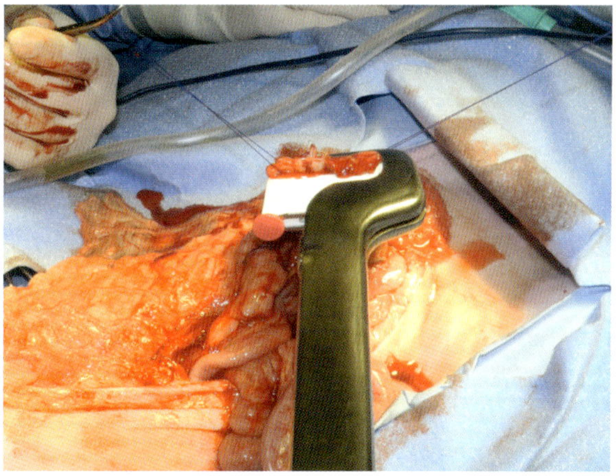

I-i)

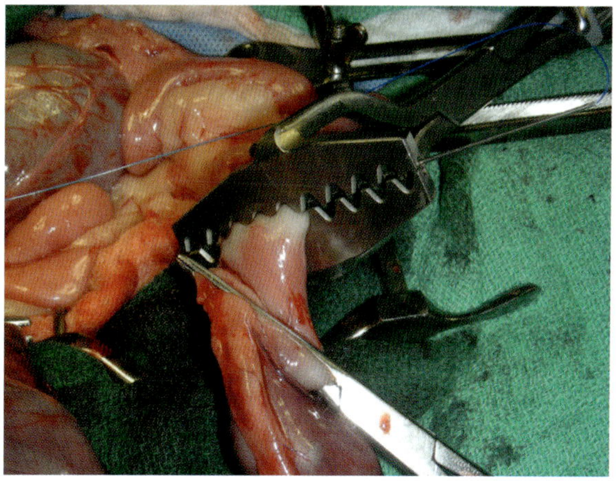

Courtesy of Dr. Eric Monnet

I-ii)

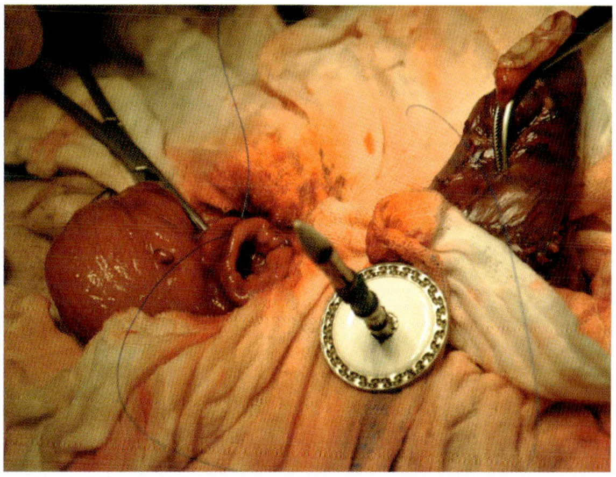

Courtesy of Dr. Bart Van Goethem

I-iii)

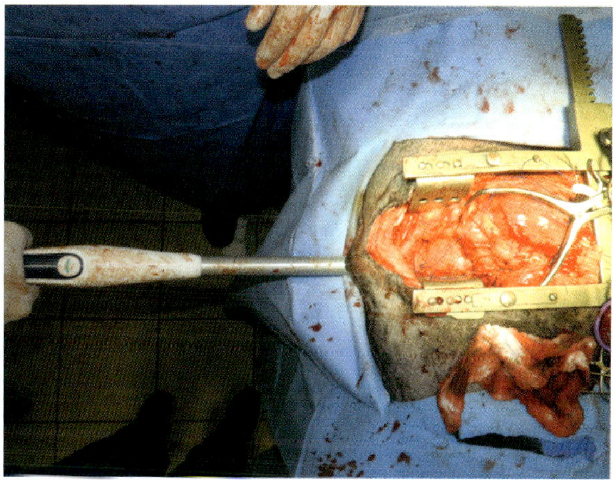

Surgical Technique [1, 2] (See Plate 24A–E, G–L) *continued*

The purse-string suture on the orad side of the resection is loosened, the anvil of the EEA stapler is advanced through the end of the colonic resection site (iv), and the purse-string suture is tightened onto the shaft of the anvil (v, vi). The EEA stapler is then advanced to the purse-string on the aborad side of the resection (vii, arrow), and then the trocar (arrow) is extended until the orange band is visible (dashed arrow) (viii). The anvil shaft is then slid over the trocar until seated in position (ix).

Plate 24

Colorectal Resection and Anastomosis *continued*

I-iv)
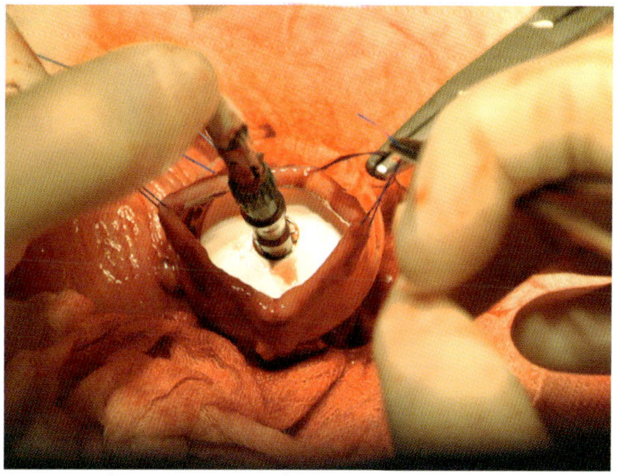
Courtesy of Dr. Bart Van Goethem

I-v)
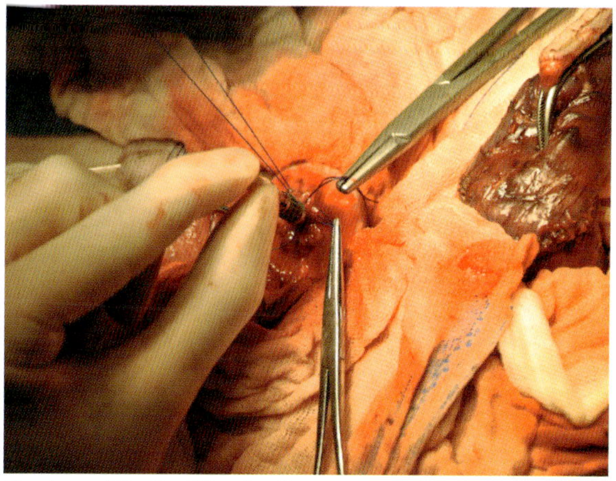
Courtesy of Dr. Bart Van Goethem

I-vi)
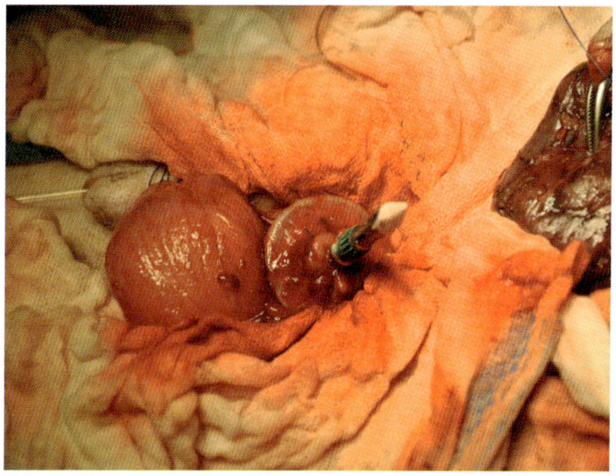
Courtesy of Dr. Bart Van Goethem

I-vii)
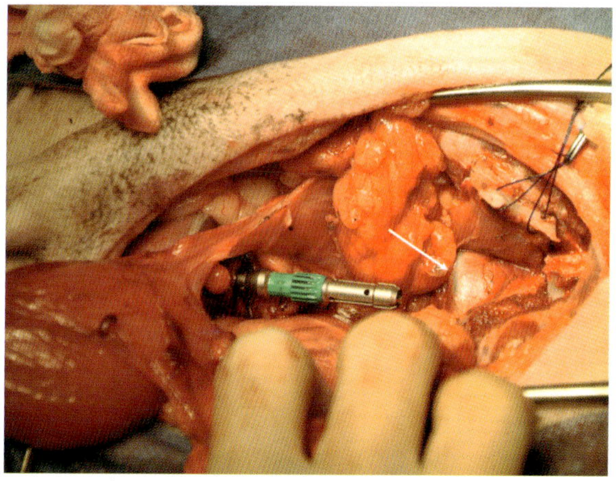
Courtesy of Dr. Bart Van Goethem

I-viii)
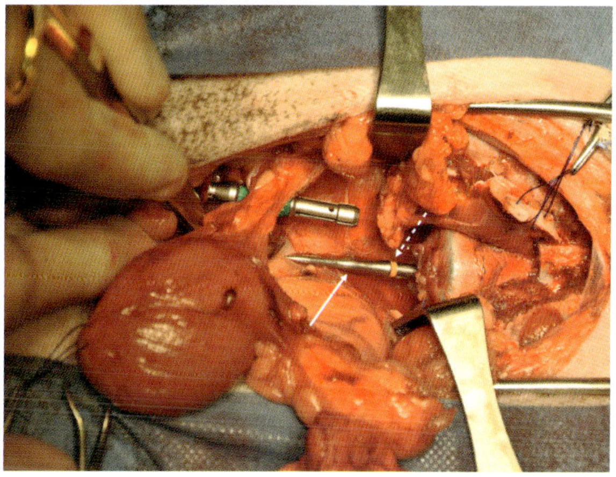
Courtesy of Dr. Bart Van Goethem

I-ix)
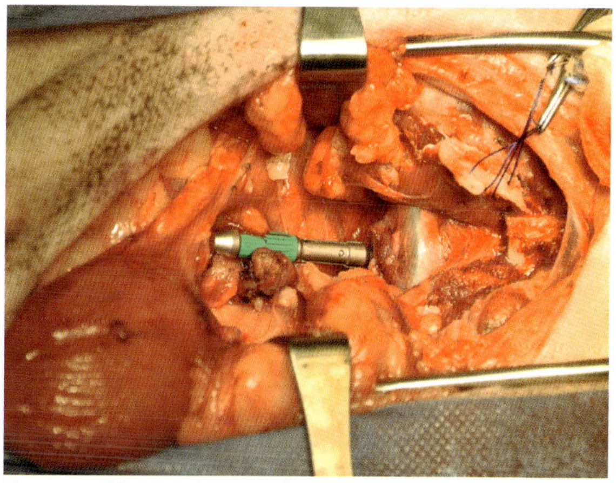
Courtesy of Dr. Bart Van Goethem

Surgical Technique [1, 2] (See Plate 24A–E, G–L) *continued*

The EEA stapler is closed (x) to an appropriate tension (please read EEA instructions) while preventing twisting of the resection ends, and the stapler is fired to complete the anastomosis (xi). The anvil is partially opened and carefully removed from the anastomosis site. The EEA stapler is then removed, and the resected tissue is examined to confirm that a circumferential, full-thickness anastomosis has been achieved (xii).

J) The patency of the anastomosis should be tested by occluding the intestines oral and aboral to the anastomosis site with an assistant's fingers (pictured) or atraumatic Doyen forceps, and then injecting sterile isotonic saline into the lumen of the anastomosed intestines. Any visible leaks should be sutured with 3-0 or 4-0 absorbable monofilament suture material in a simple interrupted pattern.

K) The anastomosis should be wrapped in omentum.

L) The abdominal cavity should be systematically explored for metastatic disease. The most common metastatic sites for large intestinal tumors include the regional lymph nodes (pictured, LN) and liver, and carcinomatosis for large intestinal carcinomas. After completion of the intestinal resection and anastomosis and abdominal exploration, the abdominal cavity should be lavaged with warmed, sterile isotonic saline.

Plate 24

Colorectal Resection and Anastomosis *continued*

I-x)

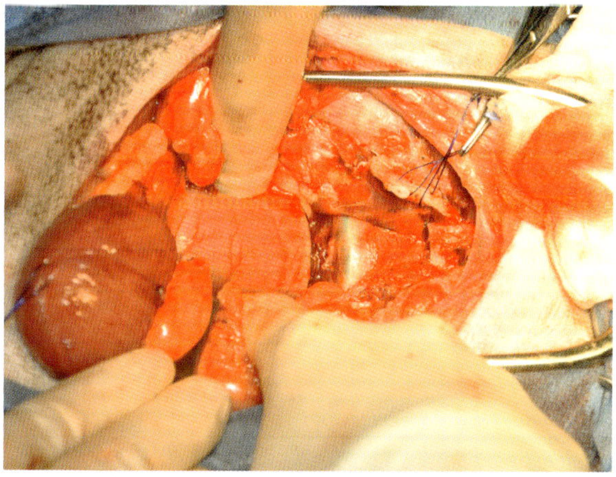

Courtesy of Dr. Bart Van Goethem

I-xi)

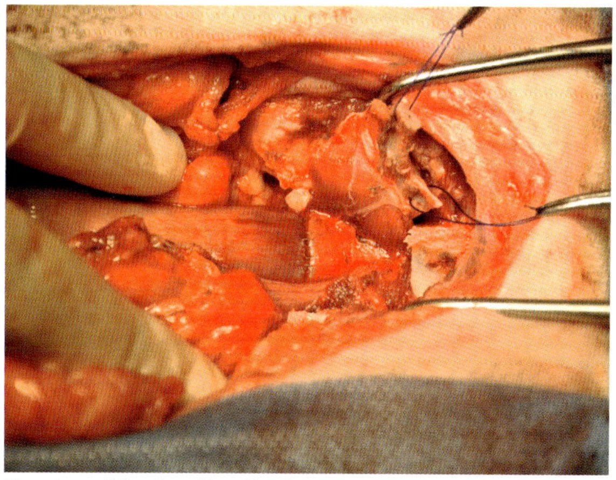

Courtesy of Dr. Bart Van Goethem

I-xii)

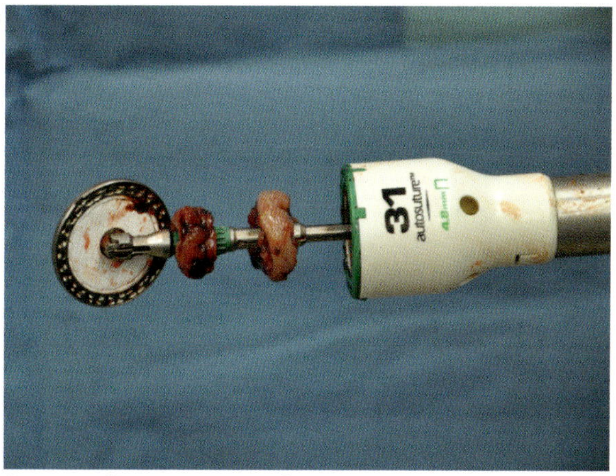

Courtesy of Dr. Bart Van Goethem

J)

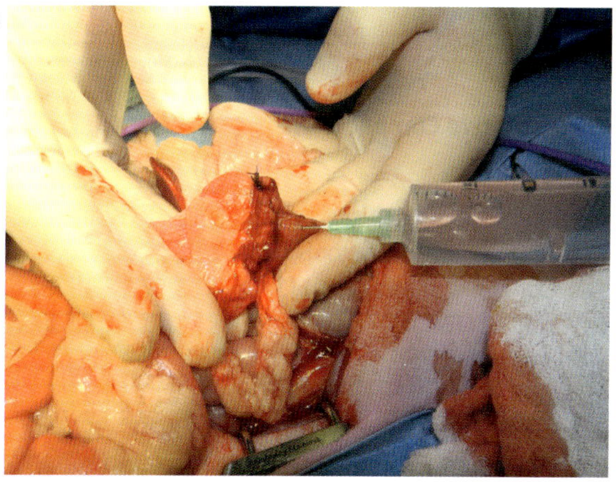

K)

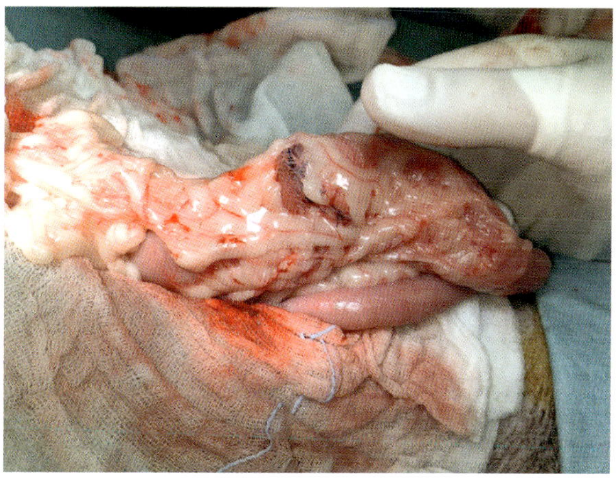

L)

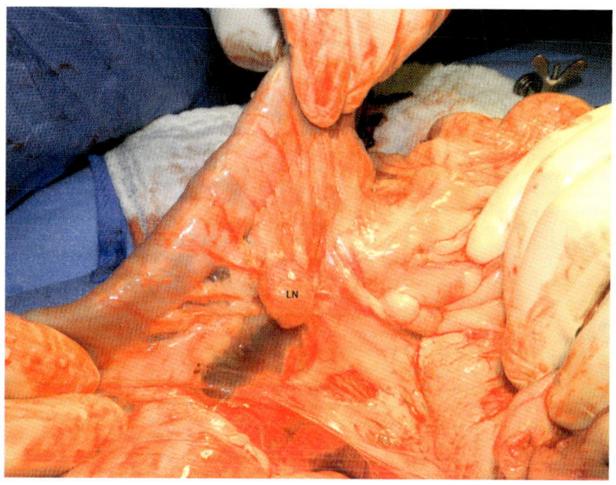

References

1 Stoloff, D., Snider, T.G., Crawford, M.P. et al. (1984). End-to-end colonic anastomosis. A comparison of techniques in normal dogs. *Vet. Surg.* 13 (2): 76–82.

2 Athar, M., Chaudhry, N.I., Shakoor, A. et al. (1996). Studies on end-to-end colonic anastomosis in the dog: a comparison of techniques. *Acta Vet. Hung.* 44 (3): 349–356.

3 Banz, W.J., Jackson, J., Richter, K. et al. (2008). Transrectal stapling for colonic resection and anastomosis (10 cases). *J. Am. Anim. Hosp. Assoc.* 44 (4): 198–204.

4 Kudisch, M. and Pavletic, M.M. (1993). Subtotal colectomy with surgical stapling instruments via a trans-cecal approach for treatment of acquired megacolon in cats. *Vet. Surg.* 22 (6): 457–463.

5 Latimer, C.R., Lux, C.N., Grimes, J.A. et al. (2019). Evaluation of short-term outcomes and potential risk factors for death and intestinal dehiscence following full-thickness large intestinal incisions in dogs. *J. Am. Vet. Med. Assoc.* 255 (8): 915–925.

6 Cohen, M., Post, G.S., and Wright, J.C. (2003). Gastrointestinal leiomyosarcoma in 14 dogs. *J. Vet. Intern. Med.* 17 (1): 107–110.

7 Russell, K.N., Mehler, S.J., Skorupski, K.A. et al. (2007). Clinical and immunohistochemical differentiation of gastrointestinal stromal tumors from leiomyosarcomas in dogs: 42 cases (1990-2003). *J. Am. Vet. Med. Assoc.* 230 (9): 1329–1333.

8 Maas, C.P.H.J., ter Haar, G., van der Gaag, I. et al. (2007). Reclassification of small intestinal and cecal smooth muscle tumors in 72 dogs: clinical, histologic, and immunohistochemical evaluation. *Vet. Surg.* 36 (4): 302–313.

9 Nucci, D.J., Liptak, J.M., Selmic, L.E. et al. (2014). Complications and outcomes following rectal pull-through surgery in dogs with rectal masses: 74 cases (2000-2013). *J. Am. Vet. Med. Assoc.* 245 (6): 684–695.

10 Morello, E., Martano, M., Squassino, C. et al. (2008). Transanal pull-through rectal amputation for treatment of colorectal carcinoma in 11 dogs. *Vet. Surg.* 37 (5): 420–426.

11 Arteaga, T.A., McKnight, J., and Bergman, P.J. (2012). A review of 18 cases of feline colonic adenocarcinoma treated with subtotal colectomies and adjuvant carboplatin. *J. Am. Anim. Hosp. Assoc.* 48 (6): 399–404.

12 Slawienski, M.J., Mauldin, G.E., Mauldin, G.N. et al. (1997). Malignant colonic neoplasia in cats: 46 cases (1990-1996). *J. Am. Vet. Med. Assoc.* 211 (7): 878–881.

13 Gouldin, E.D., Mullin, C., Morges, M. et al. (2017). Feline discrete high-grade gastrointestinal lymphoma treated with surgical resection and adjuvant CHOP-based chemotherapy: retrospective study of 20 cases. *Vet. Comp. Oncol.* 15 (2): 328–335.

14 Barrett, L.E., Skorupski, K., Brown, D.C. et al. (2018). Outcome following treatment of feline gastrointestinal mast cell tumours. *Vet. Comp. Oncol.* 16 (2): 188–193.

Chapter 25: Rectal Resection and Anastomosis

The surgical treatment of rectal tumors is largely dependent on tumor type and tumor location. Proximal rectal tumors can be treated with resection and anastomosis through an abdominal approach, with or without a pubic symphysiotomy (see *15.5. Pubic Symphysiotomy*) or pubic flap (see *15.6. Pubic Flap*) to improve exposure. Midrectal tumors, particularly those involving the dorsal aspect of the rectum, can be approached via an inverted dorsal U-shaped incision. Distal rectal tumors are treated with either a rectal eversion and submucosal resection technique if benign or low-grade malignant, or a rectal pull-through technique if malignant.

Suggested Diagnostic Workup and Clinical Staging

- Digital rectal examination
- ± Incisional biopsy via either rectal eversion or colonoscopy
- ± Transrectal or ultrasound-guided fine-needle aspirates
- Colonoscopy
- Precontrast and postcontrast computed tomography (CT) scan of the pelvis and abdomen
- Three-view thoracic radiographs or thoracic CT scan for assessment of lung metastasis

Suggested Adjuvant Treatments

- Chemotherapy for dogs with rectal lymphoma [1]
- ± Nonsteroidal anti-inflammatory drugs for rectal polyps, rectal carcinomas in situ, and rectal carcinomas
- ± Tyrosine kinase inhibitors for gastrointestinal stromal tumors

Color Atlas of Canine and Feline Surgical Oncology, First Edition. Julius M. Liptak, Paolo Buracco, William T. N. Culp, and Nicholas J. Bacon.

Prognosis and Oncologic Outcome – Dogs

	Local Recurrence Rate	Metastatic Rate	Disease-Free Interval (d)	Median Survival Time (d)	1-Year Survival Rate	2-Year Survival Rate
			Polyp [2]			
Overall	17%	8%[a]	318	–	–	–
			Carcinoma In Situ [2, 3]			
Overall	0%[b]–55%[c]	23%[a]	80	1006	–	–
			Carcinoma [3, 4]			
Overall	18%–19%	0%–23%	356[d]–417[e]	696 to NR	–	–
			Leiomyosarcoma and Gastrointestinal Stromal Tumor[f] [5, 6]			
Overall	10%	54%	–	238–650	75%	66%
			Gastrointestinal Stromal Tumor[f] [6]			
Overall	0%	7%	–	354	–	–
			Lymphoma [1]			
Overall	14%	0%	–	1697[g]	–	–
			Chemotherapy			
Yes	–	–	–	2352[g]	–	–
No	–	–	–	28	–	–

[a] These represent malignant transformation to either carcinoma in situ or carcinoma rather than metastasis.
[b] Local recurrence rate after treatment with rectal pull-through surgery.
[c] Local recurrence rate after treatment with rectal eversion and submucosal resection.
[d] Disease-free interval for metastasis.
[e] Disease-free interval for local tumor recurrence.
[f] Includes all gastrointestinal sites (stomach, small intestines, cecum, and colon).
[g] Mean overall survival time, including seven dogs treated with surgery ± chemotherapy and two dogs treated with chemotherapy alone.
NR, not reached.

References

1 Van den Steen, N., Berlato, D., Polton, G. et al. (2012). Rectal lymphoma in 11 dogs: a retrospective study. *J. Small Anim. Pract.* 53 (10): 586–591.

2 Valerius, K.D., Powers, B.E., McPherron, M.A. et al. (1997). Adenomatous polyps and carcinoma in situ of the canine colon and rectum: 34 cases (1982–1994). *J. Am. Anim. Hosp. Assoc.* 33 (2): 156–160.

3 Nucci, D.J., Liptak, J.M., Selmic, L.E. et al. (2014). Complications and outcomes following rectal pull-through surgery in dogs with rectal masses: 74 cases (2000-2013). *J. Am. Vet. Med. Assoc.* 245 (6): 684–695.

4 Morello, E., Martano, M., Squassino, C. et al. (2008). Transanal pull-through rectal amputation for treatment of colorectal carcinoma in 11 dogs. *Vet. Surg.* 37 (5): 420–426.

5 Cohen, M., Post, G.S., and Wright, J.C. (2003). Gastrointestinal leiomyosarcoma in 14 dogs. *J. Vet. Intern. Med.* 17 (1): 107–110.

6 Russell, K.N., Mehler, S.J., Skorupski, K.A. et al. (2007). Clinical and immunohistochemical differentiation of gastrointestinal stromal tumors from leiomyosarcomas in dogs: 42 cases (1990-2003). *J. Am. Vet. Med. Assoc.* 230 (9): 1329–1333.

25.1 Rectal Eversion and Submucosal Resection

Indication

1) Resection of rectal masses involving only the rectal mucosa (e.g. rectal polyps, rectal carcinomas in situ) and located in the mid-to-caudal rectum

Suggested Diagnostic Workup and Clinical Staging

See *25. Rectal Resection and Anastomosis.*

Patient Positioning

The patient is positioned in sternal recumbency with the tail secured dorsally and cranially. The perineal area can be elevated by either flexing the pelvic limbs underneath the pelvis and caudal abdomen or placing padding between the pelvic limbs with the pelvic limbs hanging over the padded end of the surgical table. The anal sacs should be expressed before surgery.

Surgical Technique (See Plate 25.1A–C)

A) Two to six stay sutures are inserted into the rectal wall 1–2 cm cranial to the anorectal line and the anorectal tumor. Caudal traction is then applied to the stay sutures to evert the rectal mucosa and expose the rectal mass (i, leiomyosarcoma; ii, rectal cyst; iii, plasmacytoma). Further stay sutures can be inserted cranial to the original stay sutures if further eversion is required (iv, carcinoma in situ).
B) **Submucosal resection technique [1]:** The rectal mucosa and submucosa are incised around the rectal mucosal mass with 5- to 10-mm surgical margins with either a scalpel blade (i) or Metzenbaum scissors (ii). The submucosa is undermined to isolate the mass and ensure a partial-thickness resection (iii), and then the resection is completed with

Color Atlas of Canine and Feline Surgical Oncology, First Edition. Julius M. Liptak, Paolo Buracco, William T. N. Culp, and Nicholas J. Bacon.

Plate 25.1

Rectal Eversion and Submucosal Resection

A-i)

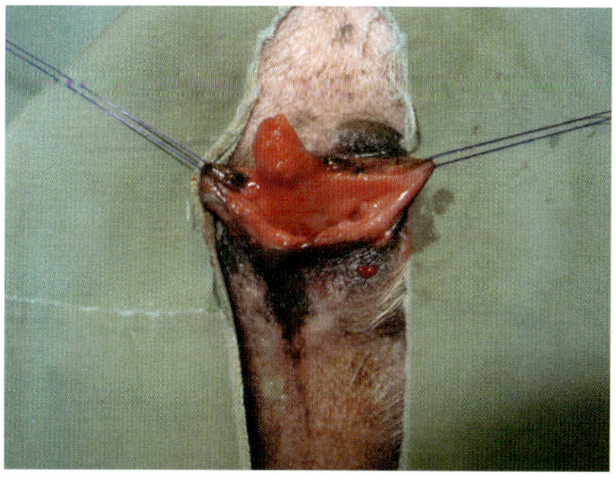

A-ii)

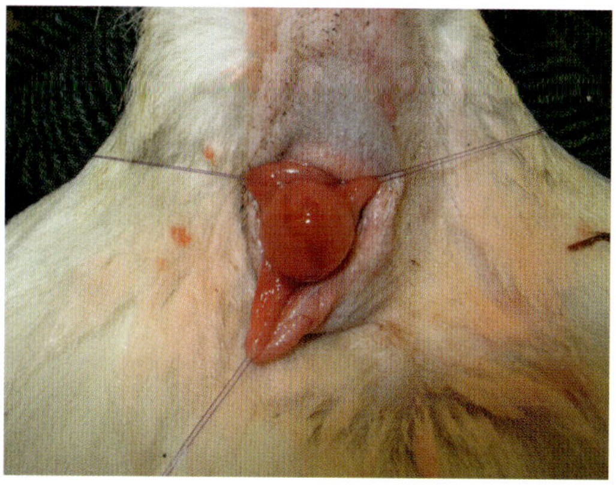

A-iii)

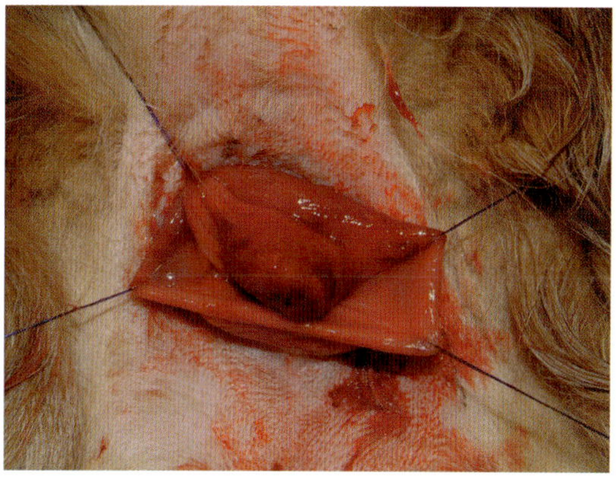

A-iv)

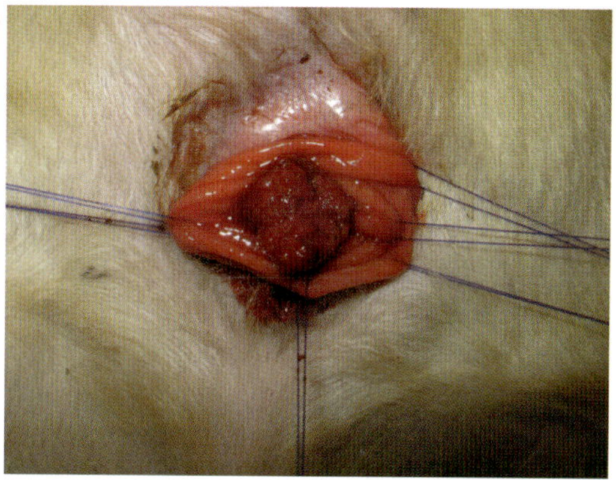

B-i)

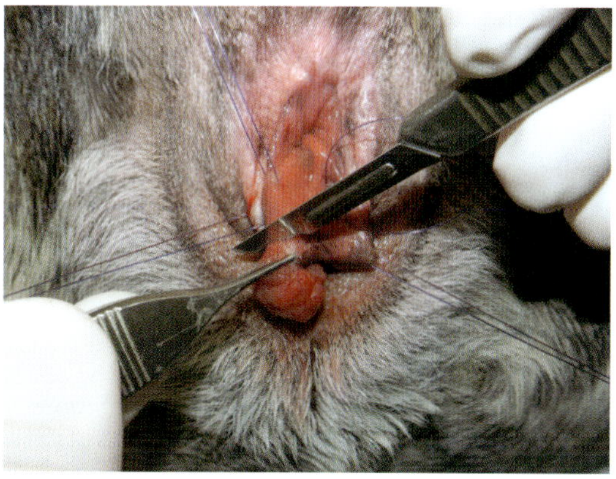

B-ii)

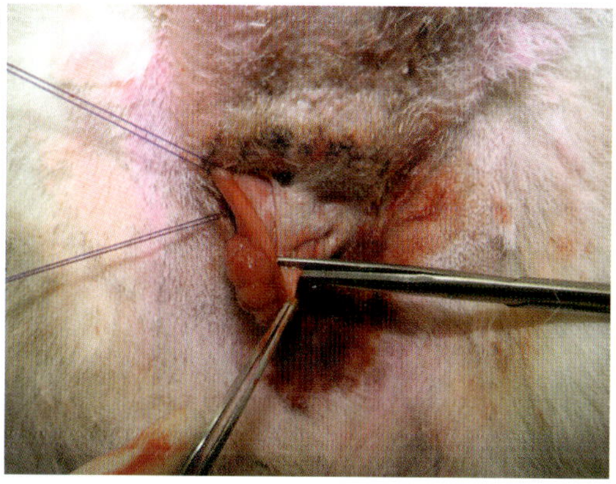

B-iii)

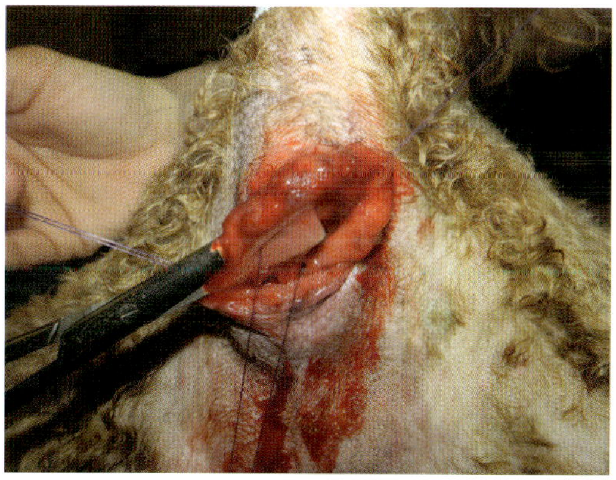

B-iii)

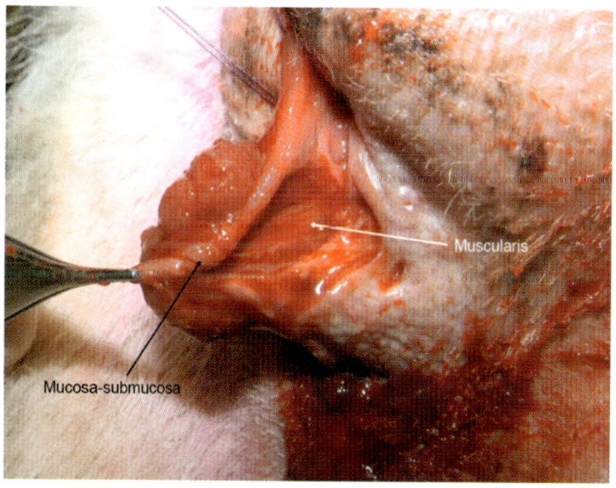

Surgical Technique (See Plate 25.1A–C) *continued*

Metzenbaum scissors (iv). Once the mass is resected, the rectal mucosa and submucosa are closed with 3-0 or 4-0 absorbable monofilament suture material in a simple continuous (v, vi) or simple interrupted suture pattern (vii).

C) **Thoracoabdominal (TA) stapler technique [2]:** An appropriately sized TA stapler (usually a 30-mm TA stapler) is placed across the base of the rectal mass (i). Additional stay sutures can be placed at the base of the mass to facilitate positioning of the TA stapler. The TA stapler is then locked and fired. The rectal mucosa-submucosa is incised with a scalpel blade between the TA stapler and rectal mass (ii), and the rectal mass is removed from the surgical field (iii). The staple line should be inspected and reinforced with a continuous suture pattern, using 3-0 to 4-0 monofilament absorbable material, if necessary; however, this is rarely required.

Postoperative Management

1) Multimodal analgesia, but consider avoiding the use of steroids and nonsteroidal anti-inflammatory drugs because of negative effects on intestinal healing
2) ± Elizabethan collar
3) Feed normal diet

Complications

Postoperative Complications [1]

- Transient rectal bleeding (22%)
- Tenesmus (17%)
- Local tumor recurrence (0%–8%) [1, 2]
- Mucosal dehiscence (4%)

Suggested Adjuvant Treatments

- See *25. Rectal Resection and Anastomosis.*

Prognosis and Oncologic Outcome

- See *25. Rectal Resection and Anastomosis.*

References

1 Danova, N.A., Robles-Emanuelli, J.C., and Bjorling, D.E. (2006). Surgical excision of primary canine rectal tumors by an anal approach in twenty-three dogs. *Vet. Surg.* 35 (4): 337–340.

2 Swiderski, J. and Withrow, S.J. (2009). A novel surgical stapling technique for rectal mass removal: a retrospective analysis. *J. Am. Anim. Hosp. Assoc.* 45 (2): 67–71.

Plate 25.1

Rectal Eversion and Submucosal Resection *continued*

B-iv)

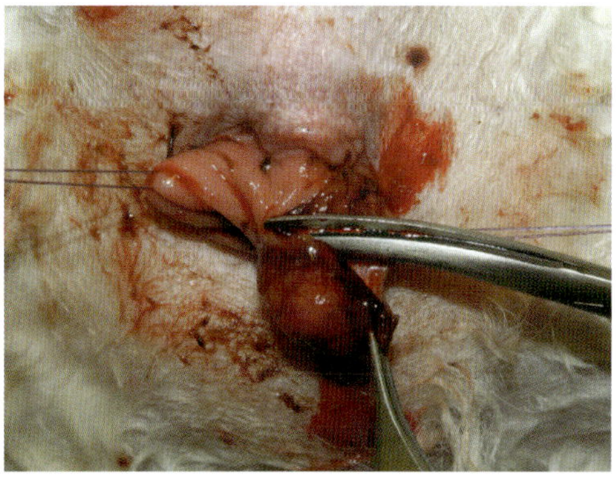

B-v)

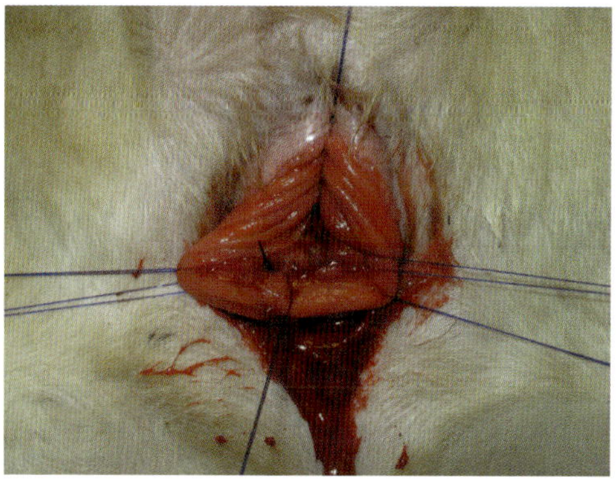

B-vi)

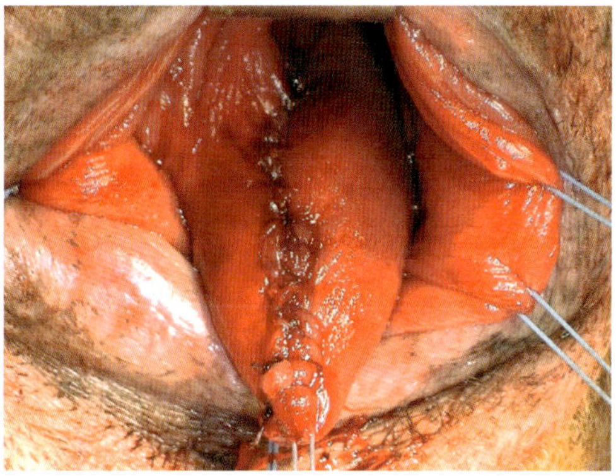

B-vii)

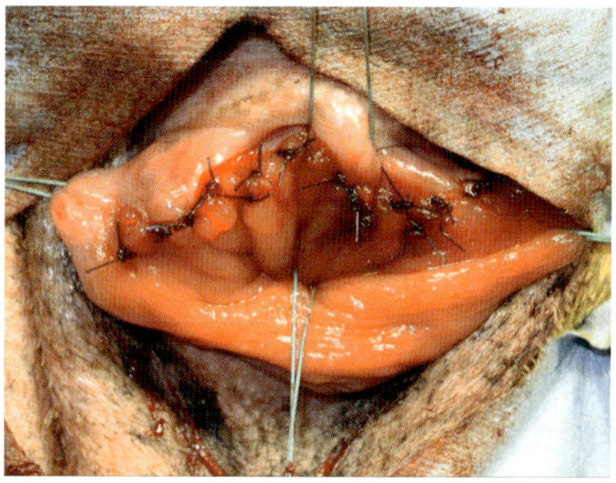

C-i)

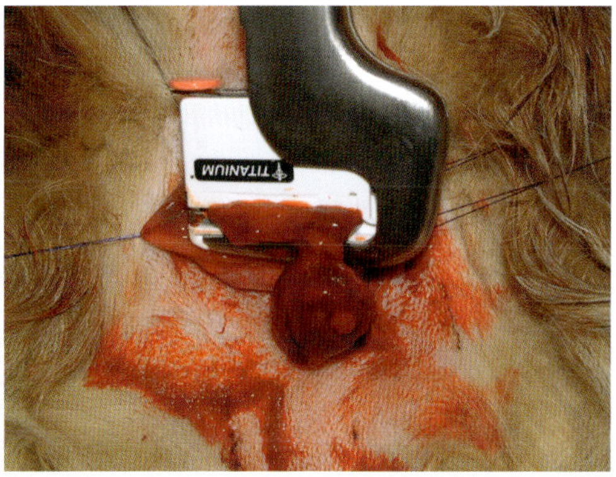

C-ii)

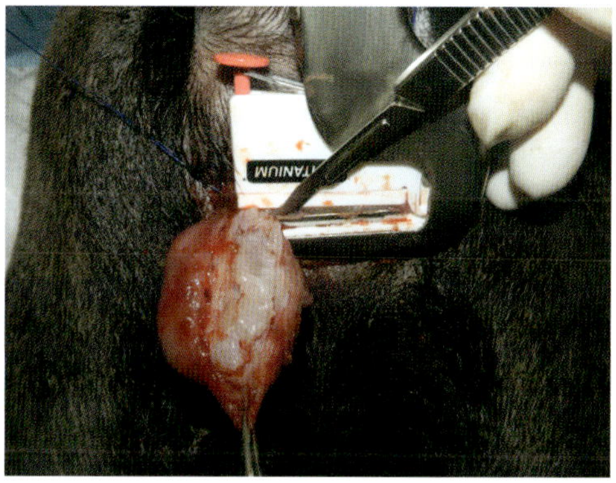

C-iii)

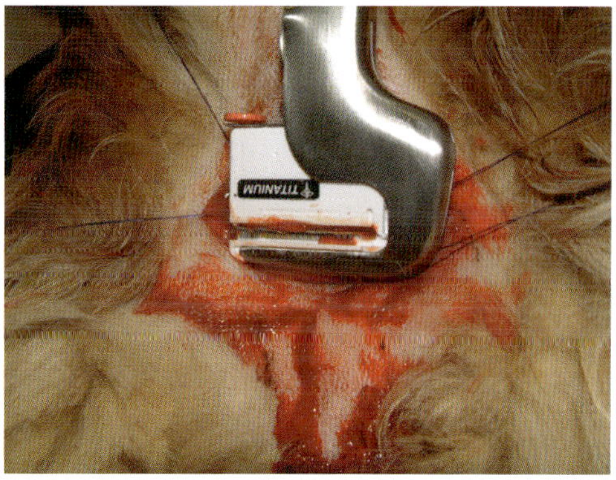

25.2 Rectal Pull-Through

Indications (See Plate 25.2 – 1, 2)

1) Resection of rectal masses in the mid-to-caudal rectum with more extensive circumferential involvement of the rectum or invasion deeper than the submucosal layer of the rectal wall (pictured, rectal adenocarcinoma in a dog)
2) Resection of perianal tumors invading into the anocutaneous junction or distal rectum (pictured, squamous cell carcinoma in a cat)

Suggested Diagnostic Workup and Clinical Staging

See *25. Rectal Resection and Anastomosis.*

Patient Positioning

The patient is positioned in sternal recumbency with the tail secured dorsally and cranially. The perineal area can be elevated by either flexing the pelvic limbs underneath the pelvis and caudal abdomen or placing padding between the pelvic limbs with the pelvic limbs hanging over the padded end of the surgical table. The anal sacs should be expressed before surgery.

Surgical Technique (See Plate 25.2A–H)

A) Stay sutures are inserted into the rectal wall cranial to the planned caudal resection site to facilitate retraction and manipulation of the rectum.
B) A circumferential incision is made with appropriate surgical margins caudal to the rectal mass or around the perianal mass. The incision may be in the rectal tissue cranial to the anocutaneous junction, along the anocutaneous junction (i), or in the perianal tissue (ii). Note that postoperative fecal incontinence is significantly more likely when the distal 2 cm of the rectum is resected (unpublished data, Dr. Dan Nucci) or the anocutaneous junction is circumferentially resected [1].
C) The anal sacs can be preserved if the caudal circumferential incision is cranial to the opening of the anal sac ducts, or resected en bloc with the rectal pull-through if the caudal circumferential incision includes the opening of the anal sac ducts (i, anal sac malignant melanoma; ii, rectal carcinoma).

Color Atlas of Canine and Feline Surgical Oncology, First Edition. Julius M. Liptak, Paolo Buracco, William T. N. Culp, and Nicholas J. Bacon.

Plate 25.2

Rectal Pull-Through

1)

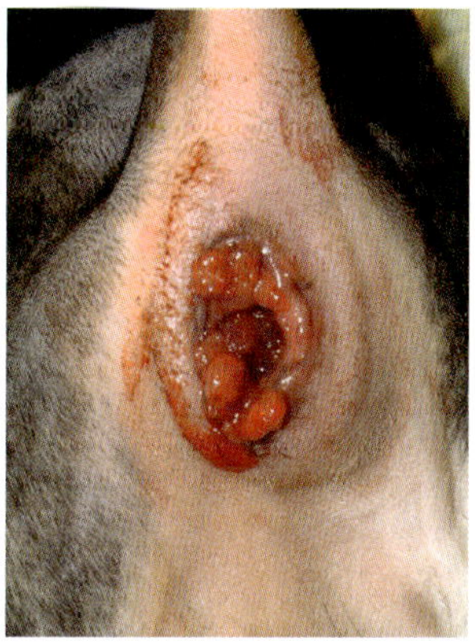

2)

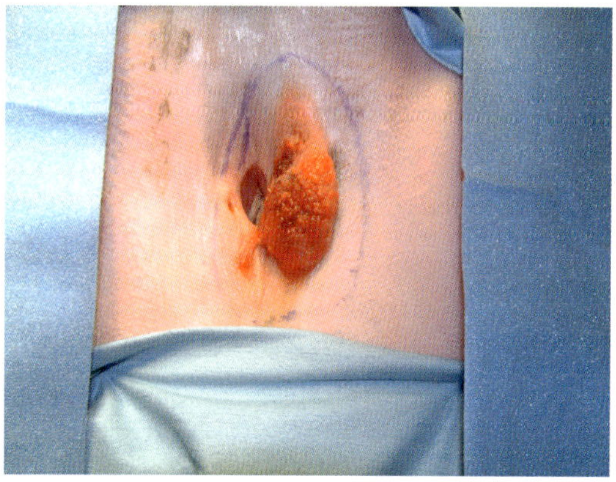

A)

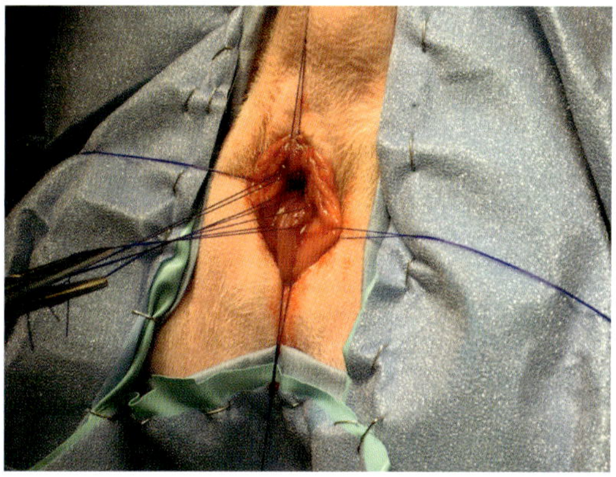

B-i)

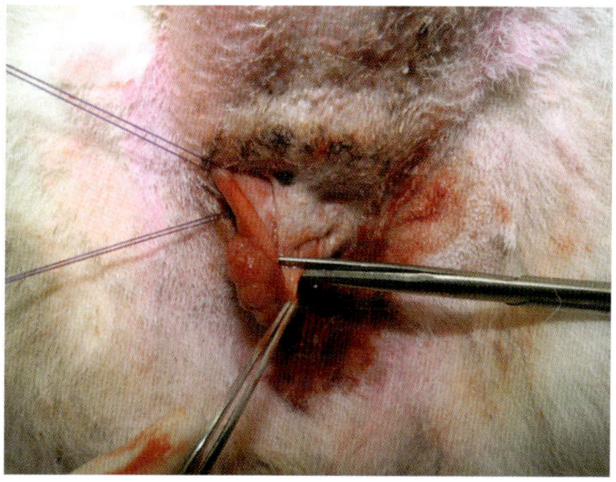

B-ii)

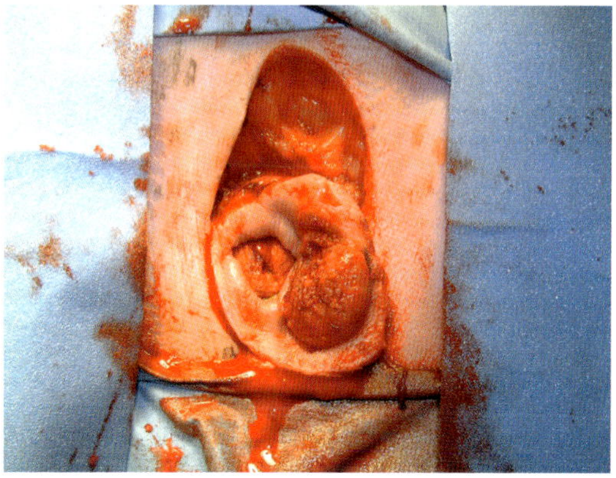

C-i)

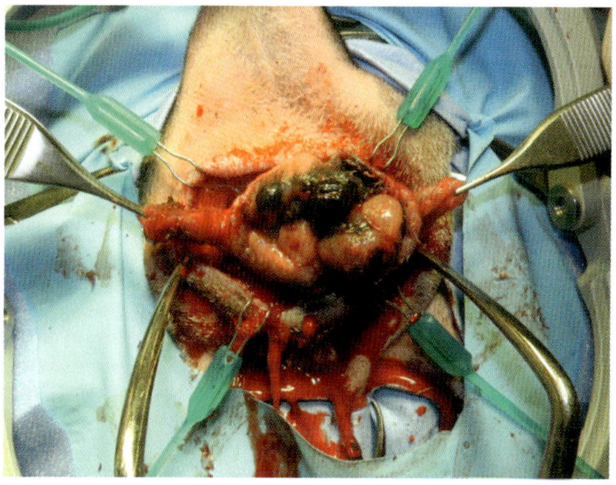

C-ii)

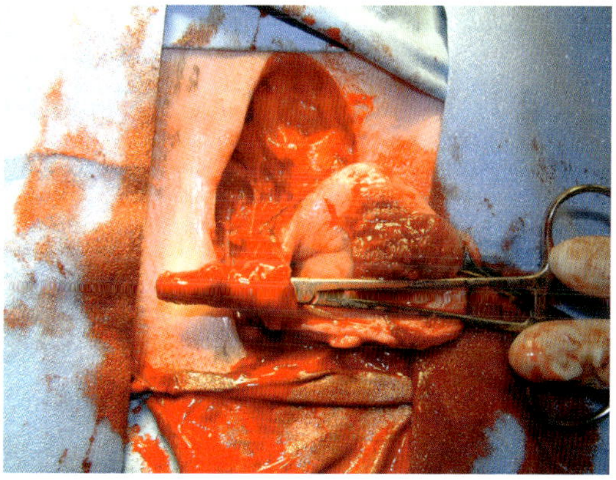

Surgical Technique (See Plate 25.2A–H) *continued*

D) After completion of the caudal circumferential incision, caudal traction is applied to Allis tissue forceps (i, iv) or the stay sutures (ii, iii), and dissection of the rectal wall is continued cranially with either blunt or digital dissection (ii–iv). The external anal sphincter and other intrapelvic structures should be preserved if possible.

E) Transection of the dorsal rectococcygeus muscle (RCM) is often required to adequately exteriorize the rectal segment.

F) A cranial rectal resection is made with appropriate surgical margins cranial to the rectal mass (i). If the cranial extent of the tumor cannot be palpated extraluminally, then the cranial extent of the tumor can be determined by dividing the rectum longitudinally provided that the tumor does not have circumferential involvement of the rectum and this incision is not done through neoplastic tissue (ii).

G) **Cranial rectal resection technique 1:** Stay sutures are inserted into the rectal wall cranial to the planned cranial resection site (i) to prevent the rectal stump from retracting into the abdominal cavity after the cranial rectal resection (ii).

Plate 25.2

Rectal Pull-Through *continued*

D-i)

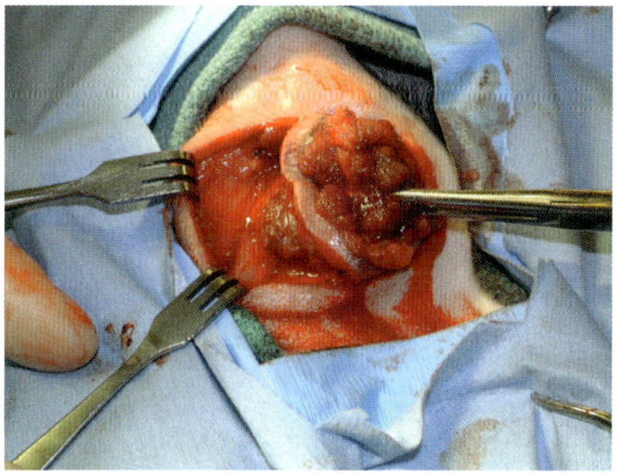

D-ii)

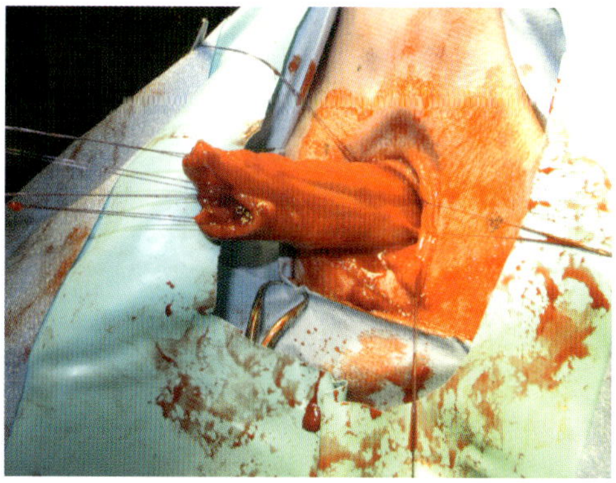

D-iii)

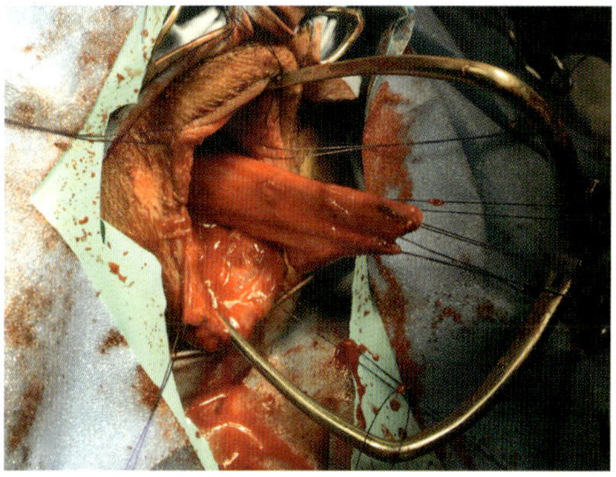

D-iv)

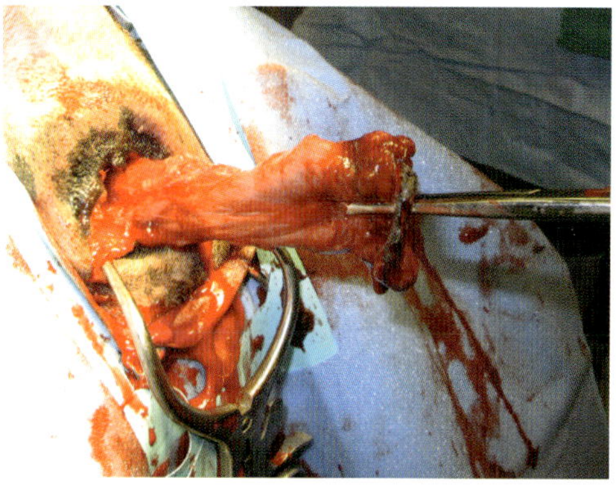

E)

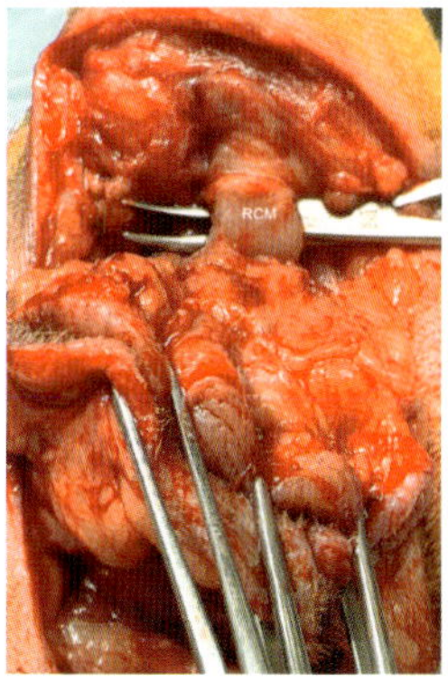

F-i)

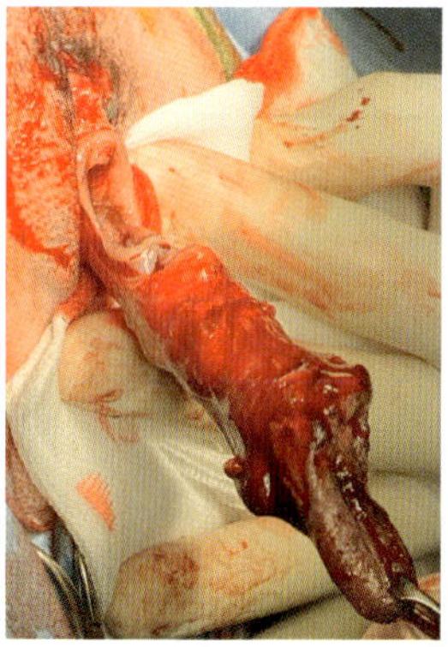

F-ii)

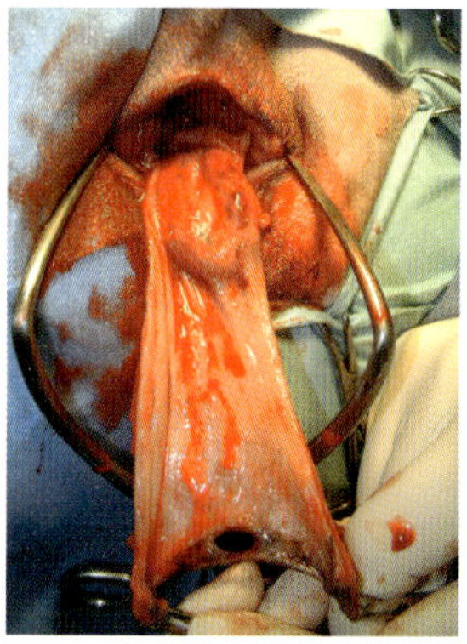

G-i)

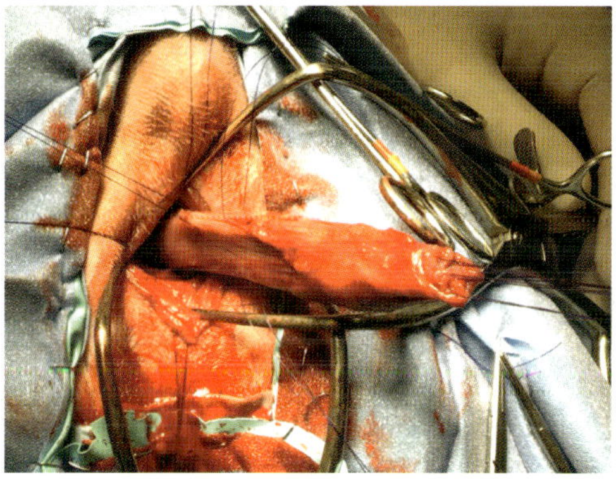

G-ii)

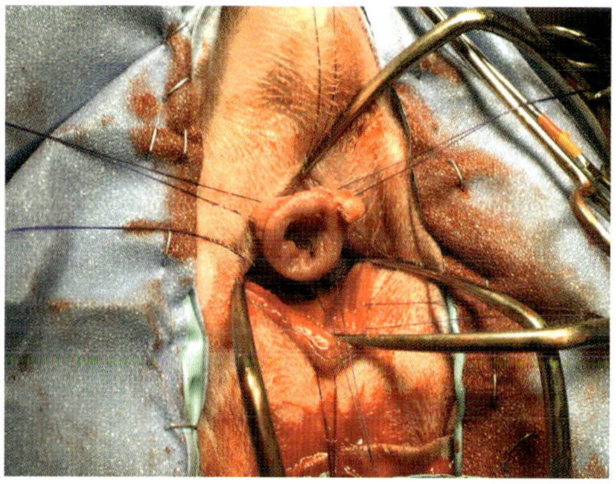

Surgical Technique (See Plate 25.2A–H) *continued*

H) **Cranial rectal resection technique 2:** Alternatively, the dorsal portion of the circumferential incision can be performed, and this is then sutured to either the caudal rectum or perianal tissue (i, see later Closure section) to prevent retraction of the rectal stump into the abdominal cavity. The ventral portion of the circumferential incision is then completed (ii), and this is then sutured to either the caudal rectum or perianal tissue (iii, see Closure section).

Closure (See Plate 25.2I–K)

The cranial rectum is sutured to either the caudal rectum or perianal tissue in one or two layers. The adventitia-muscularis layer of the cranial rectum is sutured to either the adventitia-muscularis layer of the caudal rectum or subcutaneous perianal tissue with 2-0 to 4-0 absorbable monofilament suture material in a simple interrupted or simple continuous suture pattern. The cranial rectal mucosa-submucosa is sutured to the caudal rectal mucosa-submucosa with 3-0 to 4-0 absorbable monofilament suture material in a simple interrupted (I) or simple continuous suture pattern, or to the perianal skin with 3-0 to 4-0 nonabsorbable monofilament suture material in either a simple interrupted (J) or simple continuous suture pattern (K). Simple continuous suture pattern closures should be done with two overlapping 180-degree continuous suture patterns to minimize the risk of iatrogenic stricture of the rectal anastomosis.

Postoperative Management

1) Multimodal analgesia, but consider avoiding the use of steroids and nonsteroidal anti-inflammatory drugs because of their negative effects on intestinal healing
2) Elizabethan collar
3) Feed normal diet if dog has fecal continence

Complications – Dogs [1]

- 78% overall
- Fecal incontinence (57%)
  - Transient fecal incontinence (45% of incontinent dogs)
  - Permanent fecal incontinence (55% of incontinent dogs)
- Diarrhea (43%)
- Tenesmus (31%)
- Rectal stricture (22%)
- Rectal bleeding (transient or intermittent) (11%)
- Constipation (associated with stricture and tenesmus) (9%)
- Dehiscence (8%)
- Infection (5%)

Suggested Adjuvant Treatments

- See *25. Rectal Resection and Anastomosis*.

Prognosis and Oncologic Outcome

- See *25. Rectal Resection and Anastomosis*.

Reference

1 Nucci, D.J., Liptak, J.M., Selmic, L.E. et al. (2014). Complications and outcomes following rectal pull-through surgery in dogs with rectal masses: 74 cases (2000-2013). *J. Am. Vet. Med. Assoc.* 245 (6): 684–695.

Plate 25.2

Rectal Pull-Through *continued*

H-i)

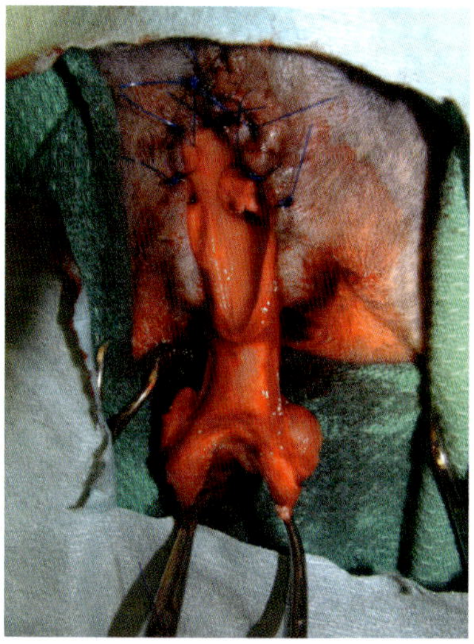

H-ii)

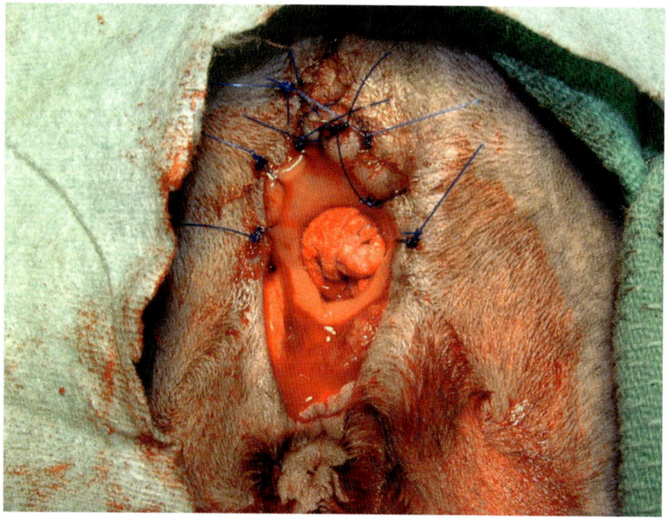

H-iii)

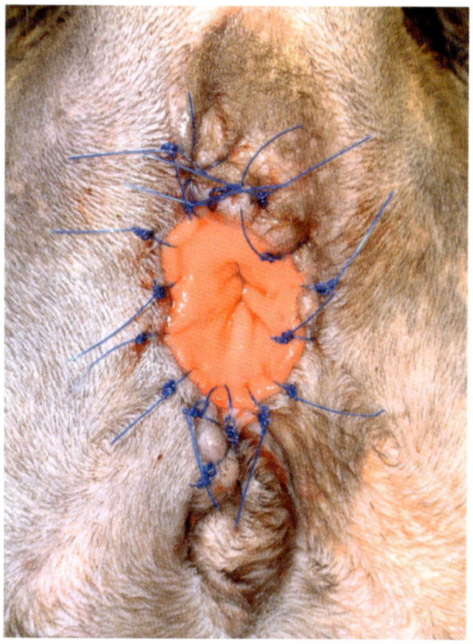

I)

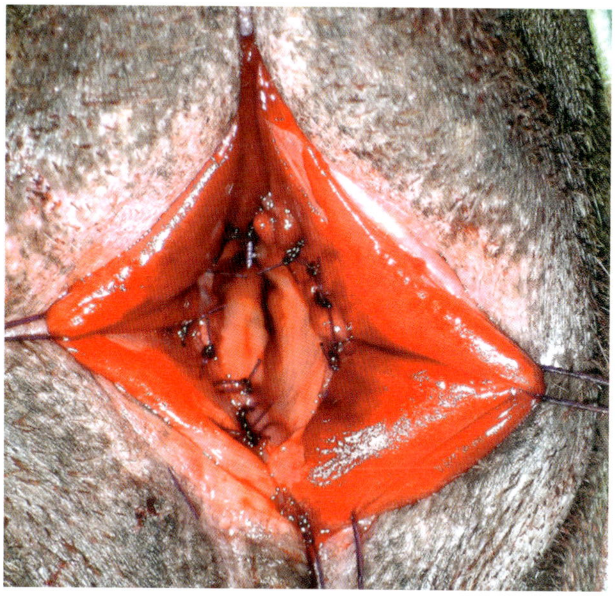

J)

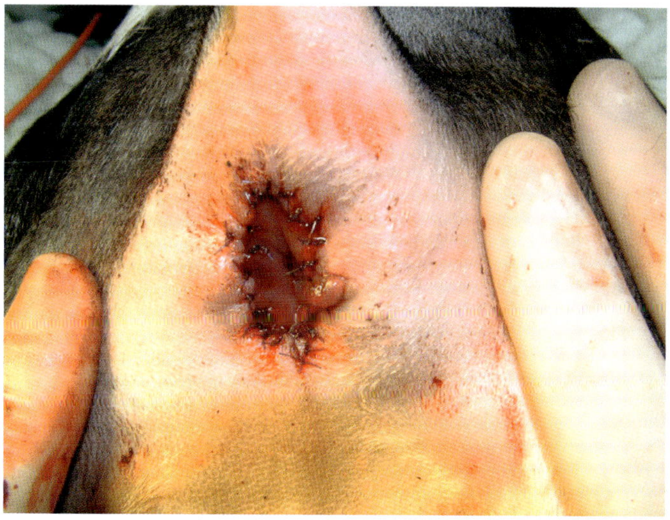

K)

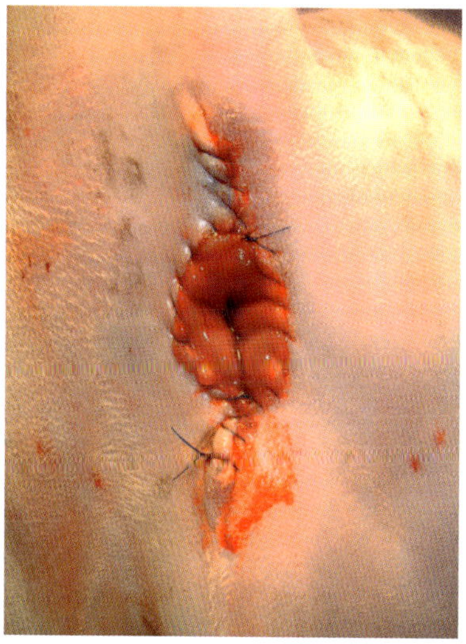

25.3 Dorsal Inverted U Approach

Indications

1) Marginal resection of benign or low-grade malignant rectal masses involving the dorsal rectal wall
2) Resection of midrectal tumors and end-to-end rectal anastomosis (see *24. Colorectal Resection and Anastomosis*)

Suggested Diagnostic Workup and Clinical Staging

See *25. Rectal Resection and Anastomosis.*

Patient Positioning

The patient is positioned in sternal recumbency with the tail secured dorsally and cranially. The perineal area can be elevated by either flexing the pelvic limbs underneath the pelvis and caudal abdomen or placing padding between the pelvic limbs with the pelvic limbs hanging over the padded end of the surgical table. The anal sacs should be expressed before surgery. The rectum should be packed with moist gauze swabs or moistened laparotomy sponges. An anal purse-string suture should also be placed (see step A).

Surgical Technique [1] (See Plate 25.3A–E, G–I)

A) An inverted U-shaped skin incision made over and parallel to the dorsal aspect of the anus, starting and finishing medial to the left and right tuber ischii.
B) The subcutaneous tissues are dissected caudally and laterally to expose the caudal aspect of the rectal mass. Stay sutures can be used to apply caudal traction to the rectum to facilitate this dissection and exposure.
C) The dorsal rectococcygeus muscle (i) is transected (ii, iii) to facilitate exposure of the rectal mass (iv, arrow, rectal leiomyoma).

Color Atlas of Canine and Feline Surgical Oncology, First Edition. Julius M. Liptak, Paolo Buracco, William T. N. Culp, and Nicholas J. Bacon.

Plate 25.3

Dorsal Inverted U Approach

A)

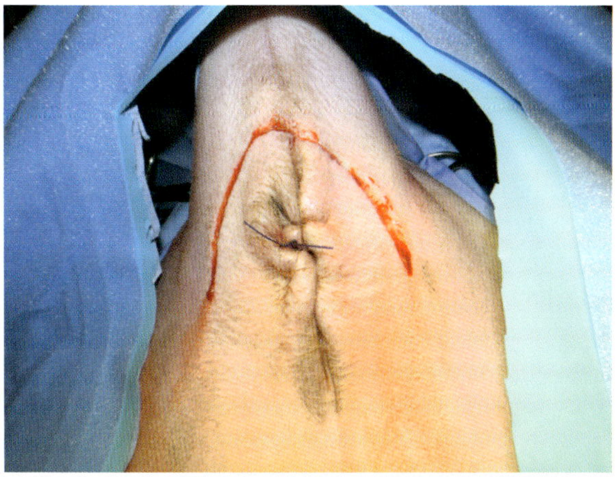

B)

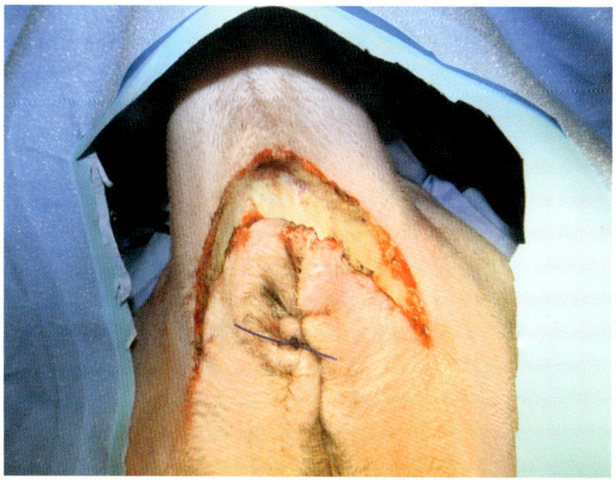

C-i)

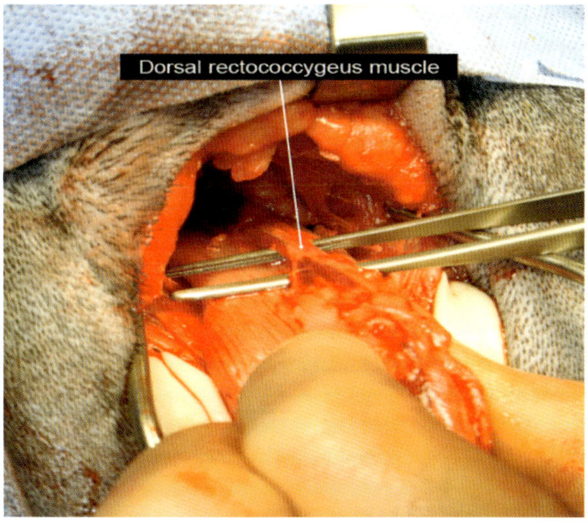

Courtesy of Dr. Laurent Findji

C-ii)

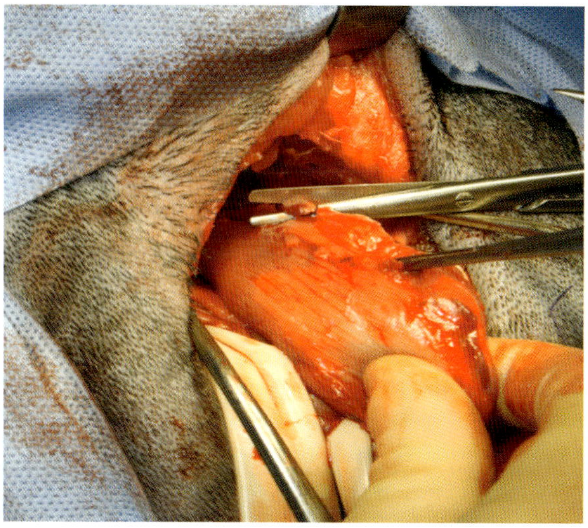

Courtesy of Dr. Laurent Findji

C-iii)

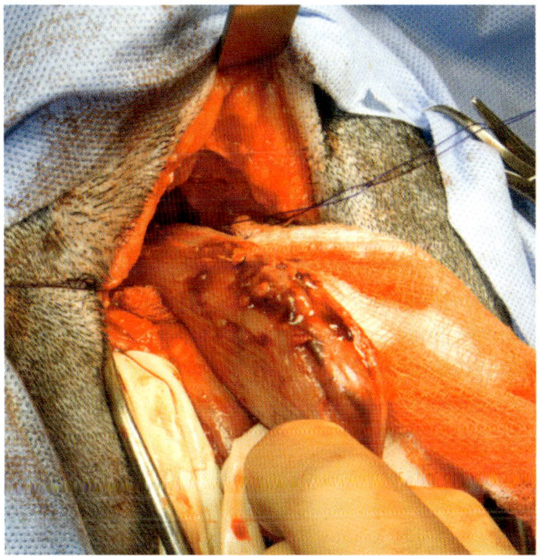

Courtesy of Dr. Laurent Findji

C-iv)

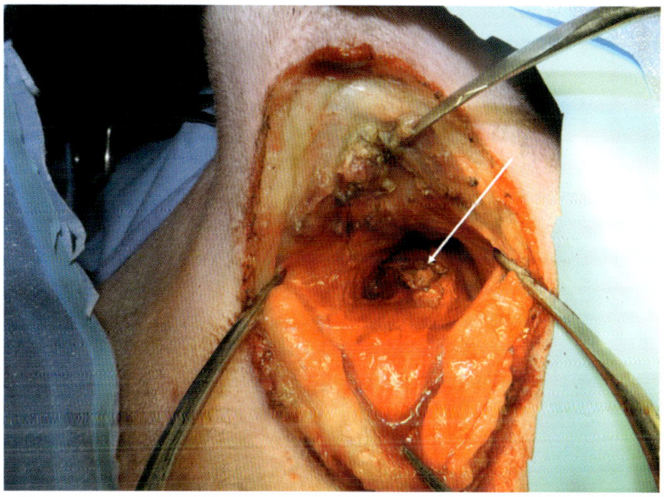

Surgical Technique [1] (See Plate 25.3A–E, G–I) *continued*

D) **Marginal rectal tumor resection technique:** The rectal adventitia is incised over the mass (i, arrow), taking care not to compromise the tumor capsule, and a marginal resection of the mass is performed with digital and blunt dissection (ii). Sharp dissection or a vessel sealing device (pictured) may occasionally be required to complete the resection (iii).

E) The partial-thickness rectal wall defect (i) is closed with a single layer of 3-0 or 4-0 absorbable monofilament suture material in a simple continuous or interrupted suture pattern (ii).

F) **End-to-end anastomosis (EEA) technique [2]:** The rectum is isolated by blunt dissection circumferentially between the rectum and the external sphincter and levator ani muscles. The left and right pudendal and caudal rectal nerves should be identified and protected. If necessary, the levator ani muscles can be transected to increase surgical exposure. The dissection is continued caudally and circumferentially to the level of the caudal peritoneal reflection (not pictured).

G) Stay sutures can be inserted into both the rectal segment to be resected and the cranial rectum to be preserved. These stay sutures facilitate traction and manipulation of the rectal segment and prevent retraction of the cranial rectum into the abdominal cavity after completion of the cranial rectal transection.

H) The rectum is transected caudally first (i–iii) with appropriate surgical margins using either a scalpel or Metzenbaum scissors. This allows the rectum to be tractioned caudally to expose the cranial resection site (iv).

Plate 25.3

Dorsal Inverted U Approach *continued*

D-i)

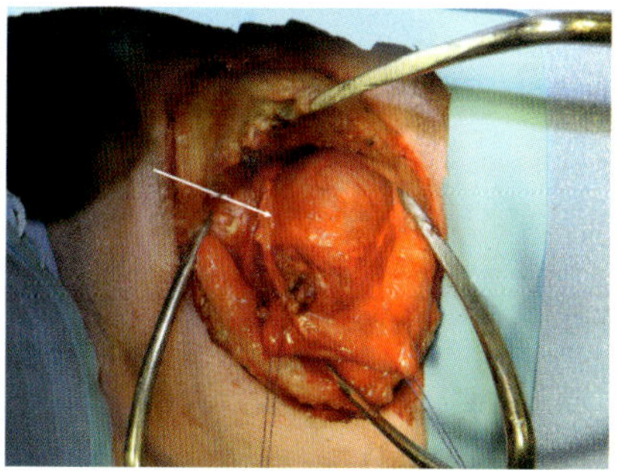

D-ii)

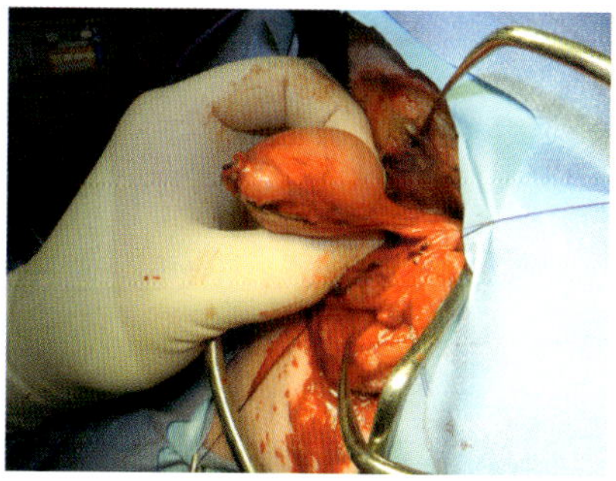

D-iii)

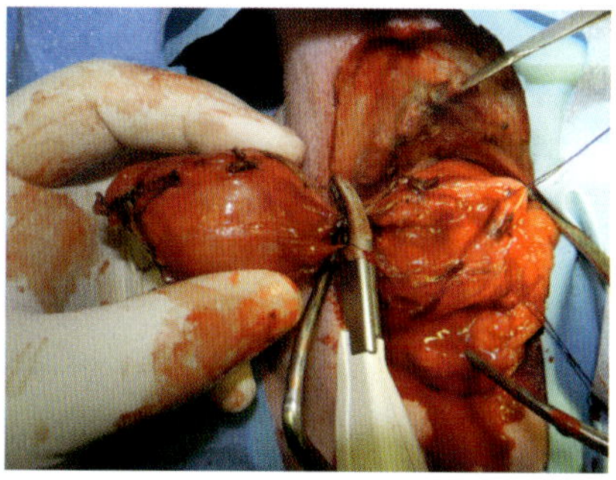

E-i)

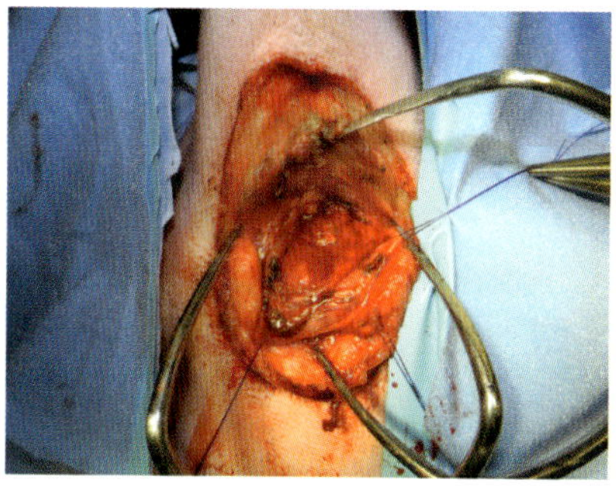

E-ii)

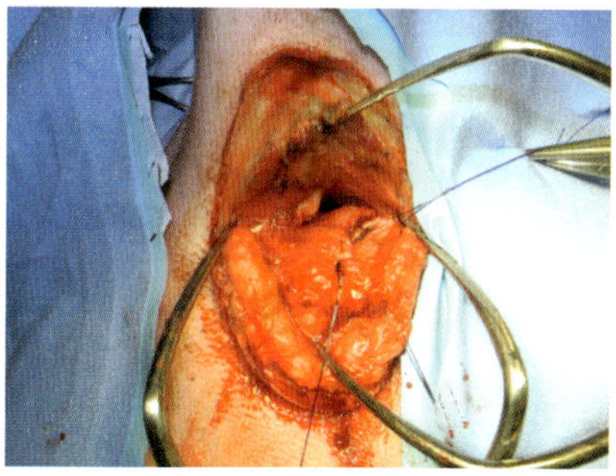

G/H-i)

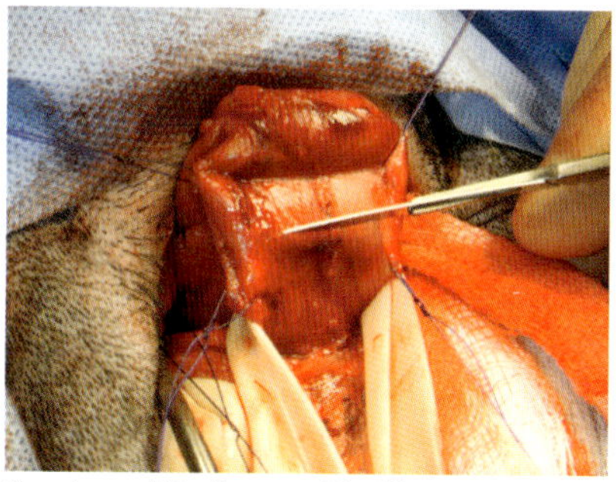

Courtesy of Dr. Laurent Findji

H-ii)

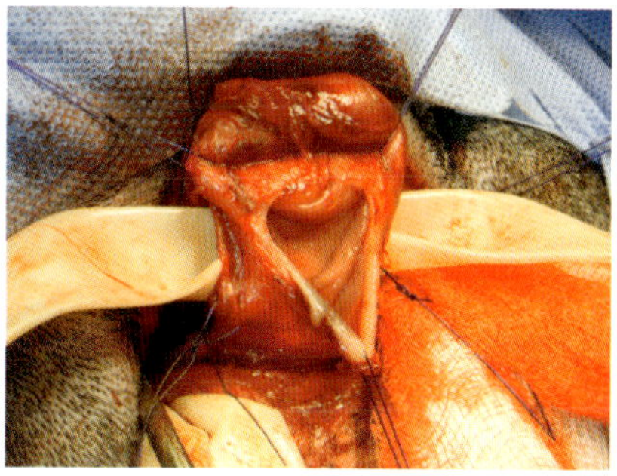

Courtesy of Dr. Laurent Findji

H-iii)

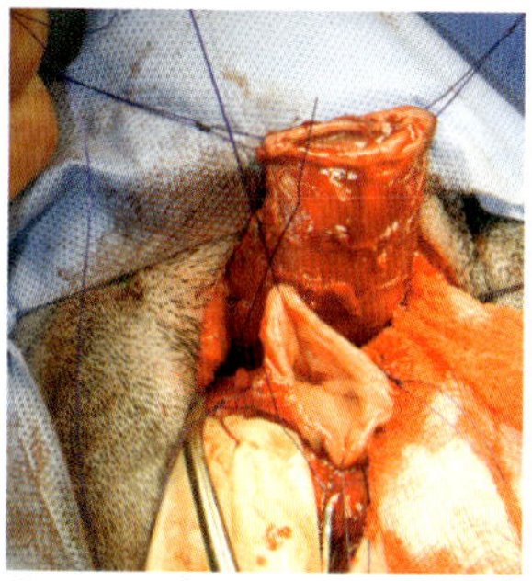

Courtesy of Dr. Laurent Findji

H-iv)

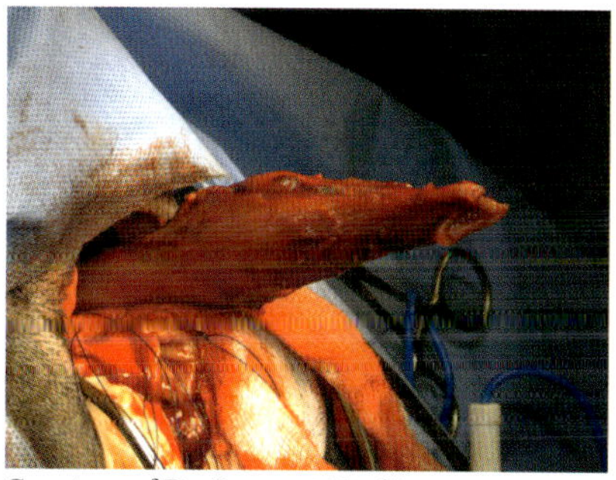

Courtesy of Dr. Laurent Findji

Surgical Technique (See Plate 25.3A–E, G–I) *continued*

I) The transected intestinal ends (i) can be anastomosed using a suture technique or an EEA stapler (see step I in *24. Colorectal Resection and Anastomosis*). For sutured anastomoses, simple interrupted, modified Gambee, or simple continuous suture pattern (pictured) can be used with 3-0 or 4-0 absorbable monofilament suture material. An EEA with a simple continuous suture pattern should be done with two overlapping 180-degree continuous suture patterns (ii–v) to minimize the risk of iatrogenic stricture of the rectal anastomosis.

Closure (See Plate 25.3J, K)

The levator ani and rectococcygeus muscles are apposed, if necessary, using 0 to 3-0 absorbable monofilament suture material in a horizontal mattress suture pattern. The wound is then closed routinely in two to three layers. The deeper subcutaneous tissue can be closed with absorbable monofilament suture material in an interrupted or continuous suture pattern. A simple continuous suture pattern using monofilament absorbable suture material is used to close the subcutis (J). An interrupted or continuous suture pattern using monofilament nonabsorbable suture material is used to close the skin (K).

Postoperative Management

- Multimodal analgesia, but consider avoiding the use of steroids and nonsteroidal anti-inflammatory drugs because of their negative effects on intestinal healing
- Elizabethan collar
- Feed normal diet

Complications

Marginal Rectal Tumor Resection [1]

- None reported

Resection and End-to-End Anastomosis [2]

- Fecal incontinence in dogs with resection of ≥6 cm of rectum and resection of the peritoneal reflection (100%)
- Tenesmus (transient) (92%)
- Anastomotic dehiscence (31%)
- Rectal bleeding (transient or intermittent) (23%)
- Surgical-site infection (15%)
- Rectal prolapse (7%)

Suggested Adjuvant Treatments

- See *25. Rectal Resection and Anastomosis.*

Prognosis and Oncologic Outcome

- See *25. Rectal Resection and Anastomosis.*

References

1 McKeown, D.B., Cockshutt, J.R., Partlow, G.D. et al. (1984). Dorsal approach to the caudal pelvic canal and rectum. Effect on normal dogs. *Vet. Surg.* 13 (3): 181–184.

2 Anderson, G.I., McKeown, D.B., Partlow, G.D. et al. (1987). Rectal resection in the dog. A new surgical approach and the evaluation of its effect on fecal continence. *Vet. Surg.* 16 (2): 119–125.

Plate 25.3

Dorsal Inverted U Approach *continued*

I-i)

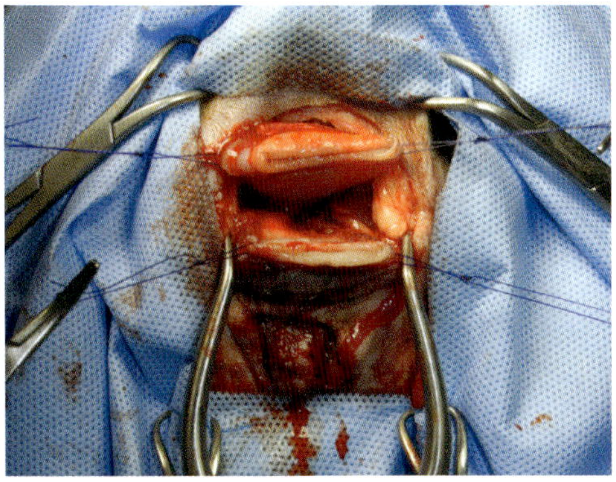

Courtesy of Dr. Laurent Findji

I-ii)

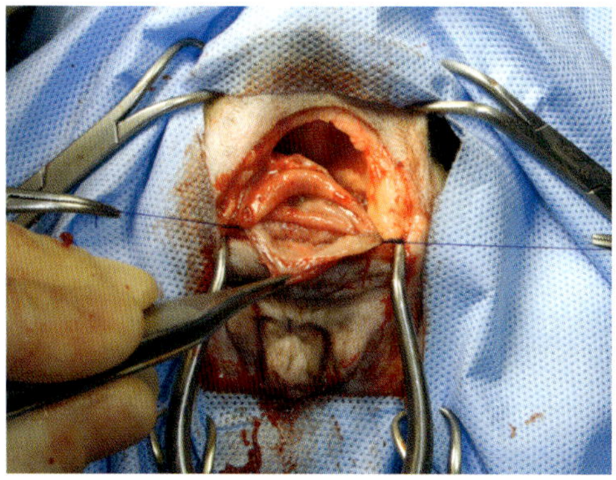

Courtesy of Dr. Laurent Findji

I-iii)

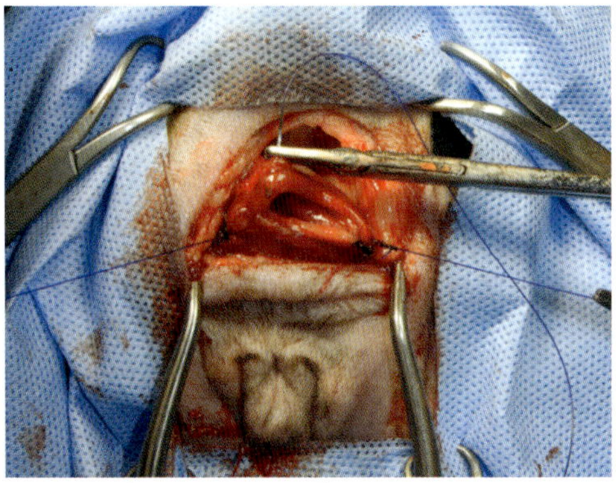

Courtesy of Dr. Laurent Findji

I-iv)

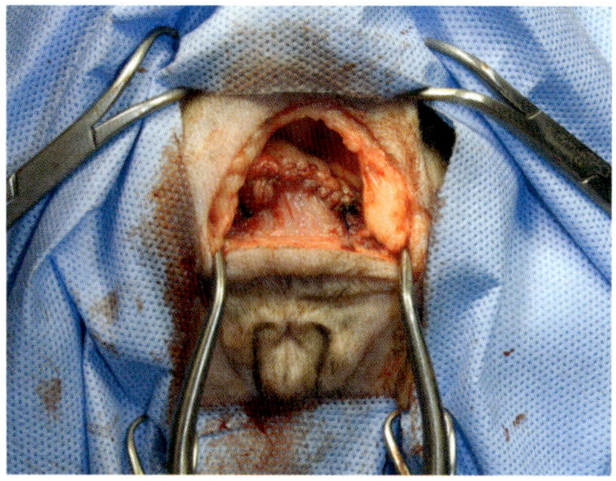

Courtesy of Dr. Laurent Findji

I-v)

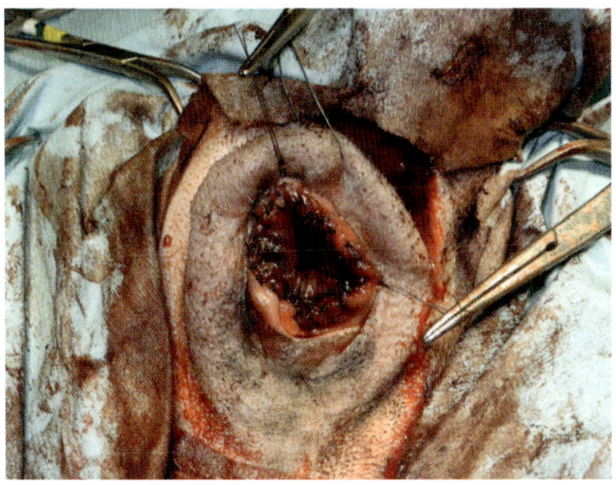

J)

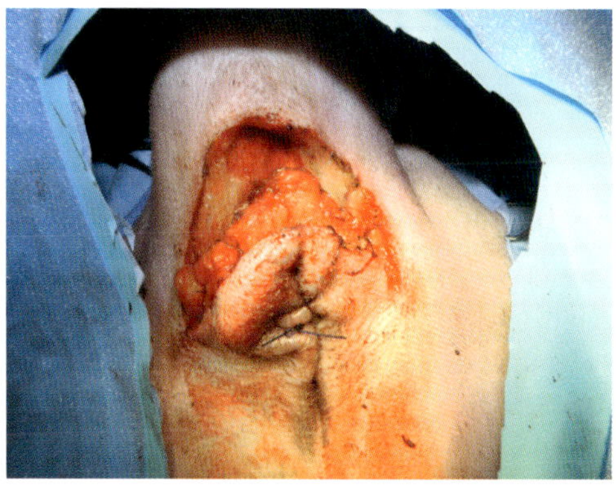

K)

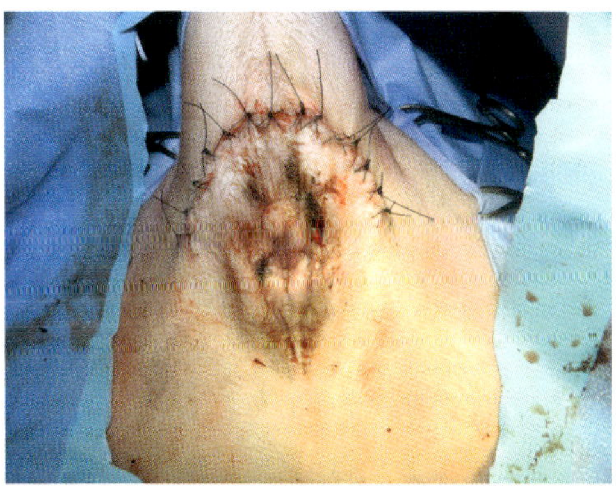

Chapter 26: Anal Sacculectomy

Indications (See Plate 26 – 1)

1) Resection of benign and malignant tumors directly or indirectly involving the anal sac. A closed anal sacculectomy is recommended for resection of anal sac tumors.
2) Anal sacculectomy can be combined with partial rectal pull-through (see *25.2. Rectal Pull-Through*) for tumors invading into the rectal wall or after intraoperative iatrogenic rectal perforation.
3) Anal sacculectomy can be combined with sublumbar lymph node resection (see *20.1. Open Sublumbar Lymph Node Resection* and *20.2. Laparoscopic Sublumbar Lymph Node Resection*) when enlarged or metastatic sublumbar lymph nodes are present.

Suggested Diagnostic Workup and Clinical Staging

- Complete blood count, serum biochemistry, and urinalysis
- Rectal examination
- Ionized calcium blood test
- ± Fine-needle aspirate cytology of the anal sac mass ± enlarged sublumbar lymph nodes
- Abdominal ultrasound or precontrast and postcontrast computed tomography (CT) scan of the abdomen and pelvis for assessment of sublumbar lymph nodes and other intra-abdominal metastasis; abdominal CT scan is preferred because of better imaging of the sacral lymph nodes within the pelvic canal [1, 2]
- Three-view thoracic radiographs or thoracic CT scan for assessment of lung metastasis

Patient Positioning

The patient is positioned in sternal recumbency with the tail secured dorsally and cranially. The perineal area can be elevated by either flexing the pelvic limbs underneath the pelvis and caudal abdomen or placing padding between the pelvic limbs with the pelvic limbs hanging over the padded end of the surgical table (see Plate 26.1). The anal sacs should be expressed before surgery. The rectum should be packed with moist gauze swabs or moistened laparotomy sponges.

Surgical Technique (See Plate 26A–F)

A) A skin incision is performed over the anal sac tumor (pictured, bilateral anal sac tumors).
B) Identifying the anal sac duct with a probe or mosquito hemostats can facilitate a closed anal sacculectomy in cats and dogs with small anal sac tumors (i, ii).

Color Atlas of Canine and Feline Surgical Oncology, First Edition. Julius M. Liptak, Paolo Buracco, William T. N. Culp, and Nicholas J. Bacon.

Plate 26

Anal Sacculectomy

1)

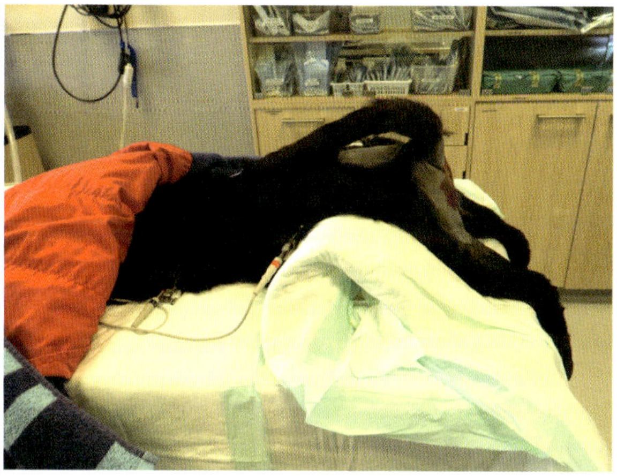

A)

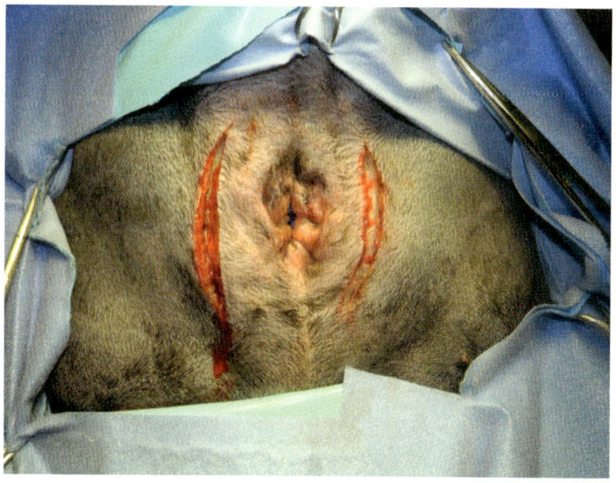

B-i)

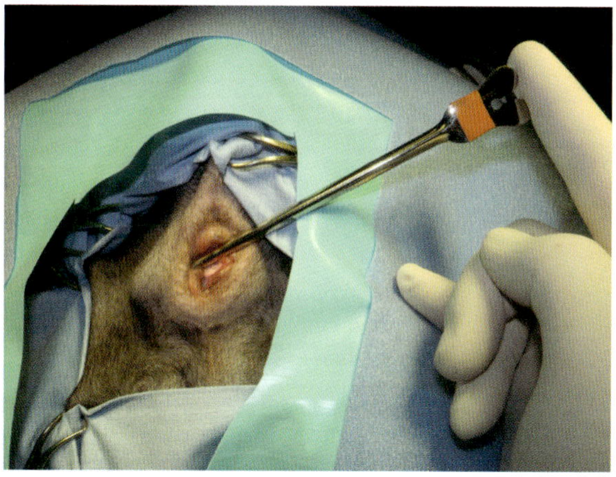

B-ii)

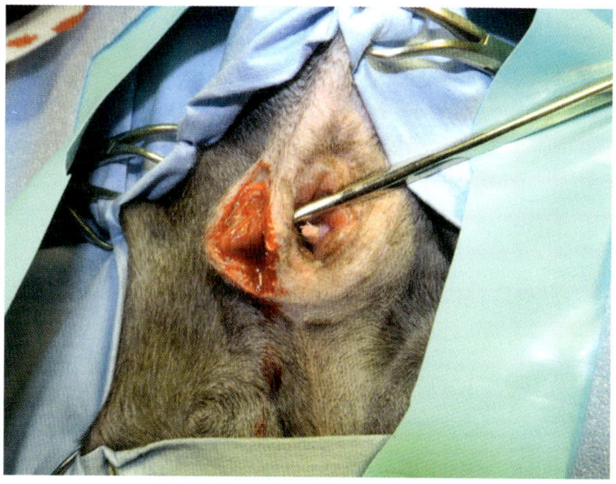

Surgical Technique (See Plate 26A–F) *continued*

C) Alternatively, instead of an incision over the anal sac tumor, an elliptical incision is performed around the opening of the anal sac duct [3, 4]. The advantage of the alternative approach is that the entire anal sac and duct are resected (which may decrease the risk of incomplete histologic excision and local tumor recurrence), the medial dissection between the anal sac and rectum is subjectively easier, and the risk of complications (e.g. rectocutaneous fistula) may be decreased.

D) The use of self-retaining retractors (e.g. Gelpi [pictured], Weitlaner, or ring retractors) can improve visualization and exposure during dissection of the anal sac mass. Note that the perianal skin and anocutaneous junction is relatively thin and can be traumatized by self-retaining retractors.

E) Marginal resection of the anal sac and anal sac tumor is performed with a combination of blunt and sharp dissection. The anal sac is adhered to the external anal sphincter muscle, and hence careful dissection is required to minimize damage to the external anal sphincter. A vessel sealing device is useful for hemostasis (i, ventral dissection; ii, cranial dissection); however, it should be used sparingly between the anal sac mass and rectum because of the risk of lateral thermal damage causing iatrogenic rectal trauma.

Plate 26

Anal Sacculectomy *continued*

C)

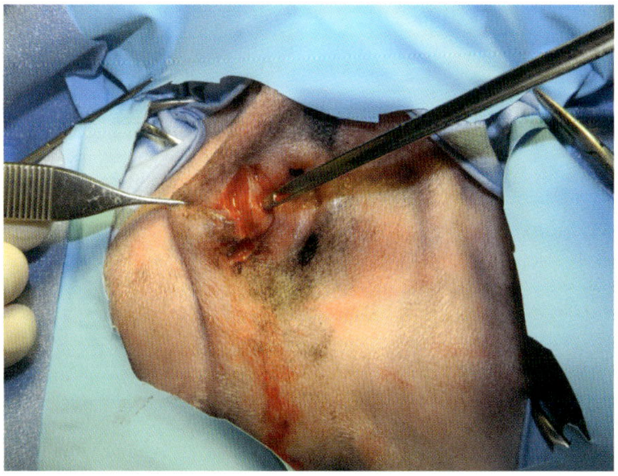

D)

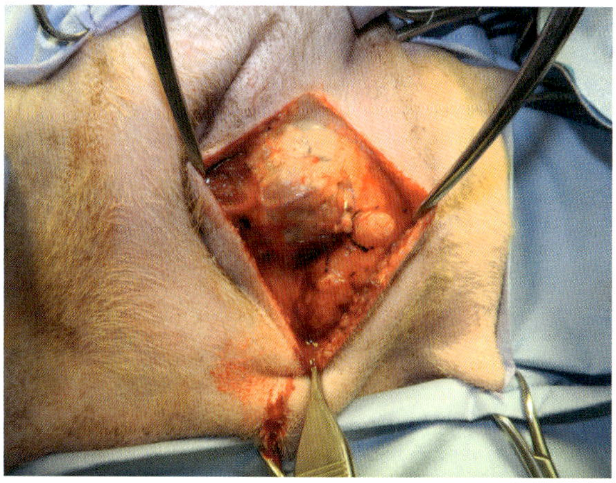

E-i)

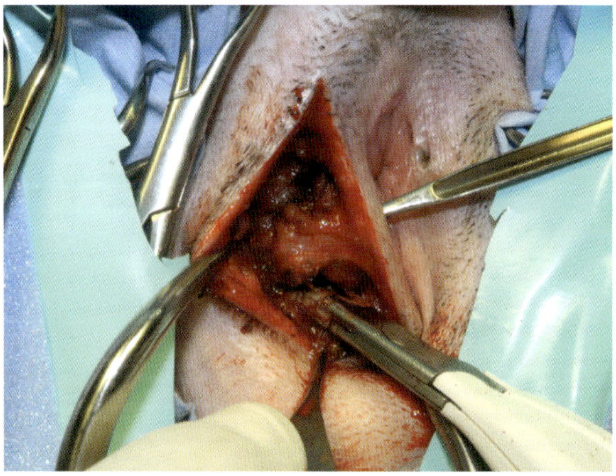

E-ii)

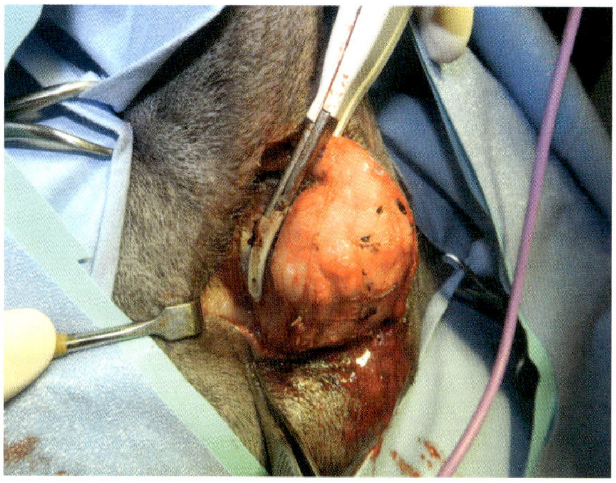

Surgical Technique (See Plate 26A–F) *continued*

F) If an incision has been performed over the anal sac tumor, then the anal sac duct should be isolated (i). Once isolated, the duct should be ligated with 3-0 or 4-0 simple or transfixion ligatures as close to the anal sac duct opening as possible (ii, iii). The anal sac duct is clamped, and the duct is transected between the clamp and ligature(s) with either a scalpel blade (iv) or Metzenbaum (v) or iris scissors. The anal sac mass is then removed from the surgical field (vi).

Plate 26

Anal Sacculectomy *continued*

F-i)

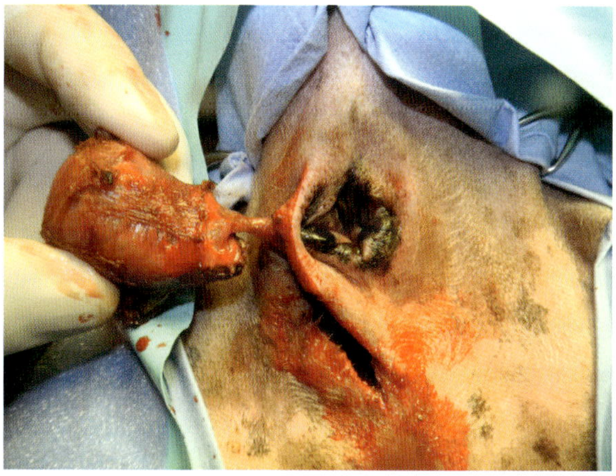

F-ii)

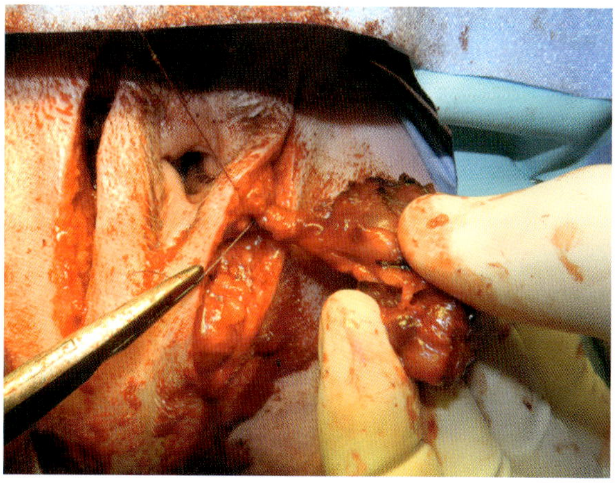

F-iii)

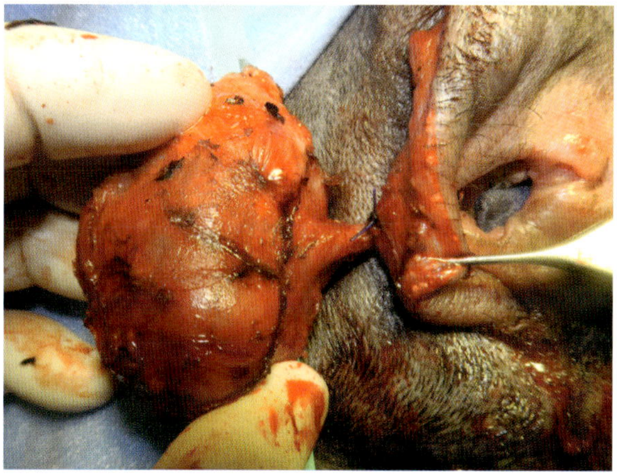

F-iv)

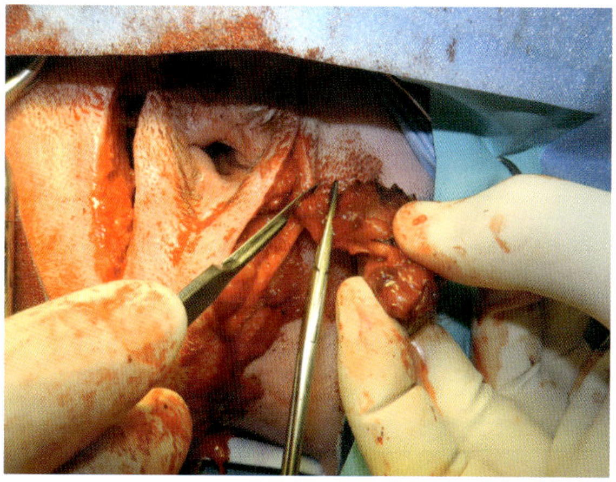

F-v)

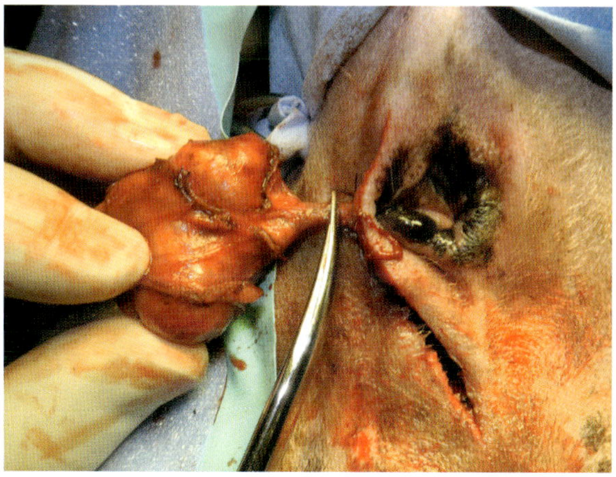

F-vi)

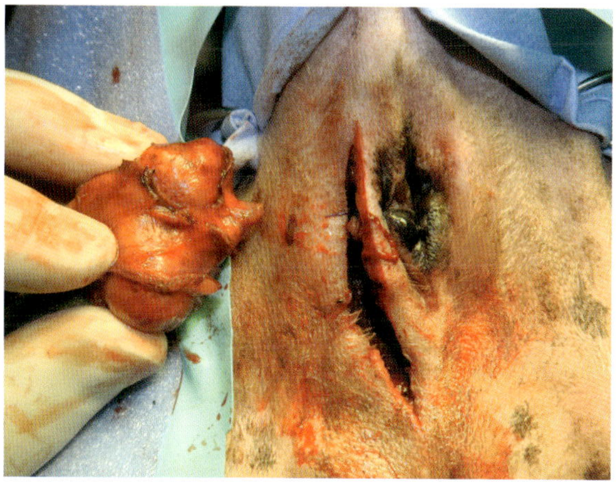

Closure (See Plate 26G)

The wound is then closed routinely in two to three layers. The deeper subcutaneous tissue can be closed with absorbable monofilament suture material in an interrupted or cruciate suture pattern. A simple continuous suture pattern using monofilament absorbable suture material is used to close the subcutis. An interrupted or continuous suture pattern using monofilament nonabsorbable suture material is used to close the skin (G).

Postoperative Management

- Multimodal analgesia, but consider avoiding the use of steroids and nonsteroidal anti-inflammatory drugs because of their negative effects on intestinal healing
- Elizabethan collar
- Feed normal diet
- ± Prophylactic antibiotics

Complications – Dogs

- Overall: 5%–42% [3–10]

Intraoperative Complications (See Plate 26H)

- Overall: 9% [7, 10]
- Rectal perforation (H, arrow) (1.2%–5%) [5, 9, 10]
  - 55% postoperative complication rate if intraoperative rectal perforation [10]
  - 14% postoperative complication rate if no intraoperative rectal perforation [10]

Postoperative Complications (See Plate 26I)

- Overall: 12%–39% [7, 9, 10] and 36% for tumors >5 cm [8]
- Incisional dehiscence (0%–23%) [3, 4, 5, 7, 9–12]
- Surgical-site infection (0%–15%) [3–7, 9, 10]
  - 63% if intraoperative rectal perforation [10]
  - 10% if no intraoperative rectal perforation [10]
- Incisional seroma (0%–1.8%) [5, 9]
- Fecal incontinence (0%–16%) [3–5, 9, 10]
  - 3.3% overall
  - 2.5% transient
  - 0.8% permanent
- Rectocutaneous fistula (I – i, ii) (0%–3.0%) [4, 6, 12]
- Neuropraxia (0.3%) [5]
- Hypocalcemia (0.1%–1.2%) [5, 12]

Suggested Adjuvant Treatments

- ± Radiation therapy for cats with apocrine gland anal sac adenocarcinoma
- ± Radiation therapy for dogs with metastatic apocrine gland anal sac adenocarcinoma
- ± Chemotherapy for dogs with metastatic apocrine gland anal sac adenocarcinoma
- Melanoma vaccine for dogs with primary anal sac melanoma

Plate 26

Anal Sacculectomy *continued*

G)

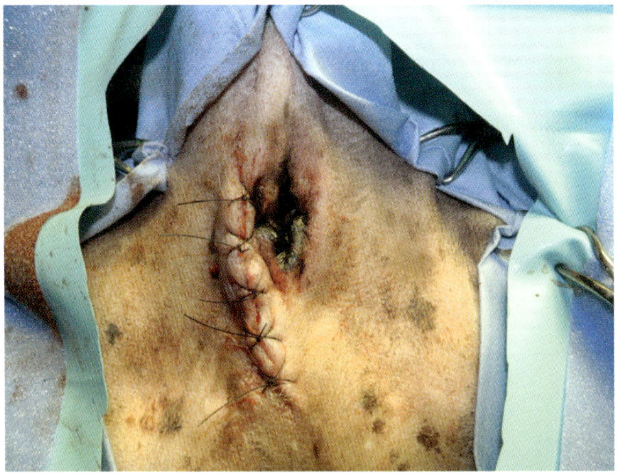

H)

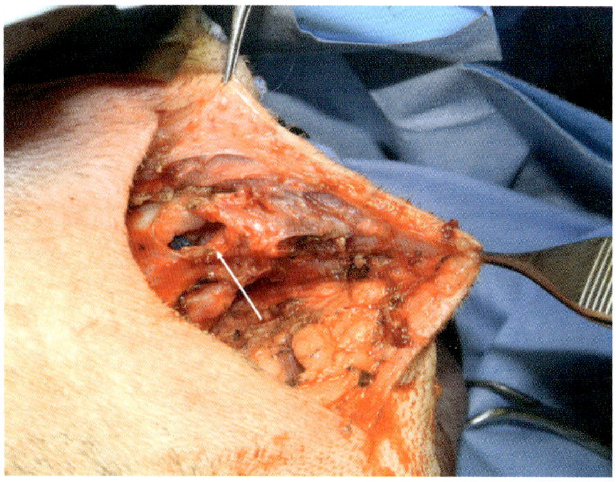

I-i)

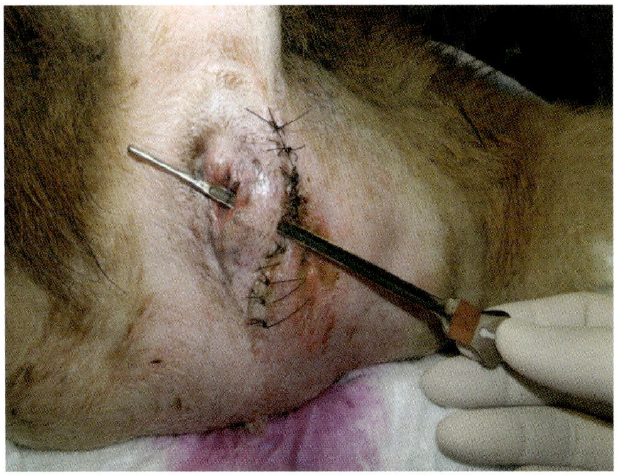

I-ii)

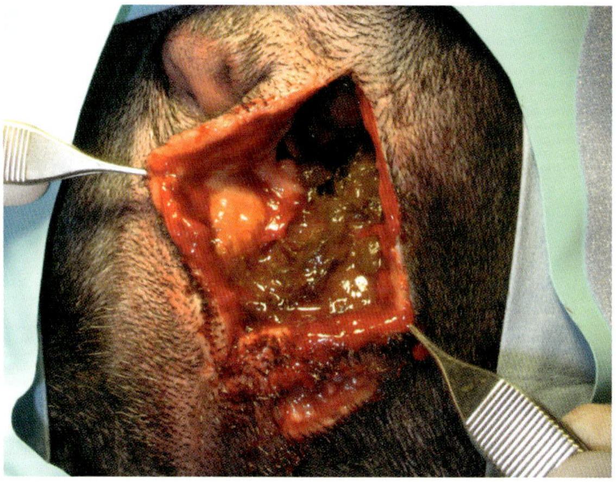

Prognosis and Oncologic Outcome – Dogs

	Local Recurrence rate	Metastatic Rate	Disease-Free Interval (d)	Median Survival Time (d)	1-Year Survival Rate	2-Year Survival Rate
Apocrine Gland Anal Sac Adenocarcinoma – Overall						
Overall [5, 6, 11–14]	5%–44%: local recurrence 6%: contralateral disease	31%–66%: sublumbar lymph nodes 14%–18%: distant sites	384–443	404–960	–	–
Clinical signs [13, 15]						
Yes	–	–	430	773	–	–
No	–	–	1609	1001	–	–
Tumor size – 10 cm^2 [6]						
<10 cm^2	–	–	–	584	–	–
≥10 cm^2	–	–	–	292	–	–
Tumor size – 2.5 cm [16]						
<2.5 cm	–	–	–	1205	–	–
≥2.5 cm	–	–	–	722	–	–
Tumor size – 4.0 cm [13]						
<4.0 cm	–	–	518	773	–	–
≥4.0 cm	–	–	251	433	–	–
Lymph node and/or distant metastasis [14, 17]						
Yes	–	–	134	183–448	–	–
No	–	–	594	471–761	–	–
Lymph node metastasis [5, 11, 13, 14]						
Yes	–	–	134–197	293–540	–	–
No	–	–	529–760	529 to >1745	–	–
Distant metastasis [5, 6]						
Yes	–	–	–	219	–	–
No	–	–	–	548	–	–
Hypercalcemia [6, 17]						
Yes	–	–	–	183–256	–	–
No	–	–	–	350–584	–	–
Histology – growth pattern [13]						
Solid	–	–	377	471	–	–
Other	–	–	1609	949	–	–
Histology – peripheral infiltration [13]						
None or mild	–	–	2164	1001	–	–
Moderate or marked	–	–	412	590	–	–

	Local Recurrence rate	Metastatic Rate	Disease-Free Interval (d)	Median Survival Time (d)	1-Year Survival Rate	2-Year Survival Rate
Histology – necrosis [13]						
Yes	–	–	378	834	–	–
No	–	–	1609	555	–	–
Histology – mitotic rate [13]						
<8/10 hpf	–	–	760	–	–	–
≥8/10 hpf	–	–	419	–	–	–
Histology – lymphovascular invasion [13]						
Yes	–	–	142	293	–	–
No	–	–	469	733	–	–
Immunohistochemistry – E-cadherin [18]						
>75% E-cadherin expression	–	–	–	1168	–	–
≤75% E-cadherin expression	–	–	–	448	–	–
Apocrine Gland Anal Sac Adenocarcinoma – Nonmetastatic						
Overall [5, 15, 16]	20%–21%	26%: sublumbar lymph nodes	354–644: local recurrence	722 to NR	–	–
		7%: distant sites	589: metastasis		–	–
Local tumor recurrence [5]						
Yes	–	–	–	809	82%	57%
No	–	–	–	1928	94%	83%
Treatment of local tumor recurrence [5]						
Yes	–	–	–	538	–	–
No	–	–	–	58	–	–
Bilateral disease [5]						
No	–	–	–	1928	91%	77%
Yes – simultaneous	–	–	–	723	87%	46%
Yes – staged	–	–	–	1233	95%	81%
Lymph node metastasis [5]						
Yes	–	–	–	794	83%	56%
No	–	–	–	NR	96%	88%
Treatment of lymph node metastasis [5]						
Yes	–	–	–	485	–	–
No	–	–	–	84	–	–
Distant metastasis [5]						
Yes	–	–	–	897	85%	65%
No	–	–	–	1670	92%	78%

(Continued)

	Local Recurrence rate	Metastatic Rate	Disease-Free Interval (d)	Median Survival Time (d)	1-Year Survival Rate	2-Year Survival Rate
Treatment of distant metastasis [5]						
Yes	–	–	–	277	–	–
No	–	–	–	27	–	–
Apocrine Gland Anal Sac Adenocarcinoma – Lymph Node Metastasis						
Overall [5, 16]	–	66%: sublumbar lymph nodes	–	294–551	–	–
	–	17%: distant sites	–		–	–
Treatment – surgery and chemotherapy [5]						
Anal sacculectomy	–	–	–	358	–	–
Anal sacculectomy and sublumbar lymph node resection	–	–	–	546	–	–
Anal sacculectomy, sublumbar lymph node resection, and chemotherapy	–	–	–	1927	–	–
Treatment – hypofractionated radiation therapy [19]						
Sublumbar lymph node resection	–	–	159	182	–	–
Hypofractionated radiation therapy	–	–	347	447	–	–
Melanoma						
Overall [20]	55%[a]	36%: sublumbar lymph nodes 18%: distant sites	–	107	9%	9%
Squamous Cell Carcinoma						
Overall [21]	75%	0%	42	100	0%	0%

[a] Includes both local recurrence in surgically treated dogs and disease progression in conservatively treated dogs.
hpf, high-power fields; NR, not reached.

Prognosis and Oncologic Outcome – Cats

	Local Recurrence rate	Metastatic Rate	Disease-Free Interval (d)	Median Survival Time (d)	1-Year Survival Rate	2-Year Survival Rate
			Apocrine Gland Anal Sac Adenocarcinoma [22]			
Overall	37%	13%	96: local recurrence 234: metastasis	360	42%	27%
			Histologic margins			
Incomplete	–	–	196	–	–	–
Complete	–	–	555	–	–	–
			Nuclear pleomorphic score (NPS)			
NPS = 2	–	–	–	909	–	–
NPS = 3	–	–	–	187	–	–

References

1 Palladino, S., Keyerleber, M.A., King, R.G. et al. (2016). Utility of computed tomography versus abdominal ultrasound examination to identify iliosacral lymphadenomegaly in dogs with apocrine gland adenocarcinoma of the anal sac. *J. Vet. Intern. Med.* 30 (6): 1858–1863.

2 Pollard, R.E., Fuller, M.C., and Steffey, M.A. (2017). Ultrasound and computed tomography of the iliosacral lymphatic centre in dogs with anal sac gland carcinoma. *Vet. Comp. Oncol.* 15 (2): 299–306.

3 Davey, E.L. and Prpich, C.Y. (2024). Outcomes of dogs with apocrine gland anal sac adenocarcinoma treated via modified closed anal sacculectomy (2015–2022). *Vet Surg.* 53: 973–979.

4 Chen, C.L., Lapsley, J.M., and Selmic, L.E. (2021). Minimal complications observed with a modified surgical approach for treatment of canine anal sac neoplasia. *J Am Vet Med Assoc.* 260: S59–S64.

5 Liptak, J.M., Selmic, L., Amsellem, P. et al. (2015). Apocrine gland anal sac adenocarcinoma and sublumbar lymph node metastasis: A VSSO retrospective study. *Am. Coll. Vet. Surg. Annu. Meeting.*

6 Williams, L.E., Gliatto, J.M., Dodge, R.K. et al. (2003). Carcinoma of the apocrine glands of the anal sacs in dogs: 113 cases (1985–1995). *J. Am. Anim. Hosp. Assoc.* 223 (6): 825–831.

7 Franca, A., Stamenova, P., and Thompson, J.L. (2024). Histopathological diagnosis and surgical complications following bilateral anal sacculectomy for the treatment of unilateral canine apocrine gland anal sac adenocarcinoma: 35 cases (2019–2023). *J Small Anim Pract.* 65: 394–401.

8 Griffin, M.A., Mayhew, P.D., Culp, W.T.N. et al. (2023). Short- and long-term outcomes associated with anal sacculectomy in dogs with massive apocrine gland anal sac adenocarcinoma. *J Am Vet Med Assoc.* 261: 1–8.

9 Tanis, J.B., Simlett-Moss, A.B., Ossowksa, M. et al. (2022). Canine anal sac gland carcinoma with regional lymph node metastases treated with sacculectomy and lymphadenectomy: outcome and possible prognostic factors. *Vet Comp Oncol.* 20: 276–292.

10 Sterman, A., Butler, J.R., Chambers, A. et al. (2021). Post-operative complications following apocrine gland anal sac adenocarcinoma resection in dogs. *Vet Comp Oncol.* 19: 743–749.

11 Ross, T.J., Scavelli, T.D., Matthiesen, D.T. et al. (1991). Adenocarcinoma of the apocrine glands of the anal sac in dogs: a review of 32 cases. *J. Am. Anim. Hosp. Assoc.* 27 (3): 349–355.

12 Barnes, D.C. and Demetriou, J.L. (2017). Surgical management of primary, metastatic and recurrent anal sac adenocarcinoma in the dog: 52 cases. *J. Small Anim. Pract.* 58 (5): 263–268.

13 Pradel, J., Berlato, D., Dobromylskyj, M. et al. (2018). Prognostic significance of histopathology in canine anal sac gland adenocarcinomas: Preliminary results in a retrospective study of 39 cases. *Vet. Comp. Oncol.* 16 (4): 518–528.

14 Wouda, R.M., Borrego, J., Keuler, N.S. et al. (2016). Evaluation of adjuvant carboplatin chemotherapy in the management of surgically excised anal sac apocrine gland adenocarcinoma in dogs. *Vet. Comp. Oncol.* 14 (1): 67–80.

15 Skorupski, K.A., Alarcón, C.N., de Lorimier, L.P. et al. (2018). Outcome and clinical, pathological, and immunohistochemical factors associated with prognosis for dogs with early-stage anal sac adenocarcinoma treated with surgery alone: 34 cases (2002-2013). *J. Am. Vet. Med. Assoc.* 253 (1): 84–91.

16 Polton, G.A. and Brearley, M.J. (2007). Clinical stage, therapy, and prognosis in canine anal sac gland carcinoma. *J. Vet. Intern. Med.* 21 (2): 274–280.

17 Potanas, C.P., Padgett, S., and Gamblin, R.M. (2015). Surgical excision of anal sac apocrine gland adenocarcinomas with and without adjunctive chemotherapy in dogs: 42 cases (2005-2011). *J. Am. Vet. Med. Assoc.* 246 (8): 877–884.

18 Polton, G.A., Brearley, M.J., Green, L.M. et al. (2007). Expression of E-cadherin in canine anal sac gland carcinoma and its association with survival. *Vet. Comp. Oncol.* 5 (4): 232–238.

19 Meier, V., Polton, G., Cancedda, S. et al. (2017). Outcome in dogs with advanced (stage 3b) anal sac carcinoma treated with surgery or hypofractionated radiation therapy. *Vet. Comp. Oncol.* 15 (3): 1073–1086.

20 Vinayak, A., Frank, C.B., Gardiner, D.W. et al. (2017). Malignant anal sac melanoma in dogs: eleven cases (2000 to 2015). *J. Small Anim. Pract.* 58 (4): 231–237.

21 Esplin, D.G., Wilson, S.R., and Hullinger, G.A. (2003). Squamous cell carcinoma of the anal sac in five dogs. *Vet. Pathol.* 40 (3): 332–334.

22 Amsellen, P.M., Cavanaugh, R.P., Po-Yen, C. et al. (2019). Apocrine gland anal sac adenocarcinoma in cats: 30 cases (1994-2015). *J. Am. Vet. Med. Assoc.* 254 (6): 716–722.

Section 6

Urogenital Tumors

Chapter 27: Ureteronephrectomy

27.1 Open Ureteronephrectomy

Indications

1) Resection of unilateral benign or malignant renal tumors.
2) Ureteronephrectomy can be combined with adrenalectomy (see *19.1. Open Adrenalectomy*) if the adrenal tumor is invasive into the kidney.
3) Ureteronephrectomy can be combined with partial cystectomy (see *28.1. Partial Cystectomy*) if the urinary bladder tumor involves one of the ureterovesicular junctions.

Suggested Diagnostic Workup and Clinical Staging

- Complete blood count, serum biochemistry, and urinalysis to test for renal function
- Abdominal ultrasound or precontrast and postcontrast computed tomography (CT) scan of the abdomen for assessment of the contralateral kidney, intra-abdominal metastasis, and tumor thrombus in the caudal vena cava
- Preoperative ultrasound-guided fine-needle aspirate cytology of the renal mass
- Three-view thoracic radiographs or thoracic CT scan for assessment of lung metastasis

Patient Positioning

The patient is positioned in dorsal recumbency.

Surgical Technique (See Plate 27.1A–F)

A) A ventral midline celiotomy is performed (i) (see *15.1. Ventral Midline Celiotomy*). The left kidney is exposed by retracting the descending colon and mesocolon toward the right side, and the right kidney (RK) is exposed by retracting the duodenum (D) and mesoduodenum (MD) to the left side (ii).
B) The affected kidney is dissected from the retroperitoneal space in a lateral-to-medial direction, preferably with a vessel sealing device (i, ii). The ipsilateral adrenal gland should be preserved if possible.
C) Once freed from the retroperitoneal space and mobilized (i), the perirenal tissue adjacent to the renal pelvis is carefully dissected to expose the renal artery and vein (and ureter) (ii). Note that the vascular anatomy of the kidney is highly variable (e.g. paired [iii] or multiple left renal arteries are reported in up to 15% of dogs, the left ovarian vein drains into the left renal vein rather than the caudal vena cava in dogs, and cats often have multiple renal veins), and that all arteries and veins should be identified before ligation and transection.

Color Atlas of Canine and Feline Surgical Oncology, First Edition. Julius M. Liptak, Paolo Buracco, William T. N. Culp, and Nicholas J. Bacon.

Plate 27.1

Open Ureteronephrectomy

A-i)

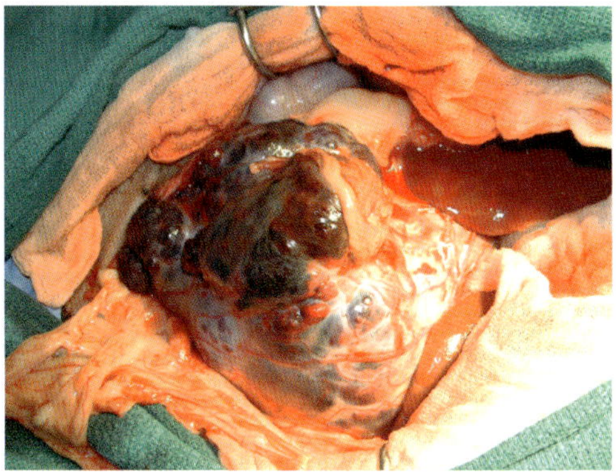

A-ii)

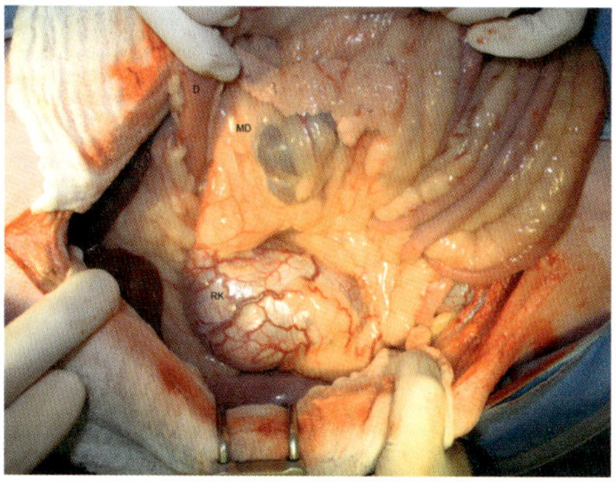

B-i)

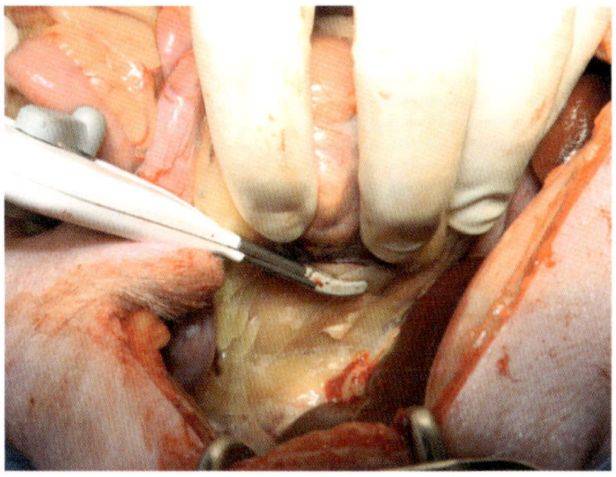

B-ii)

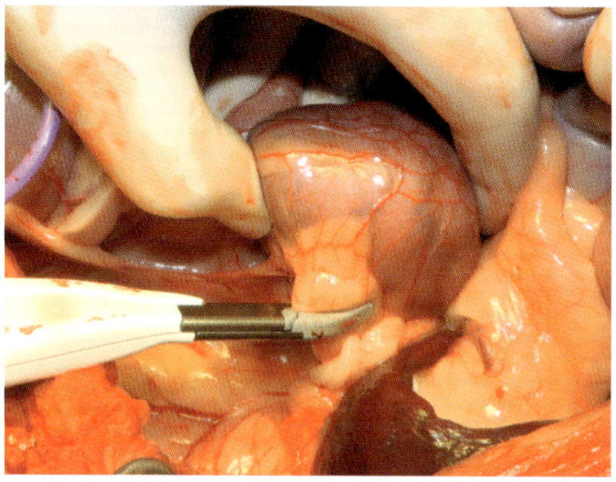

C-i)

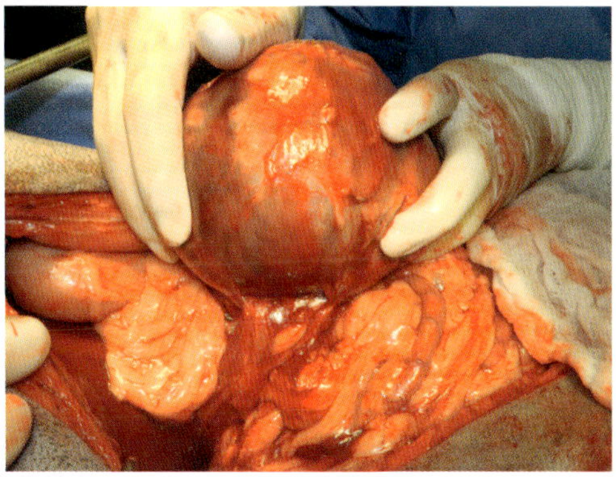

C-ii)

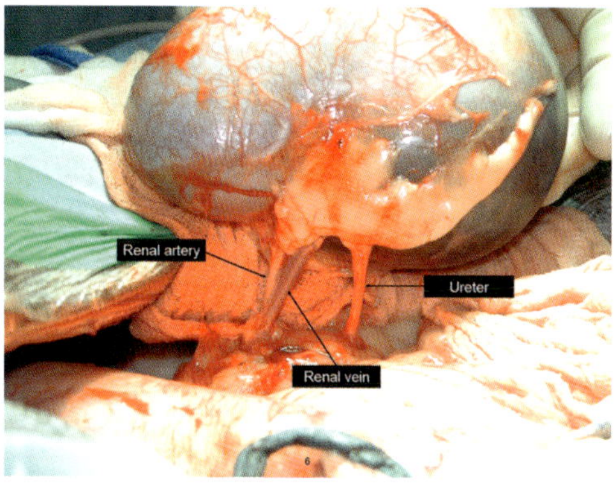

C-iii)

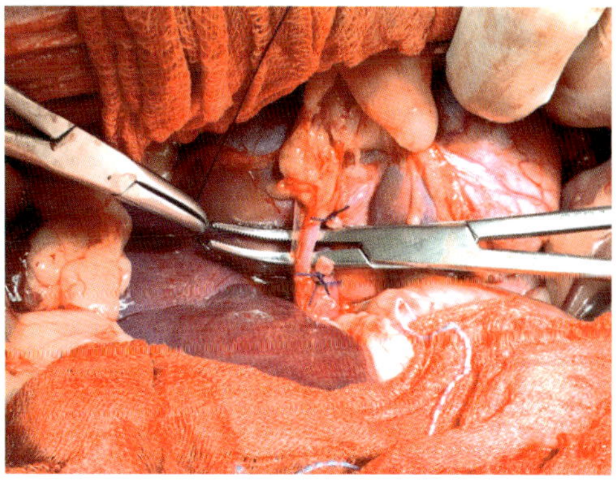

Surgical Technique (See Plate 27.1A–F) *continued*

D) The renal vessels are individually ligated with one to two simple or transfixion ligatures using 4-0 to 2-0 absorbable suture material (i, ii). Alternatively, the renal vessels can be ligated with hemoclips (iii) or sealed en bloc with a vascular 30-mm vascular thoracoabdominal stapler (iv). The vessels are then sealed and transected with a vessel sealing device between the ligatures and kidney (v) or clamped (vi) and transected with Metzenbaum scissors (vii).

Plate 27.1

Open Ureteronephrectomy *continued*

D-i)

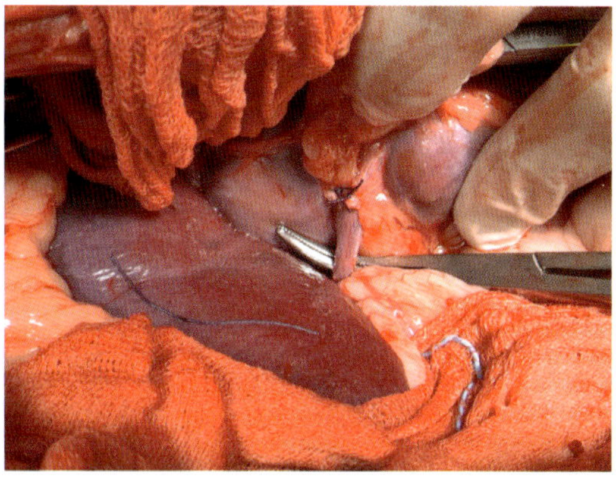

D-ii)

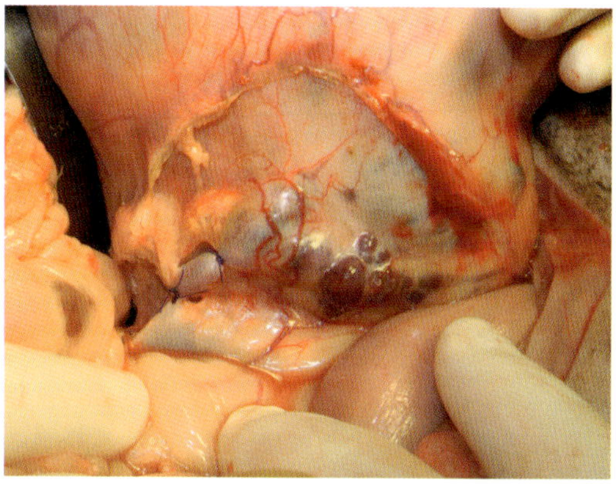

D-iii)

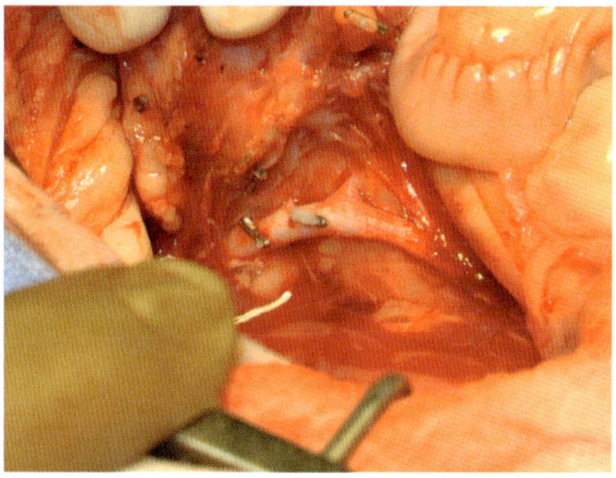

D-iv)

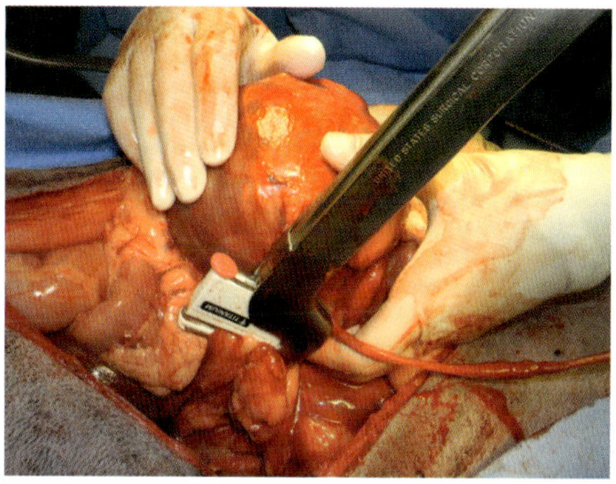

D-v)

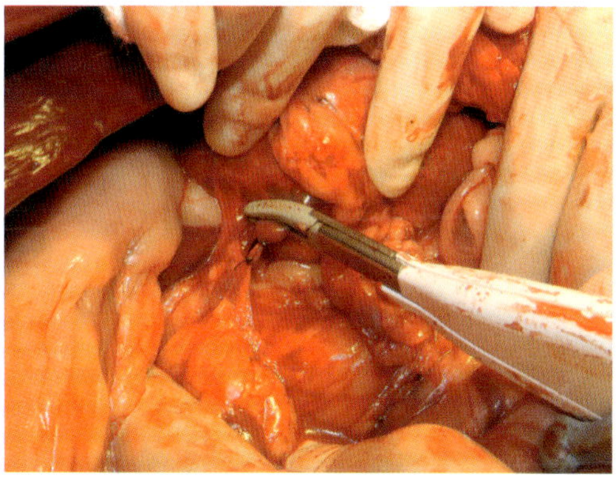

D-vi)

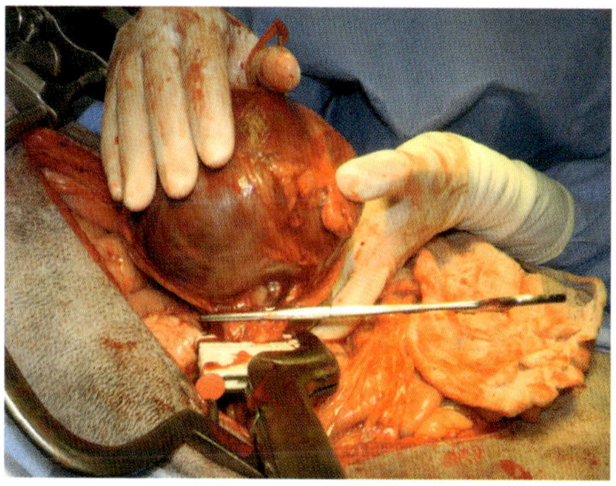

D-vii)

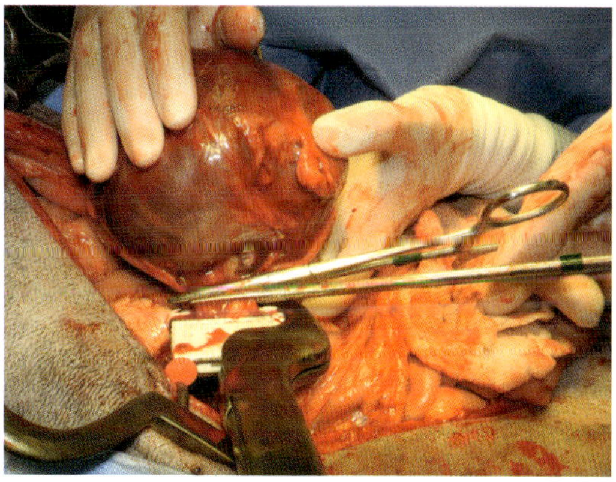

Surgical Technique (See Plate 27.1A–F) *continued*

E) The ureter is identified and dissected free from the retroperitoneal space to the level of the urinary bladder (i). The ureter is ligated as close as possible to the urinary bladder with one to two simple or transfixion ligatures using 4-0 to 2-0 absorbable suture material (ii). The ureter is then clamped (iii) and transected cranial to the ligatures (dashed line).

F) See *19.1. Open Adrenalectomy* for management of renal tumors with a tumor thrombus extending into the renal vein or caudal vena cava.

Closure

The linea alba, subcutaneous tissue, and skin are closed as described in *15.1. Ventral Midline Celiotomy*.

Postoperative Management

- Multimodal analgesia
- Monitor renal function (urine production and renal biochemistry)
- Elizabethan collar or body suit

Complications

- See *15.1. Ventral Midline Celiotomy*
- Intraoperative hemorrhage because of inadequate ligation of renal vessels
- Postoperative acute renal failure

Suggested Adjuvant Treatments

- ± Chemotherapy for dogs with renal hemangiosarcoma and high-grade renal carcinoma
- Chemotherapy (as sole therapy) for cats with renal lymphoma

Plate 27.1

Open Ureteronephrectomy *continued*

E-i)

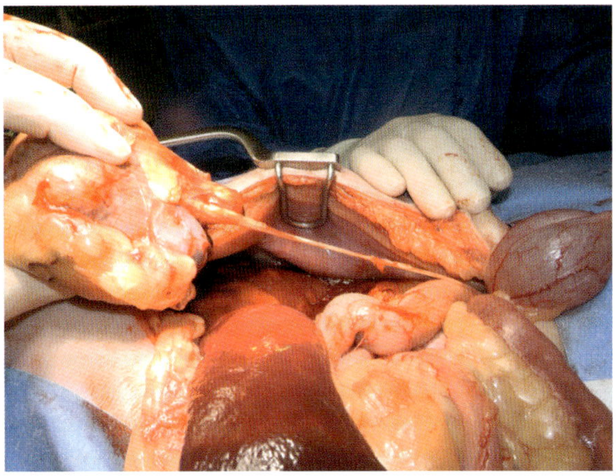

E-ii)

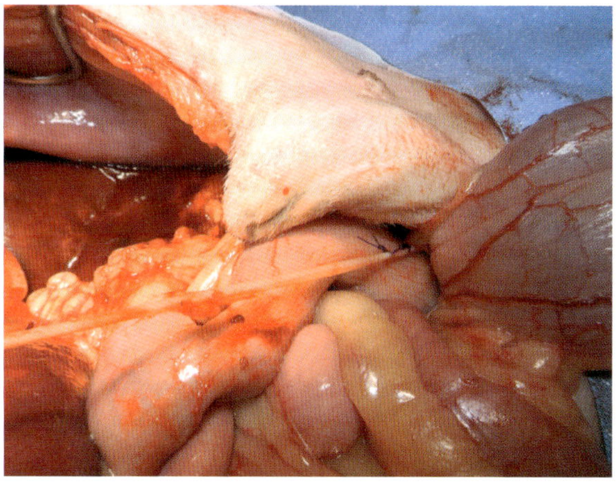

E-iii)

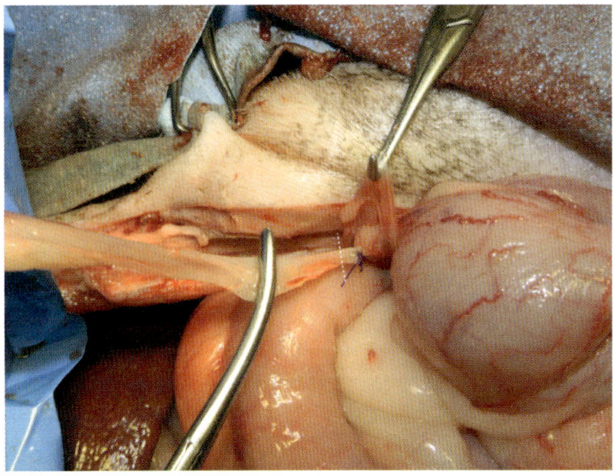

F)

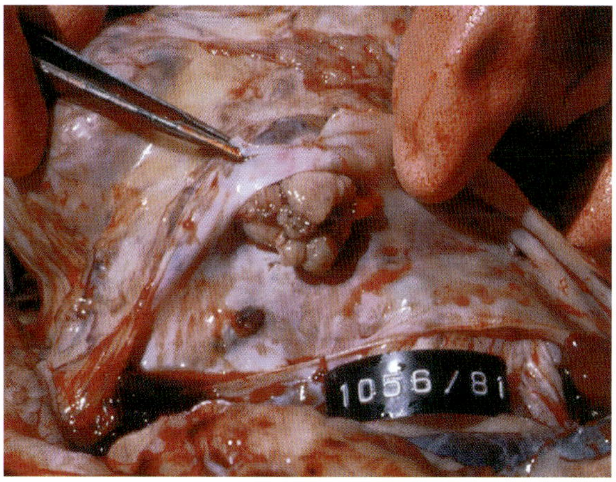

Prognosis and Oncologic Outcome – Dogs

	Local Recurrence Rate	Metastatic Rate	Disease-Free Interval (d)	Median Survival Time (d)	1-Year Survival Rate	2-Year Survival Rate
Renal Carcinoma						
Overall [1–3]	4%	36%–69%	259 (mean)	487–743	43%	25%
Age at diagnosis [2]						
<6 yr	–	–	–	187	25%	13%
≥6 yr	–	–	–	807	55%	25%
Metastasis at diagnosis [3]						
Yes	–	–	–	141	–	–
No	–	–	–	533	–	–
Tumor subtype [2]						
Tubular	–	–	–	720	77%	39%
Papillary	–	–	–	510	67%	17%
Solid	–	–	–	180	33%	20%
Poorly differentiated tubular	–	–	–	180	22%	0%
Mitotic rate [2, 3]						
<10/10 hpf	–	–	–	545–1184	50%	14%
10–30/10 hpf	–	–	–	452–532	58%	21%
>30/10 hpf	–	–	–	120–187	13%	0%
Fuhrman nuclear grade [2]						
I	–	–	–	NR	–	–
II	–	–	–	1065	–	–
III	–	–	–	379	–	–
IV	–	–	–	87	–	–
Nuclear size [2]						
10 μm	–	–	–	NR	–	–
11–15 μm	–	–	–	1184	–	–
16–20 μm	–	–	–	417	–	–
>20 μm	–	–	–	122	–	–
Nuclear pleomorphism [2]						
Mild	–	–	–	1571	–	–
Moderate	–	–	–	909	–	–
Marked	–	–	–	322	–	–
Invasiveness [2, 3]						
Mild	–	–	–	720–1065	64%	29%
Moderate	–	–	–	540–572	50%	36%
Marked	–	–	–	117–370	30%	10%

			Vascular invasion [3]			
Yes	–	–	–	210	61%	29%
No	–	–	–	545	30%	10%
			COX-2 score [3]			
≤3	–	–	–	1176	–	–
>3	–	–	–	420	–	–
			Renal Hemangiosarcoma			
Overall [1, 4]	–	77%	–	274–278	29%	–
			Hemoabdomen at diagnosis [4]			
Yes	–	–	–	62	–	–
No	–	–	–	286	–	–
			Renal Nephroblastoma			
Overall [1]	–	75%	–	183	–	–

hpf, high-power fields; NR, not reached.

Prognosis and Oncologic Outcome – Cats

	Local Recurrence Rate	Metastatic Rate	Disease-Free Interval (d)	Median Survival Time (d)	1-Year Survival Rate	2-Year Survival Rate
			Renal Carcinoma [5]			
Overall [1–3]	17%	19%	NR	1217[a]	40%	40%

[a] Median survival time for cats surviving to discharge.
NR, not reached.

References

1 Bryan, J.N., Henry, C.J., Turnquist, S.E. et al. (2006). Primary renal neoplasia of dogs. *J. Vet. Intern. Med.* 20 (5): 1155–1160.

2 Edmondson, E.F., Hess, A.M., and Powers, B.E. (2015). Prognostic significance of histologic features in canine renal cell carcinomas: 70 nephrectomies. *Vet. Pathol.* 52 (2): 260–268.

3 Carvalho, S., Stoll, A.L., Priestnall, S.L. et al. (2017). Retrospective evaluation of COX-2 expression, histological and clinical factors as prognostic indicators in dogs with renal cell carcinomas undergoing nephrectomy. *Vet. Comp. Oncol.* 15 (4): 1280–1294.

4 Locke, J.E. and Barber, L.G. (2006). Comparative aspects and clinical outcomes of canine renal hemangiosarcoma. *J. Vet. Intern. Med.* 20 (4): 962–967.

5 Kenny, S.A., Cook, M.R., Lenz, J.A. et al. (2023). Clinical outcomes in cats with renal carcinoma undergoing nephrectomy: A retrospective study. *Vet. Comp. Oncol.* 21 (4): 587–594.

27.2 Laparoscopic Ureteronephrectomy

Indications

1) Resection of unilateral benign or malignant renal tumors with no evidence of vascular invasion

Suggested Diagnostic Workup and Clinical Staging

See *27.1. Open Ureteronephrectomy*.

Patient Positioning

The patient is positioned in lateral recumbency with the affected side uppermost. An oblique positioning to the abdomen with the dorsal aspect higher than the ventral aspect improves visualization of the retroperitoneal region during dissection. The surgeon is positioned on the ventral side of the patient, and the monitor is across the table on the patient's dorsum.

Surgical Technique (See Plate 27.2A–F)

A) For ureteronephrectomy, three or four separate ports are established to perform the procedure. A skin incision is made in a subumbilical location or just lateral to the umbilicus on the affected side. Placement of the telescope cannula commences as is described in *15.3. Laparoscopic Approach*. A 5-mm 30-degree telescope is most commonly used, and this is introduced into the initial cannula after a pneumoperitoneum is established. Two to three additional cannulae are introduced to allow for placement of instrumentation. At least one of the instrument ports should be a 10-mm diameter cannula to allow for placement of an endoscopic stapling device ± retrieval bag. The first two instrument cannulae are triangulated with the telescope cannula by placing one cannula caudodorsal and one cannula craniodorsal relative to the telescope cannula. If an additional cannula is needed for retraction, this is generally placed over the affected kidney.
B) Organs covering the affected kidney need to be mobilized out of the way to allow for ureteronephrectomy to be performed. This is most easily accomplished by using a blunt probe to retract the organs off the kidney and toward the abdominal midline or opposite side of the abdomen. Dissection is usually initiated by retracting the kidney caudally (from the caudal instrument port) using a blunt probe or fan retractor. This exposes the cranial aspect of the kidney and allows the surgeon to place a J-hook electrocautery or vessel sealing device into the cranial port to begin dissection on the cranial aspect of the kidney. This dissection continues around the entire kidney until the renal vasculature is exposed.
C) Alternatively, the ureter can be dissected free first before dissecting the kidney. The advantage of this technique is that the ureter can be used to mobilize the kidney in different directions to facilitate dissection around the kidney. In addition, the ureter can be grasped to elevate the kidney during ligation or sealing of the renal vasculature. To perform this technique, the ureter is elevated with a blunt probe or grasper (pictured, i), and an endoscopic hemostat is used to create a hole in the retroperitoneal lining and the tissue surrounding the ureter (ii). Once a hole has been created, the blunt probe can be inserted into the hole, which allows the ureter to be elevated, which makes dissection around the ureter easier because the vessel sealing device can travel cranially and caudally to completely isolate the ureter. Once dissected free from surrounding tissue, the ureter can be grasped with an endoscopic hemostat and used to move the kidney in different directions to allow for dissection.

Color Atlas of Canine and Feline Surgical Oncology, First Edition. Julius M. Liptak, Paolo Buracco, William T. N. Culp, and Nicholas J. Bacon.

Plate 27.2

Laparoscopic Ureteronephrectomy

A)

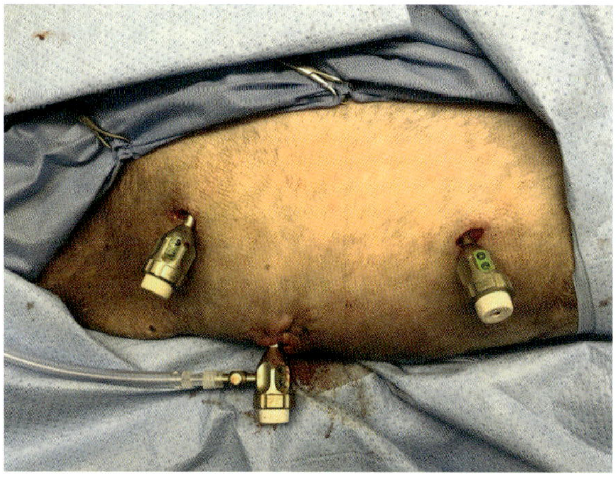

B)

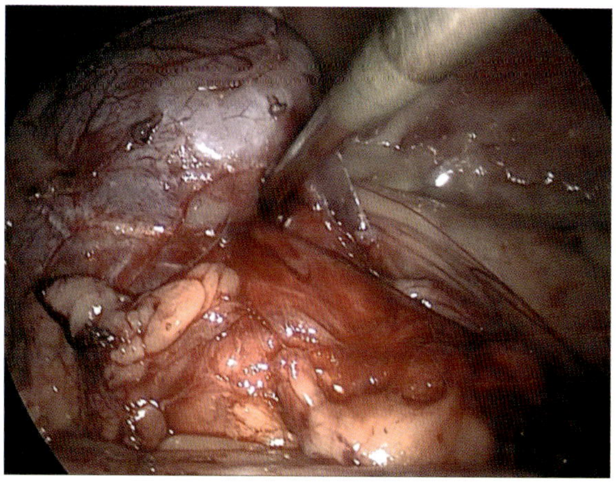

C-i)

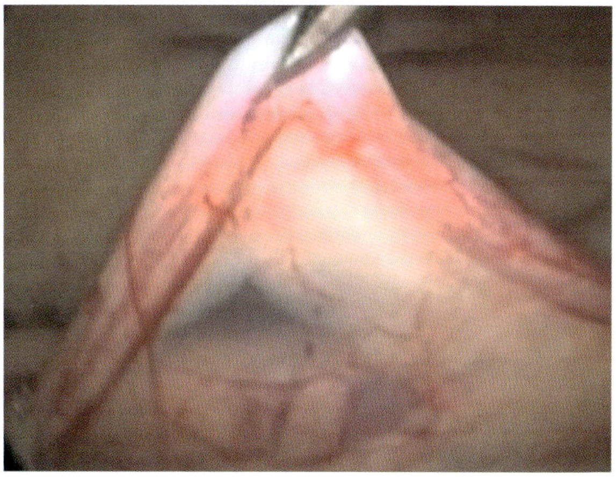

Courtesy of Dr. Philipp Mayhew

C-ii)

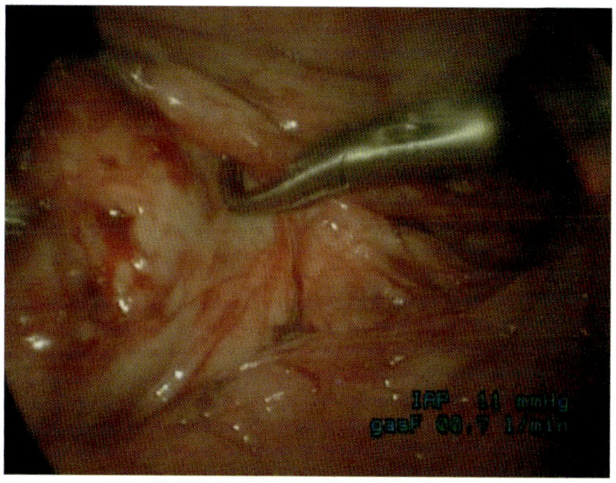

Courtesy of Dr. Philipp Mayhew

Surgical Technique (See Plate 27.2A–F) *continued*

D) The renal blood vessels are individually skeletonized with endoscopic hemostats or right-angle forceps until a length of vessel is exposed to allow for use of the vessel sealing device or the placement of laparoscopic hemoclips (i). If the renal vessels are larger than 7 mm, three laparoscopic hemoclips can be placed on the vessels and then laparoscopic scissors can be used to transect the vessel, leaving two to three hemoclips on the patient's side (ii).
E) The ureter is dissected to the level of the ureterovesicular junction. The distal ureter can be ligated with hemoclips (pictured) or sutures and then transected.
F) When the kidney has been completely separated from the surrounding tissues, the vessel sealing device is removed and a retrieval bag is introduced into the abdomen (i, ii). One of the instrument ports will likely need to be enlarged to allow for removal of the kidney in some cases.

Closure

The muscular layers are closed with 2-0 to 3-0 monofilament absorbable suture in a simple interrupted or cruciate pattern. The subcutaneous tissue is closed with 3-0 monofilament absorbable suture if needed. The dermal layer is apposed with 3-0 to 4-0 monofilament nonabsorbable suture in a simple interrupted or simple continuous pattern.

Postoperative Management

1) Multimodal analgesia
2) Elizabethan collar or body suit

Complications

Intraoperative Complications

- Splenic laceration (19%) [1]
- Subcutaneous emphysema (13%) [1]
- Conversion to an open ureteronephrectomy (22%) [2]
- For complications specific to all laparoscopic procedures, see *15.3. Laparoscopic Approach*

Suggested Adjuvant Treatments

- See *27.1. Open Ureteronephrectomy*.

Prognosis and Oncologic Outcome – Dogs

- See *27.1. Open Ureteronephrectomy*.

References

1 Kim, Y.K., Park, S.J., Lee, S.Y. et al. (2013). Laparoscopic nephrectomy in dogs: an initial experience of 16 experimental procedures. *Vet. J.* 198 (2): 513–517.
2 Mayhew, P.D., Mehler, S.J., Mayhew, K.N. et al. (2013). Experimental and clinical evaluation of transperitoneal laparoscopic ureteronephrectomy in dogs. *Vet. Surg.* 42 (5): 565–571.

Plate 27.2

Laparoscopic Ureteronephrectomy *continued*

D-i)

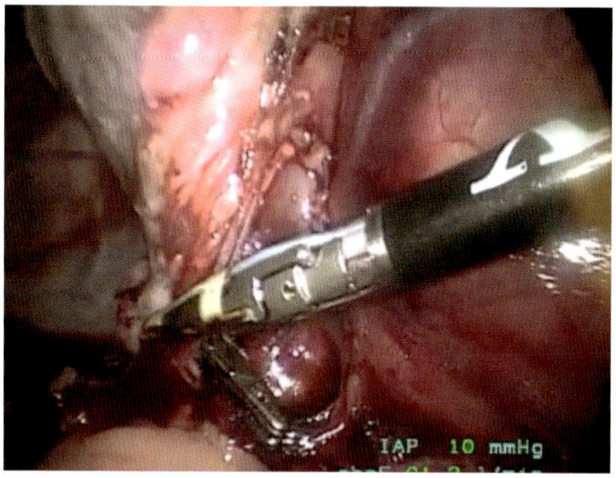

Courtesy of Dr. Philipp Mayhew

D-ii)

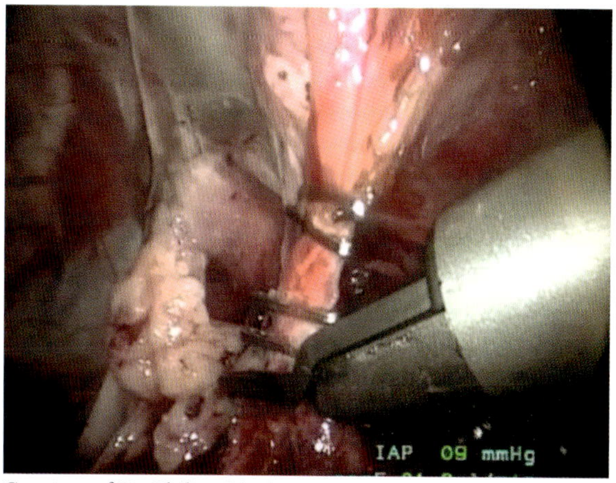

Courtesy of Dr. Philipp Mayhew

E)

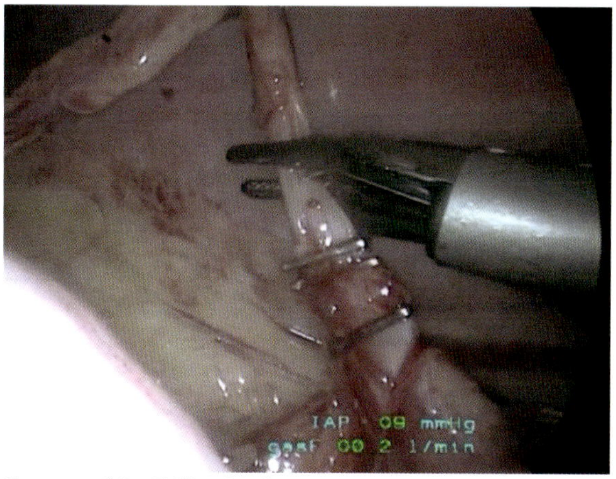

Courtesy of Dr. Philipp Mayhew

F-i)

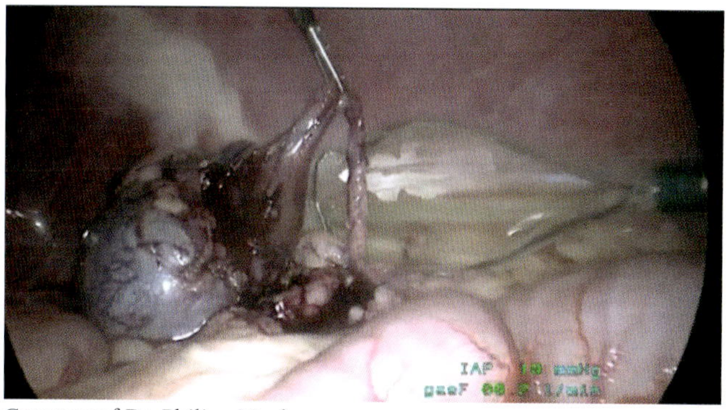

Courtesy of Dr. Philipp Mayhew

F-ii)

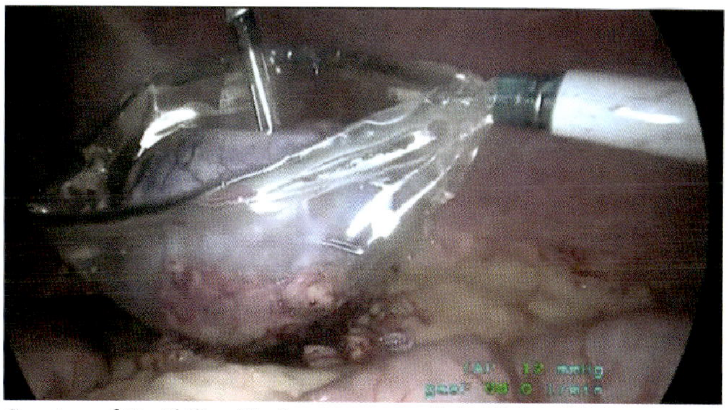

Courtesy of Dr. Philipp Mayhew

Chapter 28: Cystectomy

28.1 Partial Cystectomy

Indications

1) Resection of benign and malignant urinary bladder tumors (arrows), especially when distant to trigonal region of the urinary bladder
2) Partial cystectomy can be combined with sublumbar lymph node resection (see *20.1. Open Sublumbar Lymph Node Resection*) when enlarged or metastatic sublumbar lymph nodes are present
3) Partial cystectomy can be combined with ureteronephrectomy (see *27.1. Open Ureteronephrectomy*) if there is unilateral involvement of one of the ureterovesicular junctions

Suggested Diagnostic Workup and Clinical Staging (See Plate 28.1 – 1)

- Complete blood count, serum biochemistry, and urinalysis
- Urine sediment cytology
- Cadet BRAF mutation urine test
- ± Urethrocystoscopy for assessment and biopsy of the urethra and urinary bladder
- Abdominal ultrasound or precontrast and postcontrast computed tomography (CT) scan of the abdomen for assessment of location and extent of the urinary bladder mass (1 – i, ii) and intra-abdominal metastasis
- Three-view thoracic radiographs or thoracic CT scan for assessment of lung metastasis

Patient Positioning

The patient is positioned in dorsal recumbency.

Surgical Technique (See Plate 28.1A, C–J)

A) A ventral midline celiotomy is performed (see *15.1. Ventral Midline Celiotomy*) with the incision extending to the pubic brim. The penis or vulva should be draped into the surgical field because access may be needed for intraoperative catheterization.
B) The ventral ligament of the bladder is incised with either scissors or a vessel sealing device to allow the bladder to be mobilized to one side or the other (not pictured).

Color Atlas of Canine and Feline Surgical Oncology, First Edition. Julius M. Liptak, Paolo Buracco, William T. N. Culp, and Nicholas J. Bacon.

Plate 28.1

Partial Cystectomy

1-i)

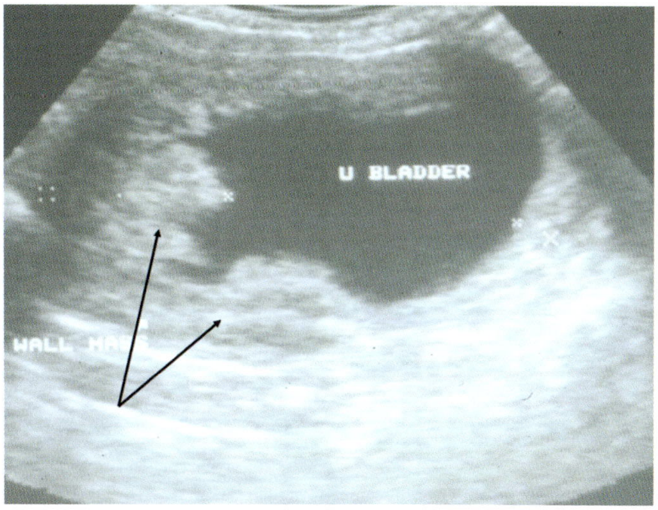

1-ii)

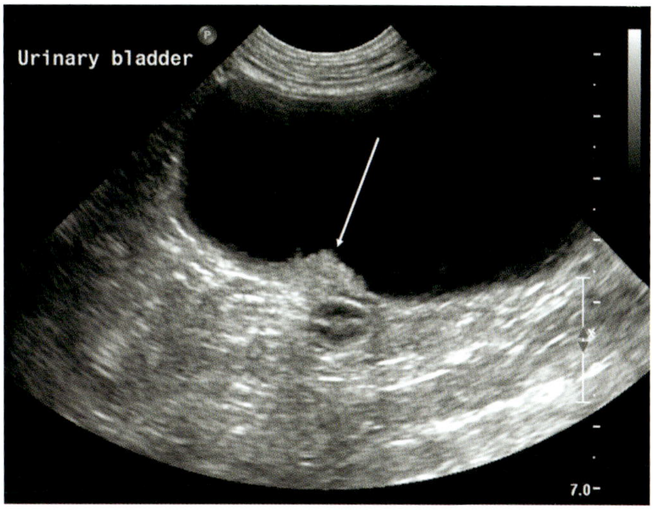

A)

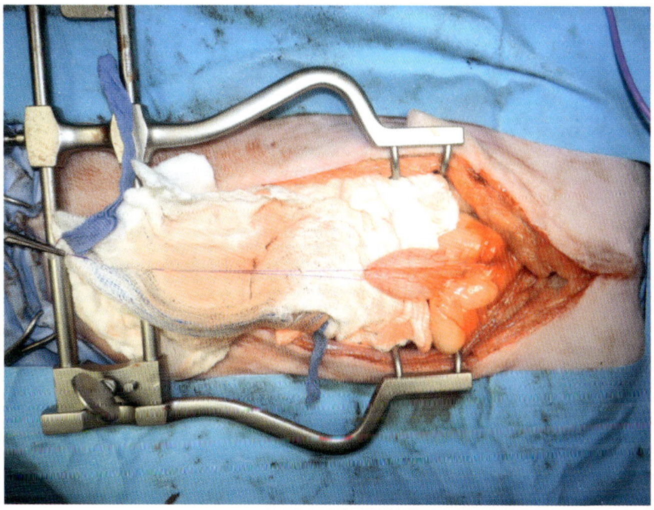

Surgical Technique (See Plate 28.1A, C–J) *continued*

C) The urinary bladder should be packed off from the rest of the abdominal contents using saline-soaked laparotomy sponges (pictured). Transitional cell carcinomas are a highly translocatable tumor, and seeding of the body wall or skin from contaminated urine, tissue, and instruments is a recognized risk with partial cystectomy (see step L).

D) A stay suture of 3-0 absorbable monofilament suture material is placed full thickness into the apex of the urinary bladder to facilitate manipulation of the urinary bladder.

E) The urinary bladder mass can usually be visualized and palpated (i), especially when the bladder is full. In some cases, cystoscopy can be done intraoperatively to transilluminate the urinary bladder wall to better visualize the extent of the mass. Further stay sutures are placed near the site of the proposed incision to help with orientation and manipulation of the urinary bladder after the bladder wall has been incised (ii, and see step C).

Plate 28.1

Partial Cystectomy *continued*

C)

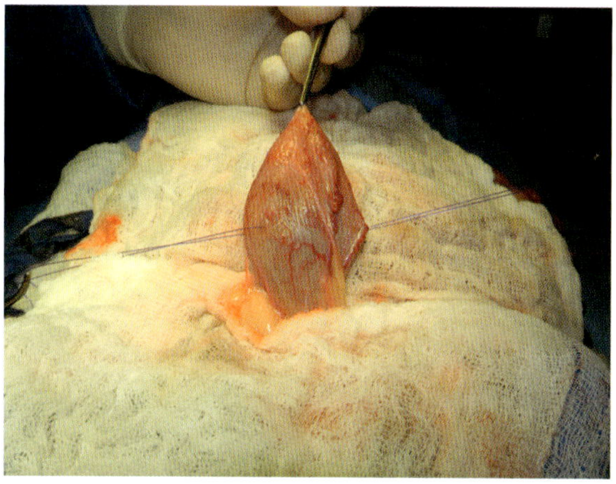

D)

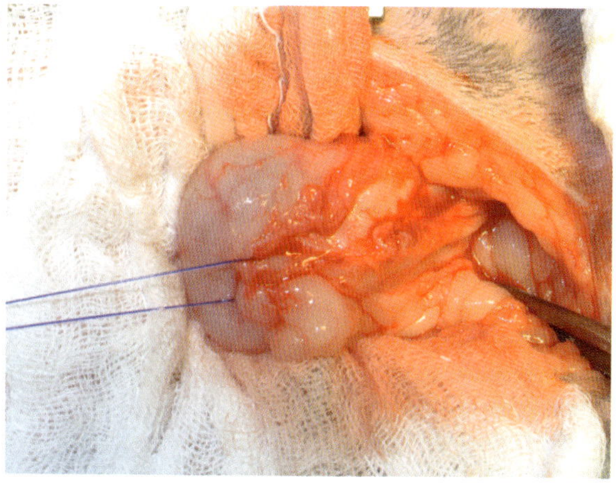

E-i)

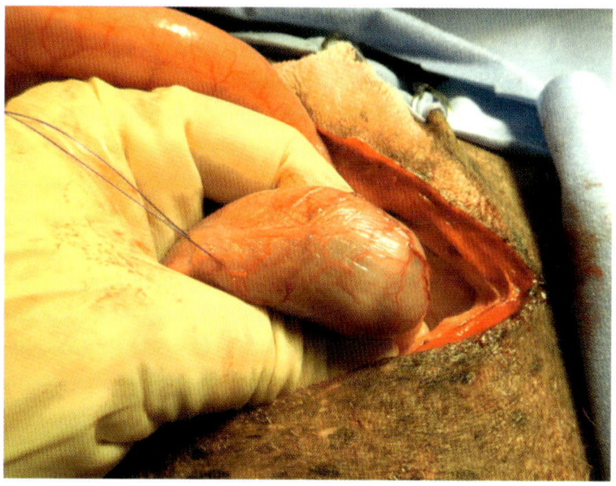

E-ii)

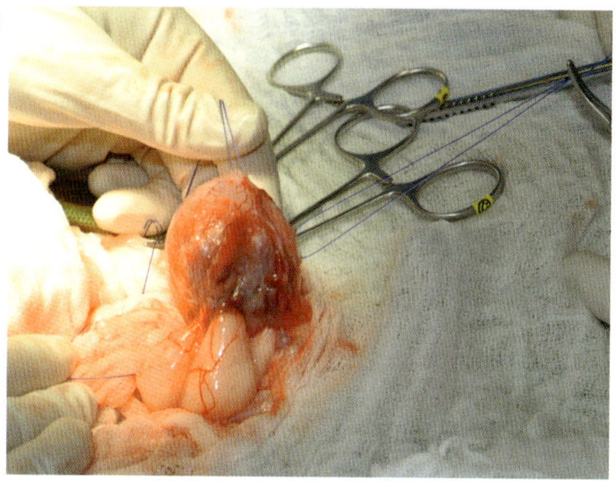

Surgical Technique (See Plate 28.1A, C–J) *continued*

F) A scalpel blade is used to incise the bladder 1–3 cm from visible and palpable margins of the tumor (i). This incision is then extended to allow intraluminal visualization of the urinary bladder mass (ii). The resection is continued circumferentially around the tumor with appropriate surgical margins to complete the resection (iii, iv). The specimen is removed from the surgical field, and instruments, gloves, and moistened laparotomy sponges are changed to minimize the risk of tumor seeding.

G) If the mass extends close to or involves the trigonal region (i), then the ureteric openings should be identified (ii). If there is unilateral involvement of one of the ureterovesicular junctions and the contralateral ureter and ureterovesicular junction can be preserved, then partial cystectomy can be combined with an ipsilateral en bloc ureteronephrectomy (see *27.1. Open Ureteronephrectomy*). If at least one ureterovesicular junction cannot be preserved, then the options include an intralesional resection that will result in preservation of the ureterovesicular junctions but macroscopic residual disease, partial cystectomy with reimplantation of the ureters (see step H), or conversion into a total cystectomy (see *28.2. Total Cystectomy*).

Plate 28.1

Partial Cystectomy *continued*

F-i)

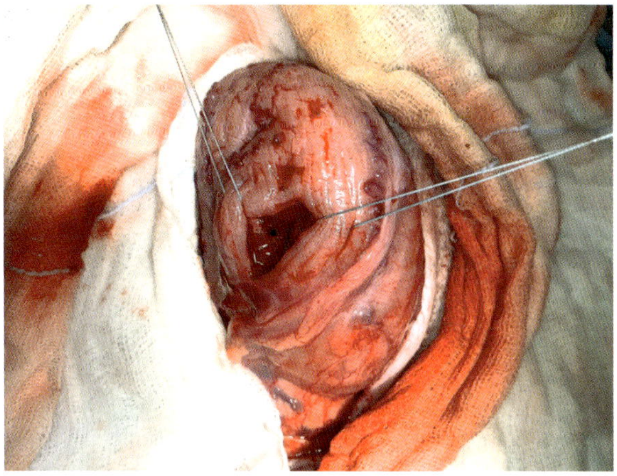

F-ii)

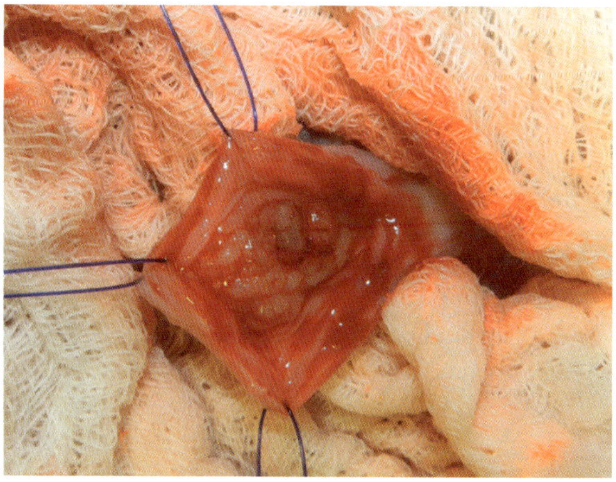

F-iii)

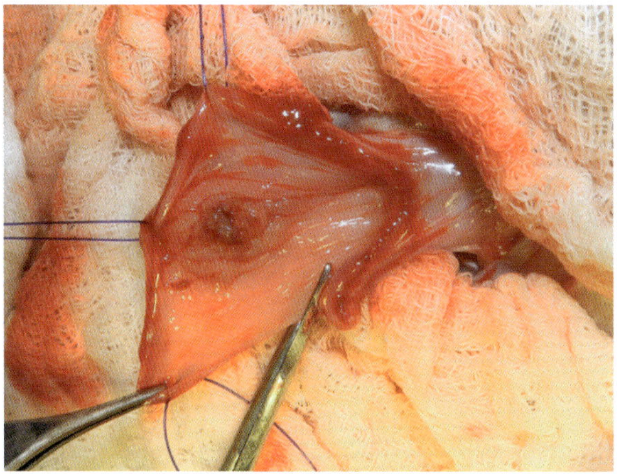

F-iv)

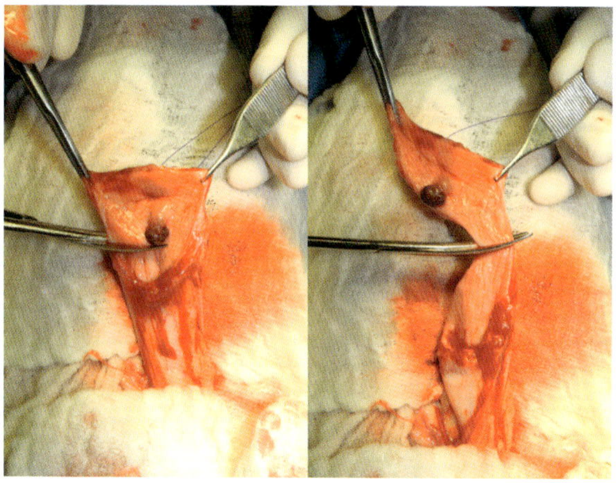

G-i)

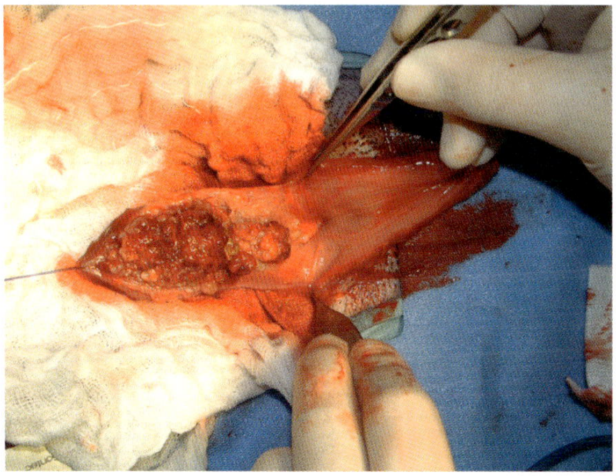

G-ii)

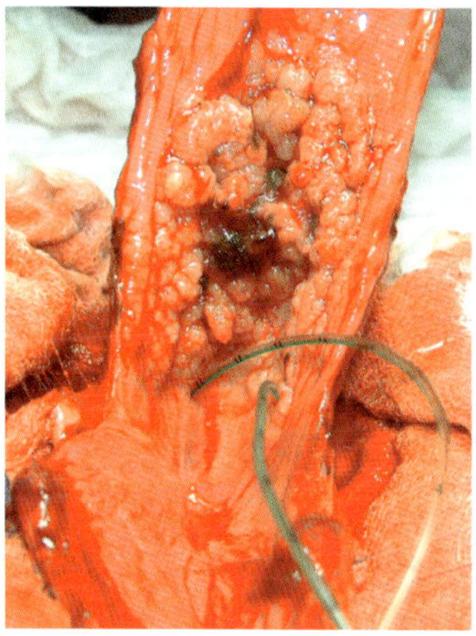

Surgical Technique (See Plate 28.1A, C–J) *continued*

H) For ureteral reimplantation, the ureter is transected 2 cm from the serosa of the urinary bladder (i, arrow, primary urinary bladder hemangiosarcoma). A stay suture of 5-0 to 3-0 absorbable monofilament suture material is placed in the ureteric wall (i, arrow), and mosquito forceps are bluntly passed through the intact bladder mucosa to grasp the suture material and pull the transected ureter through the urinary bladder wall into the lumen of the bladder (ii). The ureteral mucosa is then sutured to the urinary bladder mucosa with three to four simple interrupted sutures of 4-0 or 5-0 absorbable monofilament suture material (iii, arrow).

I) The urinary bladder wall is closed in two layers with 3-0 or 4-0 absorbable monofilament suture material in a simple continuous suture pattern in the mucosal-submucosal layer and 3-0 or 4-0 absorbable monofilament suture material in either a simple continuous or continuous Cushing suture pattern in the seromuscular layer (pictured).

J) In patients with an apical bladder mass, a partial cystectomy can be performed with a thoracoabdominal (TA) stapler. Ideally, cystoscopy will have identified the mass to be small and discrete with minimal circumferential mucosal change, and this is palpably confirmed at surgery. The TA stapler is applied transversely across the bladder caudal to the apical tumor, Doyen forceps are applied between the TA stapler and the apical bladder mass, and a scalpel blade is used to perform a partial cystectomy along the stapler cartridge. The Doyen bowel clamp can be used to minimize the risk of surgical field contamination from urine or potential tumor cells. Similar to stapled intestinal anastomoses, the stapled bladder wall should not need reinforcing.

K) The linea alba, subcutaneous tissue, and skin are closed as described in *15.1. Ventral Midline Celiotomy*.

Postoperative Management

1) Multimodal analgesia
2) Elizabethan collar or body suit
3) ± Indwelling urethral catheter for 24 hours
4) Frequent walks (every 2–4 hours) in the immediate postoperative period because of smaller bladder volume

Complications – Dogs [1]

Intraoperative Complications

- Hemorrhage (3%)

Postoperative Complications (See Plate 28.1L)

- Overall: 43%
- Transient urinary incontinence (31%)
- Tumor seeding (L) (11%)
- Stranguria (5%)
- Urethral obstruction (5%)
- Uroabdomen (3%)
- Ureteral obstruction (3%)
- Pollakiuria (3%)
- Aspiration pneumonia (3%)

Plate 28.1

Partial Cystectomy *continued*

H-i)

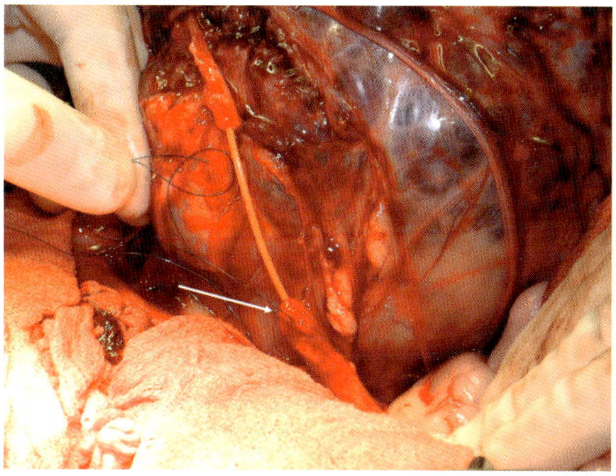

H-ii)

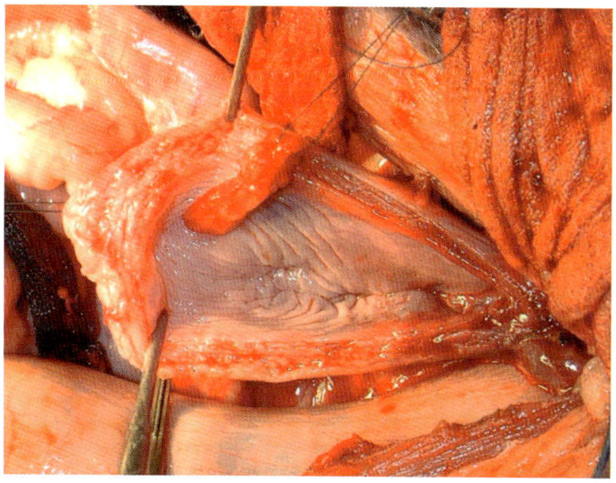

H-iii)

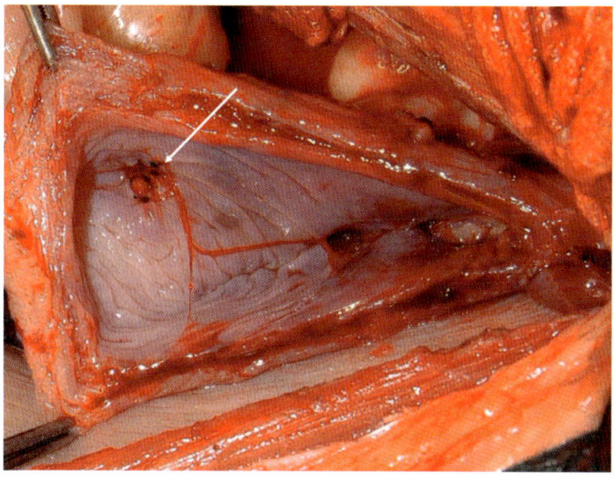

I)

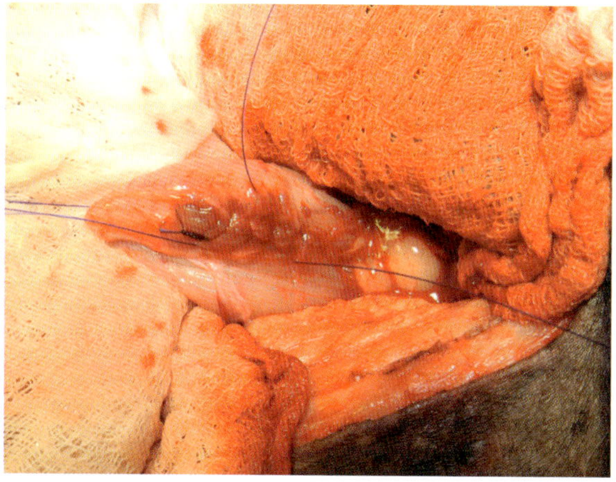

L)

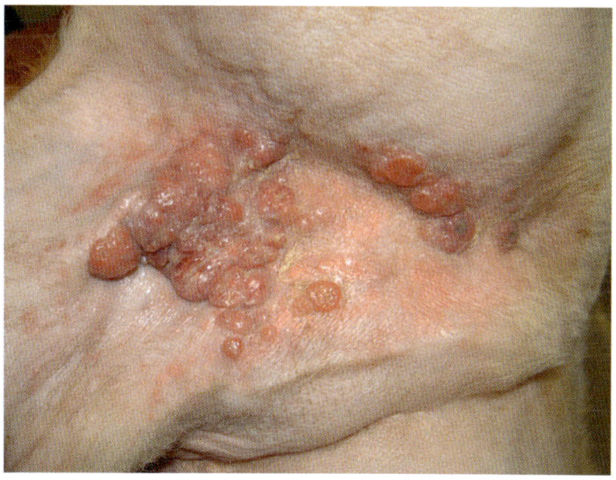

Complications – Cats [2, 3]

Postoperative Complications

- Septic peritonitis (10%)
- Uroabdomen (7%)
- Transient urinary incontinence (3%)
- Hematuria (3%)
- Stranguria (3%)

Suggested Adjuvant Treatments

- Nonsteroidal anti-inflammatory drug [1, 2]
- ± Chemotherapy [1, 2]
- ± Intensity-modulated radiation therapy in dogs with local recurrence [4]

Prognosis and Oncologic Outcome – Dogs

	Local Recurrence Rate	Metastatic Rate	Disease-Free Interval (d)	Median Survival Time (d)	1-Year Survival Rate	2-Year Survival Rate
			Transitional Cell Carcinoma [1]			
Overall	76% – local recurrence	36%–69%	235	348	–	–
	11% – tumor seeding	–	–	–	–	–
	19% – local extension into urethra or prostate	–	–	–	–	–
			Age at diagnosis			
≤11 yr	–	–	–	292	–	–
>11 yr	–	–	–	616	–	–
			Tumor location			
Trigone	–	–	–	353	–	–
Other location	–	–	–	235	–	–
			Depth of resection			
Partial	–	–	–	220	–	–
Full	–	–	–	418	–	–
			Piroxicam frequency			
Every 24 hr	–	–	–	772	–	–
Every 48 hr	–	–	–	254	–	–

Prognosis and Oncologic Outcome – Cats

	Local Recurrence Rate	Metastatic Rate	Disease-Free Interval (d)	Median Survival Time (d)	1-Year Survival Rate	2-Year Survival Rate
			Transitional Cell Carcinoma [2, 3]			
Overall	56%	21%	116 – local recurrence or progression	155	–	–
	–	–	176 – metastasis	–	–	–
			Treatment type			
Untreated	29%	–	–	46	7%	2%
Medical	79%	–	–	176	0%	0%
Partial cystectomy	64%	–	–	294	28%	8%

References

1 Marvel, S.J., Séguin, B., Dailey, D.D. et al. (2017). Clinical outcome of partial cystectomy for transitional cell carcinoma of the canine bladder. *Vet. Comp. Oncol.* 15 (4): 1417–1427.

2 Griffin, M.A., Culp, W.T.N., Giuffrida, M.A. et al. (2020). Lower urinary tract transitional cell carcinoma in cats: clinical findings, treatments, and outcomes in 118 cases. *J. Vet. Intern. Med.* 34 (1): 274–282.

3 Wilson, H.M., Chun, R., Larson, V.S. et al. (2007). Clinical signs, treatments, and outcome in cats with transitional cell carcinoma of the urinary bladder: 20 cases (1990–2004). *J. Am. Vet. Med. Assoc.* 231 (1): 101–106.

4 Nolan, M.W., Kogan, L., Griffin, L.R. et al. (2012). Intensity-modulated and image-guided radiation therapy for treatment of genitourinary carcinomas in dogs. *J. Vet. Intern. Med.* 26 (4): 987–995.

28.2 Total Cystectomy

Indications (See Plate 28.2 – 1)

1) Resection of extensive urinary bladder tumors, typically involving the body and neck of the urinary bladder ± proximal urethra ± prostate (i, ii, both transitional cell carcinomas)
2) Total cystectomy can be combined with sublumbar lymph node resection (see *20.1. Open Sublumbar Lymph Node Resection*) when enlarged or metastatic sublumbar lymph nodes are present

Suggested Diagnostic Workup and Clinical Staging

- See *28.1. Partial Cystectomy*.

Patient Positioning

The patient is positioned in dorsal recumbency.

Surgical Technique (See Plate 28.2A, C)

A) A ventral midline celiotomy is performed (see *15.1. Ventral Midline Celiotomy*) with the incision extending to the pubic brim. The penis or vulva should be draped into the surgical field because access may be needed for intraoperative catheterization.

B) The ventral ligament of the bladder is incised with either scissors or a vessel sealing device to allow the bladder to be mobilized to one side or the other (not pictured).

C) The ureters are transected at a macroscopically and palpably normal level, at least 2 cm from the serosa of the urinary bladder. Stay sutures of 5-0 suture are placed in each of the ureters (i), and the open ends of the ureters are wrapped in moistened laparotomy sponges. Alternatively, if an end-to-end ureterovaginal anastomosis is to be performed (see step I), the ureters should be catheterized to aid in spatulation, side-to-side ureteral anastomosis, and end-to-end ureterovaginal anastomosis (ii, long forceps being passed through the cervix and exiting the vagina to grasp two catheters; iii, the catheters are drawn into the abdominal cavity and inserted into the lumens of both ureters). The catheters can also be used as ureteral stents in the immediate postoperative period.

Color Atlas of Canine and Feline Surgical Oncology, First Edition. Julius M. Liptak, Paolo Buracco, William T. N. Culp, and Nicholas J. Bacon.

Plate 28.2

Total Cystectomy

1-i)

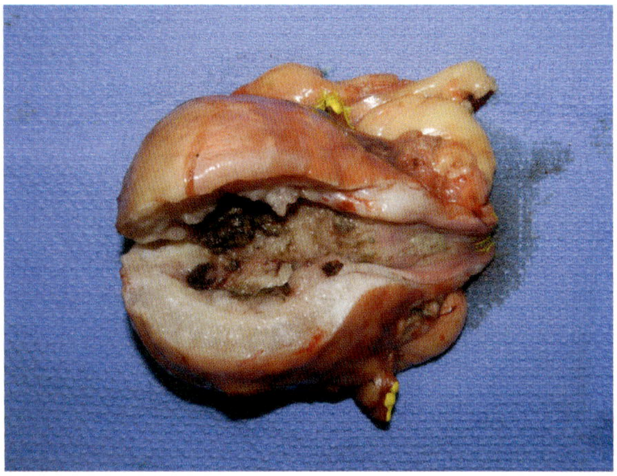

1-ii)

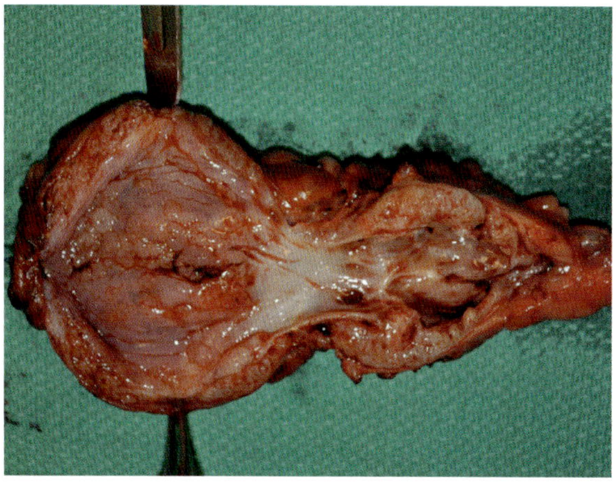

A)

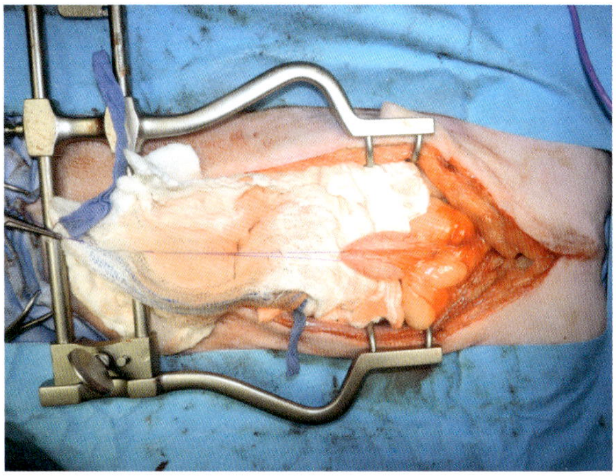

C-i)

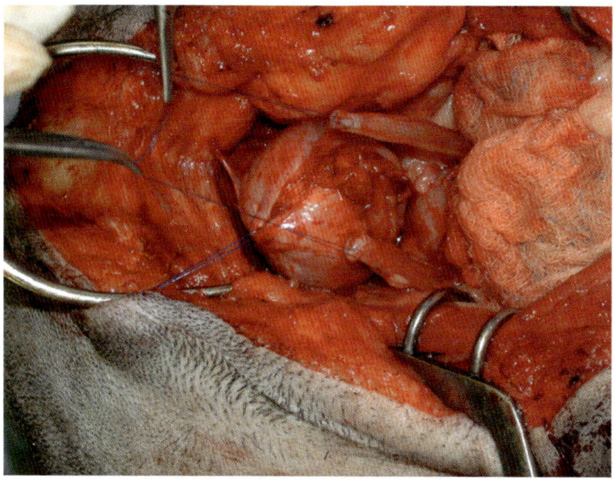

C-ii)

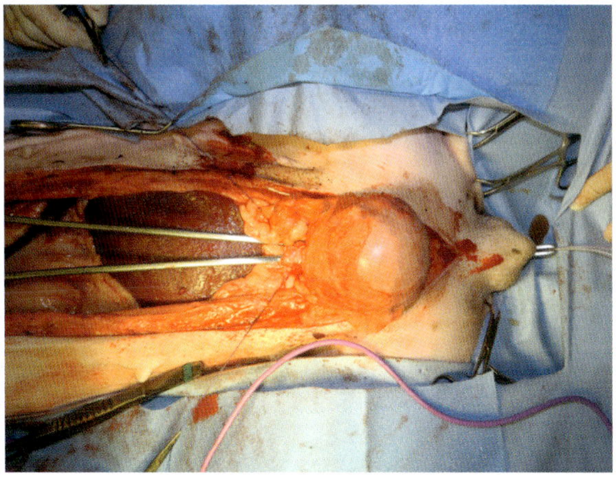

C-iii)

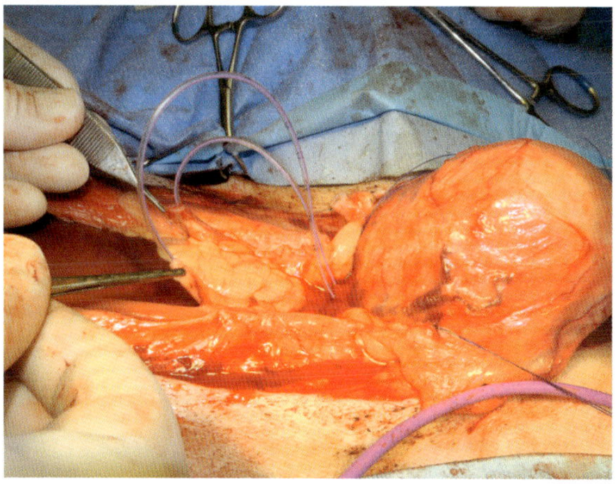

Total Cystectomy with Uretero-Vaginal Anastomosis in Female Dogs [1] (See Plate 28.2D, F, I)

D) The urethra is dissected free of local attachments in the pelvic canal with blunt dissection or a vessel sealing device as far caudally as the vestibule (arrow).
E) The urethra is clamped, ligated, and transected at this level if the urethra is palpably normal (not pictured). The vaginal branch of the internal iliac artery should be preserved. The bladder and urethra are removed from the surgical field. Instruments, gloves, and moistened laparotomy sponges are changed to minimize the risk of tumor seeding.
F) If the dog is intact (i), then an ovariohysterectomy is performed to the level of the cervix (ii, two stay sutures are placed in the cervix; iii, a scalpel blade is used to complete the ovariohysterectomy; iv, completed ovariohysterectomy).
G) Two openings are made through the vaginal wall with a 3-mm punch biopsy (not pictured).
H) The ureters are passed through these openings and anastomosed to the vagina using 5-0 absorbable monofilament suture material in a simple interrupted pattern (not pictured).
I) Alternatively, the medial aspects of the distal ureters are spatulated for approximately 1 cm (i, arrow) and sutured side to side to create a larger-diameter distal opening in a Y shape (ii). The single distal end of the cojoined ureters is either passed through a single opening into the vagina and anastomosed to the vagina using 5-0 absorbable monofilament suture material in a simple interrupted pattern, or an end-to-end ureterovaginal anastomosis is performed using 5-0 to 3-0 absorbable monofilament suture material in a simple interrupted pattern (iii).

Total Cystectomy in Male Dogs (See Plate 28.2J–T)

J) A stay suture of 3-0 absorbable monofilament suture material is placed full thickness into the apex of the urinary bladder, and the urinary bladder is then tractioned cranially. The lateral ligaments of the urinary bladder are transected bilaterally with Metzenbaum scissors or a vessel sealing device; the cranial vesicular vessels are ligated with a simple ligature using 4-0 to 3-0 absorbable monofilament suture material or a vessel sealing device; and each vas deferens is transected close to the prostate with a vessel sealing device or cautery (pictured).

Plate 28.2

Total Cystectomy *continued*

D)

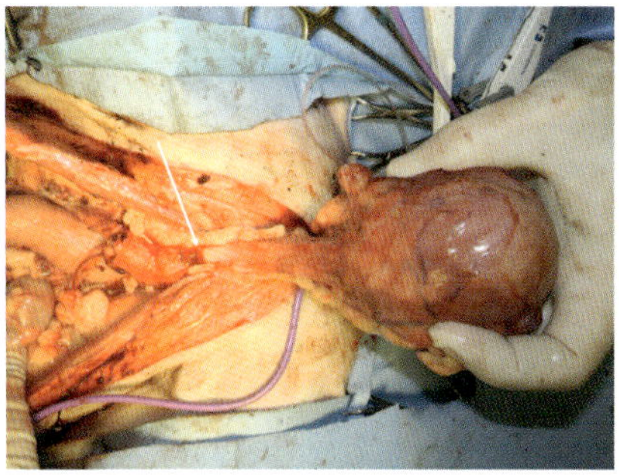

F-i)

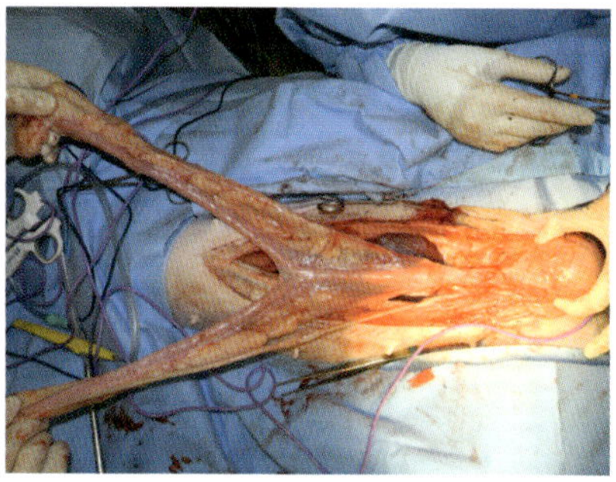

F-ii)

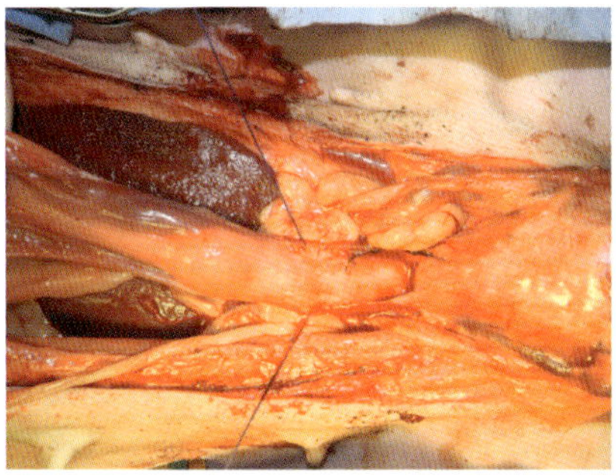

F-iii)

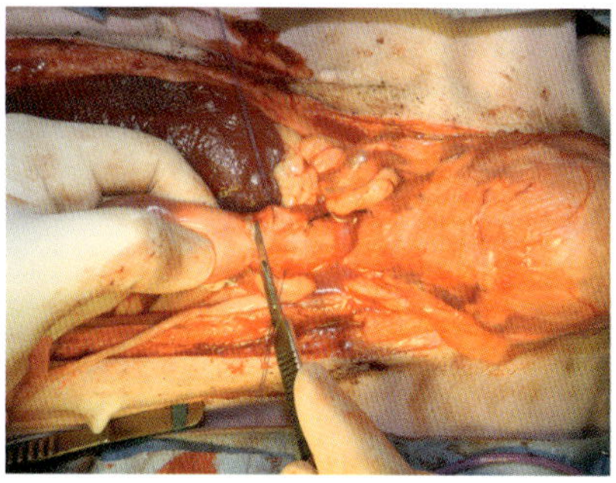

F-iv)

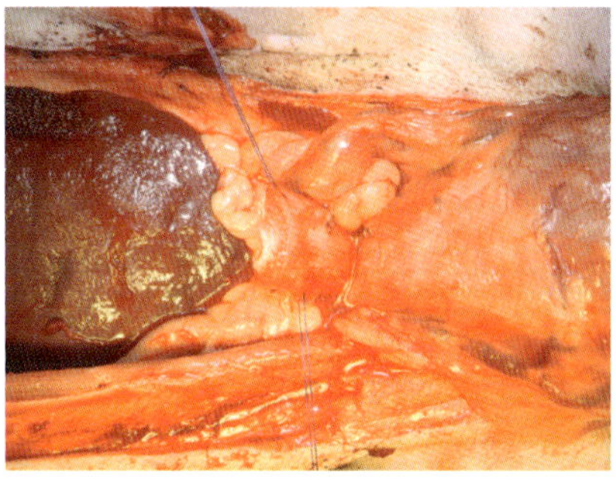

I-i)

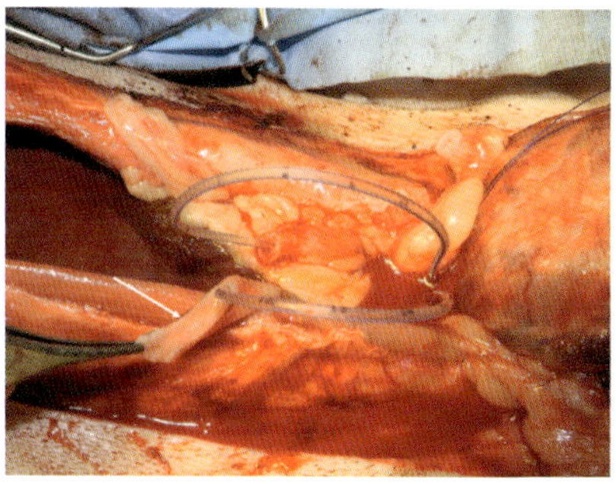

I-ii)

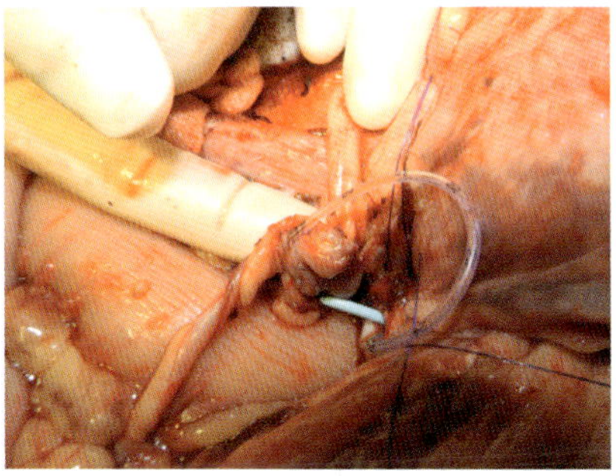

I-iii)

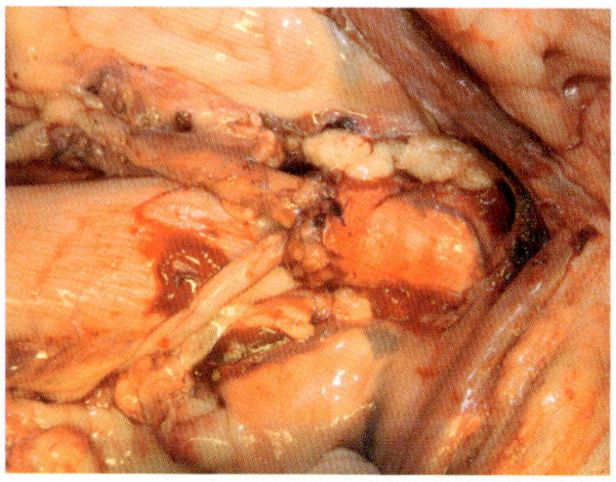

J)

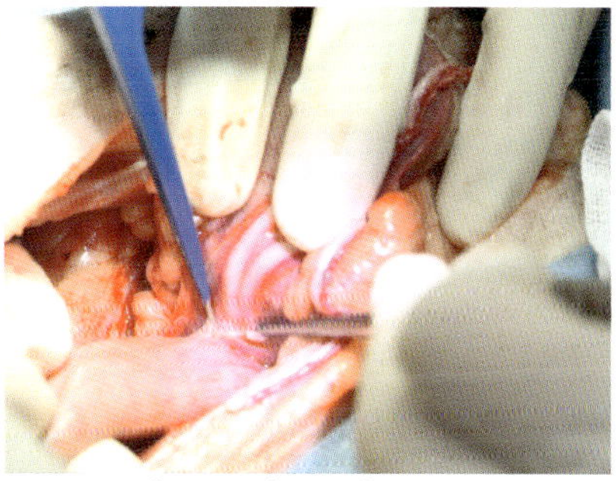

Courtesy of Dr. Ryohei Nishimura

Total Cystectomy in Male Dogs (See Plate 28.2J–T) *continued*

K) The pelvic urethra and prostate are dissected caudally, separating the peritoneal attachments between the prostate and rectum with blunt dissection or a vessel sealing device. This is continued as far caudally into the pelvic canal as possible.

L) **Total cystectomy with uretero-preputial anastomosis in male dogs [1]:** The ventral midline of the prepuce is incised caudally to the level of the perineum (i). The bladder, prostate, urethra, and penis are removed en bloc (ii, iii). A castration is performed if the dog is intact.

M) Two openings are made through the dorsal aspect of the prepuce with a 3-mm punch biopsy. The location of these openings is determined by the length of the remaining ureters gently arcing across the abdominal cavity.

Plate 28.2

Total Cystectomy *continued*

K)

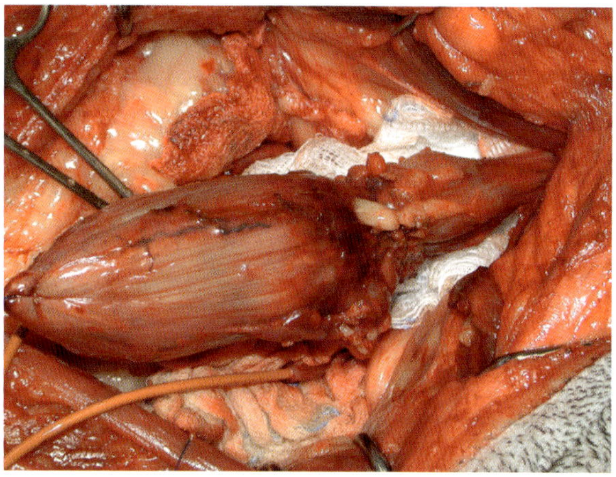

L-i)

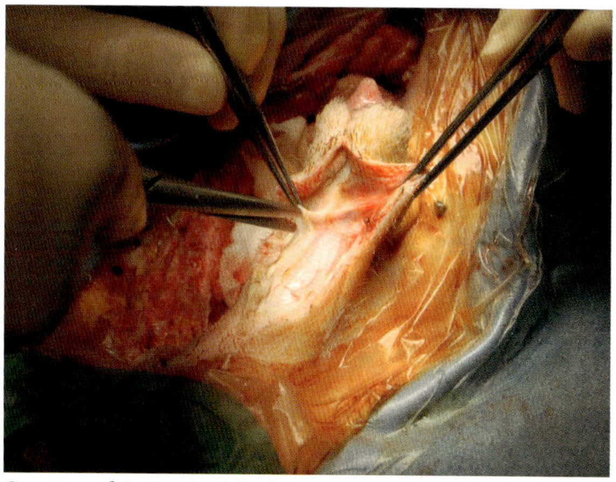

Courtesy of Dr. Ryohei Nishimura

L-ii)

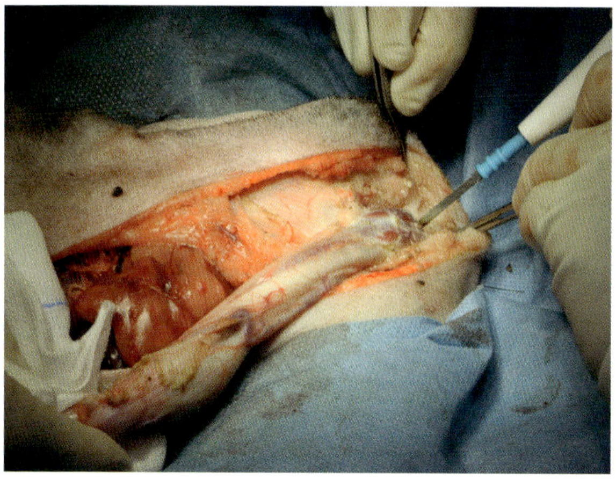

L-iii)

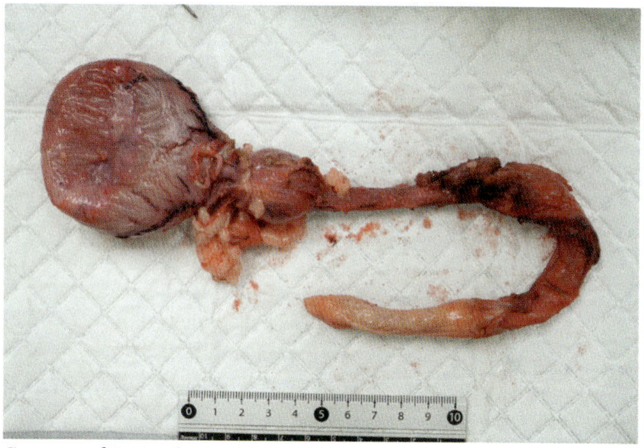

Courtesy of Dr. Ryohei Nishimura

M)

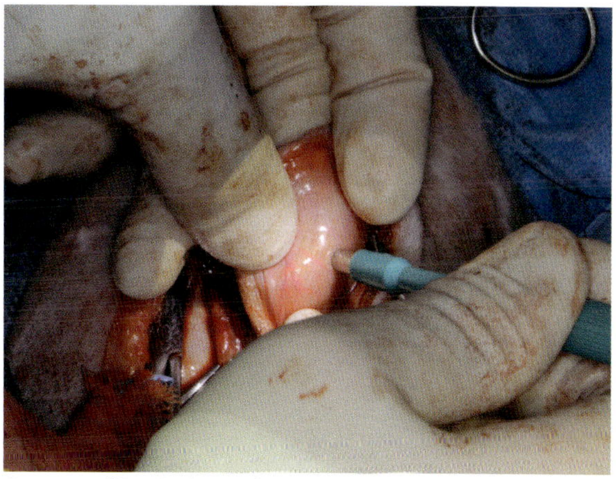

Courtesy of Dr. Ryohei Nishimura

Total Cystectomy in Male Dogs (See Plate 28.2J–T) *continued*

N) Two paramedian openings are created in the abdominal wall with a combination of sharp and blunt dissection (i, arrows). The ends of the ureters are gently grasped and pulled through the openings in the abdominal wall (i) and into the preputial orifice (ii, iii). The ureters are sutured to the preputial mucosa using 5-0 absorbable monofilament suture material in a simple interrupted pattern (iv, v).

O) **Total cystectomy with uretero-preputial anastomosis in male dogs [2]:** The retractor penis, bulbospongiosus, and ischiocavernosus muscles are identified through a perineal skin incision, and the ischiocavernosus muscles are elevated off the ischiatic tuberosities with a periosteal elevator (pictured).

P) The deep artery and vein of the penis are identified and preserved in the pelvic floor as they exit the pelvic canal caudally on either side of the midline (arrows).

Q) The penis is dissected free with blunt dissection (i, ii) or a vessel sealing device to the level of the os penis, but the penis within the prepuce and prepuce are untouched to preserve the dorsal penile vessels.

Plate 28.2

Total Cystectomy *continued*

N-i)

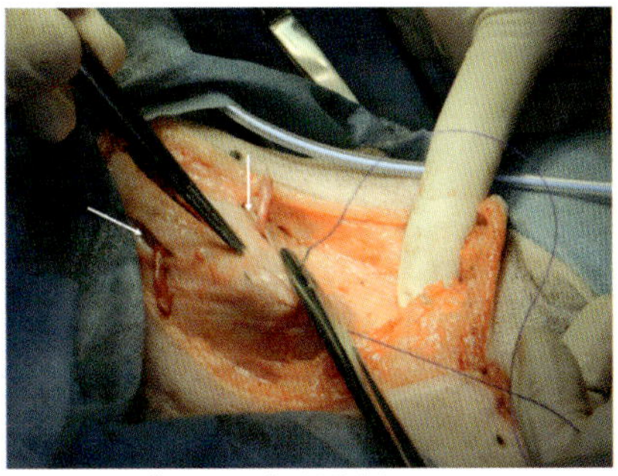

Courtesy of Dr. Ryohei Nishimura

N-ii)

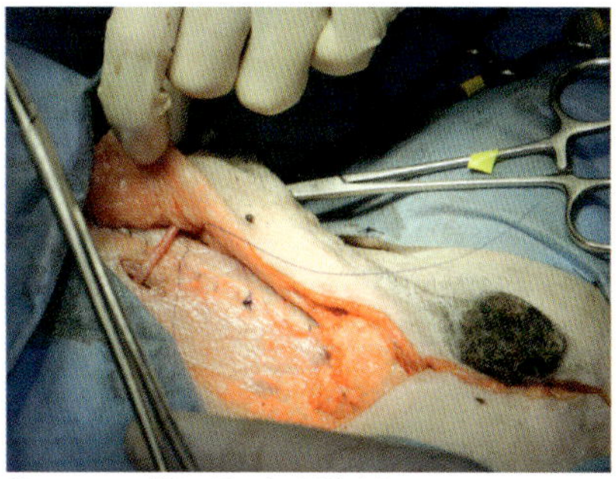

Courtesy of Dr. Ryohei Nishimura

N-iii)

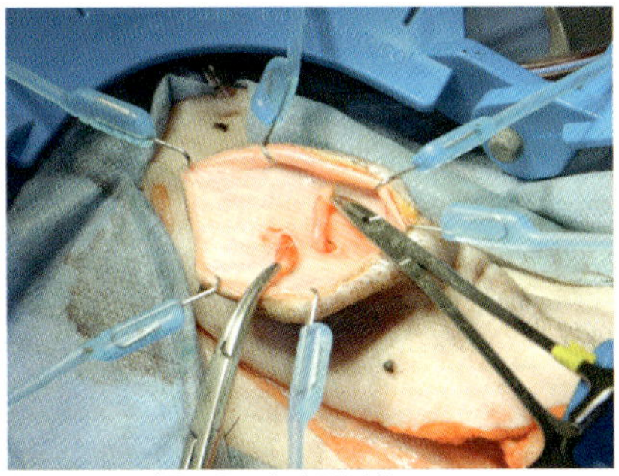

Courtesy of Dr. Ryohei Nishimura

N-iv)

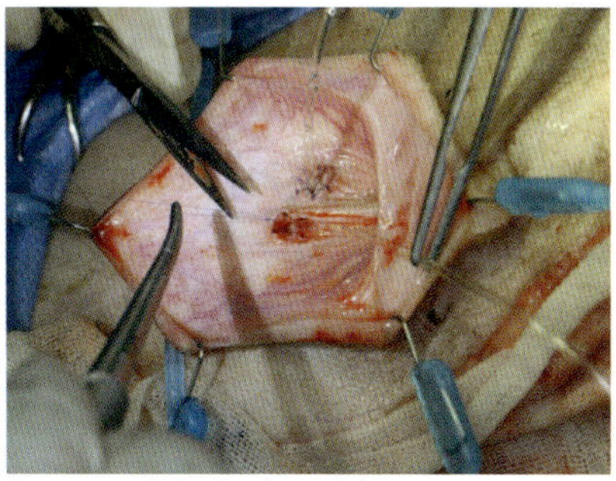

Courtesy of Dr. Ryohei Nishimura

N-v)

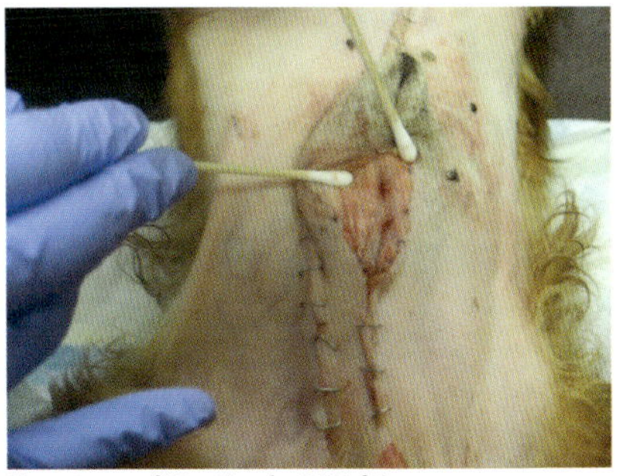

Courtesy of Dr. Ryohei Nishimura

O)

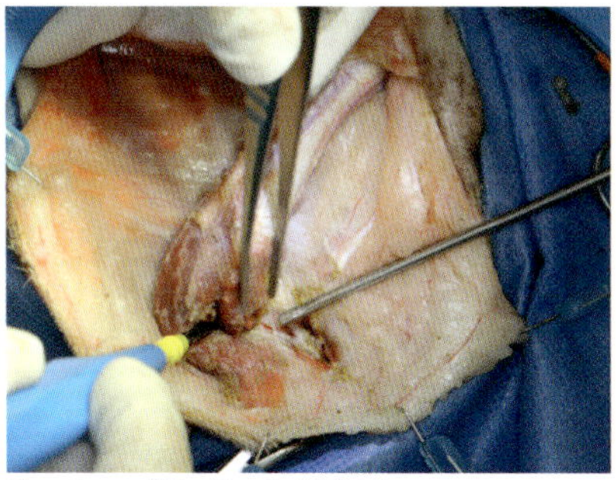

Courtesy of Dr. Ryohei Nishimura

P)

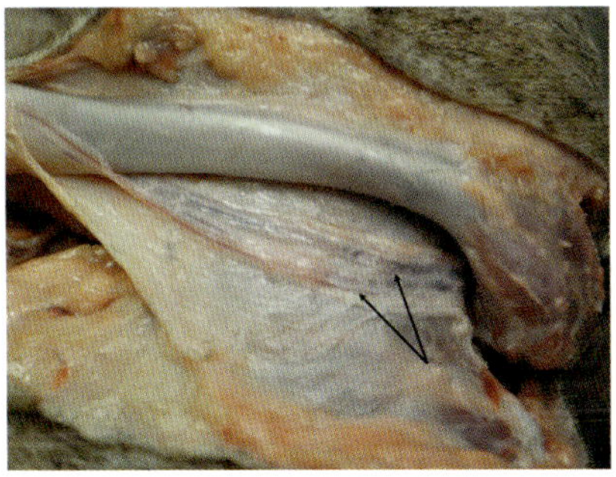

Q-i)

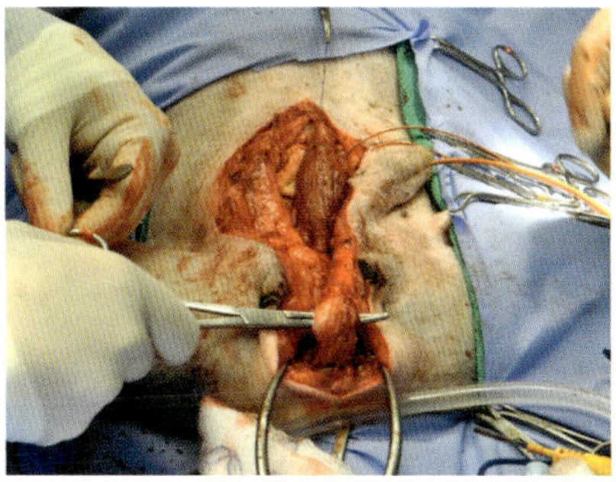

Q-ii)

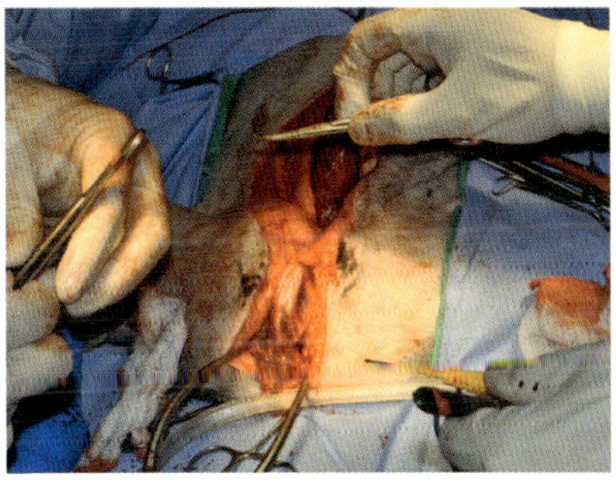

Total Cystectomy in Male Dogs (See Plate 28.2J–T) *continued*

R) The penile body is transected caudal to the scrotal remnant (i), and the urinary bladder, prostate, urethra, and penis are removed en bloc (ii).
S) The medial aspects of the distal ureters are spatulated for approximately 1 cm and sutured side to side to create a larger-diameter distal opening in a Y shape (i). The penile remnant is then diverted into the abdomen across the abdominal wall (ii, arrow). The single distal end of the cojoined uereters is anastomosed to the penile urethra using 5-0 absorbable monofilament suture material in a simple interrupted pattern (ii).
T) The connective sheath of the penis is anchored to the linea alba (arrow), and the uretero-urethral anastomosis is omentalized within the abdominal cavity.

Total Cystectomy with Cutaneous Ureterostomy [3]

U) The abdominal wall is incised bilaterally with a scalpel blade lateral to the rectus abdominus muscle. An oblique tunnel of 3–4 cm in length is created parallel to the line alba with hemostats (arrows), and the skin is incised over the end of the hemostats.
V) The ureters are passed through these tunnels, and the distal ends are spatulated and sutured to the skin (arrows) using 5-0 absorbable or nonabsorbable monofilament suture material in a simple interrupted pattern.
W) A total cystectomy is then performed as described earlier for female (see steps D and E) or male (see steps J and K) dogs.

Closure

The linea alba, subcutaneous tissue, and skin are closed as described in *15.1. Ventral Midline Celiotomy*. For male dogs with a uretero-preputial anastomosis, the preputial orifice is sutured to the ventral abdominal skin to create a wide drainage board.

Postoperative Management

1) Multimodal analgesia
2) Elizabethan collar or body suit
3) ± Indwelling urethral catheter for 72–96 hours
4) Skin care and daily cleaning due to complete urinary incontinence

Complications – Dogs [1–6]

Postoperative Complications

- Urinary incontinence (100%)
- Hematuria (26%)
- Ureterostomy dehiscence with subsequent uroabdomen (21%)
- Pyelonephritis (16%)
- Oliguria (11%)
- Azotemia (11%) [1, 5]
- Urine scald (5%) [3]

Suggested Adjuvant Treatments

- See *28.1. Partial Cystectomy*.
- Dogs treated with total cystectomy will have urinary incontinence, and hence treatment with chemotherapeutic agents that are excreted through the urinary system are not recommended because of environmental contamination and risk to the owner.

Plate 28.2

Total Cystectomy *continued*

R-i)

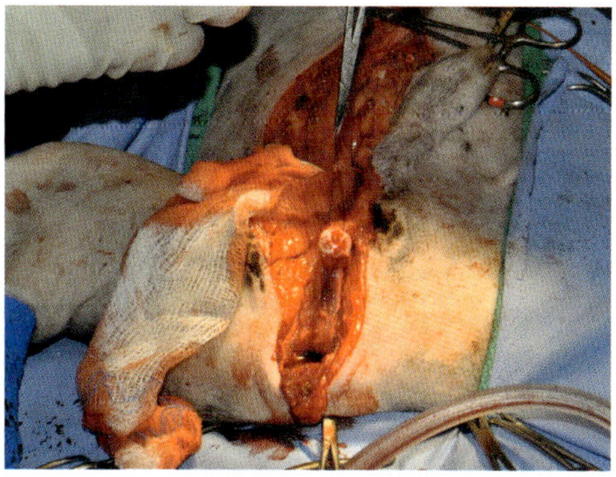

R-ii)

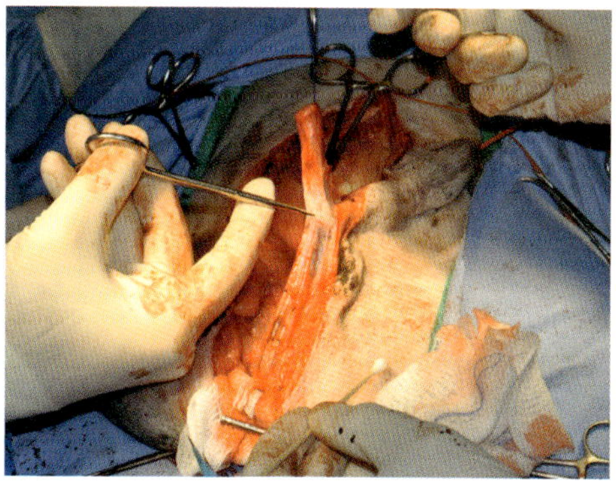

S-i)

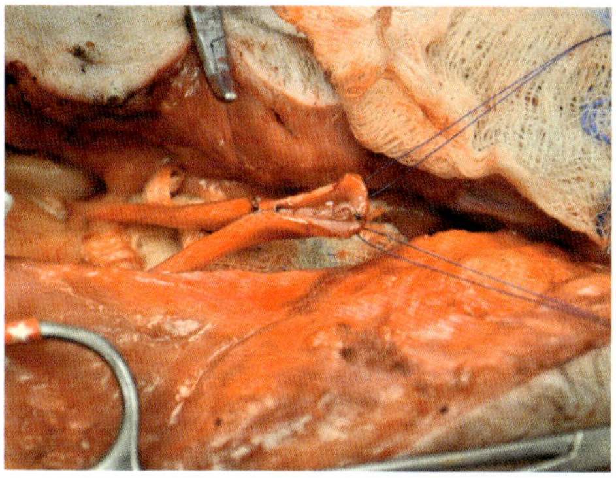

S-ii)

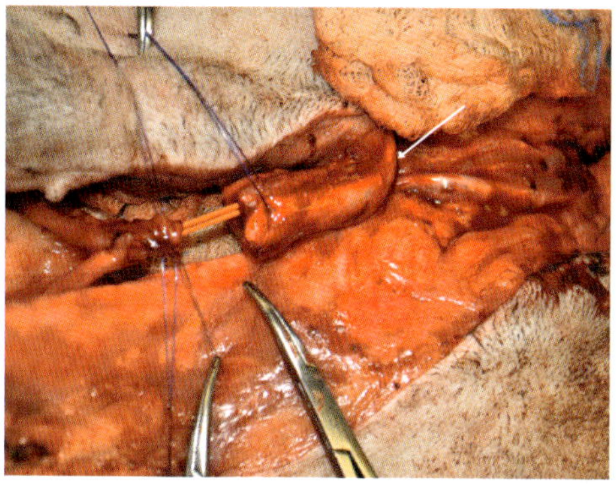

T)

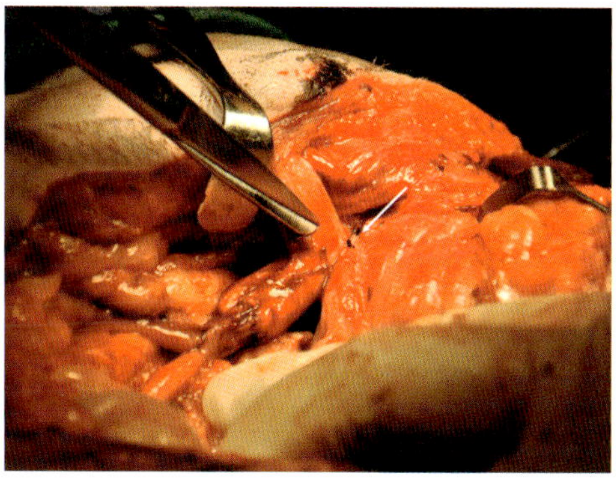

U)

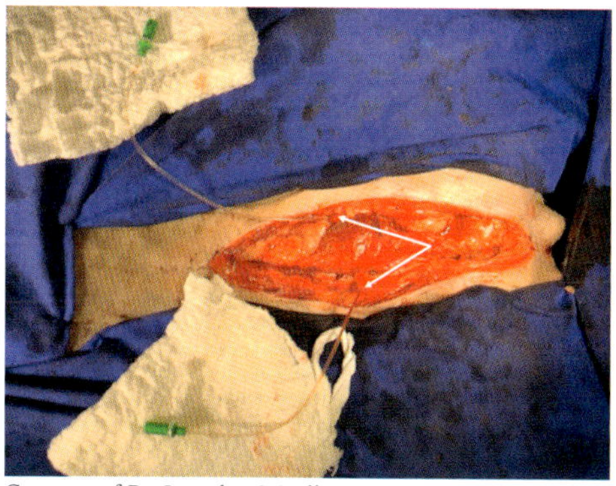

Courtesy of Dr. Leandro Crivellenti

V)

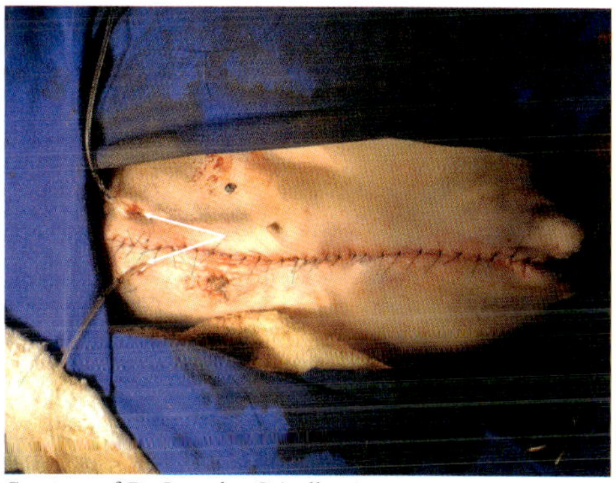

Courtesy of Dr. Leandro Crivellenti

Chapter 29: Cystostomy Tube

Indications

1) Palliation of obstruction of the urinary bladder, prostate, or urethra, typically due to neoplasia or uroliths
2) Temporary urinary diversion after significant lower urinary trauma or surgery
3) Bladder decompression to manage reduced contractile function or to treat long-standing detrusor atony, reflex dyssynergia, or other neurologic conditions

Suggested Diagnostic Workup and Clinical Staging

- Complete blood count and serum biochemistry
- Urinalysis and urine culture
- Urethroscopy and cystoscopy for assessment of the location and extent of obstructive disease
- Retrograde urethrography for assessment of the location and extent of obstructive disease
- Abdominal ultrasound or precontrast and postcontrast computed tomography (CT) scan of the abdomen and pelvis for assessment of the obstructive disease and intra-abdominal metastasis
- Three-view thoracic radiographs or thoracic CT scan for assessment of lung metastasis

Patient Positioning

The patient is positioned in dorsal recumbency.

Surgical Technique – Open Approach (See Plate 29A, C, F–K)

A) A ventral midline celiotomy is performed (see *15.1. Ventral Midline Celiotomy*). The incision is typically from the umbilicus to the pubic brim with a parapenile incision in male dogs. When the linea alba is incised, it is extended caudally to the periosteum of the pubic brim.
B) The ventral ligament of the bladder is incised to allow the bladder to be mobilized (not pictured).
C) A full-thickness purse-string suture is preplaced toward the apex of the urinary bladder in the ventrolateral bladder wall with 3-0 (cats and small dogs) to 2-0 (medium to large dogs) monofilament absorbable material. The diameter of the purse-string suture is approximately 15–20 mm. The suture is not tightened and the ends are left loose.
D) At the level of the purse-string suture in the urinary bladder, large blunt-ended forceps are directed from the internal abdominal wall externally lateral to the ventral midline celiotomy (not pictured). They should punch through the body wall to the skin so that the skin is tented by the forceps, and then a scalpel blade is used to incise over the tented skin.
E) The forceps are then exited through the skin incision, opened to grasp the end of an appropriately sized Pezzer or Foley catheter (8–24 Fr) [1], and then drawn through the abdominal wall stoma and into the abdominal cavity (not pictured).
F) A stab incision is made in the center of the purses-string suture with a no. 11 scalpel blade, and the catheter tip is pushed into the lumen of the urinary bladder (i). If using a Foley catheter, the bulb is inflated with saline (ii, arrow). The purse-string is then gently tightened around the catheter (iii, arrow).

Color Atlas of Canine and Feline Surgical Oncology, First Edition. Julius M. Liptak, Paolo Buracco, William T. N. Culp, and Nicholas J. Bacon.

Plate 29

Cystostomy Tube

A)

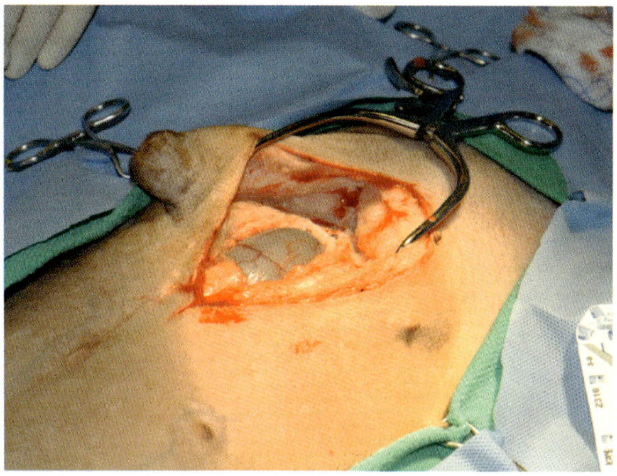

C)

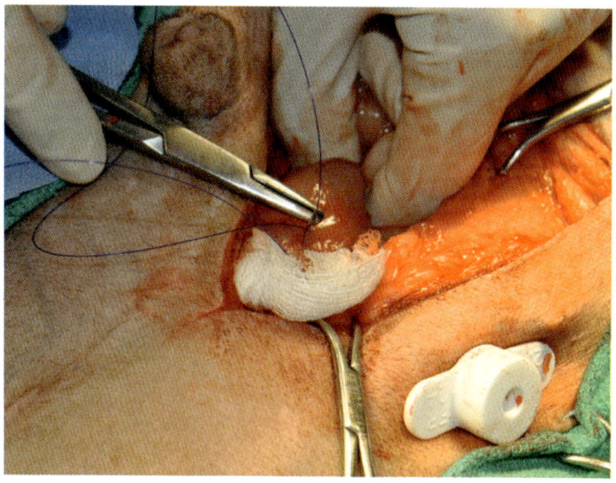

F-i)

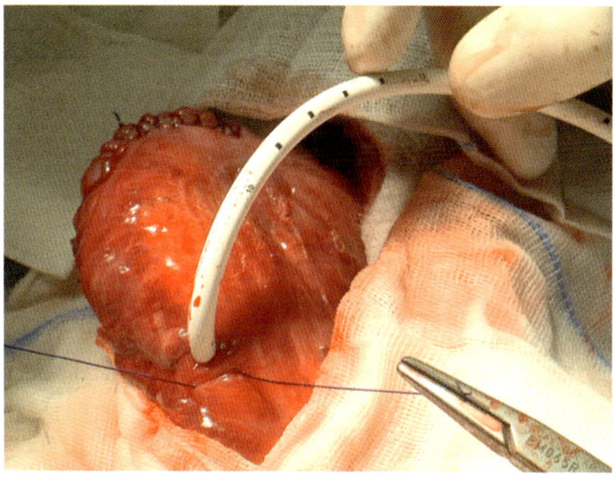

F-ii)

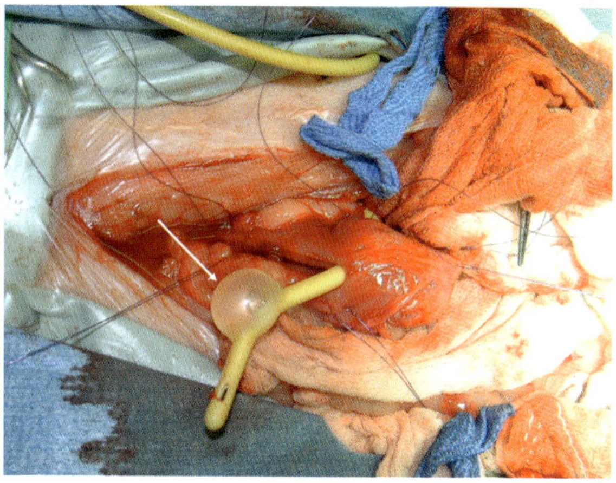

F-iii)

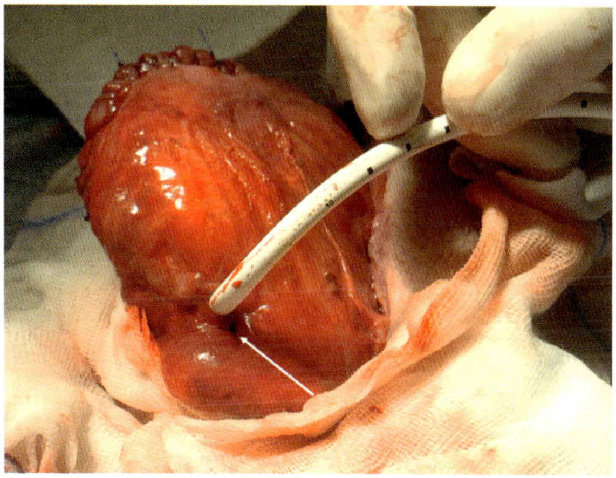

Surgical Technique – Open Approach (See Plate 29A, C, F–K) *continued*

G) The catheter is gently tractioned from externally to bring the urinary bladder up against the abdominal wall.

H) The urinary bladder is sutured to the abdominal wall using absorbable monofilament suture material in a simple interrupted or continuous suture pattern (see G). Omentum is then wrapped around the cystopexy site between the urinary bladder and abdominal wall.

I) The catheter is then fixed to the skin using a Chinese fingertrap suture pattern.

J) The catheter is connected to a passive closed-drainage urine collection bag or an active intermittent system (e.g. a three-way stopcock) and protected with a bandage.

K) For animals where a cystostomy tube is expected to be used for a long period of time, a commercially available low-profile gastrostomy tube can be used as a low-profile cystostomy tube instead of a Pezzer or Foley catheter (also see step C).

Plate 29

Cystostomy Tube *continued*

G)

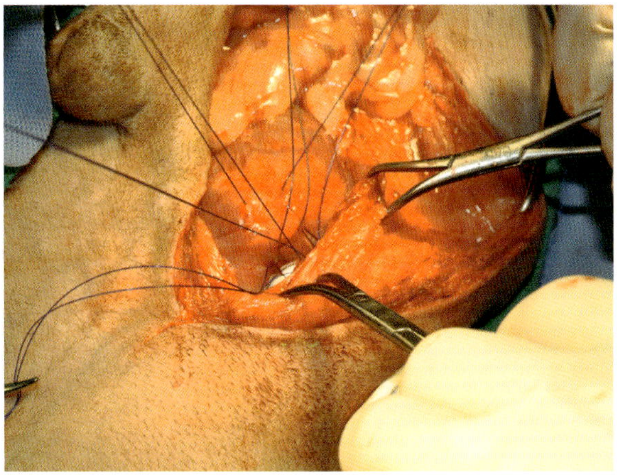

I)

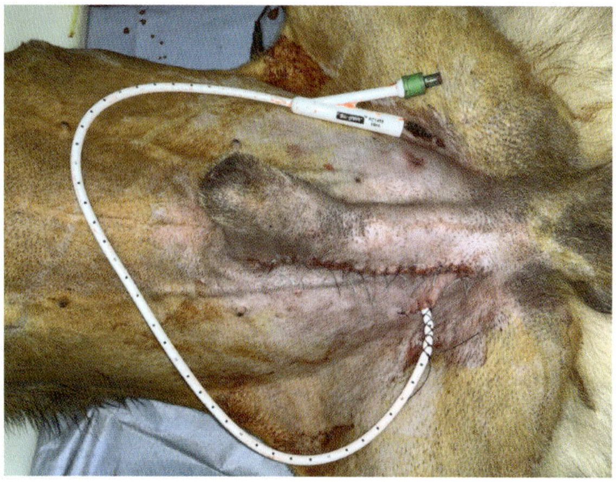

J)

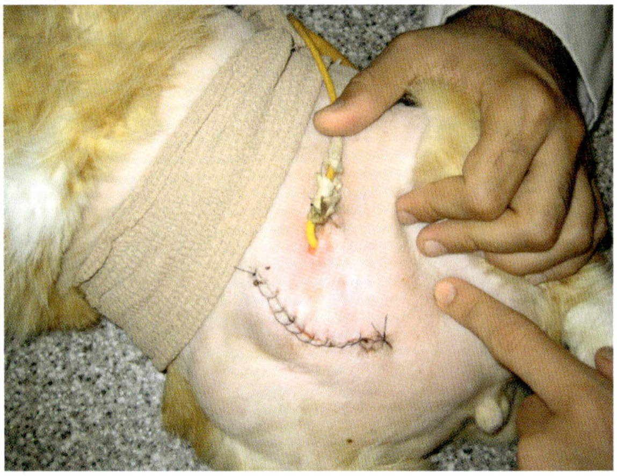

K)

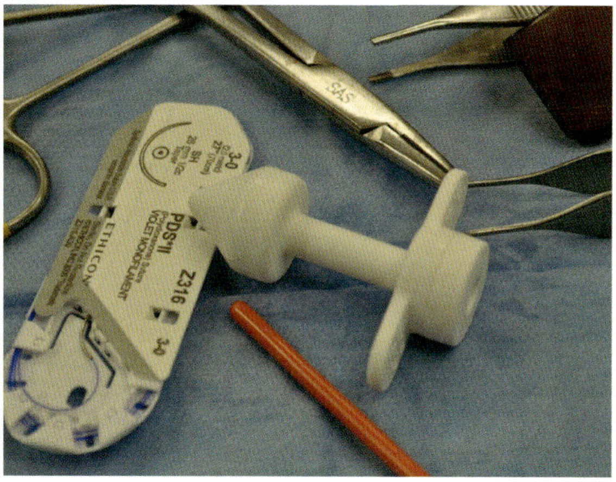

Surgical Technique – Minimally Invasive Inguinal Approach [2] (See Plate 29L–S)

L) The patient is positioned in lateral recumbency with the uppermost pelvic limb retracted caudally and secured. In larger dogs, the limb may also need to be abducted.

M) The caudal abdomen is balloted to find the urinary bladder, and then an oblique 2- to 3-cm-long skin incision is made over the site in the inguinal area, cranial to the inguinal flank fold.

N) The subcutaneous fat is dissected, and then the external fascia of the external abdominal oblique muscle is incised to expose the internal abdominal oblique muscle.

O) The underlying internal abdominal oblique and transversus abdominis muscles are then bluntly split in the directions of their fibers to expose the peritoneum. Paired orthogonal Gelpi retractors help with this dissection, including holding the surgical field open once the peritoneum is incised (pictured). The distended urinary bladder wall is typically pressed against the open peritoneal incision at this point (arrow); if not, it should be inflated with sterile saline via a urethral catheter.

P) A stab incision in the skin is made over a pair of forceps passed from the internal body wall (pictured), approximately 2–3 cm away from the existing surgical wound. A Foley catheter of adequate size is then passed through the skin into the abdomen.

Plate 29

Cystostomy Tube *continued*

L)

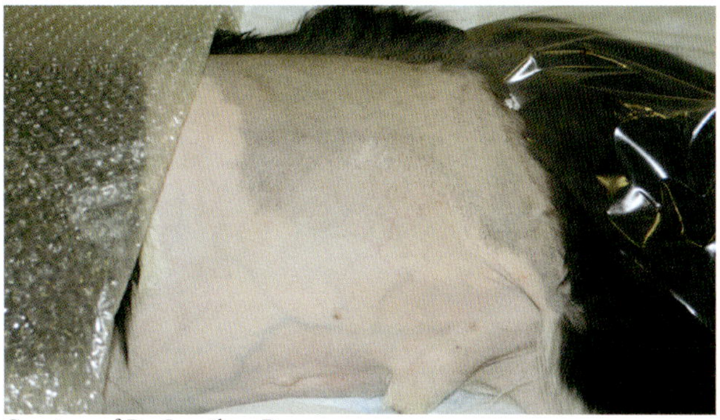

Courtesy of Dr. Jonathan Bray

M)

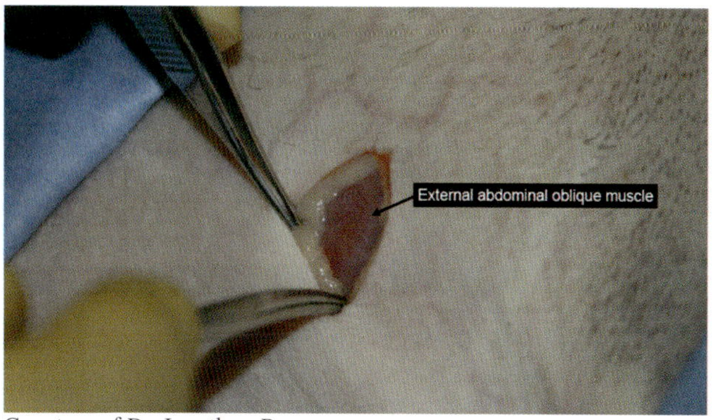

Courtesy of Dr. Jonathan Bray

N)

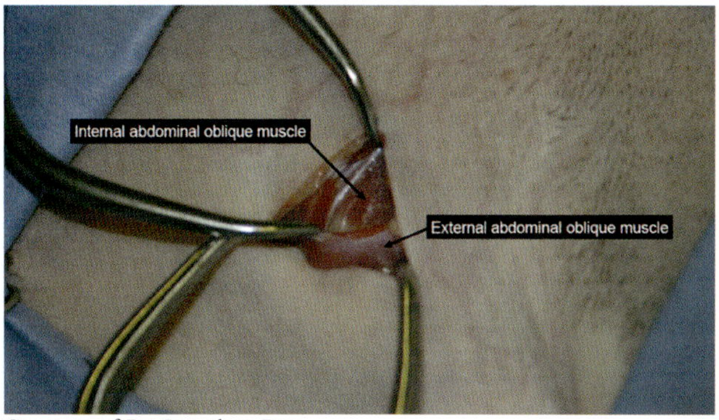

Courtesy of Dr. Jonathan Bray

O)

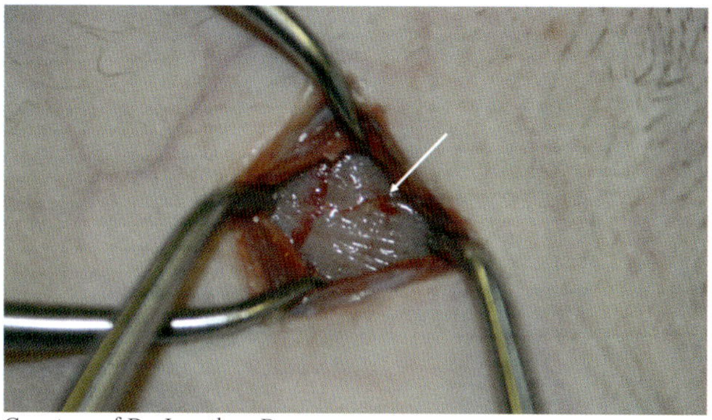

Courtesy of Dr. Jonathan Bray

P)

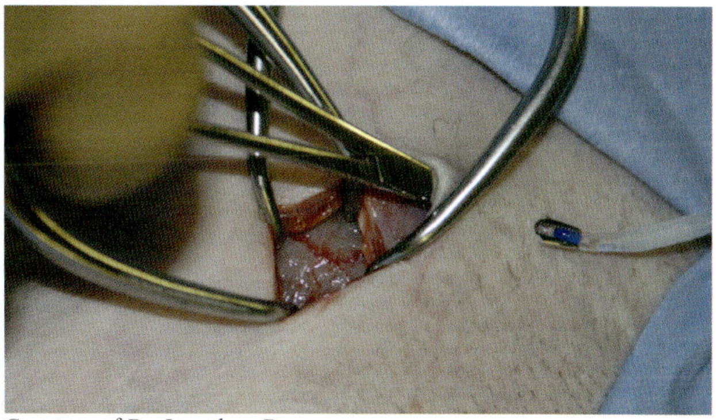

Courtesy of Dr. Jonathan Bray

Surgical Technique – Minimally Invasive Inguinal Approach [2] (See Plate 29L–S) *continued*

Q) A purse-string suture is placed in the exposed bladder wall as previously described (see earlier steps C–F), a stab incision is made into the urinary bladder in the middle of the purse-string suture (i) and the Foley catheter is inserted into the urinary bladder via a stab incision (ii), and the bulb of the Foley catheter is inflated.

R) The abdominal wound is then sutured. When closing the innermost muscle layer, a cystopexy is accomplished by incorporating the urinary bladder wall with a partial-thickness bite into the submucosa of the bladder. The muscle layers are closed separately or in a single layer depending on the size of the patient.

S) The catheter is secured to the skin as described earlier, including drainage system and protective bandage (see earlier steps I and J).

Postoperative Management

1) Multimodal analgesia.
2) A closed collection system can be used in the hospital or the cystostomy is drained three to four times per day [3].
3) Nonsterile latex gloves should be used when handling or draining urine from the cystostomy tube.
4) The cystostomy tube should be protected from self-trauma with an Elizabethan collar, T-shirt, stockinette dressings, or body suit.
5) Animals should be encouraged to urinate normally with the tube in situ, if possible.
6) Cystostomy tubes are removed when required by cutting the Chinese fingertrap suture, deflating the Foley bulb, and then applying steady, firm traction on the cystostomy tube through the stoma. The resulting stoma will heal by second intention over 3–5 days [3]. Minor urine leakage from the stoma typically occurs for a few hours after removal of the cystostomy tube [1].

Complications

- Overall: 49% [1]
- Urinary tract infection (33%–86%) [1, 2], often *Escherichia coli* or *Escherichia faecalis*
- Inadvertent tube removal (16%) [1]
- Macroscopic and microscopic hematuria
- Peristomal irritation and granuloma formation (9%) [1]
- Urine leakage around the tube (9%) [1]
- Decreased urine drainage because of overtightening of the Chinese fingertrap suture pattern [2]
- Fistula formation after tube removal (1%) [1]

References

1 Beck, A.L., Grierson, J.M., Ogden, D.M. et al. (2007). Outcome of and complications associated with tube cystostomy in dogs and cats: 76 cases (1995-2006). *J. Am. Vet. Med. Assoc.* 230 (8): 1184–1189.

2 Bray, J.P., Doyle, R.S., and Burton, C.A. (2009). Minimally invasive inguinal approach for tube cystostomy. *Vet. Surg.* 38 (3): 411–416.

3 Hayashi, K. and Hardie, R.J. (2003). Use of cystostomy tubes in small animals. *Compend. Contin. Educ. Pract. Vet.* 25 (12): 928–935.

Plate 29

Cystostomy Tube *continued*

Q-i)

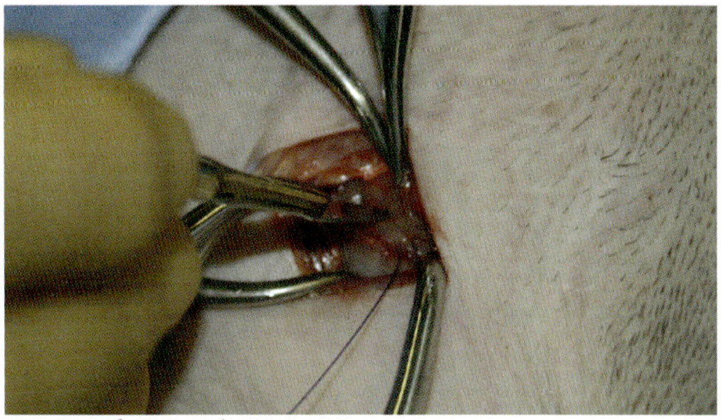

Courtesy of Dr. Jonathan Bray

Q-ii)

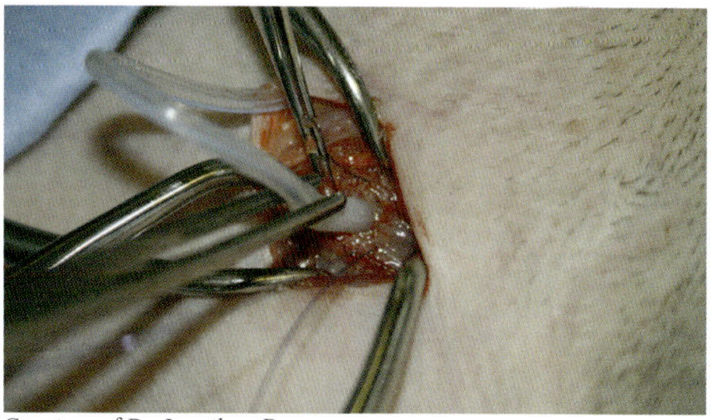

Courtesy of Dr. Jonathan Bray

R)

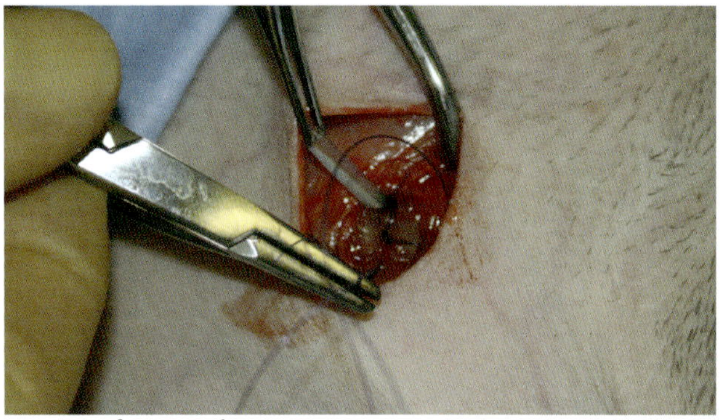

Courtesy of Dr. Jonathan Bray

S)

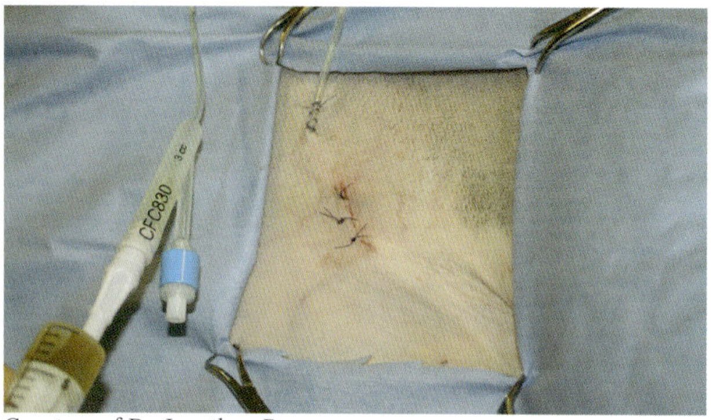

Courtesy of Dr. Jonathan Bray

Chapter 30: Prostatectomy

30.1 Partial Prostatectomy

Indications

1) Palliation of prostatic tumors causing urethral obstruction
2) Partial prostatectomy can be combined with sublumbar lymph node resection (see *20.1. Open Sublumbar Lymph Node Resection*) when enlarged or metastatic sublumbar lymph nodes are present

Suggested Diagnostic Workup and Clinical Staging

- Complete blood count, serum biochemistry, and urinalysis
- Urine sediment cytology
- Cadet BRAF mutation urine test
- ± Urethrocystoscopy for assessment and biopsy of the urethra and prostate
- Abdominal ultrasound or precontrast and postcontrast computed tomography (CT) scan of the abdomen for assessment of location and extent of the prostate mass and intra-abdominal metastasis
- Three-view thoracic radiographs or thoracic CT scan for assessment of lung metastasis

Patient Positioning

The patient is positioned in dorsal recumbency. An appropriately sized urinary catheter should be inserted to protect the urethra during the partial prostatectomy.

Surgical Technique [1, 2] (See Plate 30.1B–F)

A) A ventral midline celiotomy is performed (see *15.1. Ventral Midline Celiotomy*) with the incision extending to the pubic brim. The penis should be draped into the surgical field because access may be needed for intraoperative catheterization.
B) A stay suture of 3-0 absorbable monofilament suture material is placed full thickness into the apex of the urinary bladder, and the urinary bladder is retracted cranially.
C) The periprostatic fat (PPF) is dissected away from the prostate and retracted laterally (pictured). This should be done in a ventral-to-dorsal direction. The dorsolateral neurovascular structures, in particular the hypogastric nerve, should be preserved.

Color Atlas of Canine and Feline Surgical Oncology, First Edition. Julius M. Liptak, Paolo Buracco, William T. N. Culp, and Nicholas J. Bacon.

Plate 30.1

Partial Prostatectomy

B)

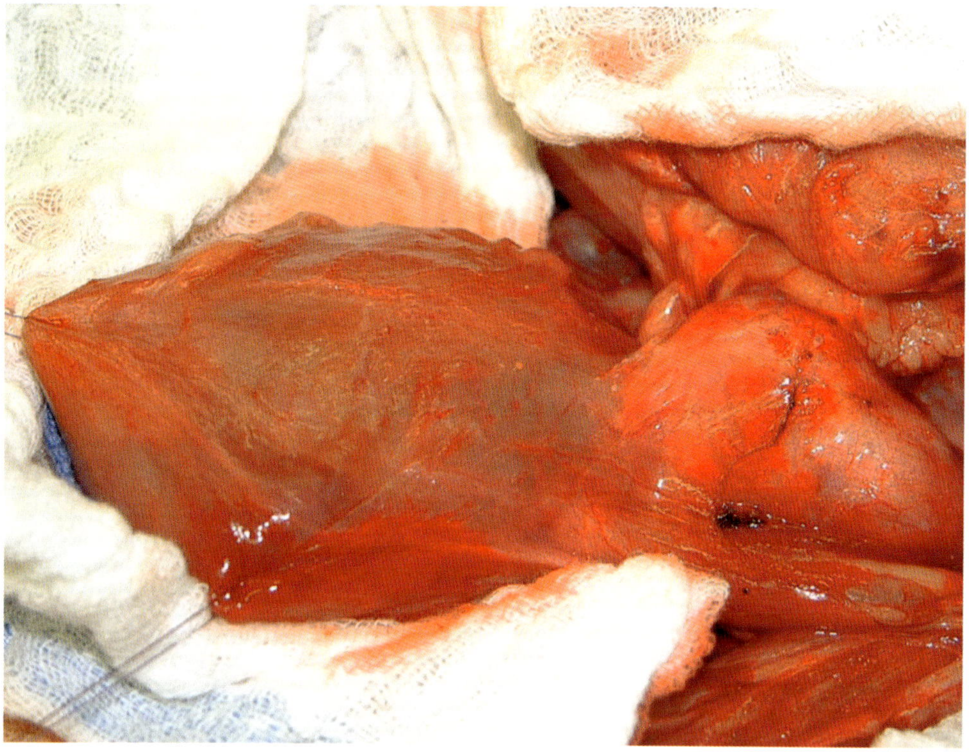

C)

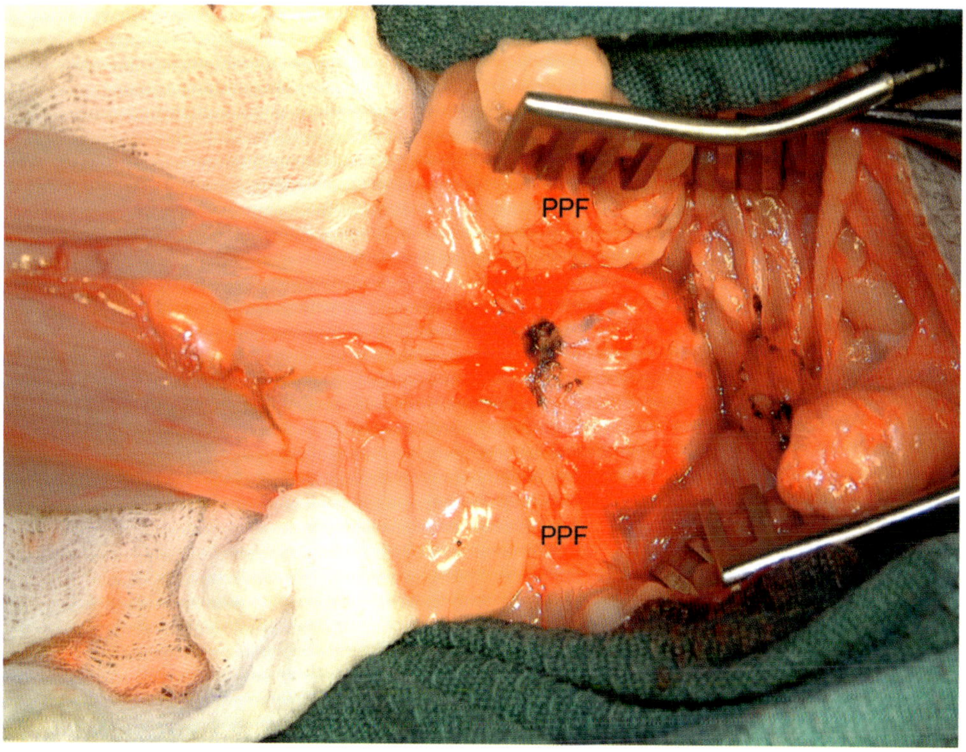

Surgical Technique [1, 2] (See Plate 30.1B–F) *continued*

D) The ventral aspect of the prostatic capsule is then incised with a scalpel blade, electrosurgery, or a laser, and retracted with self-retaining retractors.
E) The prostatic parenchyma is removed piecemeal using either electrosurgery or a laser. Up to 85% of the prostate can be removed, but the dorsal capsule and urethra should be preserved.
F) The ventral prostatomy is closed with a single layer of 3-0 absorbable monofilament suture material in a simple interrupted or simple continuous suture pattern (pictured). The linea alba, subcutaneous tissue, and skin are closed as described in *15.1. Ventral Midline Celiotomy*.

Postoperative Management

1) Multimodal analgesia
2) Elizabethan collar or body suit
3) Indwelling urethral catheter for 24–72 hours

Complications – Dogs [1, 2]

- Intermittent urinary incontinence (11%)
- Progressive local disease (common because this is a palliative procedure)

Suggested Adjuvant Treatments

- Nonsteroidal anti-inflammatory drugs [3, 4]
- Chemotherapy [3, 4]
- ± Radiation therapy or intensity-modulated radiation therapy [3–5]
- ± Prostatic artery embolization [6]

Prognosis and Oncologic Outcome – Dogs [1, 2]

	Local Recurrence rate	Metastatic Rate	Disease-Free Interval (d)	Median Survival Time (d)	1-Year Survival Rate	2-Year Survival Rate
Overall [1, 2]	100%	25%	–	103–112	0%	0%

References

1 L'Eplattenier, H.F., van Nimwegen, S.A., van Sluijs, F.J. et al. (2006). Partial prostatectomy using Nd:YAG laser for management of canine prostatic carcinoma. *Vet. Surg.* 35 (4): 406–411.
2 Vlasin, M., Rauser, P., Fichtel, T. et al. (2006). Subtotal intracapsular prostatectomy as a useful treatment for advanced-stage prostatic malignancies. *J. Small Anim. Pract.* 47 (9): 512–516.
3 Ravicini, S., Baines, S.J., Taylor, A. et al. (2018). Outcome and prognostic factors in medically treated canine prostatic carcinomas: a multi-institutional study. *Vet. Comp. Oncol.* 16 (4): 450–458.
4 Clerc-Renaud, B., Gieger, T.L., Larue, S.M. et al. (2021). Treatment of genitourinary carcinoma in dogs using nonsteroidal anti-inflammatory drugs, mitoxantrone, and radiation therapy: a retrospective study. *J. Vet. Intern. Med.* 35 (2): 1052–1061.
5 Walz, J.Z., Desai, N., Van Asselt, N. et al. (2020). Definitive-intent intensity-modulated radiation therapy for treatment of canine prostatic carcinoma: a multi-institutional retrospective study. *Vet. Comp. Oncol.* 18 (3): 381–388.
6 Culp, W.T.N., Johnson, E.G., Giuffrida, M.A. et al. (2021). Procedural description and prospective evaluation of short-term outcome for the use of prostatic artery embolization in dogs with carcinoma of the prostate. *J. Am. Vet. Med. Assoc.* 259 (10): 1154–1162.

Plate 30.1

Partial Prostatectomy *continued*

D)

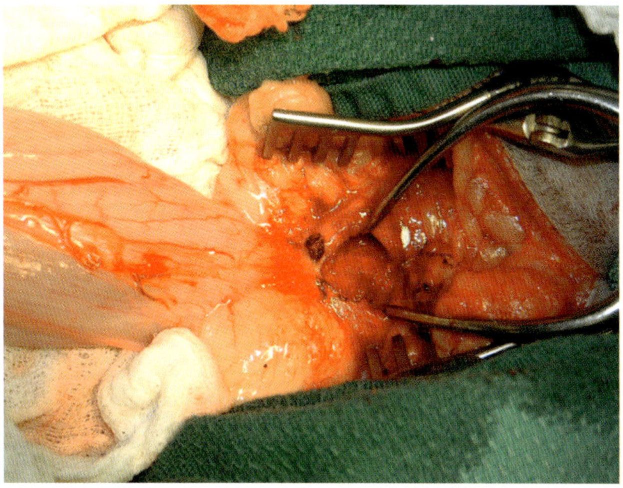

E)

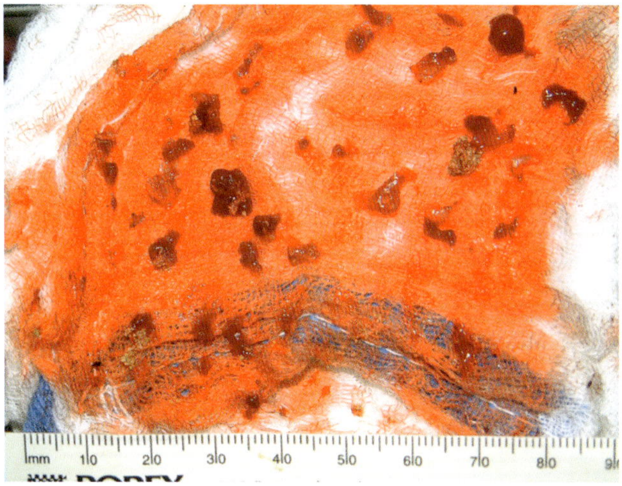

F)

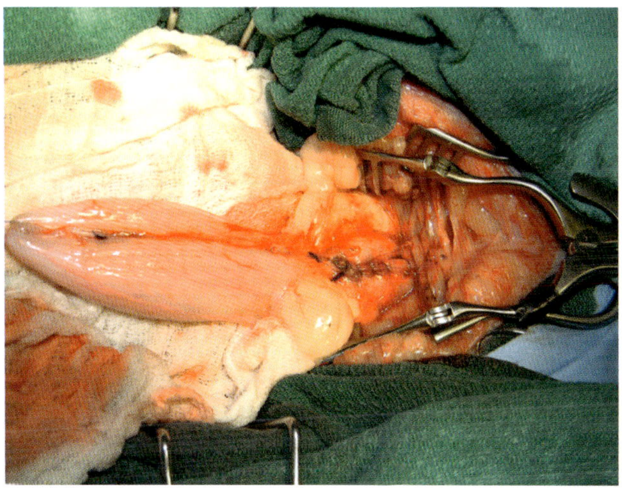

30.2 Total Prostatectomy

Indications

1) Resection of benign and nonmetastatic malignant prostatic tumors. Tumors confined to the prostate with no evidence of extension into the bladder neck, urethra, or adjacent soft tissues are the ideal candidates for total prostatectomy.
2) Total prostatectomy can be combined with either a pubic symphysiotomy (see *15.5. Pubic Symphysiotomy*) or pubic flap (see *15.6. Pubic Flap*) for caudal exposure.
3) Total prostatectomy can be combined with sublumbar lymph node resection (see *20.1. Open Sublumbar Lymph Node Resection*) when enlarged or metastatic sublumbar lymph nodes are present.

Suggested Diagnostic Workup and Clinical Staging

- Complete blood count, serum biochemistry, and urinalysis
- Urine sediment cytology
- Cadet BRAF mutation urine test
- ± Urethrocystoscopy for assessment and biopsy of the urethra and prostate
- Abdominal ultrasound or precontrast and postcontrast computed tomography (CT) scan of the abdomen for assessment of location and extent of the prostate mass, and intra-abdominal metastasis
- Three-view thoracic radiographs or thoracic CT scan for assessment of lung metastasis

Patient Positioning

The patient is positioned in dorsal recumbency.

Surgical Technique (See Plate 30.2A–G)

A) A ventral midline celiotomy is performed (see *15.1. Ventral Midline Celiotomy*) with the incision extending to the pubic brim. The penis should be draped into the surgical field to allow intraoperative catheterization of the urethra. The perineum should also be draped into the surgical field in the event that either a pubic symphysiotomy (see *15.5. Pubic Symphysiotomy*) or pubic flap (see *15.6. Pubic Flap*) is required for caudal exposure.
B) A stay suture of 3-0 absorbable monofilament suture material is placed full thickness into the apex of the urinary bladder, and the urinary bladder is retracted cranially (see step A).
C) Both vas deferens are either ligated with a single simple ligature of 2-0 to 3-0 absorbable monofilament suture material (solid black lines) and transected or sealed and transected with a vessel sealing device close to the prostate (white dashed lines).

Color Atlas of Canine and Feline Surgical Oncology, First Edition. Julius M. Liptak, Paolo Buracco, William T. N. Culp, and Nicholas J. Bacon.

Plate 30.2

Total Prostatectomy

A)

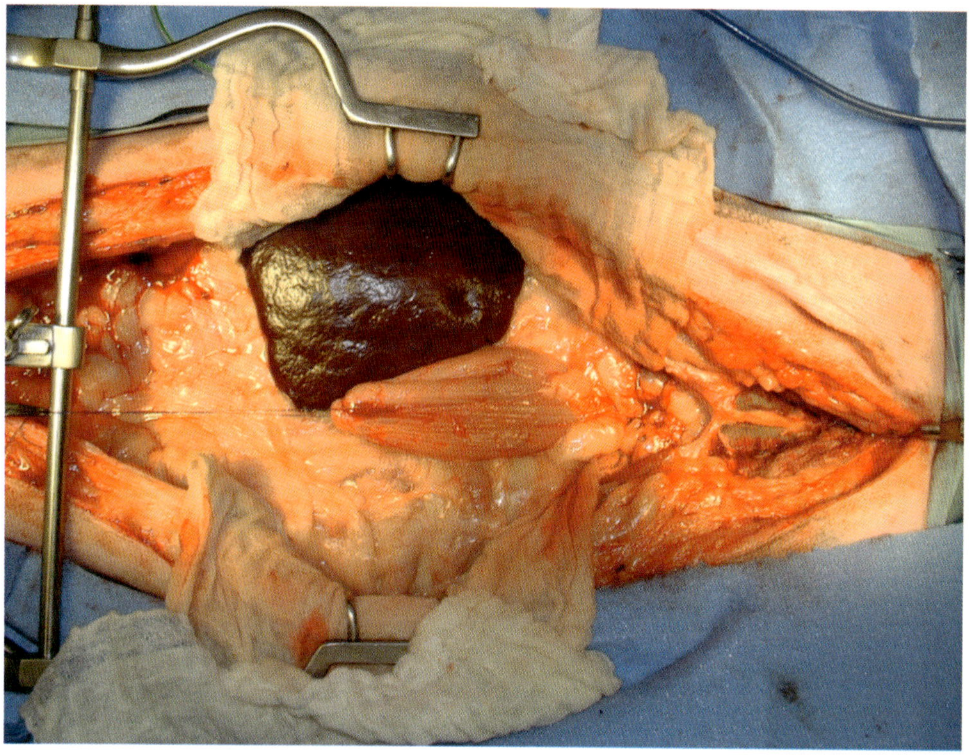

C)

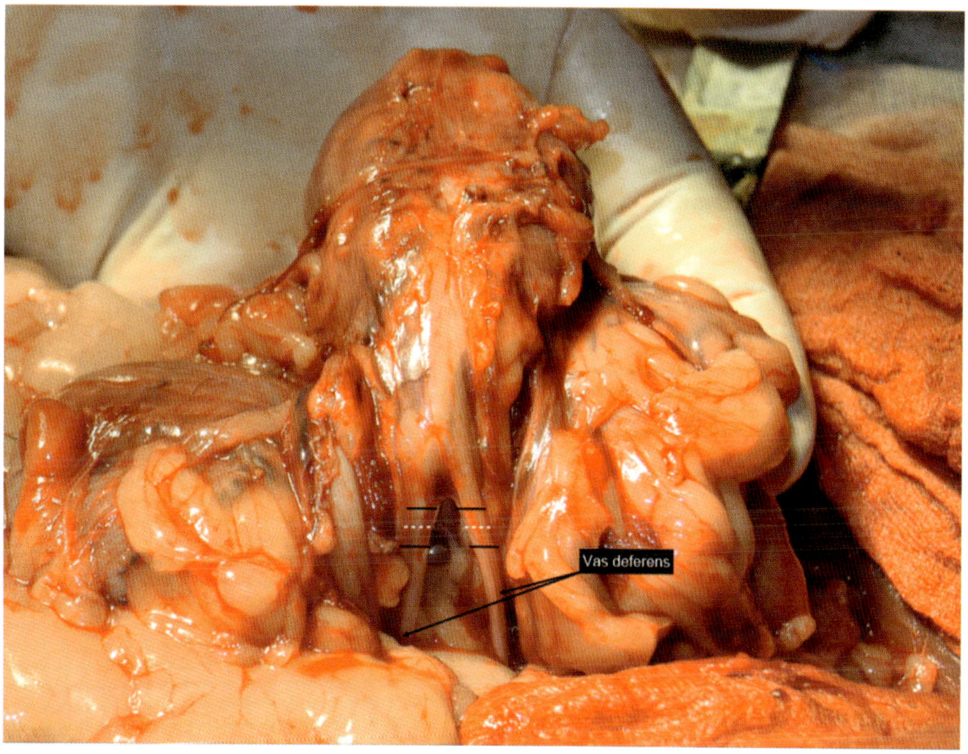

Surgical Technique (See Plate 30.2A–G) *continued*

D) The periprostatic fat (PPF) is dissected away from the prostate and retracted laterally (i, without pubic sympysiotomy or pubic flap; ii, pubic symphysiotomy has been performed to improve exposure of the prostate within the pelvic canal). Dissection can be done digitally, with blunt dissection, or with a vessel sealing device. Once the PPF is retracted, the neurovascular structures dorsolateral to the prostate should be identified, if possible (iii, arrows). Dissection is continued close to the prostatic capsule to preserve these neurovascular structures, particularly the hypogastric nerve (iv), whereas other prostatic vessels are cauterized or ligated as close as possible to the prostate. The prostate is then isolated (v) and protected from the remainder of the abdominal cavity with moistened laparotomy sponges (vi). A stay suture of 3-0 absorbable monofilament suture material is placed in the urethra immediately caudal to the planned caudal urethral transection site to prevent retraction of the urethra into the pelvic canal (vii).

Plate 30.2

Total Prostatectomy *continued*

D-i)

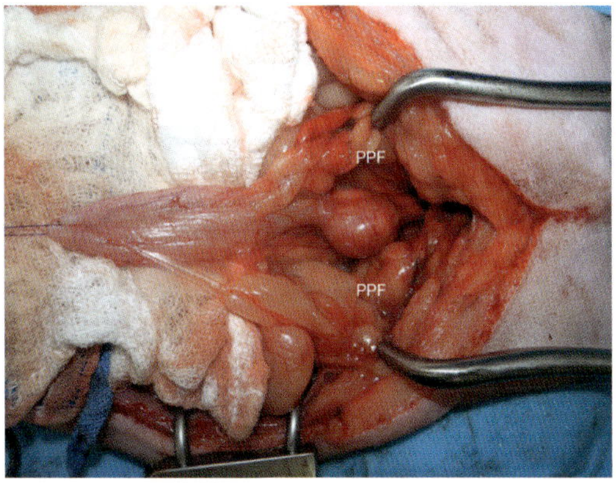

D-ii)

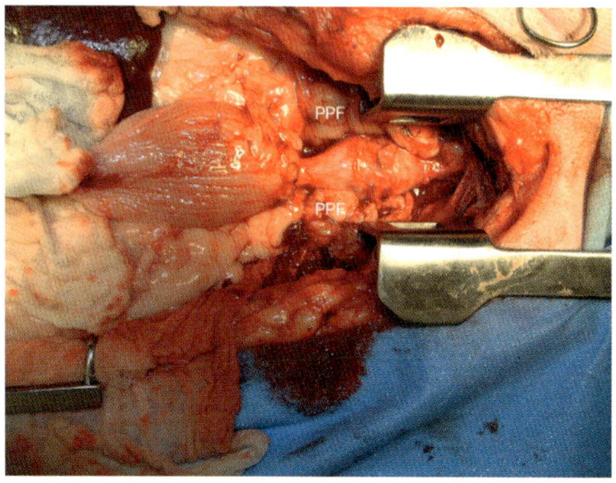

D-iii)

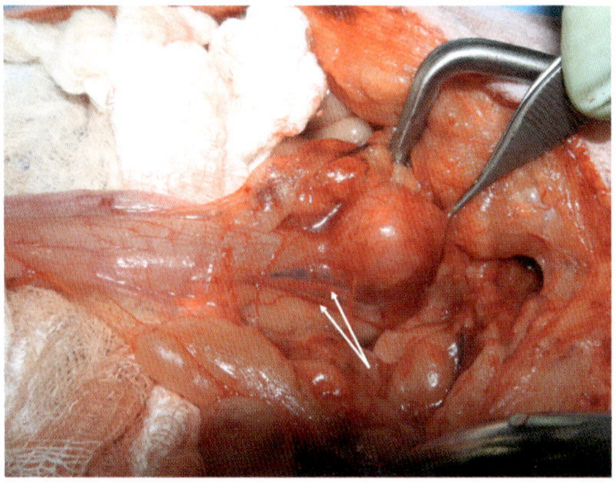

D-iv)

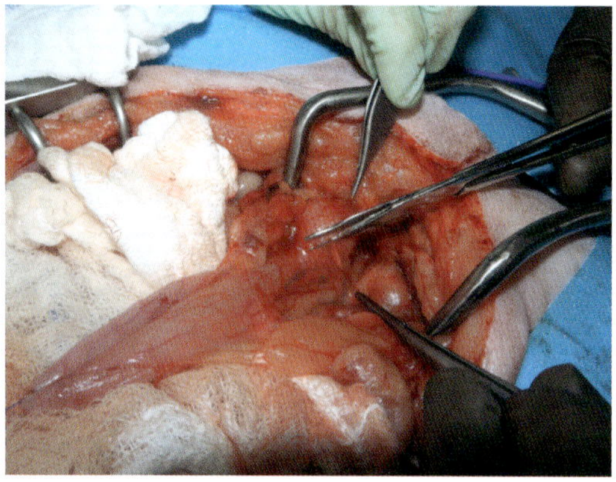

D-v)

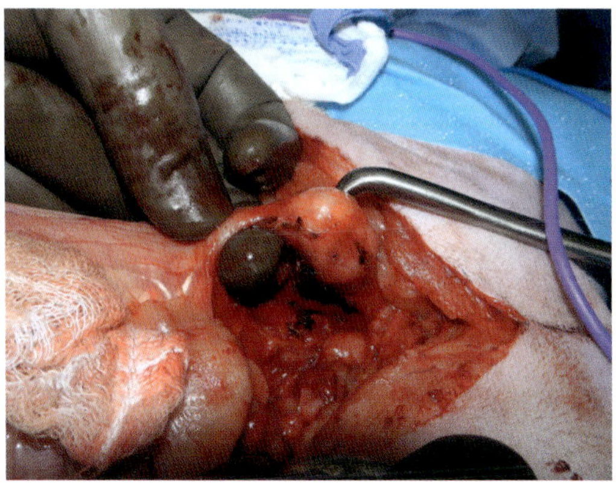

D-vi)

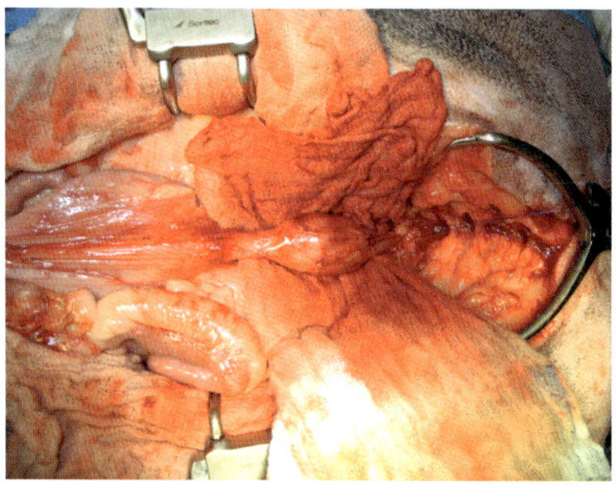

D-vii)

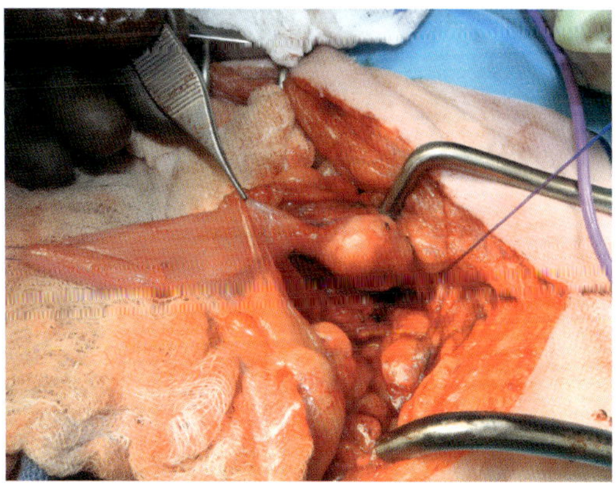

Surgical Technique (See Plate 30.2A–G) *continued*

E) The caudal (i, ii) and cranial (iii, iv) urethral transections are performed with a scalpel blade within 5–10 mm of the cranial and caudal extents of the prostate, respectively. This can either be done with the indwelling urinary catheter in situ (pictured) or after withdrawal of the indwelling urinary catheter caudal to the planned caudal urethral transection site. If the urethral resections have been performed with the indwelling urinary catheter in situ, then the urinary catheter is withdrawn to allow removal of the prostate from the surgical field (v). Instruments, gloves, and moistened laparotomy sponges are changed to minimize the risk of tumor seeding.

F) The indwelling urethral catheter is advanced into the urinary bladder. Some surgeons prefer a Foley catheter at this stage.

G) The resected ends of the urethra are approximated with stay sutures, and an end-to-end urethral anastomosis or vesicourethral anastomosis is performed with 3-0 or 4-0 absorbable monofilament suture material using either a simple interrupted (pictured) or simple continuous suture pattern. If using a simple continuous suture pattern, then this should be done with two overlapping continuous suture patterns to minimize the risk of iatrogenic stricture of the anastomosis.

Closure (See Plate 30.2H)

H) The linea alba, subcutaneous tissue, and skin are closed as described in *15.1. Ventral Midline Celiotomy*. If a pubic symphysiotomy or pubic flap has been performed, then this is closed as described in *15.5. Pubic Symphysiotomy* or *15.6. Pubic Flap*, respectively.

Postoperative Management

1) Multimodal analgesia
2) Elizabethan collar or body suit
3) Indwelling urethral catheter for 24–96 hours

Complications – Dogs [1]

- Urinary incontinence (52% overall)
  - Transient urinary incontinence (13%)
  - Permanent urinary incontinence (35%)
    - Grade I–II urinary incontinence (22%)
    - Grade III–IV urinary incontinence (13%)
- Urinary tract infection (24%)
- Minor incisional dehiscence (8%)
- Surgical-site infection (8%)
- Prepubic tendon herniation (4%)
- Dehiscence of the urethral anastomosis with subsequent uroabdomen (4%)

Suggested Adjuvant Treatments [2, 3]

- Nonsteroidal anti-inflammatory drugs
- Chemotherapy

Plate 30.2

Total Prostatectomy *continued*

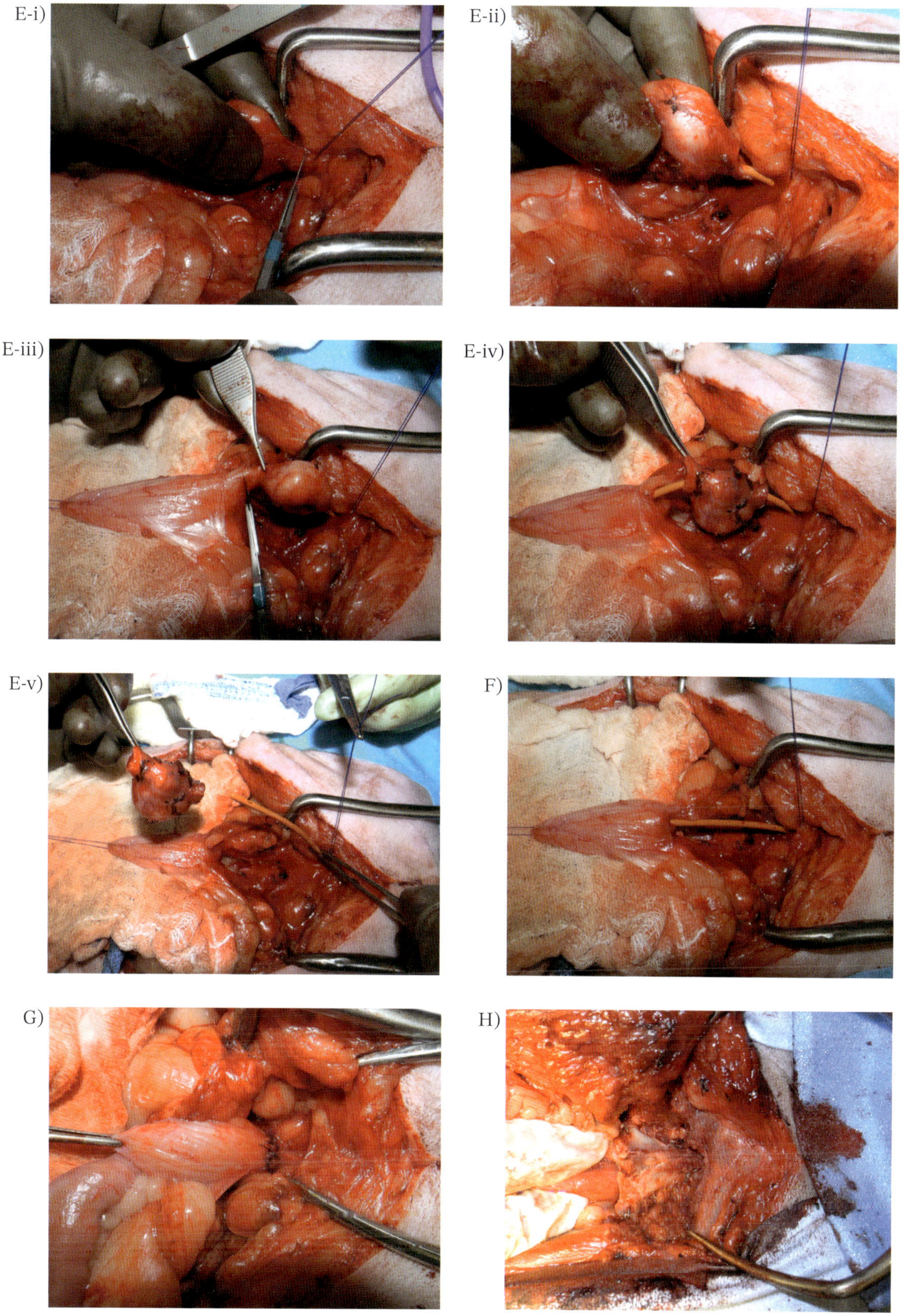

Prognosis and Oncologic Outcome – Dogs

	Local Recurrence Rate	Metastatic Rate	Disease-Free Interval (d)	Median Survival Time (d)	1-Year Survival Rate	2-Year Survival Rate
Overall	32%	52%	82	231	32%	12%
			Extracapsular extension			
Yes	–	–	–	138	–	–
No	–	–	–	248	–	–

References

1 Bennett, T.C., Matz, B.M., Henderson, R.A. et al. (2018). Total prostatectomy as a treatment for prostatic carcinoma in 25 dogs. *Vet. Surg.* 47 (3): 367–377.

2 Ravicini, S., Baines, S.J., Taylor, A. et al. (2018). Outcome and prognostic factors in medically treated canine prostatic carcinomas: a multi-institutional study. *Vet. Comp. Oncol.* 16 (4): 450–458.

3 Clerc-Renaud, B., Gieger, T.L., Larue, S.M. et al. (2021). Treatment of genitourinary carcinoma in dogs using nonsteroidal anti-inflammatory drugs, mitoxantrone, and radiation therapy: a retrospective study. *J. Vet. Intern. Med.* 35 (2): 1052–1061.

Chapter 31: Penile Amputation

Indications

1) Resection of benign and malignant tumors involving the penile soft tissues or os penis
2) Resection of malignant preputial tumors

Suggested Diagnostic Workup and Clinical Staging

- Complete blood count, serum biochemistry, and urinalysis
- Preoperative biopsy
- ± Abdominal ultrasound or precontrast and postcontrast computed tomography (CT) scan of the abdomen for assessment of intra-abdominal metastasis
- ± Three-view thoracic radiographs or thoracic CT scan for assessment of lung metastasis

Patient Positioning

The patient is positioned in dorsal recumbency.

Surgical Technique (See Plate 31A–I)

A) Castration ± scrotal ablation is performed in intact dogs.
B) An elliptical incision is made around the penis and prepuce with appropriate surgical margins.
C) The caudal epigastric and external pudendal arteries and veins (arrow) should be ligated with a single simple ligature of 2-0 to 3-0 absorbable monofilament suture material and transected or sealed and transected with a vessel sealing device.
D) The penis should be dissected away from the from the abdominal wall using either a combination of blunt and sharp dissection or a vessel sealing device (i–iv).
E) The retractor penis muscle is identified on the ventral aspect of the urethra (pictured) and transected with electrosurgery or a vessel sealing device.
F) The urethra is catheterized, and a ventral midline urethrotomy is performed in the scrotal region over the catheter with a scalpel blade. The urethrotomy is then extended with iris scissors for a length of 2.5–4.0 cm, depending on the size of the dog, to the cranial aspect of the ischiatic urethral curvature.

Color Atlas of Canine and Feline Surgical Oncology, First Edition. Julius M. Liptak, Paolo Buracco, William T. N. Culp, and Nicholas J. Bacon.

Plate 31

Penile Amputation

A)

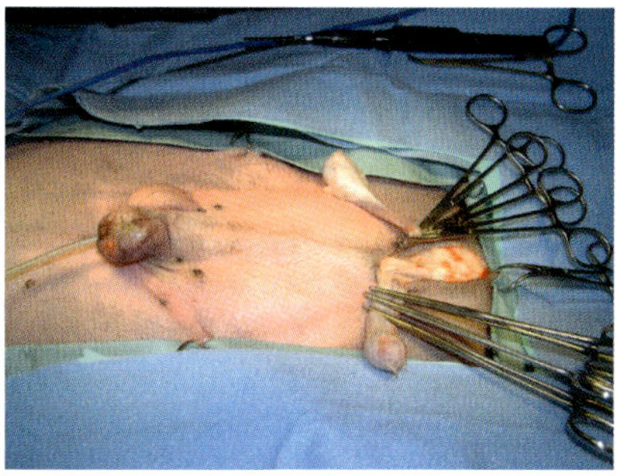

B)

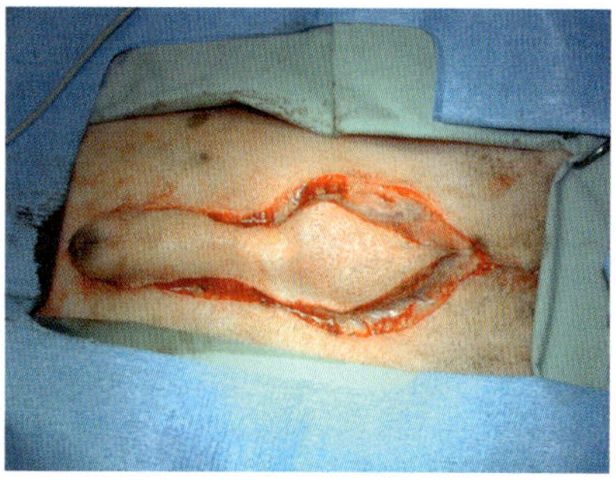

C)

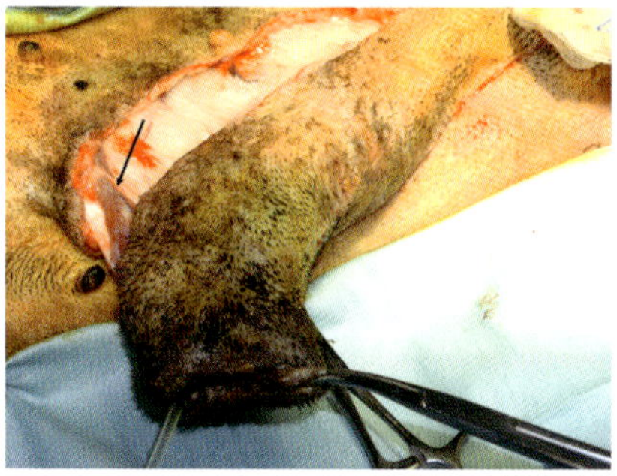

D-i)

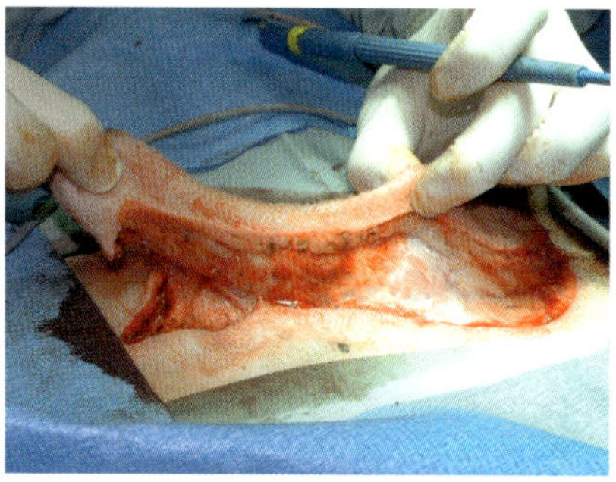

D-ii)

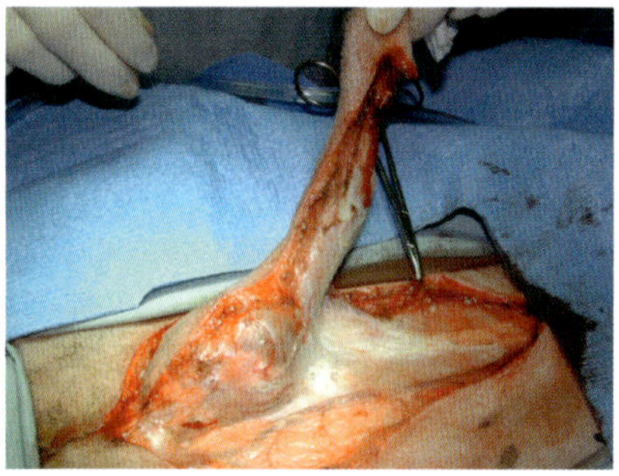

D-iii)

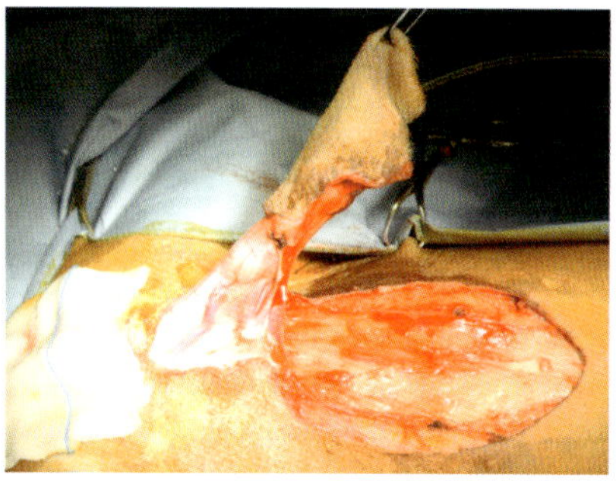

D-iv)

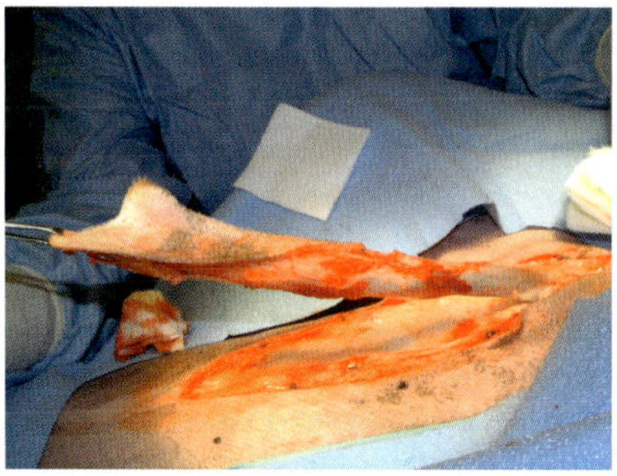

E)

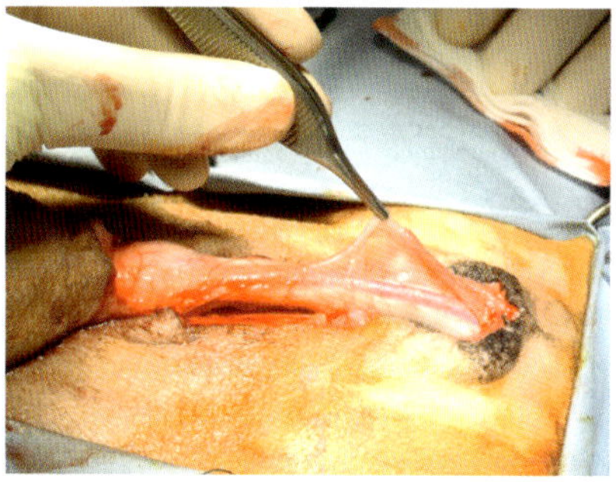

F)

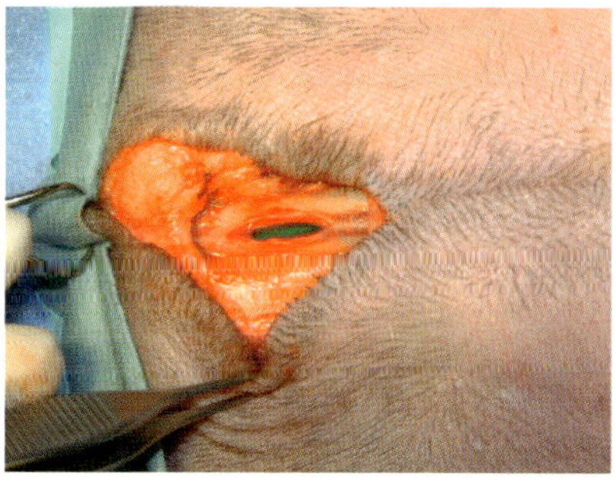

Surgical Technique (See Plate 31A–I) *continued*

G) The scrotal urethrostomy is closed in one to two layers. The subcutaneous-urethral submucosal layer is closed in with 3-0 to 4-0 absorbable monofilament suture material in a simple continuous suture pattern (i). The cutaneous-urethral mucosal layer is closed in with 3-0 to 5-0 absorbable monofilament suture material in a simple interrupted or simple continuous suture pattern (ii). A simple continuous suture pattern is preferred because it results in significantly less postoperative bleeding.
H) A tourniquet can be used at the base of the penis caudal to the planned level of the penile amputation (i). The penis is amputated with appropriate surgical margins with a scalpel blade (ii). Bleeding will be brisk and should be controlled with cautery, ligatures, hemoclips, or a vessel sealing device.
I) Suture the tunica albuginea over the penile stump.

Closure (See Plate 31J)

The skin incision is closed routinely in two layers with a simple continuous suture pattern using monofilament absorbable suture material in the subcutis and either an interrupted or continuous suture pattern using monofilament nonabsorbable suture material in the skin (J).

Postoperative Management

1) Multimodal analgesia
2) Elizabethan collar or body suit
3) ± Vaseline around the urethrostomy site to protect against urine scalding

Complications – Dogs [1] (See Plate 31K, L)

- Mild spontaneous ± posturination hemorrhage (K) (100%)
- Incisional dehiscence (11%)
- Bruising and swelling (K) (11%)
- Stricture of the urethrostomy site (L – i, immediate postoperative radiograph following penile amputation and scrotal urethrostomy for a preputial mast cell tumor; ii, urethrostomy stricture 71 days postoperatively) (6%)

Suggested Adjuvant Treatments

- ± Chemotherapy, depending on tumor type and histologic grade
- ± Radiation therapy, depending on tumor type and completeness of excision

Prognosis and Oncologic Outcome

The only published studies of penile amputation for the management of penile or preputial tumors are individual case reports and hence the prognosis and oncologic outcome after penile amputation are unknown.

Reference

1 Burrow, R.D., Gregory, S.P., Giejda, A.A., and White, R.N. (2011). Penile amputation and scrotal urethrostomy in 18 dogs. *Vet. Rec.* 169 (25): 657.

Plate 31

Penile Amputation *continued*

G-i)

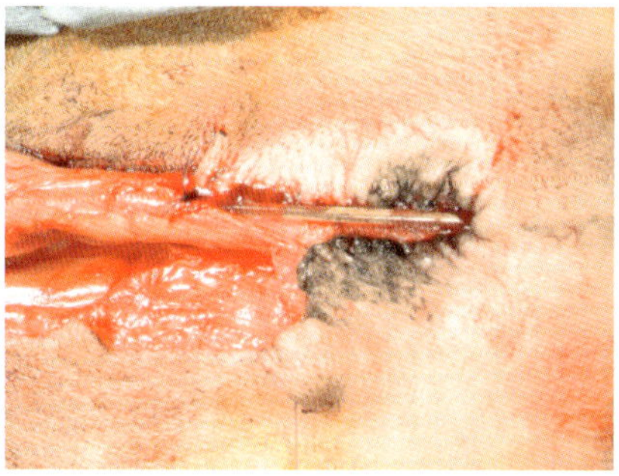

G-ii)

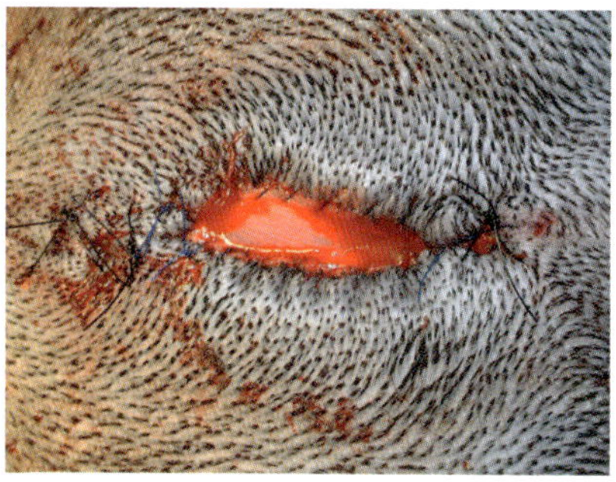

H-i)

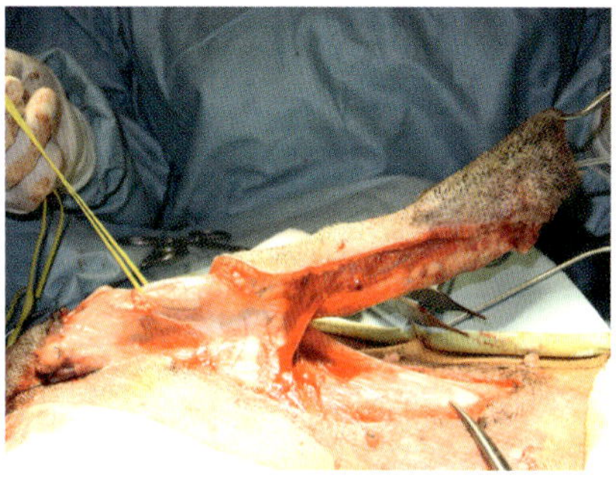

H-ii)

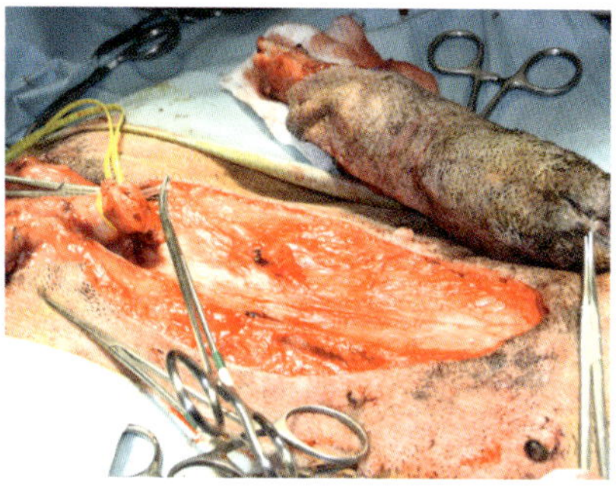

I)

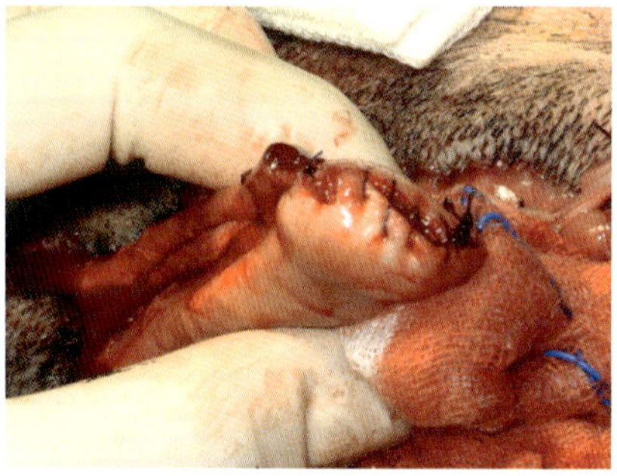

J)

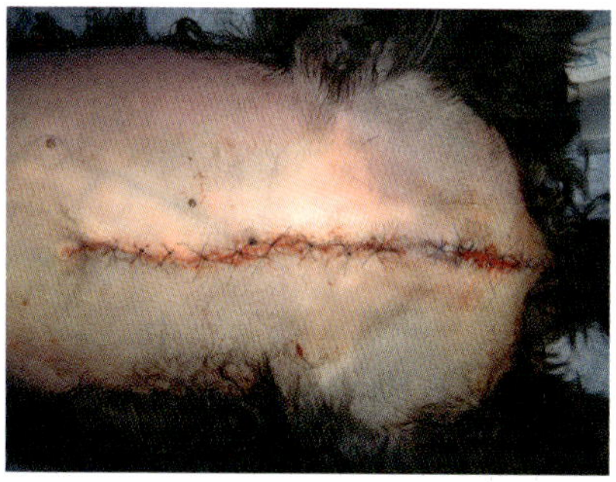

K)

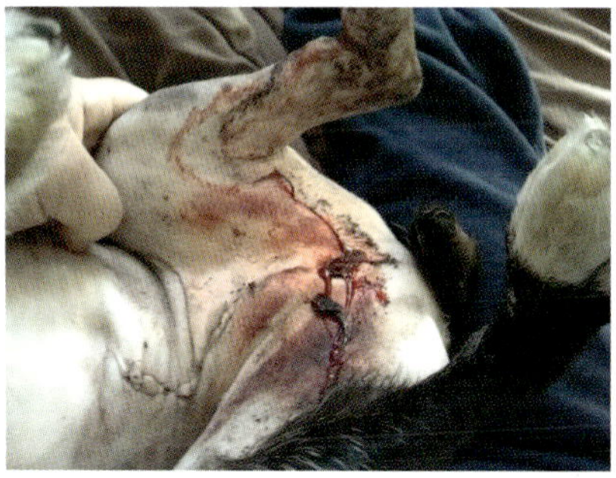

L-i)

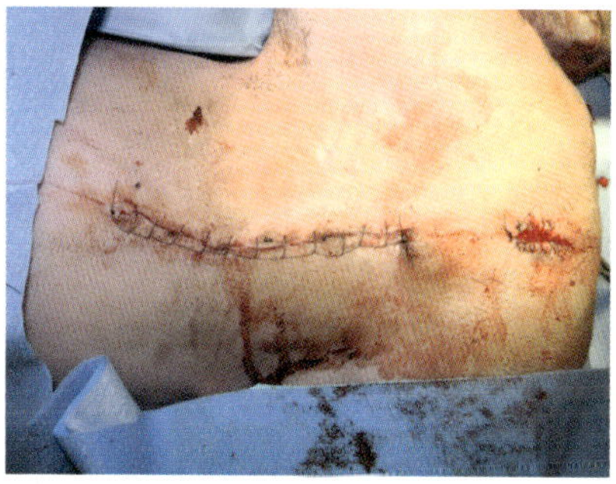

L-ii)

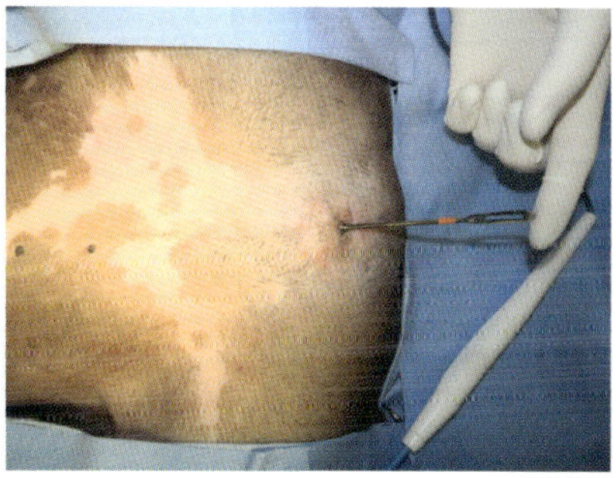

Chapter 32: Vulvovaginectomy

Indications

1) Resection of benign and malignant tumors involving the vagina, vestibule, and/or vulva

Suggested Diagnostic Workup and Clinical Staging

- Complete blood count, serum biochemistry, and urinalysis
- Rectal examination
- Vaginal examination
- ± Vaginoscopy
- ± Abdominal ultrasound or precontrast and postcontrast computed tomography (CT) scan of the abdomen for assessment of intra-abdominal metastasis
- ± Three-view thoracic radiographs or thoracic CT scan for assessment of lung metastasis

Patient Positioning

1) The patient is positioned in dorsal recumbency if a ventral midline celiotomy is planned (see step H).
2) The patient is positioned in sternal recumbency with the tail secured dorsally and cranially (see step I). The perineal area can be elevated by either flexing the pelvic limbs underneath the pelvis and caudal abdomen or placing padding between the pelvic limbs with the pelvic limbs hanging over the padded end of the surgical table. The anal sacs should be expressed before surgery. An anal purse-string suture should also be placed.

Surgical Technique [1, 2] (See Plate 32A–U)

A) **Abdominal approach for vaginectomy:** A ventral midline celiotomy is performed (see *15.1. Ventral Midline Celiotomy*) with the incision extending to the pubic brim. The vulva should be draped into the surgical field because access may be needed for intraoperative catheterization (not pictured).
B) The ventral ligament of the bladder is incised with either scissors or a vessel sealing device (i). A stay suture of 3-0 absorbable monofilament suture material is placed full thickness into the apex of the urinary bladder, and the bladder is reflected caudally (ii).
C) If the dog is intact, then an ovariohysterectomy is performed.
D) The cervix is then tractioned cranially (with either a stay suture [i] or Allis tissue forceps) as the soft tissue connections between the vagina and the rectum (ii) and urethra (iii) and the rectogenital and vesicogenital reflections are dissected off the wall of the vagina with a combination of sharp, blunt, and electrosurgery dissection, or a vessel sealing device.

Color Atlas of Canine and Feline Surgical Oncology, First Edition. Julius M. Liptak, Paolo Buracco, William T. N. Culp, and Nicholas J. Bacon.

Plate 32

Vulvovaginectomy

B-i)

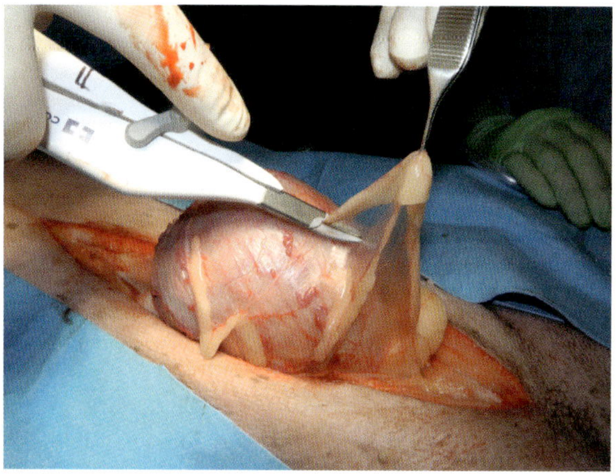

B-ii)

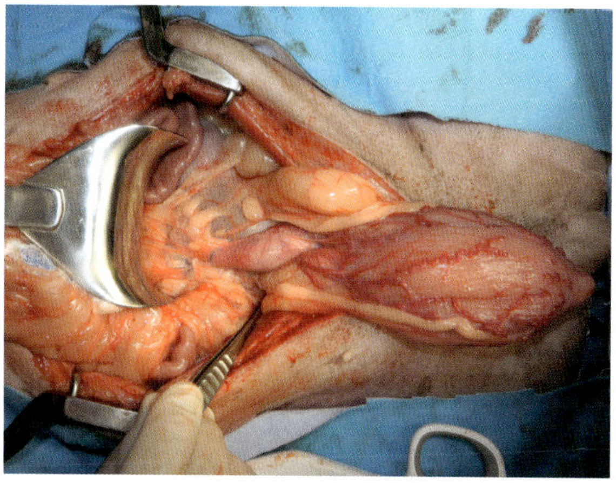

C)

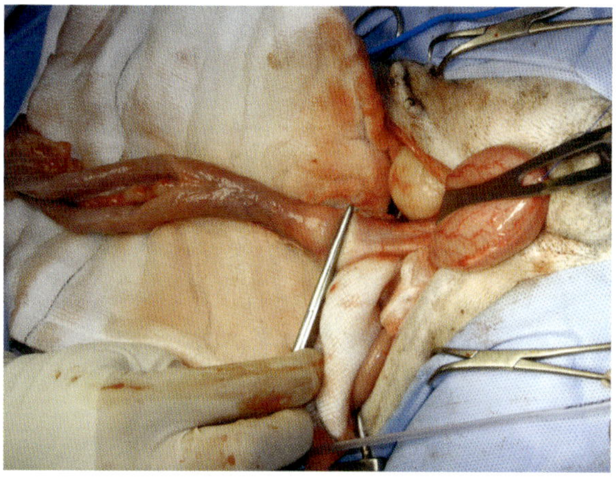

D-i)

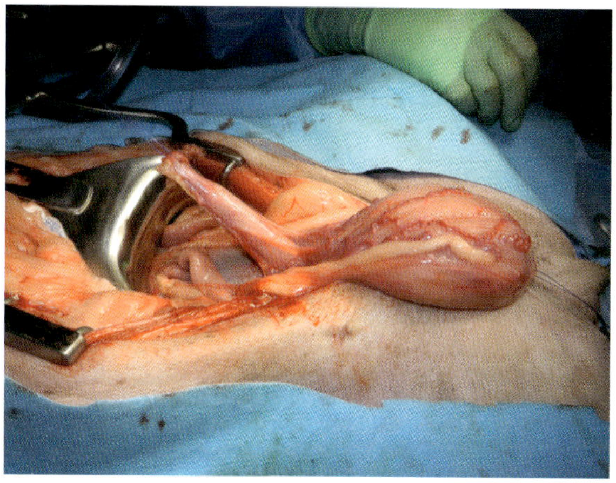

D-ii)

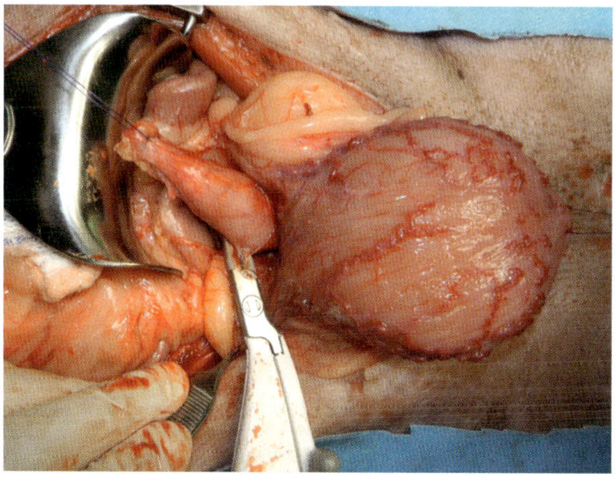

D-iii)

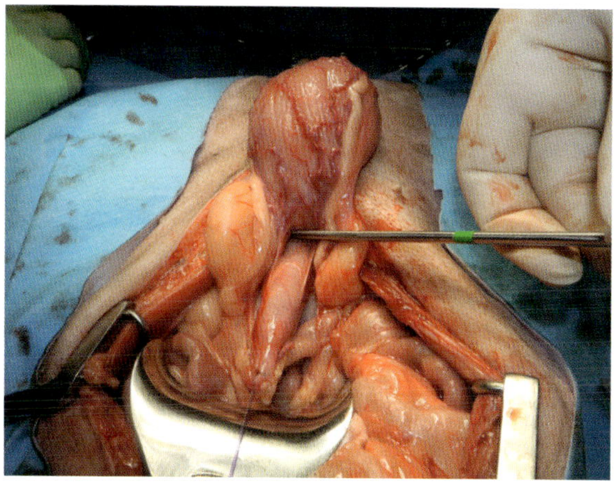

Surgical Technique [1, 2] (See Plate 32A–U) *continued*

E) The branches of the vaginal artery and vein coursing laterally are ligated, cauterized, or sealed and transected with a vessel sealing device.
F) Dissection is continued as far caudally as possible until the vagina is freely mobile.
G) A stab incision is made into the cranioventral vaginal wall (i), and a long catheter is passed caudally through the stab incision (ii) and exited through the vulva. The abdominal end of the catheter is secured to the vaginal wall with 2-0 non-absorbable monofilament suture material and then the catheter is cut flush with the vaginal wall (iii).
H) The linea alba, subcutaneous tissue, and skin are closed as described in *15.1. Ventral Midline Celiotomy*.

Plate 32

Vulvovaginectomy *continued*

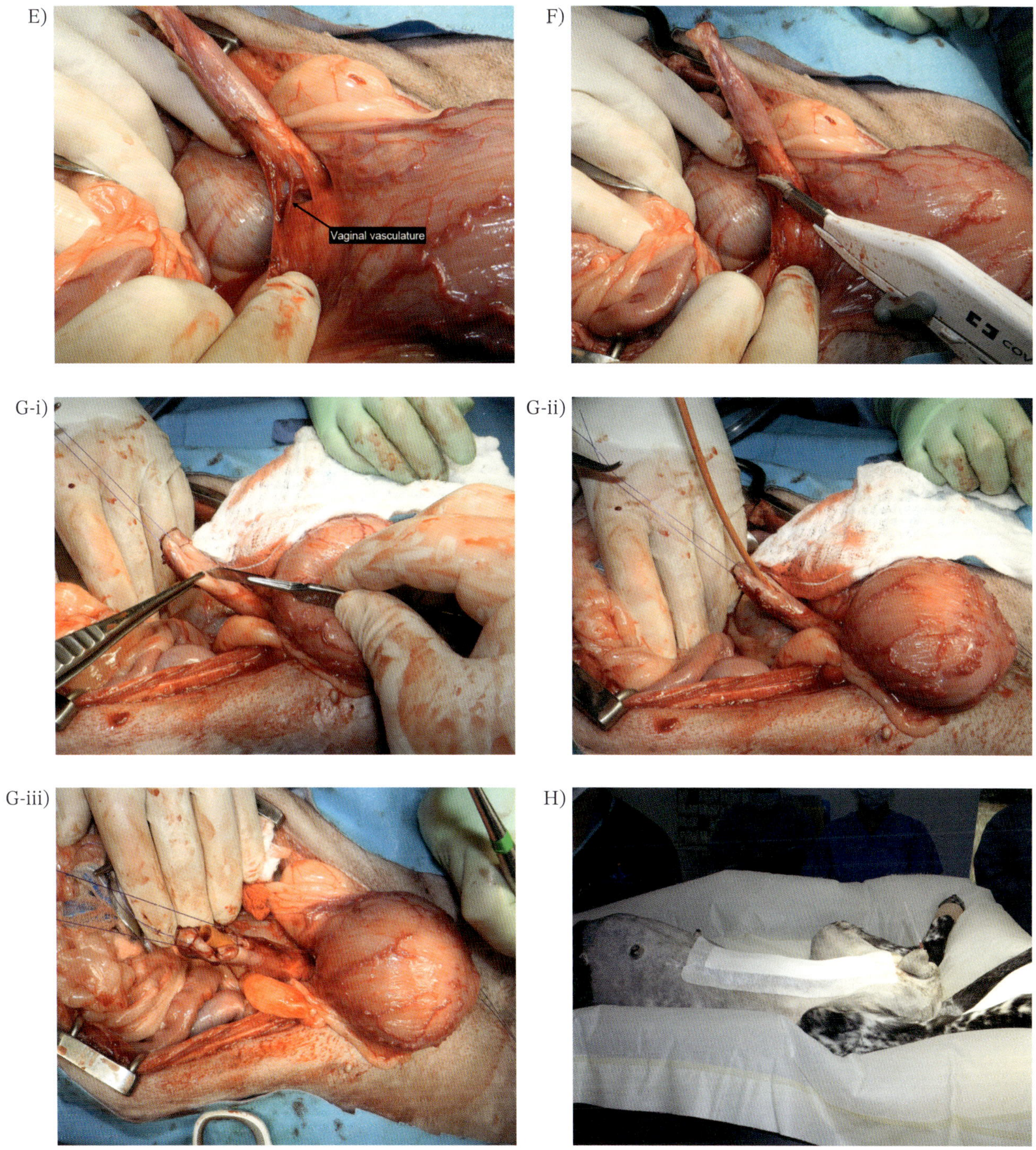

Surgical Technique [1, 2] (See Plate 32A–U) *continued*

I) The patient is then repositioned in sternal recumbency as described earlier in *Patient Positioning*.

J) **Perineal approach for vulvovaginectomy:** The catheter placed via the abdominal approach should be visible. For hemostasis, two Doyen clamps can be placed vertically either side of the median raphe of the vestibular hood as far dorsally as possible and closed, one arm in the vestibule and one arm on the skin.

K) An episiotomy is performed in a ventral-to-dorsal direction between the Doyen clamps. This incision is continued through the skin, muscle, and vestibular mucosa, and extended as far dorsally as possible, typically 2–4 cm ventral to the anus (i, ii).

L) The Doyen clamps are then rolled laterally by an assistant to open the vestibule (i). Alternatively, if not using Doyen clamps, then self-retaining retractors (i.e. Gelpi [ii] or Weitlaner retractors) or stay sutures (iii) can be used.

Plate 32

Vulvovaginectomy *continued*

I)

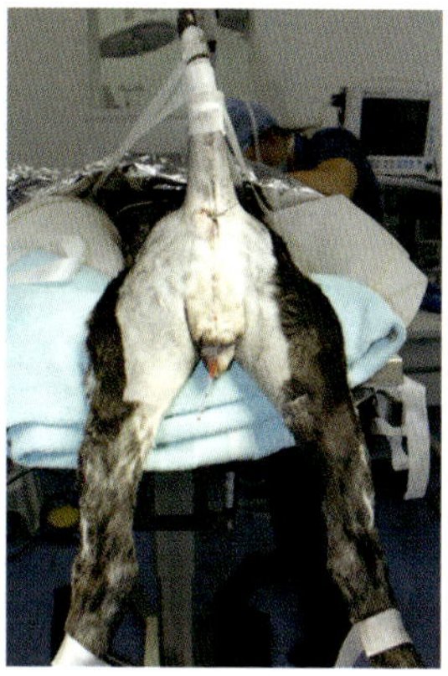

J)

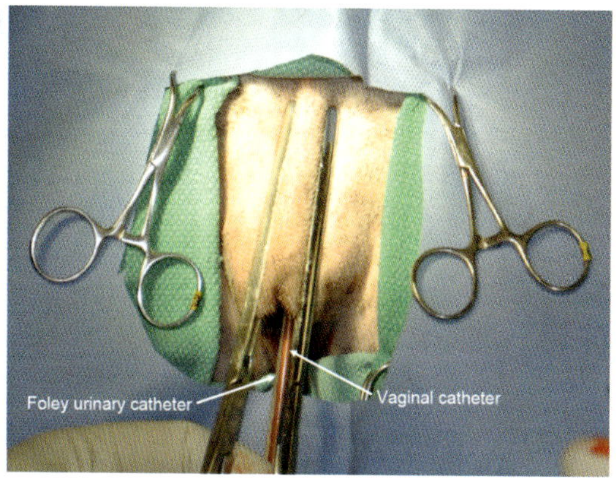

K-i)

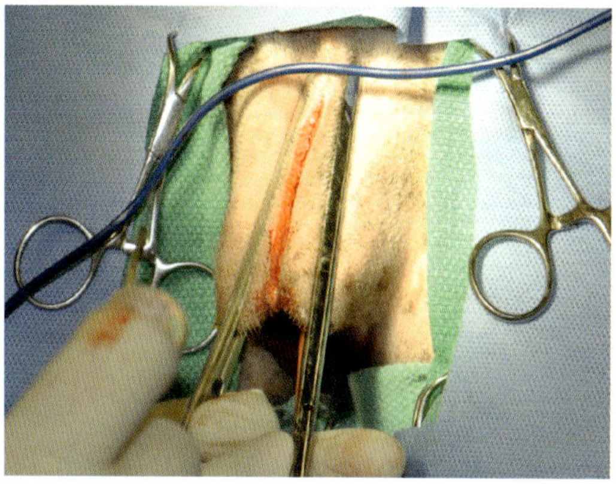

K-ii)

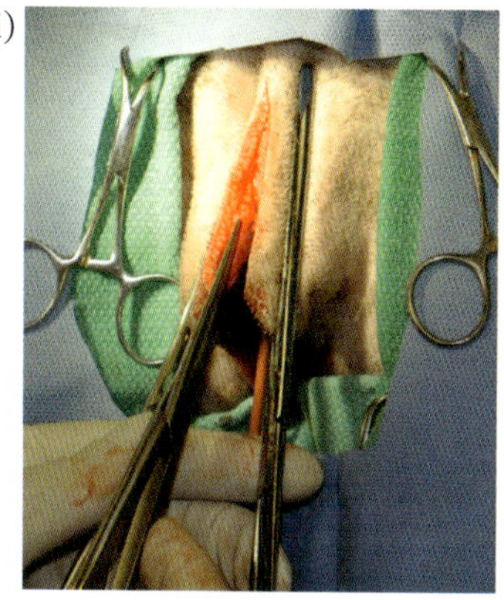

L-i)

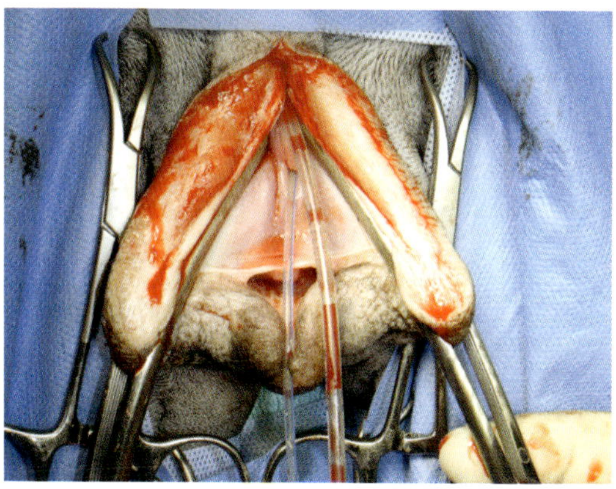

L-ii)

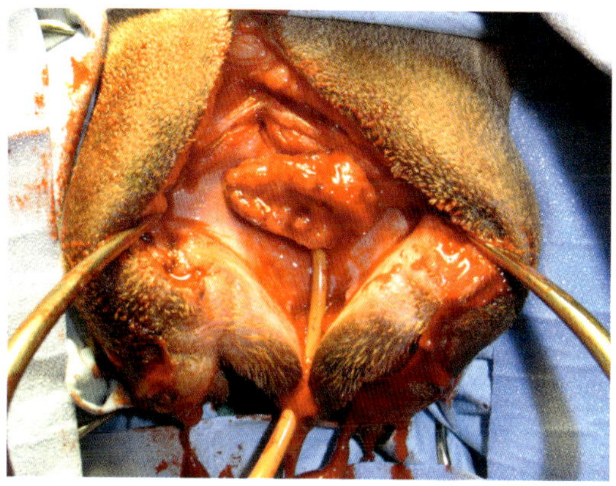

L-iii)

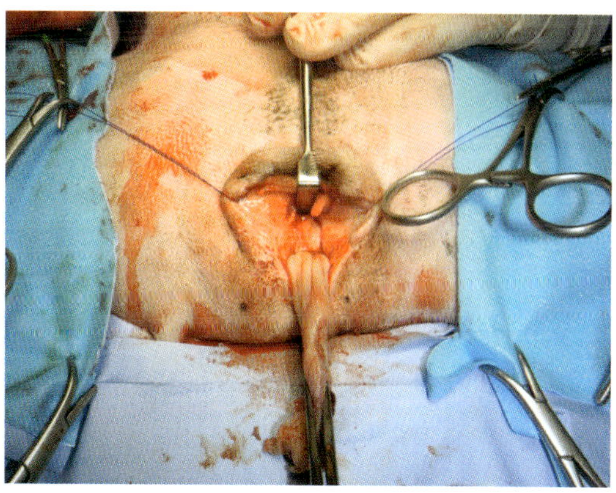

Surgical Technique [1, 2] (See Plate 32A–U) *continued*

M) A Foley urinary catheter is inserted into the urethral opening by direct visualization (arrow).

N) The vaginal catheter is then tractioned caudally, everting the cranial vagina and bringing the bulk of the vagina into the vestibule.

O) A circumferential mucosal incision is made at the junction of the vagina and vestibule from 9 o'clock dorsally to 3 o'clock with a scalpel or electrosurgery (i) and extended full thickness with Metzenbaum scissors (ii).

P) Digital palpation is then used to determine the cranial edge of the inverted vagina, and sharp and blunt dissection are used to free the remaining pelvic and retroperitoneal attachments (i, ii).

Plate 32

Vulvovaginectomy *continued*

M)

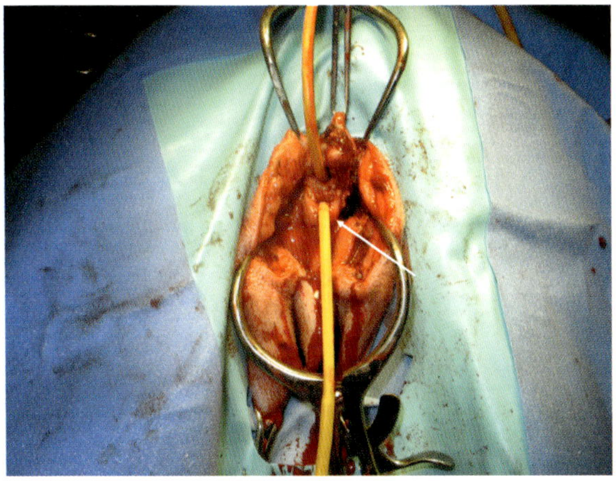

N)

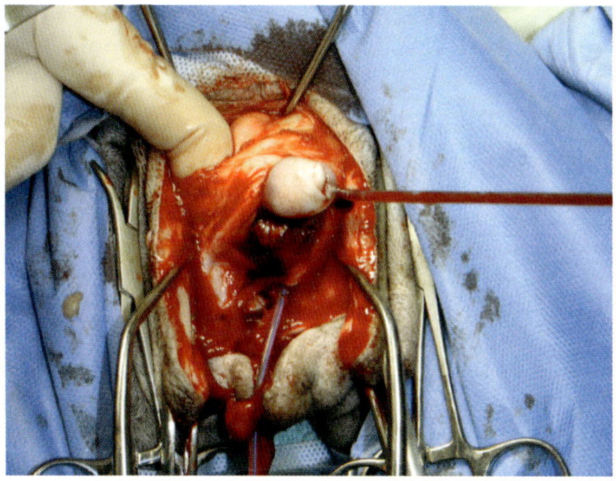

O-i)

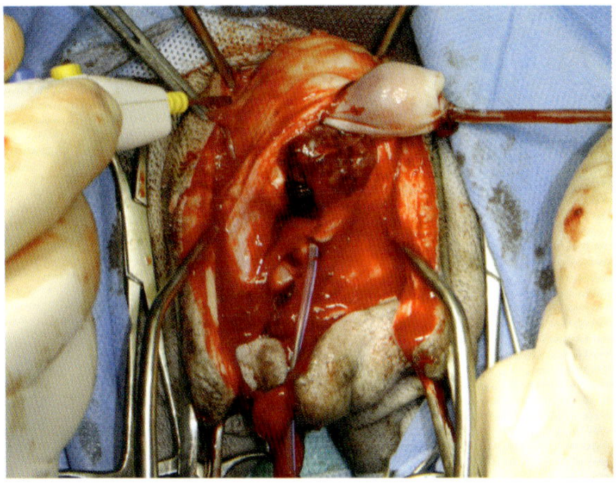

O-ii)

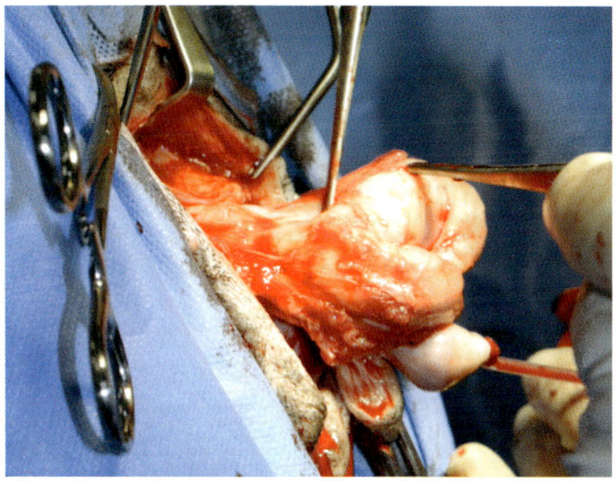

P-i)

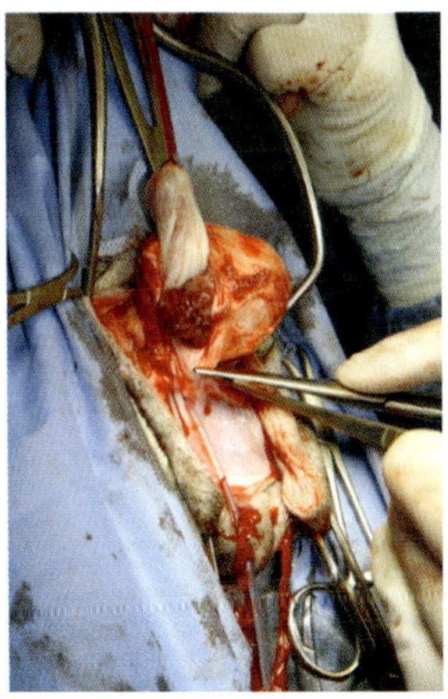

P-ii)

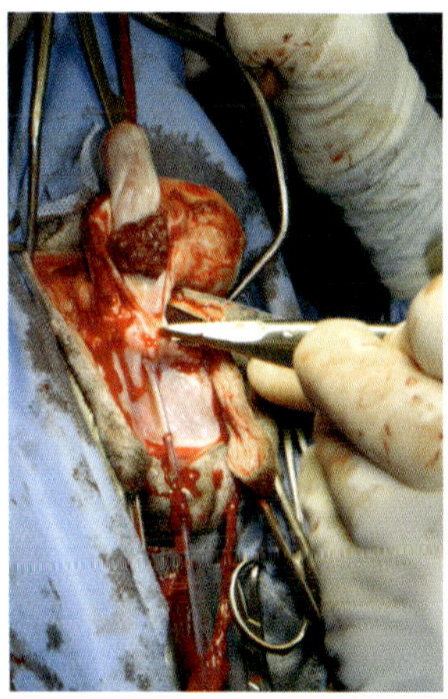

Surgical Technique [1, 2] (See Plate 32A–U) *continued*

Q) Once the dorsal attachments are freed and the vagina is falling ventrally into the vestibule, the ventral half of the mucosa can be incised (i). The urethra should be identified along the ventral border of this dissection (arrow) and preserved. The incision is continued full thickness until the entire vagina can be removed (ii).

R) If the vaginal disease also involves the terminal urethra, then the urethral orifice and affected section of urethra are included in the vaginal resection. A urethral pullout is then performed by circumferentially mobilizing the sectioned end of the urethra (i) and retracting this caudally (ii). A stay suture of 3-0 absorbable monofilament suture material should be placed in the urethra immediately cranial to the planned transection site (ii, arrow) to prevent retraction of the urethra into the pelvic canal. The distal urethra is transected and removed from the surgical field. The urethra is then sutured to the vestibular mucosa with 4-0 absorbable monofilament suture material in a simple interrupted suture pattern (iii, arrow).

S) The dead space is closed dorsally above the urethra with 2-0 to 3-0 absorbable monofilament suture material in a simple interrupted suture pattern (i, ii).

Plate 32

Vulvovaginectomy *continued*

Q-i)

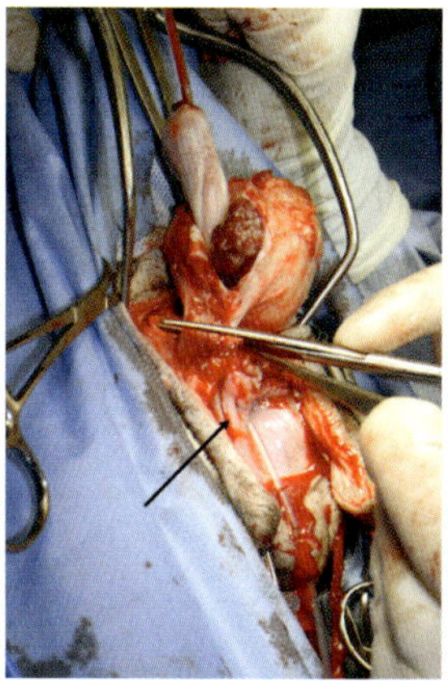

Q-ii)

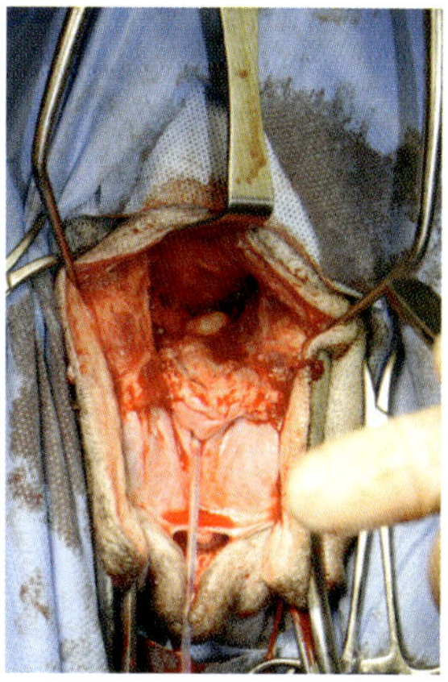

R-i)

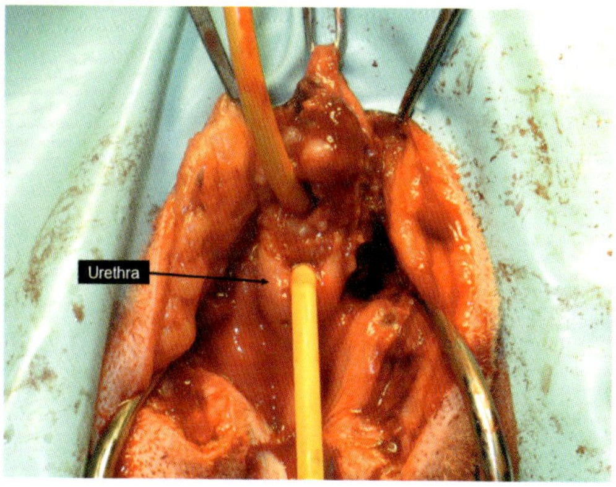

R-ii)

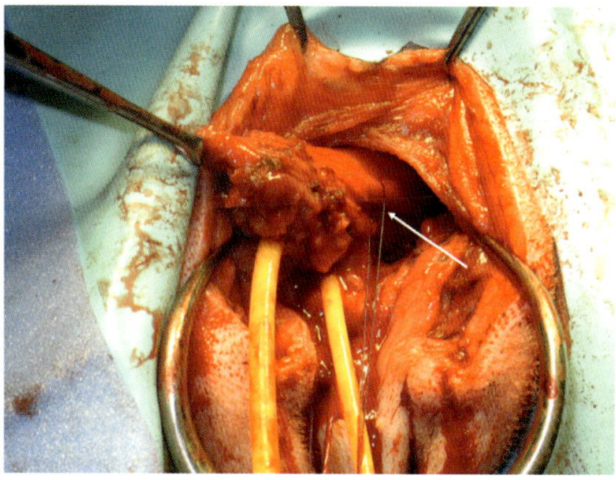

R-iii)

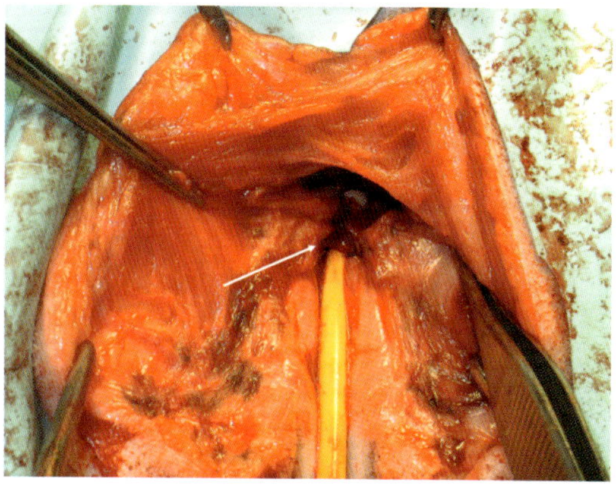

S-i)

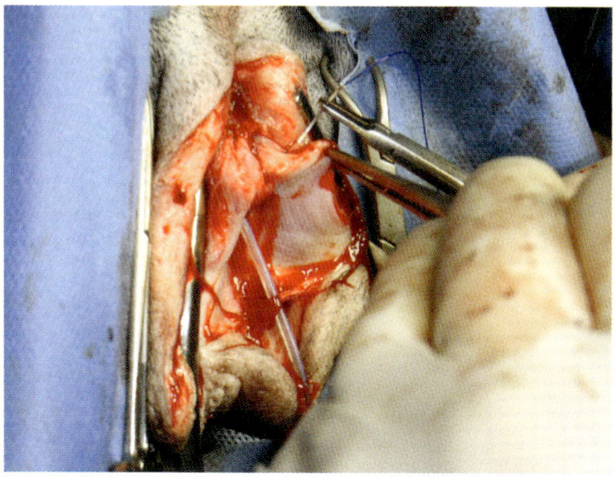

S-ii)

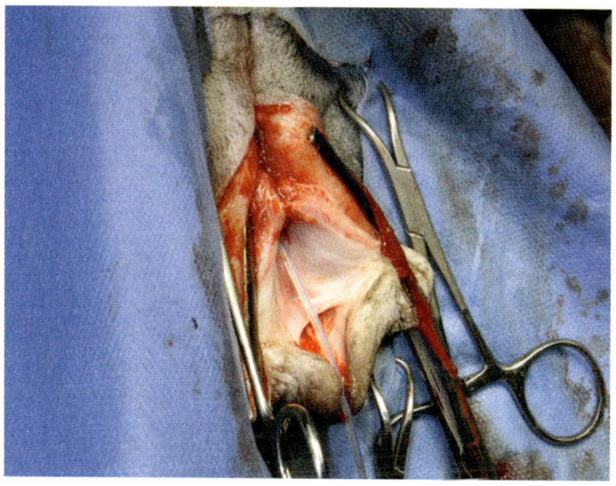

Surgical Technique [1, 2] (See Plate 32A–U) *continued*

T) A positional suture is first placed at the ventral end of the episiotomy wound to align the vulva. The episiotomy is then closed in three layers. The mucosal (i) and muscle (ii) layers are closed using 3-0 to 4-0 absorbable monofilament suture material in a simple continuous suture pattern. The skin is closed using 3-0 nonabsorbable monofilament suture material in a simple interrupted (iii) or simple continuous suture pattern.

U) If a total vulvovaginectomy has been performed (i), then the urethra (ii) will need to be sutured to the skin in two layers with urethral submucosa sutured to the subcutaneous layer with 3-0 to 4-0 absorbable monofilament suture material in a simple continuous suture pattern, and urethral mucosa sutured to the skin with 3-0 to 4-0 nonabsorbable monofilament suture material in a simple interrupted (iii) or simple continuous suture pattern. The vulvovaginectomy site is then closed routinely (iv, v).

Postoperative Management

1) Multimodal analgesia
2) Elizabethan collar or body suit
3) Vestibular tampon for 24 hours
4) Indwelling urethral catheter for 24–72 hours

Complications – Dogs

Intraoperative Complications

- Iatrogenic rectal perforation (5%) [3]
- Iatrogenic urethral trauma

Postoperative Complications [1–3]

- Urinary incontinence (25% overall)
  - Transient urinary incontinence (13%)
  - Permanent urinary incontinence (13%)
- Urine scald dermatitis (14%)
- Serosanguineous vaginal discharge (8%)
- Dyschezia (8%)
- Dysuria (3%)
- Hematuria (3%)
- Urethrostomy dehiscence (3%)
- Surgical-site infection (3%)

Suggested Adjuvant Treatments

- ± Chemotherapy, depending on tumor type and histologic grade
- ± Radiation therapy, depending on tumor type and completeness of excision

Plate 32

Vulvovaginectomy *continued*

T-i)

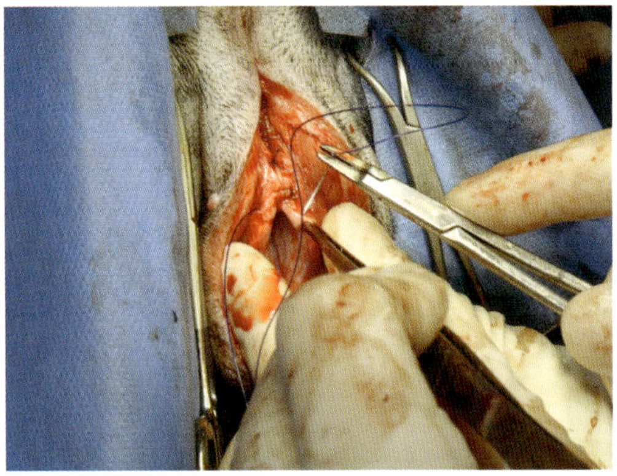

T-iii)

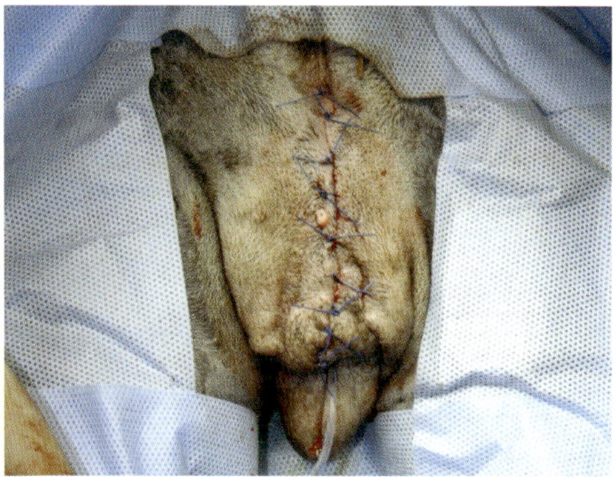

T-ii)

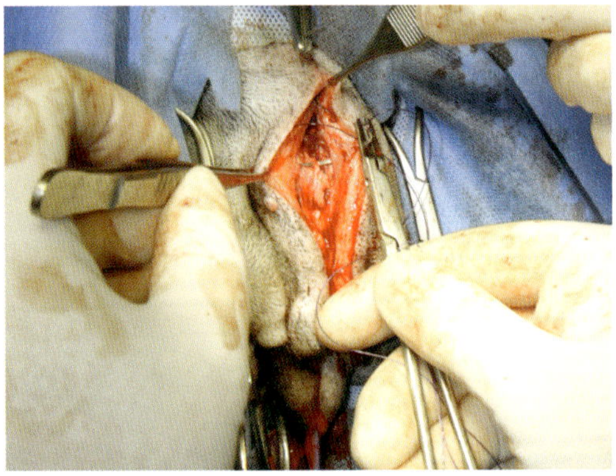

U-i)

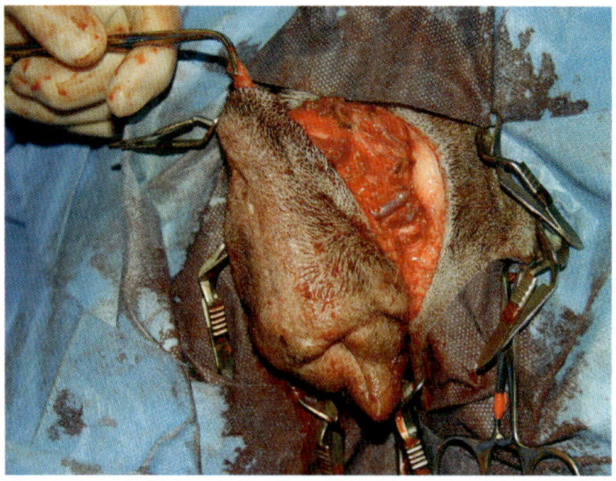

Courtesy of Dr. Bart Van Goethem

U-ii)

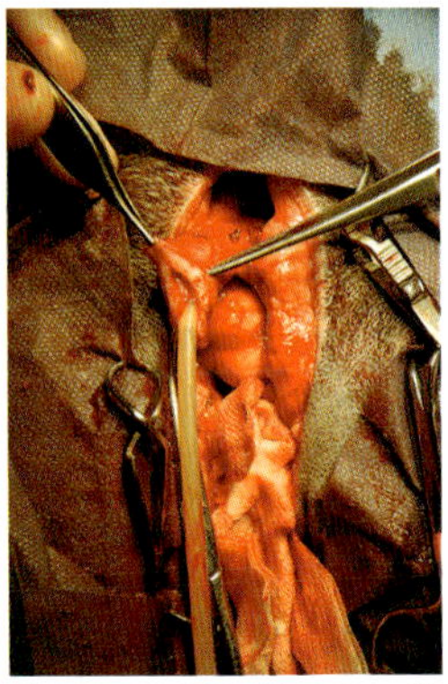

Courtesy of Dr. Bart Van Goethem

U-iii)

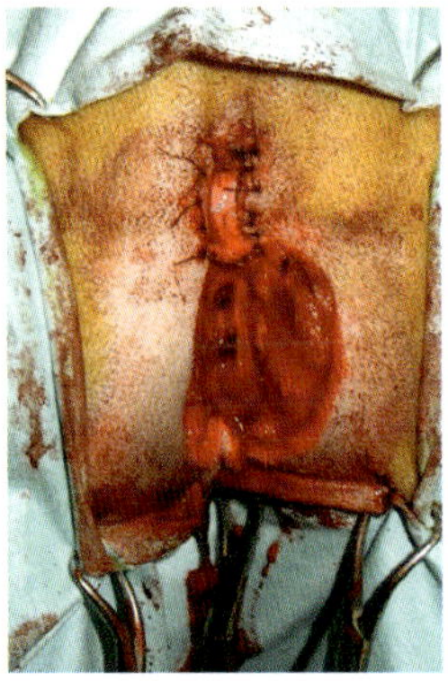

U-iv)

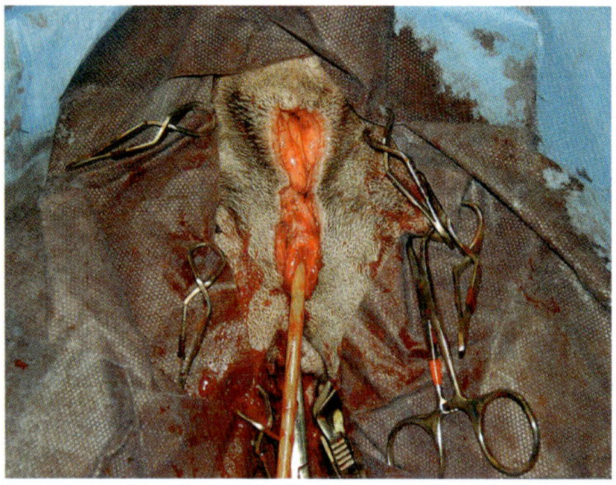

Courtesy of Dr. Bart Van Goethem

U-v)

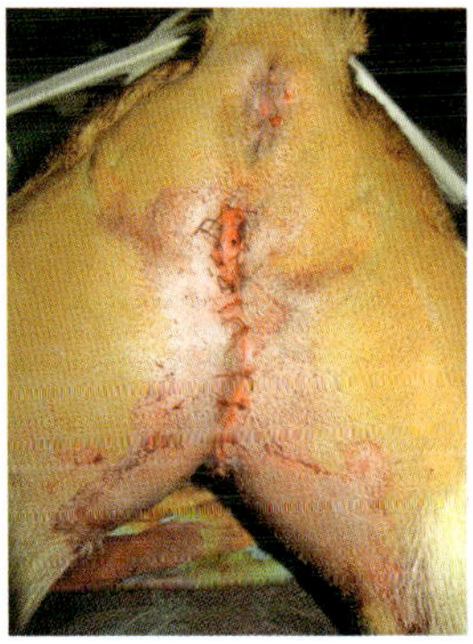

Prognosis and Oncologic Outcome

	Local Recurrence Rate	Metastatic Rate	Disease-Free Interval (d)	Median Survival Time (d)	1-Year Survival Rate	2-Year Survival Rate
			Leiomyoma [1–3]			
Overall	0%	0%	–	Not reached [3]	–	–
			Sarcomas [1, 3]			
Overall	11%	0%	308	727	83% [3]	33% [3]
			Carcinomas [1–3]			
Overall	25%	25%	80	81	0% [3]	0% [3]

References

1 Nelissen, P. and White, R.A.S. (2012). Subtotal vaginectomy for management of extensive vaginal disease in 11 dogs. *Vet. Surg.* 41 (4): 495–500.

2 Salomon, J.F., Deneuche, A., and Viguier, E. (2004). Vaginectomy and urethroplasty as a treatment for non-peduculated vaginal tumours in four bitches. *J. Small Anim. Pract.* 45 (3): 157–161.

3 Ogden, J.A., Selmic, L.E., Liptak, J.M. et al. (2020). Outcomes associated with vaginectomy and vulvovaginectomy in 21 dogs. *Vet. Surg.* 49 (6): 1132–1143.

Section 7

Musculoskeletal

Chapter 33: Primary Bone and Periarticular Tumors

The surgical management of primary musculoskeletal tumors, including appendicular and axial bone tumors and periarticular tumors, includes amputation and limb-sparing techniques. Although limb amputation can be performed at various levels, only forequarter amputation and coxofemoral disarticulation will be described in this section. Limb-sparing techniques are divided into reconstructive (distal radius) and nonreconstructive (scapulectomy, ulnectomy, ischiectomy) procedures. The distal radius is the most amenable site for limb-sparing surgery, and numerous techniques and materials have been reported. Cortical allografts [1], pasteurized [2] or irradiated [3] autografts, and commercially available [4, 5] and customized patient-specific 3D-printed endoprostheses [6, 7] have been described to reconstruct the distal radial defect. Alternative distal radial limb-sparing techniques include lateral manus translation [8], ulnar rollover [9], and bone transport osteogenesis [10]; the latter two techniques will not be described in this section. Other limb-sparing surgical procedures that have been reported but will not be described in this chapter include limb salvage for proximal humeral [11] and proximal femoral tumors [12, 13], and distal limb salvage with intraosseous transcutaneous amputation prostheses [14].

Suggested Diagnostic Workup and Clinical Staging

- Complete blood count, serum biochemistry, and urinalysis
- Fine-needle aspirate, core aspirate, or needle-core biopsy, with alkaline phosphatase (ALP) staining of fine-needle or core aspirates for appendicular bone tumors
- Limb radiographs, computed tomography (CT) scan, or magnetic resonance imaging (MRI) for planning limb-sparing surgery
- ± Regional lymph node fine-needle aspirate cytology
- ± Nuclear scintigraphy for assessment of bone metastasis
- Abdominal ultrasound for dogs with suspected periarticular histiocytic sarcomas
- Three-view thoracic radiographs or thoracic CT scan for assessment of lung metastasis

Suggested Adjuvant Treatments

- Chemotherapy for dogs with appendicular osteosarcomas
- Chemotherapy for dogs with appendicular hemangiosarcomas
- Chemotherapy for dogs with periarticular histiocytic sarcoma
- Chemotherapy for dogs with grade III periarticular synovial cell sarcomas

Color Atlas of Canine and Feline Surgical Oncology, First Edition. Julius M. Liptak, Paolo Buracco, William T. N. Culp, and Nicholas J. Bacon.

Prognosis and Oncologic Outcome – Dogs

	Local Recurrence Rate	Metastatic Rate	Disease-Free Interval (d)	Median Survival Time (d)	1-Year Survival Rate	2-Year Survival Rate
Appendicular Osteosarcoma – Amputation Alone [15]						
Overall	0%	73%	–	134	12%	2%
Appendicular Osteosarcoma – Surgery and Chemotherapy [16–25]						
Overall	0%–2%	53%–87%	137–292	258–479	28%–49%	19%–24%
Body weight [25]						
40 kg	–	–	337	>400	–	–
≥40 kg	–	–	109	242	–	–
Tumor location [19]						
Radius	–	–	468	596	–	–
Other locations	–	–	187	232	–	–
Preoperative total ALP [16, 17]						
Normal	–	–	366	381–496	53%	29%
Increased	–	–	170	168–177	0%	0%
Preoperative bone-specific ALP [16, 17]						
Normal	–	–	431	506–546	60%	48%
Increased	–	–	147	218–290	34%	6%
Preoperative proteinuria [23]						
Yes	–	–	–	149	–	–
No	–	–	–	372	–	–
Lymph node metastasis [26]						
Yes	–	–	48	59	–	–
No	–	–	238	318	–	–
Histology – vascular invasion [23]						
Yes	–	–	–	175	–	–
No	–	–	–	273	–	–
Histology – mitotic rate [23]						
<5/3 hpf	–	–	–	415	–	–
≥5/3 hpf	–	–	–	177	–	–
Histologic grade [23]						
Grade I	–	–	–	415	–	–
Grade II	–	–	–	298	–	–
Grade III	–	–	–	162	–	–

(Continued)

	Local Recurrence Rate	Metastatic Rate	Disease-Free Interval (d)	Median Survival Time (d)	1-Year Survival Rate	2-Year Survival Rate
Chemotherapy course completed [19, 23]						
Yes	–	–	295	393–507	–	–
No	–	–	106	152–156	–	–
Infection after limb-sparing surgery [4, 27]						
Yes	–	–	–	567–685	–	–
No	–	–	–	289–298	–	–
Construct failure after limb-sparing surgery [4, 28]						
Yes	–	–	–	518–685	–	–
No	–	–	–	277–322	–	–
Perioperative analgesia intensity [29]						
High	–	–	–	378	–	–
Low	–	–	–	252	–	–
Appendicular Chondrosarcoma [30]						
Overall	0%	28%	289	979	–	–
Histologic grade						
Grade I	–	–	–	2190	–	–
Grade II	–	–	–	979	–	–
Grade III	–	–	–	329	–	–
Appendicular Hemangiosarcoma [31]						
Overall	0%	49%	–	197	28%	6%
Treatment						
Amputation	–	–	103	103	–	–
Amputation and chemotherapy	–	–	129	299	–	–
Periarticular Histiocytic Sarcoma						
Overall [32, 33]	6%	91%	162	391	–	–
Clinical stage [33]						
Nonmetastatic	–	–	–	980	–	–
Metastatic	–	–	129	253	–	–
Periarticular Synovial Cell Sarcoma [34]						
Overall	7%	24%	–	>1460	–	–
Clinical stage						
Nonmetastatic	–	–	–	>1460	–	–
Metastatic	–	–	–	92	–	–

	Local Recurrence Rate	Metastatic Rate	Disease-Free Interval (d)	Median Survival Time (d)	1-Year Survival Rate	2-Year Survival Rate
Histology – mitotic rate						
<25/10 hpf	–	–	>1460	>1460	–	–
≥25/10 hpf	–	–	122	275	–	–
Histology – degree of nuclear pleomorphism						
Mild to moderate	–	–	>1460	>1460	–	–
Marked	–	–	107	214	–	–
Histology – percentage tumor necrosis						
<30%	–	–	>1460	>1460	–	–
≥30%	–	–	275	214	–	–
Histologic grade						
Grade I	–	–	>1460	>1460	–	–
Grade II	–	–	>1460	1095	–	–
Grade III	–	–	122	214	–	–
Immunohistochemistry – cytokeratin						
Negative	–	–	>1460	>1460	–	–
Positive	–	–	107	122	–	–

hpf, high-power fields.

Prognosis and Oncologic Outcome – Cats

	Local Recurrence Rate	Metastatic Rate	Disease-Free Interval (d)	Median Survival Time (d)	1-Year Survival Rate	2-Year Survival Rate
Appendicular Osteosarcoma [35–37]						
Overall	8%–9%	4%–46%	235	527–1495	–	–
Tumor location [36]						
Humerus	–	86%	–	–	–	–
Other	–	42%	–	–	–	–

References

1 LaRue, S.M., Withrow, S.J., Powers, B.E. et al. (1989). Limb-sparing treatment for osteosarcoma in dogs. *J. Am. Vet. Med. Assoc.* 195 (12): 1734–1744.

2 Morello, E., Vasconi, E., Martano, M. et al. (2003). Pasteurized tumoral autograft and adjuvant chemotherapy for the treatment of canine distal radial osteosarcoma: 13 cases. *Vet. Surg.* 32 (6): 539–544.

3 Liptak, J.M., Dernell, W.S., Lascelles, B.D.X. et al. (2004). Intraoperative extracorporeal irradiation for limb sparing in 13 dogs. *Vet. Surg.* 33 (5): 446–456.

4 Liptak, J.M., Dernell, W.S., Ehrhart, N. et al. (2006). Cortical allograft and endoprosthesis for limb-sparing surgery in dogs with distal radial osteosarcoma: a prospective clinical comparison of two different limb-sparing techniques. *Vet. Surg.* 35 (6): 518–533.

5 Mitchell, K.E., Boston, S.E., Kung, M. et al. (2016). Outcomes of limb-sparing surgery using two generations of metal endoprosthesis in 45 dogs with distal radial osteosarcoma. A veterinary society of surgical oncology retrospective study. *Vet. Surg.* 45 (1): 36–43.

6 Bray, J.P., Kersley, A., Downing, W. et al. (2017). Clinical outcomes of patient-specific porous titanium endoprostheses in dogs with tumors of the mandible, radius, or tibia: 12 cases (2013-2016). *J. Am. Vet. Med. Assoc.* 251 (5): 566–579.

7 Seguin, B., Pinard, C., Lussier, B. et al. (2020). Limb-sparing in dogs using patient-specific, three-dimensional-printed endoprosthesis for distal radial osteosarcoma: a pilot study. *Vet. Comp. Oncol.* 18 (1): 92–104.

8 Seguin, B., Walsh, P.J., Ehrhart, E.J. et al. (2019). Cortical allograft and endoprosthesis for limb-sparing surgery in dogs with distal radial osteosarcoma: a prospective clinical comparison of two different limb-sparing techniques. *Vet. Surg.* 48 (2): 247–256.

9 Seguin, B., O'Donnell, M.D., Walsh, P.J. et al. (2017). Long-term outcome of dogs treated with ulnar rollover transposition for limb-sparing of distal radial osteosarcoma: 27 limbs in 26 dogs. *Vet. Surg.* 46 (7): 1017–1024.

10 Ehrhart, N. (2005). Longitudinal bone transport for treatment of primary bone tumors in dogs: technique description and outcome in 9 dogs. *Vet. Surg.* 34 (1): 24–34.

11 Kuntz, C.A., Asselin, T.L., Dernell, W.S. et al. (1998). Limb salvage surgery for osteosarcoma of the proximal humerus: outcome in 17 dogs. *Vet. Surg.* 27 (5): 417–422.

12 Liptak, J.M., Pluhar, G.E., Dernell, W.S. et al. (2005). Limb-sparing surgery in a dog with osteosarcoma of the proximal femur. *Vet. Surg.* 34 (1): 71–77.

13 Fitzpatrick, N. and Guthrie, J.W. (2018). Hemipelvic and proximal femoral limb salvage endoprosthesis with tendon ongrowth in a dog. *Vet. Surg.* 47 (7): 963–969.

14 Fitzpatrick, N., Smith, T.J., Pendegrass, C.J. et al. (2011). Intraosseous transcutaneous amputation prosthesis (ITAP) for limb salvage in 4 dogs. *Vet. Surg.* 40 (8): 909–925.

15 Spodnick, G.J., Berg, J., Rand, W.M. et al. (1992). Use of alternating administration of carboplatin and doxorubicin in dogs with microscopic metastases after amputation for appendicular osteosarcoma: 50 cases (1999–2006). *J. Am. Vet. Med. Assoc.* 200 (7): 995–999.

16 Ehrhart, N., Dernell, W.S., Hoffmann, W.E. et al. (1998). Prognostic importance of alkaline phosphatase activity in serum from dogs with appendicular osteosarcoma: 75 cases (1990-1996). *J. Am. Vet. Med. Assoc.* 213 (7): 1002–1006.

17 Garzotto, C.K., Berg, J., Hoffmann, W.E. et al. (2000). Prognostic significance of serum alkaline phosphatase activity in canine appendicular osteosarcoma. *J. Vet. Intern. Med.* 14 (6): 587–592.

18 Kirpensteijn, J., Kik, M., Rutteman, G.R. et al. (2002). Prognostic significance of a new histologic grading system for canine osteosarcoma. *Vet. Pathol.* 39 (2): 240–246.

19 Bacon, N.J., Ehrhart, N.P., Dernell, W.S. et al. (2008). Use of alternating administration of carboplatin and doxorubicin in dogs with microscopic metastases after amputation for appendicular osteosarcoma: 50 cases (1999-2006). *J. Am. Vet. Med. Assoc.* 232 (10): 1504–1510.

20 Chun, R., Garrett, L.D., Henry, C. et al. (2005). Toxicity and efficacy of cisplatin and doxorubicin combination chemotherapy for the treatment of canine osteosarcoma. *J. Am. Anim. Hosp. Assoc.* 41 (6): 382–387.

21 Alvarez, F.J., Kisseberth, W., Hosoya, K. et al. (2014). Postoperative adjuvant combination therapy with doxorubicin and noncytotoxic suramin in dogs with appendicular osteosarcoma. *J. Am. Anim. Hosp. Assoc.* 50 (1): 12–18.

22 Phillips, B., Powers, B.E., Dernell, W.S. et al. (2009). Use of single-agent carboplatin as adjuvant or neoadjuvant therapy in conjunction with amputation for appendicular osteosarcoma in dogs. *J. Am. Anim. Hosp. Assoc.* 45 (1): 33–38.

23 Saam, D.E., Liptak, J.M., Stalker, M.J. et al. (2011). Predictors of outcome in dogs treated with adjuvant carboplatin for appendicular osteosarcoma: 65 cases (1996-2006). *J. Am. Vet. Med. Assoc.* 238 (2): 195–206.

24 Skorupski, K.A., Uhl, J.M., Szivek, A. et al. (2016). Carboplatin versus alternating carboplatin and doxorubicin for the adjuvant treatment of canine appendicular osteosarcoma: a randomized, phase III trial. *Vet. Comp. Oncol.* 14 (1): 81–87.

25 Bergman, P.J., MacEwen, E.G., Kurzman, I.D. et al. (1996). Amputation and carboplatin for treatment of dogs with osteosarcoma: 48 cases (1991 to 1993). *J. Vet. Intern. Med.* 10 (2): 76–81.

26 Hillers, K.R., Dernell, W.S., Lafferty, M.H. et al. (2005). Incidence and prognostic importance of lymph node metastases in dogs with appendicular osteosarcoma: 228 cases (1986-2003). *J. Am. Vet. Med. Assoc.* 226 (8): 1364–1367.

27 Lascelles, B.D.X., Dernell, W.S., Correa, M.T. et al. (2005). Improved survival associated with postoperative wound infection in dogs treated with limb-salvage surgery for osteosarcoma. *Ann. Surg. Oncol.* 12 (12): 1073–1083.

28 Seguin, B., Walsh, P.J., Ehrhart, E.J. 3rd et al. (2019). Lateral manus translation for limb-sparing surgery in 18 dogs with distal radial osteosarcoma in dogs. *Vet. Surg.* 48 (2): 247–256.

29 Nolan, M.W., Uzan, O.C., Green, N.A. et al. (2022). Intensity of perioperative analgesia but not pre-treatment pain is predictive of survival in dogs undergoing amputation plus chemotherapy for extremity osteosarcoma. *Vet. Comp. Oncol.* 20 (3): 568–576.

30 Farese, J.P., Kirpensteijn, J., Kik, M. et al. (2009). Biologic behavior and clinical outcome of 25 dogs with canine appendicular chondrosarcoma treated by amputation: a veterinary society of surgical oncology retrospective study. *Vet. Surg.* 38 (8): 914–919.

31 Giuffrida, M.A., Kamstock, D.A., Selmic, L.E. et al. (2018). Primary appendicular hemangiosarcoma and telangiectatic osteosarcoma in 70 dogs: a veterinary society of surgical oncology retrospective study. *Vet. Surg.* 47 (6): 774–783.

32 Craig, L.E., Julian, M.E., and Ferracone, J.D. (2002). The diagnosis and prognosis of synovial tumors in dogs: 35 cases. *Vet. Pathol.* 39 (1): 66–73.

33 Klahn, S.L., Kitchell, B.E., and Dervisis, N.G. (2011). Evaluation and comparison of outcomes in dogs with periarticular and nonperiarticular histiocytic sarcoma. *J. Am. Vet. Med. Assoc.* 239 (1): 90–96.

34 Vail, D.M., Powers, B.E., Getzy, D.M. et al. (1994). Evaluation of prognostic factors for dogs with synovial sarcoma: 36 cases (1986-1991). *J. Am. Vet. Med. Assoc.* 205 (9): 1300–1307.

35 Bitetto, W.V., Patnaik, A.K., Schrader, S.C. et al. (1987). Osteosarcoma in cats: 22 cases (1974-1984). *J. Am. Vet. Med. Assoc.* 190 (1): 91–93.

36 Heldmann, E., Anderson, M.A., and Wagner-Mann, C. (2000). Feline osteosarcoma: 145 cases (1990-1995). *J. Am. Anim. Hosp. Assoc.* 36 (6): 518–521.

37 Nakano, Y., Kagawa, Y., Shimoyama, Y. et al. (2021). Outcome of appendicular or scapular osteosarcoma treated by limb amputation in cats: 67 cases (1997-2018). *J. Am. Vet. Med. Assoc.* 260 (S1): S24–S28.

33.1 Forequarter Amputation

Indications

1) Resection of primary malignant appendicular bone tumors
2) Resection of primary benign or malignant periarticular tumors
3) Resection of extensive and infiltrative soft tissue tumors of the thoracic limb
4) Resection of brachial plexus nerve root tumors not amenable to local resection

Suggested Diagnostic Workup and Clinical Staging

- See *33. Primary Bone and Periarticular Tumors.*

Patient Positioning (See Plate 33.1A)

A) The patient is positioned in lateral recumbency with the affected limb uppermost.

Surgical Technique (See Plate 33.1B–P)

B) A skin incision is performed along the spine of the scapula, starting proximal to the dorsal margin of the scapula and extending distally to the acromion or greater tubercle of the humerus (i); then a circular incision is performed around the thoracic limb (ii). Alternatively, an elliptical incision can be performed around the thoracic limb, starting proximal to the dorsal margin of the scapula and extending distally to the axilla (iii). The advantages of this alternative approach are that there is less subcutaneous dissection and the closure is linear (see Q – v).
C) The subcutaneous tissue is dissected cranially to the spine of the scapula (SS) and caudally to the long head of the triceps brachii muscle (LH) (i). Using the alternative approach, the cranial part of the elliptical incision is positioned immediately cranial to the spine of the scapula (ii, iii) and the caudal part of the elliptical incision is positioned over the triceps muscle, hence minimizing the degree of soft tissue dissection required compared with the more traditional approach.
D) The trapezius muscle (Tr) is incised along its insertion on the spine of the scapula (SS) (pictured); this can be done with scissors, electrosurgery, or a vessel sealing device. Similarly, the omotransversarius muscle is incised at its insertion on the spine of the scapula and acromion.
E) The cleidobrachialis muscle (CB) is transected midbelly (pictured). The omobrachial and cephalic veins and branches of the cervical and suprascapular artery are deep to the cleidobrachialis muscle. These vessels need to be ligated, cauterized, or sealed and transected with a vessel sealing device during transection of the cleidobrachialis muscle.

Color Atlas of Canine and Feline Surgical Oncology, First Edition. Julius M. Liptak, Paolo Buracco, William T. N. Culp, and Nicholas J. Bacon.

Plate 33.1

Forequarter Amputation

A)

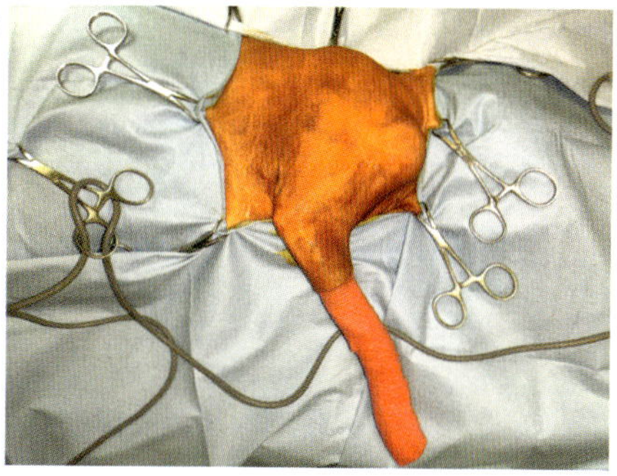

B-i)

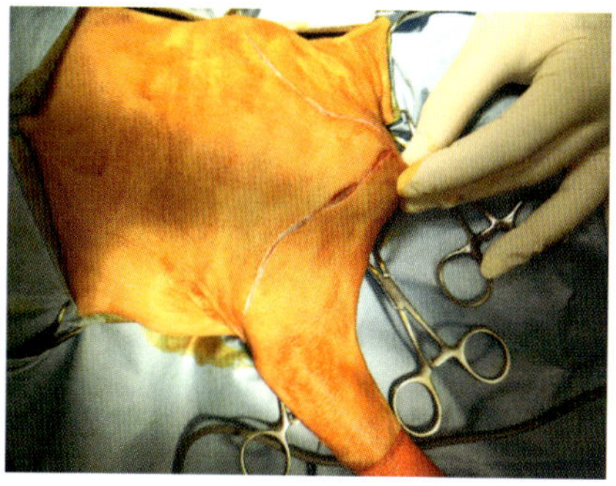

B-ii)

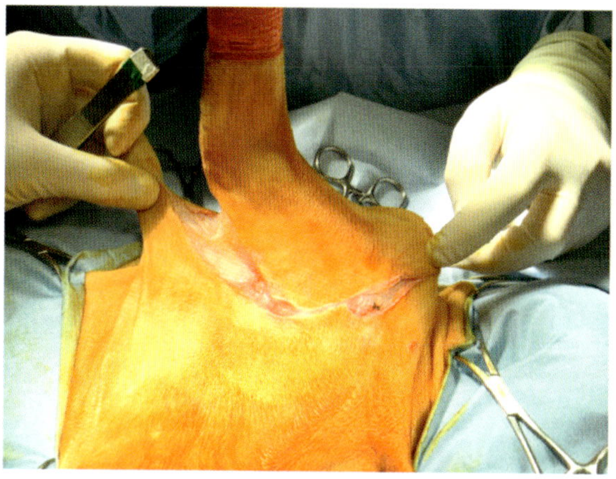

B-iii)

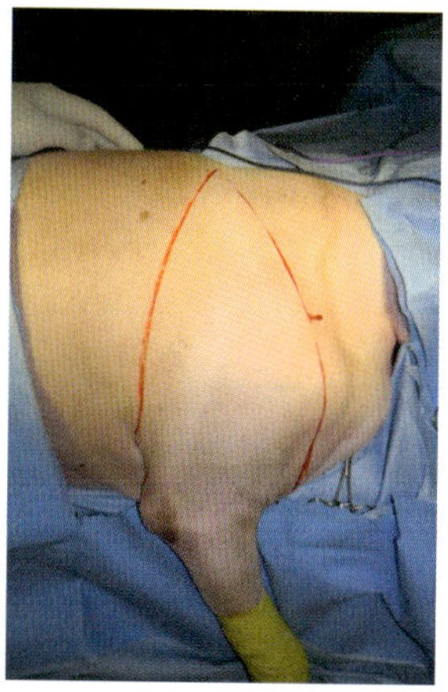

C-i)

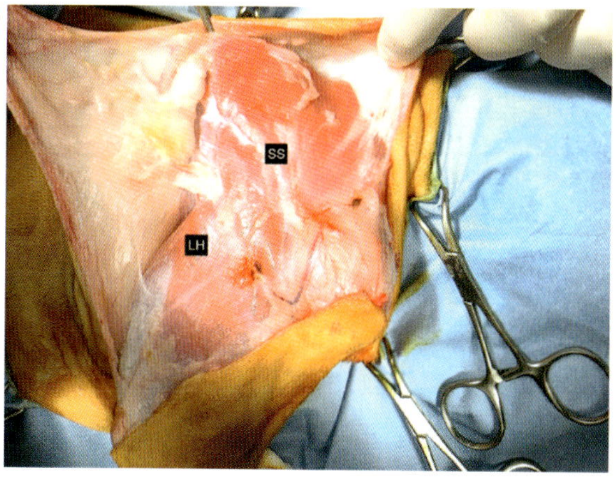

C-ii)

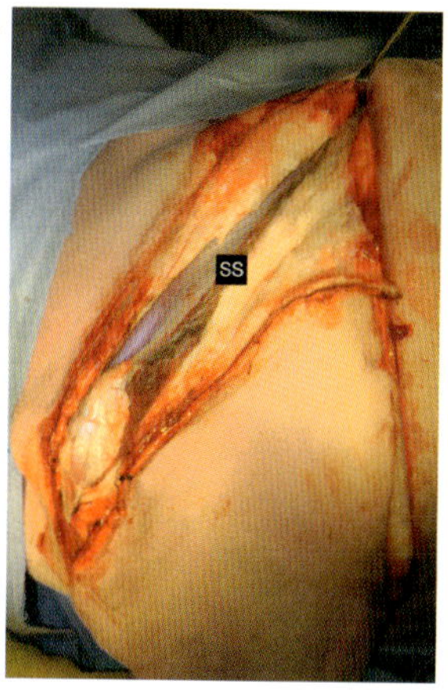

C-iii)

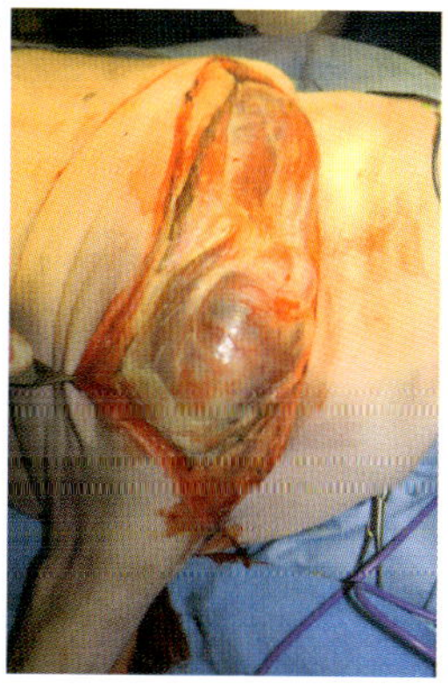

D)

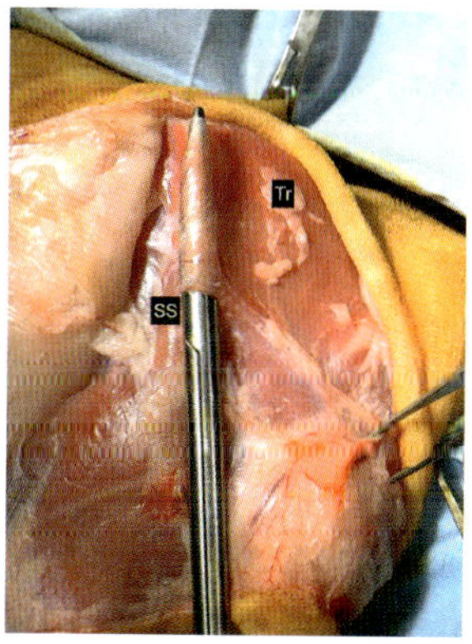

E)

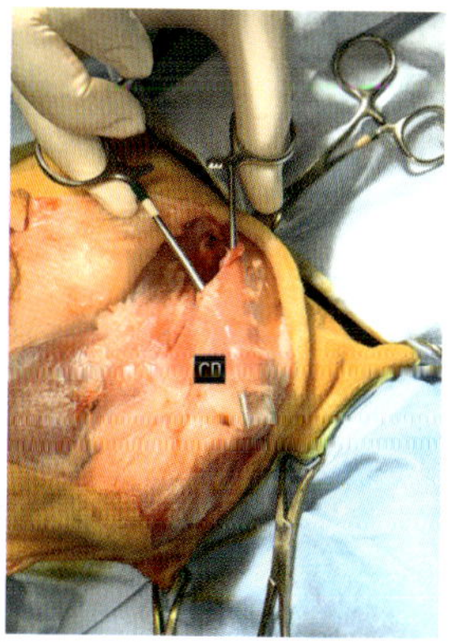

Surgical Technique (See Plate 33.1B–P) *continued*

F) Once this part of the approach is completed, the dissected muscles are retracted cranially to expose the cranial part of the scapula, which is then undermined digitally to free this portion of the scapula (SS, spine of the scapula; Tr, trapezius muscle).

G) The scapula is retracted laterally to abduct the scapula from the thoracic wall and expose the rhomboideus (RM) and serratus ventralis muscles (i). The rhomboideus muscle is then incised close to its insertion on the dorsal scapula with scissors (pictured), electrosurgery, or a vessel sealing device (ii).

H) The serratus ventralis (SV) muscle is dissected from the dorsomedial aspect of the scapula with a periosteal elevator, scissors, electrosurgery, or vessel sealing device (pictured).

I) Working caudally, the fascia caudal to the long head of triceps brachii muscle (LH) is incised to expose the latissimus dorsi muscle.

J) The scapula is retracted cranially to apply tension to the latissimus dorsi muscle (LD) (i). The latissimus dorsi muscle is then transected close to the triceps brachii muscle. The lateral thoracic artery and vein (ii, arrows) are ligated and transected (iii), and the lateral thoracic nerve is sharply transected, ventral to the latissimus dorsi muscle. The thoracodorsal artery and vein are ligated and transected, and the thoracodorsal nerve is sharply transected, medial to the latissimus dorsi muscle.

K) The scapula is retracted laterally to expose the brachial plexus. Blunt dissection is required to isolate and identify the axillary artery and vein, individual nerves of the brachial plexus, and the axillary lymph node.

Plate 33.1

Forequarter Amputation *continued*

F)

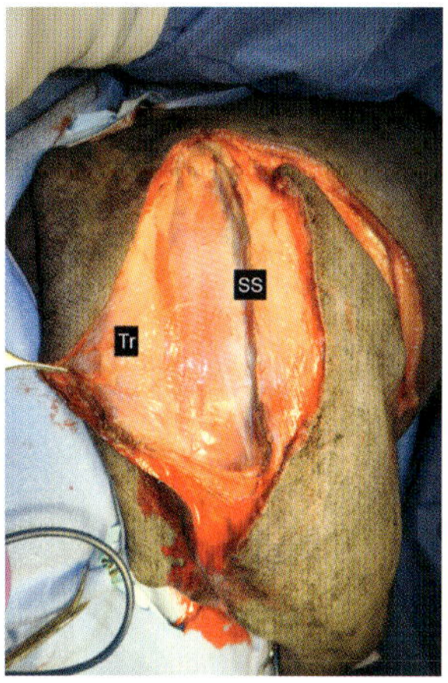

G-i)

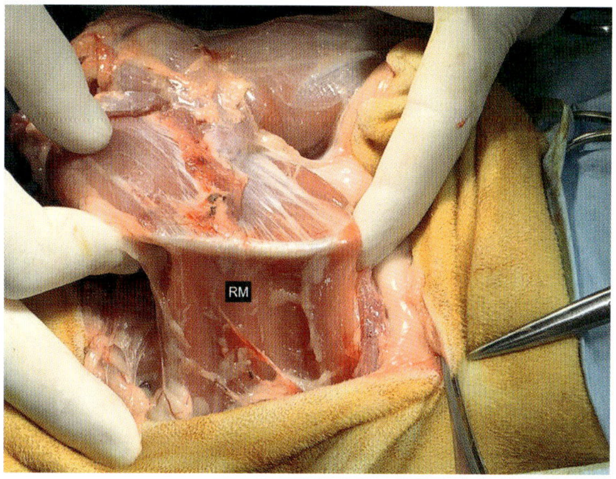

G-ii)

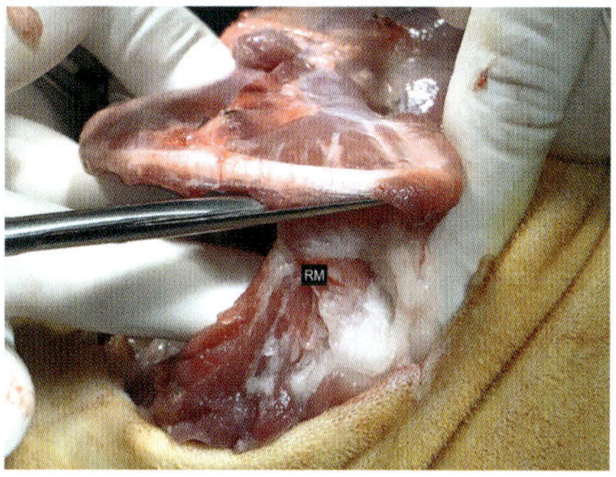

H)

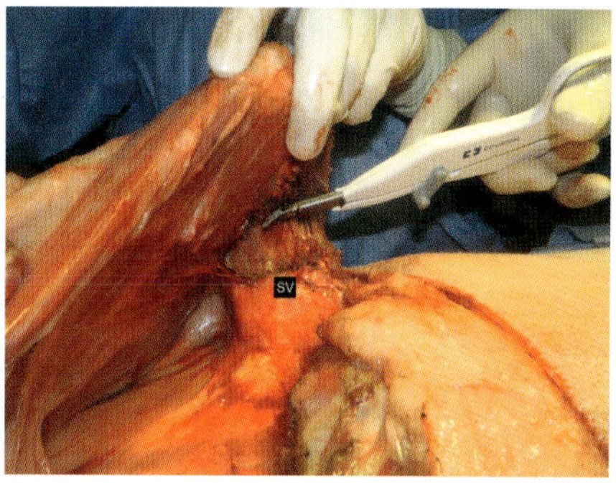

I)

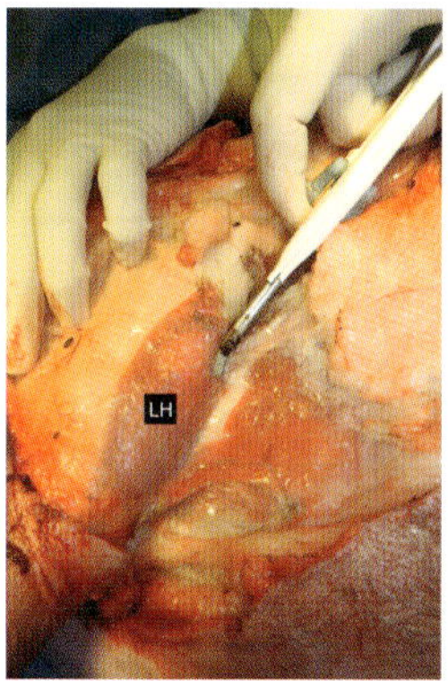

J-i)

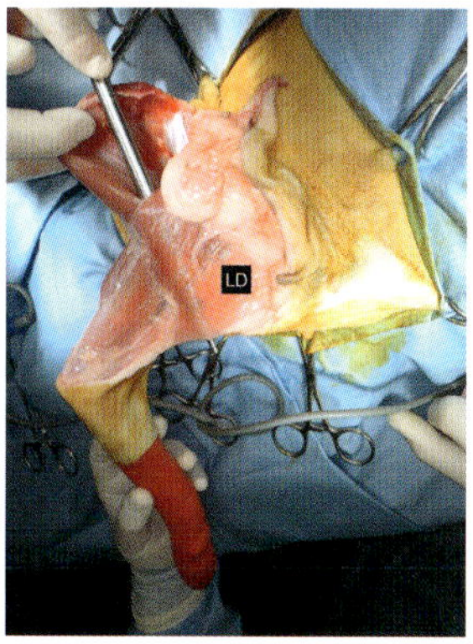

J-ii)

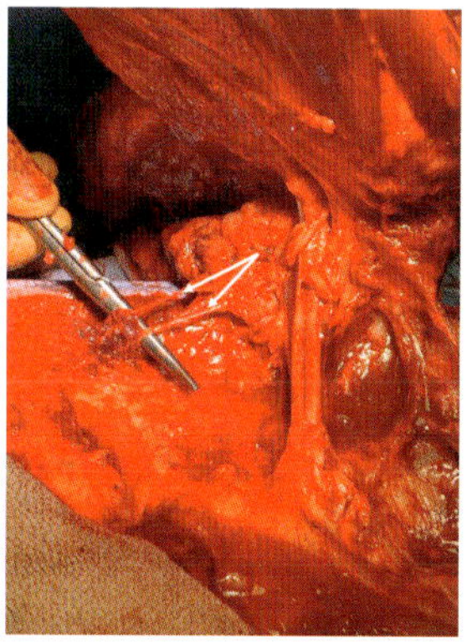

J-iii)

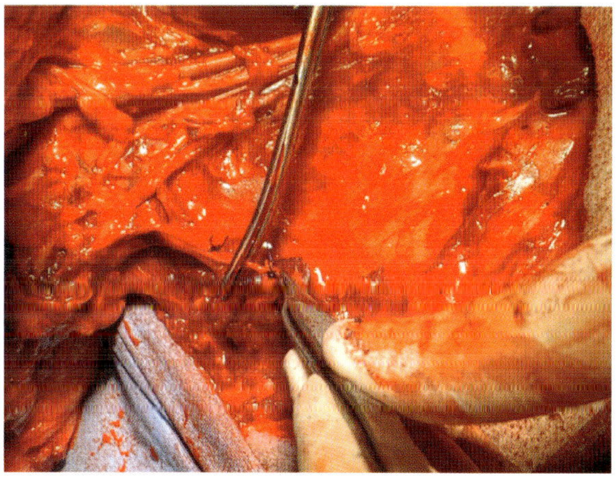

K)

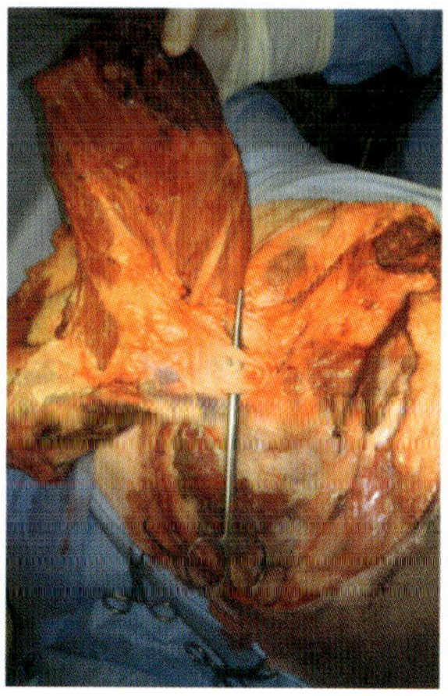

Surgical Technique (See Plate 33.1B–P) *continued*

L) The individual nerves of the brachial plexus are infiltrated with a local anesthetic (i). These nerves are transected with a scalpel blade, scissors, or a vessel sealing device (ii) after a minimum of 1 minute for the local anesthetic to adequately infiltrate the nerve.
M) The axillary vein is ligated with two simple ligatures of 2-0 or 3-0 absorbable monofilament suture material (i). The axillary vein closest to the limb is then either clamped with mosquito forceps or ligated, and then the axillary vein is transected between the ligatures and clamp with a vessel sealing device (ii) or Metzenbaum scissors.
N) The axillary artery is ligated with one simple ligature and one transfixion ligature (i) of 2-0 or 3-0 absorbable monofilament suture material. The axillary artery closest to the limb is then either clamped with mosquito forceps or ligated, and then the axillary artery is transected between the ligatures and clamp with a vessel sealing device (ii) or Metzenbaum scissors.
O) The axillary lymph node (arrow) is then identified along the dorsal border of the deep pectoral muscle and extirpated using either a vessel sealing device or a combination of blunt and sharp dissection.
P) The limb is abducted, and the superficial (i) and deep pectoral muscles (ii) are transected midbelly. The external thoracic artery is located at the cranial part of the superficial pectoral muscle, and a branch of the lateral thoracic artery is encountered during dissection of the deep pectoral muscle. These vessels need to be ligated or cauterized. After transection of the pectoral muscles, the amputated limb is removed from the surgical field.

Plate 33.1

Forequarter Amputation *continued*

L-i)

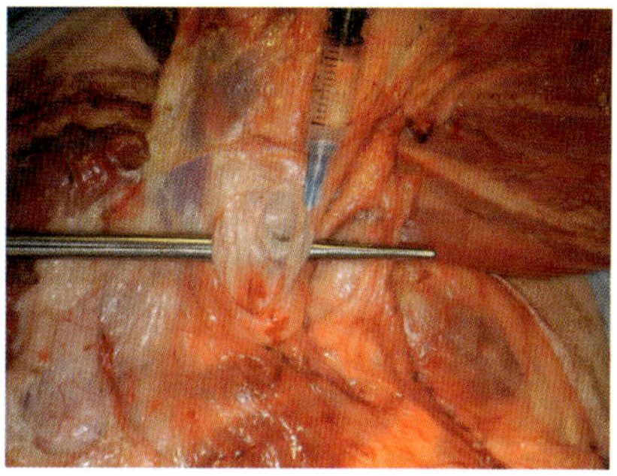

L-ii)

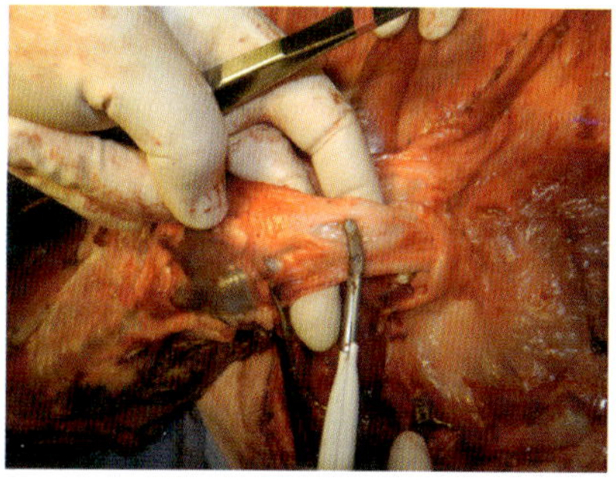

M-i)

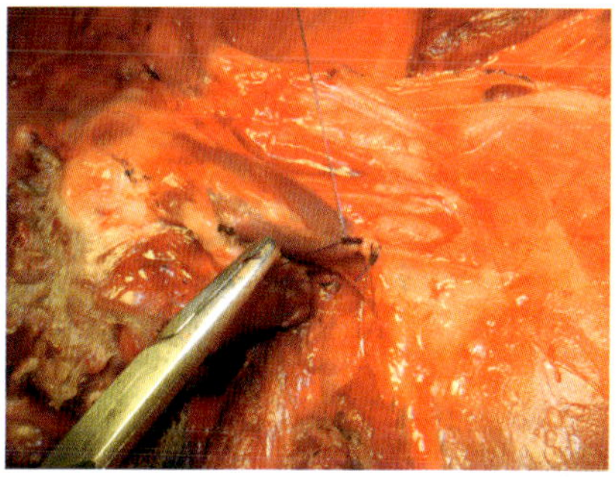

M-ii)

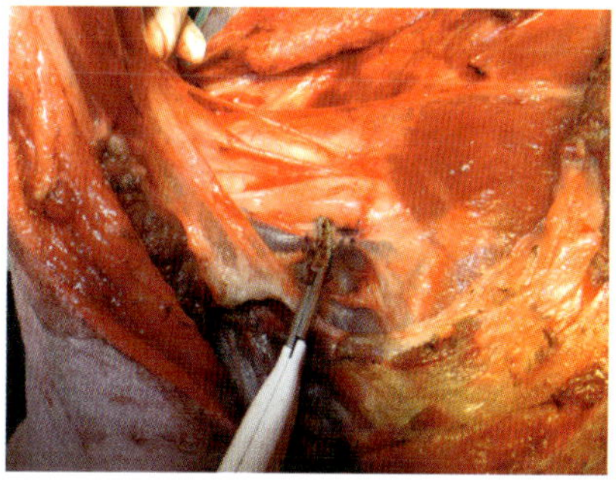

N-i)

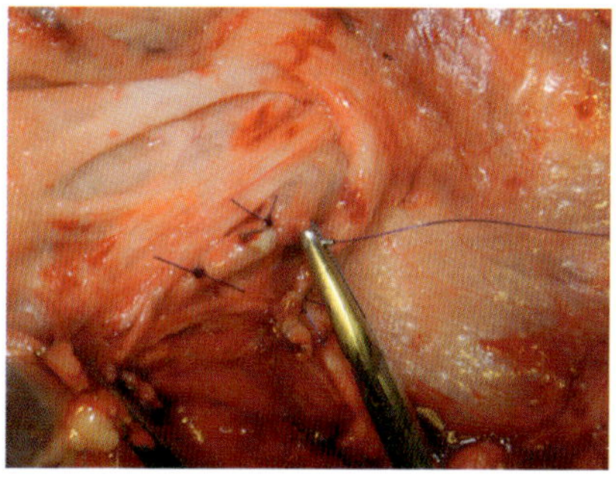

N-ii)

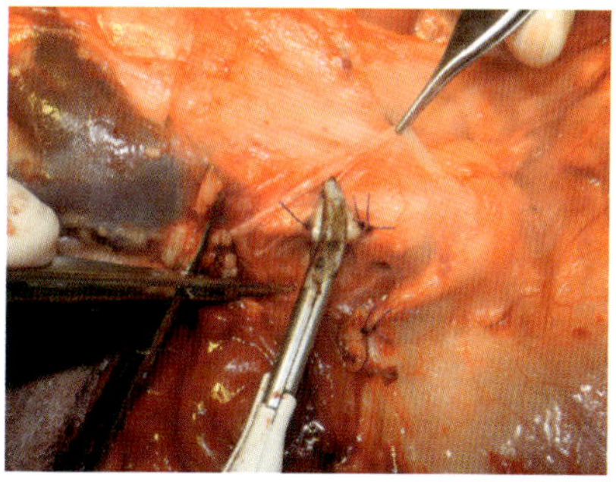

O)

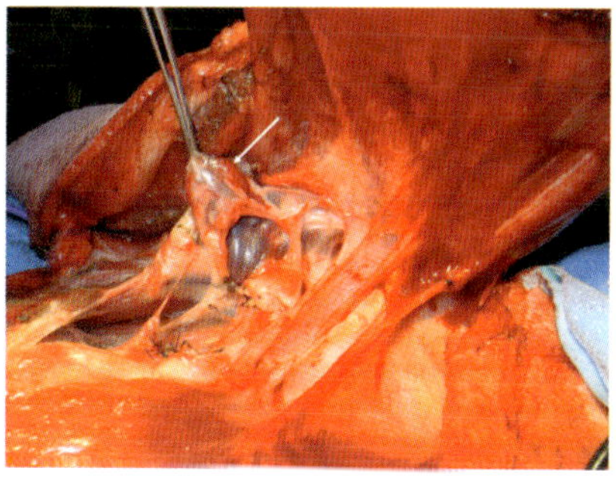

P-i)

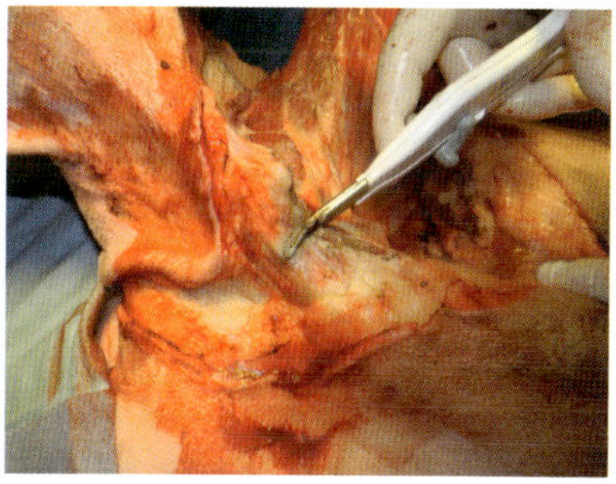

P-ii)

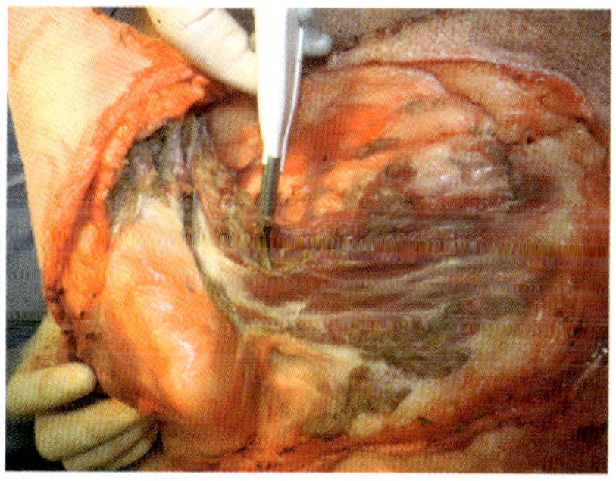

Closure (See Plate 33.1Q)

The trapezius (Tr), omotransversarius, brachiocephalicus, and pectoral muscles (PM) are sutured to the latissimus dorsi muscle (LD) using 0 to 3-0 absorbable monofilament suture material in a simple continuous suture pattern (Q – i, ii). The cutaneous trunci muscle is sutured with 2-0 to 3-0 absorbable monofilament suture material in a simple continuous suture pattern (Q – iii).

For the traditional approach, the subcutaneous tissue and skin are closed routinely in an inverted T or reversed L pattern (Q – iv). For the alternative approach, the subcutaneous tissue and skin are closed routinely in a linear fashion (Q – v).

Postoperative Management

1) Multimodal analgesia
2) Elizabethan collar or body suit
3) Sling support if necessary

Complications

Postoperative Complications

- Surgical-site infection (2%–13% in dogs [1, 2] and 4% in cats [2])
- Seroma
- Phantom limb syndrome (rare to 36% [3])
- Difficult adaption to ambulation on three limbs (rare) [4]

Suggested Adjuvant Treatments

- See *33. Primary Bone and Periarticular Tumors.*

Prognosis and Oncologic Outcome

- See *33. Primary Bone and Periarticular Tumors.*

References

1 Kirpensteijn, J., van den Bos, R., and Endenburg, N. (1999). Adaption of dogs to the amputation of a limb and their owners' satisfaction with the procedure. *Vet. Rec.* 144: 115–118.

2 Raske, M., McClaran, J.K., and Mariano, A. (2015). Short-term wound complications and predictive variables for complication after limb amputation in dogs and cats. *J. Small Anim. Pract.* 56: 247–252.

3 Boesch, J.M., Roinestad, K., Lopez, D.J. et al. (2021). The Canine Postamputation Pain (CAMPPAIN) initiative: a retrospective study and development of a diagnostic scale. *Vet. Anaesth. Analg.* 48 (6): 861–870.

4 Dickerson, V.M., Coleman, K.D., Ogawa, M. et al. (2015). Outcomes of dogs undergoing limb amputation, owner satisfaction with limb amputation procedures, and owner perceptions regarding postsurgical adaptation: 64 cases (2005-2012). *J. Am. Vet. Med. Assoc.* 247: 786–792.

Plate 33.1

Forequarter Amputation *continued*

Q-i)

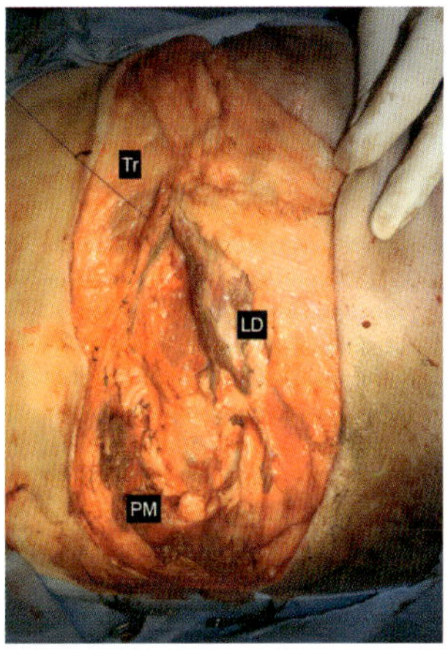

Q-ii)

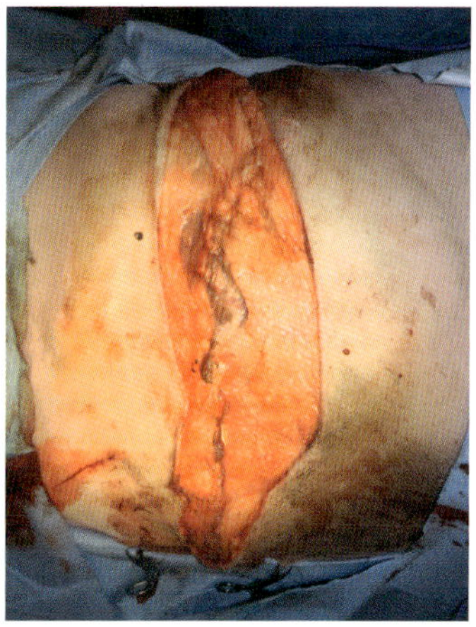

Q-iii)

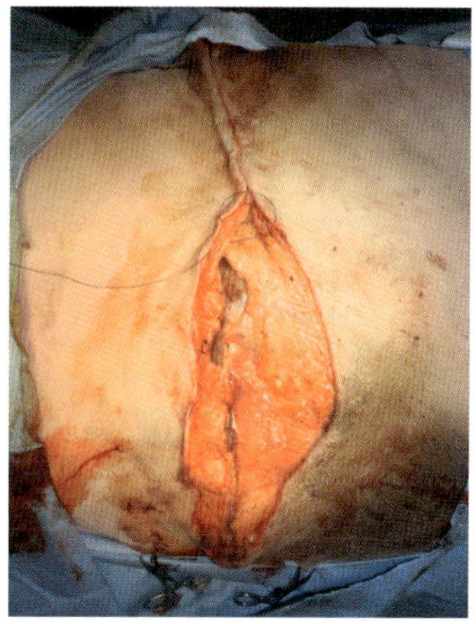

Q-iv)

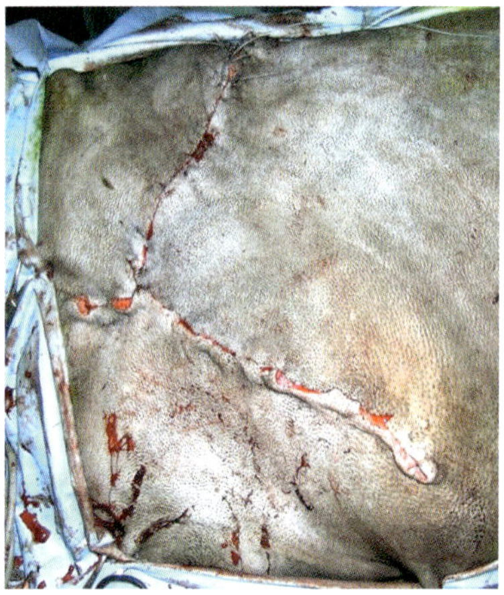

Q-v)

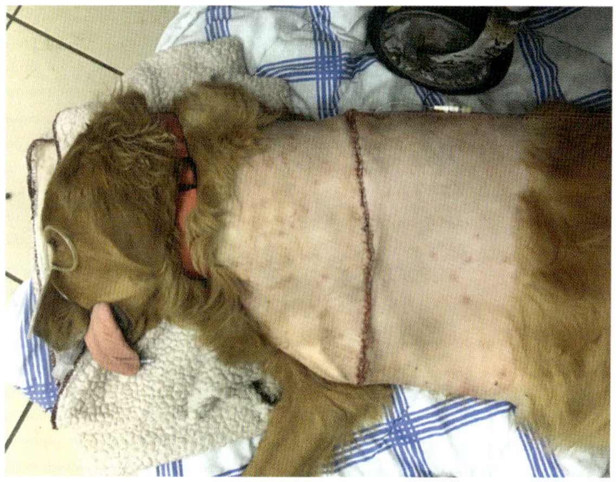

33.2 Distal Radial Limb-Sparing Surgery

Indication

1) Resection of localized and nonmetastatic primary distal radial tumors that involve <50% of the length of the radius and are compartmentalized with no evidence of extension into either the adjacent soft tissues or radiocarpal joint

Suggested Diagnostic Workup and Clinical Staging

- See *33. Primary Bone and Periarticular Tumors.*

Patient Positioning

The patient is positioned in dorsal recumbency or lateral recumbency with the affected limb uppermost.

Surgical Technique [1] (See Plate 33.2A, B, D–U)

A) A dorsal approach to the antebrachium and carpus is made with an incision extending along the dorsal aspect of the antebrachium from the elbow, over the dorsal aspect of the antebrachiocarpal joint and the third metacarpal bone, to the metacarpophalangeal joint of the third digit. This incision is lateral to the cephalic vein, which should be preserved, and extends over the accessory cephalic veins, which should be ligated as necessary. If a preoperative biopsy has been performed, then the biopsy tract is excised en bloc with the bone segment (arrow).
B) The incision is continued deeply through the subcutaneous and deep antebrachial fascia midway between the tendons of the extensor carpi radialis and common digital extensor muscles. These muscles are retracted to expose the diaphysis of the radius and distal radial tumor (arrow).
C) The supinator and pronator muscles are elevated from their insertions on the proximal radius with a periosteal elevator (not pictured).
D) The dissection is continued distally along the pseudocapsule of the distal radial tumor. The pseudocapsule should not be compromised.
E) The origin of the abductor pollicus longus muscle and the involved extensor (extensor carpi radialis, common digital extensor, and lateral digital extensor) muscles are transected at the level of the planned radial osteotomy site (arrow). If possible, the ulnaris lateralis muscle should be preserved to provide some soft tissue coverage of the construct used to reconstruct the radial defect.
F) A transverse arthrotomy of the radiocarpal joint is performed with the joint in a flexed position (i–iv). The cartilage of the distal radius is inspected for pathologic fracture and intra-articular extension of the distal radial tumor (v). If there is evidence of intra-articular extension, then the limb-sparing surgery can either be converted to an amputation (see *33.1. Forequarter Amputation*) or the distal margin can be extended farther distally to include the radiocarpal, ulnar carpal, and proximal portion of the accessory carpal bone.

Color Atlas of Canine and Feline Surgical Oncology, First Edition. Julius M. Liptak, Paolo Buracco, William T. N. Culp, and Nicholas J. Bacon.

Plate 33.2

Distal Radial Limb-Sparing Surgery

A)

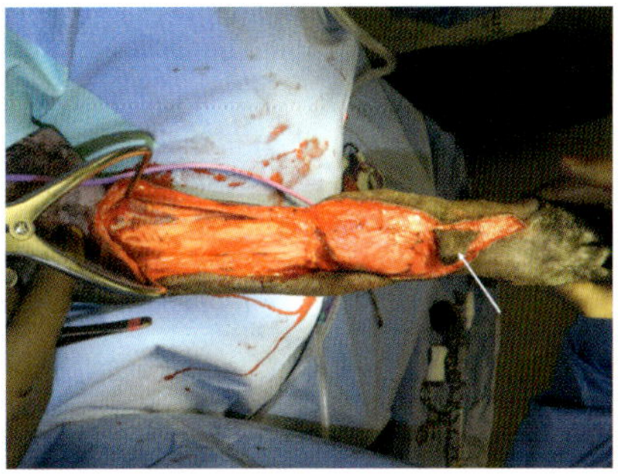

B)

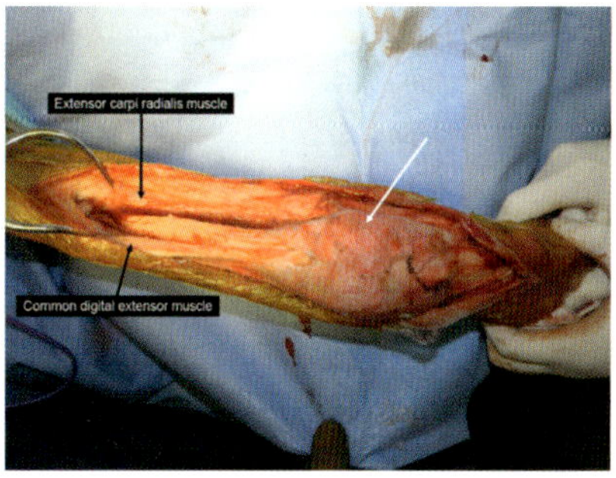

D)

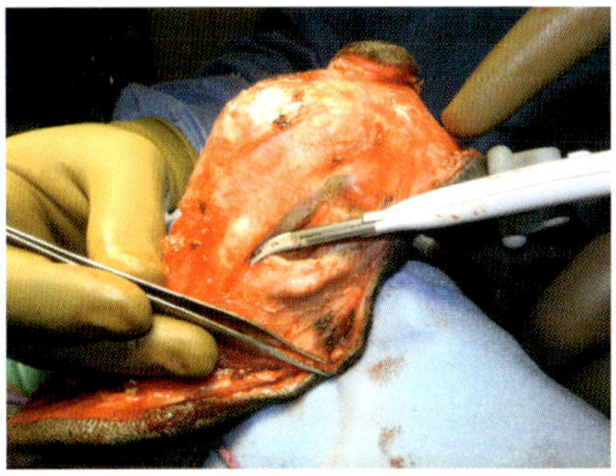

E)

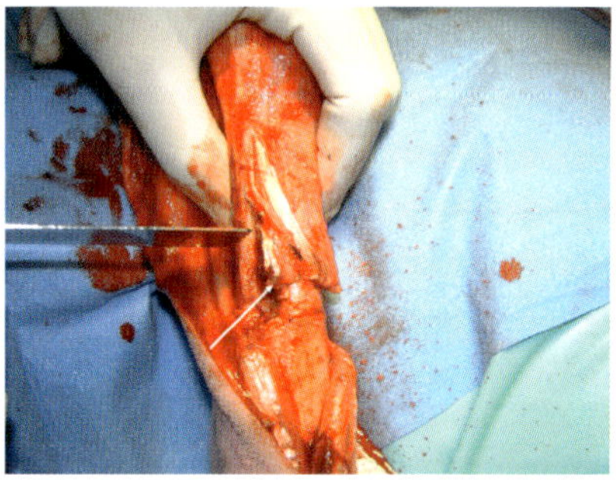

F-i)

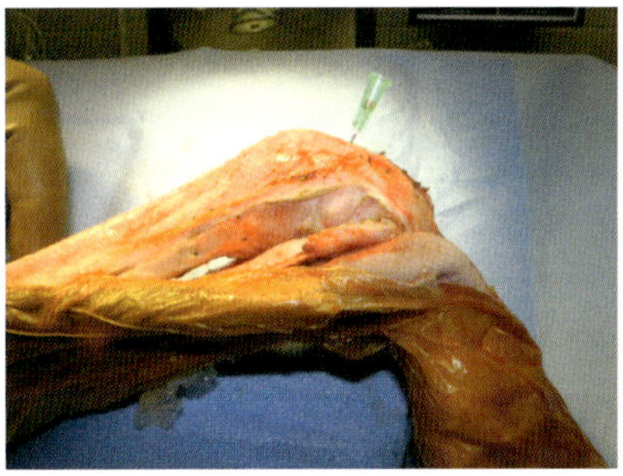

F-ii)

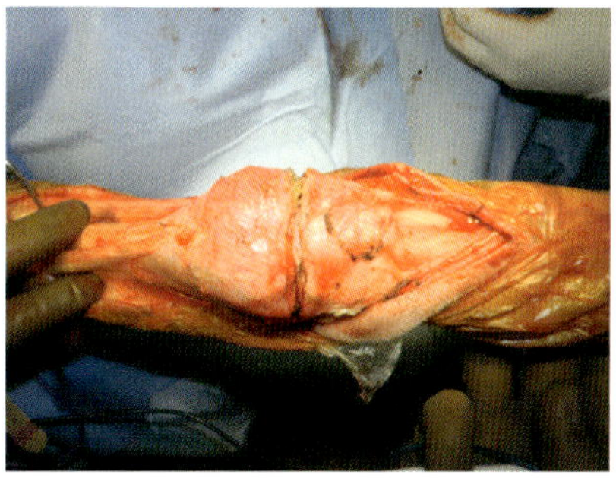

F-iii)

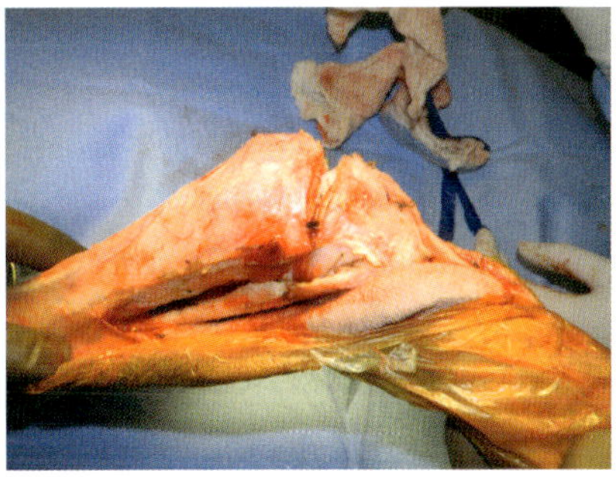

F-iv)

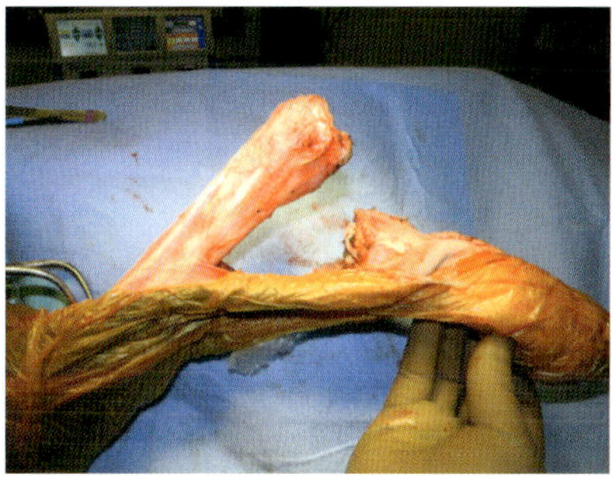

F-v)

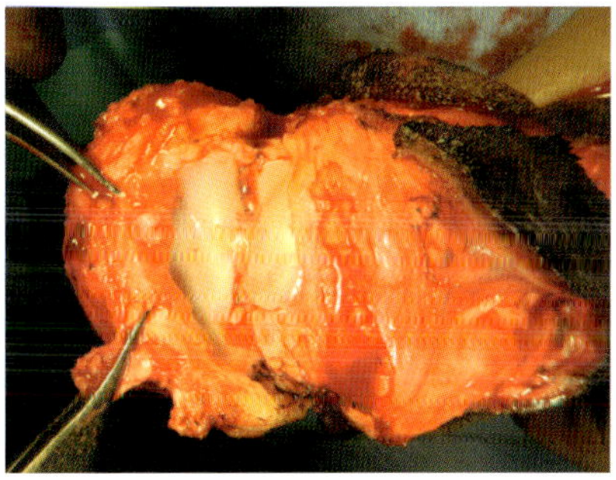

Surgical Technique [1] (See Plate 33.2A, B, D–U) *continued*

G) If a segment of the distal ulna is planned to be resected en bloc with the distal radial tumor, then the transverse arthrotomy is continued laterally, including division of the lateral collateral ligament, and medially, including division of the medial collateral ligament and transection of the insertion of the extensor carpi radialis tendon.

H) If preservation of the ulna is planned (pictured, arrow), then the transverse arthrotomy is continued laterally to the styloid process of the ulna and medially, including division of the medial collateral ligament and transection of the insertion of the extensor carpi radialis tendon.

I) The medial fascia caudal to the radius at the approximate level of the planned radial osteotomy site is incised. The soft tissues caudal to the distal radius are assessed visually and with digital palpation to ensure that the tumor pseudocapsule is intact adjacent to the flexor muscles. If the tumor is invasive into the flexor muscles, then conversion to an amputation (see *33.1. Forequarter Amputation*) should be considered.

J) A transverse osteotomy of the radial diaphysis is then performed. This osteotomy should be located with minimum bone margins of 3 cm (i) from the proximal extent of the tumor as determined from preoperative imaging. If using an endoprosthesis, then the radial osteotomy will often be performed with >3-cm bone margins because the level of this osteotomy is also dependent on the length of the endoprosthesis to be used to reconstruct the radial defect (98 or 122 mm). The osteotomy should be performed with an oscillating or sagittal saw (ii). A true transverse osteotomy is ideal to maximize contact at the bone–construct interface.

K) The ulna can be osteotomized at the same level as the radial osteotomy (i), ≥2 cm distal to the radial osteotomy (ii, iii), or preserved for its complete length (see step H). Preservation of part or all of the distal ulna can provide additional stability to the construct if a cortical allograft is used for reconstruction of the antebrachium; however, this is not necessary when using an endoprosthesis. The ulnar osteotomy can be performed in a lateral-to-medial or dorsal-to-palmar direction with an oscillating or sagittal saw (ii). If the ulnar osteotomy is planned at the same level as the radial osteotomy, which is best suited when reconstructing the radial defect with an endoprosthesis, then the radial osteotomy is continued laterally through the diaphysis of the ulna. If the ulna is to be preserved in part or completely, then every effort should be made to avoid trauma to the medial cortex of the ulna during osteotomy of the radius.

Plate 33.2

Distal Radial Limb-Sparing Surgery *continued*

G)

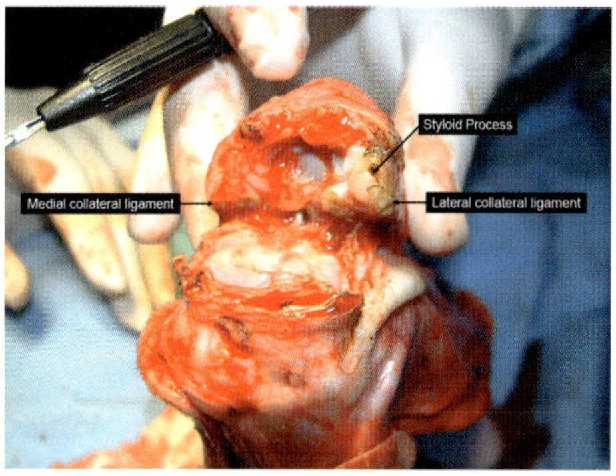

H)

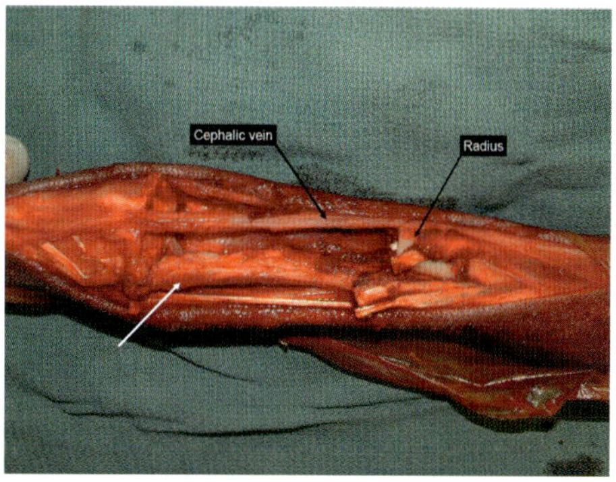

I)

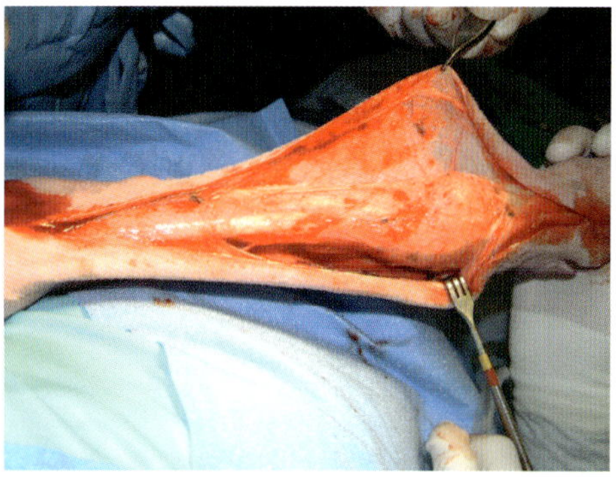

J-i)

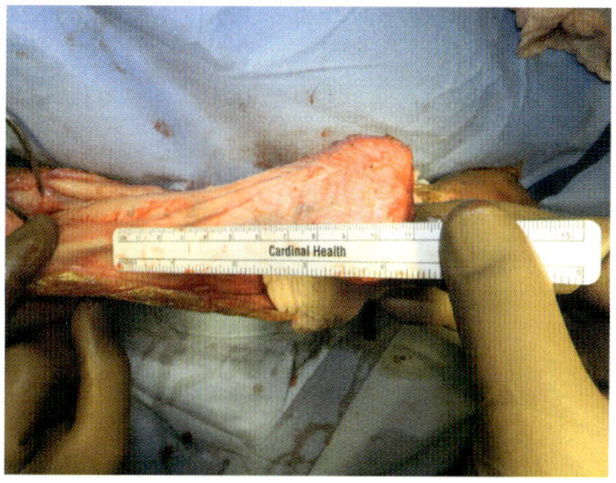

J-ii)

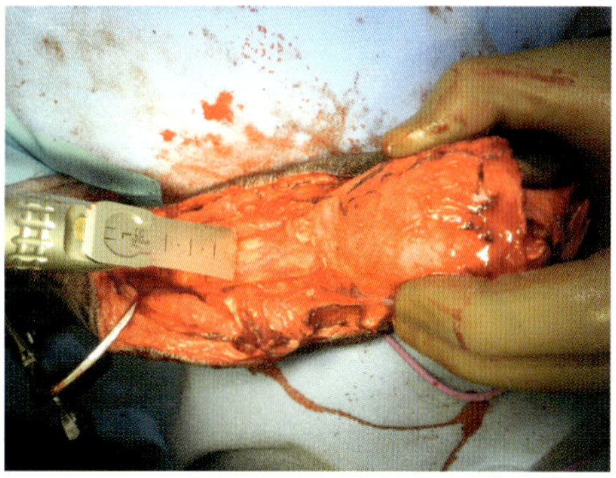

K-i)

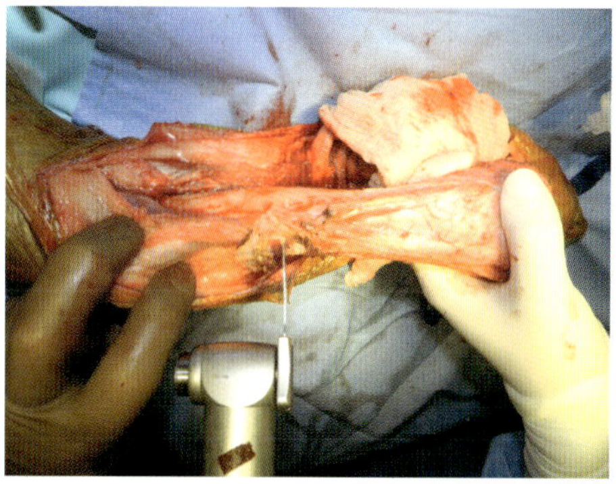

K-ii)

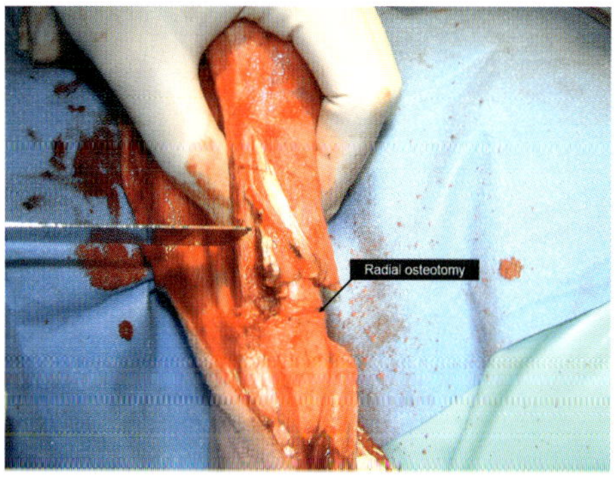

K-iii)

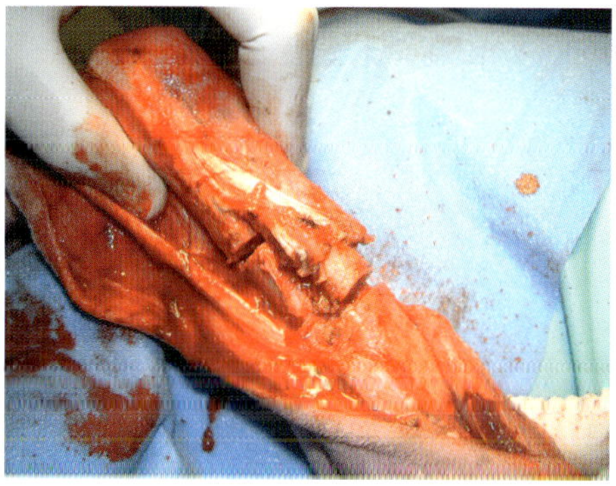

Surgical Technique [1] (See Plate 33.2A, B, D–U) *continued*

L) The fascial dissection is continued distally along the medial and caudal aspects of the radius and pseudocapsule of the distal radial tumor to the level of the radiocarpal joint. Noncontiguous flexor muscles should be preserved. Large vessels are commonly encountered during this dissection, and these should be ligated with suture material or metallic clips, or alternatively a vessel sealing device can be used.

M) The caudal aspect of the antebrachiocarpal joint is incised and the intra-articular ligaments are transected to complete the antebrachiocarpal joint disarticulation.

N) If preservation of the complete length of the ulna is planned, the disarticulated antebrachiocarpal joint is flexed to expose the distal aspect of the styloid process of the ulna. A short longitudinal osteotomy of the styloid process is performed in a distal-to-proximal direction with either an osteotome and mallet (i) or an oscillating saw (ii) such that the medial third of the distal ulna is removed en bloc with the distal radial bone segment and the lateral two-thirds of the styloid process and ulna are preserved.

O) The distal radial segment is removed from the surgical field. This bone specimen is radiographed to evaluate surgical margins before closure of the surgical site (pictured).

Plate 33.2

Distal Radial Limb-Sparing Surgery *continued*

L)

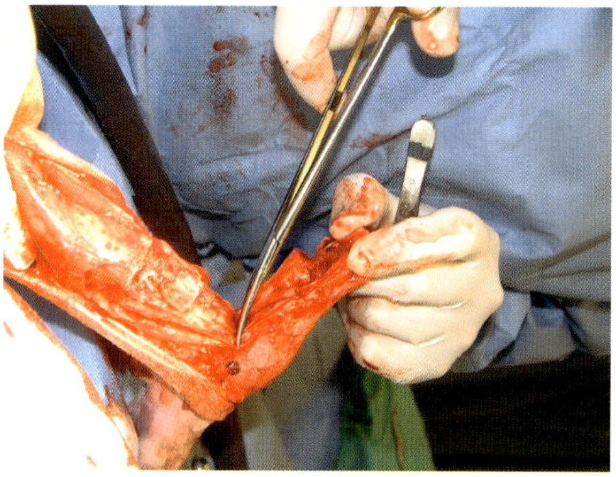

M)

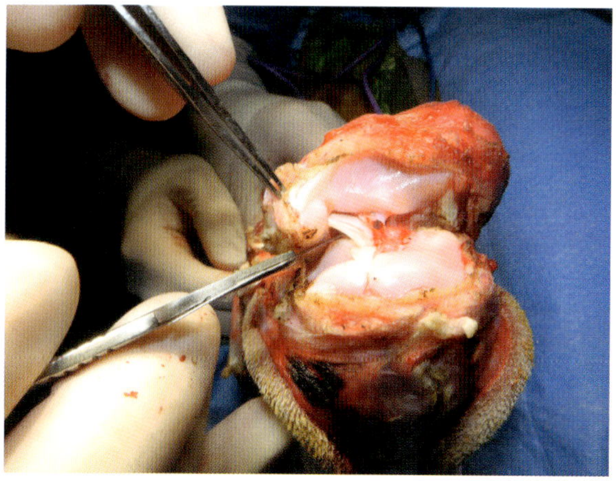

N-i)

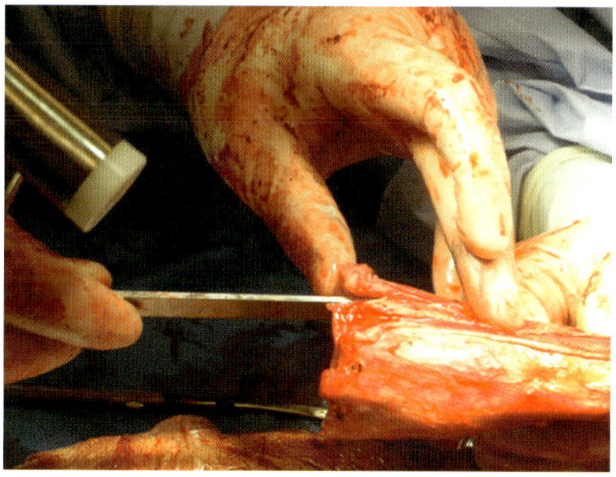

Courtesy of Dr. Bernard Séguin

N-ii)

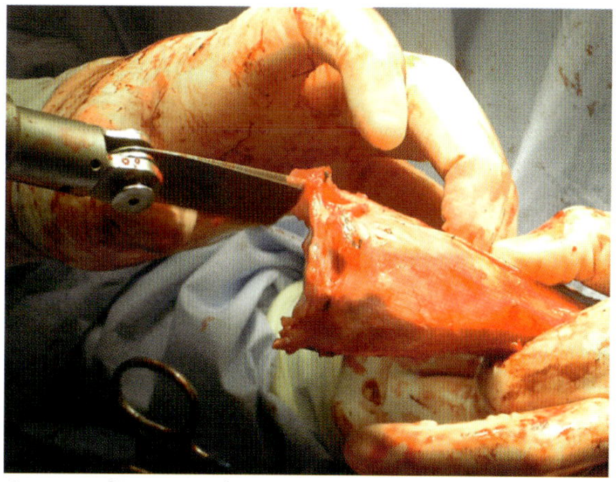

Courtesy of Dr. Bernard Séguin

O)

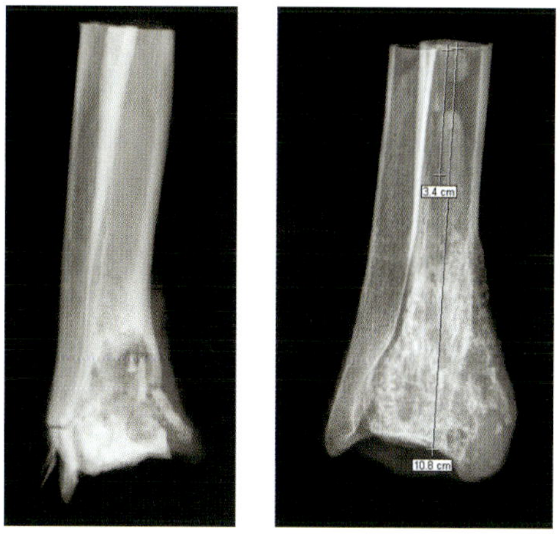

Surgical Technique [1] (See Plate 33.2A, B, D–U) *continued*

P) The proximal aspect of the radial and ulnar carpal bones is osteotomized with an oscillating saw (i, ii) or a pneumatic burr (iii) to provide a flat surface (iv, v) to abut the distal aspect of the construct used to reconstruct the radial defect.

Q) Bone marrow is collected from the radial medullary cavity at the osteotomy site for determination of histologic margins.

R) **Reconstruction technique 1 – cortical allograft [2]:** A size-matched cortical allograft is obtained preoperatively from either an institutional or commercial bone bank. The cortical allograft is thawed in a 1-l solution of sterile isotonic saline containing 1000 mg neomycin, 3000 mg ampicillin, and 500 000 U polymyxin B at room temperature. Once thawed, the bone marrow is then removed from the medullary cavity with a curette. Transverse osteotomies of the distal articular surface of the allograft and proximal allograft are done with an oscillating saw, ensuring maximal contact at the host bone–allograft interface and that the length of the allograft is appropriate for the radial defect. A hybrid limb-sparing plate is temporarily fixed to the cortical allograft with proximal and distal 3.5-mm cortical bone screws (i).

Plate 33.2

Distal Radial Limb-Sparing Surgery *continued*

P-i)

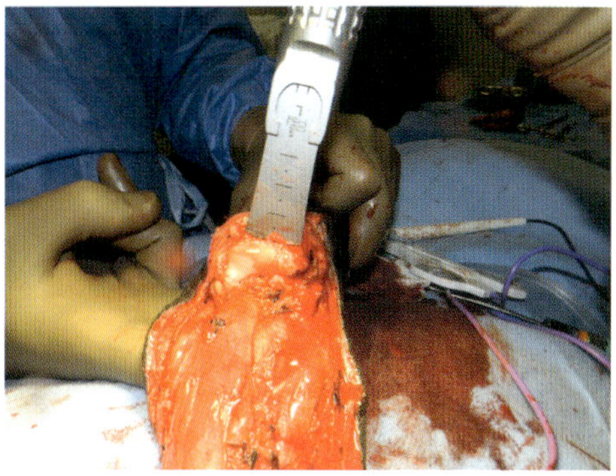

P-ii)

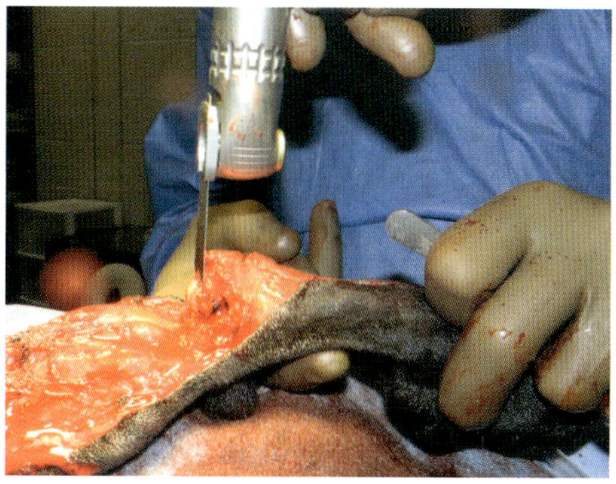

P-iii)

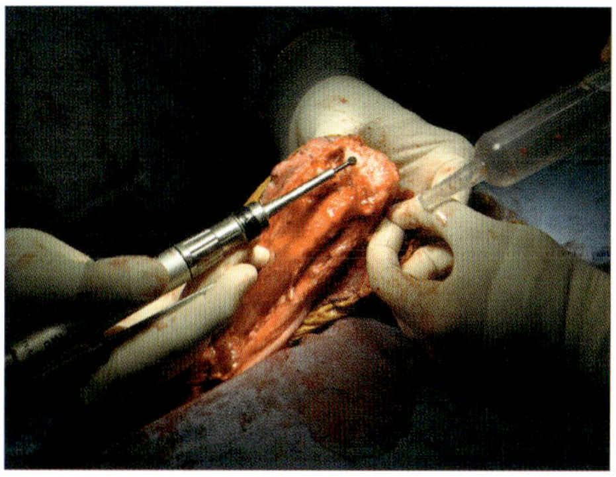

P-iv)

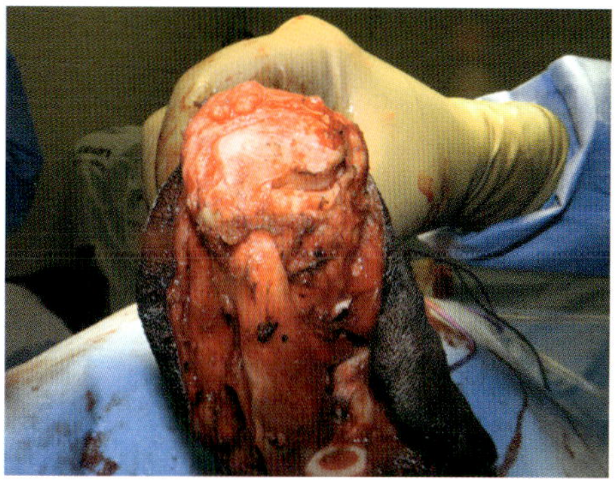

P-v)

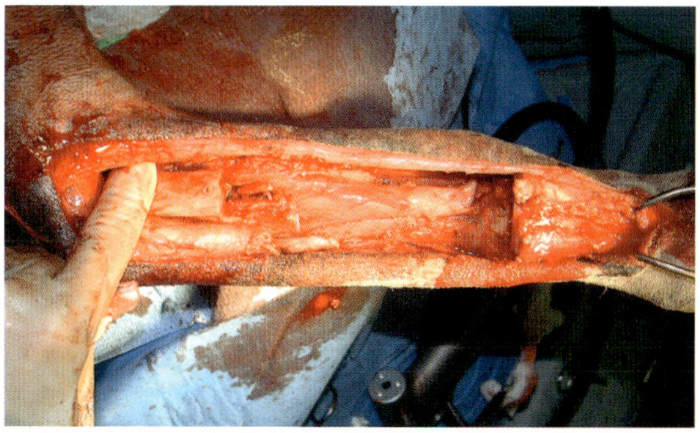

Q)

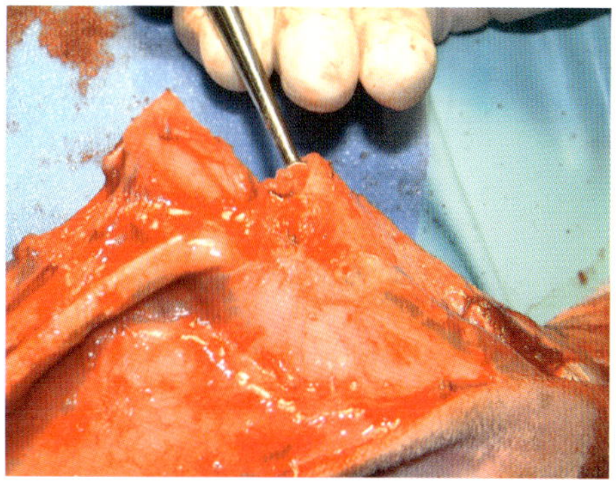

R-i)

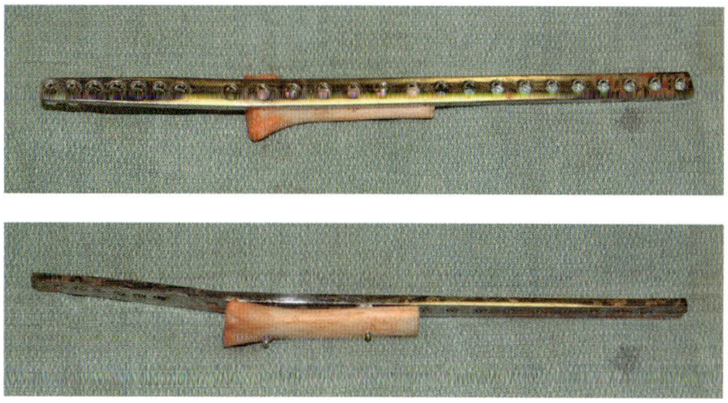

Surgical Technique [1] (See Plate 33.2A, B, D–U) *continued*

The distal 3.5/4.5-mm plate hole should be positioned immediately distal to the distal aspect of the cortical allograft because this distal 3.5/4.5-mm plate hole will be used to engage the radial carpal bone (ii, arrow). The screws and plate are then removed, and the medullary cavity of the cortical allograft is filled with polymethylmethacrylate (PMMA) impregnated with 1000 mg amikacin. The limb-sparing plate can either be applied straight or bent to 10 to 15 degrees at the distal allograft–radial carpal bone interface. If the latter is selected, then a large plate press is used to bend the hybrid limb-sparing plate at the junction between the 2.7/3.5- and 3.5/4.5-mm plate holes. As the PMMA begins to harden, the cortical bone screws are then reinserted to secure the limb-sparing plate to the cortical allograft. The cortical allograft is then inserted into the distal radial defect and secured proximally to the radius with 3.5- or 4.5-mm cortical or locking bones screws and distally to the radial carpal bone and third metacarpal bone with 2.7- or 3.5-mm cortical or locking bone screws (ii, iii). A minimum of 80% of the third metacarpal bone should be covered by the plate to minimize the risk of metacarpal fracture at the distal end of the plate. If possible, the screws on either side of the cortical allograft–host bone interface should be loaded to minimize gap formation.

S) **Reconstruction technique 2 – endoprosthesis [2]:** An appropriately sized endoprosthesis (98 or 122 mm) is selected for reconstruction of the radial defect. The hybrid limb-sparing plate can either be applied straight or bent to 10 to 15 degrees at the distal allograft–radial carpal bone interface. If the latter is selected, then a large plate press is used to bend the hybrid limb-sparing plate at the junction between the 2.7/3.5- and 3.5/4.5-mm plate holes. The limb-sparing plate is fixed to the endoprosthesis with dedicated machined screws. The distal 3.5/4.5-mm plate hole should be positioned immediately distal to the distal aspect of the endoprosthesis because this distal 3.5/4.5-mm plate hole will be used to later engage the radial carpal bone. The endoprosthesis is then inserted into the distal radial defect and secured proximally to the radius with 3.5- or 4.5-mm cortical or locking bones screws and distally to the radial carpal bone and third metacarpal bone with 2.7- or 3.5-mm cortical or locking bone screws (i, ii). A minimum of 80% of the third metacarpal bone should be covered by the plate to minimize the risk of metacarpal fracture at the distal end of the plate. If possible, the screws in the radius and radial carpal bone adjacent to the endoprosthesis should be loaded to minimize gap formation.

T) **Reconstruction technique 3 – lateral manus translation [3]:** For the lateral manus translation technique, the length of the ulna is largely preserved. A short longitudinal osteotomy of the styloid process is performed as described earlier in step O, and then a transverse osteotomy of the styloid process is performed immediately proximal to the distal articular cartilage. The manus is translated laterally so that the distal end of the ulna is in contact with the osteotomized surface of the radial carpal bone. A hybrid limb-sparing plate is bent to 10 to 15 degrees between the 2.7/3.5- and 3.5/4.5-mm plate holes with a large plate press. The limb-sparing plate is then applied distally to the dorsal aspect of the third metacarpal bone and radial carpal bone with 2.7- or 3.5-mm cortical or locking bone screws (i, ii). The plate should be positioned such that the distal 3.5/4.5-mm plate hole is level with the radial carpal bone. A minimum of 80% of the third metacarpal bone should be covered by the plate to minimize the risk of metacarpal fracture at the distal end of the plate. A 3.5-mm string-of-pearls plate is then contoured and fixed to the dorsal aspect of the fourth metacarpal bone initially followed by the lateral aspect of the proximal ulna (iii). The proximal ulnar screws should not engage the radius.

U) After completion of the reconstruction, the surgical site is lavaged with sterile isotonic saline. A Jackson-Pratt drain can be inserted through a separate proximal stab incision.

Plate 33.2

Distal Radial Limb-Sparing Surgery *continued*

R-ii)

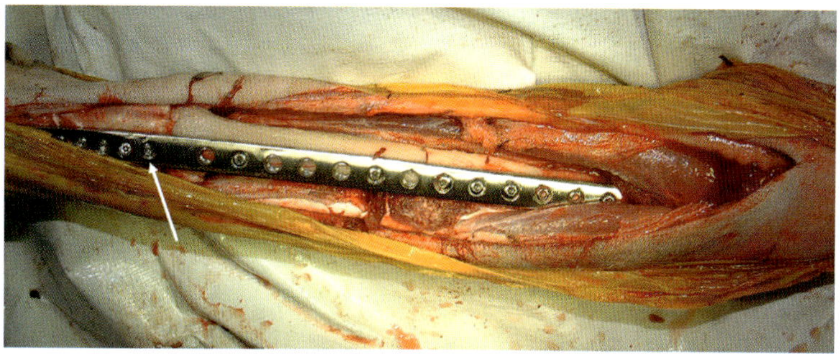

R-iii)

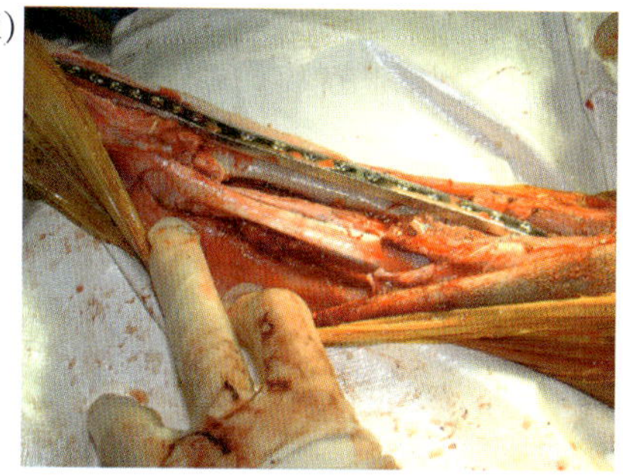

S-i)

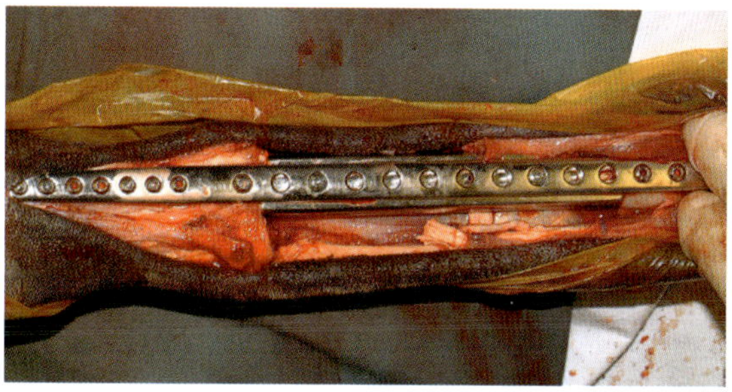

S-ii)

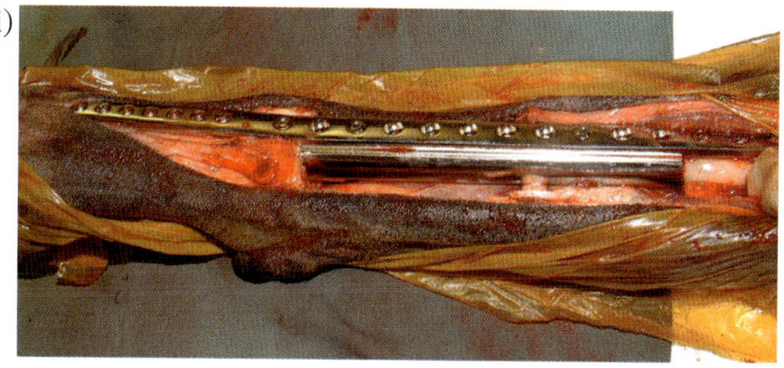

T-i)

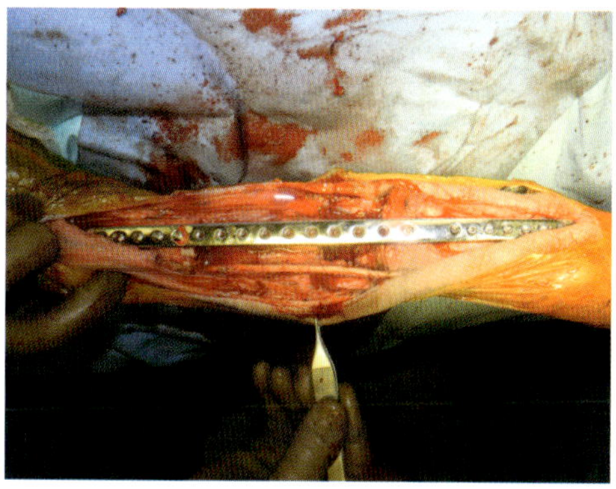

T-ii)

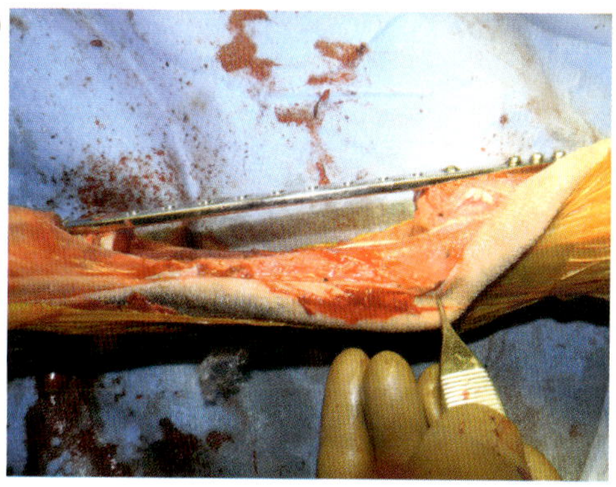

T-iii)

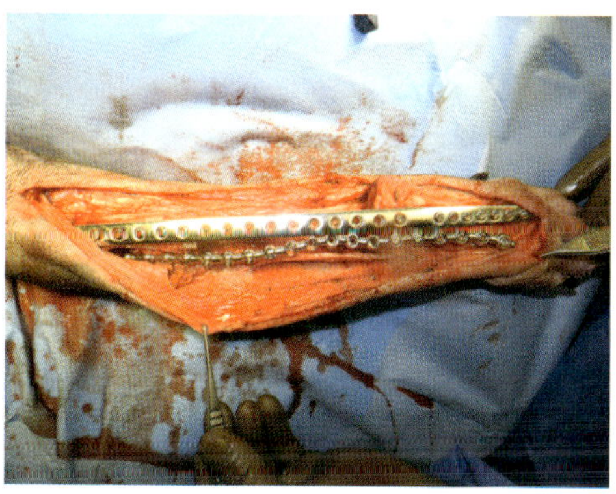

U)

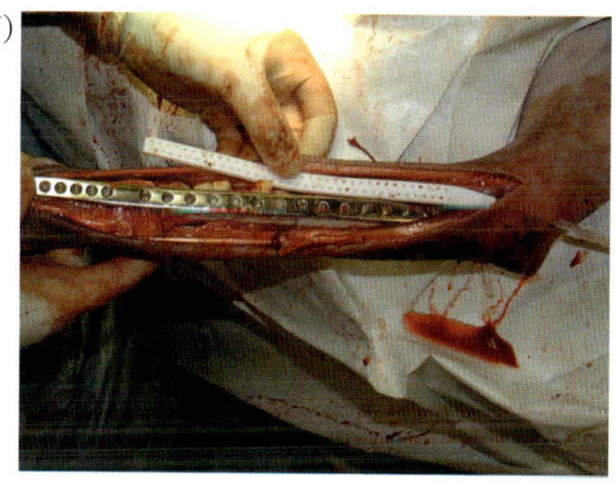

Closure

The skin incision is closed routinely in two layers with a simple continuous suture pattern using monofilament absorbable suture material in the subcutis and either an interrupted or continuous suture pattern using monofilament nonabsorbable suture material in the skin.

Postoperative Management

1) Multimodal analgesia
2) Modified Robert-Jones bandage for 14 days with or without a metasplint
3) Elizabethan collar
4) Prophylactic antibiotics for 10–21 days
5) Exercise restriction for 21 days

Complications (See Plate 33.2V, W)

	Cortical Allograft [2, 4–6]	Endoprosthesis [2, 7]	Lateral Manus Translation [3]	Bone Transport Osteogenesis [8]
Overall	78%	96%	67%	89%
• Minor	–	31%	–	44%
• Major	–	64%	–	44%
Infection (V – i, ii)	31%–68%	50%–78%	56%	0%
Construct failure (W)				
• Overall	11%–40%	36%–40%	33%	67%
• Minor	–	11%	6%	56%
• Major	–	24%	28%	11%
Local tumor recurrence	10%–28%	20%–24%	22%	22%
Limb function less than good	28%–31%	13%–20%	0%	22%

Suggested Adjuvant Treatments

- Chemotherapy for dogs with appendicular osteosarcoma
- Chemotherapy for dogs with appendicular hemangiosarcoma

Prognosis and Oncologic Outcome

- See *33. Primary Bone and Periarticular Tumors.*

References

1 Liptak, J.M., Dernell, W.S., Withrow, S.J. et al. (2012). Musculoskeletal system. In: *Veterinary Surgical Oncology*, 1e (ed. S.T. Kudnig and B. Seguin), 491–568. Wiley-Blackwell.

2 Liptak, J.M., Dernell, W.S., Ehrhart, N. et al. (2006). Cortical allograft and endoprosthesis for limb-sparing surgery in dogs with distal radial osteosarcoma: a prospective clinical comparison of two different limb-sparing techniques. *Vet. Surg.* 35 (6): 518–533.

Plate 33.2

Distal Radial Limb-Sparing Surgery *continued*

V-i)

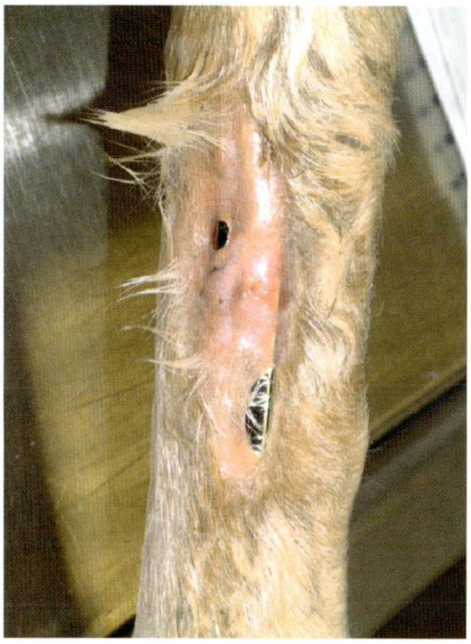

V-ii)

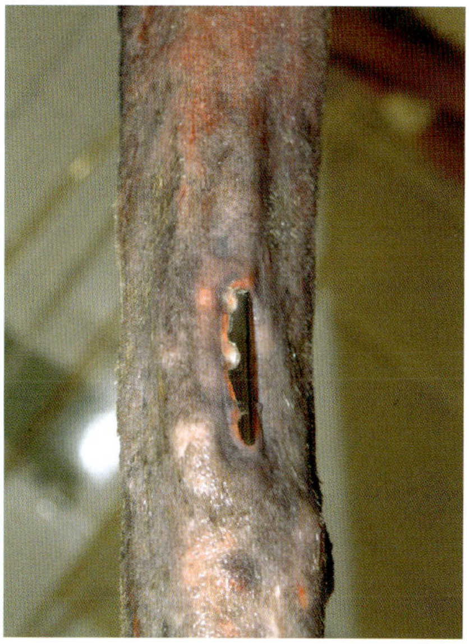

W)

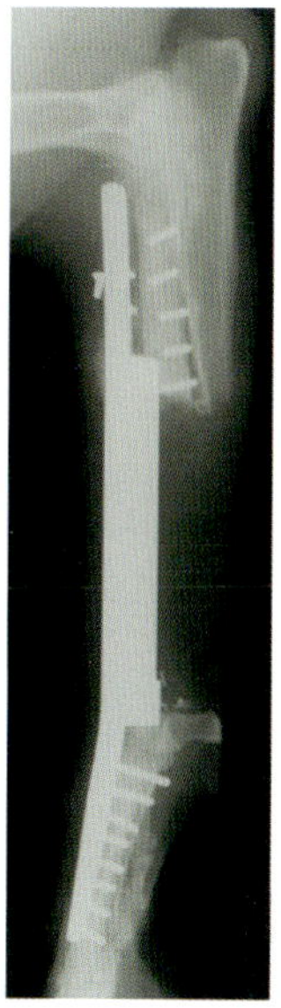

3 Seguin, B., Walsh, P.J., Ehrhart, E.J. et al. (2019). Cortical allograft and endoprosthesis for limb-sparing surgery in dogs with distal radial osteosarcoma: a prospective clinical comparison of two different limb-sparing techniques. *Vet. Surg.* 48 (2): 247–256.

4 Lascelles, B.D.X., Dernell, W.S., Correa, M.T. et al. (2005). Improved survival associated with postoperative wound infection in dogs treated with limb-salvage surgery for osteosarcoma. *Ann. Surg. Oncol.* 12 (12): 1073–1083.

5 LaRue, S.M., Withrow, S.J., Powers, B.E. et al. (1989). Limb-sparing treatment for osteosarcoma in dogs. *J. Am. Vet. Med. Assoc.* 195 (12): 1734–1744.

6 Morello, E., Buracco, P., Martano, M. et al. (2001). Bone allografts and adjuvant cisplatin for the treatment of canine appendicular osteosarcoma in 18 dogs. *J. Small Anim. Pract.* 42 (2): 61–66.

7 Mitchell, K.E., Boston, S.E., Kung, M. et al. (2016). Outcomes of limb-sparing surgery using two generations of metal endoprosthesis in 45 dogs with distal radial osteosarcoma. A veterinary society of surgical oncology retrospective study. *Vet. Surg.* 45 (1): 36–43.

8 Ehrhart, N. (2005). Longitudinal bone transport for treatment of primary bone tumors in dogs: technique description and outcome in 9 dogs. *Vet. Surg.* 34 (1): 24–34.

33.3 Partial Ulnectomy

Indication

1) Resection of localized and nonmetastatic primary bone tumors involving the mid to distal ulna

Suggested Diagnostic Workup and Clinical Staging

See *33. Primary Bone and Periarticular Tumors.*

Patient Positioning

The patient is positioned in dorsolateral recumbency with the affected limb uppermost or, in some cases, sternal oblique recumbency with the limb pulled caudally.

Surgical Technique (See Plate 33.3A–E)

A) A skin is made over the ulnar mass and extended along the length of the ulna as required (dotted line).
B) Soft tissues are dissected from the ulnar mass, taking care not to compromise the tumor capsule (i, ii). This dissection is commonly between the ulnaris lateralis and lateral digital extensor muscles, or the flexor carpi ulnaris and ulnaris lateralis muscles. The ulnar nerve should be preserved close to the lateral border of the deep digital flexor muscle and deep to the ulnar head of the flexor carpi ulnaris muscle. The ulnar artery and vein are preserved if feasible; if not, then both should be ligated and divided.
C) A transverse osteotomy of the ulnar diaphysis is then performed. This osteotomy should be located with minimum bone margins of 3 cm from the proximal extent of the tumor as determined from preoperative imaging. The osteotomy should be performed with an oscillating or sagittal saw. Every effort should be made to avoid trauma to the lateral cortex of the radius during osteotomy of the ulna (because this may predispose to fracture of the radius).
D) The osteotomized ulnar segment is then carefully dissected from the radius using a periosteal elevator and scalpel blade, taking care not to compromise the tumor capsule (i), and removed from the surgical field (ii, iii).

Color Atlas of Canine and Feline Surgical Oncology, First Edition. Julius M. Liptak, Paolo Buracco, William T. N. Culp, and Nicholas J. Bacon.

Plate 33.3

Partial Ulnectomy

A)

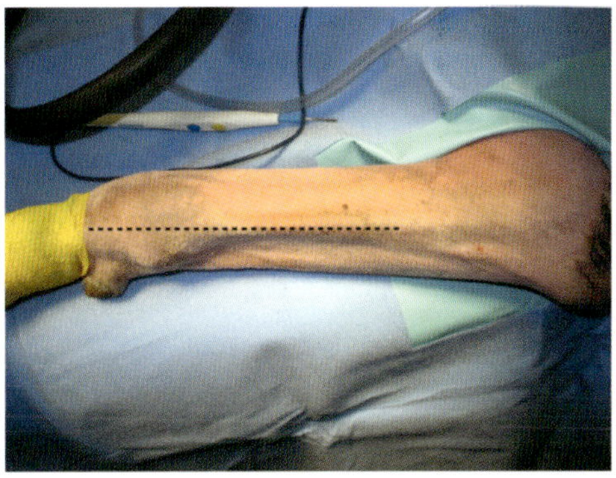

B-i)

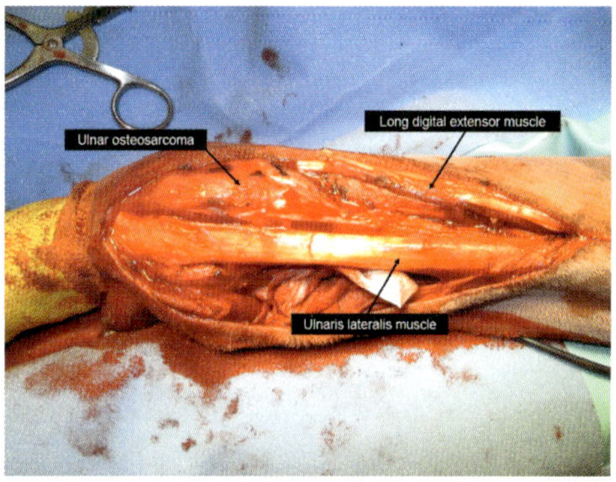

B-ii)

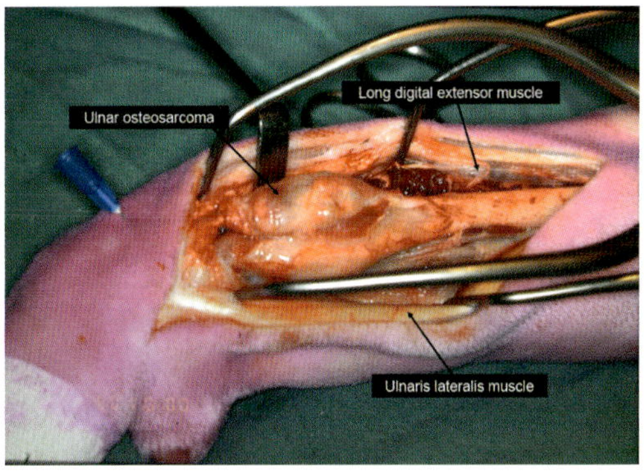

C)

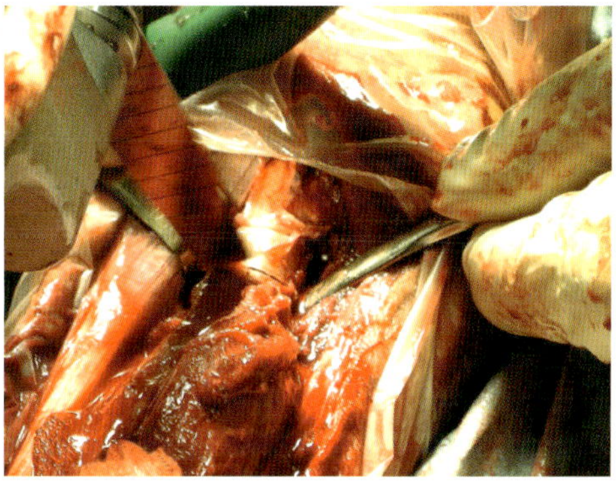

D-i)

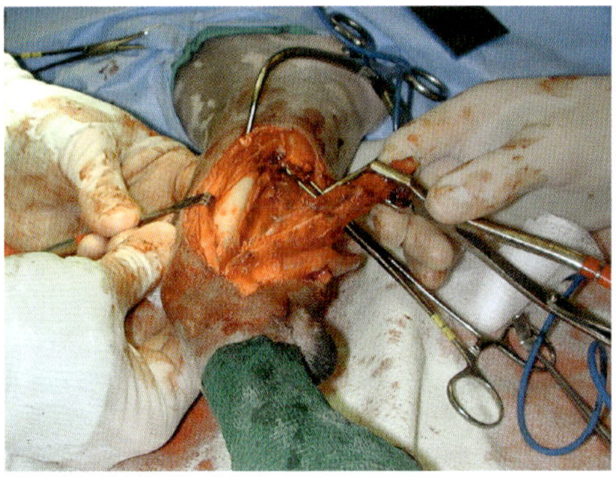

D-ii)

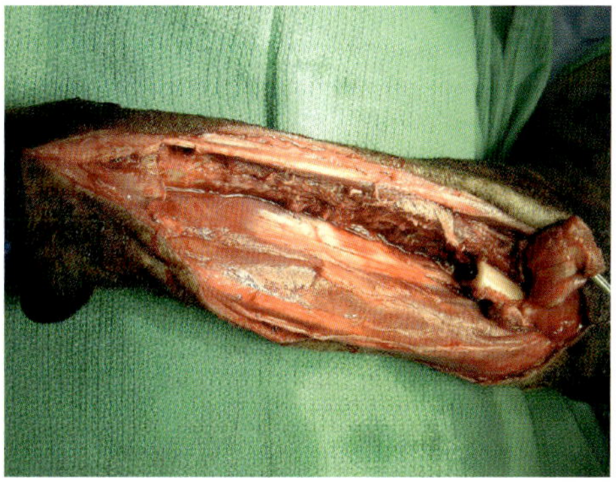

D-iii)

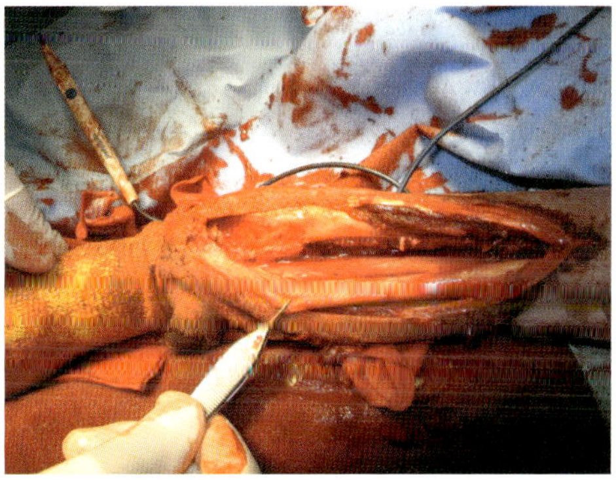

Surgical Technique (See Plate 33.3A–E) *continued*

E) For distal ulnar tumors, the styloid process can either be resected (i) or preserved (ii). If resected, the stability of the carpus should be assessed after resection. The majority of cases remain stable after resection of the styloid process and hence do not require stabilization; however, reconstruction of the lateral collateral ligament or pancarpal arthrodesis should be considered if there is residual carpal instability after distal ulnectomy.
F) After completion of the resection, the surgical site is lavaged with sterile isotonic saline. A Jackson-Pratt drain can be inserted through a separate proximal stab incision.

Closure

The skin incision is closed routinely in two layers with a simple continuous suture pattern using monofilament absorbable suture material in the subcutis and either an interrupted or continuous suture pattern using monofilament nonabsorbable suture material in the skin.

Postoperative Management

1) Multimodal analgesia
2) Modified Robert-Jones bandage for 14 days with or without a metasplint
3) Elizabethan collar
4) Exercise restriction for 21 days

Postoperative Complications [1, 2]

- Lameness [2]
  - 10–14 days: 13% no lameness, 63% mild lameness, 25% moderate lameness
  - 2–3 months: 56% no lameness, 33% mild lameness, 11% moderate lameness
- Radial fracture (18%)
- Local tumor recurrence (9%)

Suggested Adjuvant Treatments

- Chemotherapy for dogs with appendicular osteosarcoma
- Chemotherapy for dogs with appendicular hemangiosarcoma

Prognosis and Oncologic Outcome

- See *33. Primary Bone and Periarticular Tumors.*

References

1 Straw, R.C., Withrow, S.J., and Powers, B.E. (1991). Primary osteosarcoma of the ulna in 12 dogs. *J. Am. Anim. Hosp. Assoc.* 27: 323–326.
2 Sivacolundhu, R.K., Runge, J.J., Donovan, T.A. et al. (2013). Ulnar osteosarcoma in dogs: 30 cases (1992-2008). *J. Am. Vet. Med. Assoc.* 243 (1): 96–101.

Plate 33.3

Partial Ulnectomy *continued*

E-i)

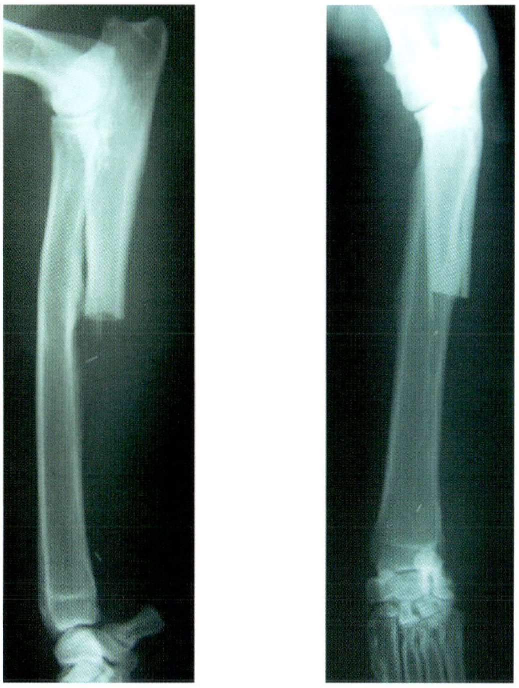

E-ii)

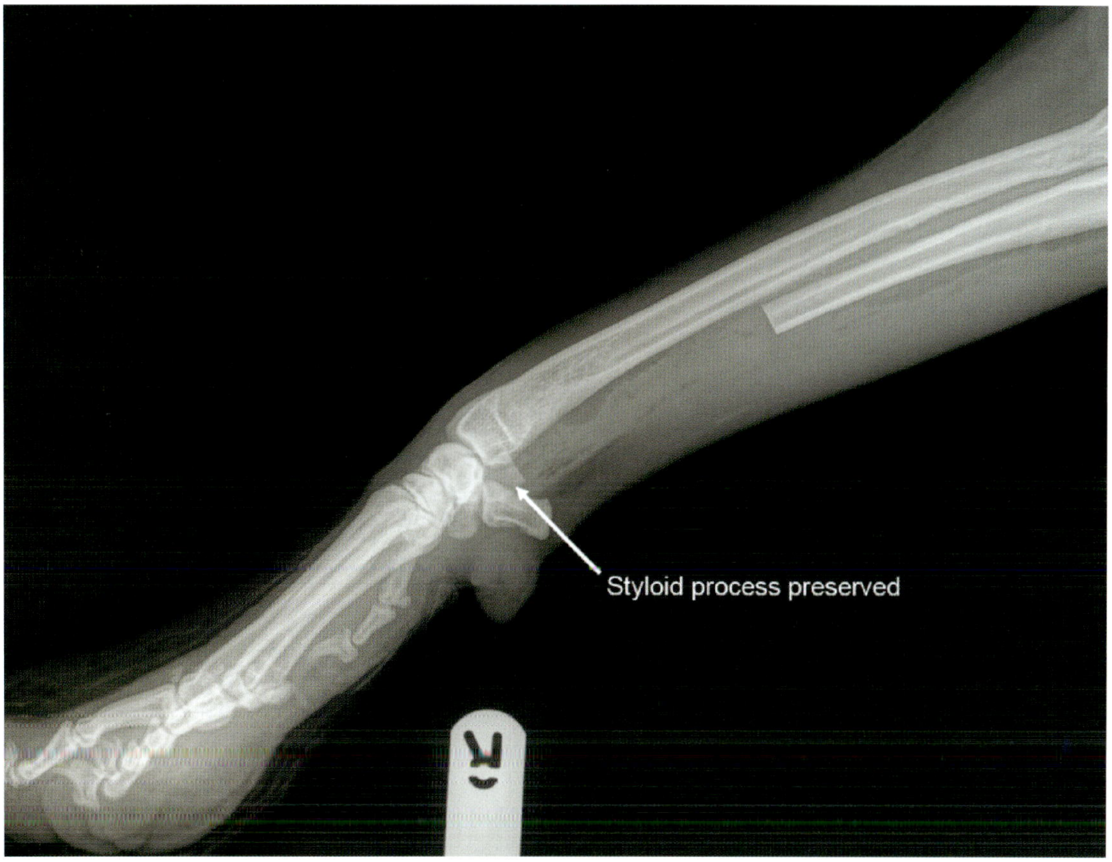

33.4 Coxofemoral Disarticulation

Indications

1) Resection of primary malignant appendicular bone tumors distal to the femoral head and neck
2) Resection of primary benign or malignant periarticular tumors distal to the coxofemoral joint
3) Resection of extensive and infiltrative soft tissue tumors of the pelvic limb
4) Resection of lumbar plexus nerve root tumors not amenable to local resection

Note that the authors recommend coxofemoral disarticulation rather than a midfemoral amputation for pelvic limb amputation. The more proximal resection with a coxofemoral disarticulation results in greater soft tissue and bone margins and greater likelihood of complete histologic excision. Coxofemoral disarticulation is also considered more cosmetic than midfemoral amputation.

Suggested Diagnostic Workup and Clinical Staging

See *33. Primary Bone and Periarticular Tumors*.

Patient Positioning (See Plate 33.4A)

A) The patient is positioned in lateral recumbency with the affected limb uppermost.

Surgical Technique (See Plate 33.4B–P, T)

B) The lateral skin incision starts at the flank, curving ventrally to the midfemur and then proximally and caudally to the ischium.
C) The medial skin incision joins the cranial and caudal ends with a flatter curve to a level halfway between midfemur and the proximal medial thigh, ensuring there is more skin on the lateral than medial aspect of the pelvic limb.
D) Dissection starts medially by isolating and ligating the femoral artery and vein cranial to the coxofemoral joint. The femoral artery and vein (i, arrows) are located between the caudal belly of the sartorius muscle (SM-Ca) and pectineus muscle (P) (AL, adductor longus muscle; Gr, gracilis muscle; SM-Cr, cranial belly of the sartorius muscle). The femoral artery and vein should be ligated distal to the lateral circumflex artery and vein as they course caudolaterally. The femoral artery is ligated with one to two simple ligatures and/or one transfixion ligature of 2-0 or 3-0 absorbable monofilament suture material (ii). Distal to this, the femoral artery is then either clamped with mosquito forceps or ligated (arrow), and then the femoral artery is transected between the ligatures and clamp with a vessel sealing device (iii, iv) or Metzenbaum scissors. The femoral vein is ligated with two simple ligatures of 2-0 or 3-0 absorbable monofilament suture material (v).

Plate 33.4

Coxofemoral Disarticulation

A)

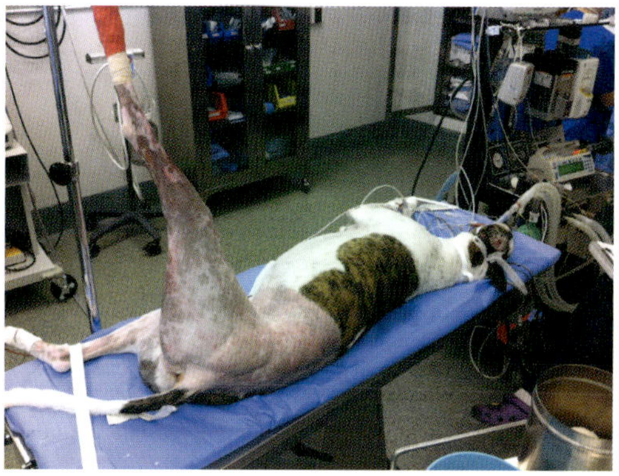

B)

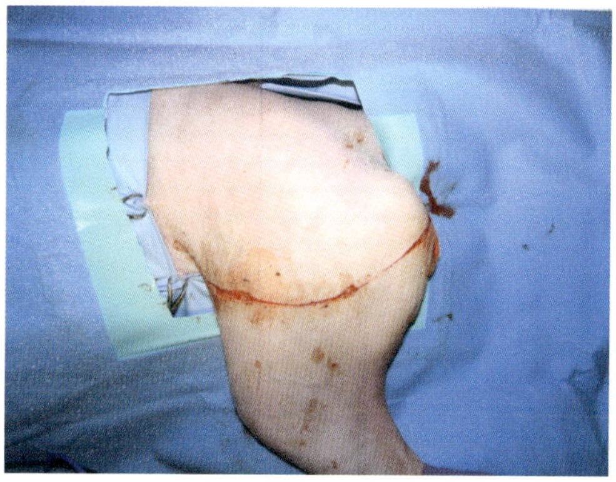

C)

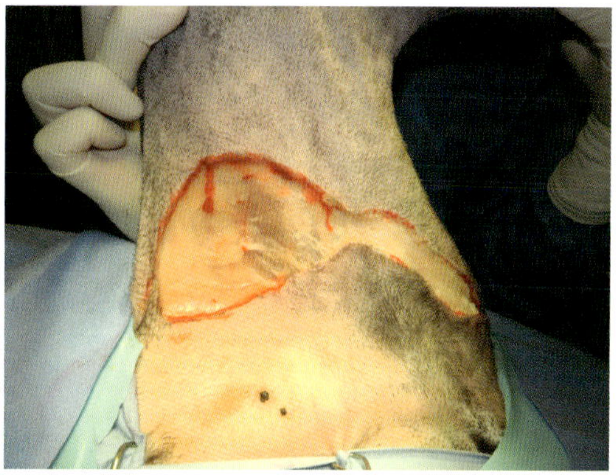

D-i)

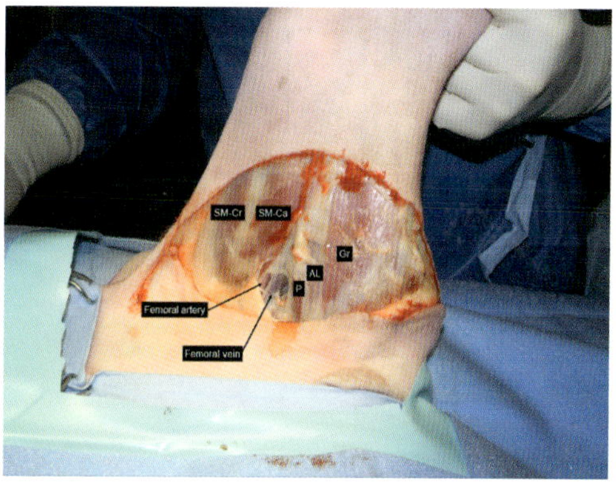

D-ii)

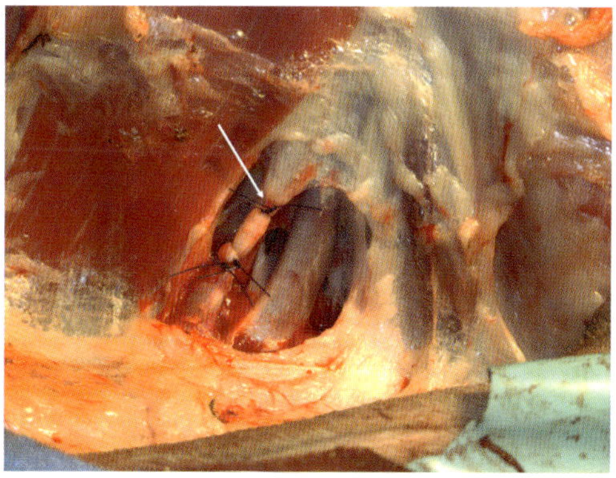

D-iii)

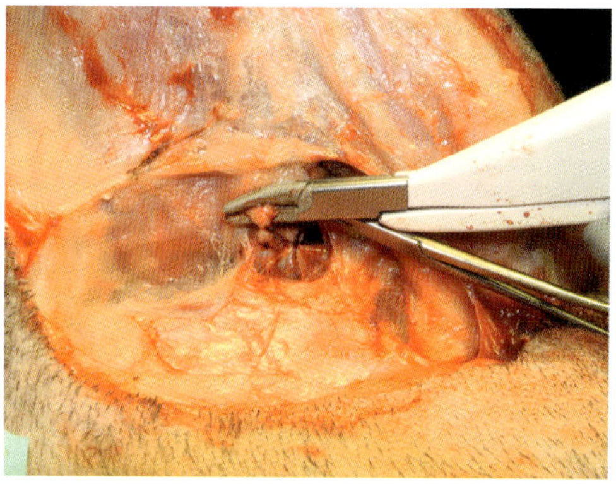

D-iv)

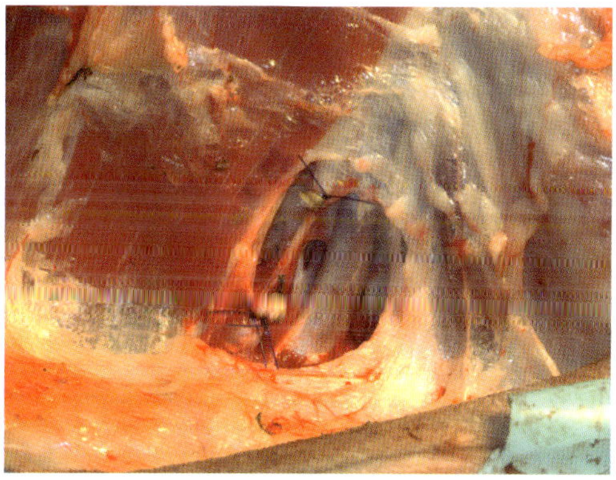

D-v)

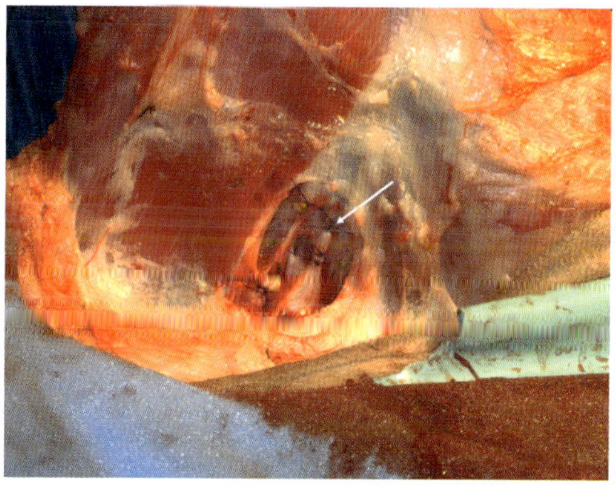

Surgical Technique (See Plate 33.4B–P, T) *continued*

Distal to this, the femoral vein closest is then either clamped with mosquito forceps or ligated (arrow), and then the femoral vein is transected between the ligatures and clamp with a vessel sealing device (vi, vii) or Metzenbaum scissors. In smaller animals, a vessel sealing device alone can be used to seal and transect the femoral artery and vein.

E) The medial femoral circumflex artery and vein (arrow) should also be ligated and divided or sealed and transected with a vessel sealing device.

F) The cranial and caudal borders of the pectineus muscle are dissected free, and the surgeon's finger is passed deep to the muscle in a cranial-to-caudal direction to aid midbody transection of the muscle with either electrosurgery or a vessel sealing device (pictured). If not done beforehand, transection of the pectineus muscle provides better exposure of the medial circumflex vessels, which are then ligated, cauterized, or sealed and transected with a vessel sealing device.

G) Cranially, the two bellies of sartorius muscle are transected several centimeters distal to the level of the coxofemoral joint. The remnant bellies of the sartorius muscle are used to reconstruct the cranial aspect of the amputation stump (P, pectineus muscle; SM-Ca, caudal belly of the sartorius muscle; SM-Cr, cranial belly of the sartorius muscle).

H) Working caudally, the flatter and broader gracilis muscle is transected midbody (i, ii) with either electrosurgery or a vessel sealing device to expose the larger adductor muscle.

I) The adductor muscle (Ad) is then transected with either electrosurgery or a vessel sealing device (SM, semimebranosus muscle; ST, semitendinosus muscle).

J) The iliopsoas muscle (ILP) is transected with either electrosurgery or a vessel sealing device. The underlying femoral and saphenous nerves are infiltrated with local anesthetic. These nerves are transected with a scalpel blade or scissors after a minimum of 1 minute for the local anesthetic to adequately infiltrate the nerve (coxofemoral joint, arrow).

Plate 33.4

Coxofemoral Disarticulation *continued*

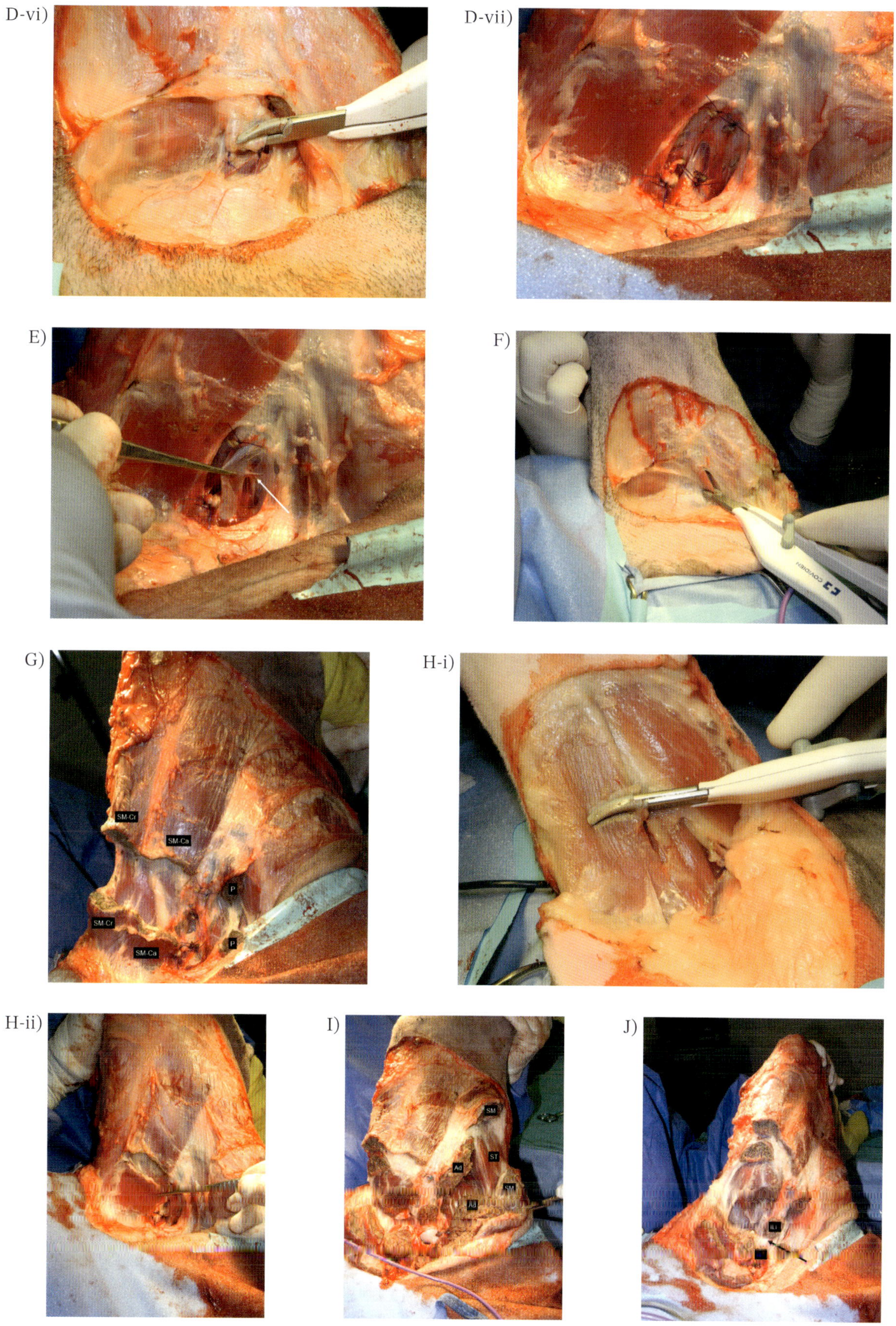

Surgical Technique (See Plate 33.4B–P, T) *continued*

K) The coxofemoral joint capsule is identified by manipulating the limb and is then incised with a scalpel blade or electrosurgery (pictured).
L) Abduction of the limb allows superior access to transect the round ligament of the femoral head (i, arrow) to disarticulate the coxofemoral joint (ii).
M) Moving to the lateral aspect of the limb (i), the skin of the proximal and lateral thigh is tightly adhered to the underlying tensor fascia lata muscle (TFL) and needs to be bluntly dissected from the tensor fascia lata muscle to the level of the greater trochanter (ii). The tensor fascia lata muscle is then transected at the level of the skin incision (iii), continuing cranially and then dorsally to expose the greater trochanter of the femur.
N) Moving caudally, the underlying bulky biceps femoris muscle (BF) is transected with either electrosurgery or a vessel sealing device (TFL, tensor fascia lata muscle).
O) Lifting the proximal body of the biceps femoris muscle (BF) dorsally, the semitendinosus (ST) and the more medial semimembranosus (SM) muscles are transected midbelly using either electrosurgery or a vessel sealing device (Ad, adductor muscle; TFL, tensor fascia lata muscle). The remnant bellies of semitendinosus and semimembranosus muscles are used to reconstruct the caudal aspect of the amputation stump.

Plate 33.4

Coxofemoral Disarticulation *continued*

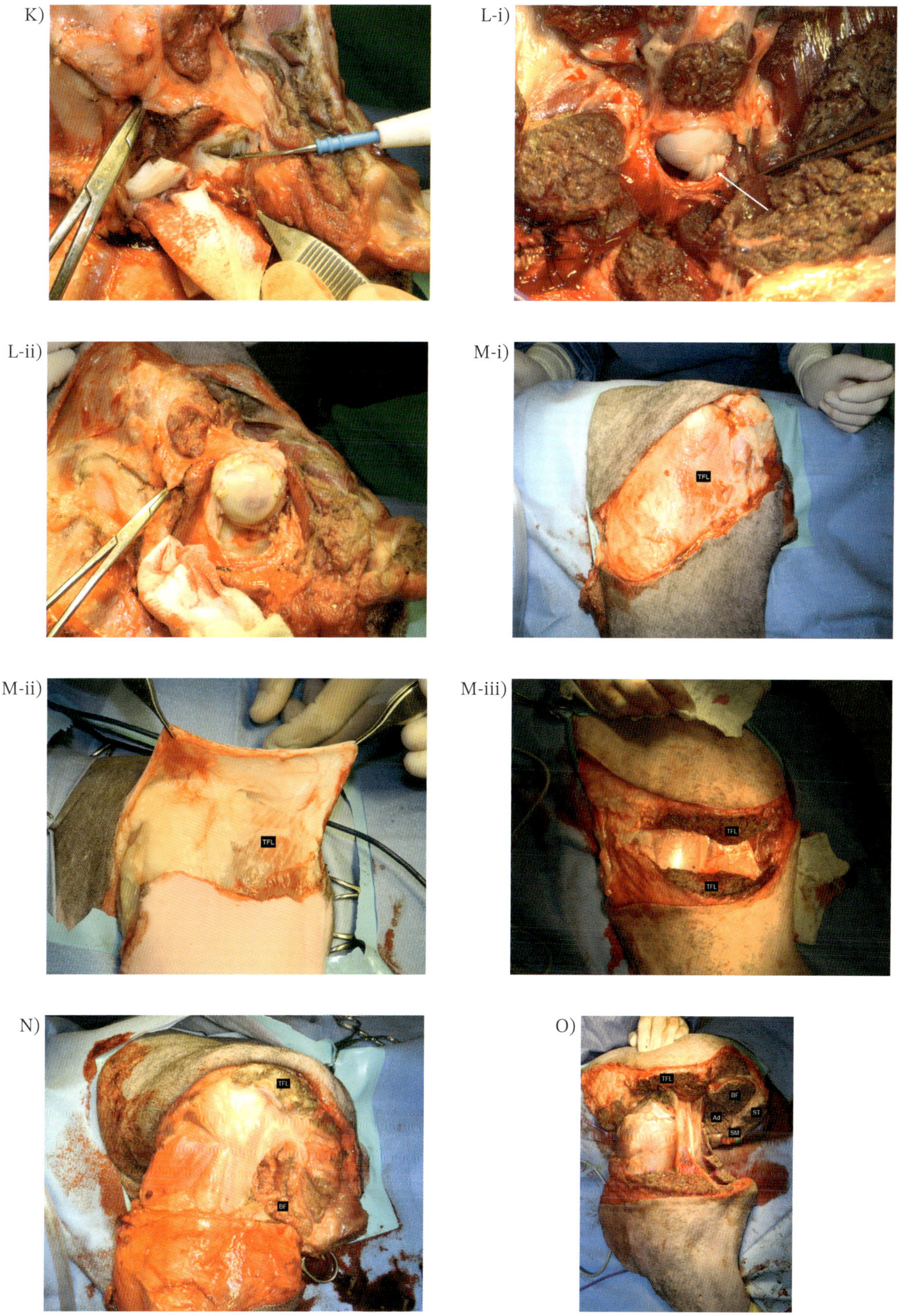

Surgical Technique (See Plate 33.4B–P, T) *continued*

P) The sciatic nerve is infiltrated with local anesthetic (i). The sciatic is transected with a scalpel blade or scissors (ii) after a minimum of 1 minute for the local anesthetic to adequately infiltrate the nerve.
Q) Caudally, the quadratus femoris muscle is now visible. An Army-Navy retractor can be passed medial to the muscle, and the qudratus femoris muscle is then transected midbelly using either electrosurgery or a vessel sealing device (not pictured).
R) The caudal rotator muscles of the coxofemoral joint are individually transected using either electrosurgery or a vessel sealing device (not pictured).
S) The gluteal muscles are transected close to their insertions on the greater trochanter (not pictured). The residual gluteal muscles are also used to reconstruct the middle aspects of the amputation stump.
T) Any remaining joint capsule or muscles are incised or transected, and the limb is removed from the surgical field.

Closure (See Plate 33.4U–W)

U) The muscles are then closed by suturing the fascia together to bring the transected muscle surfaces together (i; Ad, adductor muscle; BF, biceps femoris muscle; SM, semimembranosus muscle; SM-Ca, caudal belly of the sartorius muscle; SM-Cr, cranial belly of the sartorius muscle; ST, semitendinosus muscle). The cranial edge of biceps femoris muscle is sutured to the adductor muscle, with the semimembranosus and semitendinosus filling the caudal defect using 0 to 3-0 absorbable monofilament suture material in a cruciate or simple continuous pattern (ii).
V) The sartorius muscle bellies and tensor fascia lata are collectively sutured to the fascia of the muscle bellies caudally using 0 to 3-0 absorbable monofilament suture material in a cruciate or simple continuous pattern.
W) The subcutaneous tissue (i) and skin (ii) are closed routinely.

Postoperative Management

1) Multimodal analgesia
2) Elizabethan collar or body suit
3) Sling support if necessary

Plate 33.4

Coxofemoral Disarticulation *continued*

P-i)

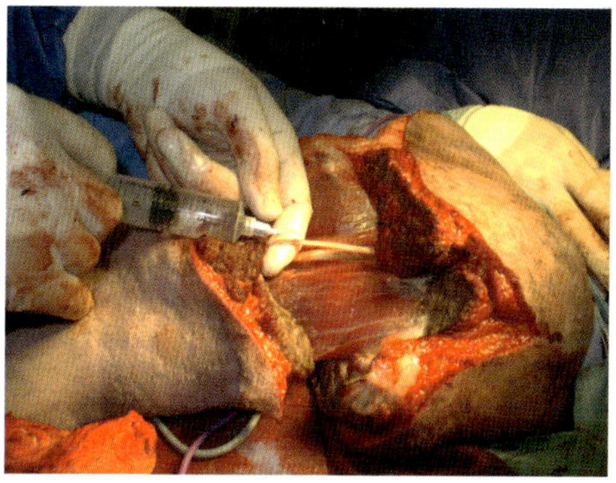

P-ii)

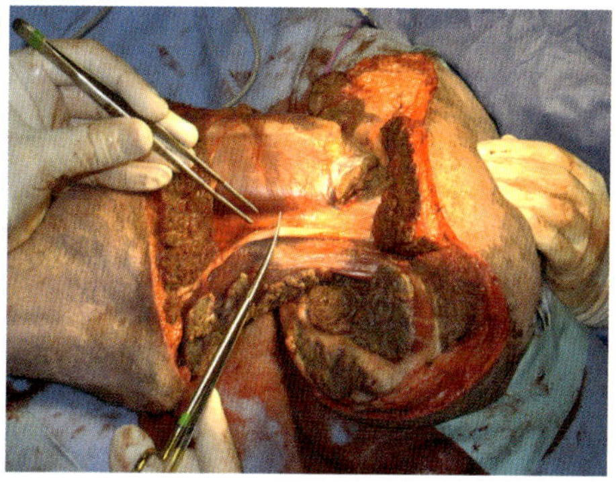

T)

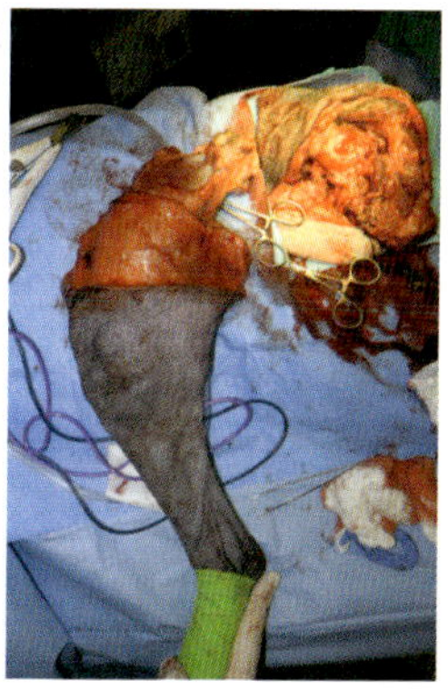

U-i)

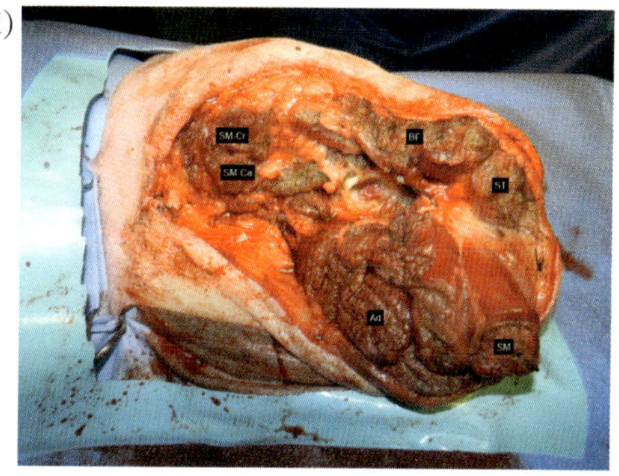

U-ii)

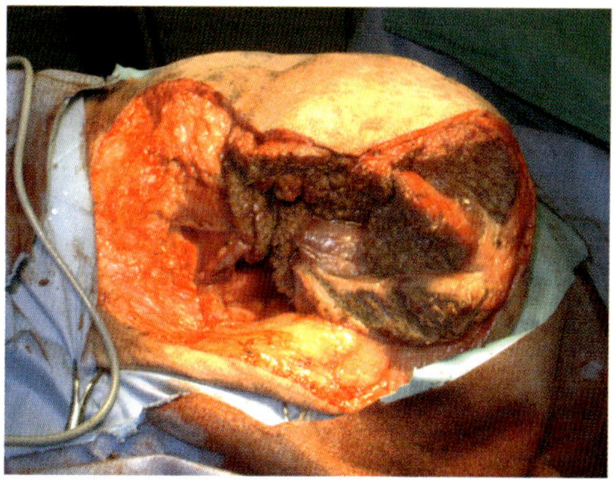

V)

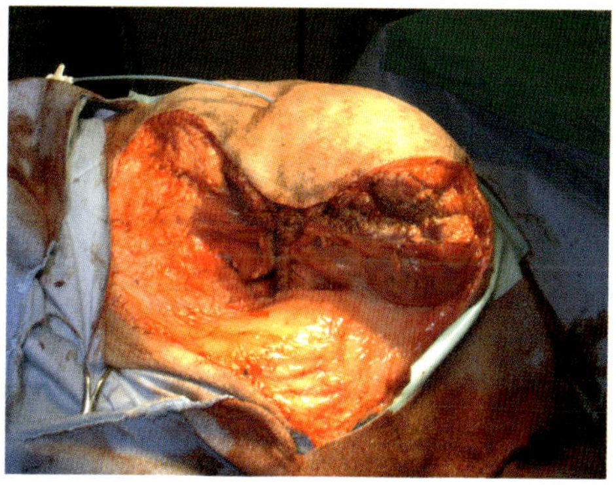

W-i)

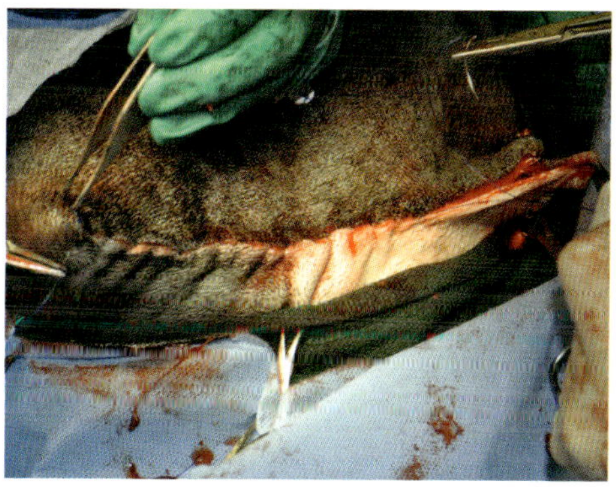

W-ii)

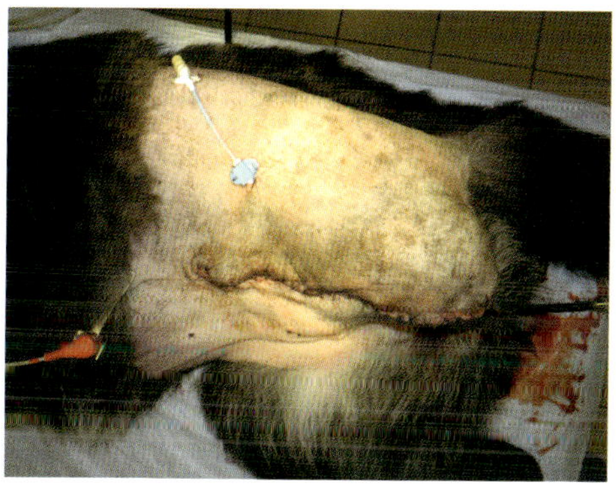

Chapter 34: Partial and Total Scapulectomy

Indication (See Plate 34 – 1)

1) Resection of benign or malignant tumors arising from the scapula or secondarily involving the scapula

Suggested Diagnostic Workup and Clinical Staging

- See *33. Primary Bone and Periarticular Tumors*
- Precontrast and postcontrast computed tomography scan of the scapula for surgical planning [1]

Patient Positioning

The patient is positioned in lateral recumbency with the affected limb uppermost.

Surgical Technique [1] (See Plate 34A–F)

A) A skin incision is made along the spine of the scapula extending from dorsal to the dorsal border of the scapula proximally to the level of the proximal to midhumerus distally. If a preoperative biopsy has been performed, then the biopsy tract is excised en bloc with the scapulectomy (arrow). The skin incision is continued deeply through the subcutaneous tissue.
B) The trapezius (Tr), omotransversarius, rhomboideus, and acromial and spinous heads of the deltoid muscle are transected close to their origin on the scapula; however, the level of transection may need to be modified to provide a compartment of normal muscle around the pseudocapsule of the scapular tumor. If the level of transection is through the muscle belly, then cautery or a vessel sealing device is recommended for hemostasis.
C) The scapula is retracted laterally to expose the serratus ventralis muscle on the medial aspect of the scapula. The serratus ventralis muscle is either elevated from the fascia serrata with a periosteal elevator (if distant to the pseudocapsule of the scapular tumor) or transected through the muscle belly (if the pseudocapsule of the scapular tumor is in close proximity to the fascia serrata). If the level of transection is through the muscle belly, then electrosurgery or a vessel sealing device is recommended for hemostasis.
D) The scapula is abducted to identify and preserve the nerves of the brachial plexus and the axillary artery and vein.
E) **Partial scapulectomy:** The supraspinatus, infraspinatus, and subscapularis muscles are transected at the level of the planned osteotomy site (i–iii). Electrosurgery or a vessel sealing device is recommended for hemostasis during transection of these muscle bellies (ii). The osteotomy should be located with minimum bone margins of 3 cm from the distal extent of the tumor as determined from preoperative imaging. The osteotomy can be performed with an

Color Atlas of Canine and Feline Surgical Oncology, First Edition. Julius M. Liptak, Paolo Buracco, William T. N. Culp, and Nicholas J. Bacon.

Plate 34

Partial and Total Scapulectomy

1)

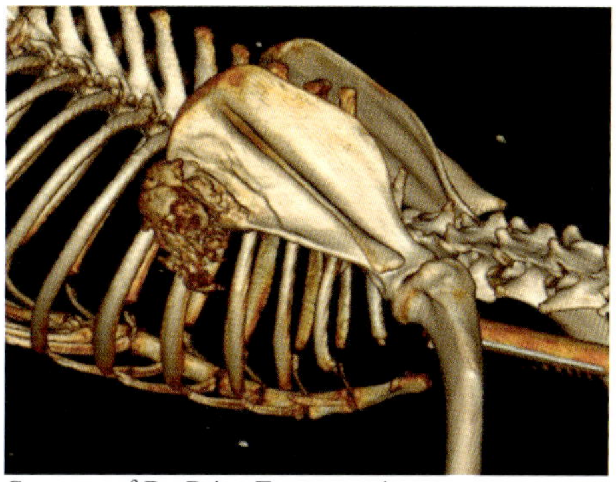

Courtesy of Dr. Brian Trumpatori

A)

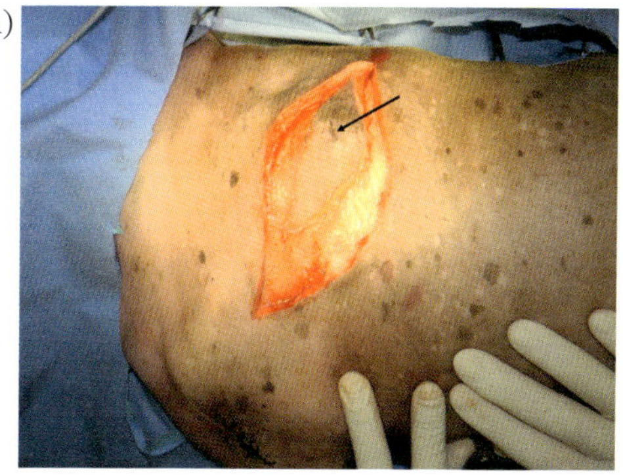

B)

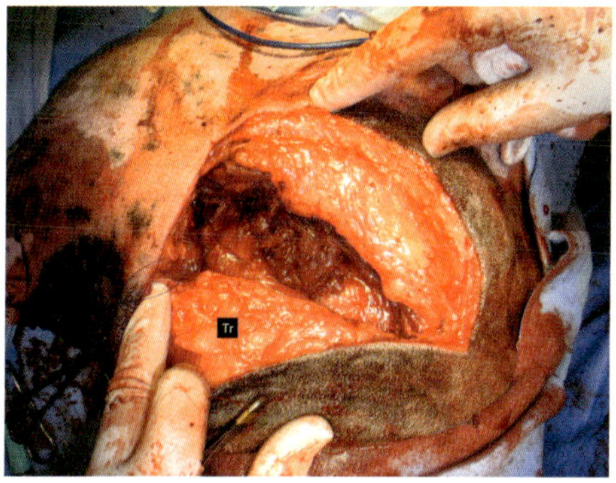

C)

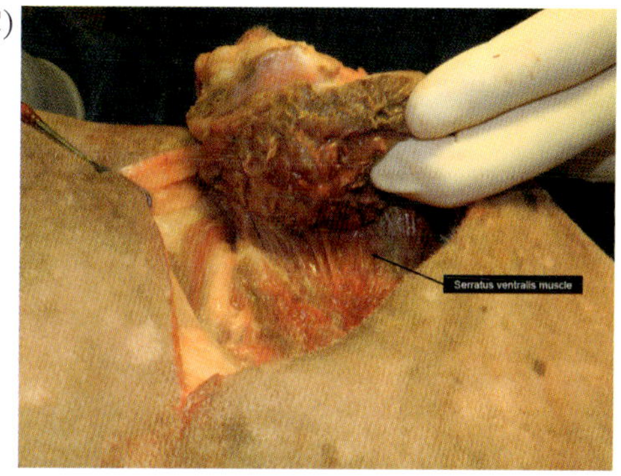

D)

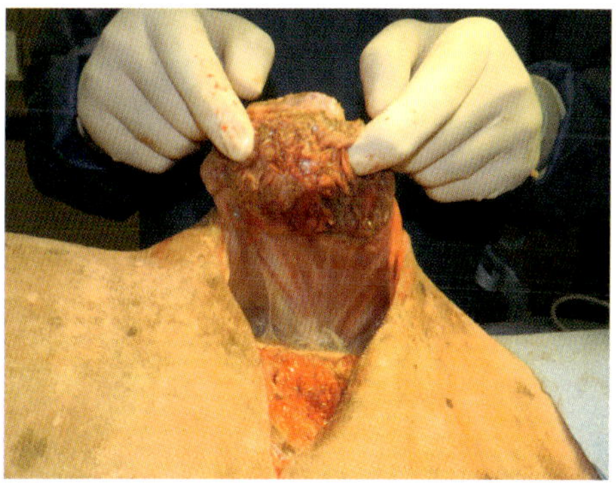

E-i)

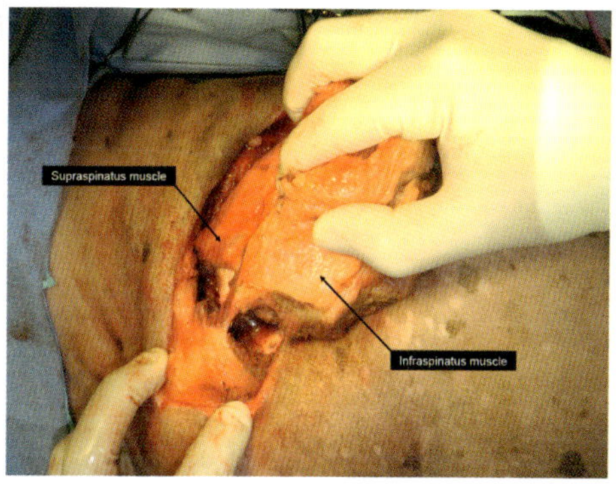

E-ii)

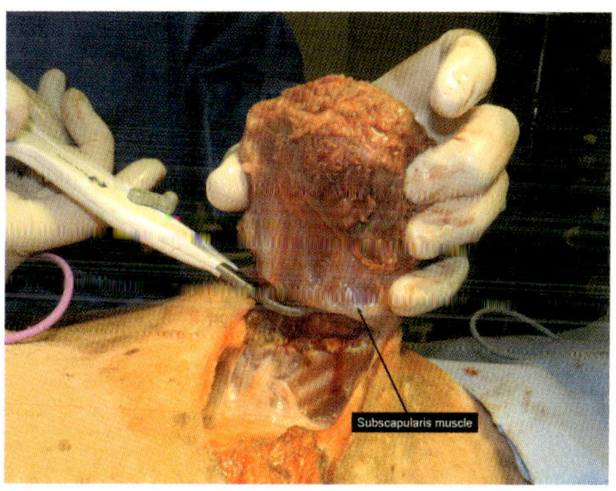

E-iii)

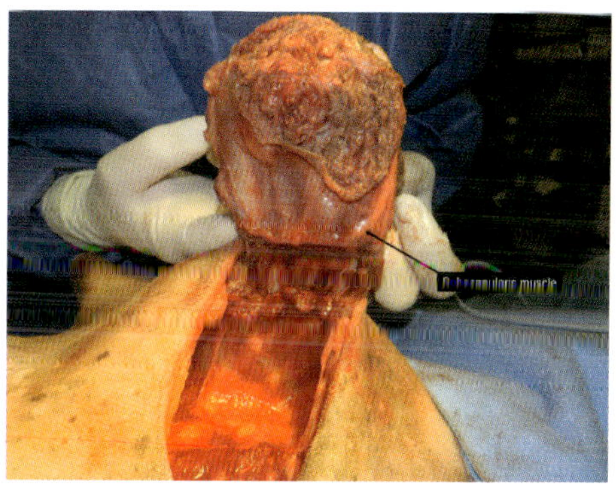

Surgical Technique [1] (See Plate 34A–F) *continued*

oscillating or sagittal saw (iv, v), or a pneumatic drill. The partial scapulectomy specimen is removed from the surgical field (vi). Bone tunnels are drilled along the proximal edge of the residual scapula (vii). The omotransversarius, trapezius, serratus ventralis, and rhomboideus muscles are reattached to the distal scapular remnant with 2-0 to 2 absorbable or nonabsorbable monofilament suture material in a simple interrupted or horizontal mattress suture pattern through the bone tunnels (viii–x). Alternatively, the remaining supraspinatus and infraspinatus muscles and the deltoid and long head of the triceps muscles are sutured to the serratus ventralis, omotransversarius, and trapezius muscles with 2-0 to 2 absorbable or nonabsorbable monofilament suture material in a horizontal mattress pattern. This alternative technique does not require bone tunnels to be drilled in the proximal edge of the residual scapula.

Plate 34

Partial and Total Scapulectomy *continued*

E-iv)

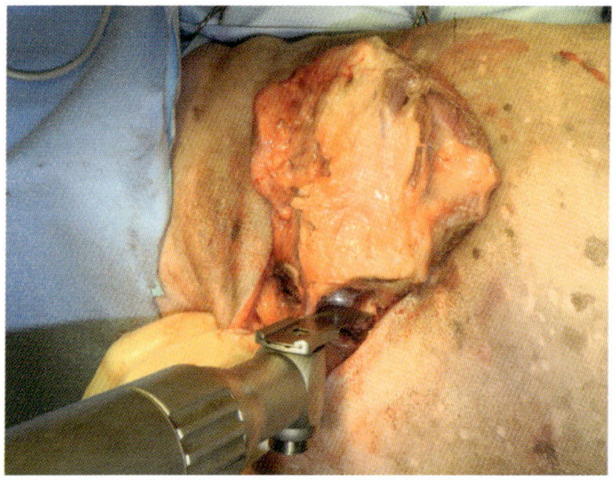

E-v)

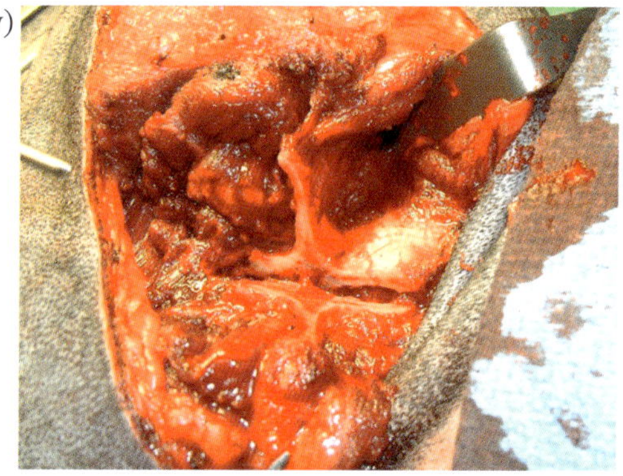

E-vi)

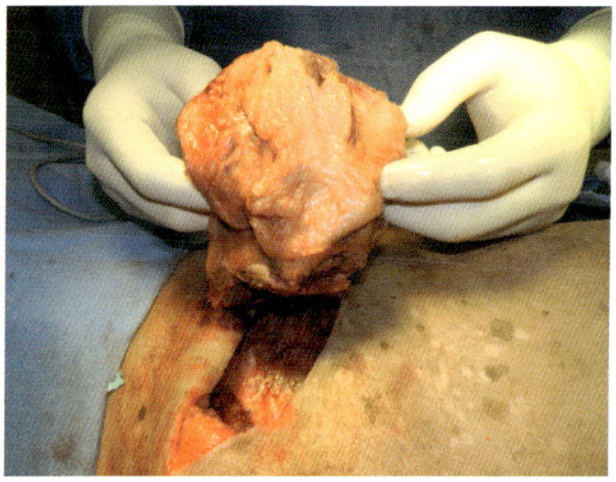

E-vii)

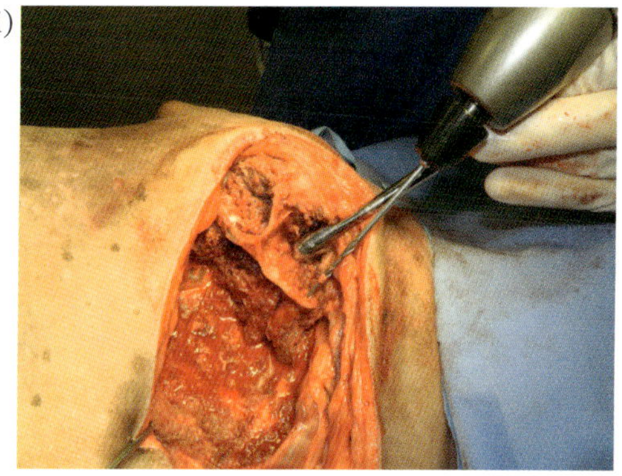

E-viii)

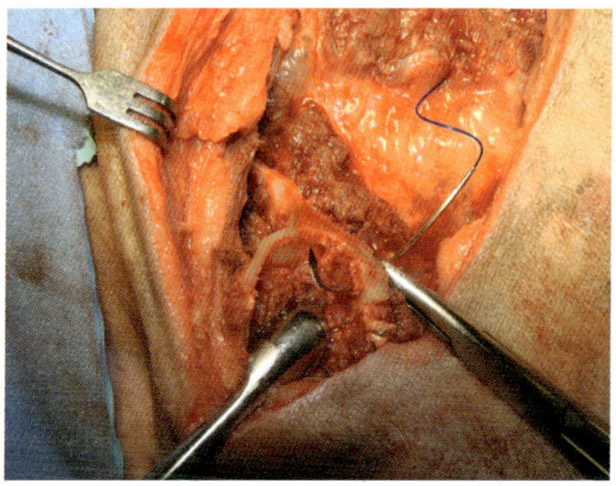

E-ix)

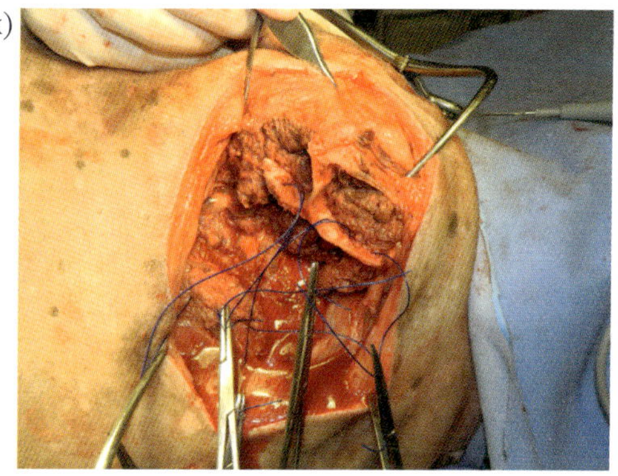

E-x)

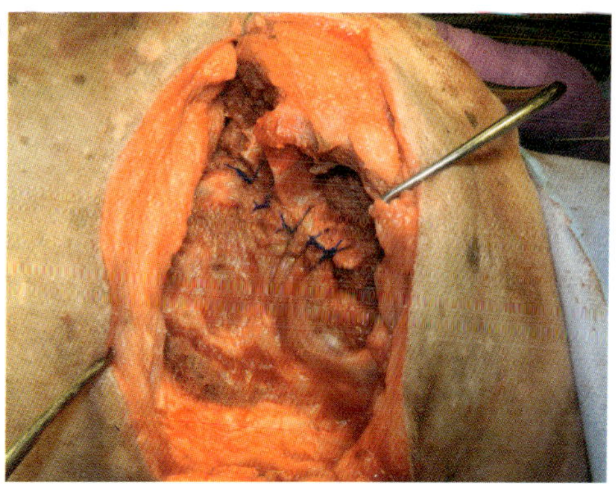

Surgical Technique [1] (See Plate 34A–F) *continued*

F) **Total scapulectomy:** The suprascapular and subscapular nerves, which are located along the ventral border of the scalenus muscle, are infused with 0.2–0.5 ml bupivacaine and, after 1–3 minutes, transected. The tendons of the coracobrachialis, teres minor, infraspinatus, supraspinatus, and subscapularis muscles are transected close to their insertions on the proximal humerus. A transverse arthrotomy of the glenohumeral joint is performed, and the insertion of the teres major muscle and the long head of the triceps muscle are transected close to their insertion on the caudal border of the scapula. The biceps tendon is transected, and the scapula is removed in its entirety from the surgical field (i). The biceps tendon is fixed to the craniolateral aspect of the proximal humerus with an appropriately sized cortical or cancellous bone screw and spiked washer (ii). The triceps muscle is reattached over the humeral head to the deltoid, omotransversarius, and trapezius (Tr) muscles. The trapezius muscle is sutured to the serratus ventralis muscle (iii). Reattachment of the muscles should be done with 2-0 to 2 absorbable or nonabsorbable monofilament suture material in a horizontal mattress pattern.

Closure

The skin incision is closed routinely in two layers with a simple continuous suture pattern using monofilament absorbable suture material in the subcutis and either an interrupted or continuous suture pattern using monofilament nonabsorbable suture material in the skin.

Postoperative Management

1) Multimodal analgesia
2) Elizabethan collar
3) Rehabilitation

Complications in Dogs [2]

Acute Complications (<1 Month)

- Overall: 35%
- Seroma (18%)
- Marked lameness (15%)
- Suture failure between scapula and adjacent muscles (3%)

Chronic Complications (>1 Month)

- Overall: 15%
- Seroma (5%)
- Marked lameness (8%)

Plate 34

Partial and Total Scapulectomy *continued*

F-i)

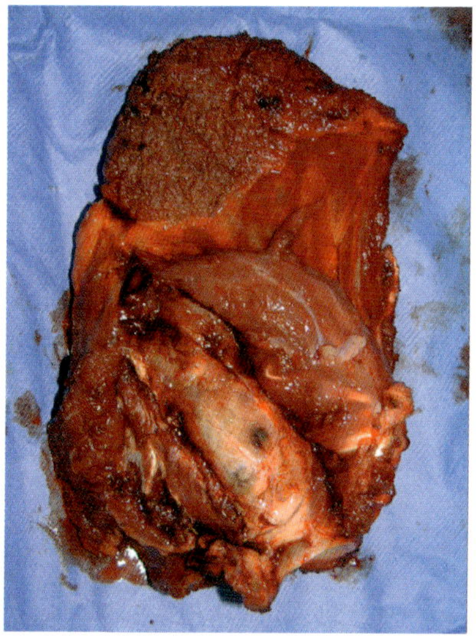

F-ii)

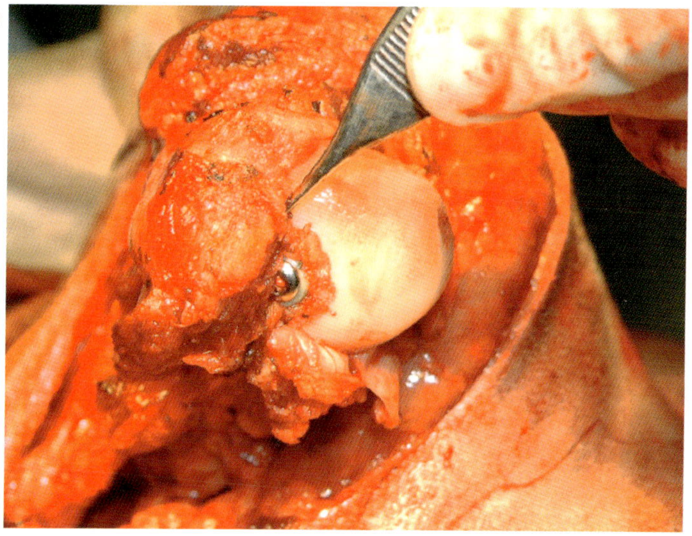

F-iii)

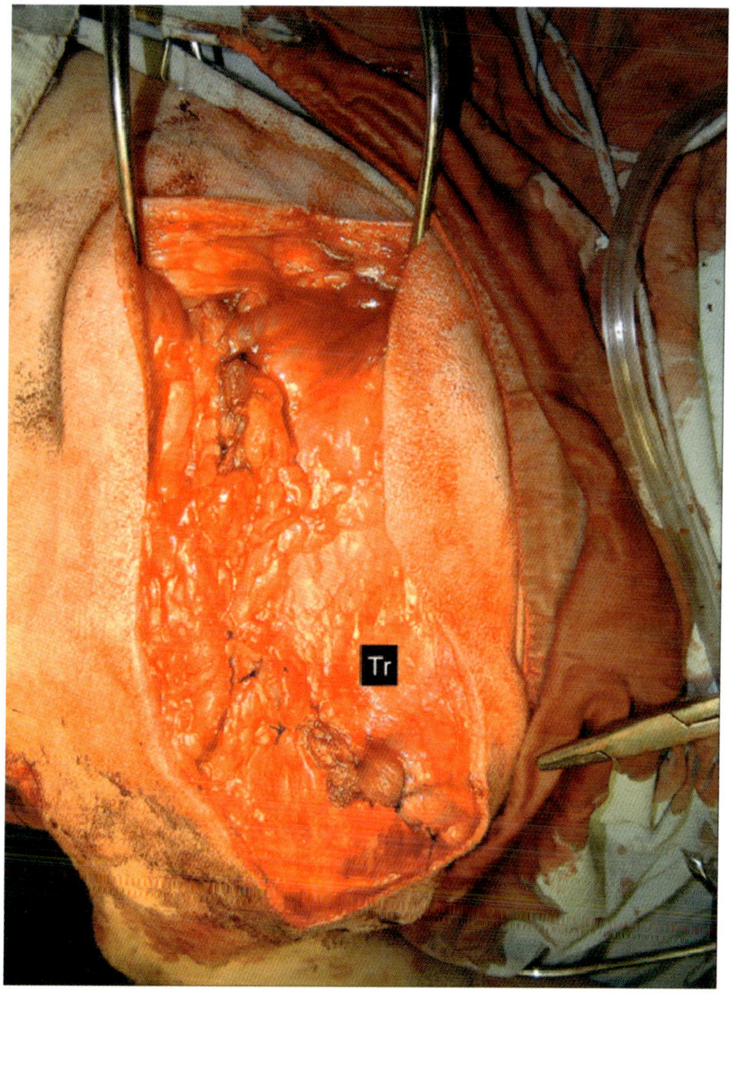

Postoperative Limb Use

Limb Use	<2 wk	<1 mo	<2 mo	<3 mo	>3 mo
Poor	37%	20%	7%	0%	0%
Fair	41%	41%	21%	0%	0%
Good	17%	29%	29%	67%	11%
Excellent	5%	10%	43%	33%	89%

Suggested Adjuvant Treatments

- Chemotherapy for dogs with scapular osteosarcoma

Prognosis and Oncologic Outcome [2]

Prognosis and Oncologic Outcome – Dogs

	Local Recurrence Rate	Metastatic Rate	Disease-Free Interval (d)	Median Survival Time (d)	1-Year Survival Rate	2-Year Survival Rate
			Osteosarcoma			
Overall	4%	59%	210	246	–	–
			Chondrosarcoma			
Overall	25%	50%	55	NR	–	–
			Soft tissue sarcoma			
Overall	14%	28%	366	413	–	–

NR, not reached.

References

1 Kirpensteijn, J., Straw, R.C., Pardo, A.D. et al. (1995). Partial and total scapulectomy in the dog. *J. Am. Anim. Hosp. Assoc.* 30 (4): 313–319.

2 Montinaro, V., Boston, S.E., Buracco, P. et al. (2013). Clinical outcome of 42 dogs with scapular tumors treated by scapulectomy: a veterinary society of surgical oncology (VSSO) retrospective study (1995-2010). *Vet. Surg.* 42 (8): 943–950.

Chapter 35: Metacarpectomy and Metatarsectomy

Indications

1) Resection of primary benign or malignant tumors of the metacarpus or metatarsus
2) Metacarpectomy or metatarsectomy can be combined with a digit amputation (see *36. Digit Amputation*)

Suggested Diagnostic Workup and Clinical Staging

See *33. Primary Bone and Periarticular Tumors.*

Patient Positioning

The patient is positioned in dorsal, dorsolateral, or lateral recumbency with the affected limb uppermost.

Surgical Technique (See Plate 35A–C)

A) A dorsal skin incision is made over the affected metacarpal or metatarsal bone.
B) Soft tissues are dissected from the affected metacarpal or metatarsal bone using a combination of blunt and sharp dissection, taking care not to compromise the tumor capsule.
C) The affected metacarpal or metatarsal bone can be resected in its entirety or segmentally. For resection of the entire metacarpal bone, the carpometacarpal (i, ii) and metacarpophalangeal joints are incised and disarticulated. Similarly, for resection of the entire metatarsal bone, the tarsometatarsal and metatarsophalangeal joints are incised and disarticulated. Digit amputation is often preferred to disarticulation of either the metacarpophalangeal or metatarsophalangeal joint (iii). The medial and lateral collateral ligaments insert onto the proximal second and fifth metacarpal and metatarsal bones, respectively. Disarticulation of the second or fifth carpometacarpal or tarsometatarsal joints can result in transection of the respective collateral ligaments and subsequent joint instability. As a result, in these cases, osteotomy of the proximal metacarpal or metatarsal bone with a pneumatic burr or bone cutters (iv) is preferred to preserve the integrity of the collateral ligament insertion and joint stability. However, this should be performed only if surgical margins are not compromised by the more distal resection of the proximal margins.

Color Atlas of Canine and Feline Surgical Oncology, First Edition. Julius M. Liptak, Paolo Buracco, William T. N. Culp, and Nicholas J. Bacon.

Plate 35

Metacarpectomy and Metatarsectomy

A)

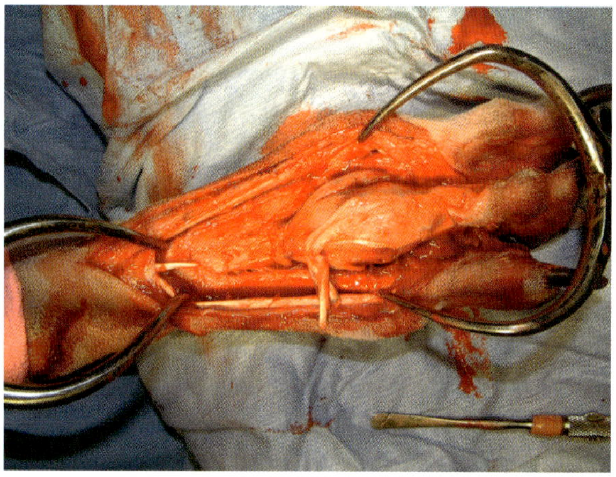

B)

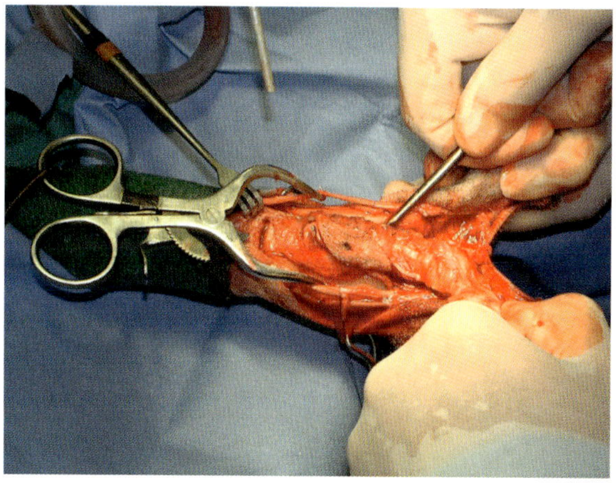

C-i)

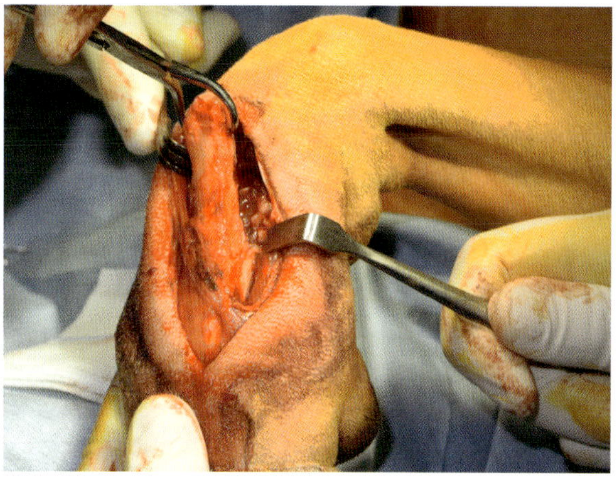

C-ii)

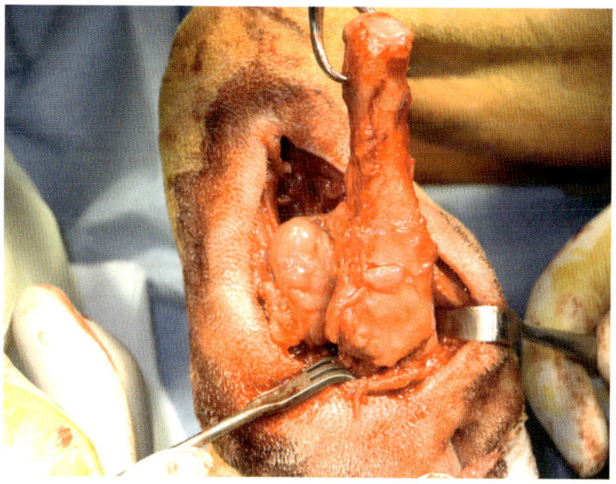

C-iii)

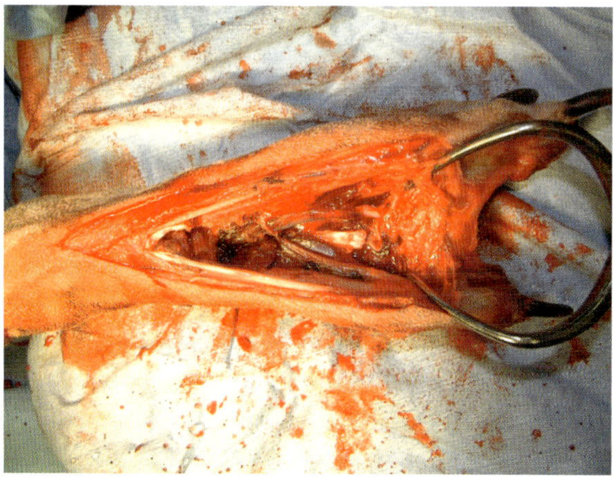

C-iv)

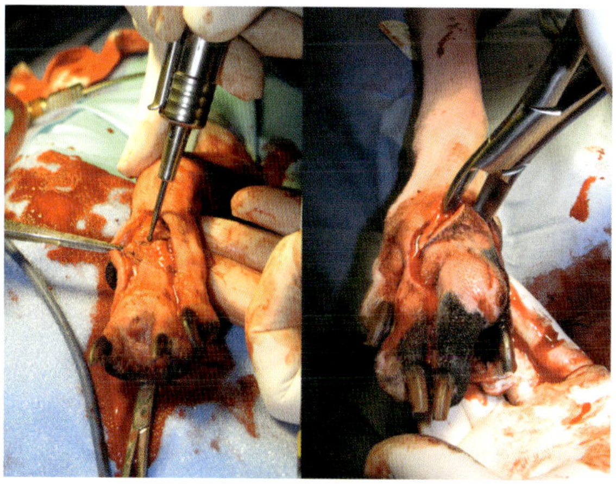

Closure

The skin incision is closed routinely in two layers with a simple continuous suture pattern using monofilament absorbable suture material in the subcutis and either an interrupted or continuous suture pattern using monofilament nonabsorbable suture material in the skin.

Postoperative Management

1) Multimodal analgesia
2) Modified Robert-Jones bandage for 14 days with or without a splint
3) Elizabethan collar
4) Exercise restriction for 14 days

Complications

- Surgical-site infection (21%) [1]

Suggested Adjuvant Treatments

- Chemotherapy for dogs with appendicular osteosarcoma
- Chemotherapy for dogs with appendicular hemangiosarcoma

Prognosis and Oncologic Outcome

	Local Recurrence Rate	Metastatic Rate	Disease-Free Interval (d)	Median Survival Time (d)	1-Year Survival Rate	2-Year Survival Rate
			Osteosarcoma [1, 2]			
Overall	14%	50%–67%	377	466–687	–	–

References

1 Tremolada, G., Thamm, D.H., Milovancev, M. et al. (2021). Biological behaviour of primary osteosarcoma of the digits, metacarpal and metatarsal bones in dogs. *Vet. Comp. Oncol.* 19: 735–742.

2 Gamblin, R.M., Straw, R.C., Powers, B.E. et al. (1995). Primary osteosarcoma distal to the antebrachiocarpal and tarsocrural joints in nine dogs (1980-1992). *J. Am. Anim. Hosp. Assoc.* 31 (1): 86–91.

Chapter 36: Digit Amputation

Tumors of the digit can arise from the subungual crest (nail bed), skin and subcutaneous tissue, and phalangeal bones. Single-digit amputation is recommended for the management of tumors confined to a single digit where adequate lateral margins are able to be achieved with subsequent primary closure of the surgical wound. Partial foot (or double-digit) amputation is recommended for the management of digit tumors that involve two adjacent digits, where adequate lateral margins with subsequent primary closure of the surgical wound is not possible with a single-digit amputation, or for resection of interdigital tumors. Digit amputation is not recommended for cats with metastatic digit tumors (acrometastasis or lung-digit syndrome). For both single-digit and partial foot amputation, the digits should be amputated at the level of the distal metacarpal or metatarsal bone rather than disarticulation of the metacarpophalangeal or metatarsophalangeal joint or more distal locations to minimize the risk of postoperative lameness.

Suggested Diagnostic Workup and Clinical Staging

- Fine-needle aspirate cytology or incisional biopsy
- Regional lymph node assessment
  - Fine-needle aspirate cytology or nonselective excision of the ipsilateral superficial cervical and axillary lymph nodes for digit tumors involving the thoracic limb, or the ipsilateral popliteal and superficial inguinal lymph nodes for digit tumors involving the pelvic limb
  - Sentinel lymph node mapping and excision of the sentinel lymph node
- Three-view thoracic radiographs for assessment of lung metastasis

Suggested Adjuvant Treatments

- Melanoma vaccine for cats and dogs with subungual or digit pad melanomas
- Chemotherapy for dogs with digit osteosarcomas
- Chemotherapy for dogs with high-grade mast cell tumors

Color Atlas of Canine and Feline Surgical Oncology, First Edition. Julius M. Liptak, Paolo Buracco, William T. N. Culp, and Nicholas J. Bacon.

Prognosis and Oncologic Outcome

Prognosis and Oncologic Outcome – Dogs

	Local Recurrence Rate	Metastatic Rate	Disease-Free Interval (d)	Median Survival Time (d)	1-Year Survival Rate	2-Year Survival Rate
			Squamous Cell Carcinoma [1–3]			
Overall	0%	5%–29%	–	–	50%–95%	18%–74%
			Subungual Malignant Melanoma [1, 4]			
Overall						
Surgery [1]	–	58%	–	365	42%	13%
Surgery and melanoma vaccine [4]	–	50%	–	476	63%	32%
Clinical stage [4]						
Stage I	–	–	–	>952	–	–
Stage II	–	–	–	>1093	–	–
Stage III	–	–	–	321	–	–
Stage IV	–	–	–	76	–	–
Lymph node metastasis at diagnosis [4]						
No	–	–	–	459	–	–
Yes	–	–	–	110	–	–
Distant metastasis at diagnosis [4]						
No	–	–	–	459	–	–
Yes	–	–	–	76	–	–
Macroscopic disease at first vaccination [4]						
No	–	–	–	533	–	–
Yes	–	–	–	76	–	–
Completion of vaccination protocol [4]						
Yes	–	–	–	418	–	–
No	–	–	–	63	–	–
Distant metastasis after vaccination					–	–
protocol completion [4]					–	–
No	–	–	–	≥1152		
Yes	–	–	–	238		
			Osteosarcoma [3]			
Overall	–	25%	–	–	33%	0%
			Mast Cell Tumor [1]			
Overall	–	–	–	610	88%	50%

Prognosis and Oncologic Outcome – Cats

	Local Recurrence Rate	Metastatic Rate	Disease-Free Interval (d)	Median Survival Time (d)	1-Year Survival Rate	2-Year Survival Rate
			Melanoma [5]			
Overall	40%	60%	–	253	20%	–
			Giant Cell Reparative Granuloma [6]			
Overall	23%	0%	–	–	–	–

References

1 Marino, D.J., Matthiesen, D.T., Stefanacci, J.D. et al. (1995). Evaluation of dogs with digit masses: 117 cases (1981-1991). *J. Am. Vet. Med. Assoc.* 207 (6): 726–728.

2 O'Brien, M.G., Berg, J., and Engler, S.J. (1992). Treatment by digital amputation of subungual squamous cell carcinoma in dogs: 21 cases (1987-1988). *J. Am. Vet. Med. Assoc.* 201 (5): 759–761.

3 Henry, C.J., Brewer, W.G.J., Whitley, E.M. et al. (2005). Canine digital tumors: a veterinary cooperative oncology group retrospective study of 64 dogs. *J. Vet. Intern. Med.* 19 (5): 720–724.

4 Manley, C.A., Leibman, N.F., Wolchok, J.D. et al. (2011). Xenogeneic murine tyrosinase DNA vaccine for malignant melanoma of the digit of dogs. *J. Vet. Intern. Med.* 25 (1): 94–99.

5 Luna, L.D., Higginbotham, M.L., Henry, C.J. et al. (2000). Feline non-ocular melanoma: a retrospective study of 23 cases (1991-1999). *J. Feline Med. Surg.* 2 (4): 173–181.

6 Dobromylskyj, M.J., Fernandes, R.A., French, A. et al. (2017). Clinical, histological and prognostic features of a novel nail-bed lesion of cats: 41 cases. *J. Feline Med. Surg.* 19 (8): 853–859.

36.1 Single-Digit Amputation

Indications (See Plate 36.1 – 1)

1) Resection of benign (i, keratocanthoma; ii, intraosseous cyst) or malignant tumors (iii, malignant melanoma; iv, squamous cell carcinoma) involving a single digit where adequate lateral margins are able to be achieved with subsequent primary closure of the surgical wound.
2) Digit amputation can be combined with metacarpectomy or metatarsectomy (see *35. Metacarpectomy and Metatarsectomy*).

Suggested Diagnostic Workup and Clinical Staging

- See *36. Digit Amputation*.

Patient Positioning

The patient can be positioned in lateral recumbency with the affected limb uppermost (especially for tumors involving the fifth digit), dorsal recumbency (especially for tumors involving the third or fourth digits), or lateral recumbency with the affected limb downmost (especially for tumors involving the second digit).

Surgical Technique (See Plate 36.1A–C, F)

A) **Approach for all digits:** An incision is made over the dorsal aspect of the affected digit extending from the midmetacarpal/metatarsal bone to the metacarpophalangeal/metatarsophalangeal joint and then medially and laterally around the base of the digit so that the incisions join on the palmar/plantar aspect of the digit and are continuous circumferentially (i). The skin incision is then continued deeply through the subcutaneous tissue (ii, iii).

Color Atlas of Canine and Feline Surgical Oncology, First Edition. Julius M. Liptak, Paolo Buracco, William T. N. Culp, and Nicholas J. Bacon.

Plate 36.1

Single-Digit Amputation

1-i)
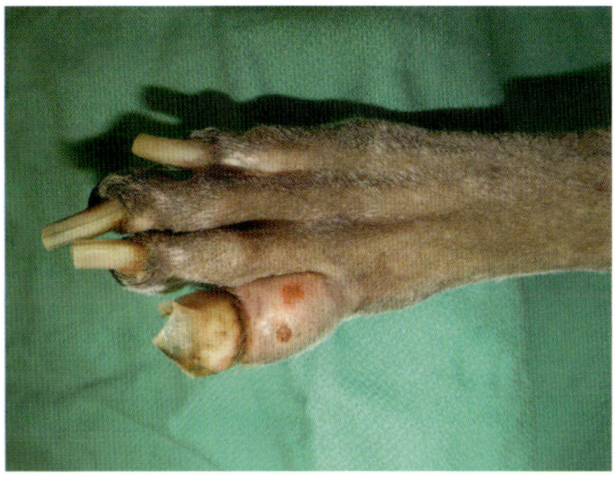

1-ii)
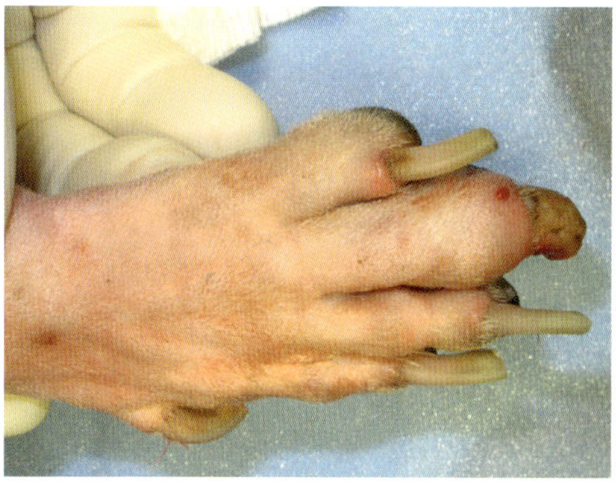

1-iii)
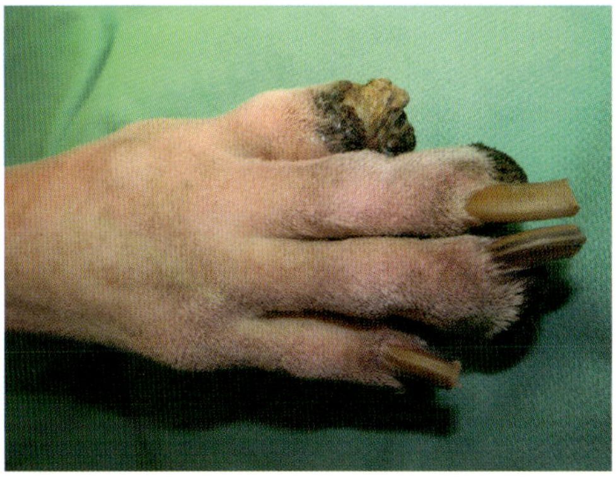

1-iv)
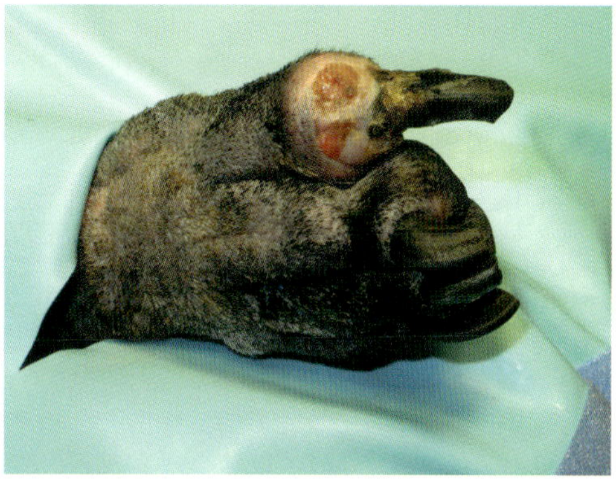

A-i)
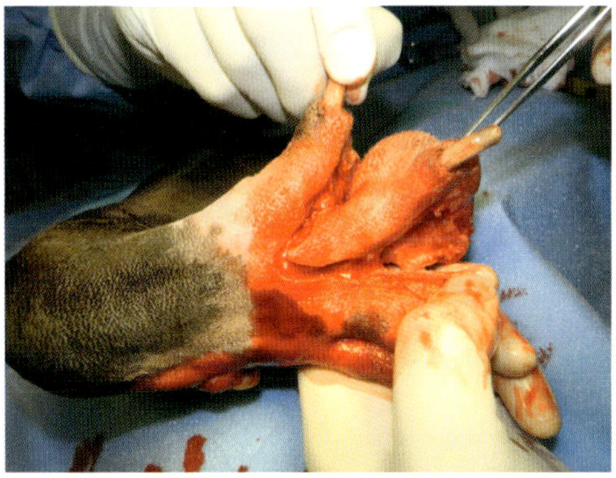

A-ii)
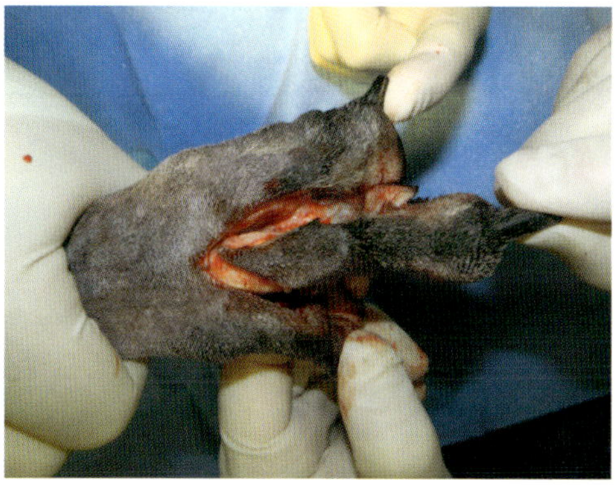

A-iii)
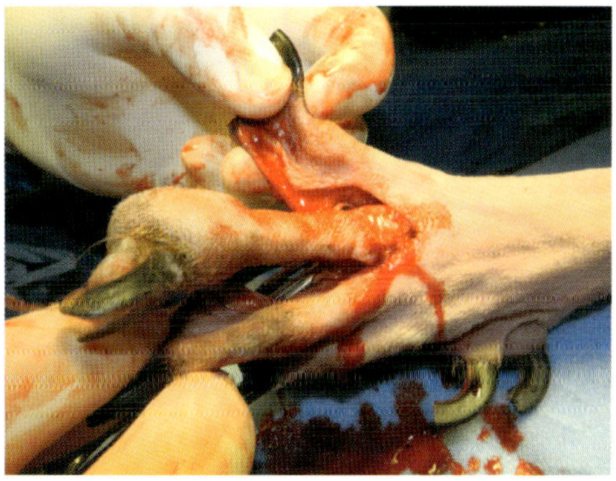

Surgical Technique (See Plate 36.1A–C, F) *continued*

B) **Alternative approach for amputation of digit II:** An incision is made over the medial aspect of digit II extending from the midmetacarpal/metatarsal bone to the metacarpophalangeal/metatarsophalangeal joint and then along the dorsal and palmar/plantar aspects of the digit around the base of the digit so that the incisions join on the lateral aspect of the digit and are continuous circumferentially (i, ii). The skin incision is then continued deeply through the subcutaneous tissue (iii).

C) **Alternative approach for amputation of digit V:** An incision is made over the lateral aspect of digit V extending from the midmetacarpal/metatarsal bone to the metacarpophalangeal/metatarsophalangeal joint and then along the dorsal and palmar/plantar aspects of the digit around the base of the digit so that the incisions join on the medial aspect of the digit and are continuous circumferentially (i, ii). The skin incision is then continued deeply through the subcutaneous tissue.

D) In the thoracic limb, the interosseous muscles and tendons of the common and lateral digital extensors and superficial and deep digital flexors are transected at the level of the planned osteotomy. The appropriate branches of the dorsal and palmar common digital and metapodial arteries and veins are cauterized or ligated and divided (not pictured).

E) In the pelvic limb, the interosseous muscles and tendons of the long and lateral digital extensors and superficial and deep digital flexor are transected at the level of the planned osteotomy. The appropriate branches of the dorsal and plantar metatarsal and common digital arteries and veins are cauterized or ligated and divided (not pictured).

F) An osteotomy of the distal aspect of the metacarpal/metatarsal bone is performed with bone cutters (i, ii). Alternatively, a pneumatic drill or oscillating or sagittal saw can be used. The amputated digit is removed from the surgical field.

Plate 36.1

Single-Digit Amputation *continued*

B-i)

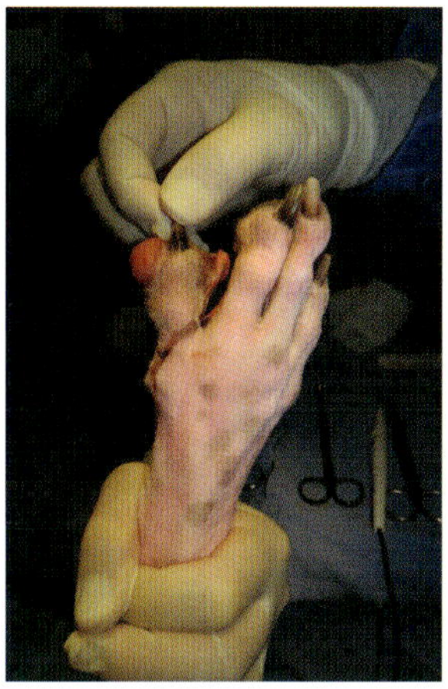

B-ii)

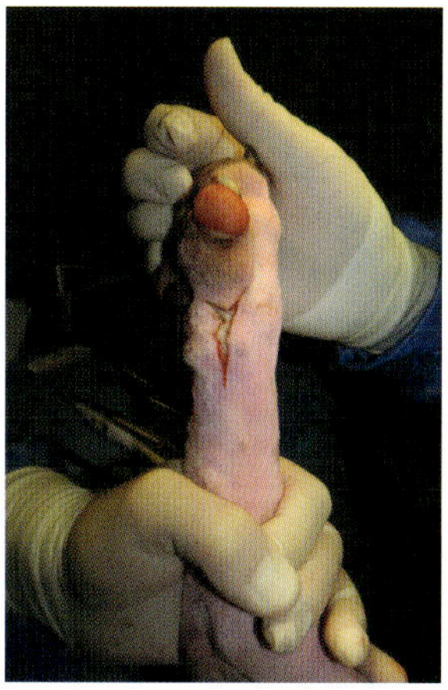

B-iii)

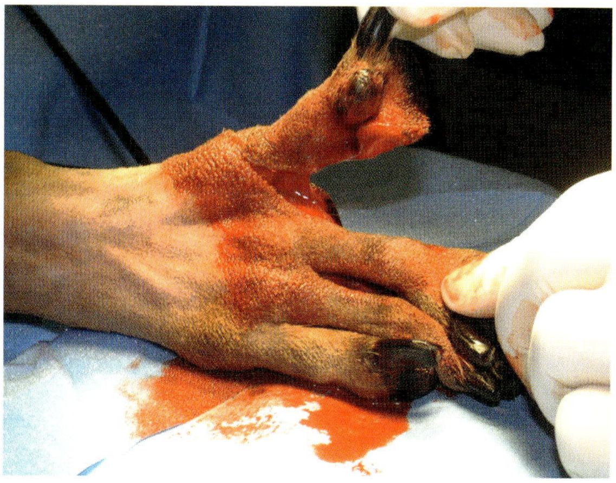

C-i)

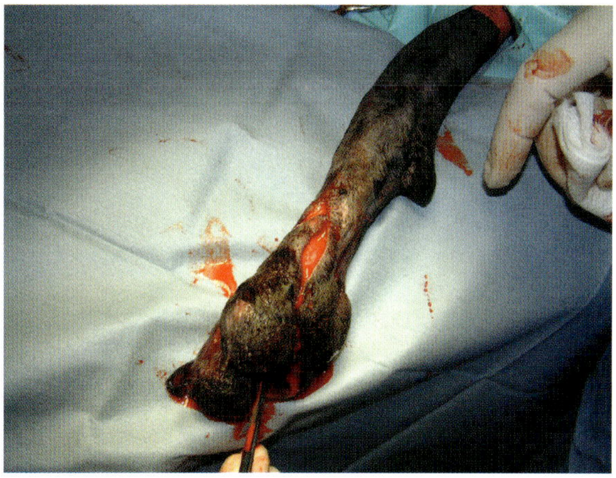

C-ii)

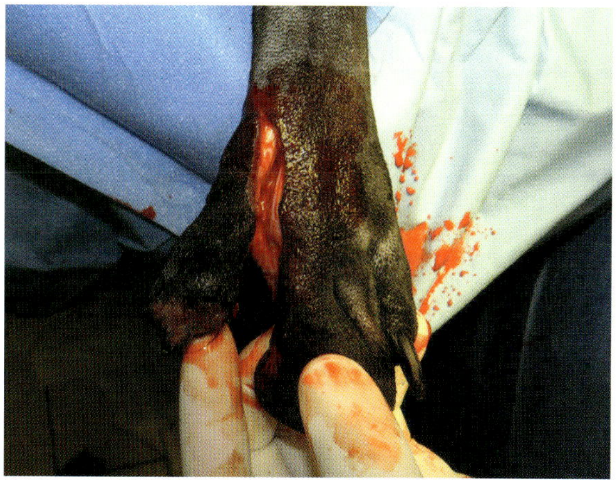

F-i)

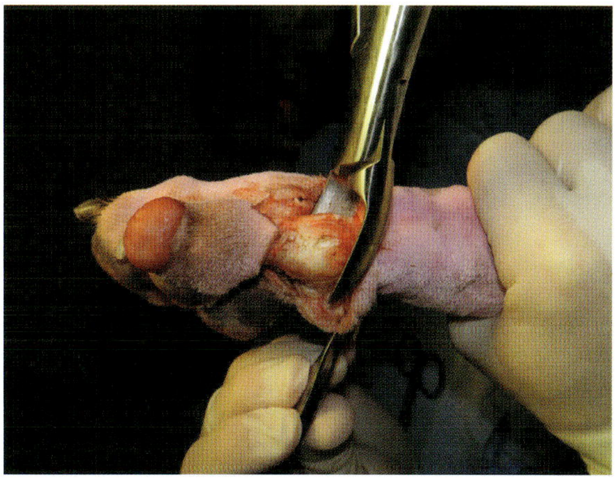

F-ii)

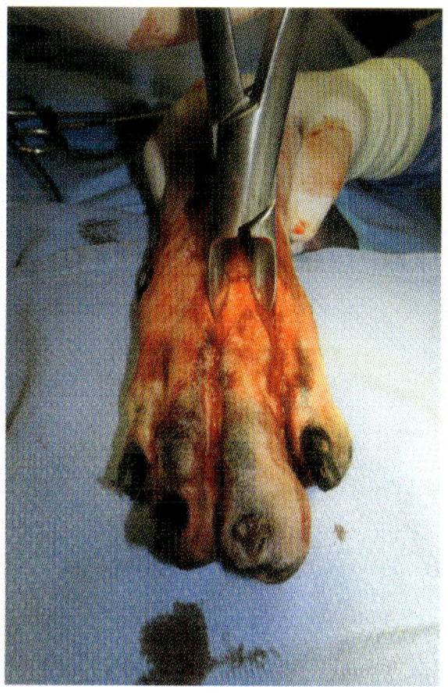

Closure (See Plate 36.1G)

G) The skin incision is closed routinely in two layers with a simple continuous suture pattern using monofilament absorbable suture material in the subcutis (i, ii) and either an interrupted or continuous suture pattern using monofilament nonabsorbable suture material in the skin (iii, iv).

Postoperative Management

1) Multimodal analgesia
2) Elizabethan collar
3) Modified Robert-Jones bandage with or without a splint
4) Exercise restriction for 14 days

Complications in Dogs [1] (See Plate 36.1H)

- Dehiscence (H) (27%)
- Surgical-site infection (H) (15%)
- Lameness >14 days postoperatively (25%), with mild or intermittent lameness in 19% and moderate to marked lameness in 6% of dogs

Suggested Adjuvant Treatments

- Melanoma vaccine for cats and dogs with subungual or digit pad melanomas
- Chemotherapy for dogs with digit osteosarcomas
- Chemotherapy for dogs with high-grade mast cell tumors

Prognosis and Oncologic Outcome

- See *36. Digit Amputation*.

Reference

1 Kaufman, K.L. and Mann, F.A. (2013). Short- and long-term outcomes after digit amputation in dogs: 33 cases (1999-2011). *J. Am. Vet. Med. Assoc.* 242 (9): 1249–1254.

Plate 36.1

Single-Digit Amputation *continued*

G-i)

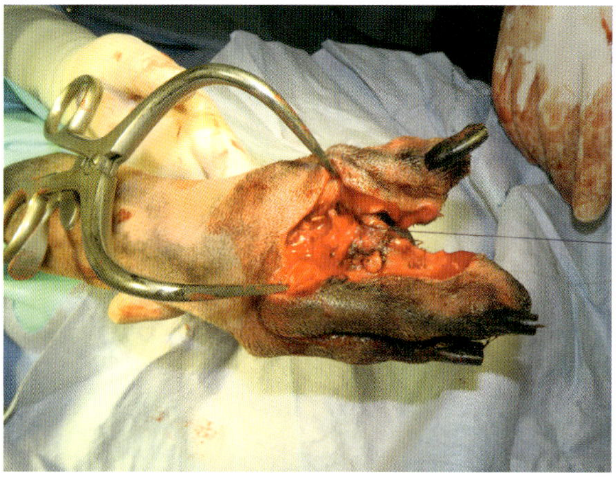

G-ii)

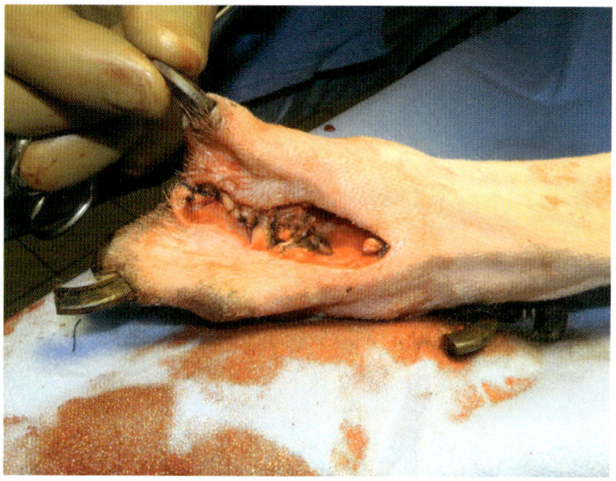

G-iii)

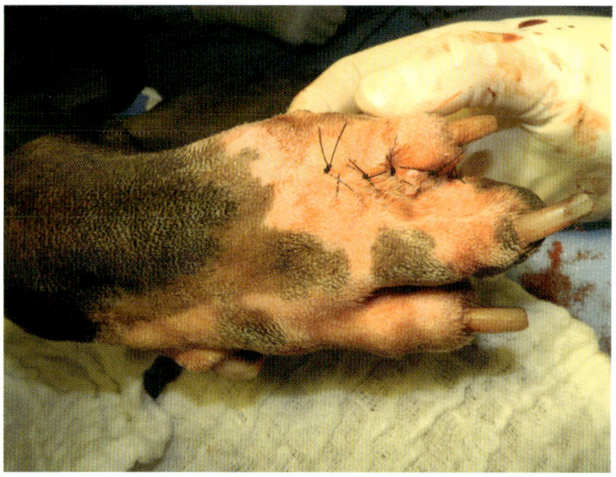

G-iv)

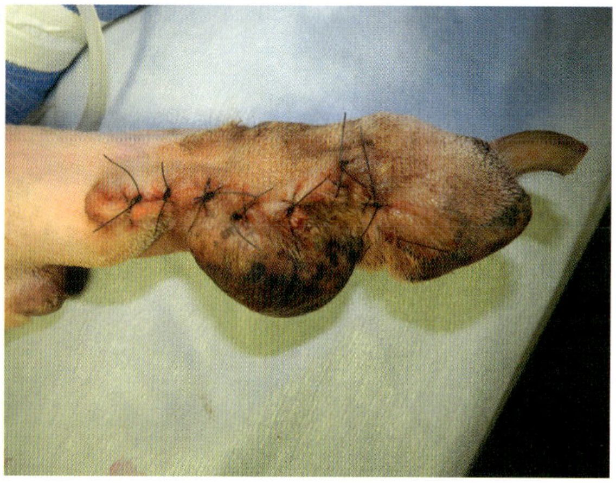

H)

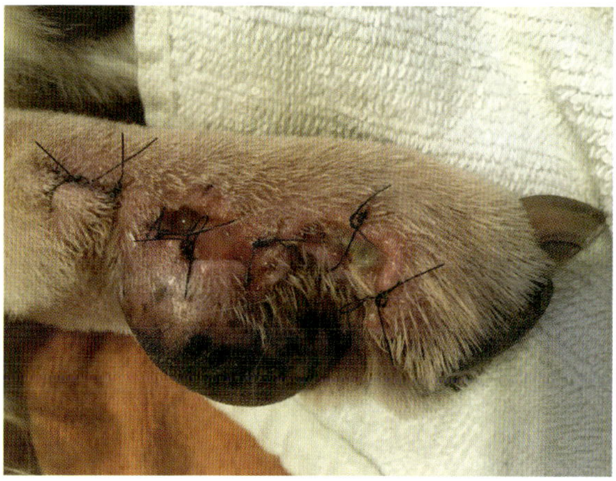

36.2 Partial Foot Amputation

Indications (See Plate 36.2 – 1)

1) Resection of benign or malignant tumors involving two adjacent digits (i, mast cell tumor), where adequate lateral margins with subsequent primary closure of the surgical wound is not possible with a single-digit amputation, or for resection of interdigital tumorssssss (ii, mast cell tumor).
2) Partial foot amputation can be combined with metacarpectomy or metatarsectomy (see *35. Metacarpectomy and Metatarsectomy*).

Suggested Diagnostic Workup and Clinical Staging

- See *36. Digit Amputation*.

Patient Positioning

The patient is positioned in dorsal recumbency.

Surgical Technique [1] (See Plate 36.2A–D)

A) An incision is made over the dorsal aspect of the paw between the two affected digits extending from the midmetacarpal/metatarsal region to the level of the metacarpophalangeal/metatarsophalangeal joints and then medially and laterally around the base of the digits (i, ii) so that the incisions join on the palmar/plantar aspect of the digit and are continuous circumferentially (iii). The skin incision is then continued deeply through the subcutaneous tissue (iv).
B) In the thoracic limb, the interosseous muscles and tendons of the common and lateral digital extensors and superficial and deep digital flexors are transected at the level of the planned osteotomy. The appropriate branches of the dorsal and palmar common digital and metapodial arteries and veins are cauterized or ligated and divided (not pictured).
C) In the pelvic limb, the interosseous muscles and tendons of the long and lateral digital extensors and superficial and deep digital flexor are transected at the level of the planned osteotomy. The appropriate branches of the dorsal and plantar metatarsal and common digital arteries and veins are cauterized or ligated and divided (not pictured).

Color Atlas of Canine and Feline Surgical Oncology, First Edition. Julius M. Liptak, Paolo Buracco, William T. N. Culp, and Nicholas J. Bacon.

Plate 36.2

Partial Foot Amputation

1-i)

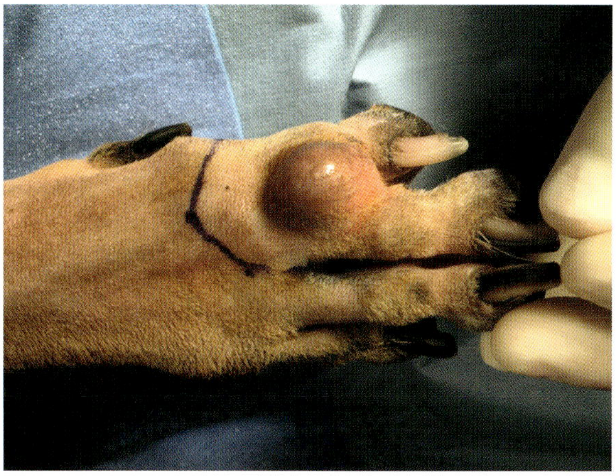

1-ii)

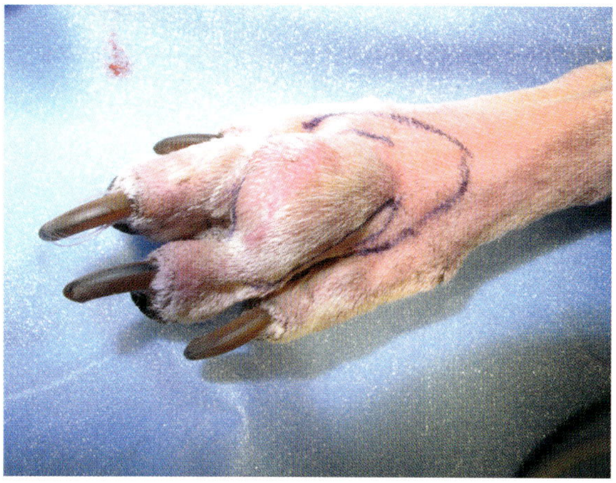

A-i)

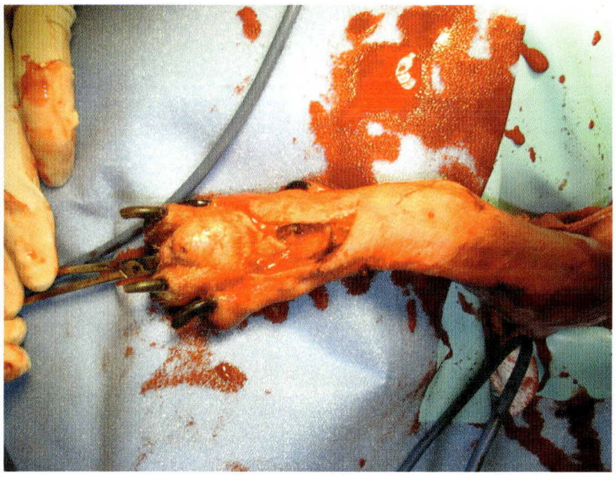

A-ii)

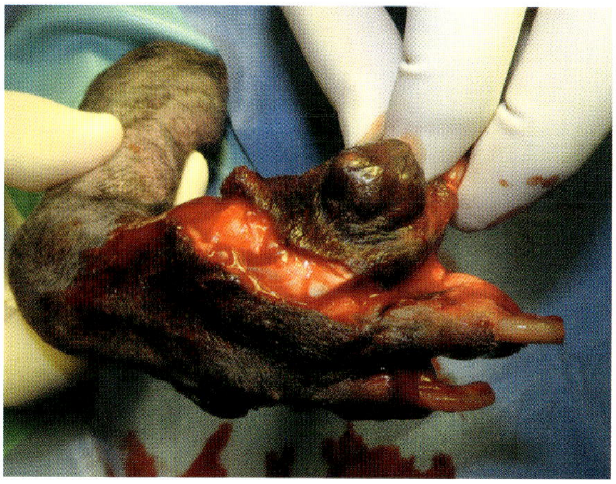

A-iii)

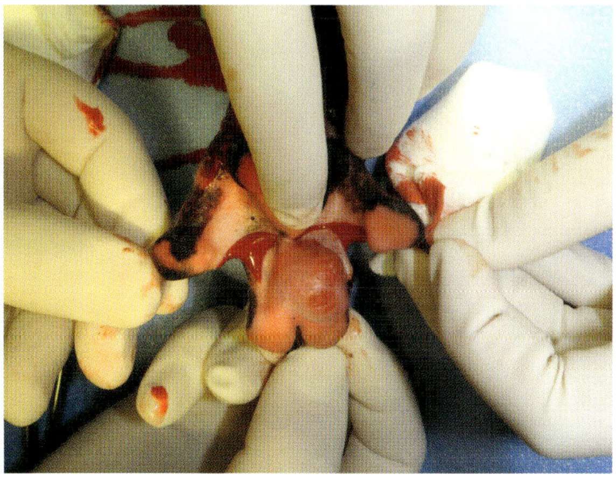

A-iv)

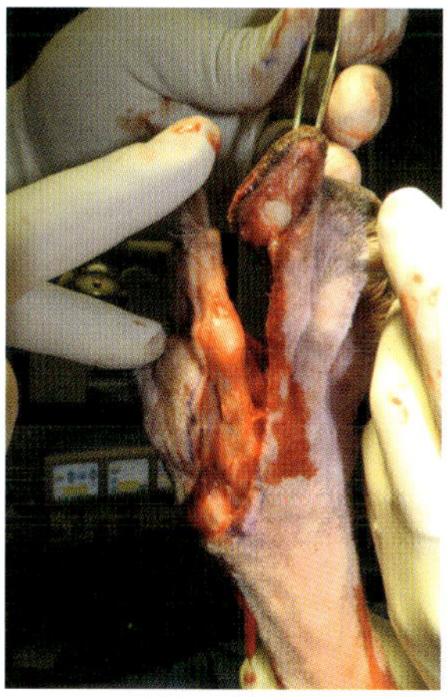

Surgical Technique [1] (See Plate 36.2A–D) *continued*

D) An osteotomy of the distal aspect of the metacarpal/metatarsal bones is performed with bone cutters (i). Alternatively, a pneumatic drill (ii) or oscillating or sagittal saw can be used. The amputated digits are removed from the surgical field (iii–v).

Closure (See Plate 36.2E)

E) The skin incision is closed routinely in two layers with a simple continuous suture pattern using monofilament absorbable suture material in the subcutis (i) and either an interrupted or continuous suture pattern using monofilament nonabsorbable suture material in the skin (ii–iv).

Postoperative Management

1) Multimodal analgesia
2) Elizabethan collar
3) Modified Robert-Jones bandage with or without a metasplint for thoracic limb partial foot amputations
4) Exercise restriction for 14 days

Complications in Dogs [1]

- Surgical-site infection (9%)
- Mild or intermittent lameness (27%)

Suggested Adjuvant Treatments

- Melanoma vaccine for cats and dogs with subungual or digit pad melanomas
- Chemotherapy for dogs with digit osteosarcomas
- Chemotherapy for dogs with high-grade mast cell tumors

Prognosis and Oncologic Outcome

- See *36. Digit Amputation*.

Reference

1 Liptak, J.M., Dernell, W.S., Rizzo, S.A. et al. (2005). Partial foot amputation in 11 dogs. *J. Am. Anim. Hosp. Assoc.* 41 (1): 47–55.

Plate 36.2

Partial Foot Amputation *continued*

D-i)

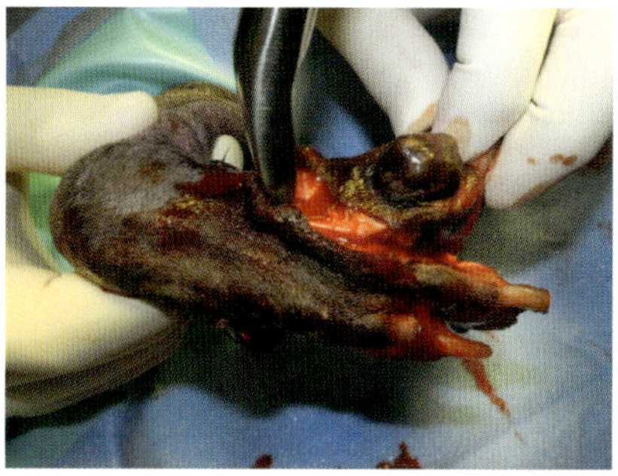

D-ii)

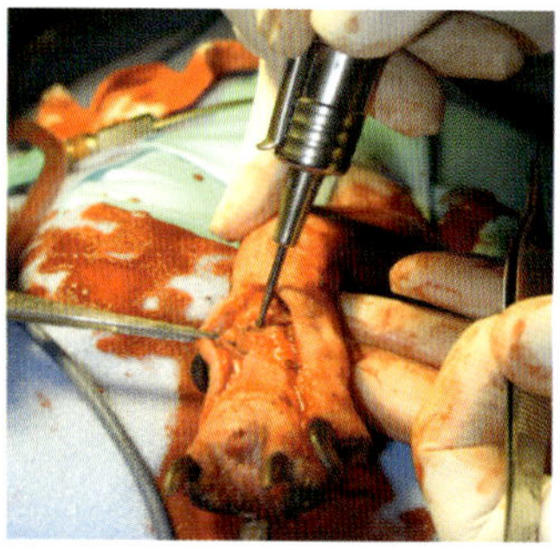

D-iii)

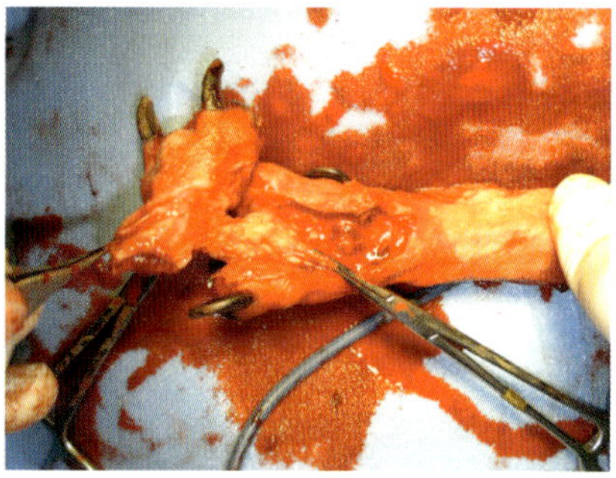

D-iv)

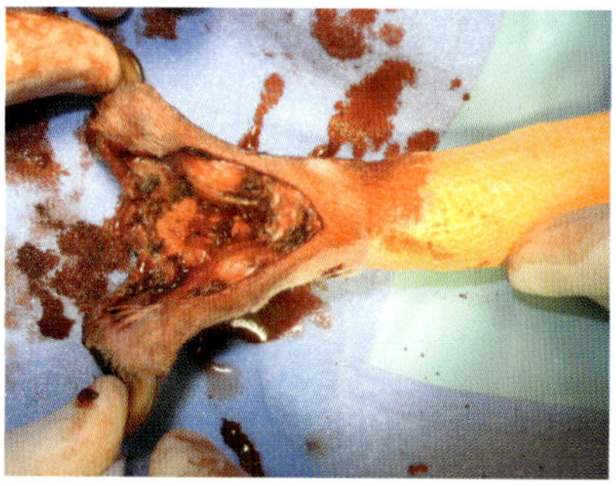

D-v)

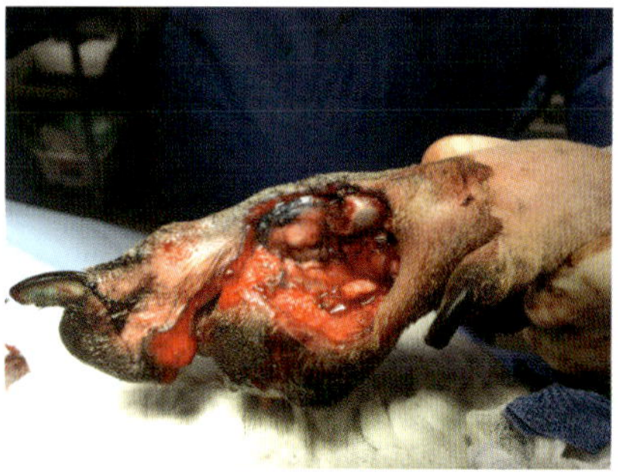

E-i)

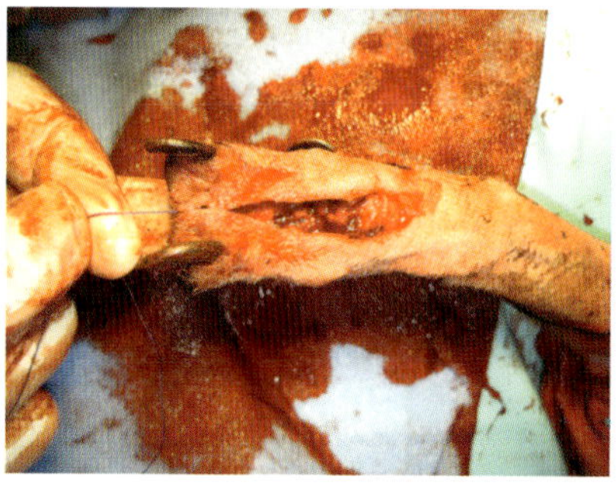

E-ii)

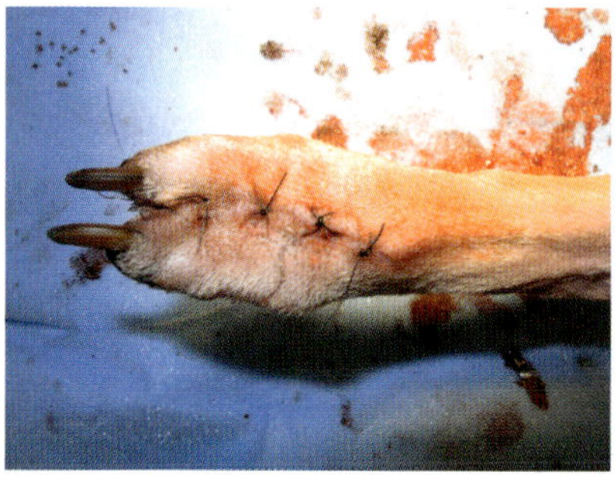

E-iii)

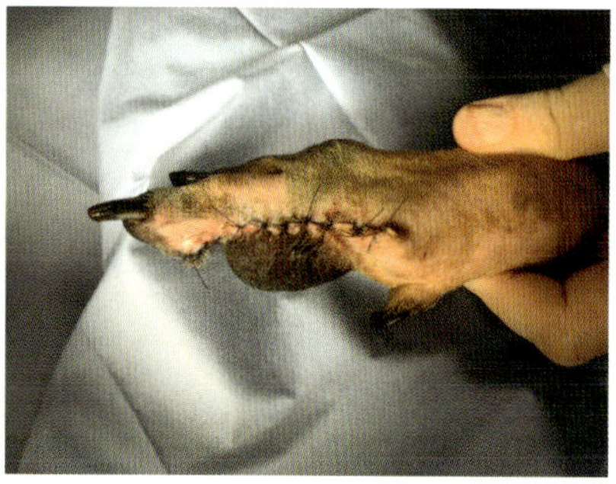

E-iv)

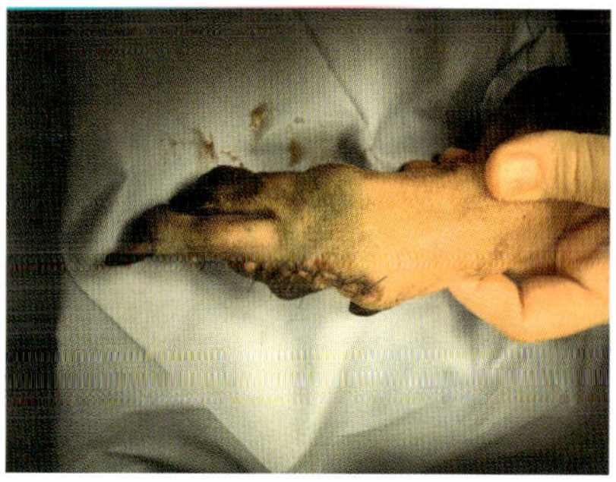

Chapter 37: Hemipelvectomy

37.1 Total Hemipelvectomy

Indications (See Plate 37.1 – 2)

1) Resection of primary malignant axial bone tumors involving the majority of the ilium, ischium, and pubis
2) Resection of extensive and infiltrative soft tissue tumors of the pelvis or vaccine-associated sarcomas in cats (computed tomography [CT] of a vaccine-associated extraskeletal osteosarcoma in a cat)

General Considerations

Total hemipelvectomy involves resection of entire hemipelvis from the sacroiliac joint to the pubic symphysis (which is the procedure described later). There are two modifications of this surgery; however, these should be performed only when the surgeon is very comfortable with the procedure, including case selection, surgical planning, operative technique, and postoperative care:

1) The authors have extended the ventral midline osteotomy into the contralateral obturator foramen (i.e. crossing midline), but very careful case selection and planning are recommended. Postoperative mobility issues should be expected in the immediate postoperative period, especially with rising from the ground.
2) The cranial osteotomy can be made through the body of the sacrum with up to one third of the lateral sacrum being resected, especially if the tumor is encroaching on the sacroiliac joint.

Suggested Diagnostic Workup and Clinical Staging

- See *33. Primary Bone and Periarticular Tumors.*
- Pelvic CT scan is highly recommended for surgical planning (see 2).

Patient Positioning

The patient is positioned in lateral recumbency with the affected limb uppermost. A urinary catheter should be placed to aid urethral identification during pelvic dissection (see step O). Depending on the size of the patient, moistened gauze swabs, moistened laparotomy sponge(s), or a syringe can be inserted into the rectum to aid identification of the rectum during pelvic dissection. A purse-string should be placed in the anus to minimize the risk of intraoperative contamination.

Color Atlas of Canine and Feline Surgical Oncology, First Edition. Julius M. Liptak, Paolo Buracco, William T. N. Culp, and Nicholas J. Bacon.

Plate 37.1

Total Hemipelvectomy

2) 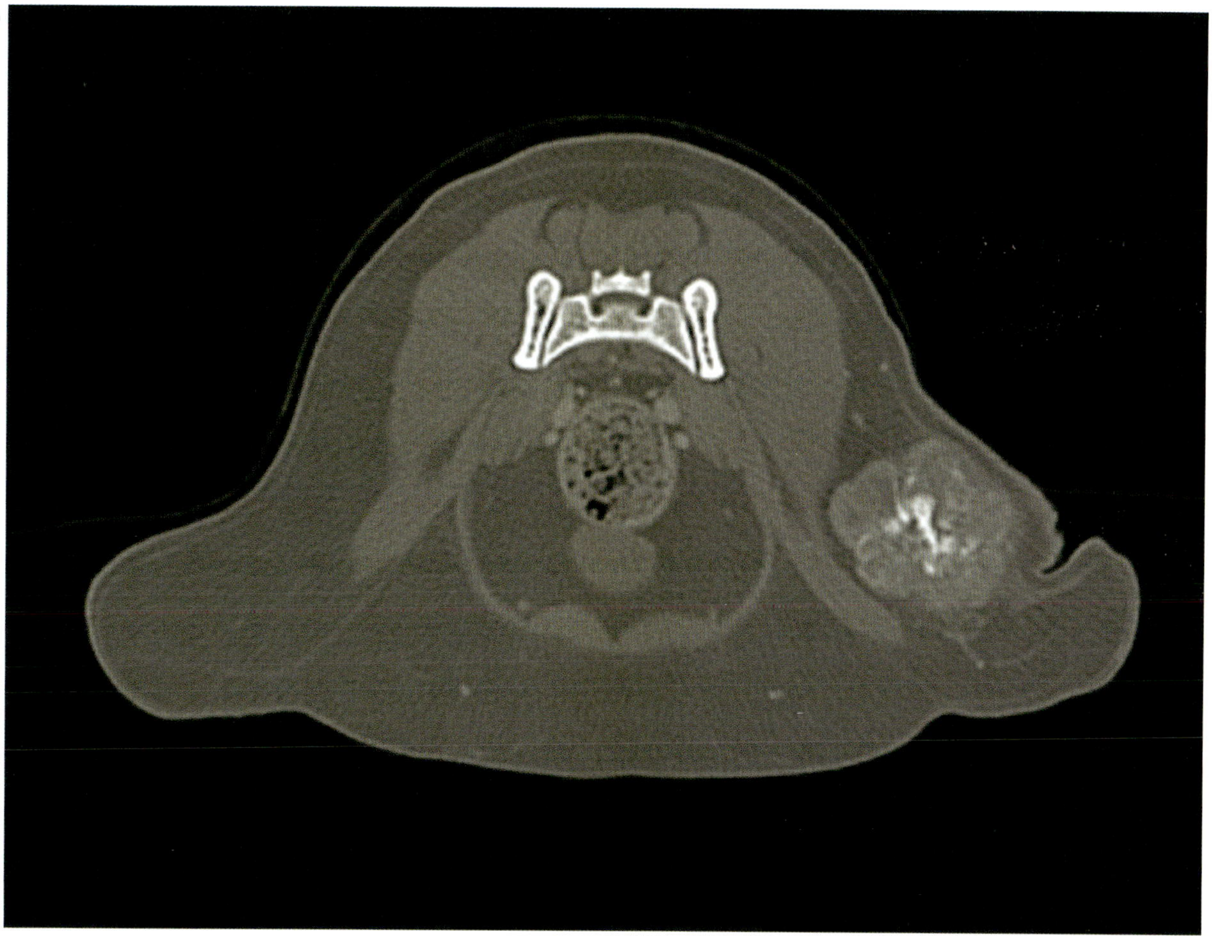

Surgical Technique – Caudal Subtotal Hemipelvectomy (See Plate 37.2A–K)

A) The skin incision is made dependent on the location of the primary tumor (i) and/or biopsy tracts (ii) but is directed as distally as possible, either laterally or medially, to ensure sufficient skin is preserved for wound closure (iii). Starting medially, the skin incision runs from the inguinal skin, curving ventrally to the midfemur and then proximally and caudally to the ischiatic tuberosity (iii).

B) During medial dissection, the goal is to preserve the sartorius muscle originating on the cranioventral ilium because this muscle is used to reconstruct the lateral pelvic wall after completion of the hemipelvectomy (i). The sartorius muscle is identified, bluntly dissected to isolate the muscle (ii), and both the cranial and the caudal bellies of the sartorius muscle are incised at their insertion at the level of the stifle (iii, iv). Penetrating vessels are ligated or sealed and transected when encountered. The sartorius muscle is then wrapped in a moist gauze swab.

C) The femoral artery and vein are located between the caudal belly of the sartorius muscle and pectineus muscle (i). The femoral artery and vein should be ligated as proximally as possible. The femoral artery is ligated with one simple ligature and one transfixion ligature of 2-0 or 3-0 absorbable monofilament suture material (ii). Distal to this, the femoral

Plate 37.2

Subtotal Hemipelvectomy *continued*

A-i)

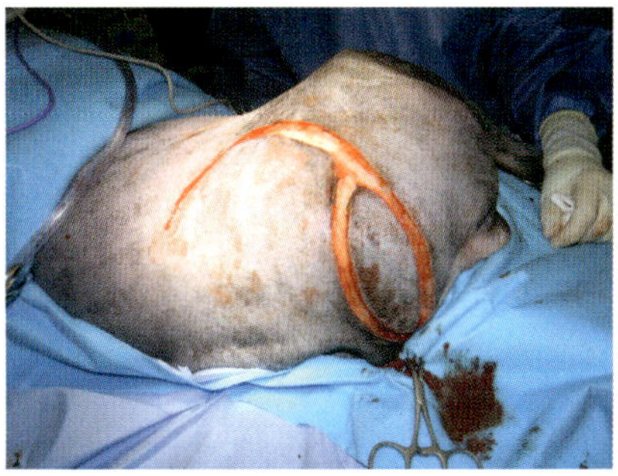

A-ii)

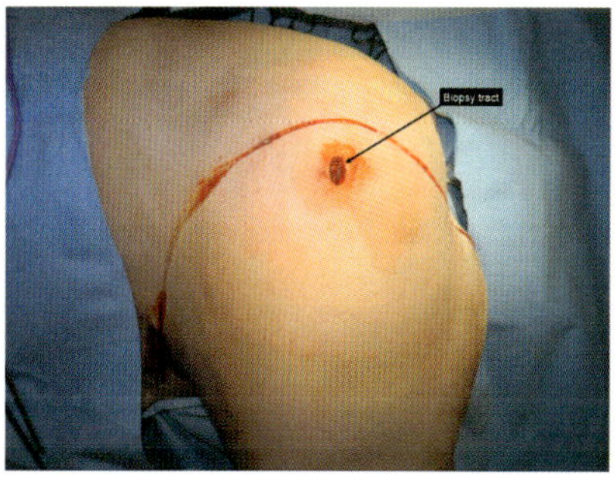

A-iii)

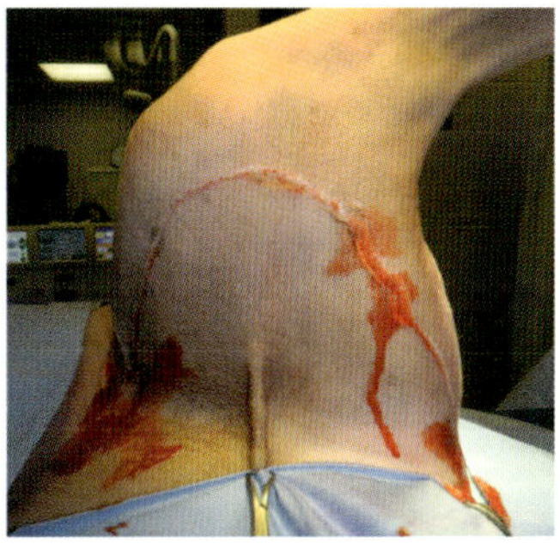

B-i)

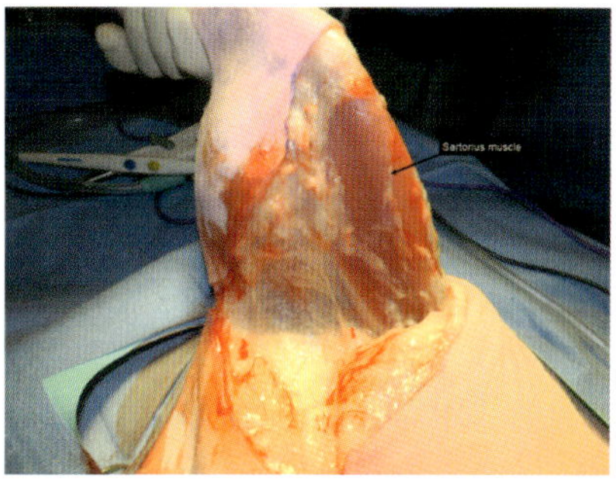

B-ii)

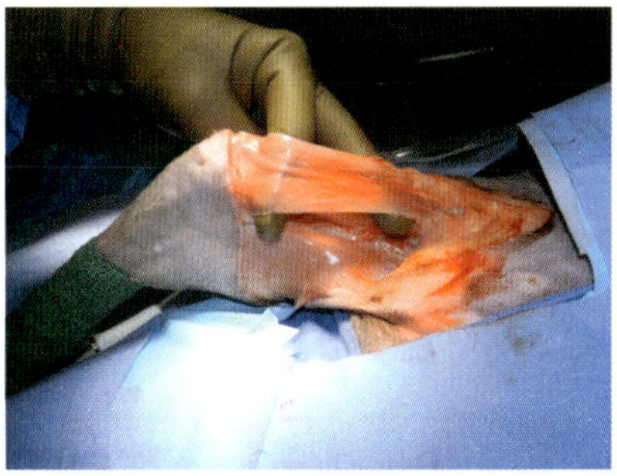

B-iii)

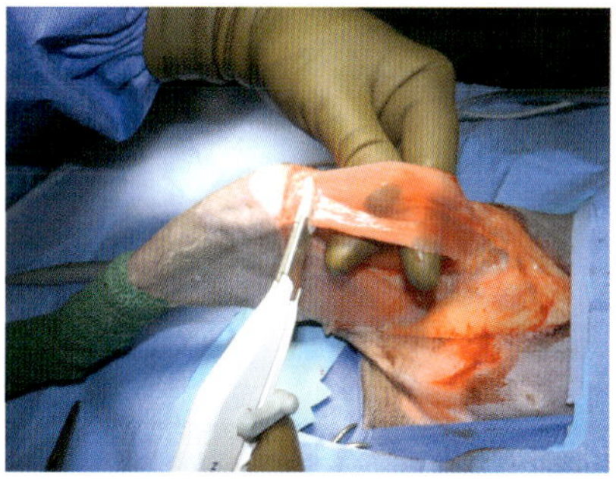

B-iv)

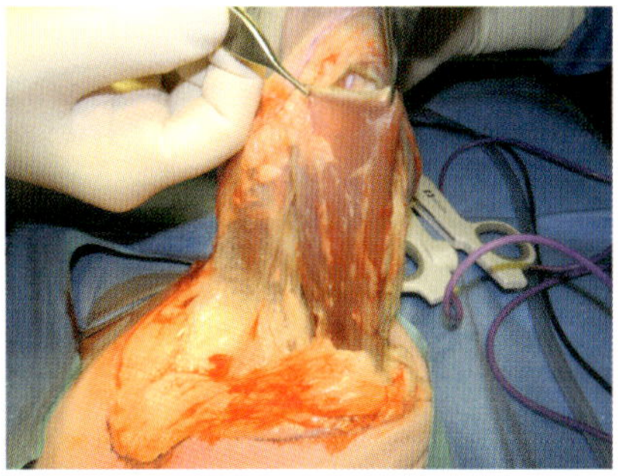

C-i)

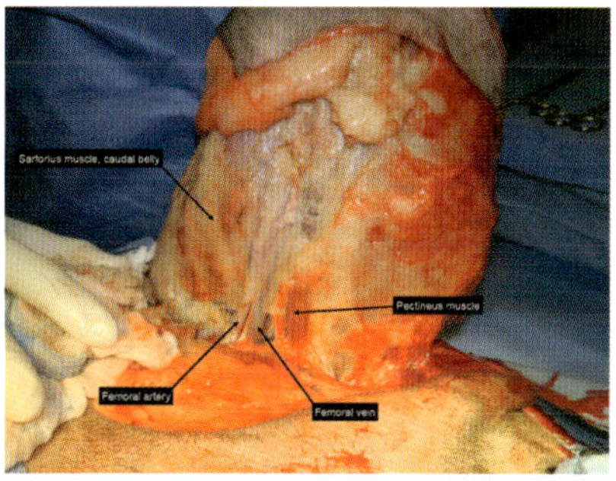

C-ii)

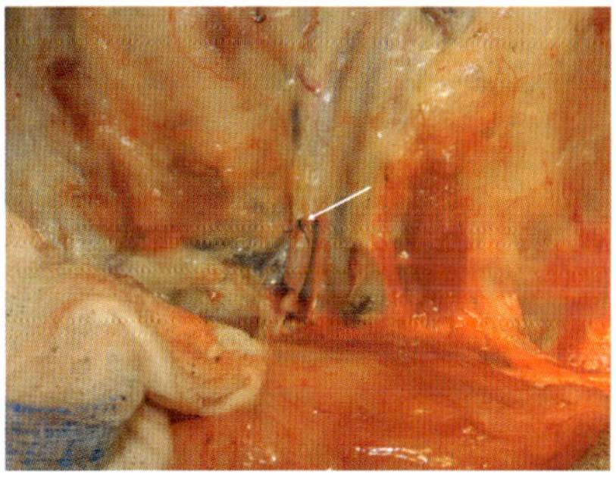

Surgical Technique – Caudal Subtotal Hemipelvectomy (See Plate 37.2A–K) *continued*

artery is then either clamped with mosquito forceps or ligated (arrow), and then the femoral artery is transected between the ligatures and clamp with a vessel sealing device (iii) or Metzenbaum scissors. The femoral vein is ligated with two simple ligatures of 2-0 or 3-0 absorbable monofilament suture material (iv). Distal to this, the femoral vein closest is then either clamped with mosquito forceps or ligated (arrow), and then the femoral vein is transected between the ligatures and clamp with a vessel sealing device (v) or Metzenbaum scissors. In smaller animals, a vessel sealing device alone can be used to seal and transect the femoral artery and vein. Small inguinal vessels may also be encountered during this dissection, and these should be ligated or sealed, and transected.

D) Medially, the subcutaneous tissues are dissected to expose the ventral midline, which is identified by a thin fascial aponeurosis between converging muscle bellies, and the pubic and ischial bones (i). If the osteotomy is to be along the symphysis, the attachments of the adductor, gracilis, and pectineus muscles are incised (ii) and gently elevated off the ridged pubic midline with a periosteal elevator (iii) or electrosurgery. These are then reflected laterally to expose the entire length of the pubic bone. The muscles on the contralateral aspect of the pubis should not be disturbed.

E) The muscular attachments of the caudal body wall are incised as they insert on the pubic brim (tumor side, from midline laterally), typically subperiosteally with electrosurgery or with a vessel sealing device (pictured). These are then allowed to retract cranially.

F) Now that the cranial pubic brim is exposed, a periosteal elevator, malleable retractor (i), or the long arm of an Army-Navy retractor should be gently rotated under the symphysis within the floor of the pelvic canal staying as close to the bone as possible. At the caudal end of the pubis, any soft tissues should be dissected off the end of the elevator or retractor. A pubic symphysiotomy is performed with a ventrally directed oscillating (pictured) or sagittal saw while protecting the structures of the pelvic canal with the elevator or retractor (i, ii).

Plate 37.2

Subtotal Hemipelvectomy *continued*

C-iii)

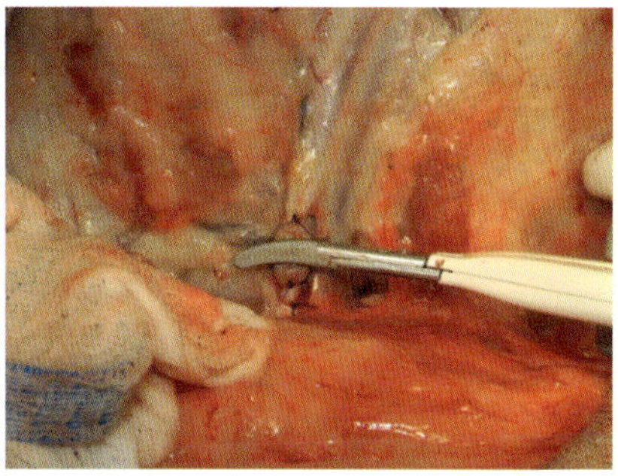

C-iv)

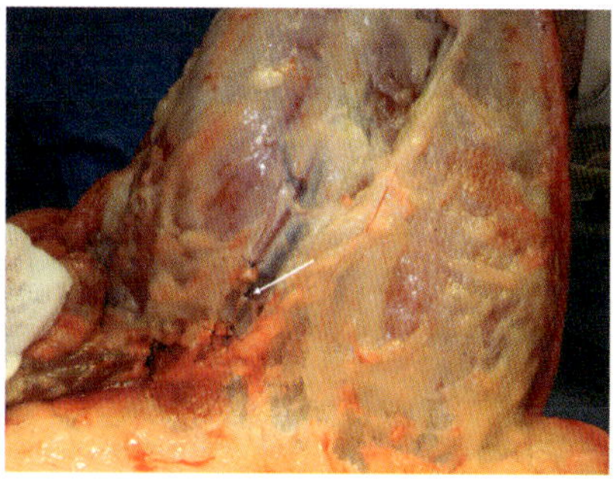

C-v)

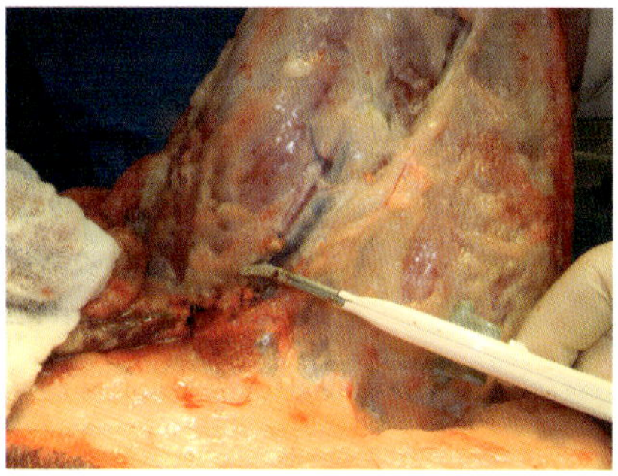

D-i)

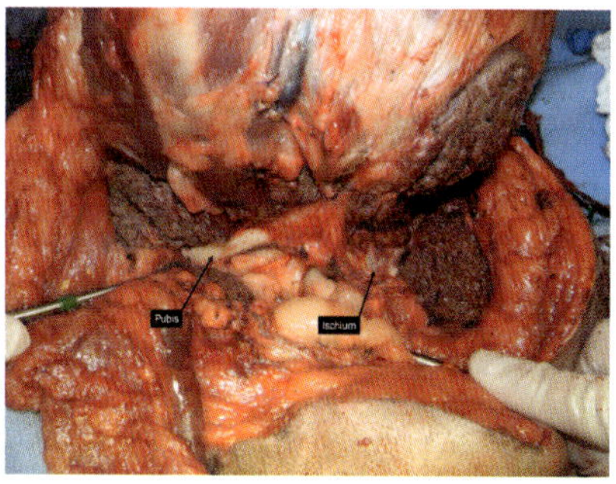

D-ii)

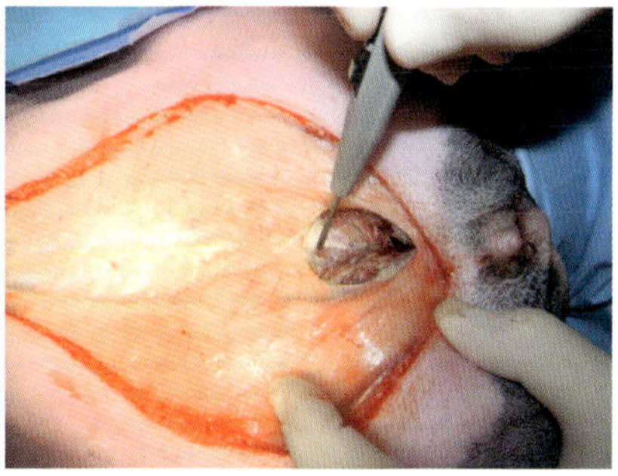

D-iii)

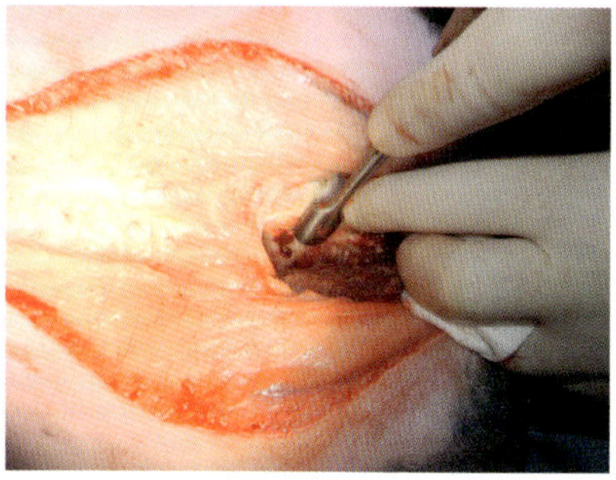

E)

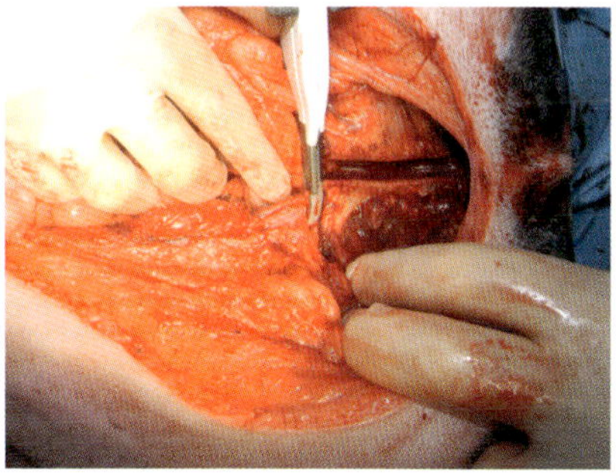

F-i)

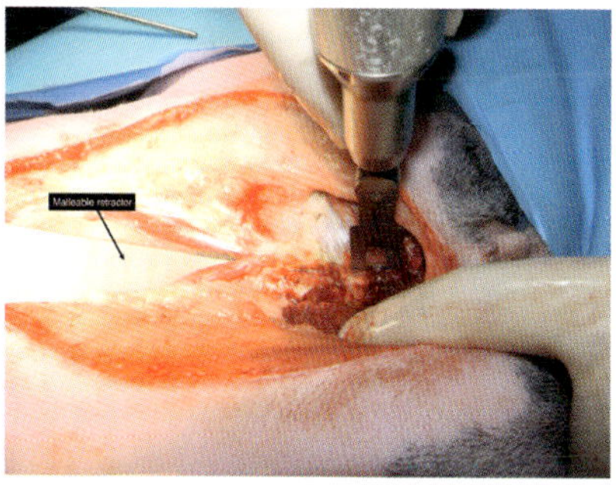

F-ii)

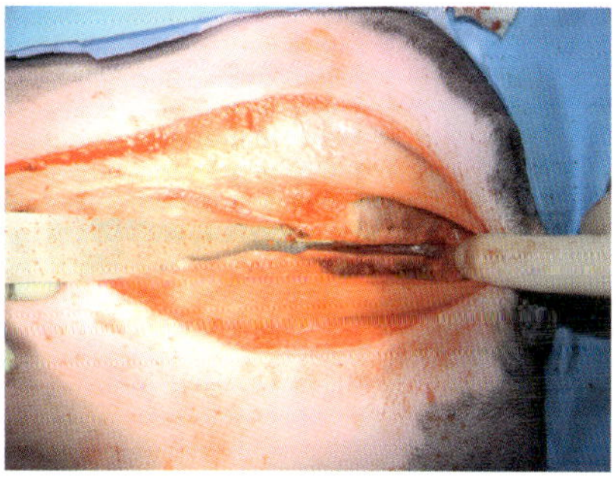

Surgical Technique – Caudal Subtotal Hemipelvectomy (See Plate 37.2A–K) *continued*

G) Paramedian pubic and ischial osteotomies are an alternative to a pubic symphysiotomy, and this retains some of the origins of the adductor and gracilis muscles. The muscles should be incised as distally as possible toward their insertion to aid in reconstruction. A periosteal elevator (i) or the long arm of an Army-Navy retractor should be gently rotated under the pubis within the floor of the pelvic canal staying as close to the bone as possible. A pubic osteotomy is performed with an oscillating or sagittal saw (ii) while protecting the structures of the pelvic canal with an elevator (iii) or retractor.

H) Moving to the lateral aspect of the limb, the lateral skin incision starts at the flank, curving ventrally to the midfemur and then proximally and caudally to the ischium (i). The skin of the proximal and lateral thigh is tightly adhered to the underlying tensor fascia lata muscle and needs to be bluntly dissected from the tensor fascia lata muscle to the level of the greater trochanter (ii).

I) Laterally, an incision is made through the middle and deep gluteal muscles to the level of the ilial body to create a soft tissue corridor (i). A retractor is passed around the medial aspect of the ilial body to protect the pelvic contents, and then an ilial osteotomy is performed with an oscillating or sagittal saw (ii, iii).

Plate 37.2

Subtotal Hemipelvectomy *continued*

G-i)

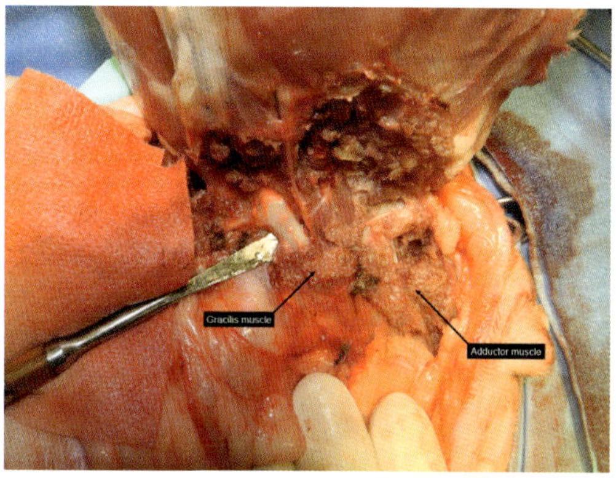

G-ii)

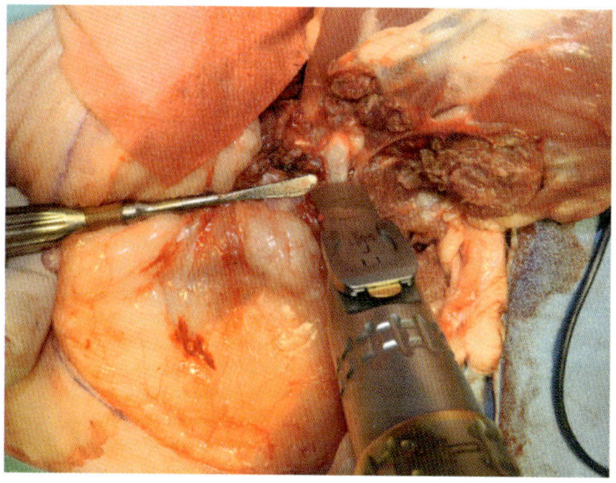

G-iii)

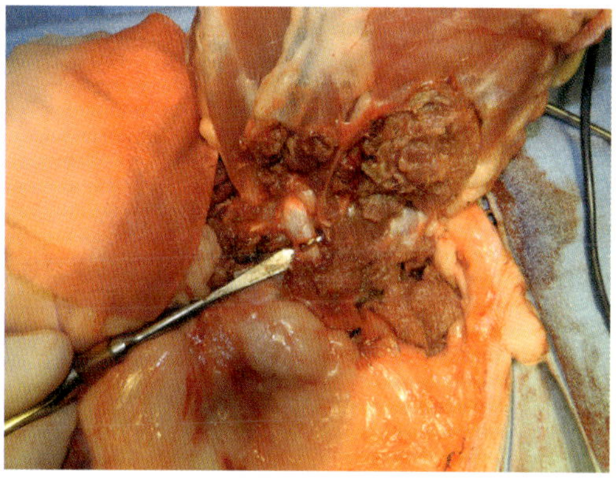

H-i)

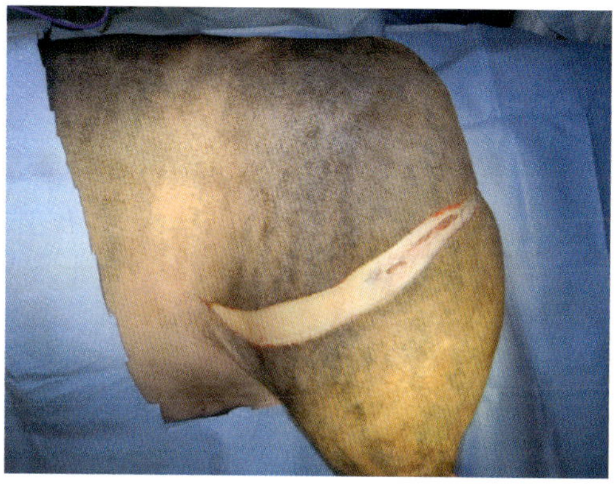

H-ii)

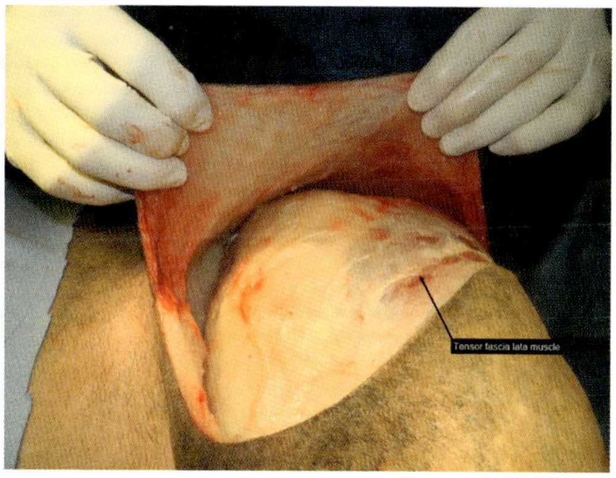

I-i)

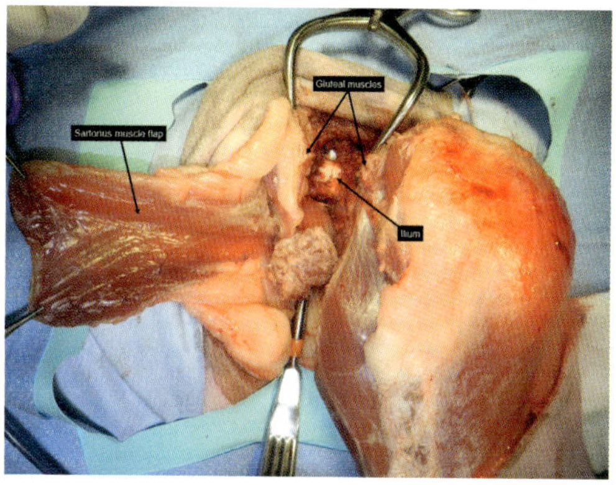

I-ii)

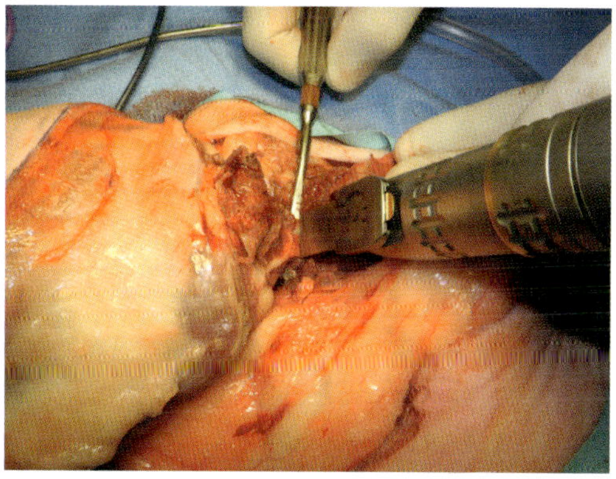

I-iii)

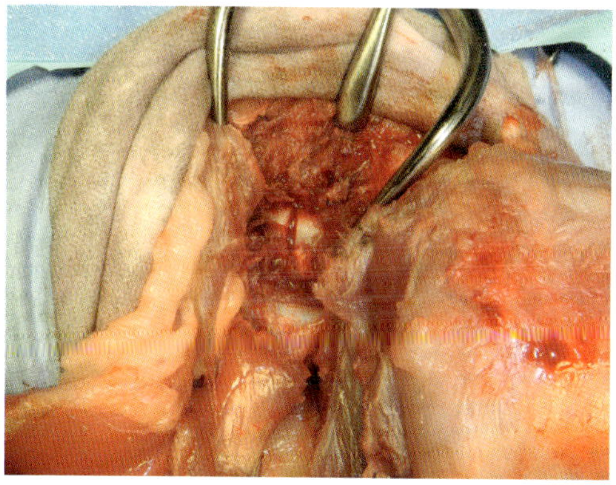

Surgical Technique – Caudal Subtotal Hemipelvectomy (See Plate 37.2A–K) *continued*

J) Muscle dissection continues caudally around the ischium, between the semitendinosus and ischiocavernosus muscles and medial to the sacrotuberous ligament. The muscles of the pelvic diaphragm can normally be left intact medially. An ischial osteotomy can be performed from either a medial or lateral approach. From a medial approach, a retractor is passed around the lateral aspect of the caudal ilial body (i) to protect the pelvic contents, and then an ilial osteotomy is performed with an oscillating or sagittal saw (ii, iii).

K) The limb is now elevated away from the patient to identify any remaining medial soft tissue attachments, which are incised if present. The lumbosacral plexus nerves must be identified, infiltrated with local anesthetic, and then transected with a scalpel blade or scissors after a minimum of 1 minute for the local anesthetic to adequately infiltrate the nerve.

Closure (See Plate 37.2L, M)

L) For closure after a caudal subtotal hemipelvectomy, the sartorius muscle flap (i) is transposed caudally (ii) and sutured in position to the abdominal muscles, pelvic diaphragm (caudally), and adductor muscles (medially) with 0 to 3-0 absorbable monofilament suture material in a cruciate or simple continuous pattern (iii).

M) The subcutaneous tissue and skin are closed routinely. The use of an active suction drain may be required.

Postoperative Management

1) Multimodal analgesia; this may include an epidural catheter and/or wound soaker catheter (see step M)
2) Elizabethan collar or body suit
3) Sling support if necessary
4) A urinary catheter should be left in situ for up to 48 hours to minimize the need to move the patient in the immediate postoperative period

Complications

- Wound infection (up to 50%) [1, 2]
- Urinary retention (5%) [3]
- Hemorrhage and hematoma formation [1]
- Incisional dehiscence (1%) [1, 3]
- Hernia formation (1%) [1, 3]
- Seroma formation [1]
- Decubital ulcer formation [1]
- Urethral and rectal trauma [1]
- Corneal ulceration (2%) [1]
- Aspiration pneumonia (1%) [3]

Suggested Adjuvant Treatments

- See *33. Primary Bone and Periarticular Tumors.*

Prognosis and Oncologic Outcome

- See *37.1. Total Hemipelvectomy.*

Plate 37.2

Subtotal Hemipelvectomy *continued*

J-i)

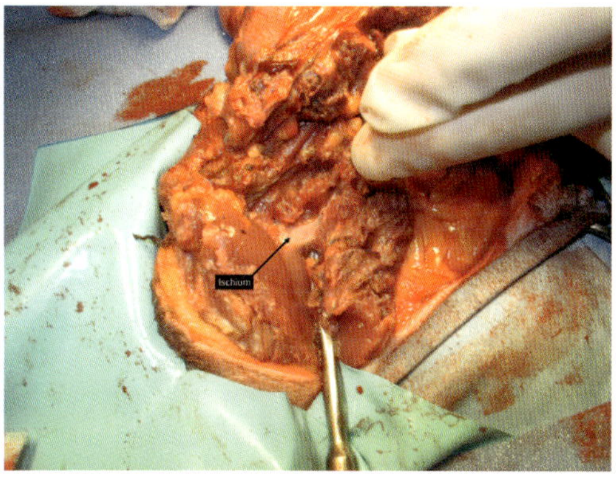

J-ii)

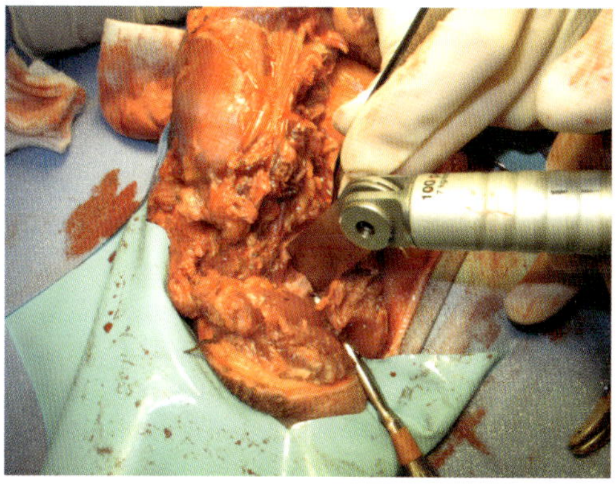

J-iii)

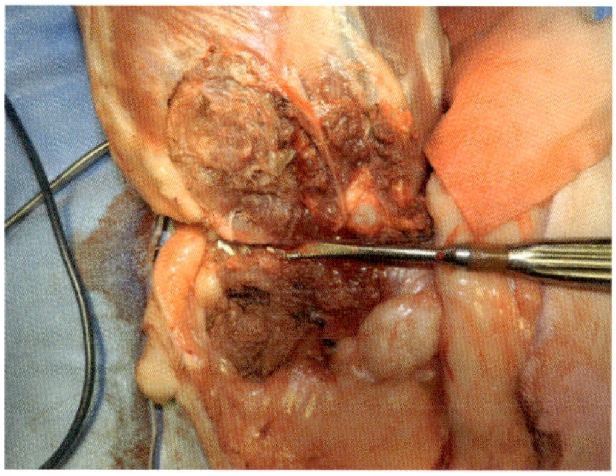

K)

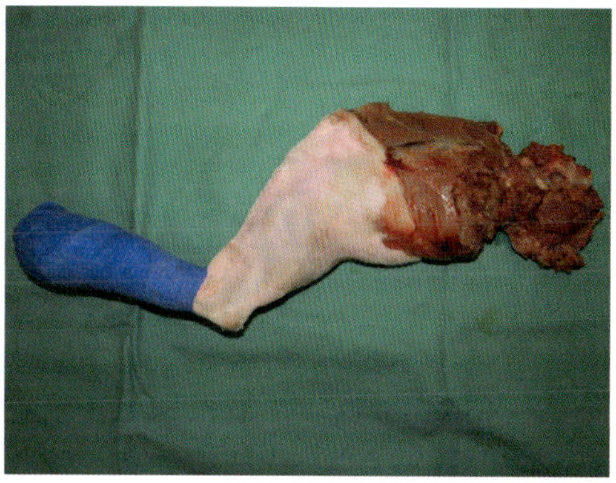

L-i)

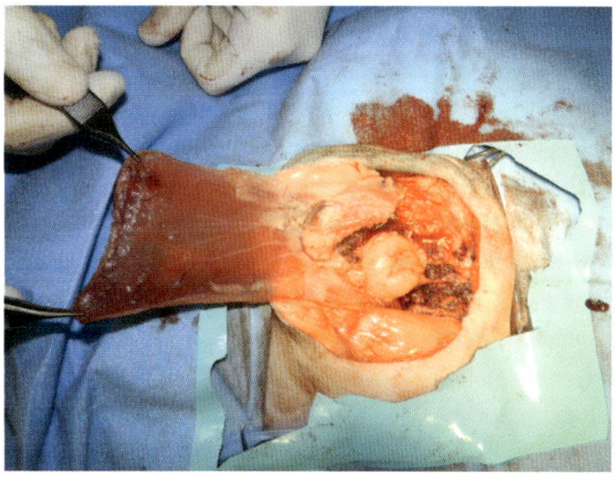

L-ii)

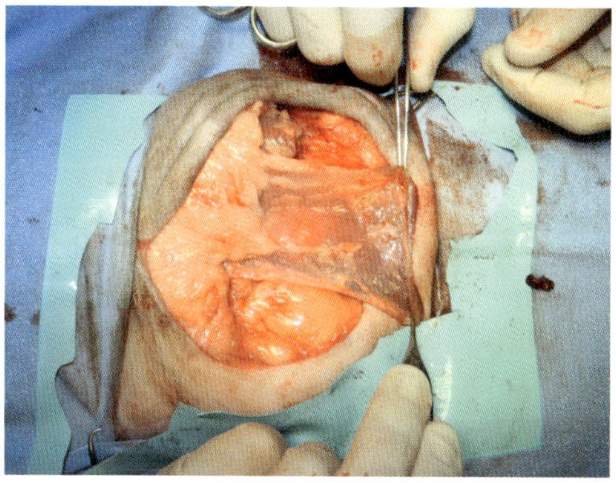

L-iii)

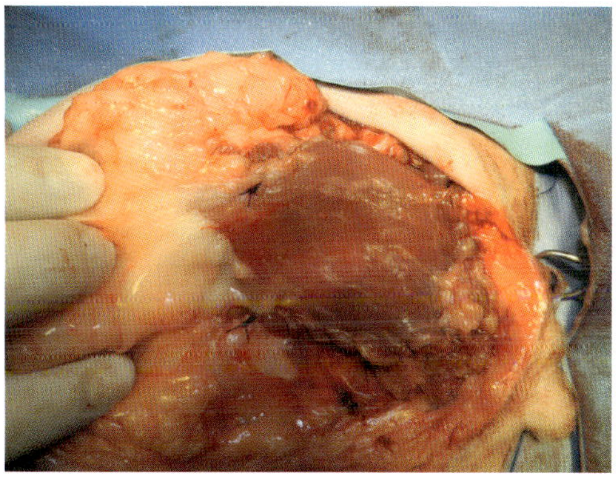

M)

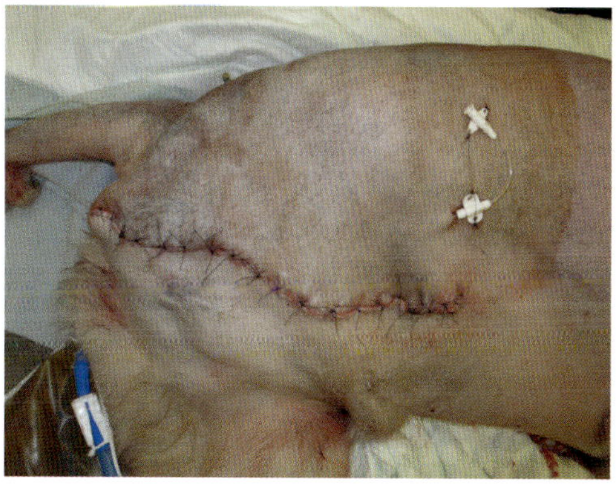

Cranial Subtotal Hemipelvectomy

A description for cranial subtotal hemipelvectomy is included in the following section; however, this is not accompanied with step-by-step images.

Surgical Technique – Cranial Subtotal Hemipelvectomy

N) The skin incision is made dependent on the location of the primary tumor but is directed as distally as possible, either laterally or medially, to ensure sufficient skin is preserved for wound closure. Starting medially, the skin incision runs from the inguinal skin, curving ventrally to the midfemur, and then proximally and caudally to the ischiatic tuberosity.

O) Medially, the subcutaneous tissues are dissected to expose the ventral midline, which is identified by a thin fascial aponeurosis between converging muscle bellies. These muscles should be transected with a vessel sealing device or electrosurgery close to the medial aspect of the acetabulum and then reflected medially to expose the ramus of the pubis. A curved retractor, such as an Army-Navy retractor, is passed around the pubic ramus to protect the pelvic contents, and an osteotomy of the midpubic ramus is performed with an oscillating or sagittal saw.

P) The muscular attachments of the caudal body wall are incised as they insert on the pubic brim (tumor side, from midline laterally), typically subperiosteally with electrosurgery. These are then allowed to retract cranially.

Q) The dissection is continued laterally, elevating the sartorius and gluteal muscles from the iliac wing until the wing of the ilium is visible.

R) This caudolateral abdominal access allows for the femoral artery and vein to be followed toward the external iliac artery and vein. The femoral artery is ligated with one simple ligature and one transfixion ligature of 2-0 or 3-0 absorbable monofilament suture material. Distal to this, the femoral artery is then either clamped with mosquito forceps or ligated, and then the femoral artery is transected between the ligatures and clamp with a vessel sealing device or Metzenbaum scissors. The femoral vein is ligated with two simple ligatures of 2-0 or 3-0 absorbable monofilament suture material. Distal to this, the femoral vein closest is then either clamped with mosquito forceps or ligated, and then the femoral vein is transected between the ligatures and clamp with a vessel sealing device or Metzenbaum scissors. In smaller animals, a vessel sealing device alone can be used to seal and transect the femoral artery and vein. Small inguinal vessels may also be encountered during this dissection, and these should be ligated or sealed, and transected.

S) Moving onto the lateral aspect, the lateral skin incision is made connecting the previous cranial and caudal point in a curvilinear fashion to mid-thigh (if possible, depending on the primary tumor). The skin should be undermined and elevated dorsally toward the lumbar fascia.

T) The muscular dissection is continued caudal to the greater trochanter of the femur and in a dorsal-to-ventral direction, including the superficial gluteal and biceps femoris muscles, staying lateral to the sacrotuberous ligament to expose the ischiatic spine. All soft tissue attachments are freed with a periosteal elevator. A curved retractor, such as an Army-Navy retractor, is passed around the exposed ischium to protect the pelvic canal structures and tissues medially, and then the ischial osteotomy is performed with an oscillating or sagittal saw.

U) The medial aspect of the ilial wing is identified and freed of all soft tissue attachments. A sacroiliac disarticulation is then performed, typically with a broad osteotome and mallet. This is best done in a dorsal-to-ventral direction, taking care to angle the strike ventrally and dorsally to account for the trapezoid shape of the canine sacrum.

V) As much of the caudal musculature as possible is preserved to aid in reconstruction of the lateral pelvic wall, especially the semimembranosus and semitendinosus muscles, which are transected as far distally toward their insertions as possible.

W) The limb is now elevated away from the patient to identify any remaining medial soft tissue attachments, which are incised if present. The lumbosacral plexus nerves must be identified, infiltrated with local anesthetic, and then transected with a scalpel blade or scissors after a minimum of 1 minute for the local anesthetic to adequately infiltrate the nerve.

X) For closure after a cranial subtotal hemipelvectomy, the semitendinosus and semimembranosus muscles are transposed cranially to cover the pelvic defect and are anchored to the adductors (medially), the abdominal muscles (cranially), and remaining soft tissue dorsally with 0 to 3-0 absorbable monofilament suture material in a cruciate or simple continuous pattern.

References

1 Kramer, A., Walsh, P.J., and Seguin, B. (2008). Hemipelvectomy in dogs and cats: technique overview, variations and description. *Vet. Surg.* 37: 413–419.

2 Barbur, L.A., Coleman, K.D., Schmeidt, C.W. et al. (2015). Description of the anatomy, surgical technique, and outcome of hemipelvectomy in 4 dogs and 5 cats. *Vet. Surg.* 44: 613–626.

3 Bray, J.P., Worley, D.R., Boston, S.E. et al. (2014). Hemipelvectomy: outcome in 84 dogs and 16 cats. A veterinary society oncology retrospective study. *Vet. Surg.* 43: 27–37.

37.3 Acetabulectomy

Indications

1) Resection of primary malignant bone tumors involving the femoral head or the coxofemoral joint
2) Resection of soft tissue tumors affecting the periarticular tissues of the coxofemoral joint

Suggested Diagnostic Workup and Clinical Staging

- See *33. Primary Bone and Periarticular Tumors.*
- Pelvic computed tomography scan is highly recommended for surgical planning.

Patient Positioning

The patient is positioned in lateral recumbency with the affected limb uppermost. A urinary catheter should be placed to aid urethral identification during pelvic dissection. Depending on the size of the patient, moistened gauze swabs, moistened laparotomy sponge(s), or a syringe can be inserted into the rectum to aid identification of the rectum during pelvic dissection. A purse-string should be placed in the anus to minimize the risk of intraoperative contamination.

Surgical Technique (See Plate 37.3A–J)

A) The lateral skin incision starts at the flank, curving ventrally to the midfemur and then proximally and caudally to the ischium.
B) The medial skin incision joins the cranial and caudal ends with a flatter curve to a level halfway between midfemur and the proximal medial thigh, ensuring there is more skin on the lateral than medial aspect of the pelvic limb.
C) Dissection starts medially by ligating the femoral artery and vein. The femoral artery and vein are located between the caudal belly of the sartorius muscle and pectineus muscle (i). The femoral artery and vein should be ligated as proximally as possible. The femoral artery is ligated with one simple ligature and one transfixion ligature of 2-0 or 3-0 absorbable monofilament suture material (ii). Distal to this, the femoral artery is then either clamped with mosquito forceps or ligated (arrow), and then the femoral artery is transected between the ligatures and clamp with a vessel sealing device (iii) or Metzenbaum scissors. The femoral vein is ligated with two simple ligatures of 2-0 or 3-0 absorbable monofilament suture material (iv). Distal to this, the femoral vein closest is then either clamped with mosquito forceps or ligated (arrow), and then the femoral vein is transected between the ligatures and clamp with a vessel sealing device (v, vi) or Metzenbaum scissors. In smaller animals, a vessel sealing device alone can be used to seal and transect the femoral artery and vein. Small inguinal vessels may also be encountered during this dissection, and these should be ligated or sealed, and transected.

Color Atlas of Canine and Feline Surgical Oncology, First Edition. Julius M. Liptak, Paolo Buracco, William T. N. Culp, and Nicholas J. Bacon.

Plate 37.3

Acetabulectomy

A)

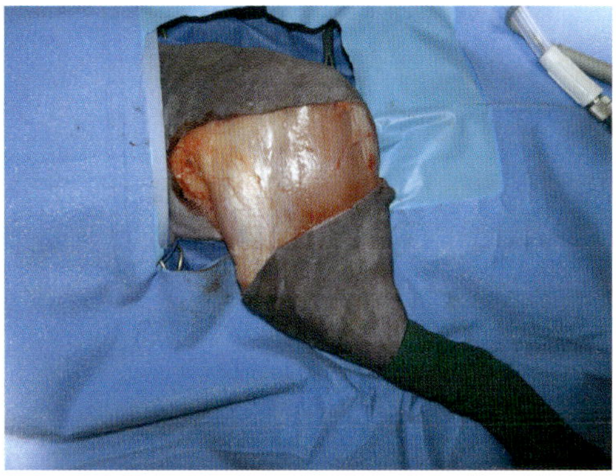

B)

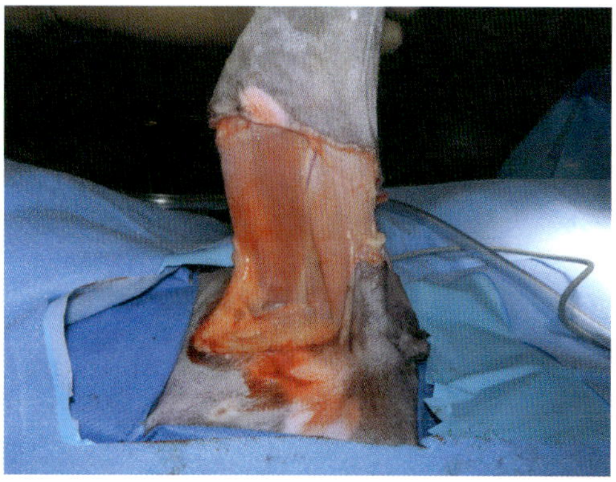

C-i)

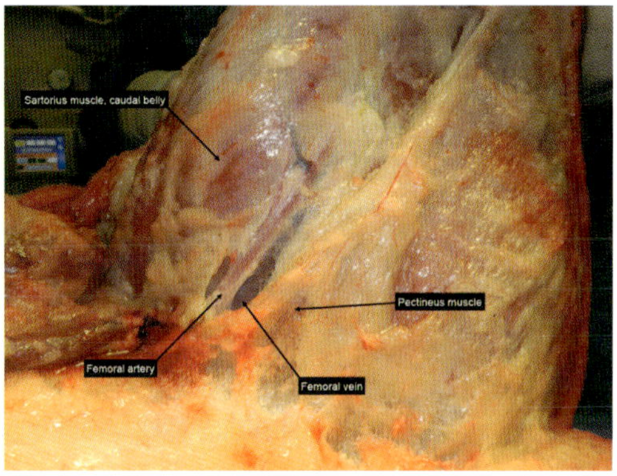

C-ii)

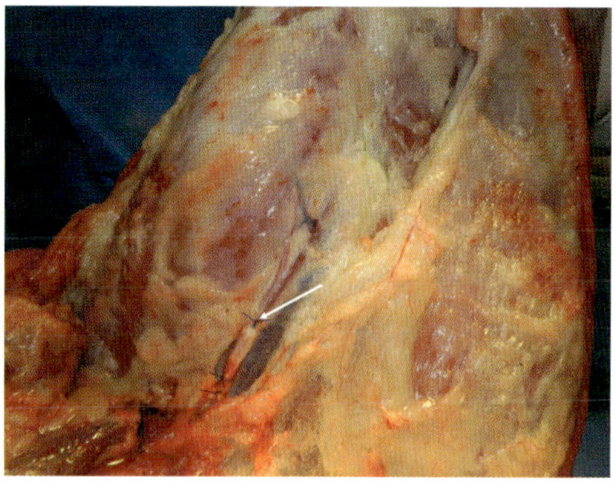

C-iii)

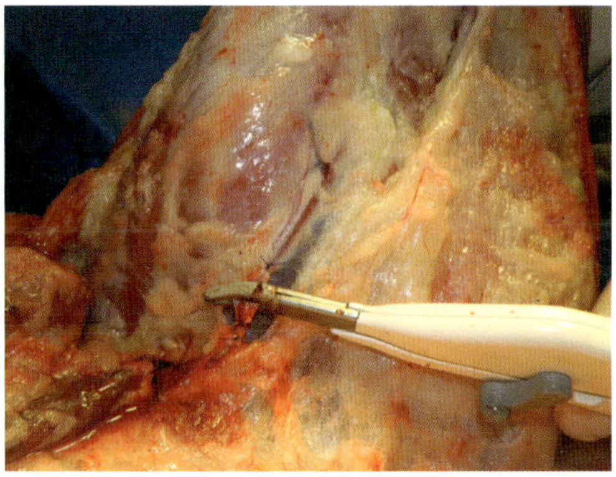

C-iv)

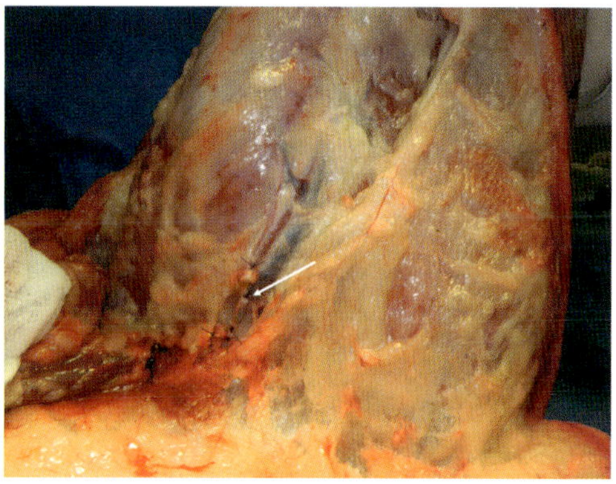

C-v)

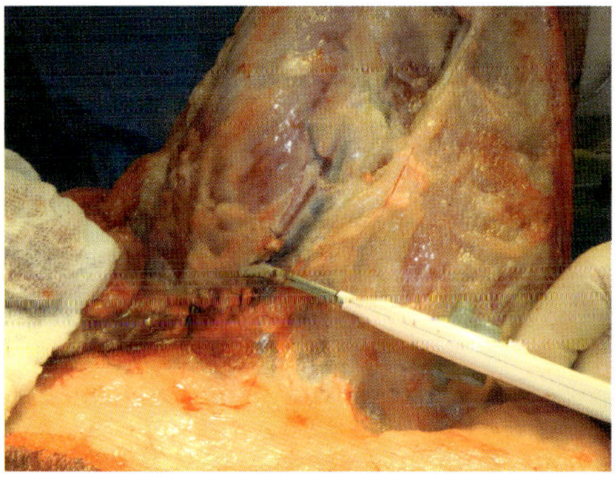

C-vi)

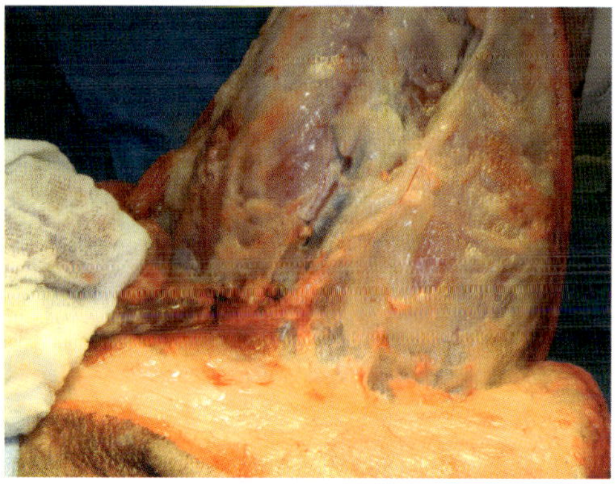

Surgical Technique (See Plate 37.3A–J) *continued*

D) Cranially, the two bellies of sartorius muscle are identified, bluntly dissected to isolate the muscle (i), and both the cranial and caudal bellies of the sartorius muscle are incised at their insertion at the level of the stifle (ii, iii). The sartorius muscle flap (iv) is used to reconstruct the cranial aspect of the amputation stump.

E) Medially, the subcutaneous tissues are dissected to expose the ventral midline, which is identified by a thin fascial aponeurosis between converging muscle bellies. These muscles should be transected with a vessel sealing device (i) or electrosurgery close to the medial aspect of the acetabulum and then reflected medially to expose the ramus of the pubis. A curved retractor, such as an Army-Navy retractor, or periosteal elevator is passed around the pubic ramus to protect the pelvic contents (ii), and an osteotomy of the midpubic ramus (arrow) is performed with an oscillating or sagittal saw (iii, iv).

Plate 37.3

Acetabulectomy *continued*

D-i)

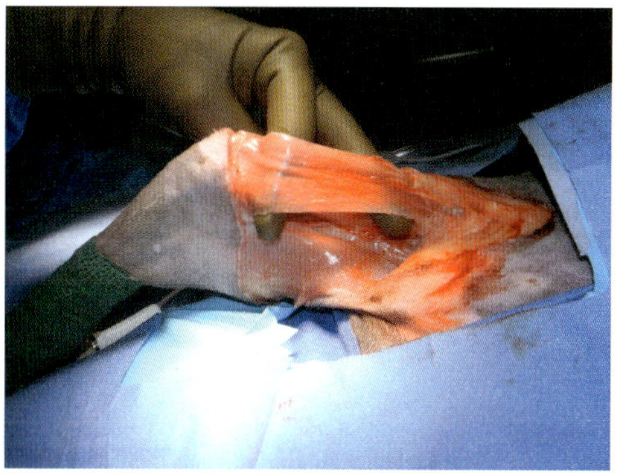

D-ii)

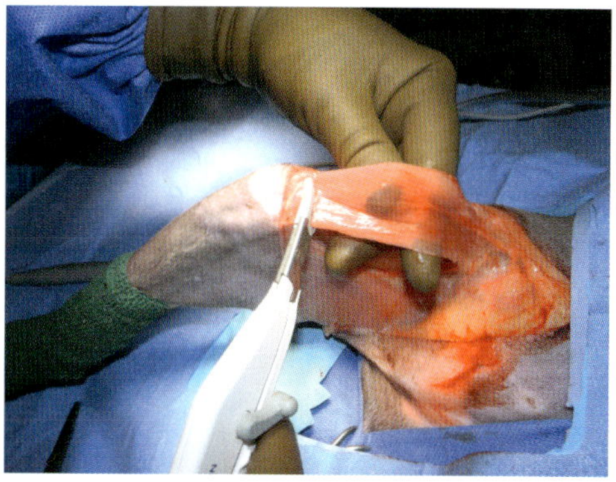

D-iii)

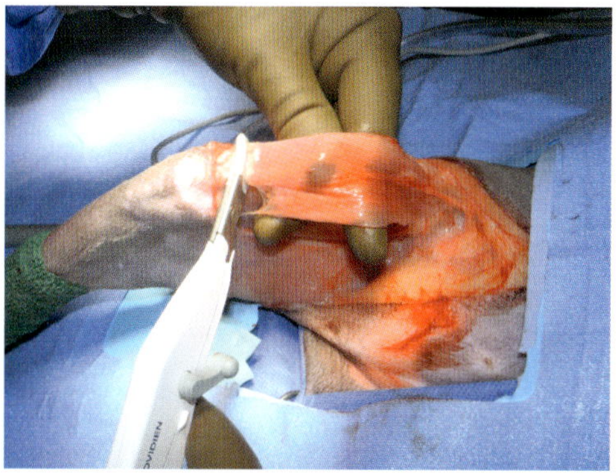

D-iv)

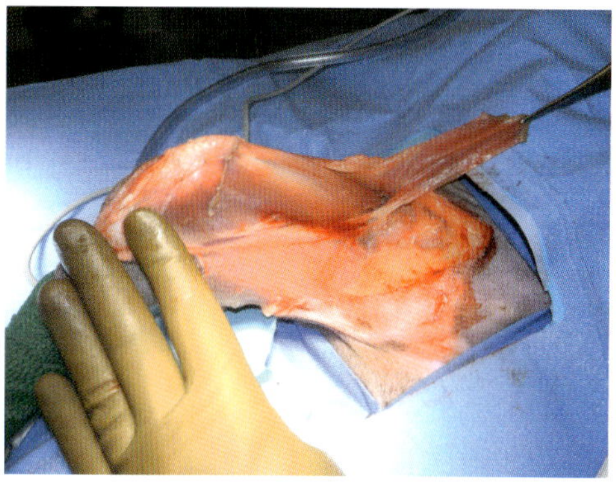

E-i)

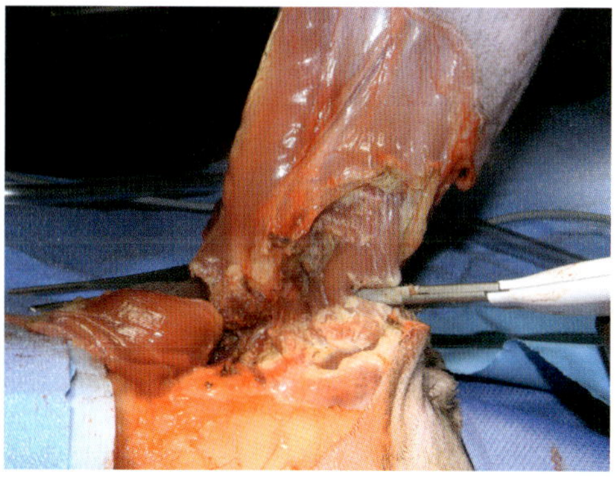

E-ii)

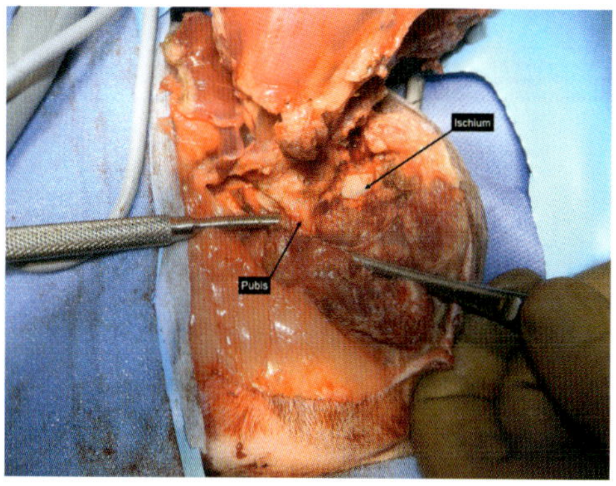

E-iii)

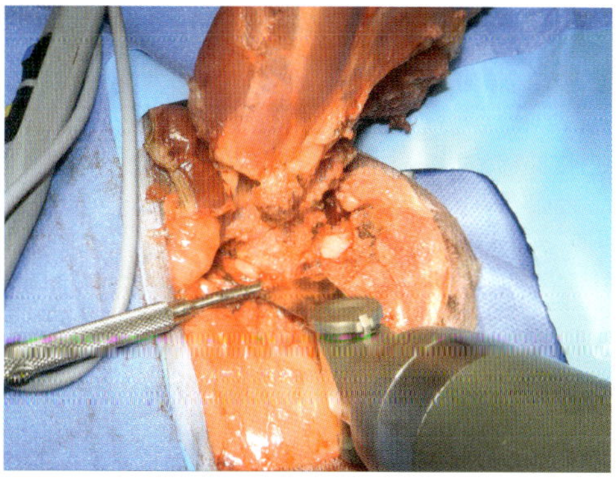

E-iv)

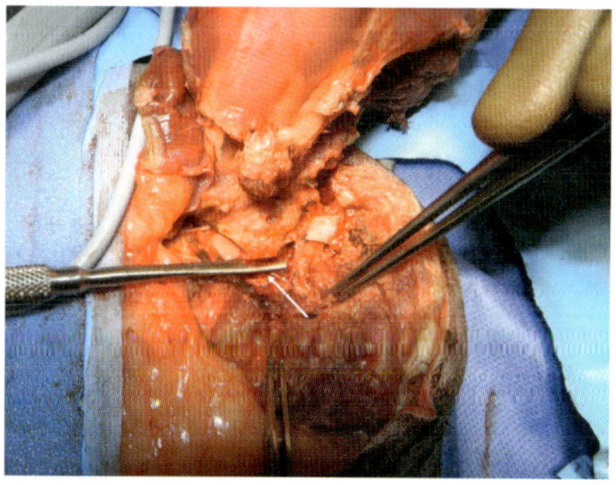

Surgical Technique (See Plate 37.3A–J) *continued*

F) Laterally, an incision is made through the middle and deep gluteal muscles to the level of the ilial body to create a soft tissue corridor. A retractor is passed around the medial aspect of the ilial body to protect the pelvic contents (i), and then an ilial osteotomy is performed with an oscillating or sagittal saw (ii, iii).

G) Moving caudally, the underlying bulky biceps femoris muscle is transected with either cautery or a vessel sealing device.

H) The muscular dissection is continued caudal to the greater trochanter of the femur in a dorsal-to-ventral direction (i), staying lateral to the sacrotuberous ligament to expose the ischiatic spine. All soft tissue attachments are freed with a periosteal elevator. A curved retractor, such as an Army-Navy retractor or a periosteal elevator, is passed around the exposed ischium to protect the pelvic canal structures and tissues medially (ii), and then the ischial osteotomy is performed with an oscillating or sagittal saw (iii, iv).

I) The sciatic nerve is infiltrated with local anesthetic. The sciatic is transected with a scalpel blade or scissors after a minimum of 1 minute for the local anesthetic to adequately infiltrate the nerve.

Plate 37.3

Acetabulectomy *continued*

F-i)

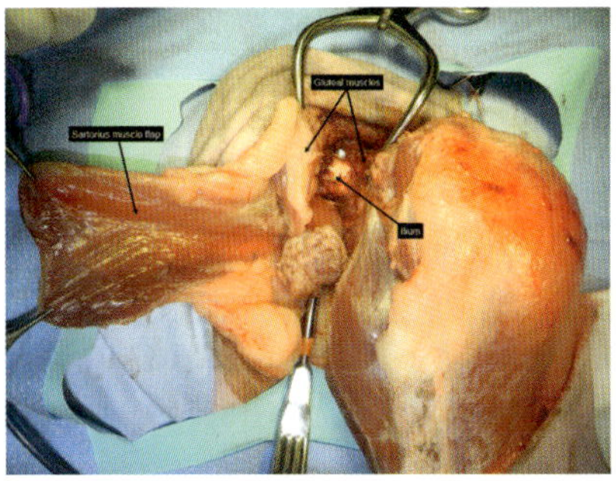

F-ii)

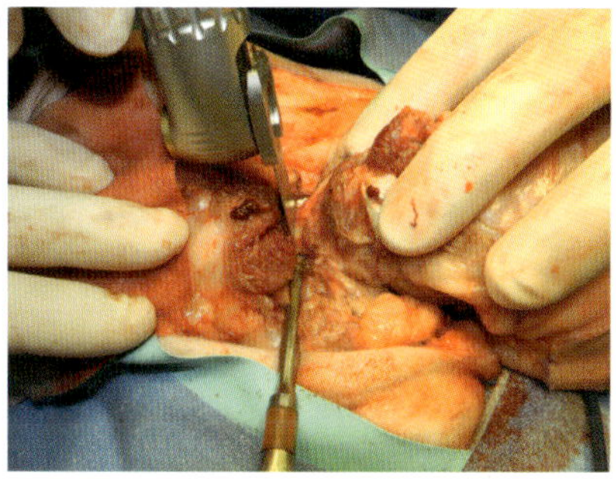

F-iii)

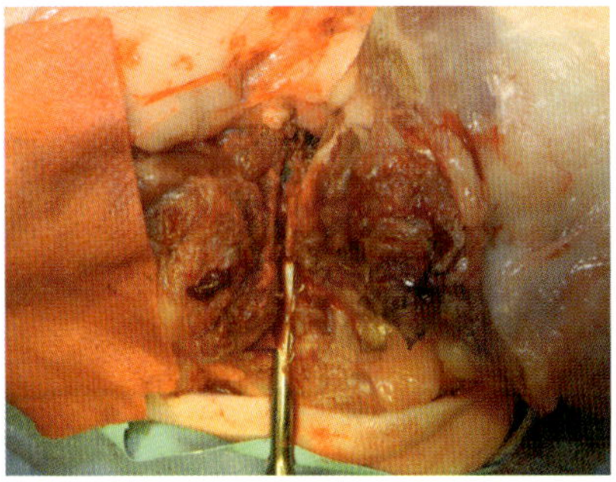

G)

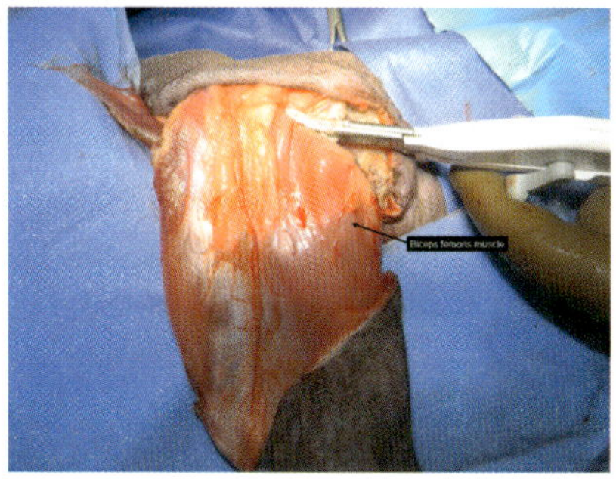

H-i)

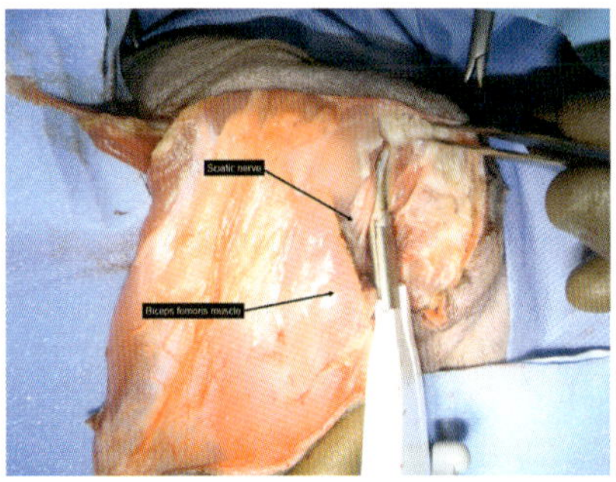

H-ii)

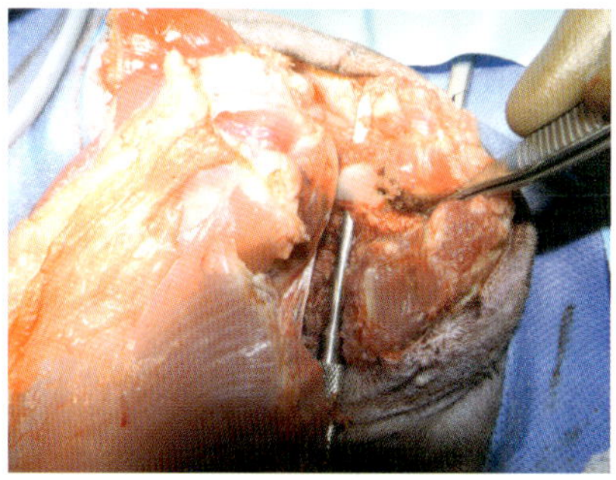

H-iii)

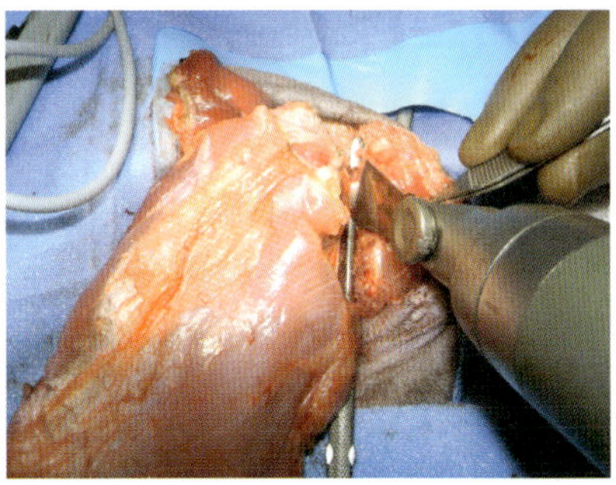

H-iv)

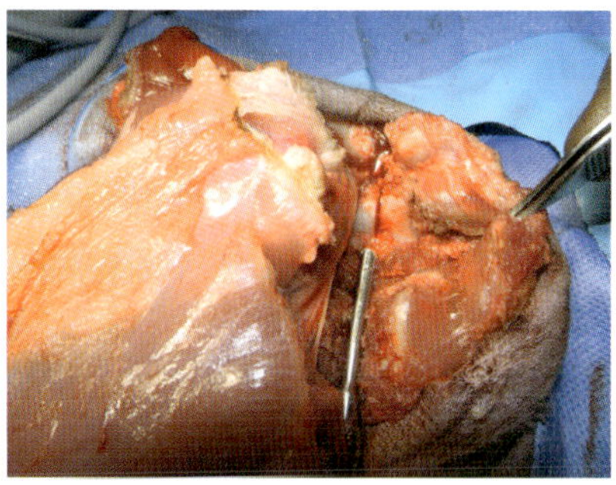

I)

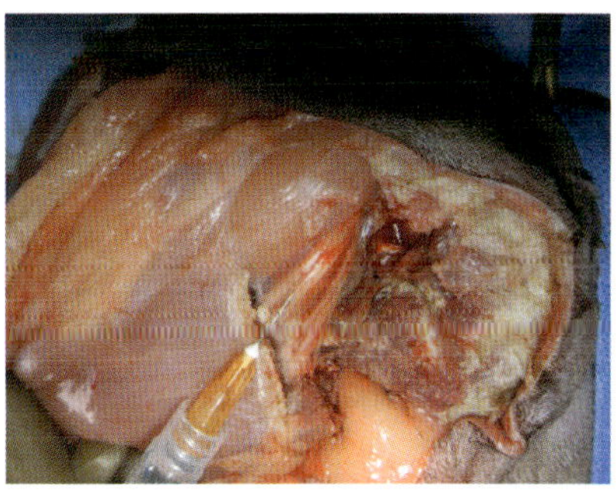

Surgical Technique (See Plate 37.3A–J) *continued*

J) The remaining dorsal (i), caudal, and medial (ii) muscle and soft tissue attachments are transected using either cautery or a vessel sealing device.

Closure (See Plate 37.3K, L)

K) The sartorius muscle flap (i) is transposed caudally and sutured in position to the abdominal muscles, pelvic diaphragm (caudally), and adductor muscles (medially) with 0 to 3-0 absorbable monofilament suture material in a cruciate or simple continuous pattern (ii).
L) The subcutaneous tissue and skin are closed routinely (i). The use of an active suction drain may be required (ii, postoperative ventrodorsal radiograph of a dog treated with an acetabulectomy and amputation for resection of a proximal femoral hemangiosarcoma).

Postoperative Management

1) Multimodal analgesia
2) Elizabethan collar or body suit
3) Sling support if necessary

Complications

- Wound infection (up to 50%) [1, 2]
- Urinary retention (5%) [3]
- Hemorrhage and hematoma formation [1]
- Incisional dehiscence (1%) [1, 3]
- Hernia formation (1%) [1, 3]
- Seroma formation [1]
- Decubital ulcer formation [1]
- Urethral and rectal trauma [1]
- Corneal ulceration (2%) [1]
- Aspiration pneumonia (1%) [3]

Suggested Adjuvant Treatments

- See *33. Primary Bone and Periarticular Tumors*.

Prognosis and Oncologic Outcome

- See *37.1. Total Hemipelvectomy*.

References

1 Kramer, A., Walsh, P.J., and Seguin, B. (2008). Hemipelvectomy in dogs and cats: technique overview, variations and description. *Vet. Surg.* 37: 413–419.
2 Barbur, L.A., Coleman, K.D., Schmeidt, C.W. et al. (2015). Description of the anatomy, surgical technique, and outcome of hemipelvectomy in 4 dogs and 5 cats. *Vet. Surg.* 44: 613–626.
3 Bray, J.P., Worley, D.R., Boston, S.E. et al. (2014). Hemipelvectomy: Outcome in 84 dogs and 16 cats. A veterinary society oncology retrospective study. *Vet. Surg.* 43: 27–37.

Plate 37.3

Acetabulectomy *continued*

J-i)

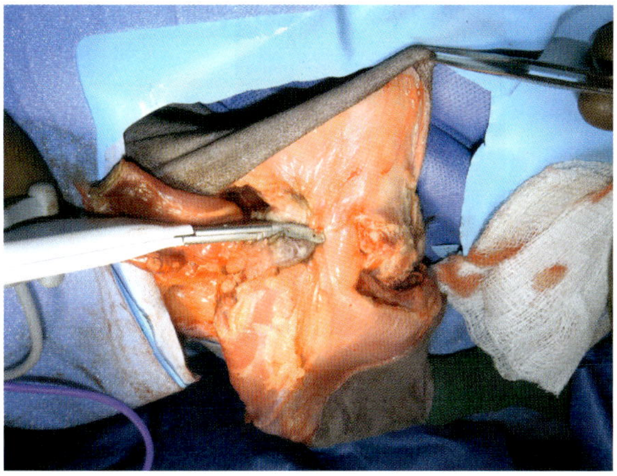

J-ii)

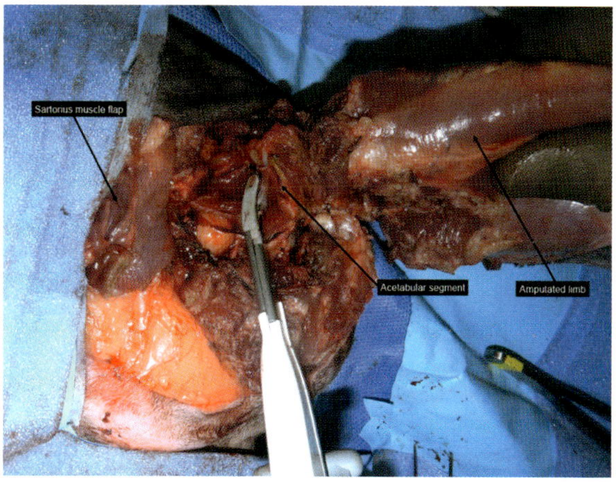

K-i)

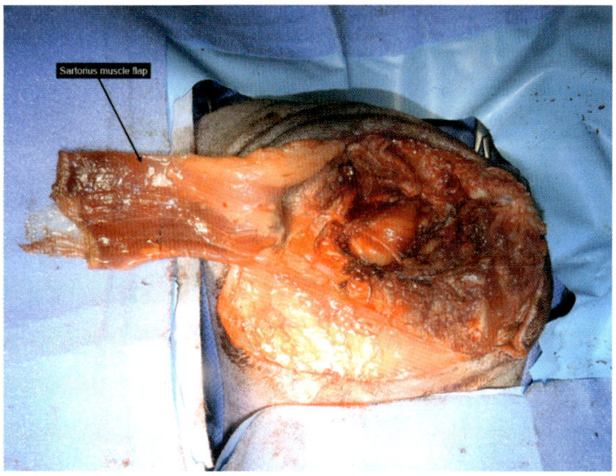

K-ii)

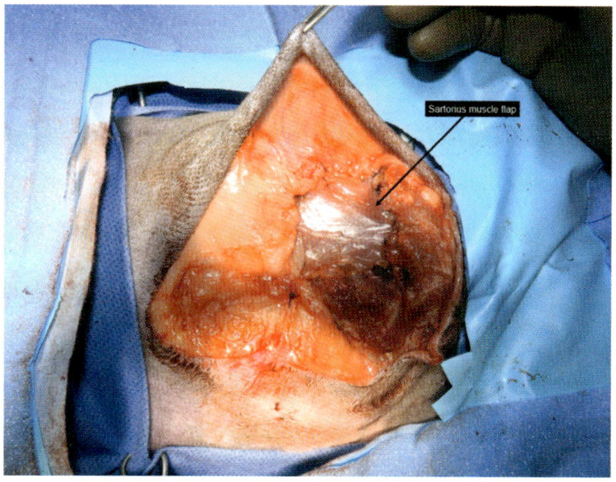

L-i)

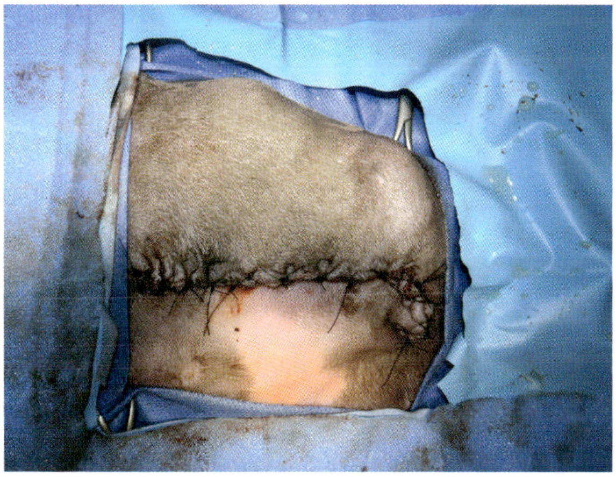

L-ii)

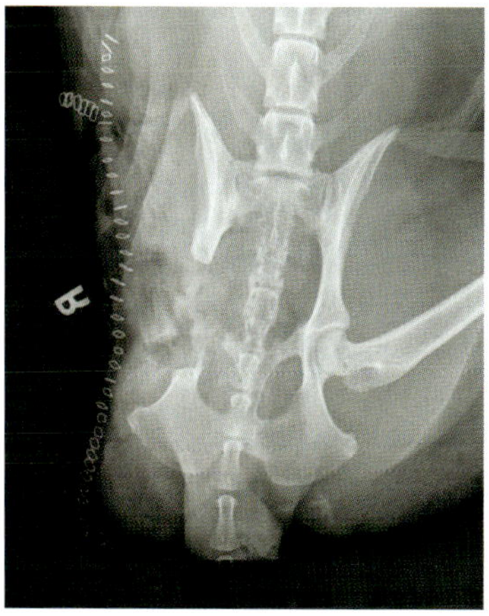

Surgical Technique – Single-Incision Approach (See Plate 37.4A–F) *continued*

E) Cranial and medial ischial osteotomies are performed with an oscillating or sagittal saw while protecting the mass and adjacent soft tissues with retractors (i; ii, ventrodorsal pelvic radiograph after internal hemipelvectomy with cranial and medial ischial osteotomies [arrowheads]). If the tumor is small, then it may be possible to resect the tumor with a single osteotomy using an appropriately sized biradial saw (iii, iv, ventrodorsal pelvic radiograph after internal hemipelvectomy with a single ischial osteotomy [arrowheads]).
F) The ischium is then elevated and freed from any remaining soft tissue attachments.

Closure (See Plate 37.4G, H)

G) The semimembranosus and semitendinosus are sutured to local soft tissues with 0 to 3-0 absorbable monofilament suture material in a cruciate pattern.
H) The subcutaneous tissues and skin are closed routinely.

Surgical Technique – Double-Incision Approach (Not Pictured)

I) Starting ventrally, a midline skin incision is made from the last mammary gland caudally to midpubic symphysis in female dogs and cats. In male dogs, this is a parapenile incision, with care being taken to avoid iatrogenic trauma to the urethra in the caudal midline.
J) Medially, the subcutaneous tissues are dissected to expose the ventral midline, which is identified by a thin fascial aponeurosis between converging muscle bellies. The attachments of the adductor, gracilis, and pectineus muscles are incised and gently elevated off the ridged pubic midline with a periosteal elevator or electrocautery. These are then reflected laterally to expose the entire length of the pubic bone. The muscles on the contralateral aspect of the pubis should not be disturbed.
K) The caudal ramus of the pubis is identified and freed of soft tissues. A retractor is passed around the caudal ramus of the pubis from the caudomedial aspect of the obturator foramen to the ipsilateral paramedian or medial ischiatic arch. An osteotomy of the caudal pubic ramus is then performed with an oscillating or sagittal saw. A more complex osteotomy involving the caudal symphysis might be required depending on the location of the tumor, and rarely contralateral osteotomies of the pubis and ischium are required [1].
L) Laterally, a skin incision is made from the mid-ilium over the greater trochanter and to the caudal aspect of the ischiatic tuberosity.
M) A dissection plane is identified between the superficial gluteal and biceps femoris muscles, and the biceps femoris muscle is retracted caudally to expose the sciatic nerve. The sciatic nerve is gently protected cranially.
N) The proximal biceps femoris muscle is incised over the ischium, and then the semitendinosus and semimembranosus muscles are transected distal to their origins with electrocautery or a vessel sealing device.
O) The quadratus femoris and adductor muscles are incised over the lesser ischial notch to expose the ischium. The sacrotuberous ligament is transected. A retractor is passed around the cranial ischium, caudal to the acetabulum, and an ischial osteotomy is then performed with an oscillating or sagittal saw.
P) The ischium is then elevated and freed from any remaining soft tissue attachments.

Closure

Q) The semimembranosus and semitendinosus cannot be reattached, but the biceps femoris is anchored proximally to local soft tissues with 0 to 3-0 absorbable monofilament suture material in a cruciate pattern.
R) Medially, the adductor, gracilis, and pectineus muscles are reattached to the midline musculature with 0 to 3-0 absorbable monofilament suture material in a cruciate pattern.
S) The subcutaneous tissues and skin are closed routinely.

Plate 37.4

Internal Hemipelvectomy *continued*

E-i)

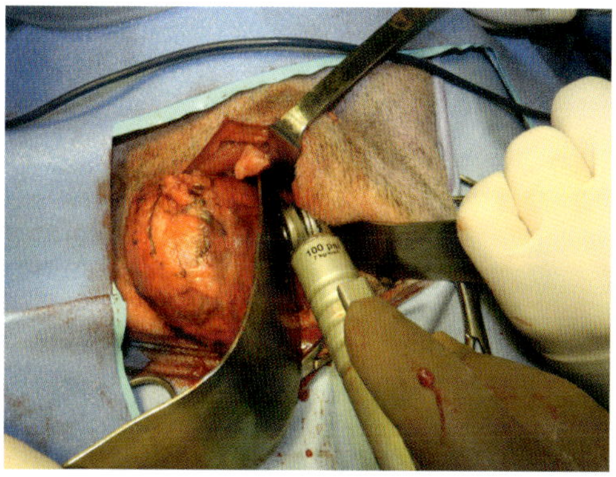

E-ii)

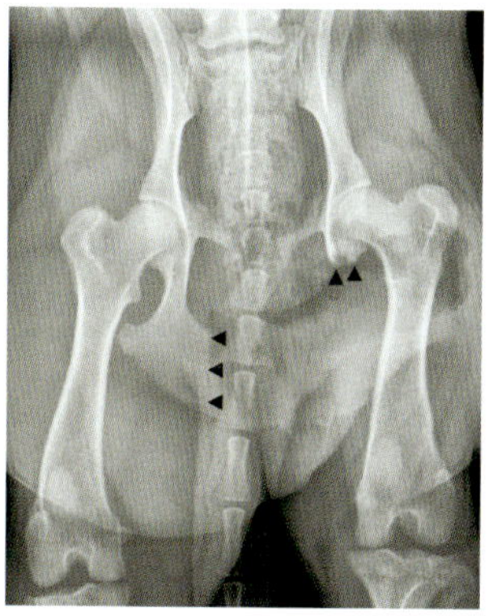

E-iii)

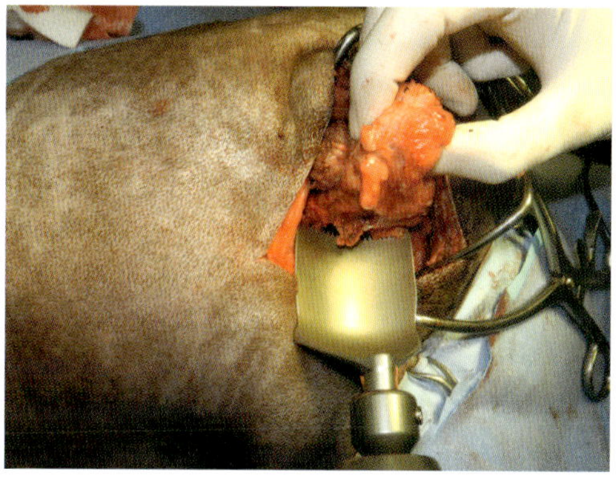

E-iv)

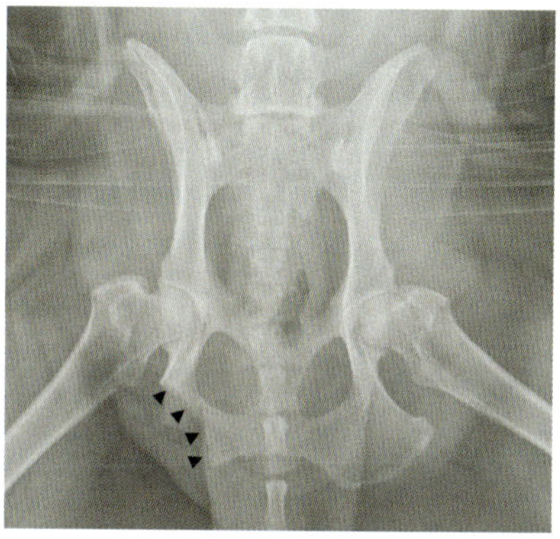

F)

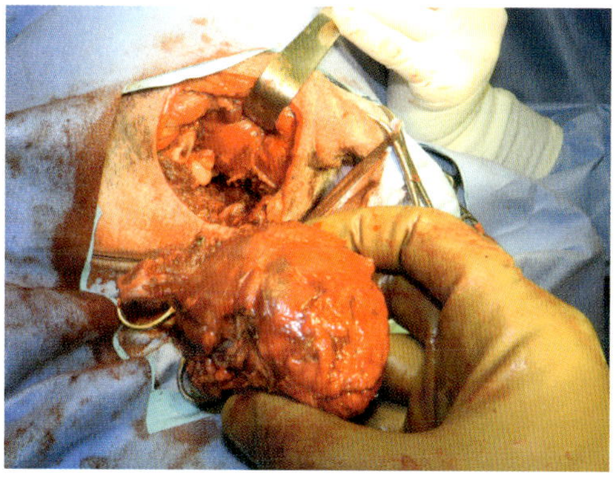

G)

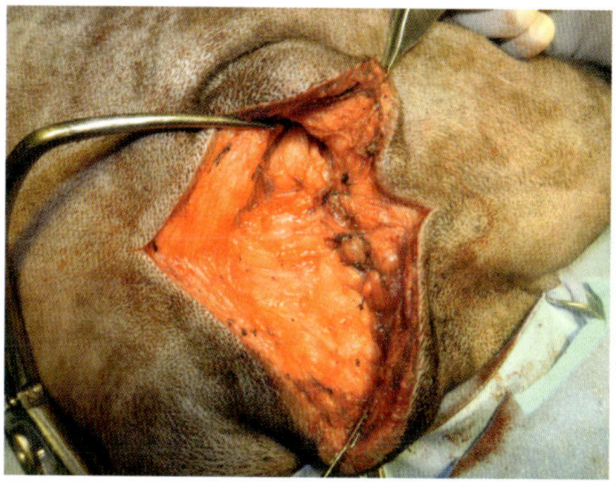

H)

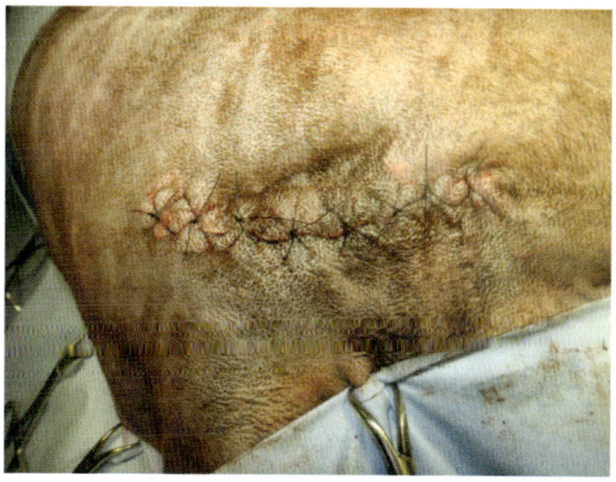

Postoperative Management

1) Multimodal analgesia
2) Elizabethan collar or body suit
3) Sling support if necessary

Complications

- Seroma [1]
- Incisional infection [1]
- Pollakiuria, hematuria [1]
- Lameness and reduced limb function [2]

Suggested Adjuvant Treatments

- See *33. Primary Bone and Periarticular Tumors*.

Prognosis and Oncologic Outcome [3]

- See *37.1. Total Hemipelvectomy*.

References

1 Sharma, S., Boston, S.E., Mosley, C. et al. (2021). Internal hemipelvectomy with ischiectomy, partial acetabulectomy, and femoral head and neck excision in a cat with a pelvic osteocondroma. *J. Am. Vet. Med. Assoc.* 259 (4): 401–405.

2 Oblak, M.L. and Boston, S.E. (2015). Ischiectomy with limb preservation for a dog with ischial chondrosarcoma: case report and surgical technique. *Vet. Surg.* 44 (5): 571–575.

3 Bray, J.P., Worley, D.R., Boston, S.E. et al. (2014). Hemipelvectomy: outcome in 84 dogs and 16 cats. A veterinary society oncology retrospective study. *Vet. Surg.* 43 (1): 27–37.

Chapter 38: Tail Amputation

Indications

1) Resection of benign or malignant tumors of the caudal vertebrae and/or soft tissues of the tail
2) Trauma, including degloving, fracture-luxation, and avulsion/traction injuries [1]
3) When using the lateral caudal axial pattern flap (see *43.11. Lateral Caudal Axial Pattern Flap*) for reconstruction of perineal defects

Suggested Diagnostic Workup and Clinical Staging

- Complete blood count, serum biochemistry, and urinalysis
- Fine-needle aspirate cytology or incisional biopsy
- ± Regional lymph node assessment
- ± Three-view thoracic radiographs (or thoracic computed tomography) for assessment of lung metastasis

Patient Positioning

The patient is positioned in ventral recumbency with the pelvic limbs positioned over the end of the operating table.

Surgical Technique (See Plate 38A, C–F)

A) The level of amputation is based on the surgical margin required (for neoplastic tail amputation, pictured with margins marked with a sterile marker pen) or health of the local soft tissues (for traumatic tail amputation). There are some minor variations in the surgical technique between partial and total tail amputation.
B) The coccygeal articulation immediately proximal to the intended level of amputation is identified by manipulation and palpation (not pictured).
C) The skin of the tail is pushed toward the base of the tail. A circumferential incision (i, dorsal incision; ii, ventral incision) or dorsally and ventrally based double V-shaped skin incisions (iii) are made an entire coccygeal vertebra distal to articulation.
D) For partial tail amputation, the skin and subcutaneous tissue are retracted cranially to expose the tail amputation site (i), and the soft tissue envelope (including muscle and tendons) are incised at the planned articulation site using a scalpel or electrosurgery (ii, iii).
E) For total tail amputation, the tail is elevated dorsally to transect the rectococcygeus muscle. The lateral levator ani and coccygeus muscles are elevated from the ventral surface of the proximal caudal vertebra. Care is taken with the dissection under the coccygeal vertebrae as the rectum is immediately ventral to the tail base. (Note that this is a tail amputation performed in preparation for a lateral caudal axial pattern flap).

Color Atlas of Canine and Feline Surgical Oncology, First Edition. Julius M. Liptak, Paolo Buracco, William T. N. Culp, and Nicholas J. Bacon.

Plate 38

Tail Amputation

A)

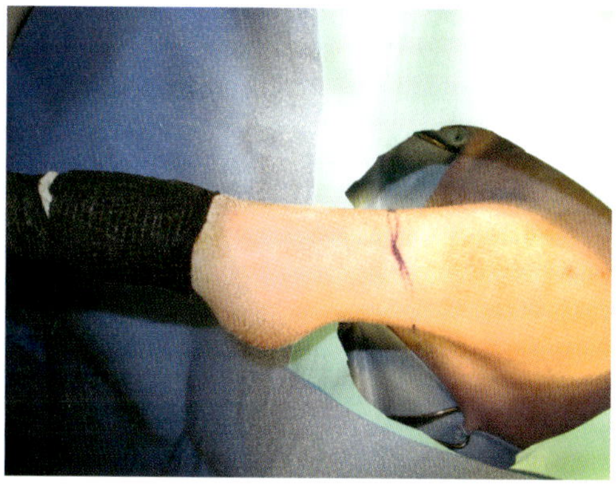

C-i)

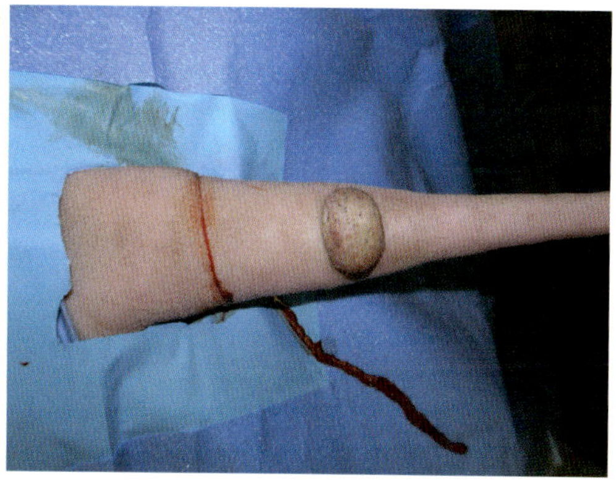

C-ii)

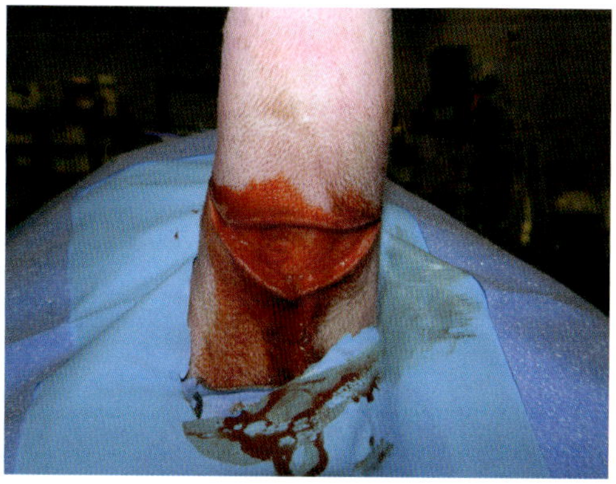

C-iii)

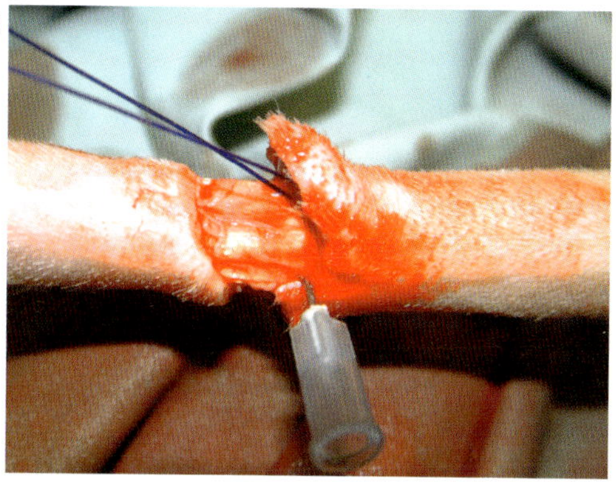

D-i)

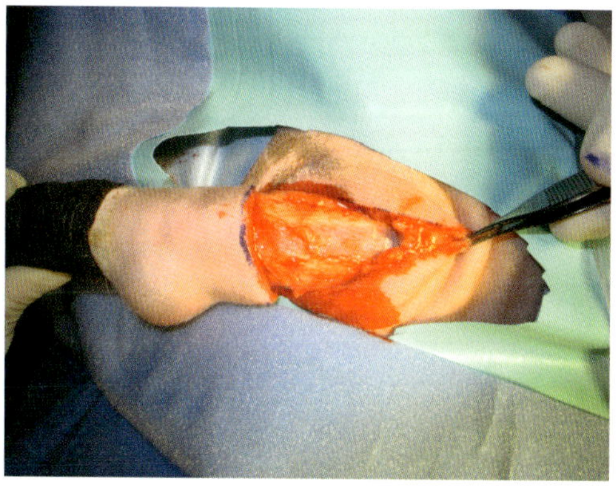

D-ii)

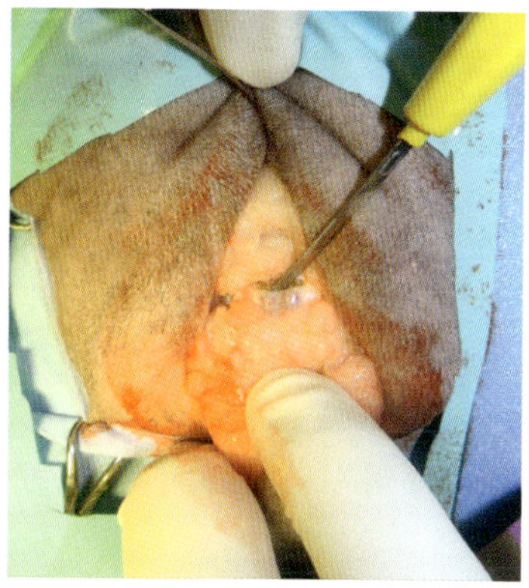

D-iii)

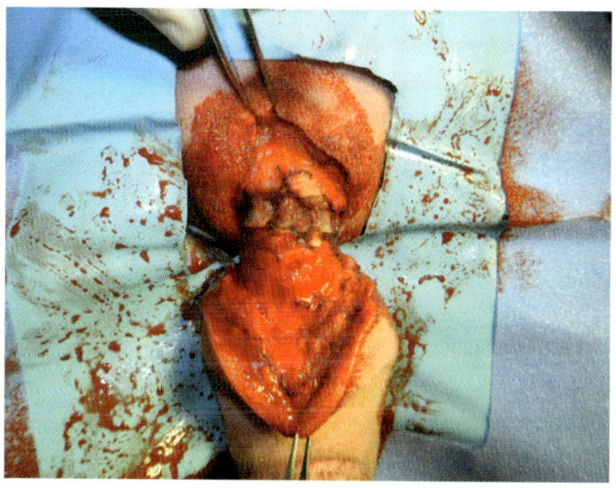

E)

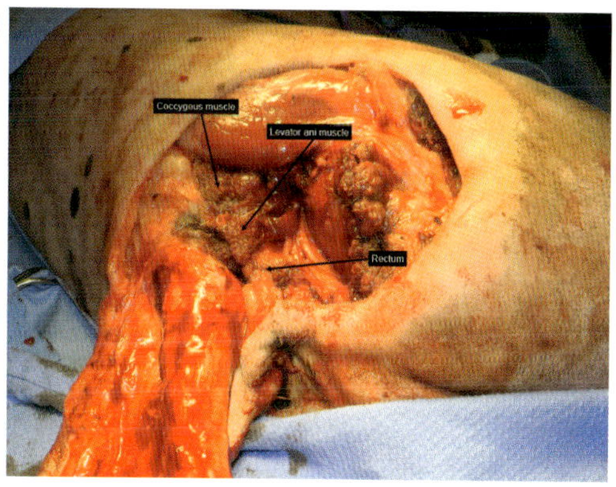

Surgical Technique (See Plate 38A, C–F) *continued*

F) The tail is disarticulated at the desired level with a no. 15 scalpel blade (i) or electrosurgery. Alternatively, bone cutters can be used (ii, partial tail amputation; iii, total tail amputation). The lateral arteries are ligated at that level, as is the medial artery ventral to the coccygeal vertebrae (iv). Alternatively, these vessels can be either ligated or cauterized before amputation.

Closure (See Plate 38G, H)

The local muscle and soft tissues are sutured over the exposed articular surface of the caudal vertebra (G) with 2-0 to 3-0 monofilament absorbable suture material using an interrupted pattern. The subcutaneous tissue and skin are closed routinely (H – i, partial tail amputation; H – ii, total tail amputation).

Postoperative Management

1) Multimodal analgesia
2) Elizabethan collar until 2 days after suture removal [2]

Complications

- Mild to severe incisional crusting (20%) [3]
- Incisional dehiscence (5%) [3]
- Rectal displacement dorsally [4]
- Surgical-site infection
- Distal skin ischemia and necrosis
- Bleeding
- Amputation neuromas [5]

References

1 Bellah, J.R. (2006). Tail and perineal wounds. *Vet. Clin. Small Anim. Pract.* 36 (4): 913–929.

2 Schoen, K. and Sweet, D.C. (2009). Canine and feline tail amputation. *Clin. Tech.* 38 (7): 232–233.

3 Simons, M.C. and Ben-Amotz, P.C. (2014). Post-operative complications and owner satisfaction following partial caudectomies: 22 cases (2008 to 2013). *J. Small Anim. Pract.* 55 (10): 509–514.

4 Gotzens, B., Medl, N.S., and Medl, S.C. (2020). Dorsal displacement of the rectum after proximal tail amputation and subsequent surgical repair by bilateral semitendinosus muscle transposition in a cat. *J. Am. Vet. Med. Assoc.* 256 (12): 1375–1378.

5 Gross, T.L. and Carr, S.H. (1990). Amputation neuroma of docked tails in dogs. *Vet. Pathol.* 27: 61–62.

Plate 38

Tail Amputation *continued*

F-i)

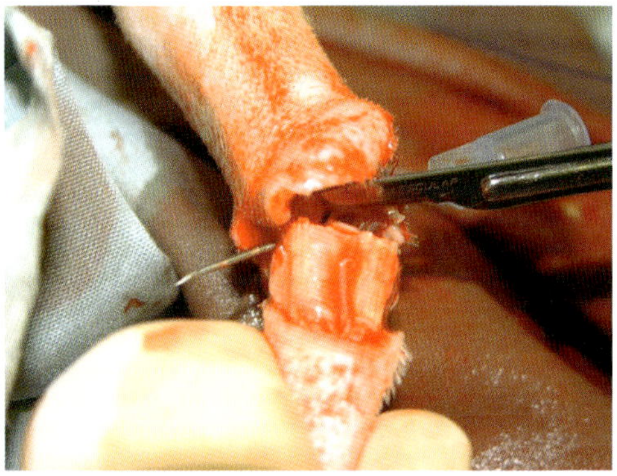

F-ii)

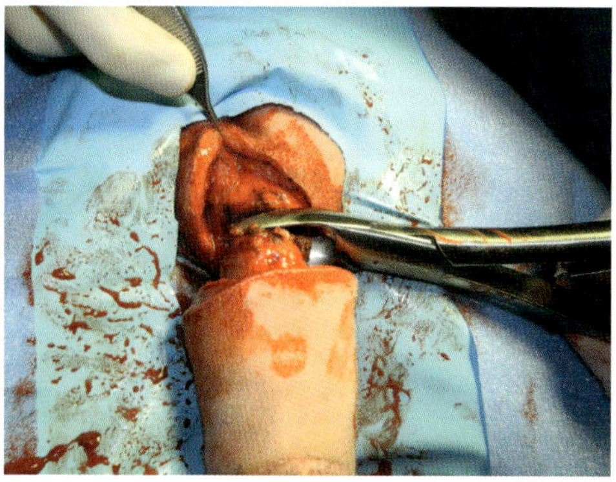

F-iii)

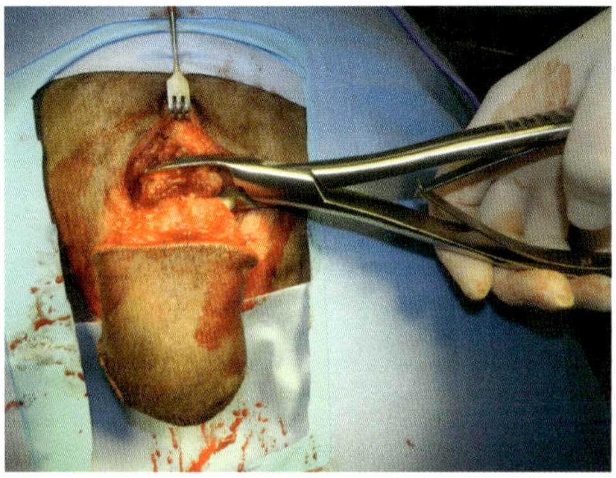

F-iv)

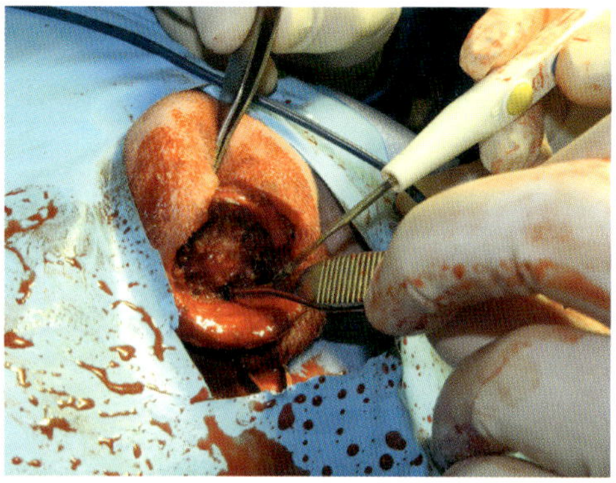

G)

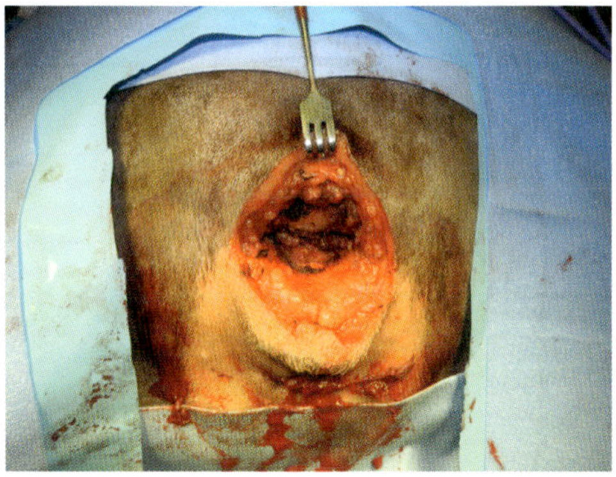

H-i)

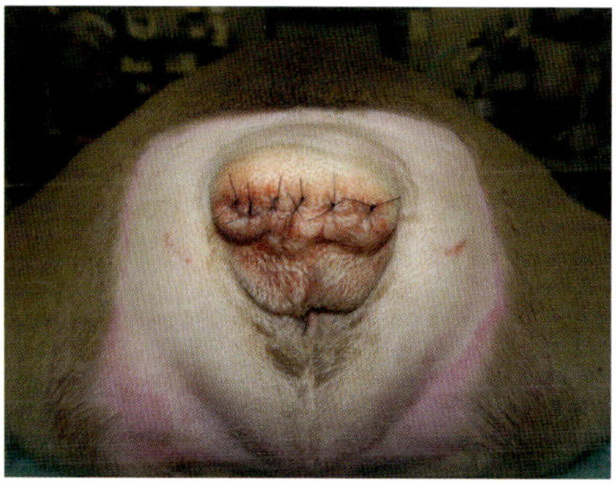

H-ii)

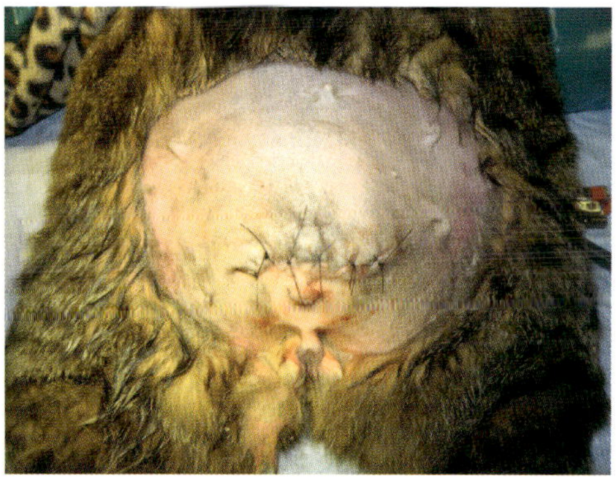

Section 8

Reconstructive Surgery

Chapter 39: Advancement Flap

39.1 General Advancement Flaps

General Considerations (See Plate 39.1A)

Subdermal plexus flaps derive their blood supply from the terminal branches of direct cutaneous vessels in the subdermal plexus at the base of the flap. Subdermal plexus flaps are classified according to their location relative to the skin defect and the method of transfer, such as advancement, transposition, and rotation flaps. These flaps are typically harvested from adjacent to the wound defect, ideally in areas with loose skin so that the flap donor site can be closed primarily with minimal tension. The donor site should not have excessive motion or tension because this may result in incisional complications (e.g. seroma, dehiscence) or decreased local mobility. The shape and size of the wound defect influences the type of subdermal plexus flap used for reconstruction of the wound. Advancement flaps are indicated for reconstruction of square or rectangular wounds (A – i, ii).

Surgical Technique – Single Advancement Flap (See Plate 39.1B–D)

B) Two parallel incisions are made starting from the base of the wound and at the same width as the defect (arrows). These incisions can diverge slightly so that the base of the advancement flap is not narrowed. The distant edge of the flap borders the defect. The length of the two incisions should correspond to the length of the defect, and the base of the flap should be proportional to its width.
C) The advancement flap is undermined starting from the distant edge of the flap bordering the wound defect. The flap should be undermined below the cutaneous trunci or platysma muscle (arrow) to preserve the subdermal plexus.
D) The distant edge of the advancement flap is advanced to the opposite side of the defect. The skin incisions are closed routinely in two layers with a simple continuous suture pattern using monofilament absorbable suture material in the subcutis and either skin staples or an interrupted or continuous suture pattern using monofilament nonabsorbable suture material in the skin (i–iii; iv, postoperative appearance of the dog in ii; v, postoperative appearance of the dog in iii). Tension-relieving sutures can be used if indicated.

Color Atlas of Canine and Feline Surgical Oncology, First Edition. Julius M. Liptak, Paolo Buracco, William T. N. Culp, and Nicholas J. Bacon.

Plate 39.1

General Advancement Flaps

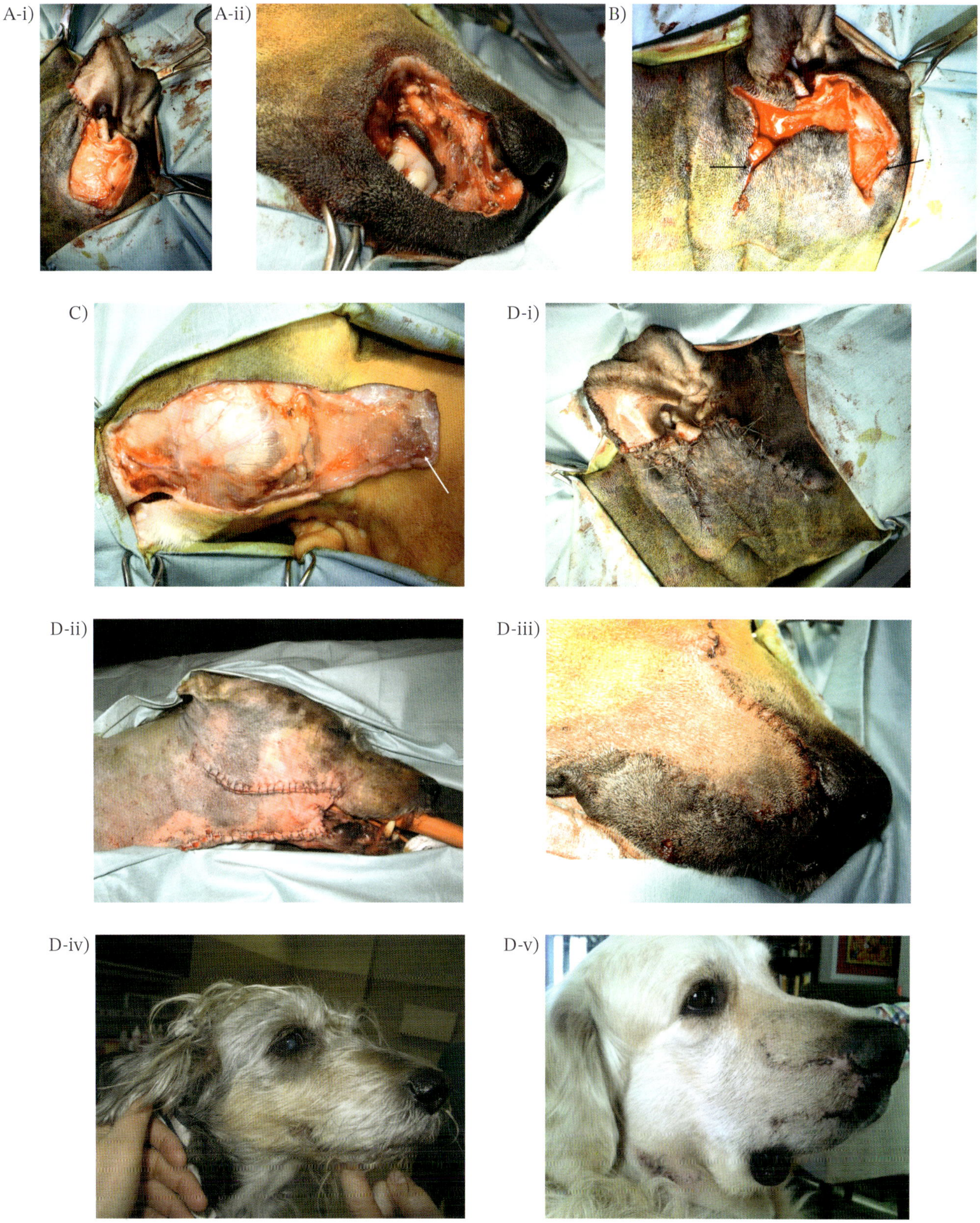

Surgical Technique – Double Advancement Flap (H-Plasty) (See Plate 39.1E)

E) An H-plasty consists of two advancement flaps on opposite sides of the wound defect. An H-plasty may be more effective because the individual length of each advancement flap is less than a single advancement flap.

Surgical Technique – Bipedicle Advancement Flap (See Plate 39.1F, H)

F) An incision is made parallel to the defect. This incision is the same length as the defect, and the width between the incision and defect should be 1.0–1.5 times the width of the defect.
G) The skin between the incision and the defect should be undermined below the cutaneous trunci or platysma muscle to preserve the subdermal plexus (not pictured).
H) The defect is closed routinely in two layers with a simple continuous suture pattern using monofilament absorbable suture material in the subcutis and either skin staples or an interrupted or continuous suture pattern using monofilament nonabsorbable suture material in the skin. The donor site can be closed primarily if feasible (pictured) or allowed to heal by second intention (see *46. Second Intention Healing*).

Postoperative Management

1) Multimodal analgesia
2) Elizabethan collar
3) ± Tie-over bandage

Complications

- Overall: 23% for advancement subdermal plexus flaps with 16% classified as minor and 6% as major [1]
- Overall: 51% for all types of subdermal plexus flap [1]
  - Dogs: 55% overall with 39% classified as minor and 16% as major
  - Cats: 43% overall with 32% classified as minor and 11% as major
- Incisional dehiscence (30%) [1]
- Seroma (12%) [1]
- Partial necrosis of the distal extent of the flap (10%–15%) [1, 2]
- Surgical-site infection (9%) [1]

References

1 Jones, C.A. and Lipscomb, V.J. (2019). Indications, complications, and outcomes associated with subdermal plexus skin flap procedures in dogs and cats: 92 cases (2000-2017). *J. Am. Vet. Med. Assoc.* 255 (8): 933–938.
2 De Carvalho Vasconcellos, C.H., Matera, J.M., and Zaidan Dagli, M.L. (2005). Clinical evaluation of random skin flaps based on the subdermal plexus secured with sutures or sutures and cyanoacrylate adhesive for reconstructive surgery in dogs. *Vet. Surg.* 34 (1): 59–63.

Plate 39.1

General Advancement Flaps *continued*

E)

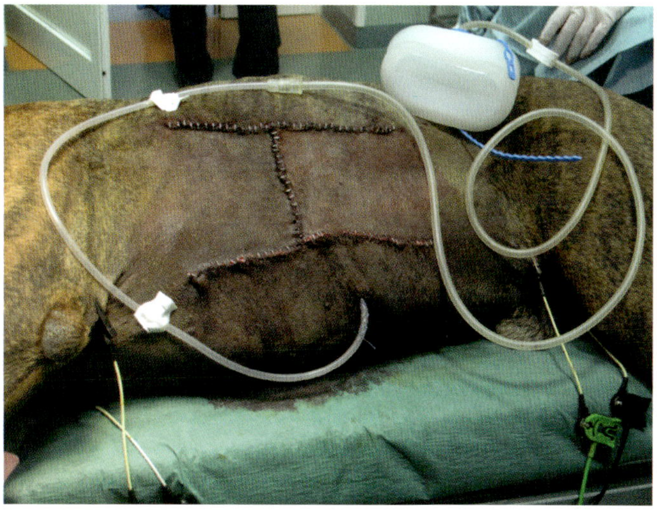

F)

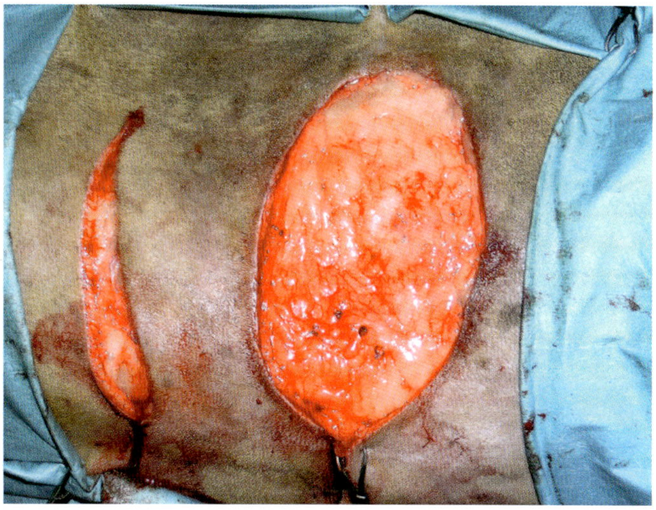

H)

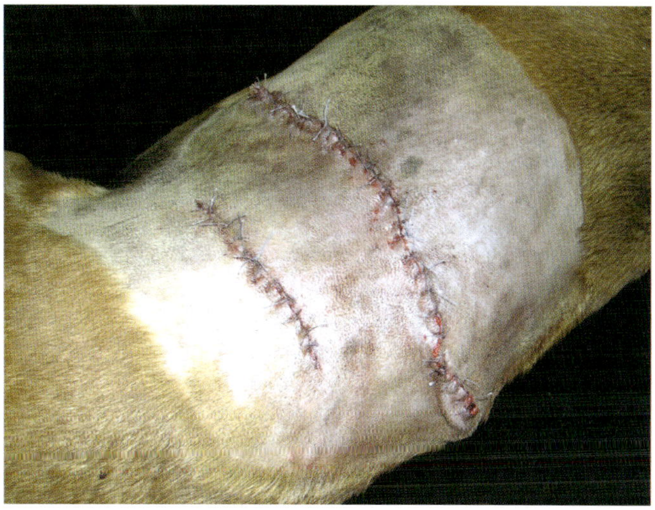

39.2 Upper Lip Advancement Flap

Indications (See Plate 39.2 – 1)

1) To reconstruct rostral upper lip defects that cannot be closed primarily (i, mucosal mast cell tumor in a dog; ii, iii, sarcoid in a cat).
2) An upper lip advancement flap can be combined with maxillary incisivectomy (see *6.10. Maxillary Incisivectomy*), unilateral rostral maxillectomy (see *6.11. Unilateral Rostral Maxillectomy*), bilateral rostral maxillectomy (see *6.12. Bilateral Rostral Maxillectomy*), or nasal planum resection (see *4.1. Nasal Planum Resection – Feline* and *4.2. Nasal Planum Resection – Canine*)

Patient Positioning

The patient is positioned in lateral recumbency with the affected lip uppermost for unilateral upper lip advancement flap. The patient is positioned in either dorsal or ventral recumbency for bilateral upper lip advancement flaps.

Surgical Technique (See Plate 39.2A–F)

A) An incision is performed starting at the caudodorsal corner of the lip defect and extended caudally, either parallel to or slightly diverging from the margin of the upper lip (dashed line; defect pictured resulted from resection of mast cell tumor in 1 – i).
B) The incision is continued through the subcutaneous/submucosal and mucosal tissue of the lip (i, ii). When performing the mucosal incision, it is important to preserve a cuff of mucosa along the maxilla to allow suturing of the mucosa of the advancement flap to the maxillary mucosa.
C) The advancement flap is undermined to allow rostral advancement. Fibrous tissue, blood vessels, and peripheral nerves will often be encountered during this dissection. If these tissues and structures cause a tethering effect on the advancement flap, then they should be sealed and transected or ligated and divided; however, blood vessels should be preserved when possible.

Plate 39.2

Upper Lip Advancement Flap

1-i)

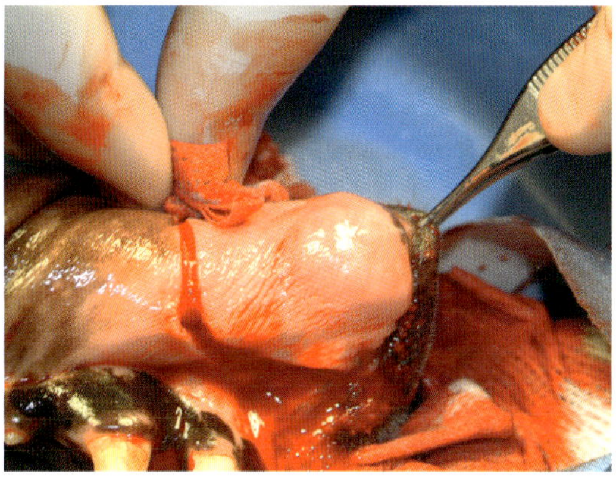

1-ii)

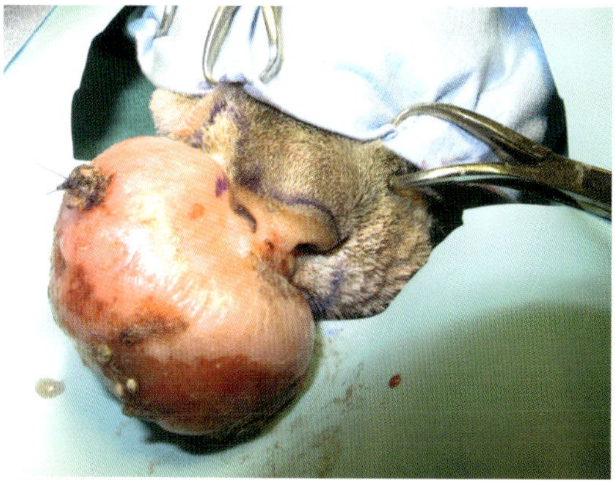

1-iii)

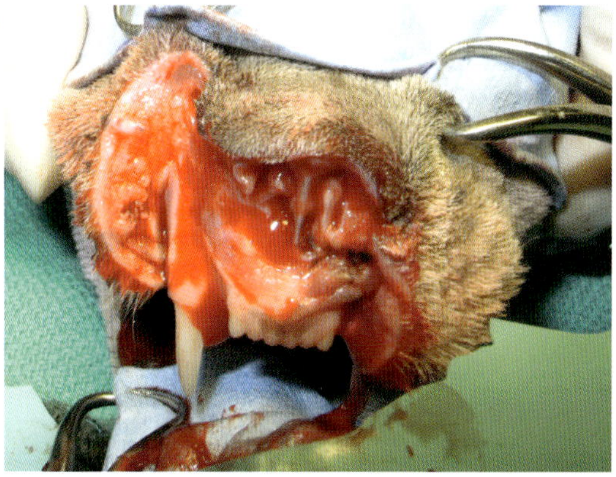

A)

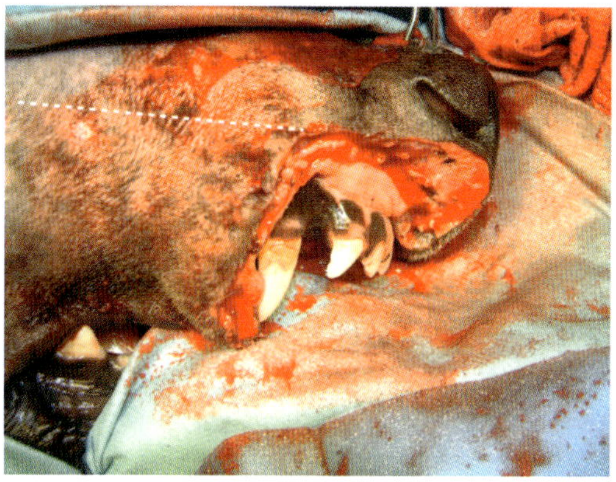

B-i)

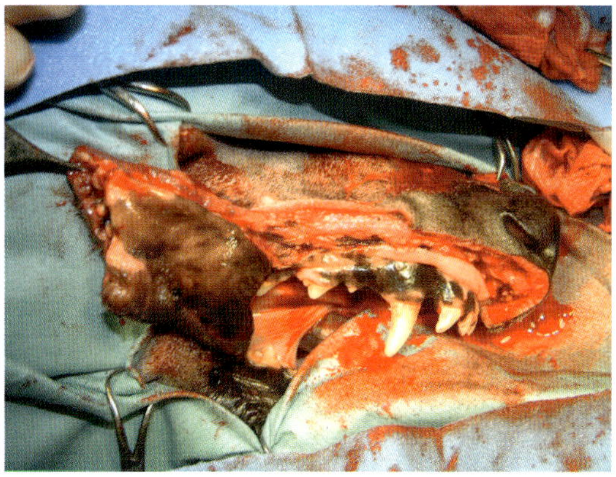

B-ii)

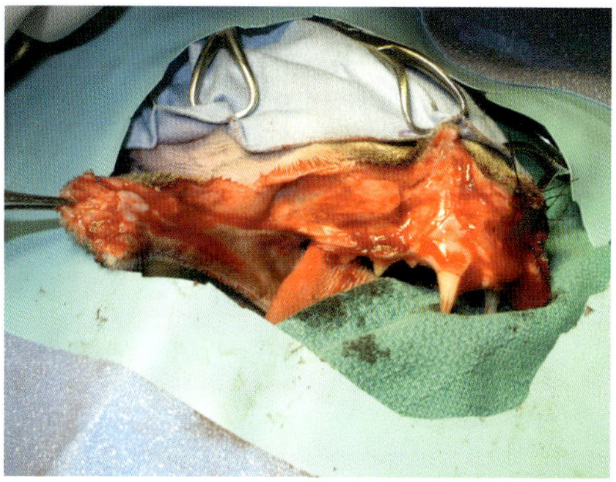

C)

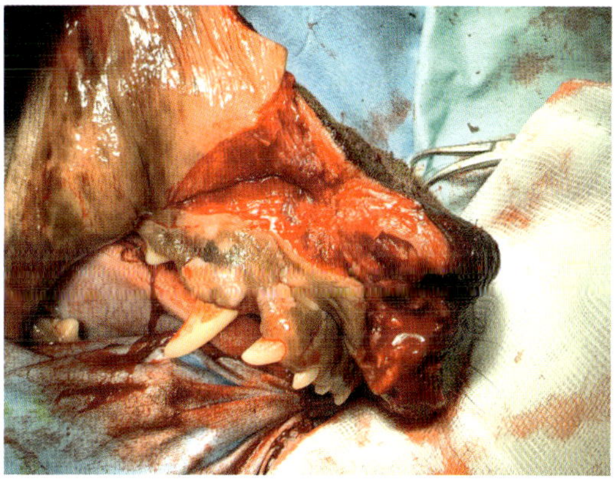

Surgical Technique (See Plate 39.2A–F) *continued*

D) The rostral edge of the advancement flap is advanced into the rostral aspect of the defect or to the philtrum of the lip (i, dog; ii, cat).

E) Closure begins with aligning the rostral margin of the lips. The incision is closed in three layers with a simple interrupted or continuous suture pattern using monofilament absorbable suture material in the mucosal layer (i, ii), a simple continuous suture pattern using monofilament absorbable suture material in the submucosal/subcutaneous layer, and either skin staples or an interrupted or continuous suture pattern using monofilament nonabsorbable suture material in the skin (iii, dog; iv, v, cat; vi, 3-month postoperative appearance in a cat). Tension-relieving sutures can be used if indicated.

Plate 39.2

Upper Lip Advancement Flap *continued*

D-i)

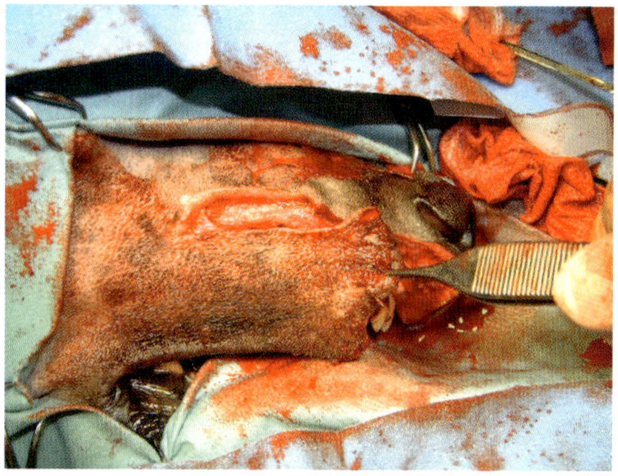

D-ii)

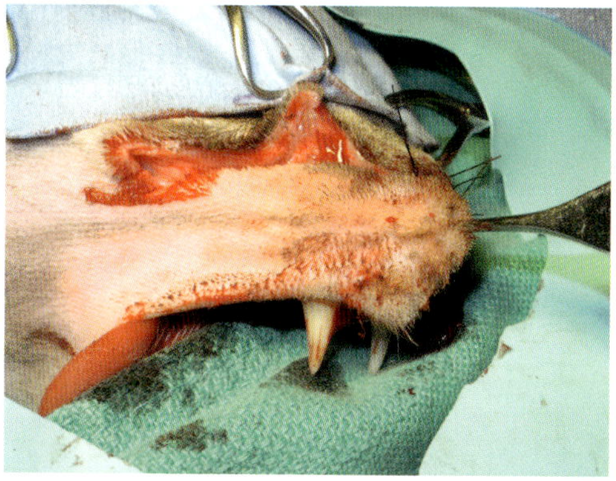

E-i)

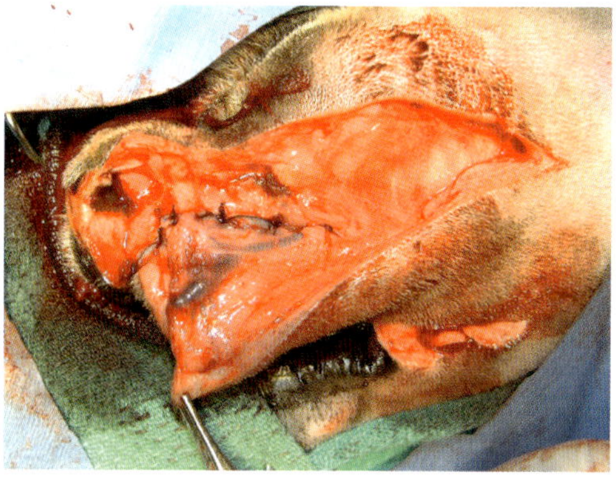

E-ii)

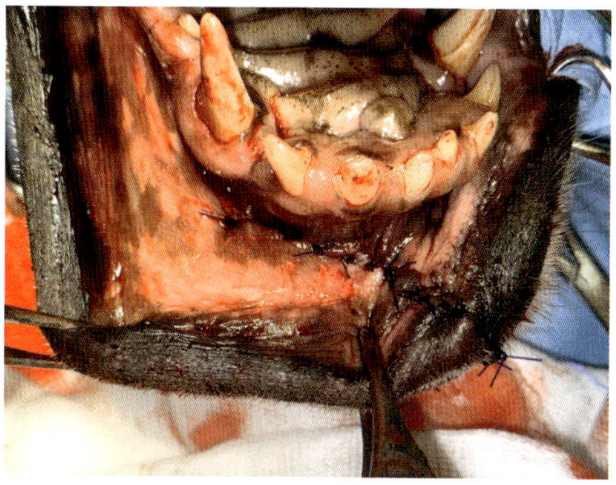

E-iii)

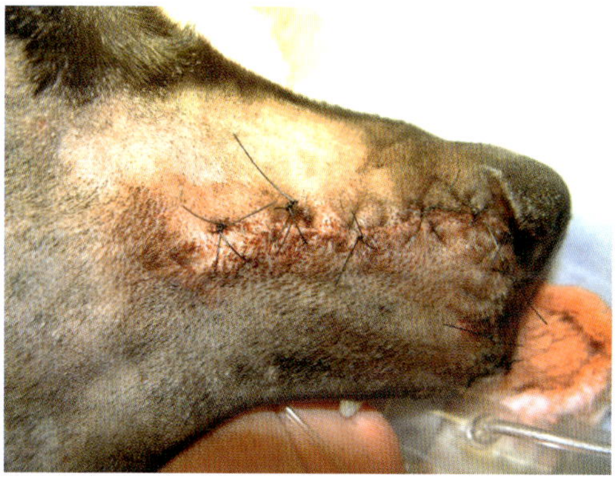

E-iv)

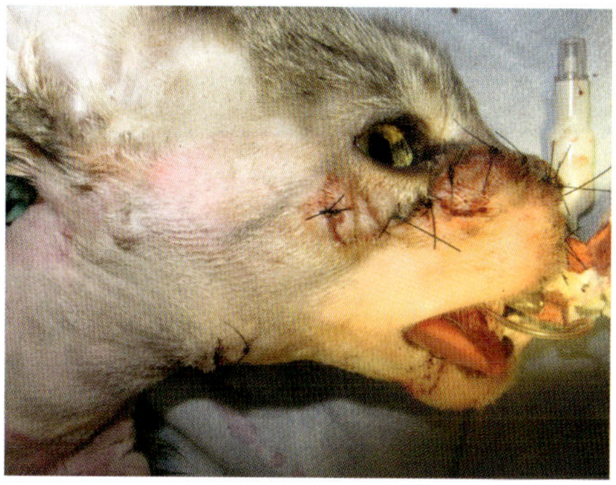

E-v)

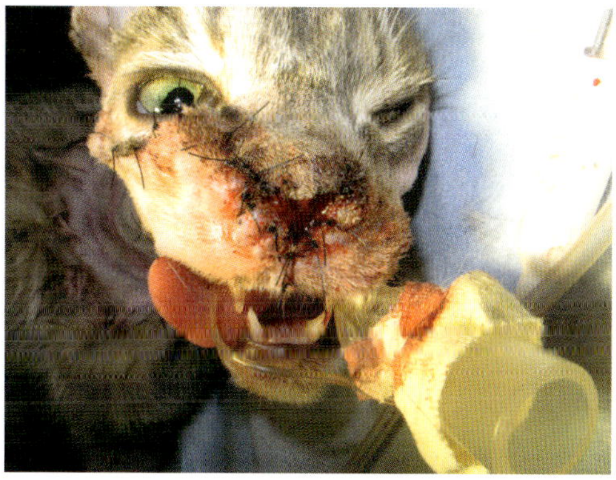

E-vi)

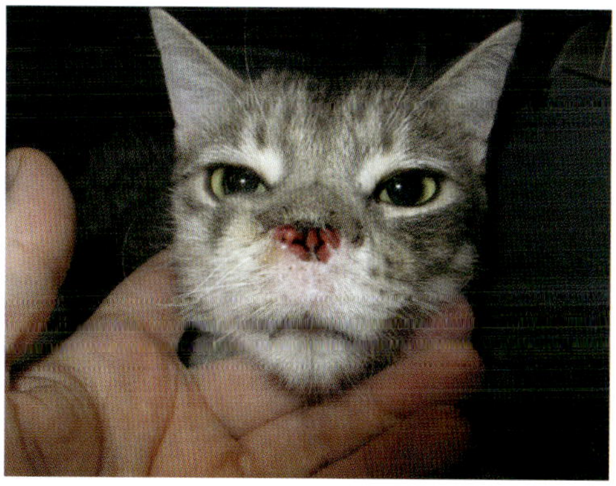

Surgical Technique (See Plate 39.2A–F) *continued*

F) If the rostral lip defect is bilateral, then bilateral advancement flaps can be used to reconstruct the defect with the rostral edges of both advancement flaps being sutured to each other in the rostral midline (i–v).

Postoperative Management

1) Multimodal analgesia
2) Elizabethan collar

Complications

- Overall: 23% for advancement subdermal plexus flaps with 16% classified as minor and 6% as major [1]
- Overall: 51% for all types of subdermal plexus flap [1]
  - Dogs: 55% overall with 39% classified as minor and 16% as major
  - Cats: 43% overall with 32% classified as minor and 11% as major
- Incisional dehiscence (30%) [1]
- Seroma (12%) [1]
- Partial necrosis of the distal extent of the flap (10%–15%) [1, 2]
- Surgical-site infection (9%) [1]

References

1 Jones, C.A. and Lipscomb, V.J. (2019). Indications, complications, and outcomes associated with subdermal plexus skin flap procedures in dogs and cats: 92 cases (2000-2017). *J. Am. Vet. Med. Assoc.* 255 (8): 933–938.
2 De Carvalho Vasconcellos, C.H., Matera, J.M., and Zaidan Dagli, M.L. (2005). Clinical evaluation of random skin flaps based on the subdermal plexus secured with sutures or sutures and cyanoacrylate adhesive for reconstructive surgery in dogs. *Vet. Surg.* 34 (1): 59–63.

Plate 39.2

Upper Lip Advancement Flap *continued*

F-i)

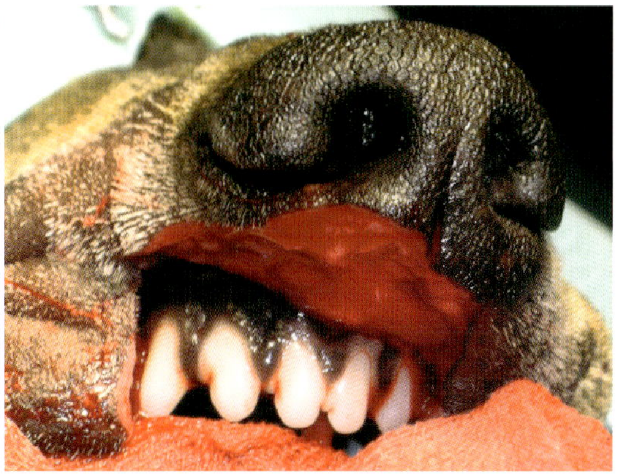

F-ii)

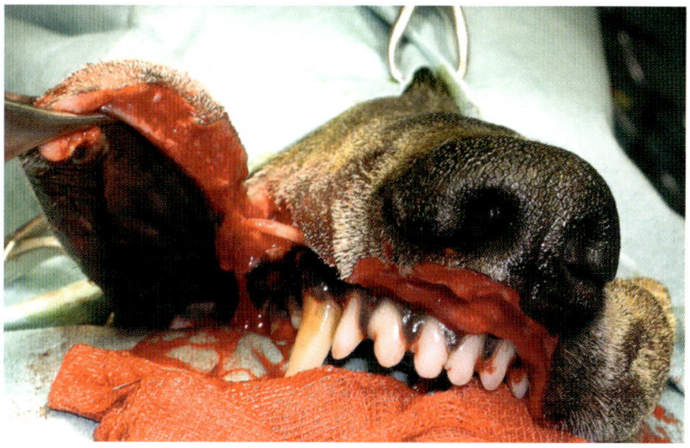

F-iii)

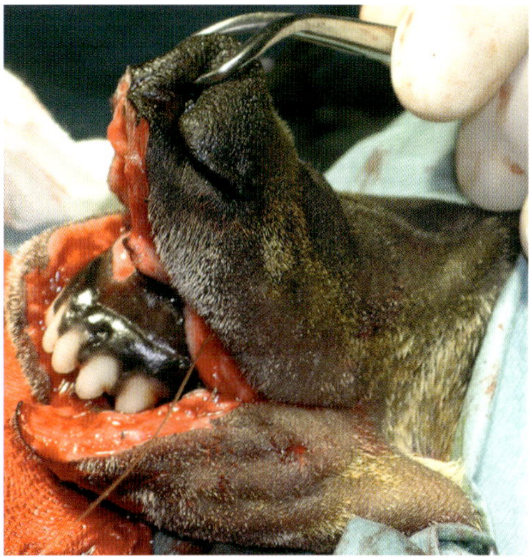

F-iv)

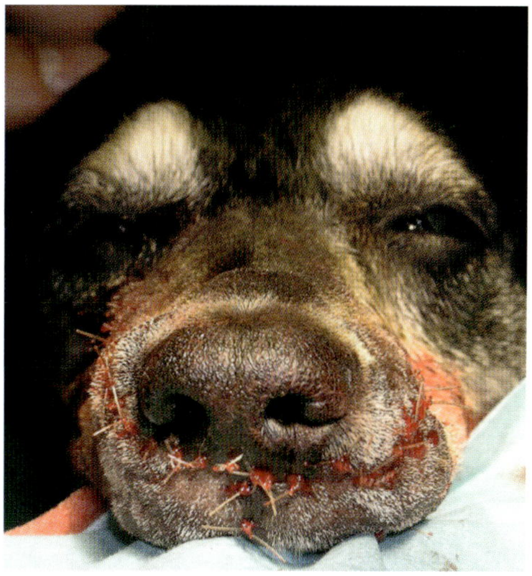

F-v)

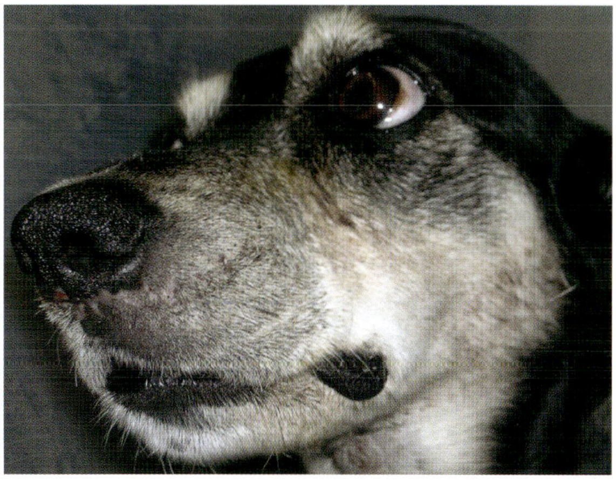

39.3 Lower Lip Advancement Flap

Indications (See Plate 39.3 – 1)

1) To reconstruct rostral lower lip defects that cannot be closed primarily (pictured, defect resulting from incisional dehiscence after wide surgical resection of a cutaneous soft tissue sarcoma)
2) A lower lip advancement flap can be combined with a mandibular incisivectomy (see *6.10. Maxillary Incisivectomy*), unilateral rostral mandibulectomy (see *6.11. Unilateral Rostral Maxillectomy*), or bilateral rostral mandibulectomy (see *6.12. Bilateral Rostral Maxillectomy*)

Patient Positioning

The patient is positioned in lateral recumbency with the affected lip uppermost for unilateral lower lip advancement flap. The patient is positioned in ventral recumbency for bilateral lower lip advancement flaps.

Surgical Technique (See Plate 39.3A–E)

A) An incision is performed starting at the caudoventral corner of the lip defect and extended caudally, either parallel to or slightly diverging from the margin of the lower lip (dashed line).
B) The incision is continued through the subcutaneous/submucosal and mucosal tissue of the lip. When performing the mucosal incision, it is important to preserve a cuff of mucosa along the mandible to allow suturing of the mucosa of the advancement flap to the mandibular mucosa.
C) The advancement flap is undermined to allow rostral advancement.
D) The rostral edge of the advancement flap is advanced into the rostral aspect of the defect.
E) Closure begins with aligning the rostral margin of the lips. The incision is closed in three layers with a simple interrupted or continuous suture pattern using monofilament absorbable suture material in the mucosal layer, a simple continuous suture pattern using monofilament absorbable suture material in the submucosal/subcutaneous layer (i), and either skin staples or an interrupted or continuous suture pattern using monofilament nonabsorbable suture material in the skin (ii). Tension-relieving sutures can be used if indicated.
F) If the rostral lip defect is bilateral, then bilateral advancement flaps can be used to reconstruct the defect with the rostral edges of both advancement flaps being sutured to each other in the rostral midline (not pictured).

Color Atlas of Canine and Feline Surgical Oncology, First Edition. Julius M. Liptak, Paolo Buracco, William T. N. Culp, and Nicholas J. Bacon.

Plate 39.3

Lower Lip Advancement Flap

1)

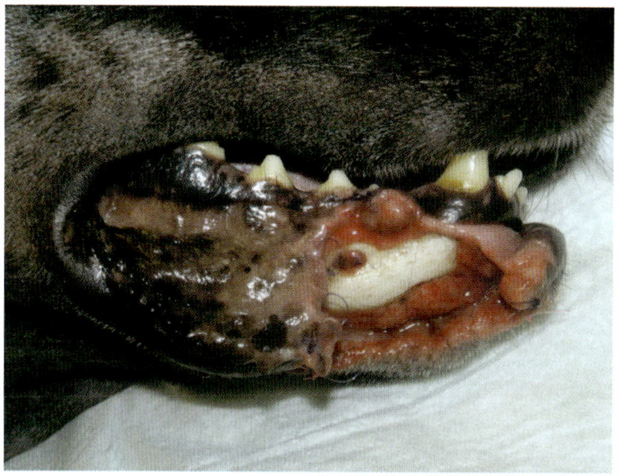

A)

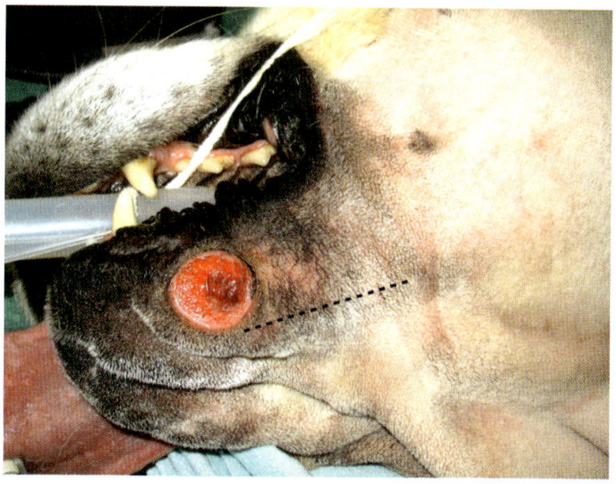

B/C)

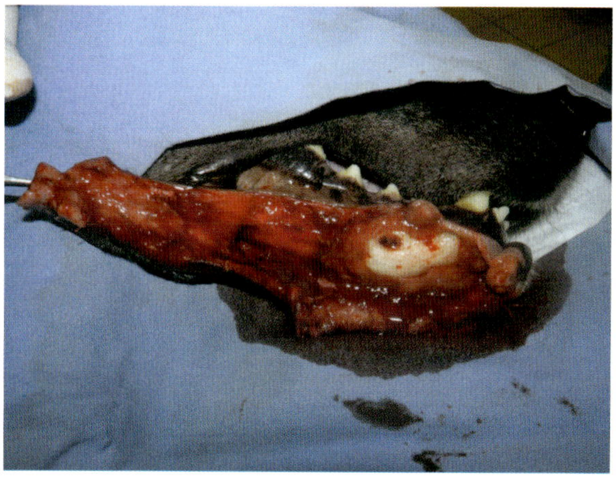

D)

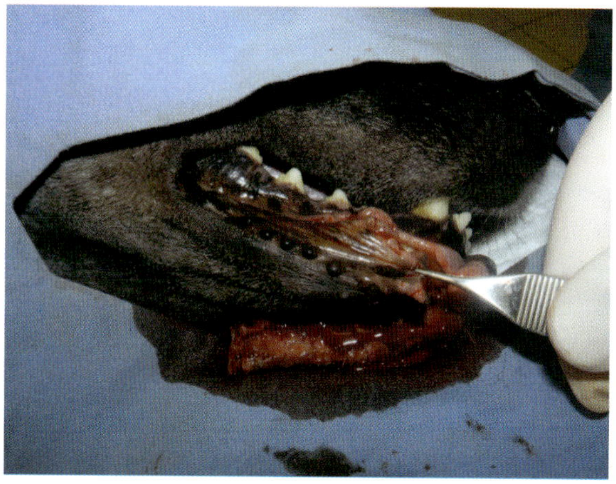

E-i)

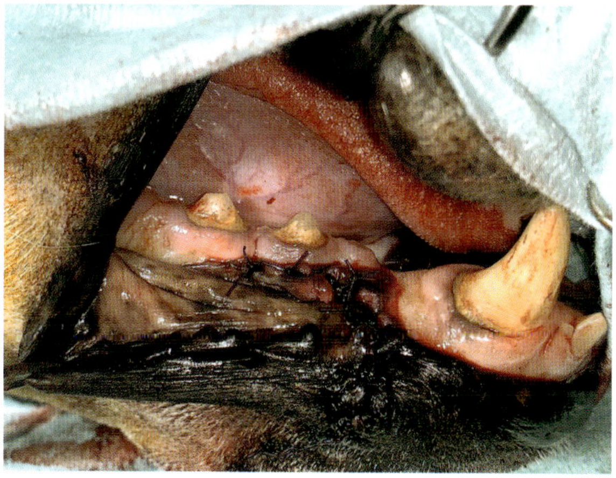

E-ii)

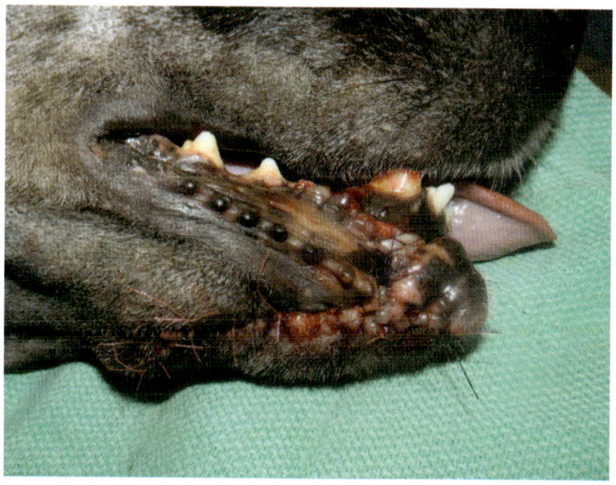

Postoperative Management

1) Multimodal analgesia
2) Elizabethan collar

Complications

- Overall: 23% for advancement subdermal plexus flaps with 16% classified as minor and 6% as major [1]
- Overall: 51% for all types of subdermal plexus flaps [1]
  - Dogs: 55% overall with 39% classified as minor and 16% as major
  - Cats: 43% overall with 32% classified as minor and 11% as major
- Incisional dehiscence (30%) [1]
- Seroma (12%) [1]
- Partial necrosis of the distal extent of the flap (10%–15%) [1, 2]
- Surgical-site infection (9%) [1]

References

1 Jones, C.A. and Lipscomb, V.J. (2019). Indications, complications, and outcomes associated with subdermal plexus skin flap procedures in dogs and cats: 92 cases (2000-2017). *J. Am. Vet. Med. Assoc.* 255 (8): 933–938.
2 De Carvalho Vasconcellos, C.H., Matera, J.M., and Zaidan Dagli, M.L. (2005). Clinical evaluation of random skin flaps based on the subdermal plexus secured with sutures or sutures and cyanoacrylate adhesive for reconstructive surgery in dogs. *Vet. Surg.* 34 (1): 59–63.

39.4 Advancement of the Commissure of the Lips

Indications (See Plate 39.4 – 1)

1) To reconstruct the caudal commissure of the lips after resection of benign (i, adenoma) or malignant tumors (ii, salivary gland carcinoma)
2) Advancement of the commissure of the lips can be combined with either unilateral subtotal (see *6.8. Unilateral Subtotal Mandibulectomy*) or total unilateral mandibulectomy (see *6.9. Unilateral Total Mandibulectomy*)

Patient Positioning

The patient is positioned in lateral recumbency with the affected side uppermost.

Surgical Technique (See Plate 39.4 A, B)

A) After tumor resection with appropriate surgical margins (i) and evaluation of the resultant defect (ii), the rostral lip margins are aligned to advance the commissure of the lips (iii).
B) The incision is closed in three layers with a simple interrupted or continuous suture pattern using monofilament absorbable suture material in the mucosal layer (i), a simple continuous suture pattern using monofilament absorbable suture material in the submucosal/subcutaneous layer, and either skin staples or an interrupted or continuous suture pattern using monofilament nonabsorbable suture material in the skin (ii, iii). Tension-relieving sutures can be used if indicated (iv).

Postoperative Management

1) Multimodal analgesia
2) Elizabethan collar

Complications

- Incisional dehiscence
- Surgical-site infection

Color Atlas of Canine and Feline Surgical Oncology, First Edition. Julius M. Liptak, Paolo Buracco, William T. N. Culp, and Nicholas J. Bacon.

Plate 39.4

Advancement of the Commissure of the Lips

1-i)

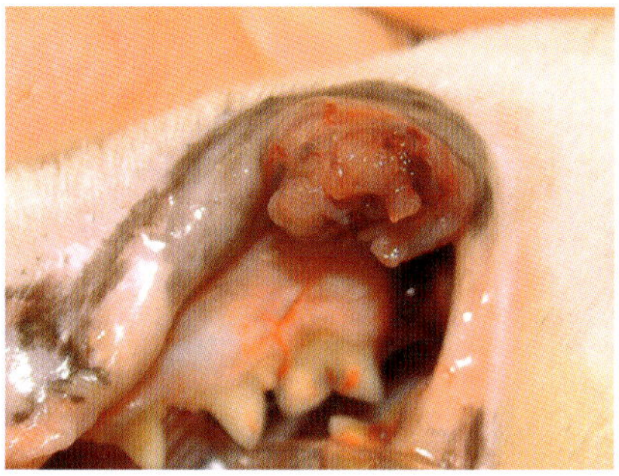

1-ii)

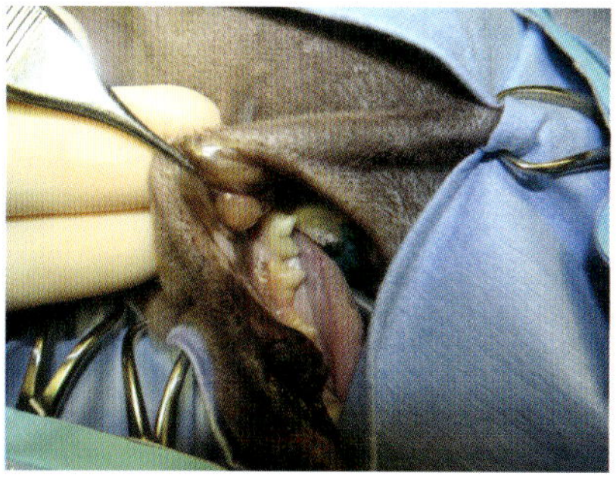

A-i)

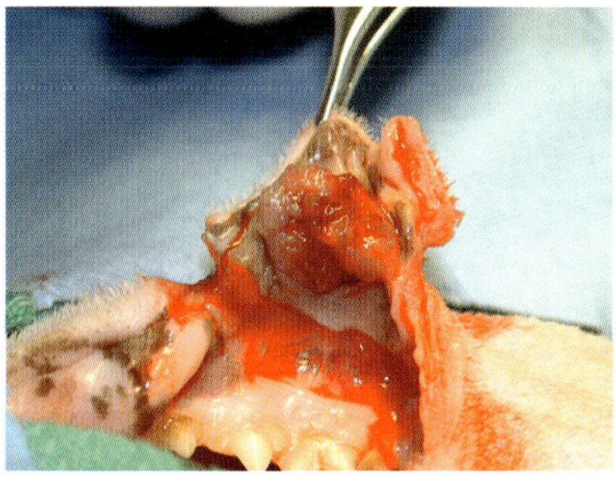

A-ii)

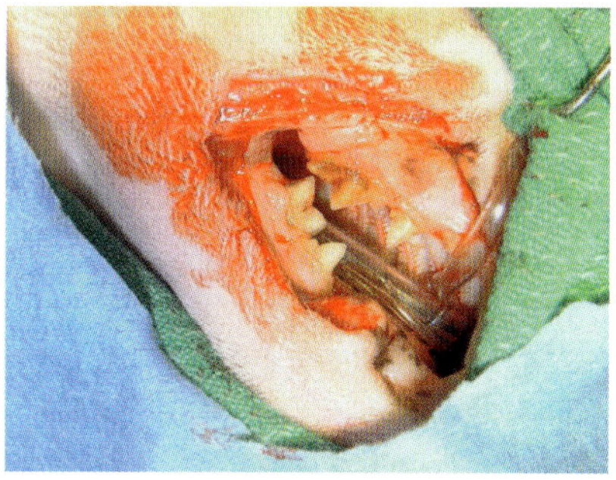

A-iii)

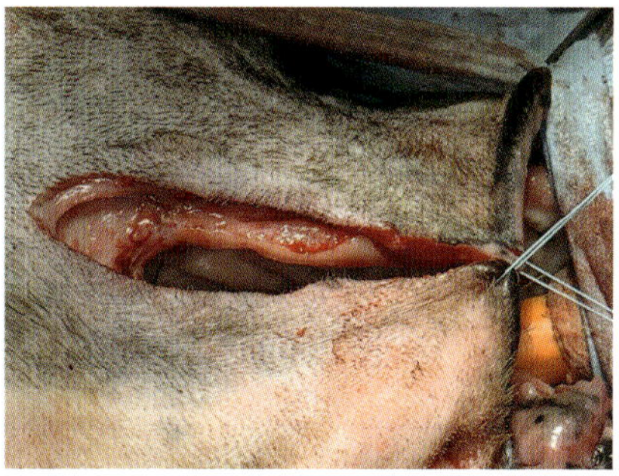

B-i)

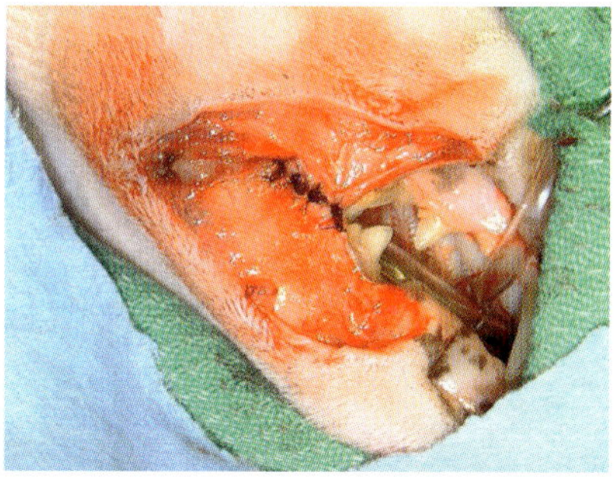

B-ii)

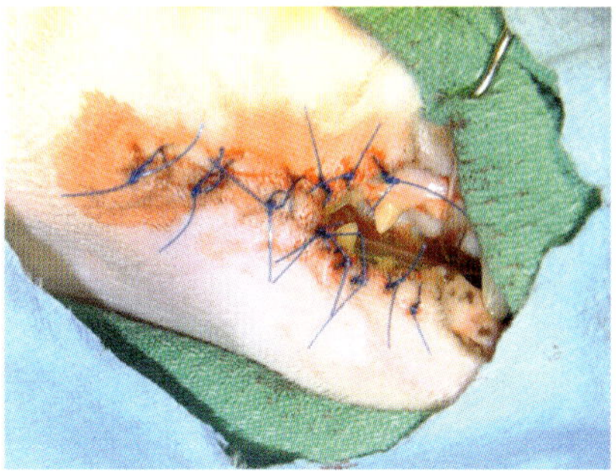

B-iii)

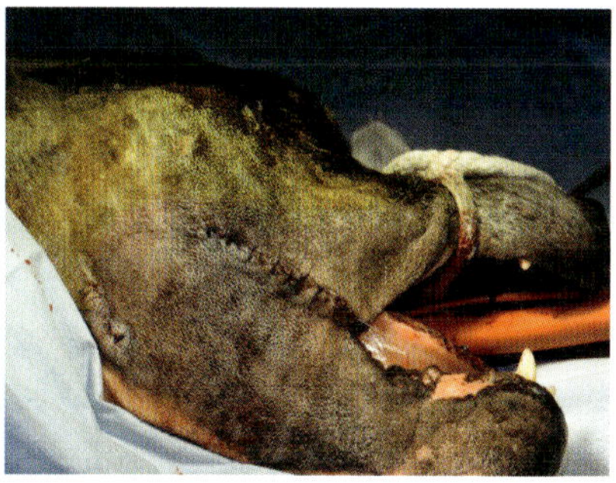

B-iv)

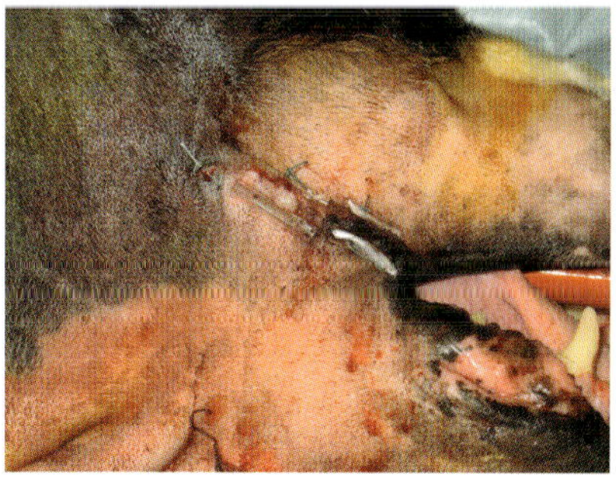

Chapter 40: Rotation Flap

General Considerations (See Plate 40A)

Subdermal plexus flaps derive their blood supply from the terminal branches of direct cutaneous vessels in the subdermal plexus at the base of the flap. Subdermal plexus flaps are classified according to their location relative to the skin defect and the method of transfer, such as advancement, transposition, and rotation flaps. These flaps are typically harvested adjacent to the wound defect, ideally in areas with loose skin so that the flap donor site can be closed primarily with minimal tension. The donor site should not have excessive motion or tension because this may result in incisional complications (e.g. seroma, dehiscence) or decreased local mobility. The shape and size of the wound defect influences the type of subdermal plexus flap used for reconstruction of the wound. Rotation flaps are indicated for reconstruction of triangular wounds, especially when skin is available on only one side of the wound (i, defect resulting from soft tissue sarcoma resection in a dog; ii, iii, preresection and postresection of a soft tissue sarcoma in a dog).

Color Atlas of Canine and Feline Surgical Oncology, First Edition. Julius M. Liptak, Paolo Buracco, William T. N. Culp, and Nicholas J. Bacon.

Plate 40

Rotation Flap

A-i)

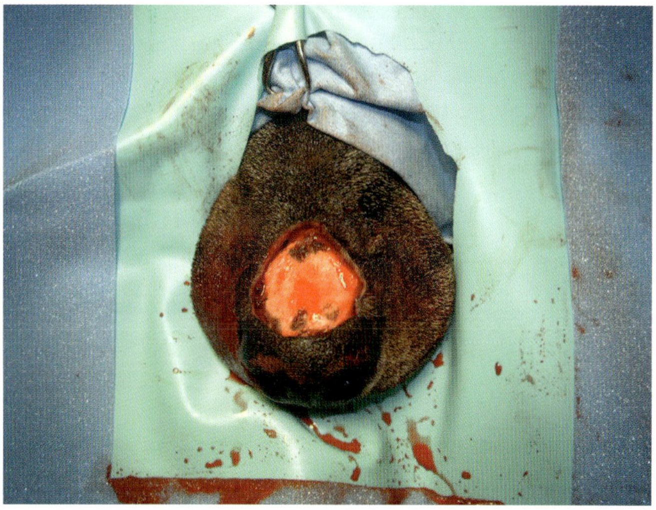

A-ii)

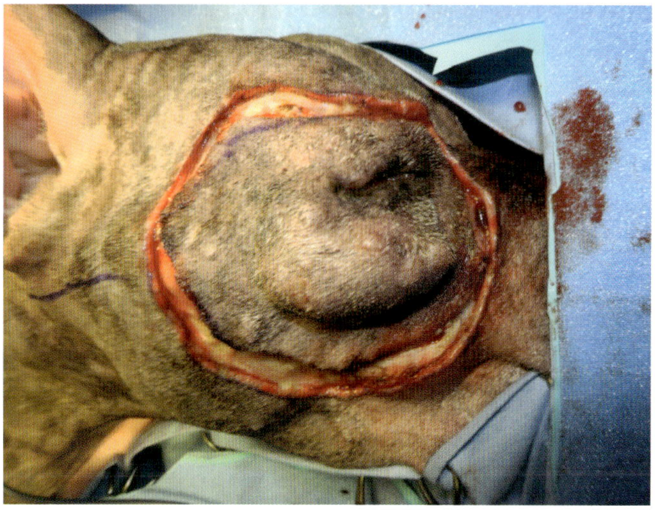

A-iii)

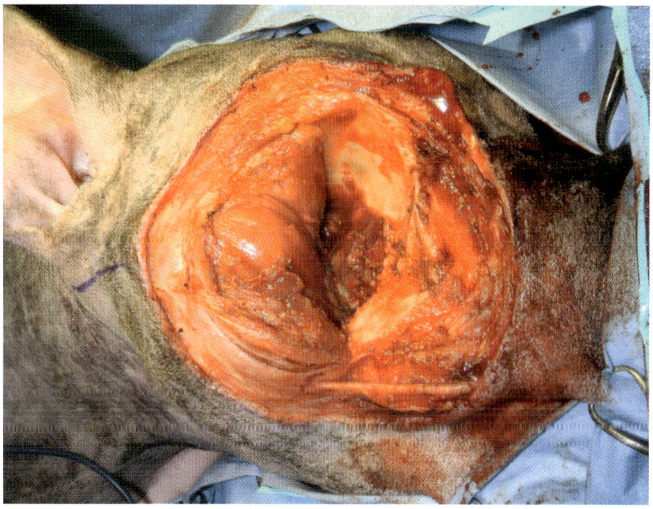

Surgical Technique (See Plate 40B–D)

B) A semicircular incision is made extending from a common border with the wound defect (i, ii).
C) The rotation flap is undermined starting from the edge of the flap bordering the wound defect. The flap should be undermined below the cutaneous trunci or platysma muscle to preserve the subdermal plexus.
D) The distant edge of the rotation flap is rotated into the opposite corner of the defect (i). The skin incisions are closed routinely in two layers with a simple continuous suture pattern using monofilament absorbable suture material in the subcutis and either skin staples or an interrupted or continuous suture pattern using monofilament nonabsorbable suture material in the skin (ii–iv). Tension-relieving sutures can be used if indicated.

Postoperative Management

1) Multimodal analgesia
2) Elizabethan collar
3) ± Tie-over bandage

Complications

- Overall: 56% overall for rotation subdermal plexus flaps with 56% classified as minor and 0% as major [1]
- Overall: 51% for all types of subdermal plexus flap [1]
  - Dogs: 55% overall with 39% classified as minor and 16% as major
  - Cats: 43% overall with 32% classified as minor and 11% as major
- Incisional dehiscence (30%) [1]
- Seroma (12%) [1]
- Partial necrosis of the distal extent of the flap (E) (10%–15%) [1, 2]
- Surgical-site infection (9%) [1]

References

1 De Carvalho Vasconcellos, C.H., Matera, J.M., and Zaidan Dagli, M.L. (2005). Clinical evaluation of random skin flaps based on the subdermal plexus secured with sutures or sutures and cyanoacrylate adhesive for reconstructive surgery in dogs. *Vet. Surg.* 34 (1): 59–63.
2 Jones, C.A. and Lipscomb, V.J. (2019). Indications, complications, and outcomes associated with subdermal plexus skin flap procedures in dogs and cats: 92 cases (2000-2017). *J. Am. Vet. Med. Assoc.* 255 (8): 933–938.

Plate 40

Rotation Flap *continued*

B-i)

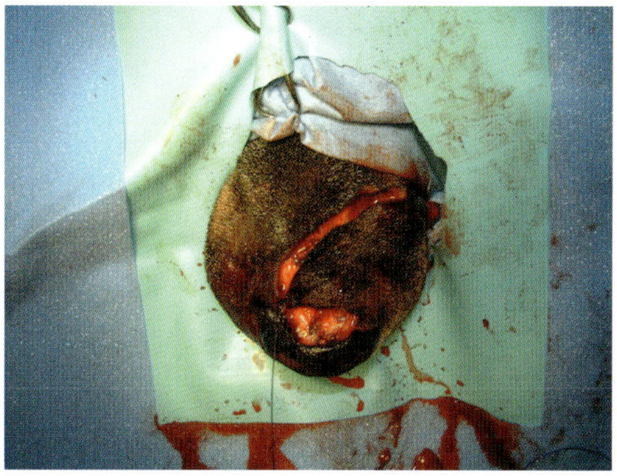

B-ii)

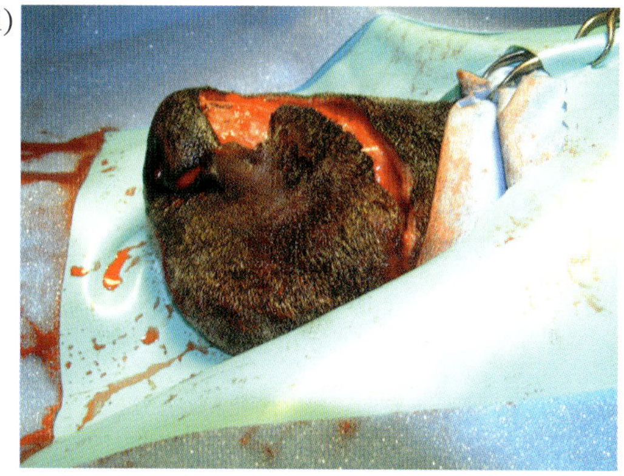

C)

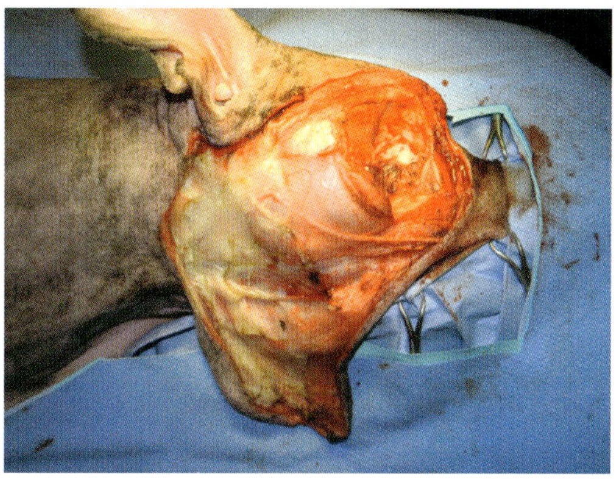

D-i)

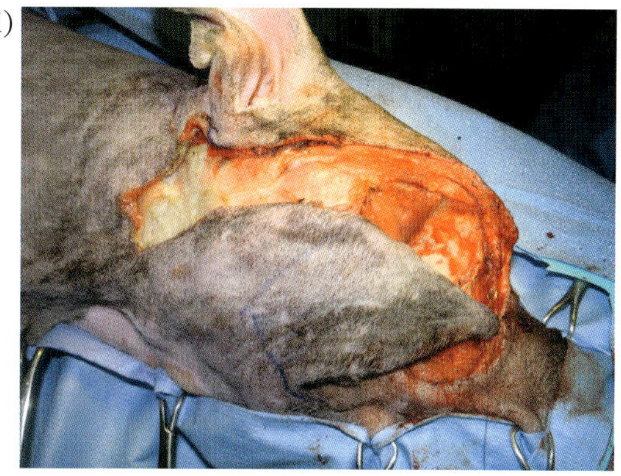

D-ii)

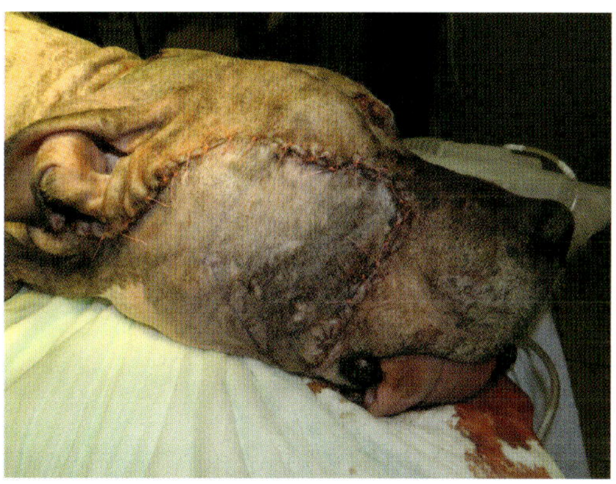

D-iii)

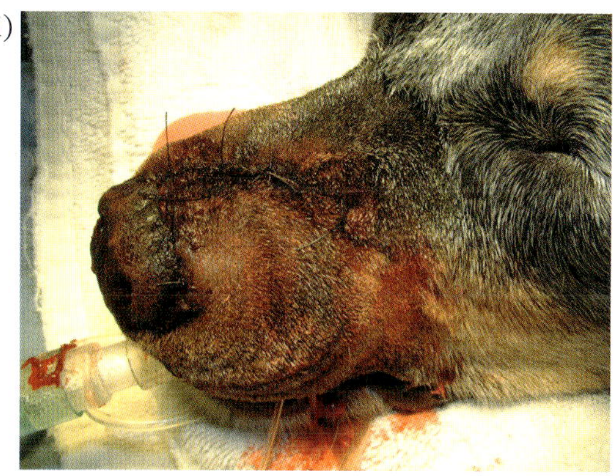

D-iv)

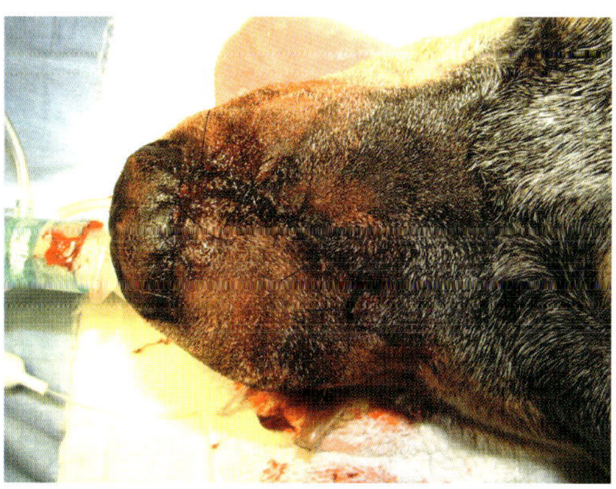

E)

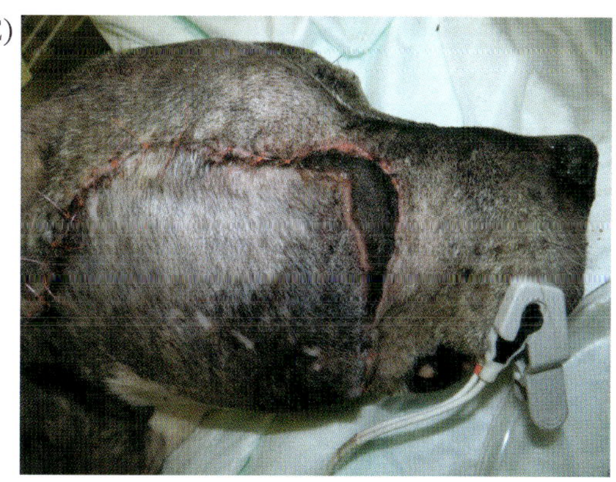

Chapter 41: Transposition Flap

41.1 General Transposition Flaps

General Considerations

Subdermal plexus flaps derive their blood supply from the terminal branches of direct cutaneous vessels in the subdermal plexus at the base of the flap. Subdermal plexus flaps are classified according to their location relative to the skin defect and the method of transfer, such as advancement, transposition, and rotation flaps. These flaps are typically harvested from adjacent to the wound defect, ideally in areas with loose skin so that the flap donor site can be closed primarily with minimal tension. The donor site should not have excessive motion or tension because this may result in incisional complications (e.g. seroma, dehiscence) or decreased local mobility. The shape and size of the wound defect influences the type of subdermal plexus flap used for reconstruction of the wound. A transposition flap is a versatile flap that can be used to reconstruct variously shaped wounds.

Surgical Technique (See Plate 41.1A–C)

A) A transposition flap is a rectangular subdermal plexus flap created within 90 degrees of the long axis of the defect. The width of the flap (dotted line) is equal to the width of the defect. The length of the flap is equal to the distance from the pivot point of the flap to the most distant point of the defect (dashed line).
B) The transposition flap is undermined starting from the edge of the flap bordering the wound defect. The flap should be undermined below the cutaneous trunci or platysma muscle to preserve the subdermal plexus (i, ii).

Color Atlas of Canine and Feline Surgical Oncology, First Edition. Julius M. Liptak, Paolo Buracco, William T. N. Culp, and Nicholas J. Bacon.

Plate 41.1

General Transposition Flaps

A)

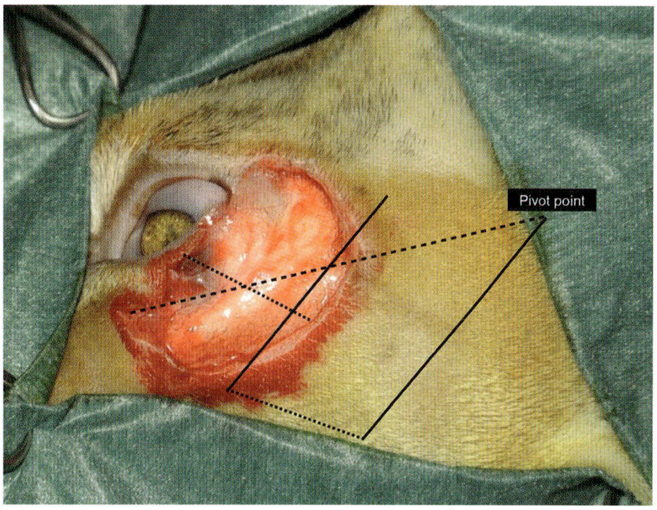

B-i)

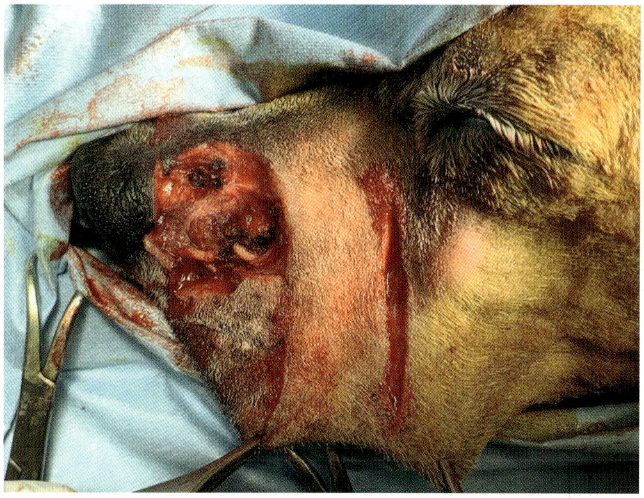

B-ii)

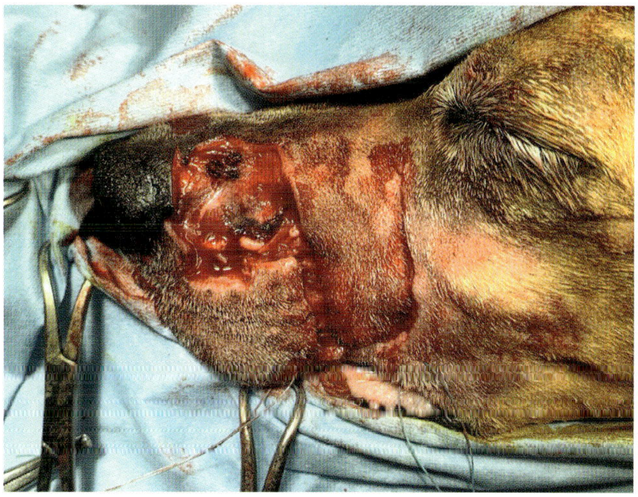

Surgical Technique (See Plate 41.1A–C) *continued*

C) The transposition flap is transposed into the wound defect (i). The skin incisions are closed routinely in two layers with a simple continuous suture pattern using monofilament absorbable suture material in the subcutis and either skin staples or an interrupted or continuous suture pattern using monofilament nonabsorbable suture material in the skin (ii, iii, 45-degree rotation; iv, postoperative appearance; v, 90-degree rotation; vi, postoperative appearance). Tension-relieving sutures can be used if indicated.

Postoperative Management

1) Multimodal analgesia
2) Elizabethan collar
3) ± Tie-over bandage

Complications

- Overall: 33% for transposition subdermal plexus flaps with 0% classified as minor and 33% as major [1]
- Overall: 51% overall for all types of subdermal plexus flaps [1]
  - Dogs: 55% overall with 39% classified as minor and 16% as major
  - Cats: 43% overall with 32% classified as minor and 11% as major
- Incisional dehiscence (30%) [1]
- Seroma (12%) [1]
- Partial necrosis of the distal extent of the flap (10–15%) [1, 2]
- Surgical-site infection (9%) [1]

References

1 Jones, C.A. and Lipscomb, V.J. (2019). Indications, complications, and outcomes associated with subdermal plexus skin flap procedures in dogs and cats: 92 cases (2000-2017). *J. Am. Vet. Med. Assoc.* 255 (8): 933–938.

2 De Carvalho Vasconcellos, C.H., Matera, J.M., and Zaidan Dagli, M.L. (2005). Clinical evaluation of random skin flaps based on the subdermal plexus secured with sutures or sutures and cyanoacrylate adhesive for reconstructive surgery in dogs. *Vet. Surg.* 34 (1): 59–63.

Plate 41.1

General Transposition Flaps *continued*

C-i)

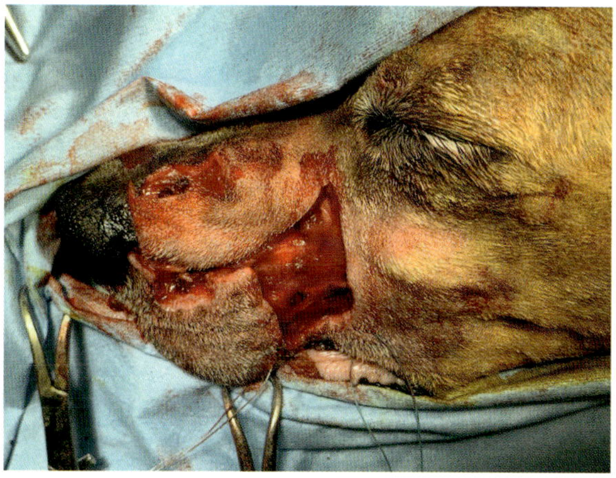

C-ii)

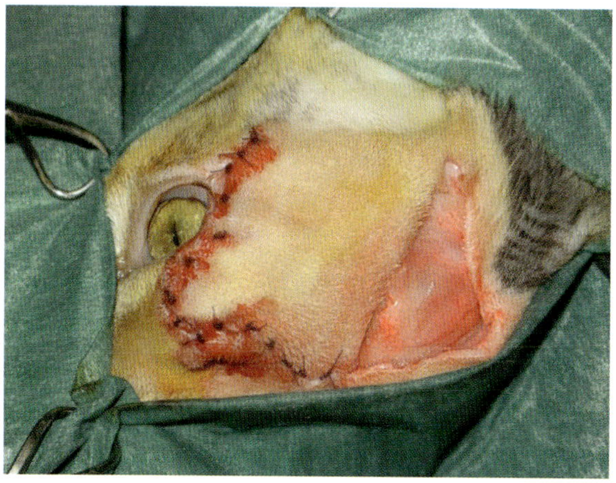

C-iii)

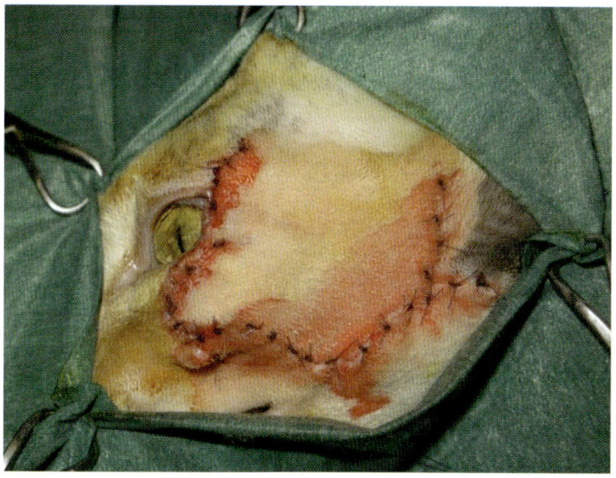

C-iv)

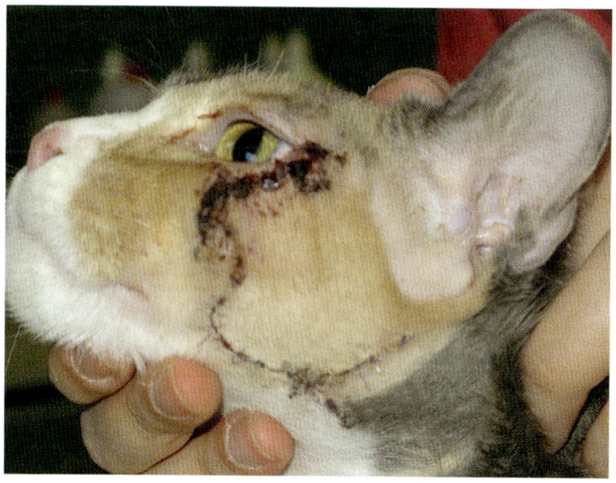

C-v)

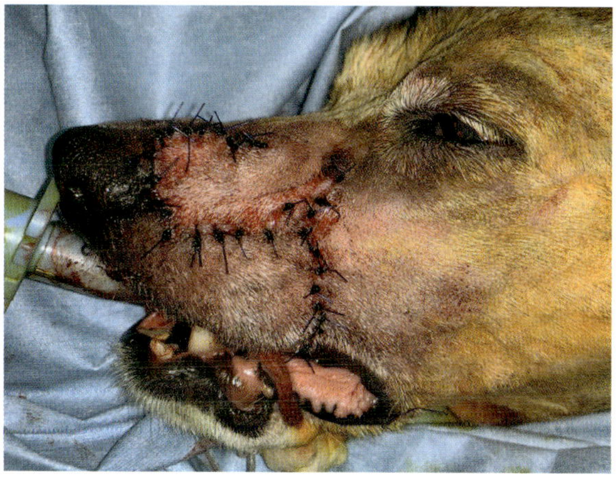

C-vi)

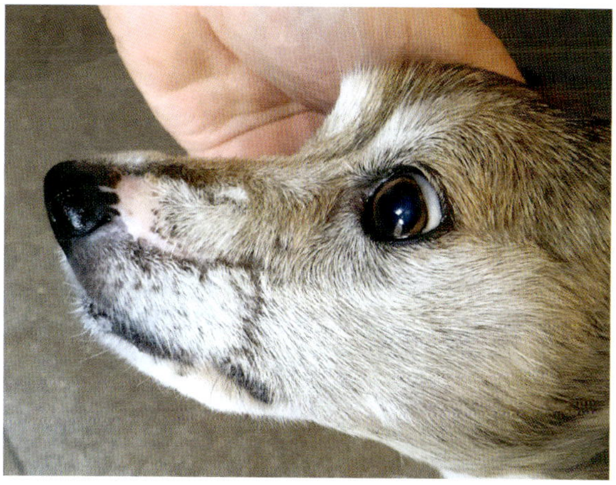

41.2 Filleted Digit Pad Transposition Flap

Indications

1) Reconstruction of the metacarpal/metatarsal pad postresection
2) Filleted digit pad transfer is combined with amputation of one or both of digits II and/or V (see *36.1. Single-Digit Amputation*)

Surgical Technique (See Plate 41.2A–E)

A) The filleted digit pad can be harvested either before or after resection of the palmar/plantar tumor and part or all of the metacarpal/metatarsal pad. The digit to be filleted depends on whether a partial or total metacarpal/metatarsal pad resection has been performed and, if partial, whether the medial or lateral aspect of the metacarpal/metatarsal pad has been resected. A medial partial metacarpal/metatarsal pad resection is reconstructed with a filleted digit pad transfer from digit II, a lateral partial metacarpal/metatarsal pad resection (i, ii) is reconstructed with a filleted digit pad transfer from digit V, and a total metacarpal/metatarsal pad resection is reconstructed with a filleted digit pad transfer from both digits II and V (iii, iv).
B) An incision is performed along the desired aspect of the appropriate digit to the level of the digit pad (i) and circumferentially around the subungual crest (ii).

Color Atlas of Canine and Feline Surgical Oncology, First Edition. Julius M. Liptak, Paolo Buracco, William T. N. Culp, and Nicholas J. Bacon.

Plate 41.2

Filleted Digit Pad Transposition Flap

A-i)

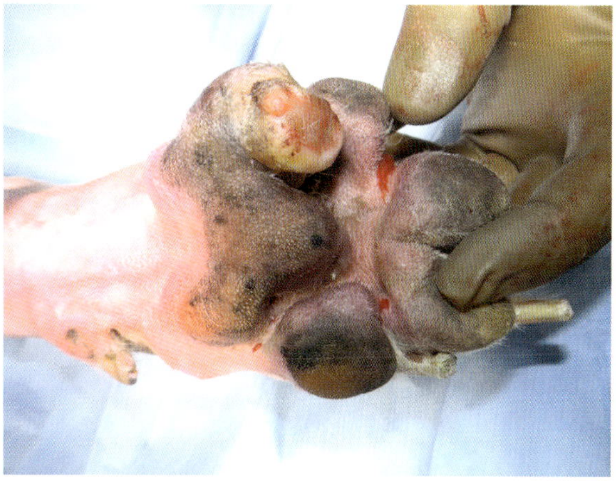

A-ii)

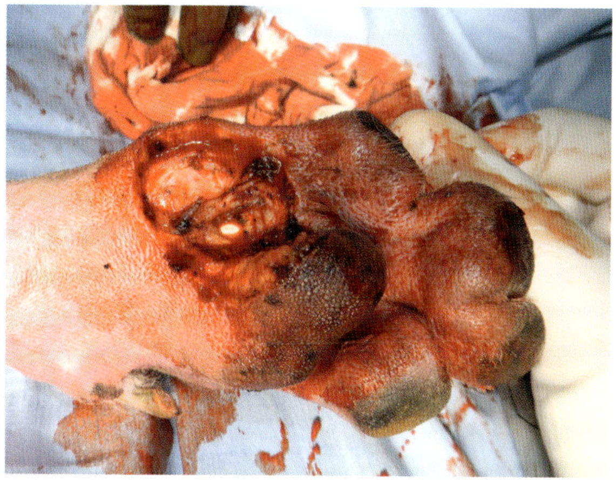

A-iii)

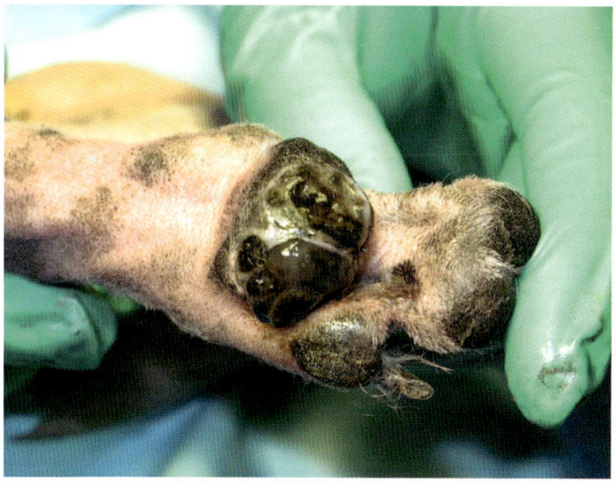

A-iv)

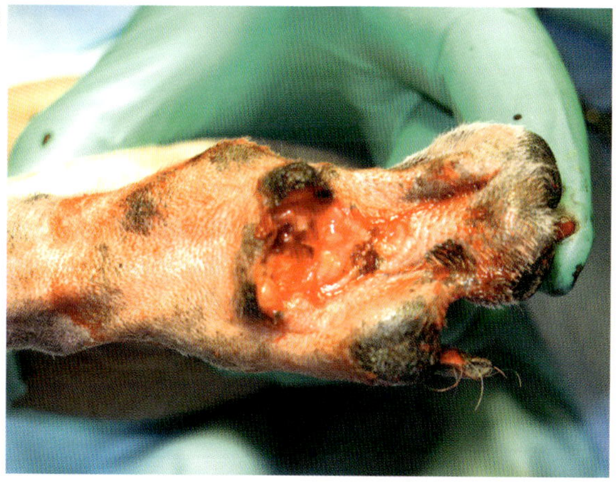

B-i)

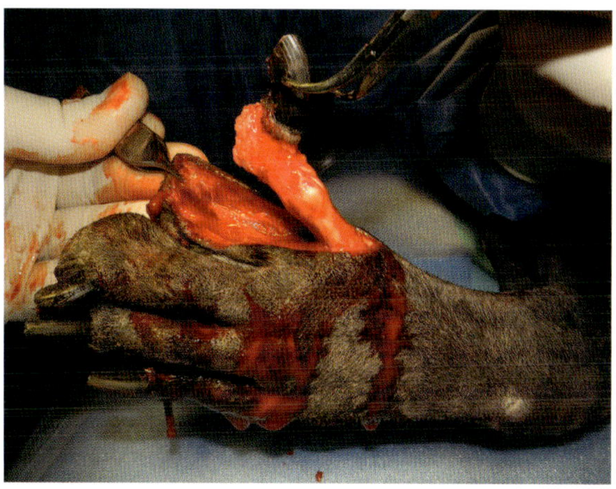

B-ii)

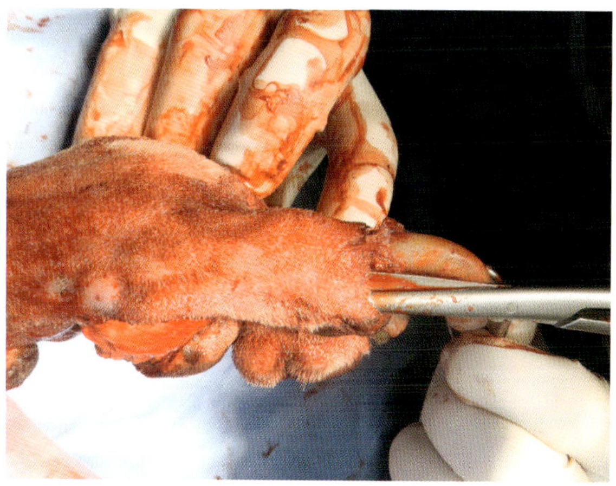

Surgical Technique (See Plate 41.2A–E) *continued*

C) The nail and first through third phalangeal bones are dissected free of all attached soft tissues (i, ii). The proximal level of the filleted bone is either disarticulation of the metacarpophalangeal/metatarsophalangeal joint or, preferably, osteotomy through the distal aspect of the appropriate metacarpal/tarsal bone (iii). The filleted bone segment is removed either en bloc or after segmental disarticulation of one or more of the interphalangeal joints. The filleted bone is removed from the surgical field (iv).

D) The digit pad is then transferred into the metacarpal/metatarsal pad defect (i, ii).

Plate 41.2

Filleted Digit Pad Transposition Flap *continued*

C-i)

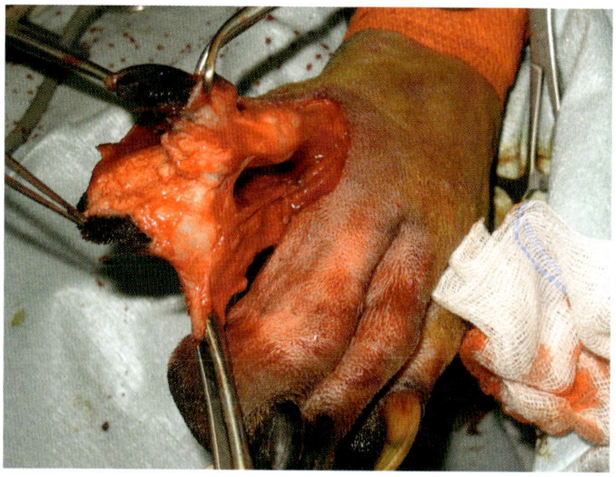

C-ii)

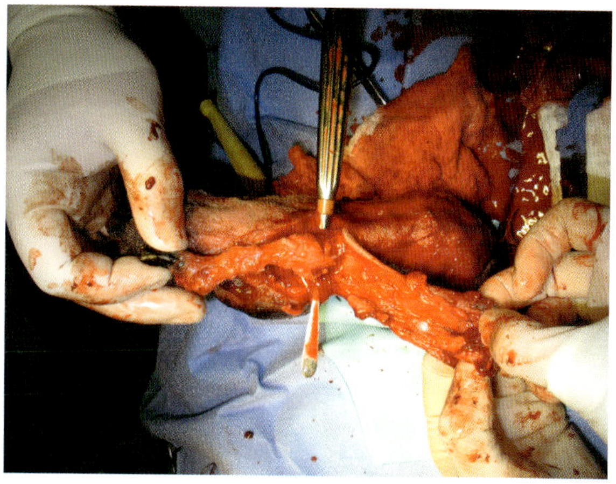

C-iii)

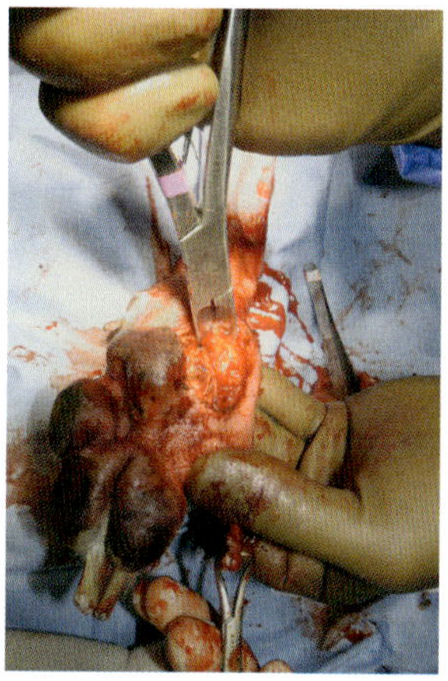

C-iv)

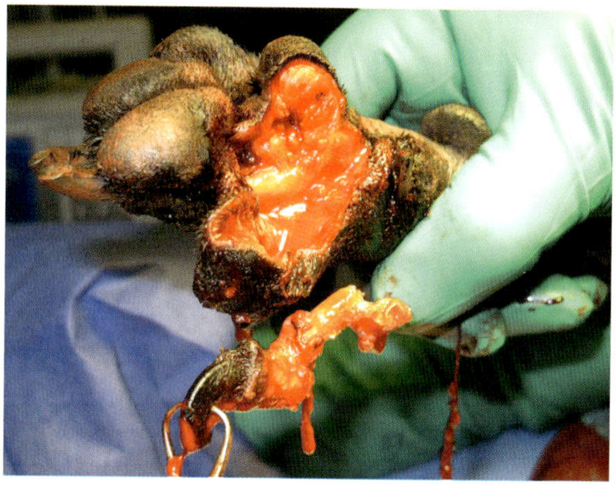

D-i)

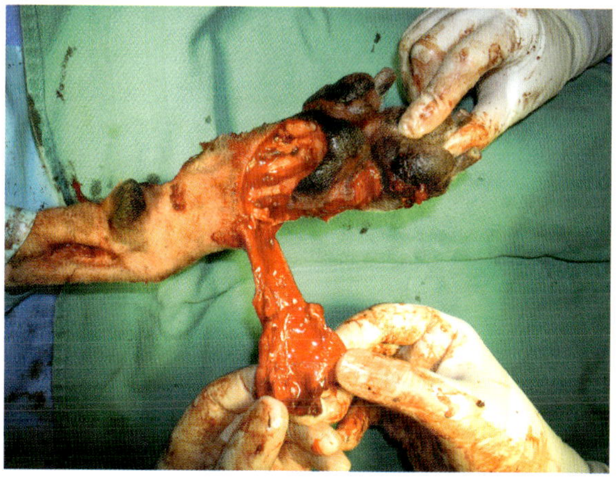

D-ii)

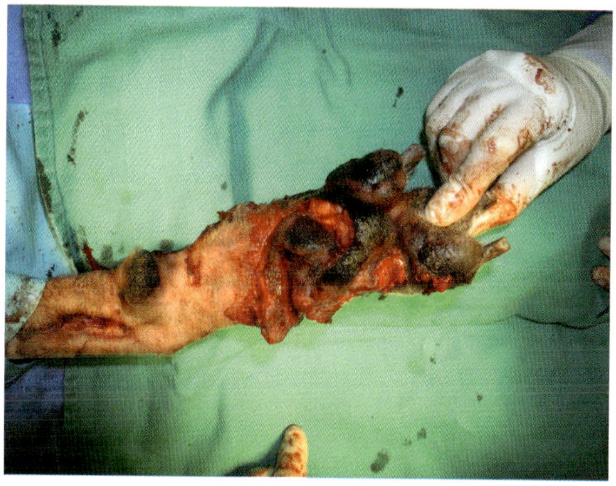

Surgical Technique (See Plate 41.2A–E) *continued*

E) The skin incision is closed routinely in two layers with a simple continuous suture pattern using monofilament absorbable suture material in the subcutis and an interrupted suture pattern using monofilament nonabsorbable suture material in the skin and/or pad (i–iv). The skin defect at the site of the nail is closed with an interrupted suture pattern using monofilament nonabsorbable suture material.

Postoperative Management

1) Multimodal analgesia
2) Elizabethan collar
3) Soft padded bandage for 14 days

Complications

- Incisional dehiscence
- Surgical-site infection
- Partial necrosis of the distal extent of the flap
- Pain and lameness

Plate 41.2

Filleted Digit Pad Transposition Flap *continued*

E-i)

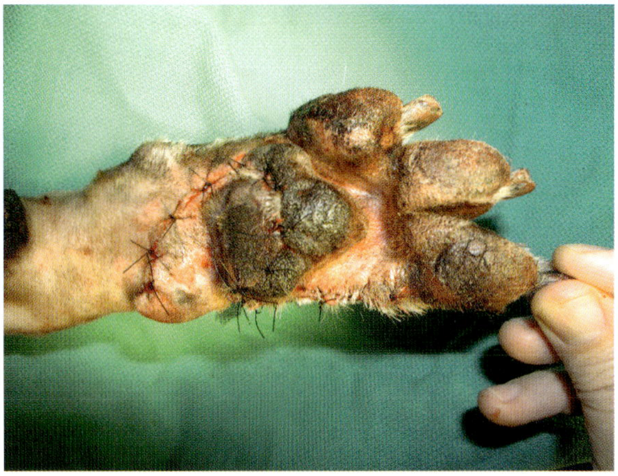

E-ii)

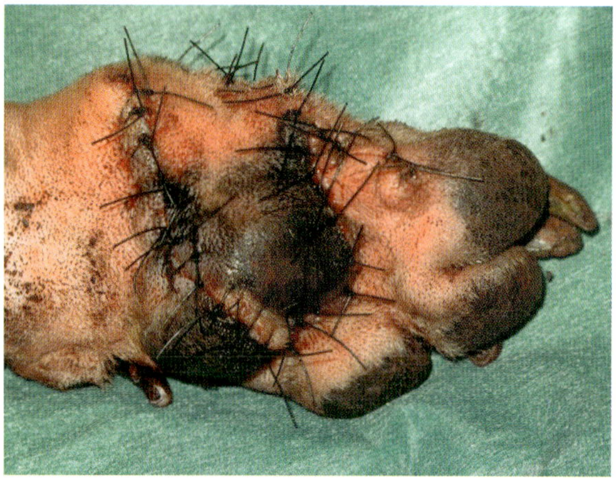

E-iii)

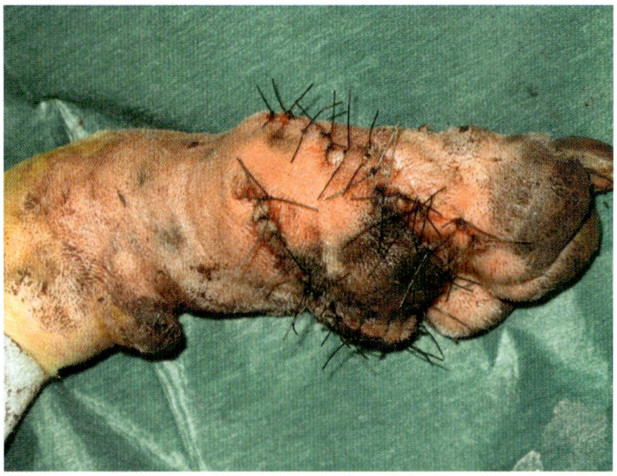

E-iv)

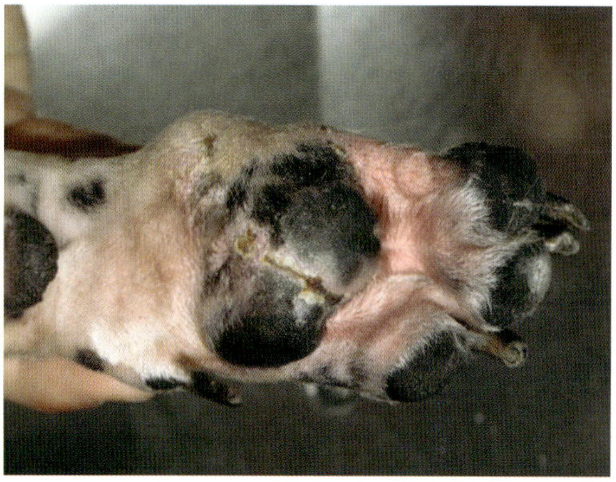

41.3 Lip-to-Eyelid Transposition Flap

Indication

1) To reconstruct part or all of the lower eyelid after en bloc resection of an eyelid tumor

Patient Positioning

The patient is positioned in lateral recumbency with the affected side uppermost.

Surgical Technique [1] (See Plate 41.3A–C, E–G, I)

A) A skin incision is made starting at (i, arrow) or rostral (ii, arrow) to the caudal commissure of the lips and angled at 45–50 degrees to a line connecting the medial and lateral canthus.
B) A second skin incision is made rostral and parallel to the first incision. The distance between these two incisions is equal to the width of the eyelid defect.
C) The mucocutaneous junction of the lip between the rostral and caudal incisions is preserved to reconstruct the eyelid. A transverse incision is made on the mucosal side of the lip dorsal to the lip margin (arrow), and the mucosa dorsal to the transverse incision is dissected away from the remainder of the flap (dashed arrow) and discarded.
D) The skin incisions are continued deeply through the labial mucosa to create a full-thickness lip flap. Alternatively, the labial mucosa can be preserved and just the skin and labial mucocutaneous junction can be used for the transposition flap (not pictured). The flap is carefully undermined in a ventral-to-dorsal direction.
E) The cranial incision is extended to the eyelid defect as a bridging incision (arrow), minimizing dissection of the submucosa to preserve the regional vasculature.
F) The flap is transposed in a rostrodorsal direction into the wound defect.

Color Atlas of Canine and Feline Surgical Oncology, First Edition. Julius M. Liptak, Paolo Buracco, William T. N. Culp, and Nicholas J. Bacon.

Plate 41.3

Lip-to-Eyelid Transposition Flap

A-i/B)

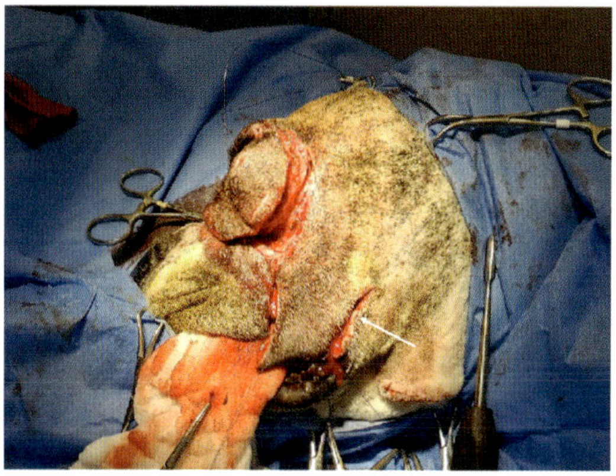

Courtesy of Dr. Bart Van Goethem

A-ii/B)

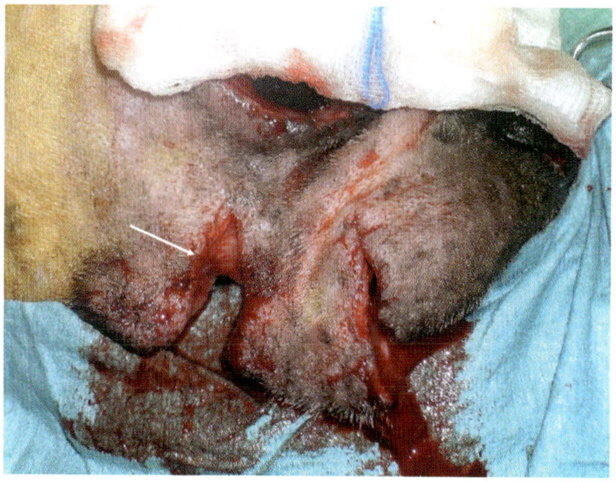

C)

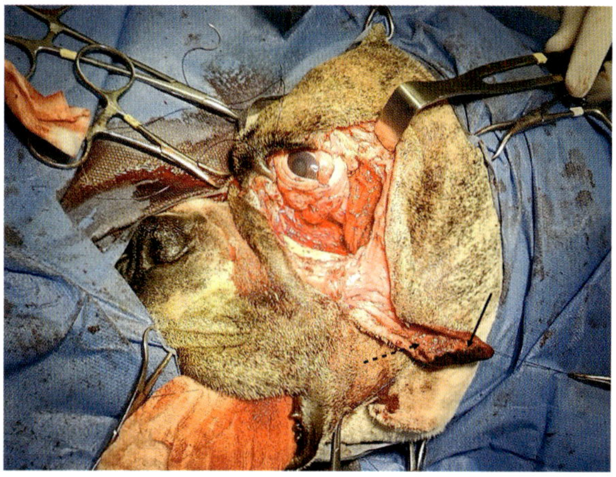

Courtesy of Dr. Bart Van Goethem

E)

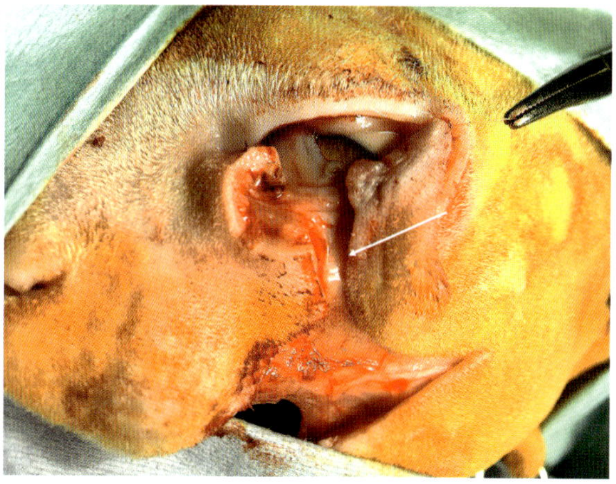

F)

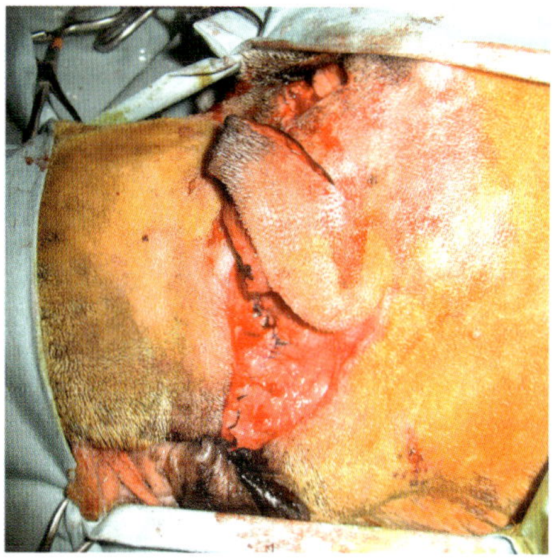

Surgical Technique [1] (See Plate 41.3A–C, E–G, I) *continued*

G) The lower eyelid is reconstructed by suturing the rostral (i) and caudal (ii) corners of the lip margin of the flap to the rostral and caudal aspects, respectively, of the lower eyelid defect with 5-0 to 3-0 monofilament or coated multifilament absorbable suture material.

H) For the donor site, the labial mucosa is closed with a submucosal simple continuous suture pattern using monofilament absorbable suture material (see step F). Ideally, suture material should not include the mucosa.

I) The skin incisions of the flap and donor site are then closed routinely in two layers with a simple continuous suture pattern using monofilament absorbable suture material in the subcutis and an interrupted or continuous suture pattern using monofilament nonabsorbable suture material in the skin (i–iii, immediately postoperatively; iv, 2 weeks postoperatively).

Postoperative Management

1) Multimodal analgesia
2) Elizabethan collar
3) Artificial tears

Complications

- Partial necrosis of the distal extent of the flap (24% in dogs [1] and 20% in cats [2])
- Partial incisional dehiscence
- Thickening of the border of the reconstructed eyelid
- Ocular discharge
- Keratoconjunctivitis sicca (rare)

References

1 Pavletic, M.M., Nafe, L.A., and Confer, A.W. (1982). Mucocutaneous subdermal plexus flap from the lip for lower eyelid restoration in the dog. *J. Am. Vet. Med. Assoc.* 180 (8): 921–926.

2 Hunt, G.B. (2006). Use of the lip-to-lid flap for replacement of the lower eyelid in five cats. *Vet. Surg.* 35 (3): 284–286.

Plate 41.3

Lip-to-Eyelid Transposition Flap *continued*

G-i)

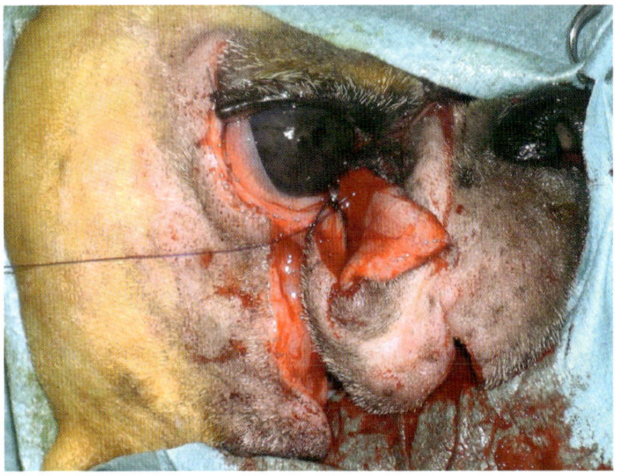

G-ii)

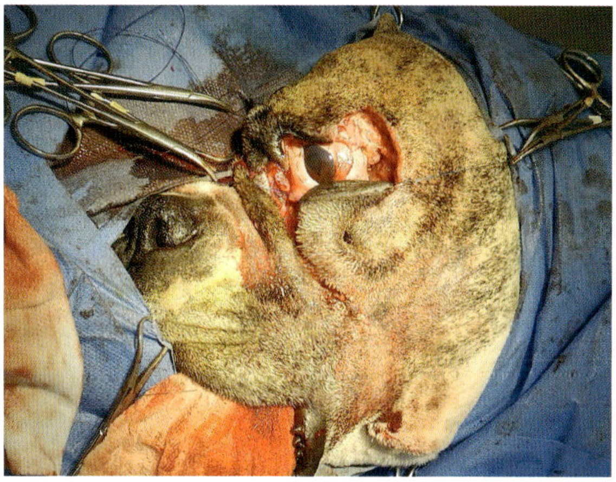

Courtesy of Dr. Bart Van Goethem

I-i)

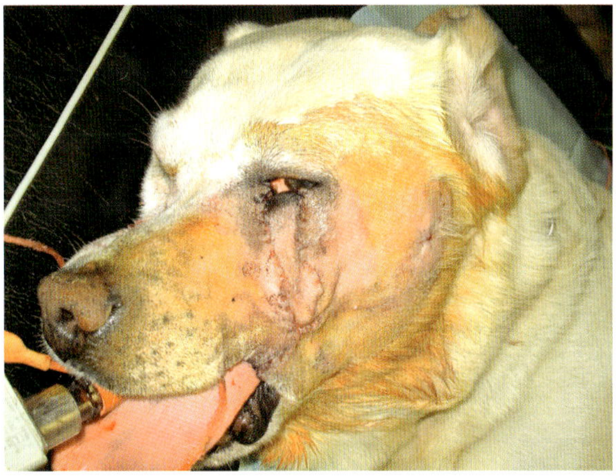

I-ii)

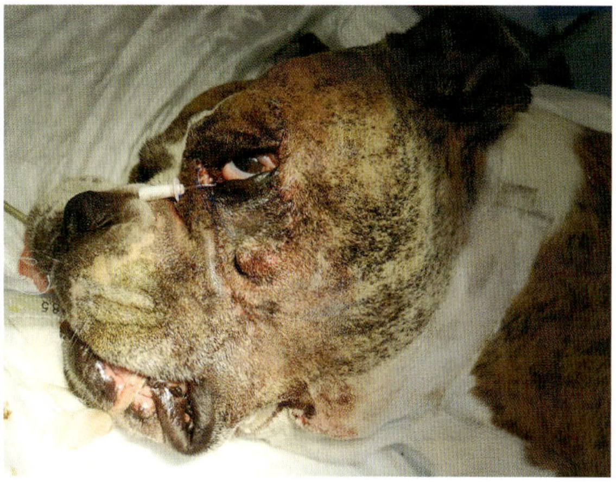

Courtesy of Dr. Bart Van Goethem

I-iii)

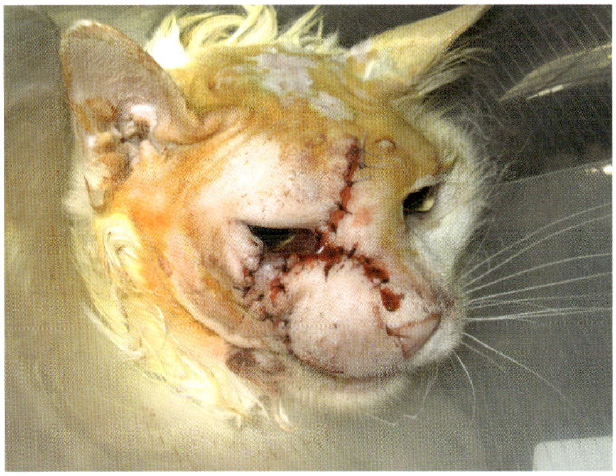

I-iv)

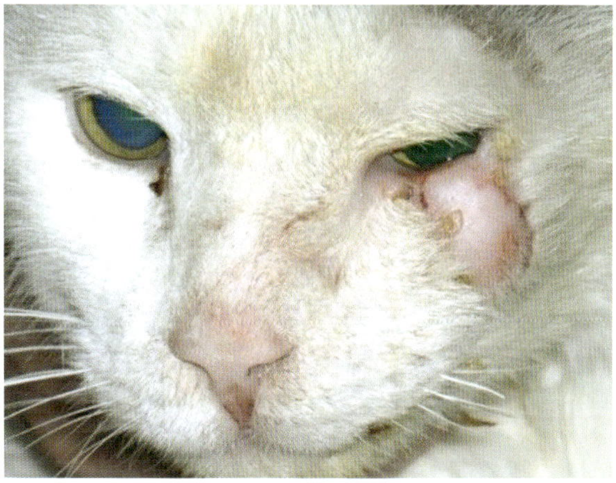

41.4 Lip-to-Nose Transposition Flap

Indication

1) Reconstruction of defects of the rostrodorsal or dorsolateral nasal planum

Patient Positioning

The patient is positioned in either sternal or lateral recumbency, depending on the location of the defect, with the affected side uppermost.

Surgical Technique [1] (See Plate 41.4A–E, G)

A) A skin incision is made, starting at the ventral lip margin and angled at 45–50 degrees (dashed line A) to a line connecting the medial and lateral canthus (dashed line B). A second skin incision is made rostral and parallel to the first incision (dashed line C). The distance between these two incisions is equal to the width of the nasal planum defect. The length of the skin is equal to the distance from the pivot point of the flap to the most distant point of the defect (see *41.1. General Transposition Flaps*).

B) The skin incisions are continued deeply through the labial mucosa to create a full-thickness lip flap. Alternatively, the labial mucosa can be preserved and just the skin can be used for the transposition flap (not pictured).

C) The mucocutaneous junction of the lip between the rostral and caudal incisions is preserved to reconstruct a nasal planum mucosal defect; however, this is not required if there is no mucosal defect to reconstruct. Preservation of the lip margin (i, ii) can be done by performing a transverse incision on the mucosal side of the lip dorsal to the lip margin (arrow), and the mucosa dorsal to the transverse incision is dissected away from the remainder of the flap and discarded.

D) The flap is carefully undermined in a ventral-to-dorsal direction and then transposed into the wound defect in a rostrodorsal direction, either directly if the donor site is adjacent to the wound defect (i) or via a bridging incision if the wound defect is not adjacent to the donor site (ii, arrow).

Color Atlas of Canine and Feline Surgical Oncology, First Edition. Julius M. Liptak, Paolo Buracco, William T. N. Culp, and Nicholas J. Bacon.

Plate 41.4

Lip-to-Nose Transposition Flap

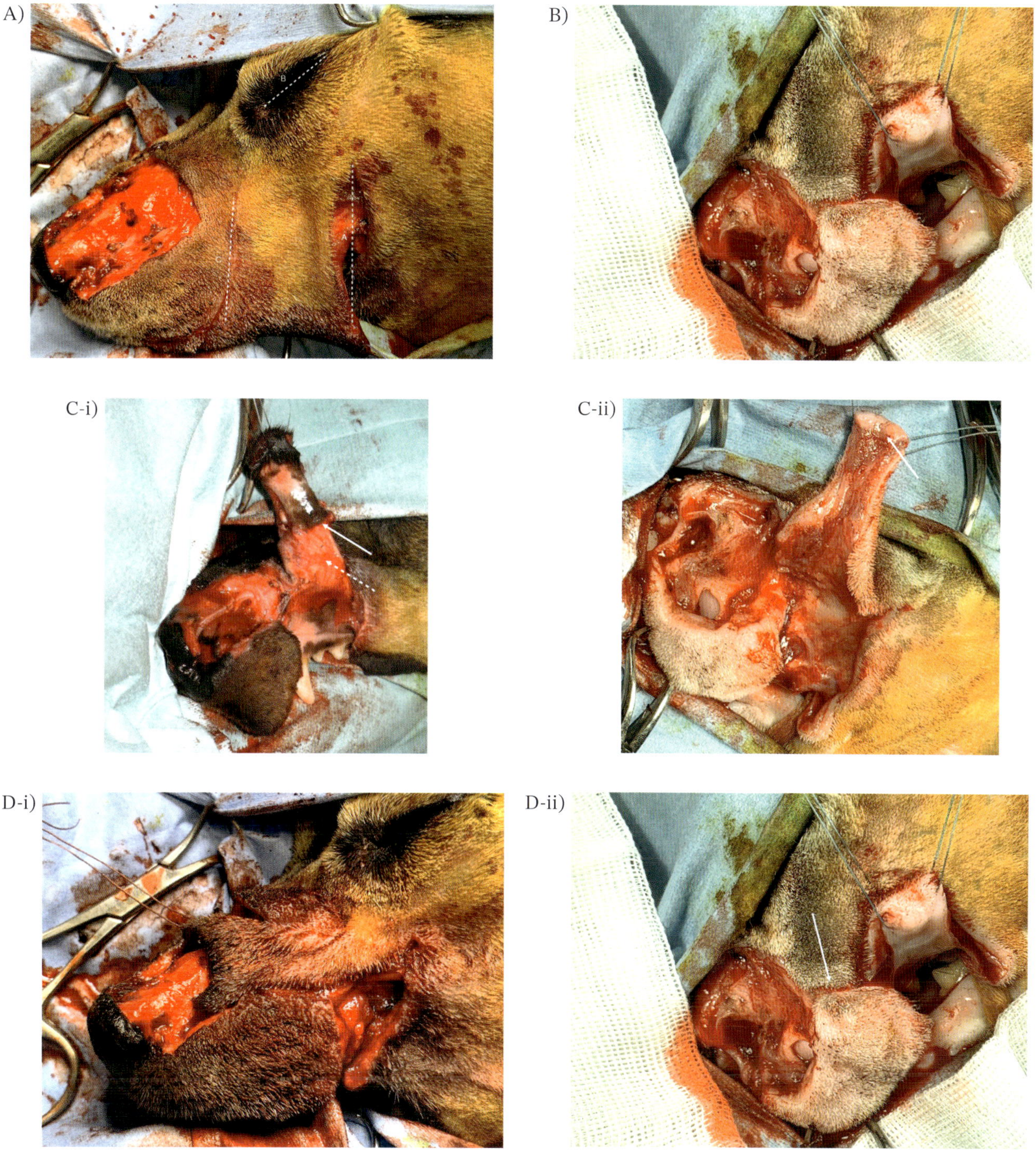

Surgical Technique [1] (See Plate 41.4A–E, G) *continued*

E) If there is a mucosal defect, then this is reconstructed by suturing the corners of the lip margin of the flap to the rostral aspect of the defect with 5-0 to 3-0 monofilament or coated multifilament absorbable suture material (arrows).
F) If the lip margin was included in the flap, then the labial mucosa at the donor site is closed with a submucosal simple continuous suture pattern using monofilament absorbable suture material (not pictured). Ideally, suture material should not include the mucosa.
G) The skin incisions of the flap and donor site are then closed routinely in two layers with a simple continuous suture pattern using monofilament absorbable suture material in the subcutis and an interrupted or continuous suture pattern using monofilament nonabsorbable suture material in the skin (i–iv, immediately postoperatively; v, vi, ≥2 weeks postoperatively).

Postoperative Management

1) Multimodal analgesia
2) Elizabethan collar

Complications – Cats [2]

- Overall: 43% with 43% classified as minor and 0% as major
  - Partial necrosis of the distal extent of the flap (43%)

References

1 Chiti, L.E., Montinaro, V., Lisi, M.L.P. et al. (2018). Lip-to-nose flap for nasal plane reconstruction in dogs: a cadaveric and in vivo feasibility study. *Vet. Surg.* 47 (8): 1101–1105.
2 Massari, F., Chiti, L.E., and Lisi, M.L.P. (2020). Lip-to-nose flap for reconstruction of the nasal planum after curative intent excision of squamous cell carcinoma in cats: description of technique and outcome in seven cases. *Vet. Surg.* 49 (2): 339–346.

Plate 41.4

Lip-to-Nose Transposition Flap *continued*

E)

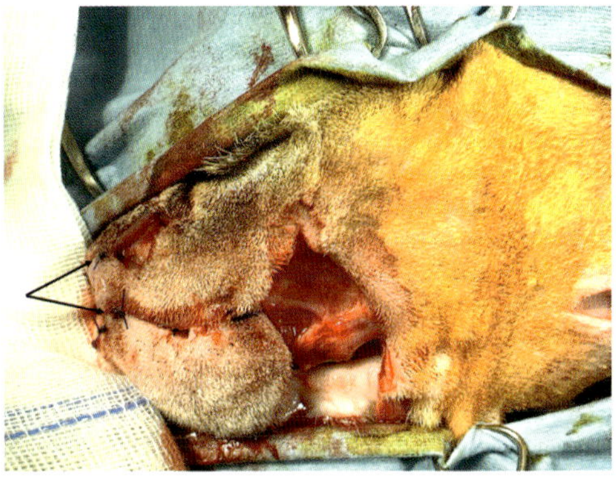

G-i)

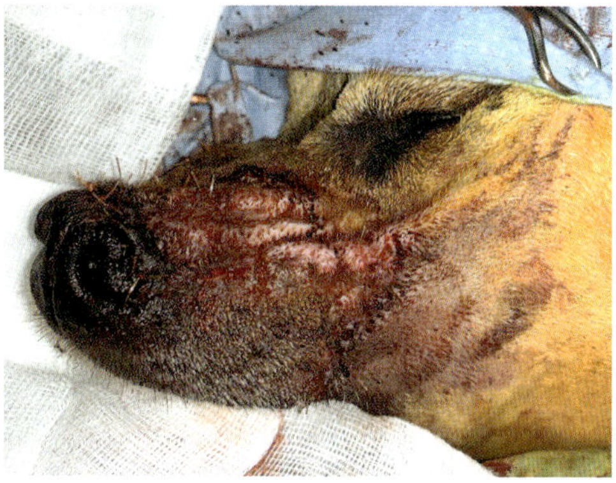

G-ii)

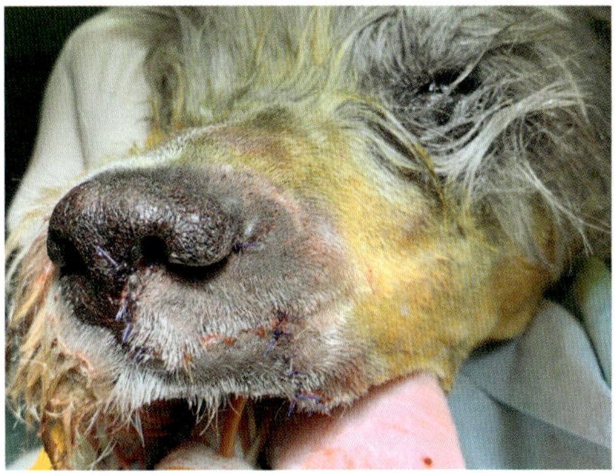

G-iii)

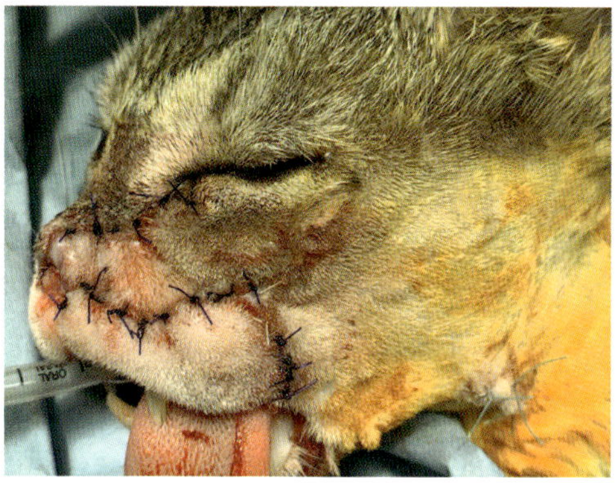

G-iv)

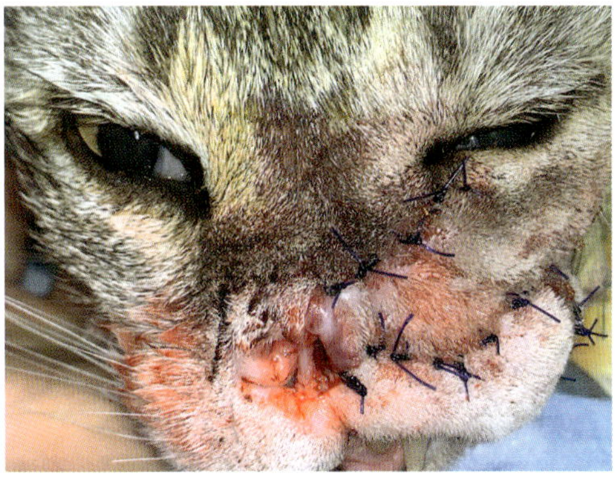

G-v)

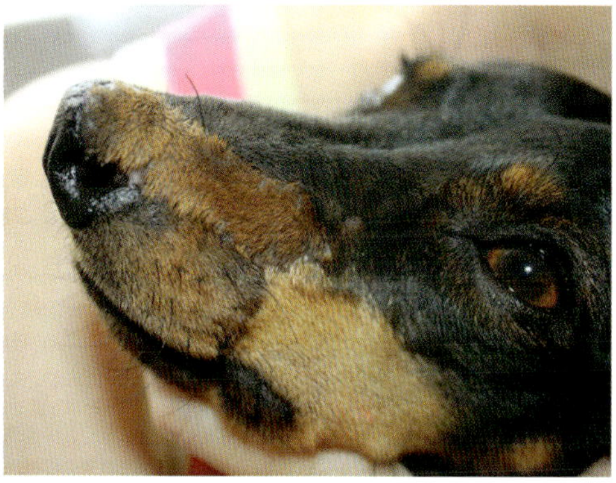

G-vi)

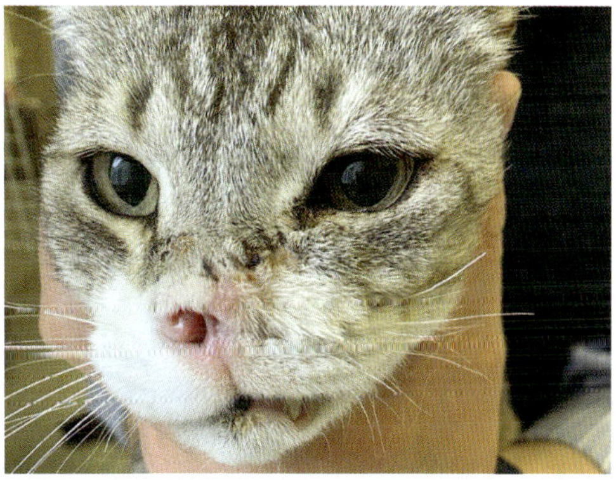

Chapter 42: Flank Fold Flaps

42.1 Axillary Flank Fold Flap

Indications

1) Reconstruction of defects from the elbow to the mid-antebrachium
2) Reconstruction of defects in the axillary and sternal region; bilateral axillary flank fold flaps can be used to reconstruct large sternal defects

Patient Positioning

The patient is positioned in lateral recumbency with the affected limb uppermost.

Surgical Technique [1] (See Plate 42.1A–E, G)

A) The axillary flank fold on the caudal aspect of the upper thoracic limb is grasped to determine the medial and lateral extents of the axillary flank fold. The medial and lateral extents of the axillary flank fold should be outlined with a sterile marker pen (i). The planned flap dimensions should be assessed to determine whether the flap donor site can be closed without excessive tension. If the donor site can be closed without excessive tension, then incisions are performed along the medial and lateral extents of the axillary flank fold (ii).
B) For reconstruction of thoracic limb defects, the medial and lateral incisions are connected with an incision along the proximal aspect of the axillary flank fold (see A – ii).
C) For reconstruction of axillary or sternal defects, the medial and lateral incisions are connected with an incision along the distal aspect of the axillary flank fold, immediately proximal to the elbow.
D) The axillary flank fold flap is carefully undermined to preserve the subdermal plexus and elevated.
E) The axillary flank fold flap is transposed into the wound defect either directly if the donor site is adjacent to the wound defect (i, ii) or via a bridging incision (iii, arrows) if the wound defect is not adjacent to the donor site.
F) Consider placement of a closed suction drain (not pictured).

Color Atlas of Canine and Feline Surgical Oncology, First Edition. Julius M. Liptak, Paolo Buracco, William T. N. Culp, and Nicholas J. Bacon.

Plate 42.1

Axillary Flank Fold Flap

A-i)

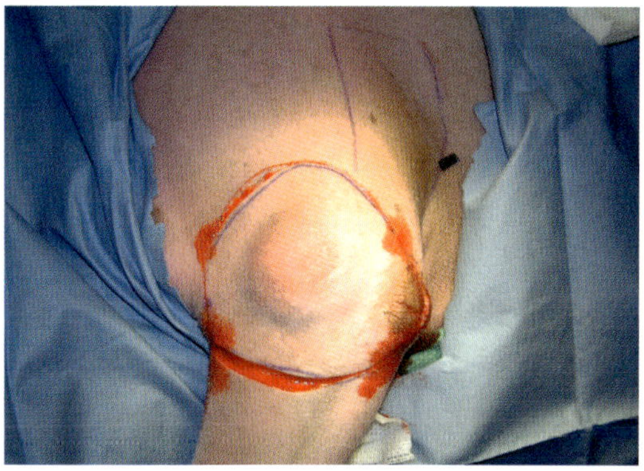

A-ii)

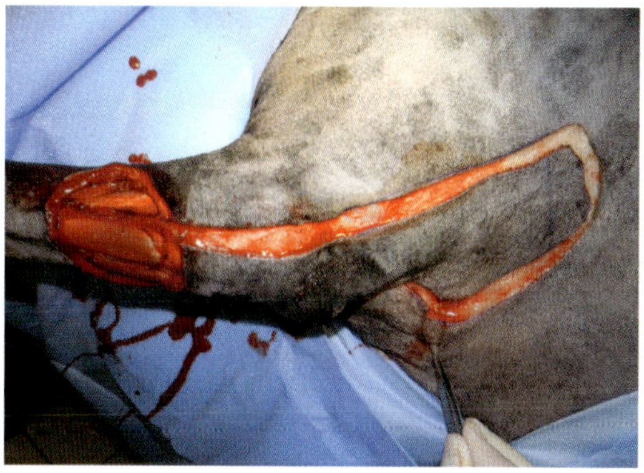

C)

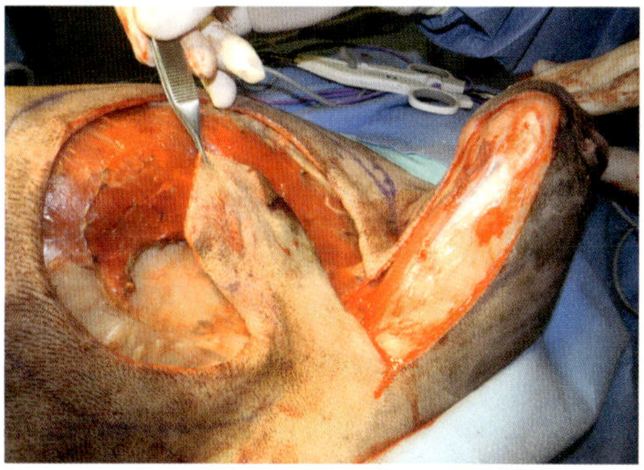

D)

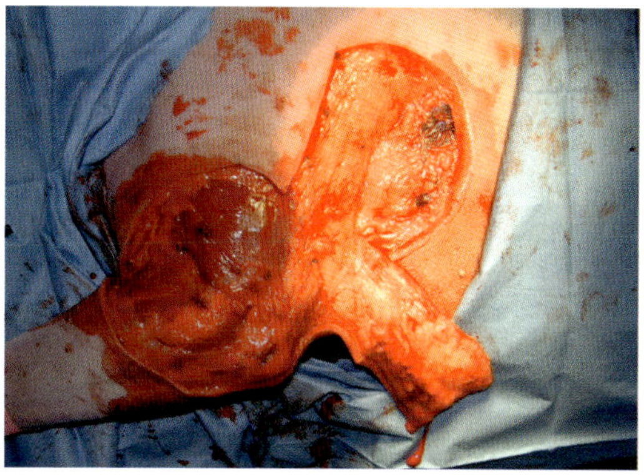

E-i)

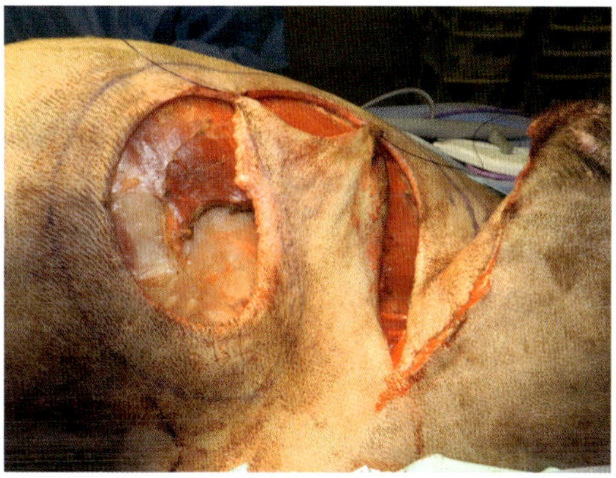

E-ii)

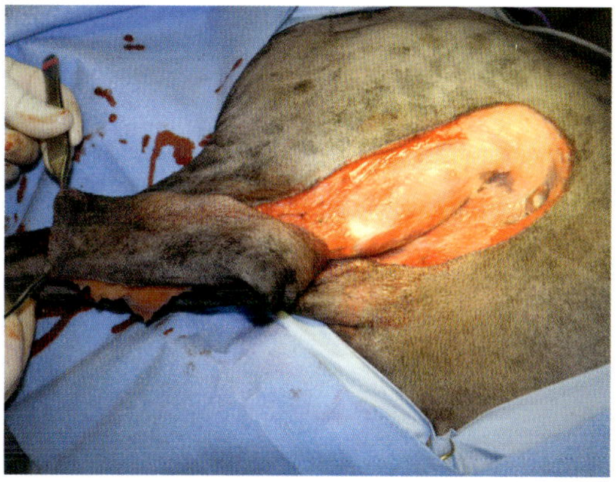

E-iii)

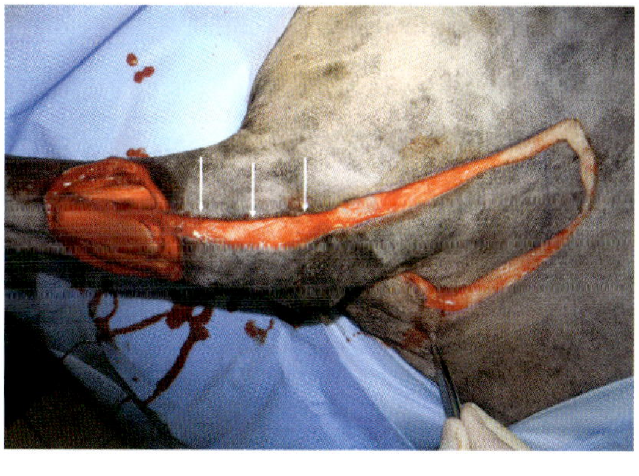

Surgical Technique [1] (See Plate 42.1A–E, G) *continued*

G) The transposed axillary flank fold flap and donor site are closed in two layers with a simple continuous suture pattern using monofilament absorbable suture material in the subcutis and either an interrupted or continuous suture pattern using monofilament nonabsorbable suture material in the skin (i, ii, immediately postoperatively; iii, iv, 1-month post-operative appearance).

Postoperative Management

1) Multimodal analgesia
2) Elizabethan collar
3) ± Closed suction drain management, if placed, for 2–5 days
4) ± Soft padded bandage for 7–14 days
5) Exercise restriction for 14 days

Complications – Dogs [1, 2] (See Plate 42.1H, I)

- Overall: 75% for axillary flank fold flap with 50% classified as minor and 25% as major [2]
- Overall: 51% for all types of subdermal plexus flap [2]
  - Dogs: 55% overall with 39% classified as minor and 16% as major
  - Cats: 43% overall with 32% classified as minor and 11% as major
- Incisional dehiscence (H) (30%) [2]
- Seroma (12%) [2]
- Partial necrosis of the distal extent of the flap (I) (10%–25%) [1, 2]
- Surgical-site infection (9%) [2]

References

1 Hunt, G.B., Tisdall, P.L., Liptak, J.M. et al. (2001). Skin-fold advancement flaps for closing large proximal limb and trunk defects in dogs and cats. *Vet. Surg.* 30 (5): 440–448.

2 Jones, C.A. and Lipscomb, V.J. (2019). Indications, complications, and outcomes associated with subdermal plexus skin flap procedures in dogs and cats: 92 cases (2000-2017). *J. Am. Vet. Med. Assoc.* 255 (8): 933–938.

Plate 42.1

Axillary Flank Fold Flap *continued*

G-i)

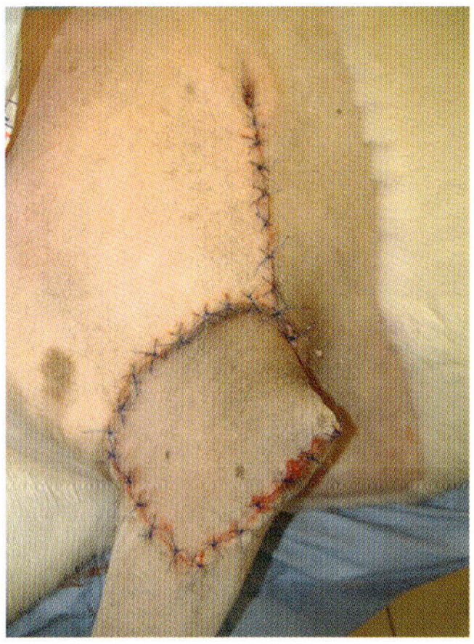

G-ii)

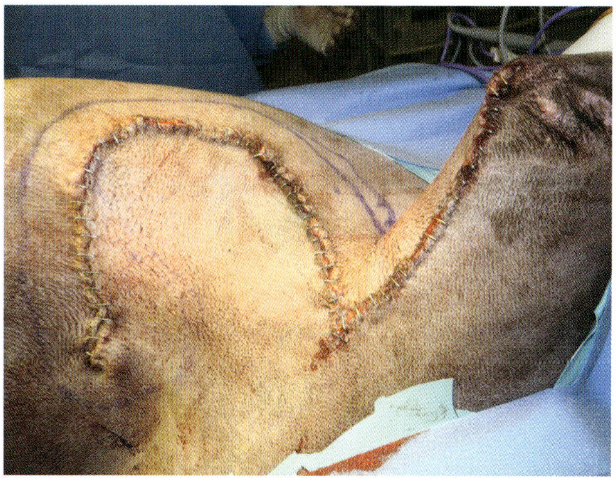

G-iii)

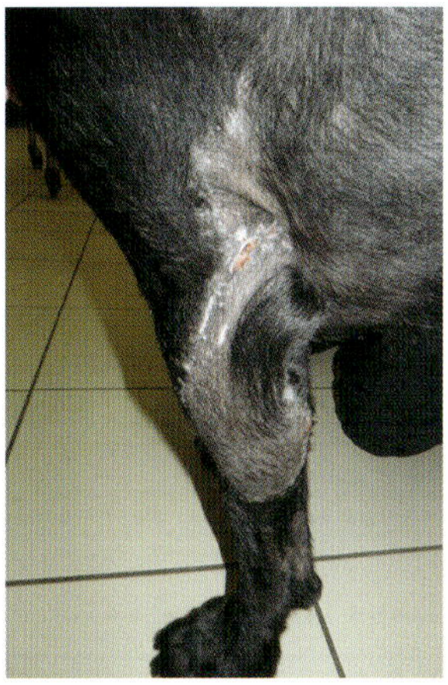

G-iv)

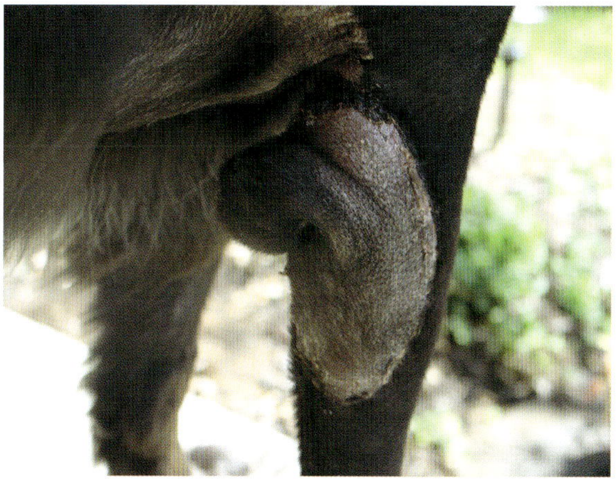

H)

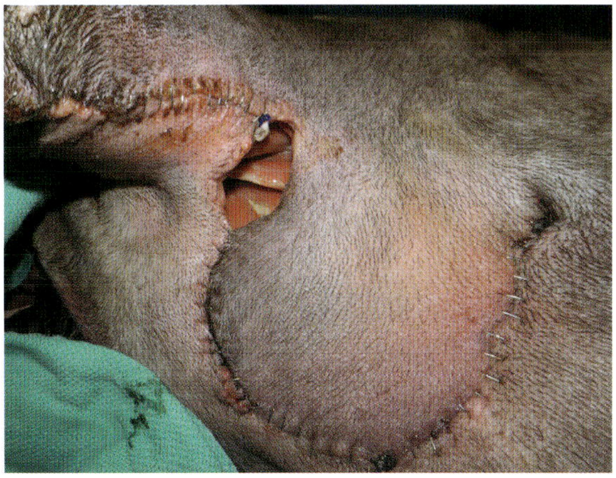

I)

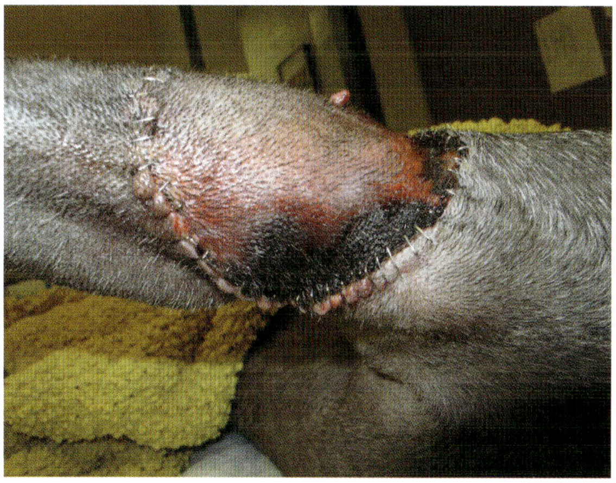

42.2 Inguinal Flank Fold Flap

Indications

1) Reconstruction of defects from the midthigh to the proximal tibia
2) Reconstruction of defects from the proximal thigh and hip region to the ventral abdomen; bilateral inguinal flank fold flaps can be used to reconstruct large ventral abdominal defects

Patient Positioning

The patient is positioned in lateral recumbency with the affected limb uppermost.

Surgical Technique [1] (See Plate 42.2A–E, G)

A) The inguinal flank fold on the cranial aspect of the thigh is grasped to determine the medial and lateral extents of the inguinal flank fold (i). The medial and lateral extents of the axillary flank fold should be outlined with a sterile marker pen (ii). The planned flap dimensions should be assessed to determine whether the flap donor site can be closed without excessive tension. If the donor site can be closed without excessive tension, then incisions are performed along the medial and lateral extents of the inguinal flank fold.
B) For reconstruction of defects between the midthigh and proximal tibia, the medial and lateral incisions are connected with an incision along the proximal aspect of the inguinal flank fold.
C) For reconstruction of defects from the proximal thigh and hip region to the ventral abdomen, the medial and lateral incisions are connected with an incision along the distal aspect of the inguinal flank fold, immediately proximal to the stifle.
D) The inguinal flank fold flap is carefully undermined to preserve the subdermal plexus and elevated (i, ii).
E) The inguinal flank fold flap is transposed into the wound defect either directly if the donor site is adjacent to the wound defect (i) or via a bridging incision (ii, dashed line) if the wound defect is not adjacent to the donor site.
F) Consider placement of a closed suction drain (not pictured).

Color Atlas of Canine and Feline Surgical Oncology, First Edition. Julius M. Liptak, Paolo Buracco, William T. N. Culp, and Nicholas J. Bacon.

Plate 42.2

Inguinal Flank Fold Flap

A-i)

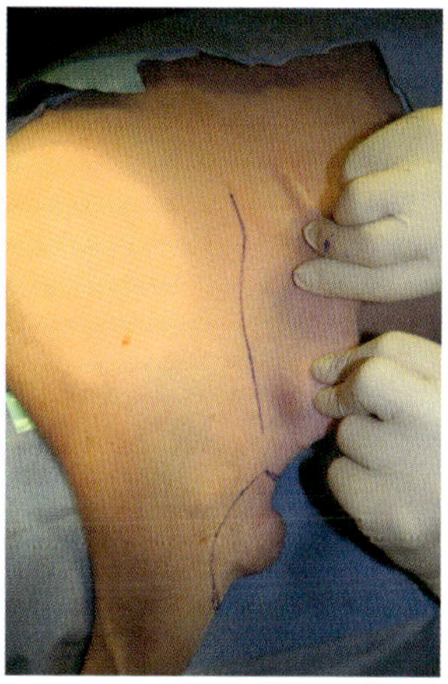

A-ii)

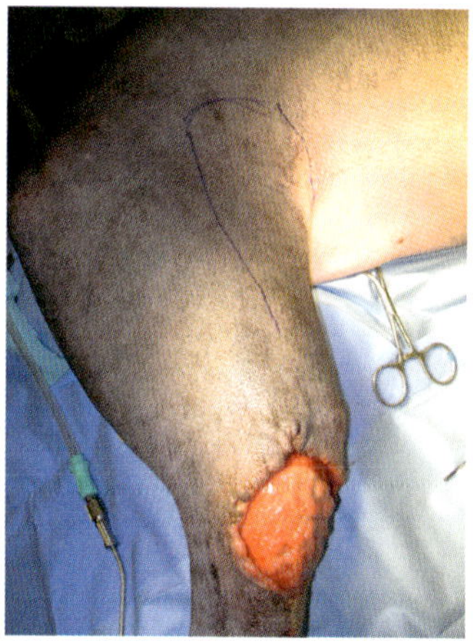

B)

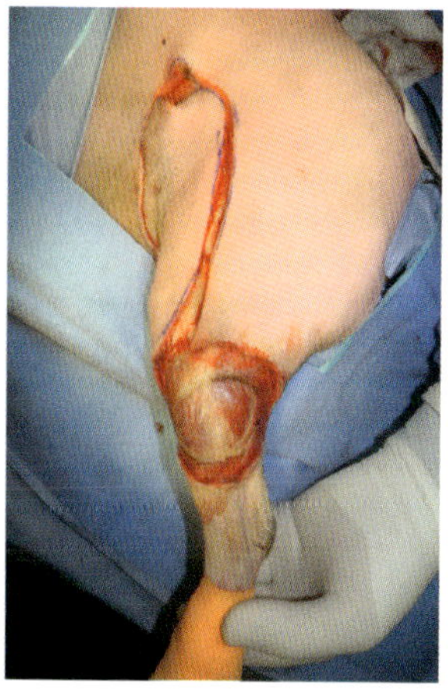

C)

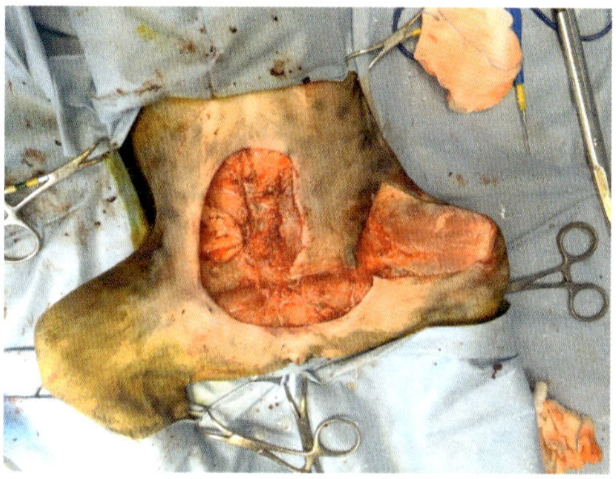

D-i)

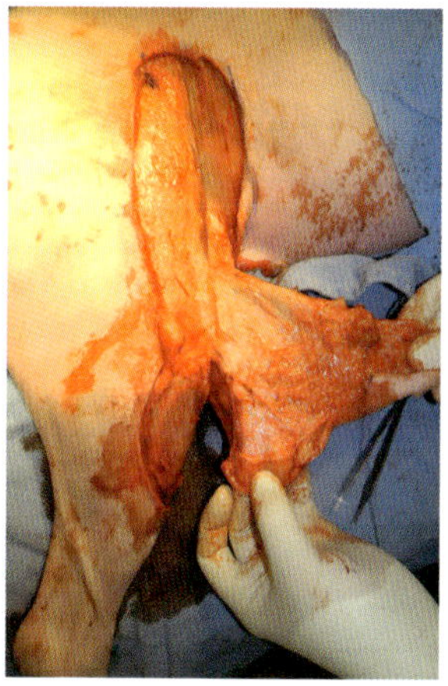

D-ii)

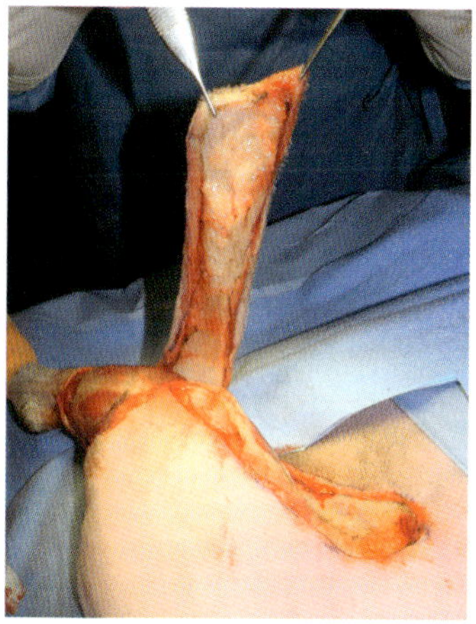

E-i)

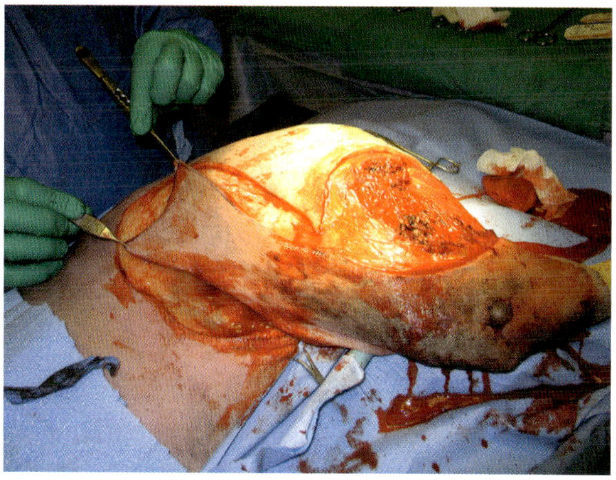

E-ii)

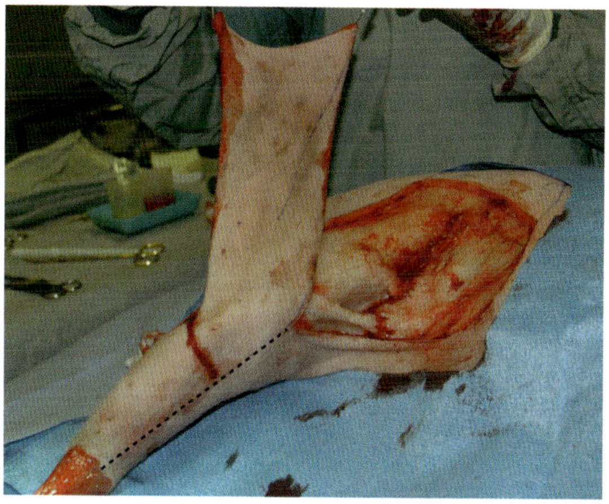

Surgical Technique [1] (See Plate 42.2A–E, G) *continued*

G) The transposed inguinal flank fold flap and donor site are closed in two layers with a simple continuous suture pattern using monofilament absorbable suture material in the subcutis and either an interrupted or continuous suture pattern using monofilament nonabsorbable suture material in the skin (i–v).

Postoperative Management

1) Multimodal analgesia
2) Elizabethan collar
3) ± Closed suction drain management, if placed, for 2–5 days
4) ± Soft padded bandage for 7–14 days
5) Exercise restriction for 14 days

Complications – Dogs [1, 2] (See Plate 42.2H, I)

- Overall: 65% for inguinal flank fold flap with 45% classified as minor and 20% as major [2]
- Overall: 51% for all types of subdermal plexus flap [2]
  - Dogs: 55% overall with 39% classified as minor and 16% as major
  - Cats: 43% overall with 32% classified as minor and 11% as major
- Incisional dehiscence (H) (30%) [2]
- Seroma (12%) [2]
- Partial necrosis of the distal extent of the flap (I) (10%–25%) [1, 2]
- Surgical-site infection (9%) [2]

References

1 Hunt, G.B., Tisdall, P.L., Liptak, J.M. et al. (2001). Skin-fold advancement flaps for closing large proximal limb and trunk defects in dogs and cats. *Vet. Surg.* 30 (5): 440–448.
2 Jones, C.A. and Lipscomb, V.J. (2019). Indications, complications, and outcomes associated with subdermal plexus skin flap procedures in dogs and cats: 92 cases (2000-2017). *J. Am. Vet. Med. Assoc.* 255 (8): 933–938.

Plate 42.2

Inguinal Flank Fold Flap *continued*

G-i)

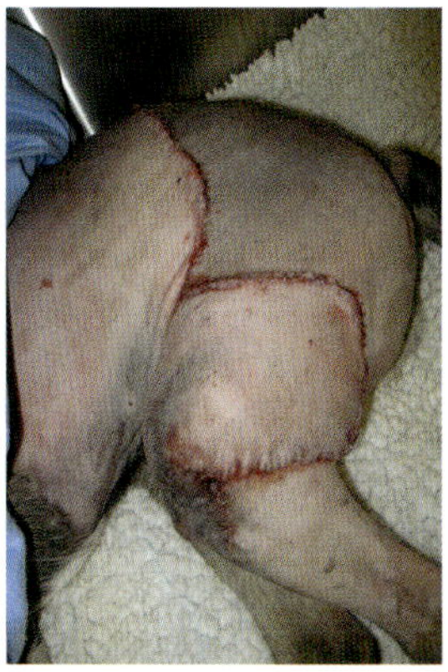

G-ii)

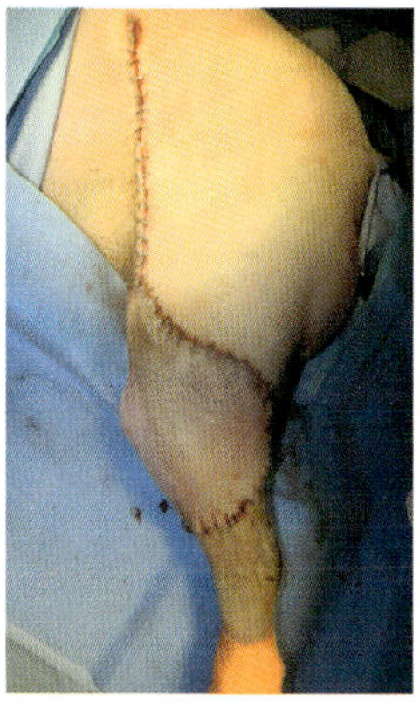

G-iii)

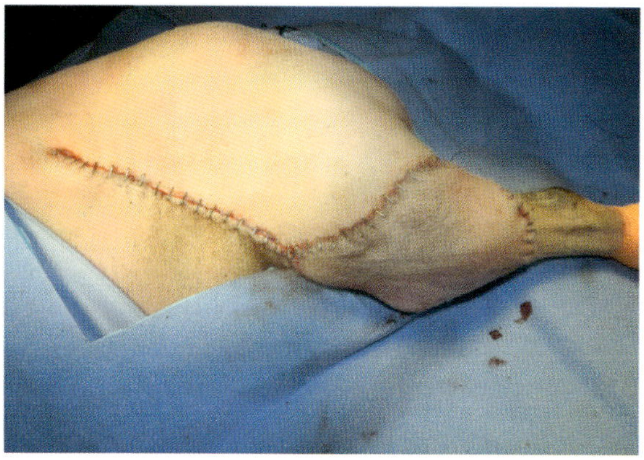

G-iv)

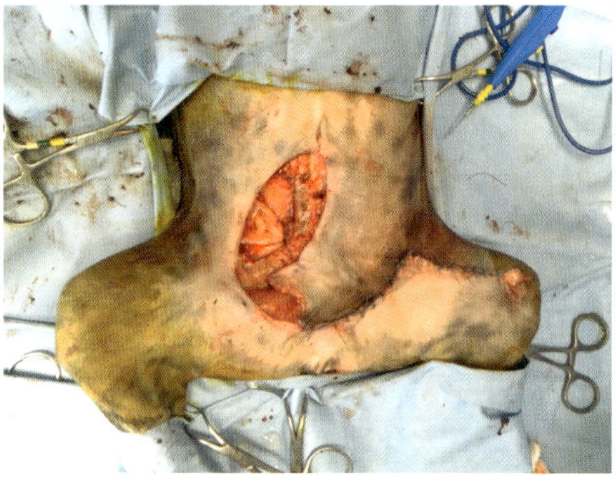

G-v)

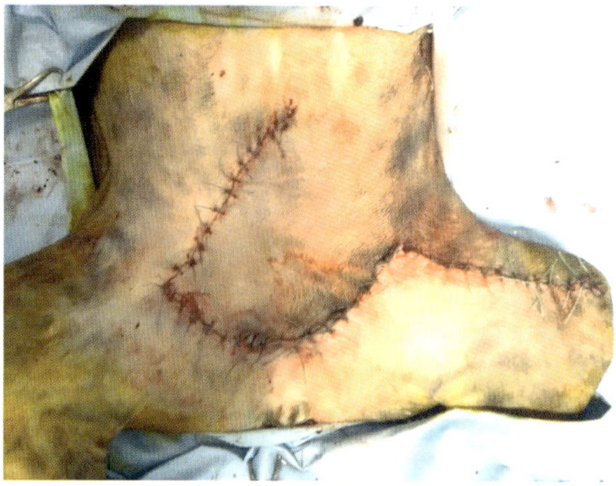

H)

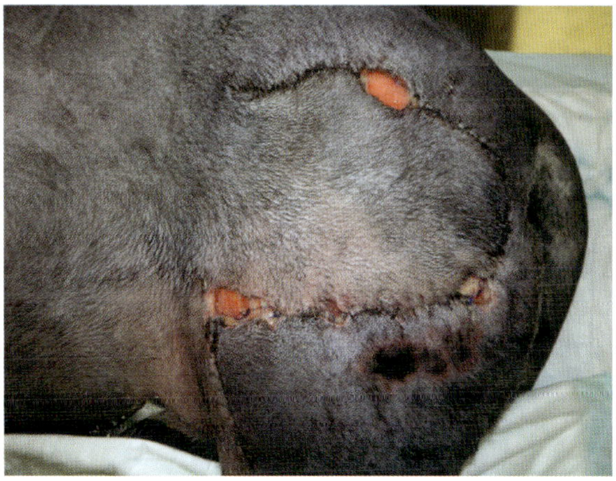

I)

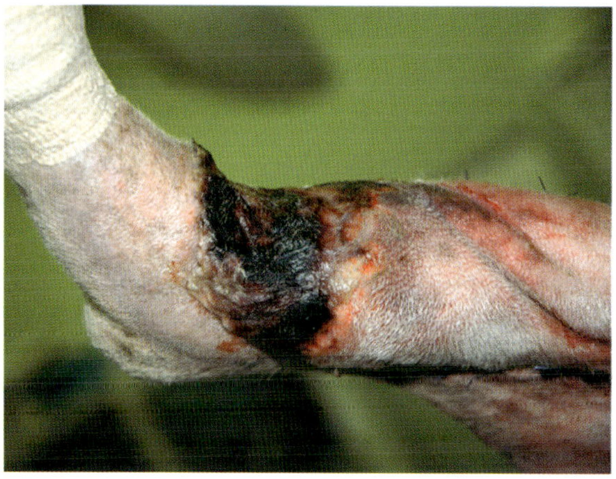

Chapter 43: Axial Pattern Flaps

43.1 Facial Axial Pattern Flap

Indications

1) Reconstruction of defects on the upper lip, cheek, and muzzle
2) Facial axial pattern flap can be combined with total unilateral maxillectomy or caudal maxillectomy for reconstruction of lateral lip and facial defects (see *6.16. Combined Approach for Caudal and Total Unilateral Maxillectomy*)

Patient Positioning

The patient is positioned in lateral recumbency with the affected side uppermost.

Surgical Technique [1] (See Plate 43.1A–D)

A) The facial axial pattern flap is based on three direct arteries arising at the commissure of the lips: angularis oris artery and superior and inferior labial arteries. A sterile marker pen should be used to indicate the dorsal (D), caudal (C), and ventral (V) borders of the facial axial pattern flap. The dorsal border is along the ventral aspect of the zygomatic arch, the ventral border is parallel to the dorsal border along the ventral border of the mandible, and the caudal border connects the dorsal and ventral borders at the level of the vertical ear canal.
B) Skin incisions are made along the marked dorsal, caudal, and ventral borders (pictured, cat with fibrosarcoma).
C) The flap is carefully undermined deep to the platysma muscle to preserve the direct cutaneous arteries and distal arterial plexus, and elevated.
D) The flap is transposed into the wound defect either directly if the donor site is adjacent to the wound defect (i) or via a bridging incision (ii, arrows) if the wound defect is not adjacent to the donor site.
E) Consider placement of a closed suction drain (not pictured).

Color Atlas of Canine and Feline Surgical Oncology, First Edition. Julius M. Liptak, Paolo Buracco, William T. N. Culp, and Nicholas J. Bacon.

Plate 43.1

Facial Axial Pattern Flap

A)

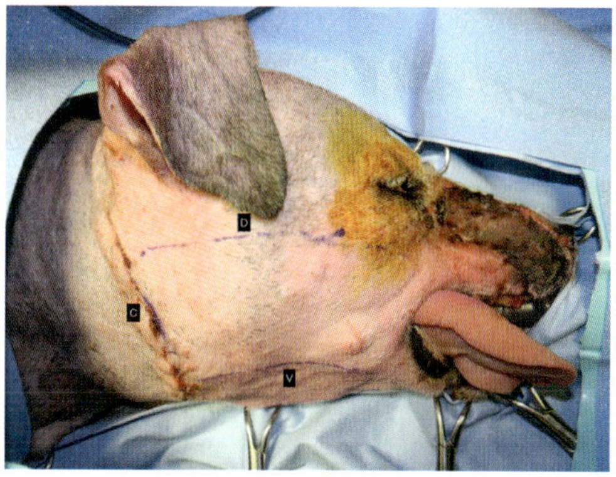

B)

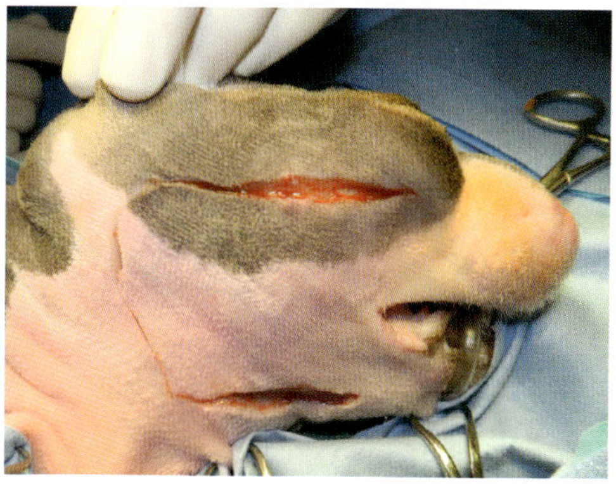

C)

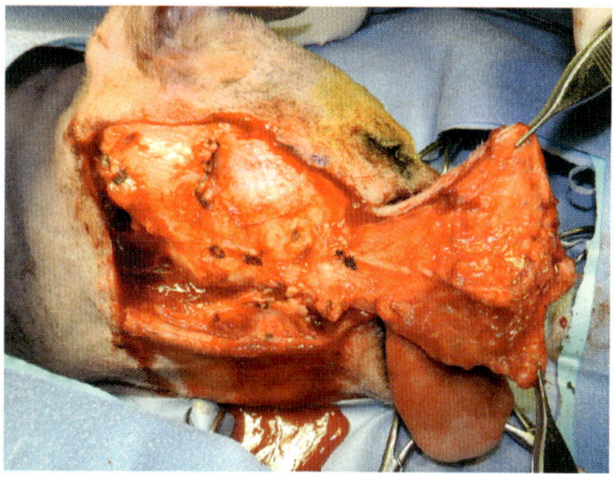

D-i)

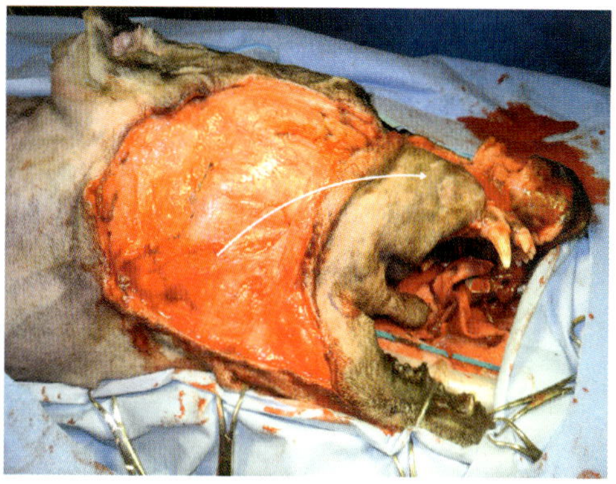

D-ii)

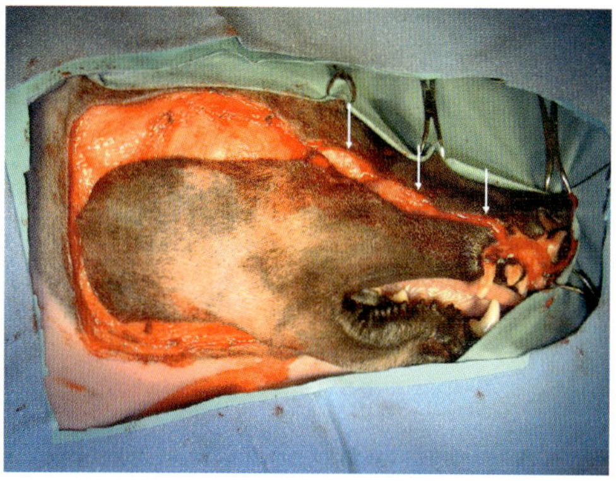

Closure (See Plate 43.1F)

F) The transposed flap and donor site are closed in two layers with a simple continuous suture pattern using monofilament absorbable suture material in the subcutis and either skin staples or an interrupted or continuous suture pattern using monofilament nonabsorbable suture material in the skin (i, ii, immediate postoperative appearance; iii–v, postoperative appearance ranging from 2 weeks to 3 months after surgery).

Postoperative Management

1) Multimodal analgesia
2) Elizabethan collar
3) ± Closed suction drain management, if placed, for 2–5 days

Complications – Dogs [1, 2] (See Plate 43.1G–I)

- Flap edema (G) (89%)
- Incisional dehiscence (33%)
- Partial necrosis of the distal extent of the flap (H, arrows) (22%)
- Oroantral fistula (11%)
- Haired skin on the mucosal aspect of the lip (I – i, ii)

Complications – Cats [3]

- Flap edema (see F – ii) (100%)
- Incisional dehiscence (30%)
- Partial necrosis of the distal extent of the flap (30%)
- Epiphora (20%)
- Frequent periocular grooming (20%)
- Corneal ulceration secondary to impaired eyelid function (10%)

References

1 Yates, G., Landon, B., and Edwards, G. (2007). Investigation and clinical application of a novel axial pattern flap for nasal and facial reconstruction in the dog. *Aust. Vet. J.* 85 (3): 113–118.
2 Losinski, S.L., Stanley, B.J., Schallberger, S.O. et al. (2015). Versatility of the angularis oris axial pattern flap for facial reconstruction. *Vet. Surg.* 44 (8): 930–938.
3 Albernaz, V.G.P., Oblak, M.L., and Quitzan, J.G. (2021). Angularis oris axial pattern flap as a reliable and versatile option for rostral facial reconstruction in cats. *Vet. Surg.* 50 (8): 1688–1695.

Plate 43.1

Facial Axial Pattern Flap *continued*

F-i)

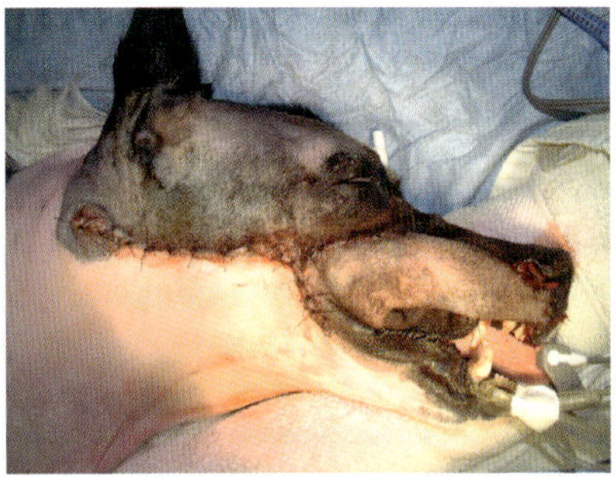

F-ii)

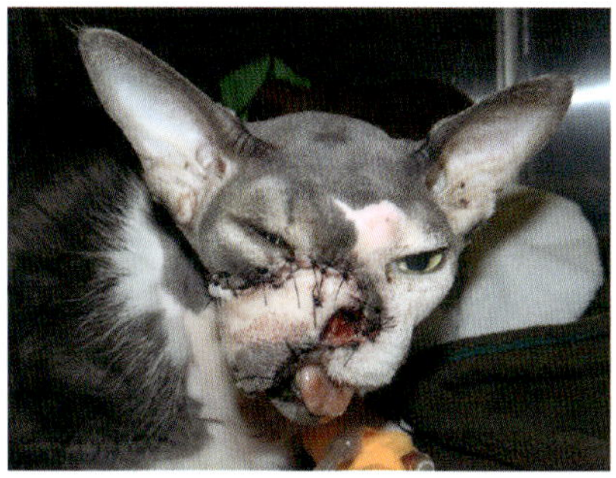

F-iii)

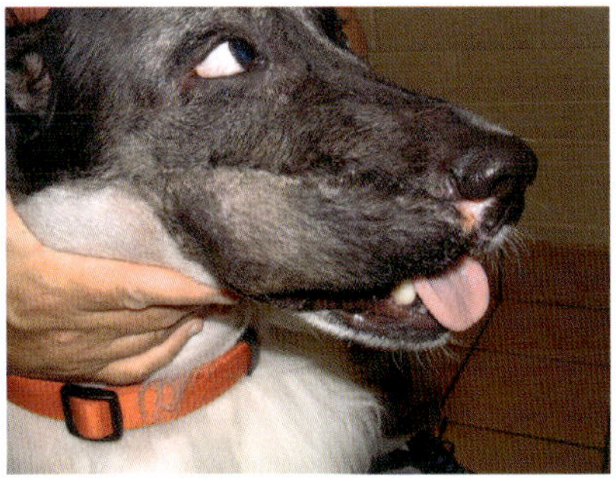

F-iv)

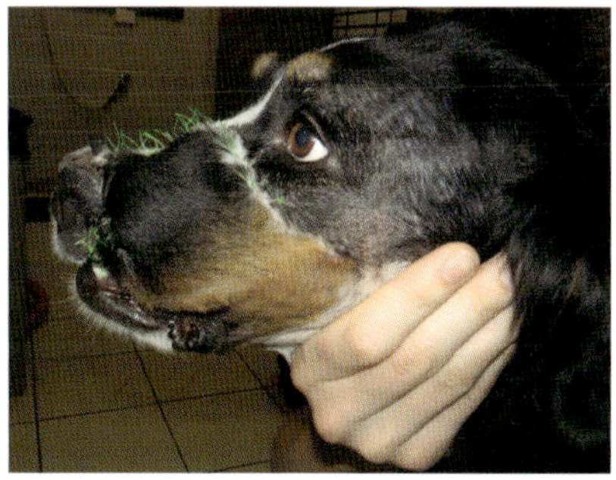

F-v)

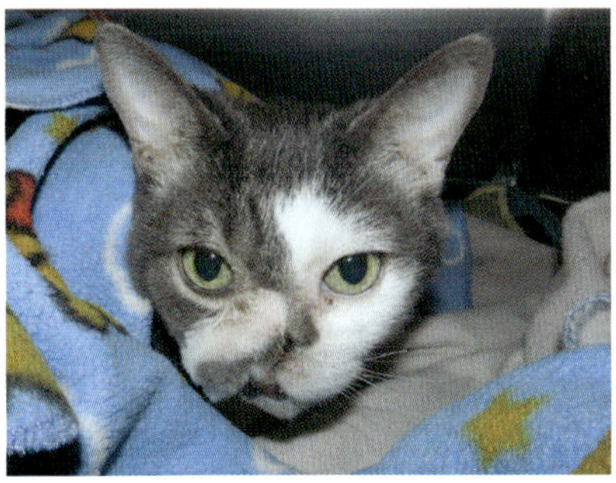

G)

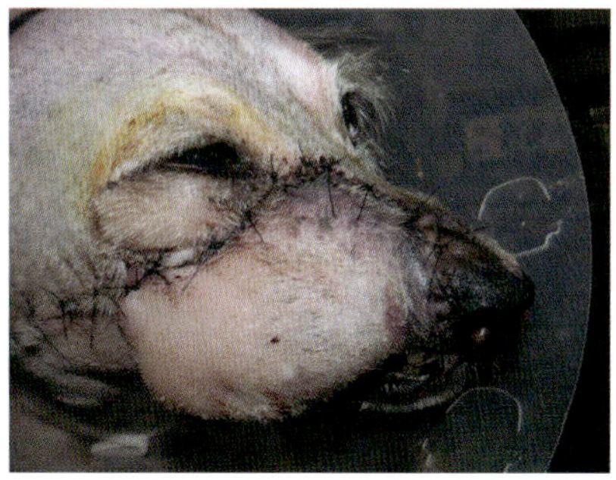

H)

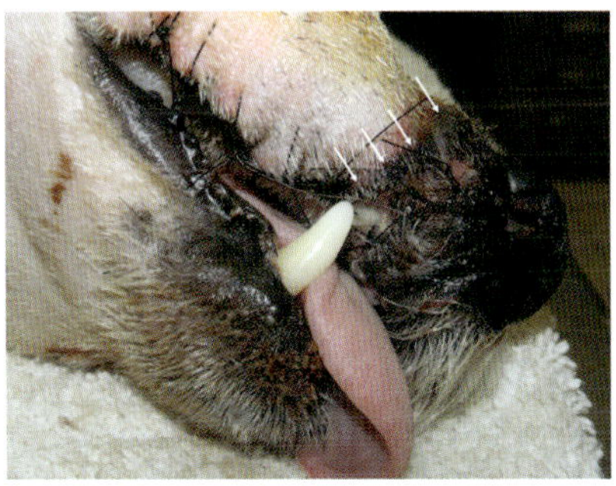

I-i)

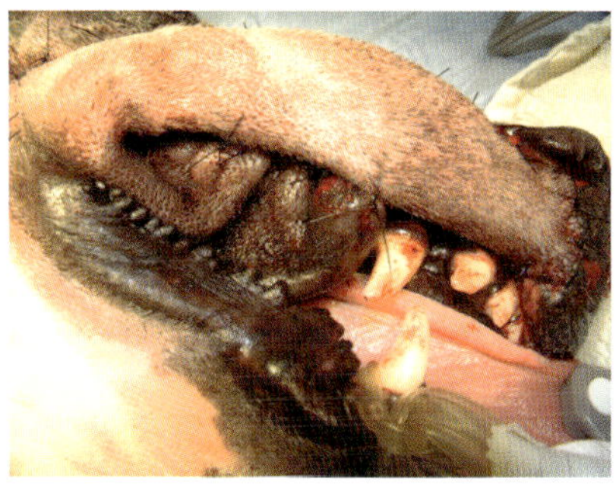

I-ii)

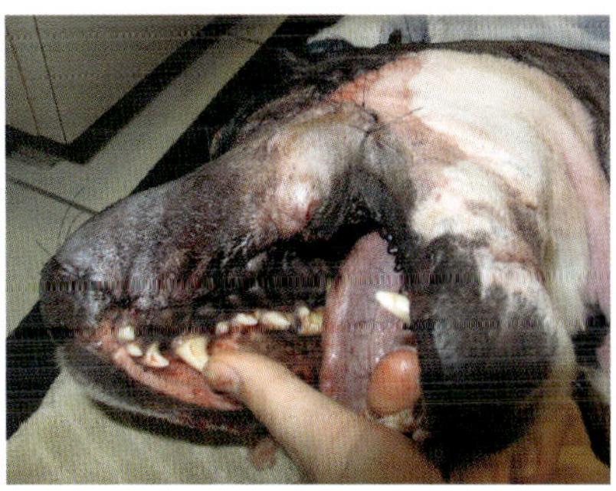

43.2 Superficial Temporal Axial Pattern Flap

Indication

1) Reconstruction of defects over the dorsal nasal and lateral facial regions

Patient Positioning

The patient is positioned in sternal recumbency.

Surgical Technique [1] (See Plate 43.2A–D)

A) The superficial temporal axial pattern flap is based on the cutaneous branch of the superficial temporal artery. The flap is based on the zygomatic arch, and the width of the flap is equivalent to the length of the zygomatic arch (ZA; double-arrowed line) (i). A sterile marker pen should be used to indicate the rostral, caudal, and lateral borders of the superficial temporal axial pattern flap. The rostral border (R) is the caudal orbital rim (i, ii), the caudal border (C) is parallel to the rostral border and at the level of the caudal aspect of the zygomatic arch (i, ii), and the lateral border (L) connects the rostral and caudal borders at the level of the contralateral middorsal orbital rim (ii).
B) Skin incisions are made along the marked rostral, caudal, and lateral borders.
C) The flap is carefully undermined to preserve the direct cutaneous artery and distal arterial plexus, and elevated.
D) The flap is transposed into the wound defect on the dorsal muzzle (i) either directly if the donor site is adjacent to the wound defect (not pictured) or via a bridging incision (ii, arrow) if the wound defect is not adjacent to the donor site.
E) Consider placement of a closed suction drain (not pictured).

Closure (See Plate 43.2F)

F) The transposed flap and donor site are closed in two layers with a simple continuous suture pattern using monofilament absorbable suture material in the subcutis and either skin staples or an interrupted or continuous suture pattern using monofilament nonabsorbable suture material in the skin (i, ii).

Color Atlas of Canine and Feline Surgical Oncology, First Edition. Julius M. Liptak, Paolo Buracco, William T. N. Culp, and Nicholas J. Bacon.

Plate 43.2

Superficial Temporal Axial Pattern Flap

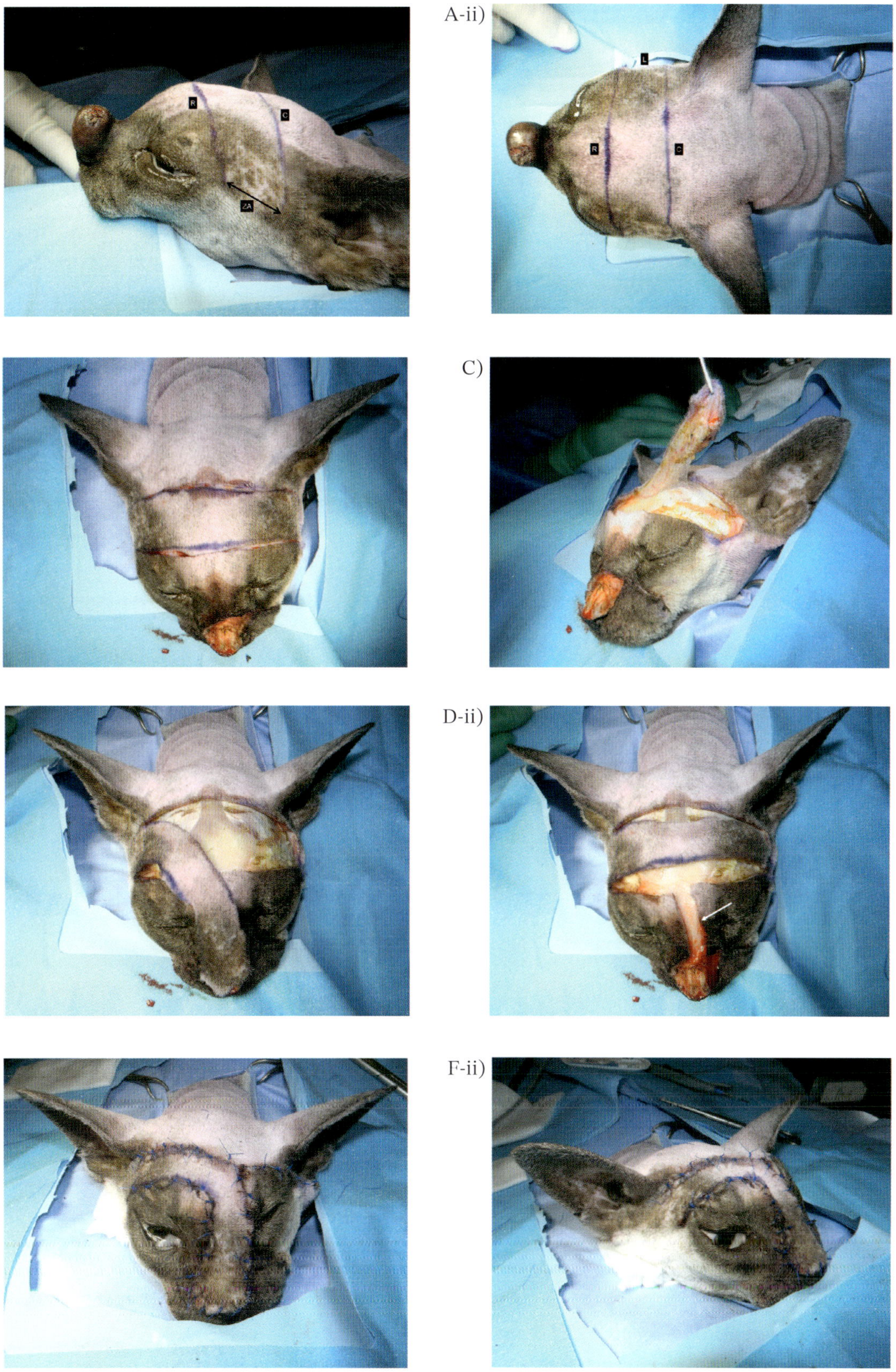

A-i) A-ii) B) C) D-i) D-ii) F-i) F-ii)

Postoperative Management

1) Multimodal analgesia
2) Elizabethan collar
3) ± Closed suction drain management, if placed, for 2–5 days

Complications – Dogs [2]

- Overall: 55%
- Partial- or full-thickness necrosis of the distal aspect of the flap (11%)
- Flap edema (11%)
- Surgical-site infection (22%)
- Mild ectropion (11%)
- Mild exposure of the eye (22%)
- Decreased palpebral reflex (11%)

Complications – Cats [2]

- Overall: 30%
- Partial- or full-thickness necrosis of the distal aspect of the flap (10%)
- Mild exposure of the eye (10%)
- Subcutaneous emphysema (10%)

References

1 Pavletic, M.M. (2018). Axial pattern skin flaps. In: *Atlas of Small Animal Wound Management*, 4e (ed. M.M. Pavletic), 417–462. Hoboken: Wiley Blackwell.

2 de la Puerta, B., Buracco, P., Ladlow, J. et al. (2021). Superficial temporal axial pattern flap for facial reconstruction of skin defects in dogs and cat. *J. Small Anim. Pract.* 62: 984–991.

43.3 Caudal Auricular Axial Pattern Flap

Indication (See Plate 43.3 – 1)

1) Reconstruction of defects of the ear, dorsal head, and orbital region (i–iii, wide resection of a periocular soft tissue sarcoma)

Patient Positioning

The patient is positioned in lateral recumbency with the affected side uppermost and the thoracic limb in relaxed extension with the scapula perpendicular to the trunk.

Surgical Technique [1] (See Plate 43.3A–D)

A) The caudal auricular axial pattern flap is based on the sternocleidomastoid branches of the caudal auricular artery and vein, located in the depression between the lateral aspect of the wing of the atlas and the vertical ear canal (arrow). A sterile marker pen should be used to indicate the dorsal (D), caudal (C), and ventral (V) borders of the caudal auricular axial pattern flap. The flap is centered over the wing of the atlas. The dorsal and ventral borders are parallel to each other along the central third of the lateral cervical region (although the dorsal border is closer to the dorsal midline in cats), and the caudal border connects the dorsal and ventral borders at the level of the scapular spine.
B) Skin incisions are made along the marked dorsal, caudal, and ventral borders.
C) The flap is carefully undermined in a caudal-to-cranial direction and deep to the sphincter coli superficialis muscle to preserve the direct cutaneous arteries and distal arterial plexus, and elevated.
D) The flap is transposed into the wound defect either directly if the donor site is adjacent to the wound defect or via a bridging incision (pictured, arrows) if the wound defect is not adjacent to the donor site.
E) Consider placement of a closed suction drain (not pictured).

Color Atlas of Canine and Feline Surgical Oncology, First Edition. Julius M. Liptak, Paolo Buracco, William T. N. Culp, and Nicholas J. Bacon.

Plate 43.3

Caudal Auricular Axial Pattern Flap

1-i)

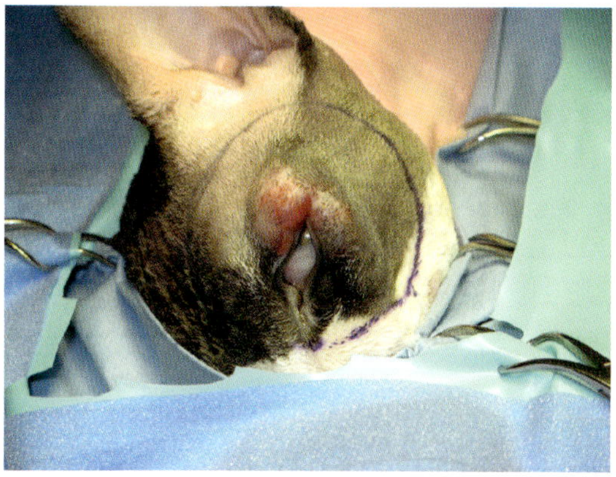

1-ii)

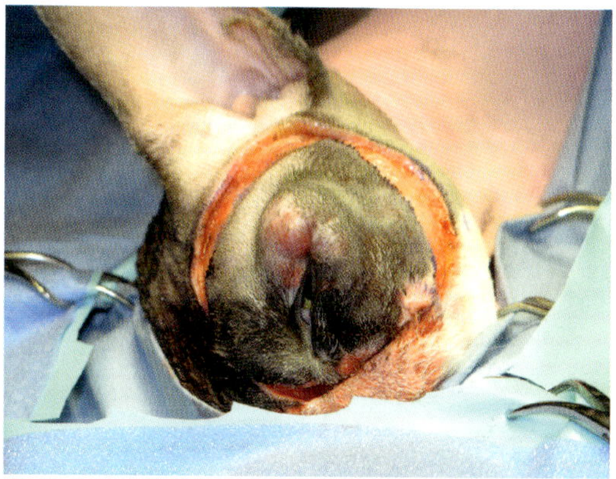

1-iii)

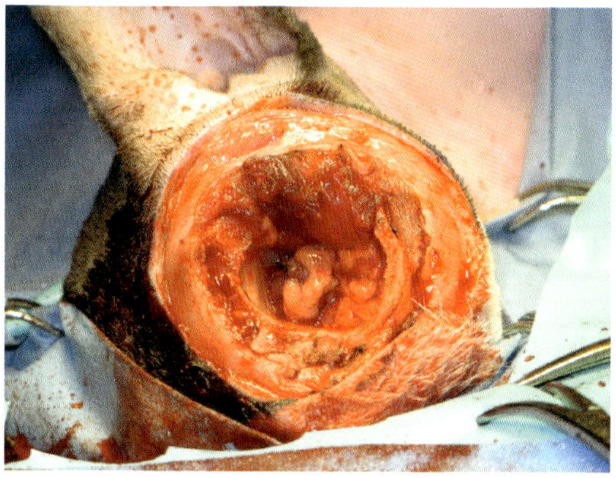

A)

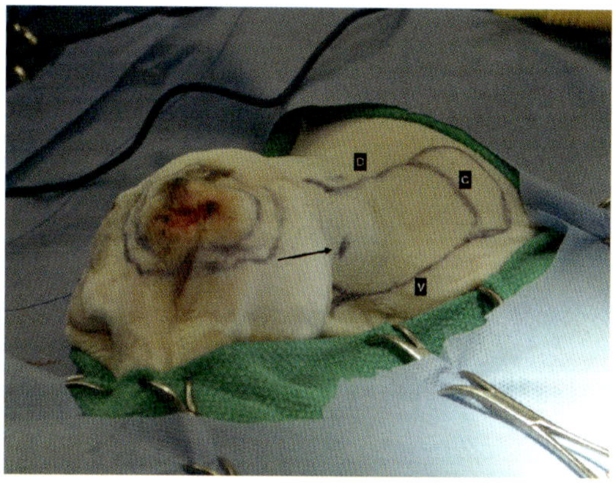

B)

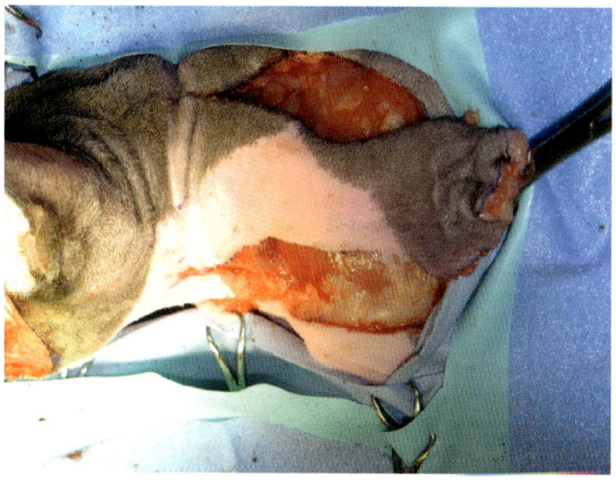

C)

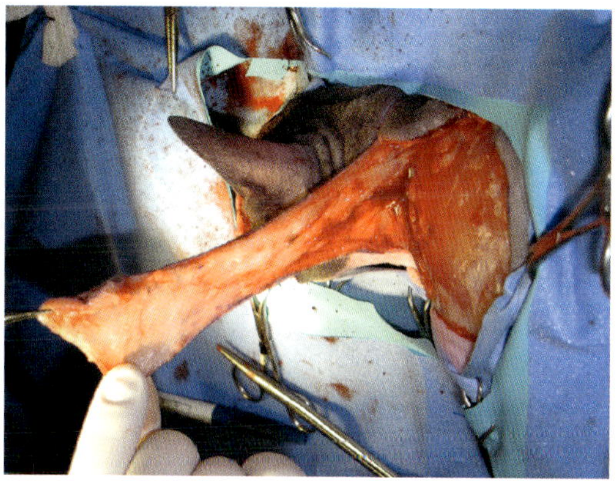

D)

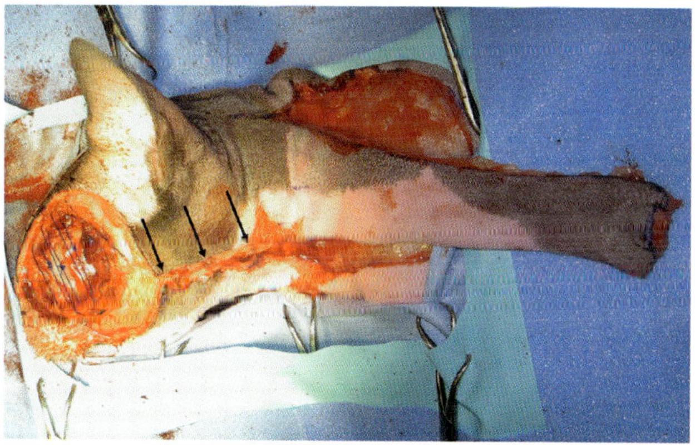

Closure (See Plate 43.3F)

F) The transposed flap and donor site are closed in two layers with a simple continuous suture pattern using monofilament absorbable suture material in the subcutis and either skin staples or an interrupted or continuous suture pattern using monofilament nonabsorbable suture material in the skin (pictured).

Postoperative Management

1) Multimodal analgesia
2) Elizabethan collar
3) ± Closed suction drain management, if placed, for 2–5 days

Complications – Dogs [2]

- Partial- or full-thickness necrosis of the distal aspect of the flap (63%)
- Incisional dehiscence (6%)

Complications – Cats [2] (See Plate 43.3G)

- Partial- or full-thickness necrosis of the distal aspect of the flap (G) (42%)
- Incisional dehiscence (8%)

References

1 Pavletic, M.M. (2018). Axial pattern skin flaps. In: *Atlas of Small Animal Wound Management*, 4e (ed. M.M. Pavletic), 417–462. Hoboken: Wiley Blackwell.

2 Proot, L.J.L., Jeffery, N., Culp, W.T.N. et al. (2019). Is the caudal auricular axial pattern flap robust? A multi-centre cohort study of 16 dogs and 12 cats (2005 to 2016). *J. Small Anim. Pract.* 60 (2): 102–106.

Plate 43.3

Caudal Auricular Axial Pattern Flap *continued*

F)

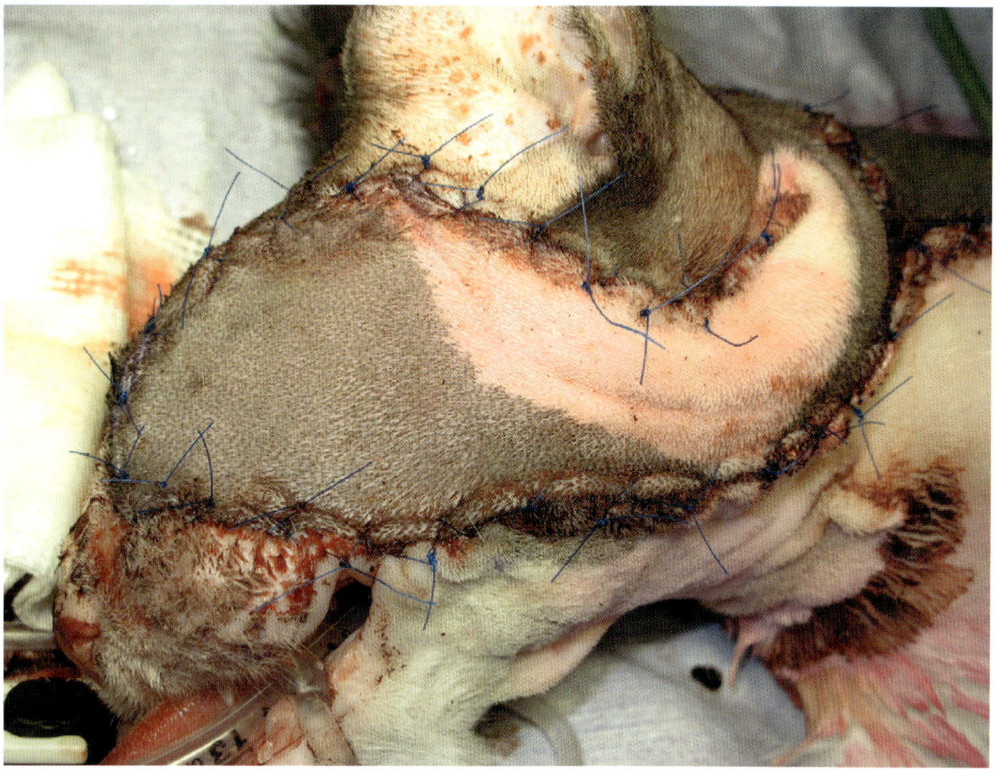

G)

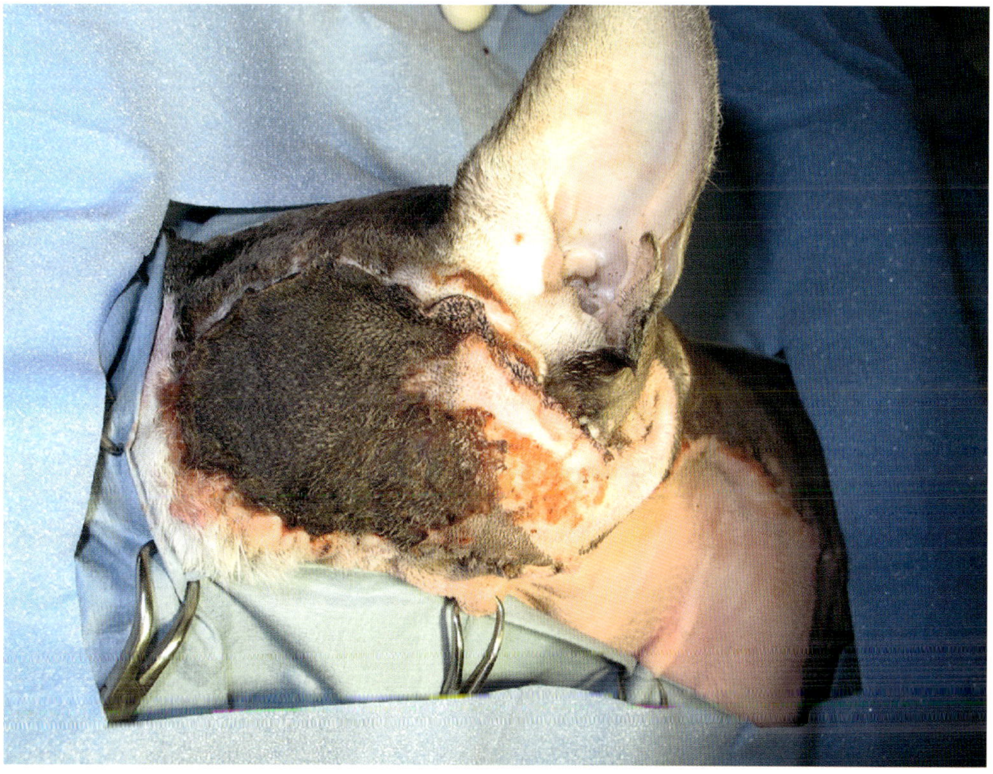

43.4 Thoracodorsal Axial Pattern Flap

Indication

1) Reconstruction of defects on the neck, thoracic wall, and thoracic limb: The thoracodorsal axial pattern flap can extend a variable length on the distal thoracic limb depending on the conformation and limb length of the dog but extends to the carpus in cats.

Patient Positioning

The patient is positioned in lateral recumbency with the affected side uppermost.

Surgical Technique [1] (See Plate 43.4A–D)

A) The thoracodorsal axial pattern flap is based on the cutaneous branch of the thoracodorsal artery. A sterile marker pen should be used to indicate the cranial (Cr), caudal (Ca), and dorsal (D) borders of the thoracodorsal axial pattern flap. The cranial border is along the spine of the scapula, and the caudal border is parallel to the cranial border and equidistant from the cranial border to the caudal shoulder depression (arrow). The cranial and caudal borders are extended to the dorsal midline and connected dorsally. Alternatively, a hockey stick configuration can be created (not pictured).
B) Skin incisions are made along the marked cranial, caudal, and dorsal borders.
C) The flap is carefully undermined in a dorsal-to-ventral direction deep to the cutaneous trunci muscle to preserve the direct cutaneous artery and distal arterial plexus, and elevated.
D) The flap is transposed into the wound defect either directly if the donor site is adjacent to the wound defect (i, wide resection of a cutaneous soft tissue sarcoma from the lateral thorax) or via a bridging incision (ii, arrows; reconstruction of a dehisced wound after wide resection of a subcutaneous soft tissue sarcoma) or a tubed flap (iii, arrow; reconstruction of a distal antebrachial wound after failure of a free-meshed skin graft to reconstruct a defect resulting from wide surgical resection of a cutaneous mast cell tumor) if the wound defect is not adjacent to the donor site.
E) Consider placement of a closed suction drain (not pictured).

Color Atlas of Canine and Feline Surgical Oncology, First Edition. Julius M. Liptak, Paolo Buracco, William T. N. Culp, and Nicholas J. Bacon.

Plate 43.4

Thoracodorsal Axial Pattern Flap

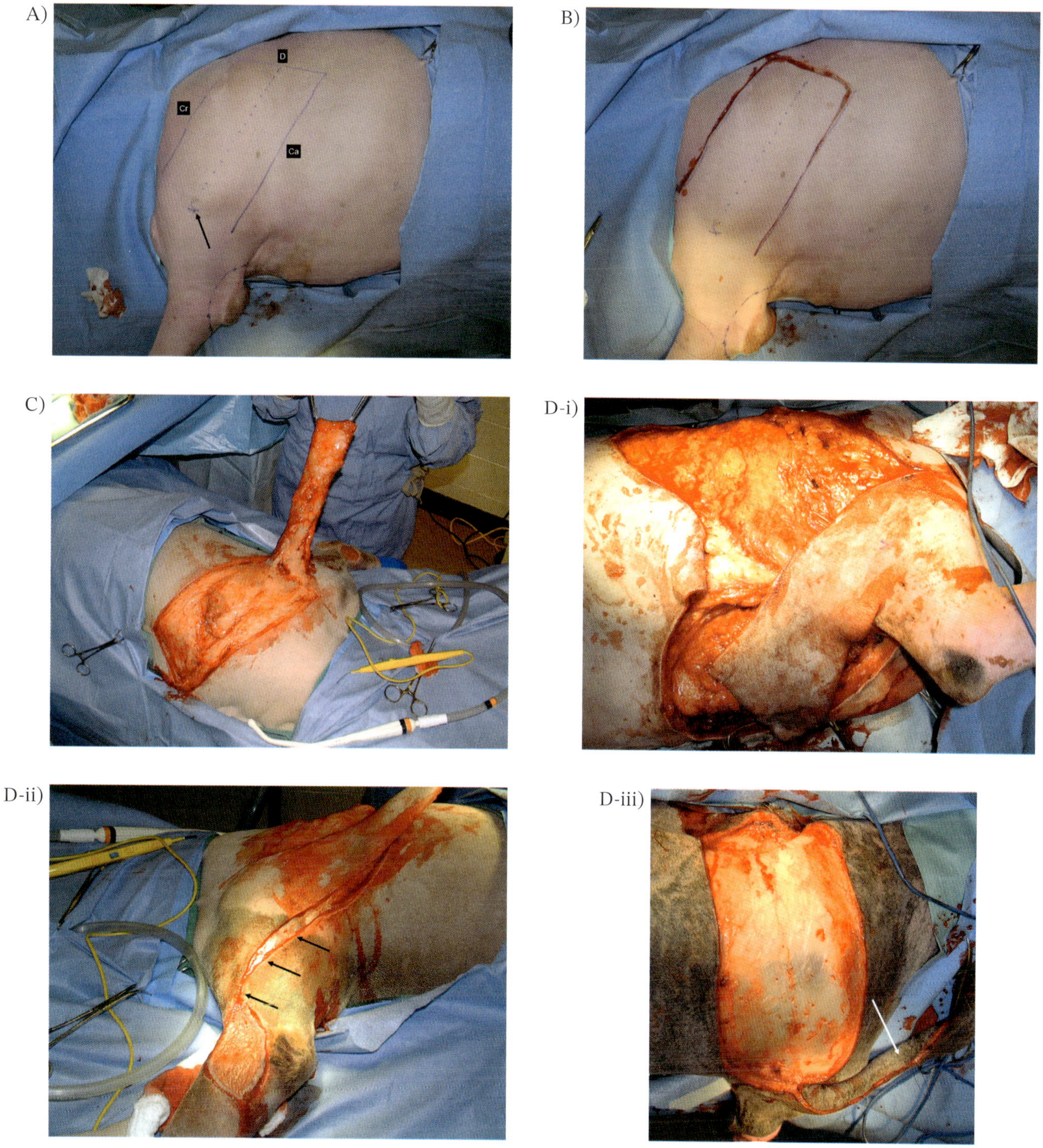

Closure (See Plate 43.4F)

F) The transposed flap and donor site are closed in two layers with a simple continuous suture pattern using monofilament absorbable suture material in the subcutis and either skin staples or an interrupted or continuous suture pattern using monofilament nonabsorbable suture material in the skin (i–iii; iv, appearance of the thoracodorsal axial pattern flap 2 years postoperatively).

Postoperative Management

1) Multimodal analgesia
2) Elizabethan collar
3) ± Closed suction drain management, if placed, for 2–5 days
4) ± Soft padded bandage

Complications – Dogs [2] (See Plate 43.4G)

- Partial- or full-thickness necrosis of the distal aspect of the flap (G) (70%)
- Flap edema (80%)
- Surgical-site infection (30%)
- Seroma (20%)

References

1 Pavletic, M.M. (2018). Axial pattern skin flaps. In: *Atlas of Small Animal Wound Management*, 4e (ed. M.M. Pavletic), 417–462. Hoboken: Wiley Blackwell.
2 Aper, R. and Smeak, D. (2004). Complications and outcome after thoracodorsal axial pattern flap reconstruction of forelimb skin defects in 10 dogs, 1989-2001. *Vet. Surg.* 32 (4): 378–384.

Plate 43.4

Thoracodorsal Axial Pattern Flap *continued*

F-i)

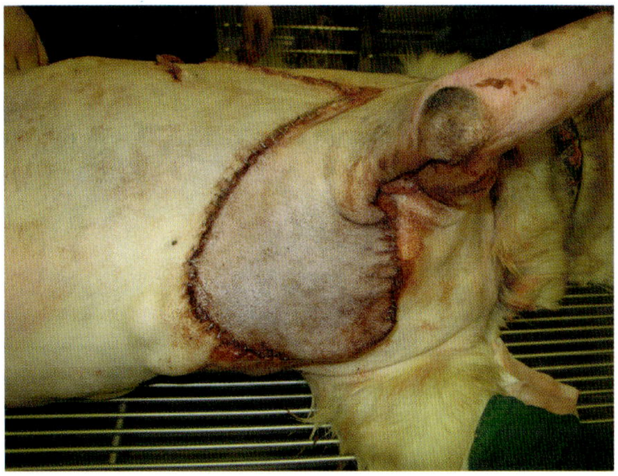

F-ii)

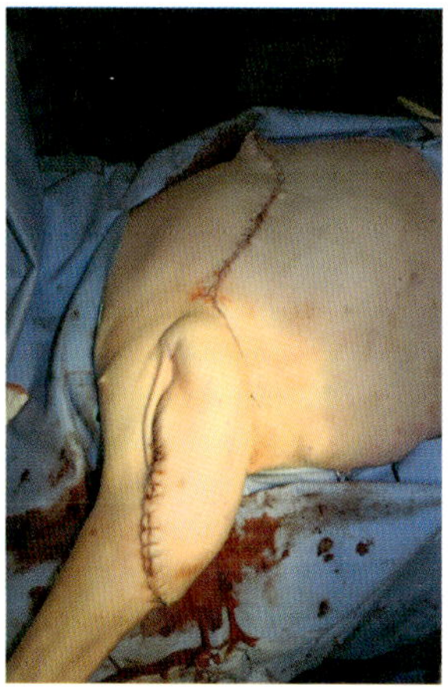

F-iii)

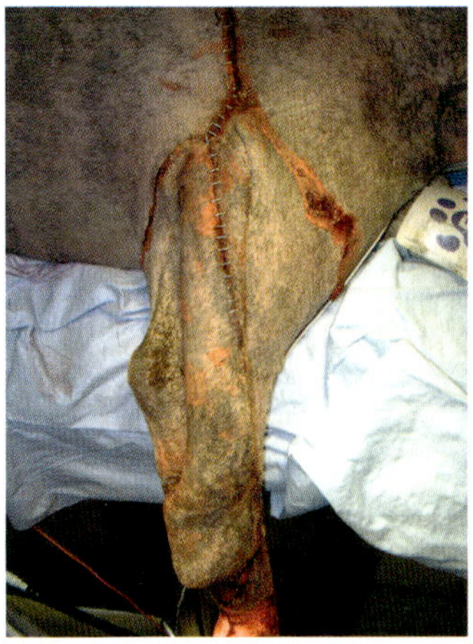

F-iv)

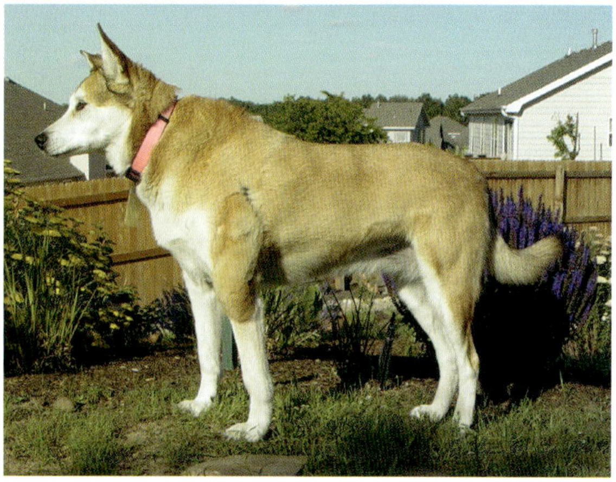

G)

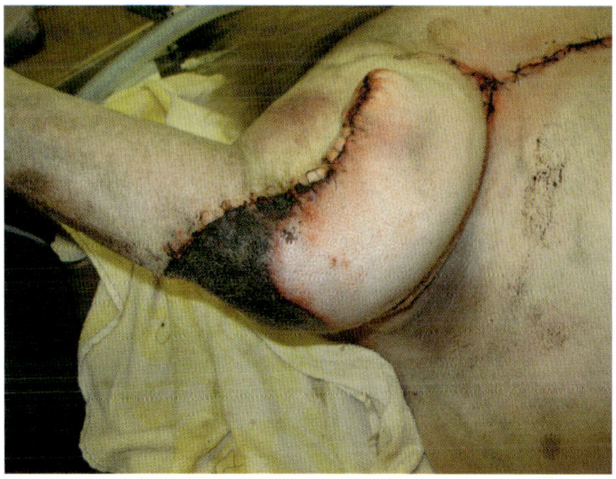

43.5 Superficial Brachial Axial Pattern Flap

Indication (See Plate 43.5 – 1)

1) Reconstruction of defects between the elbow and mid-antebrachium (i, ii)

Patient Positioning

The patient is positioned in dorsal recumbency with the affected limb elevated.

Surgical Technique [1] (See Plate 43.5A–D)

A) The superficial brachial axial pattern flap is based on the superficial brachial artery, which arises from the brachial artery proximal to the elbow joint, and courses medial to the cephalic vein. A sterile marker pen should be used to indicate the lateral (L), medial (M), and proximal (P) borders of the superficial brachial axial pattern flap. The flap is centered over the cranial third of the flexor surface of the elbow. The lateral and medial borders are parallel to the diaphysis of the humerus and are tapered proximally (to facilitate primary closure of the donor site) to the level of the proximal aspect of the greater tubercle of the humerus. The proximal border connects the proximal aspect of the lateral and medial borders.
B) Skin incisions are made along the marked medial, lateral, and proximal borders.
C) The flap is carefully undermined in a proximal-to-distal direction to preserve the direct cutaneous artery and distal arterial plexus, and elevated.
D) The flap is transposed into the wound defect either directly if the donor site is adjacent to the wound defect (i) or via a bridging incision (ii, dashed line) if the wound defect is not adjacent to the donor site.
E) Consider placement of a closed suction drain (not pictured).

Color Atlas of Canine and Feline Surgical Oncology, First Edition. Julius M. Liptak, Paolo Buracco, William T. N. Culp, and Nicholas J. Bacon.

Plate 43.5

Superficial Brachial Axial Pattern Flap

1-i)

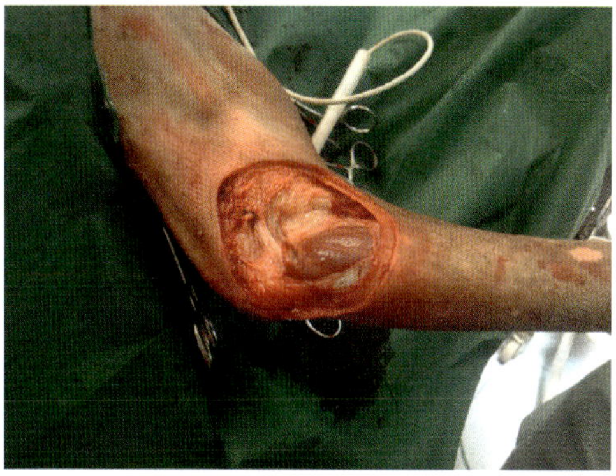

Courtesy of Dr. Maurizio Annoni

1-ii)

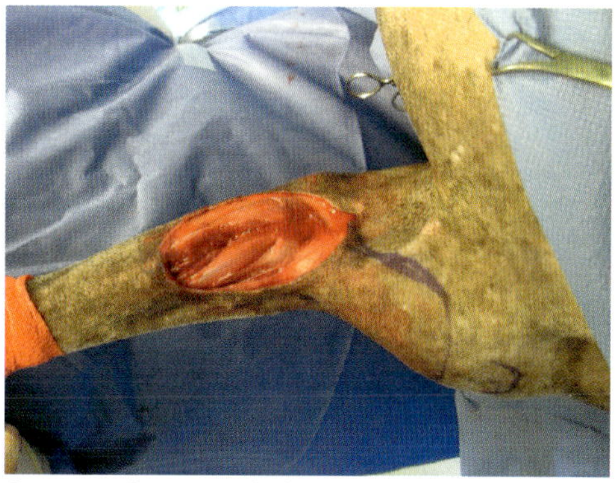

Courtesy of Dr. Ben Clarke

A)

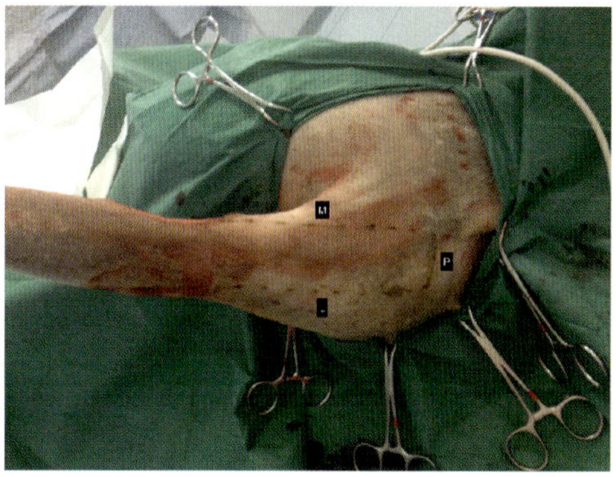

Courtesy of Dr. Maurizio Annoni

B)

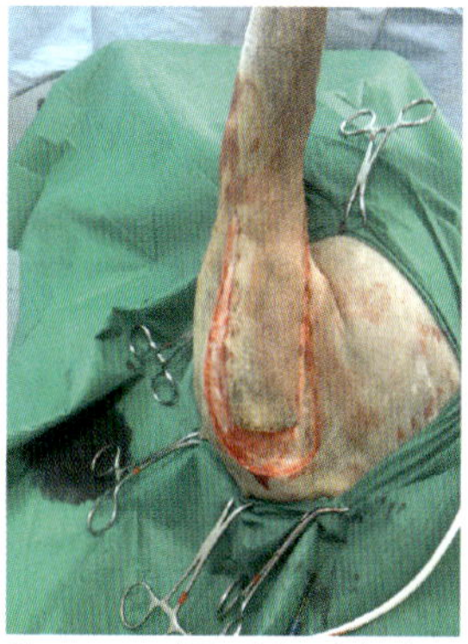

Courtesy of Dr. Maurizio Annoni

C)

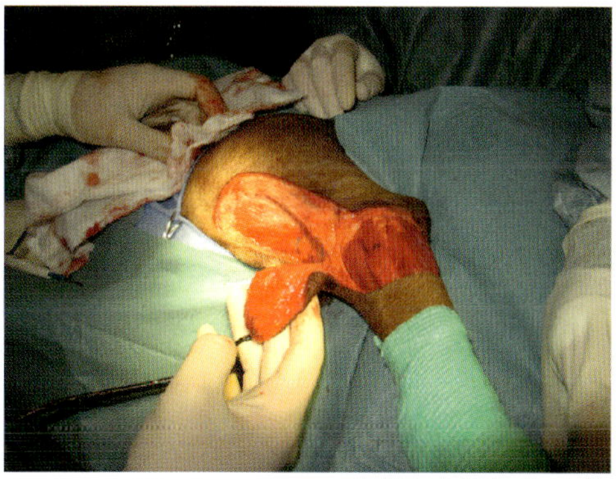

Courtesy of Dr. James Simcock

D-i)

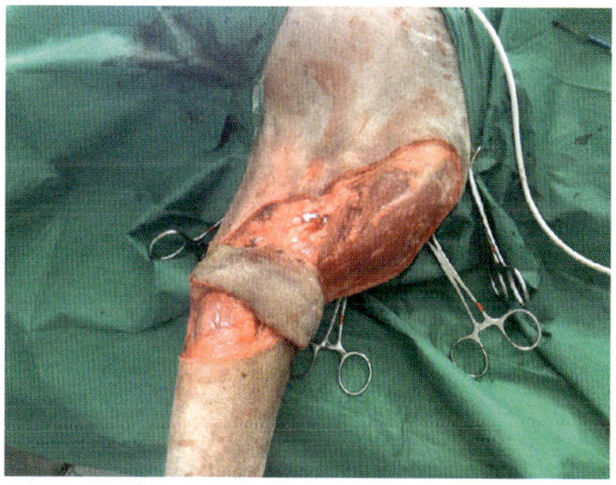

Courtesy of Dr. Maurizio Annoni

D-ii)

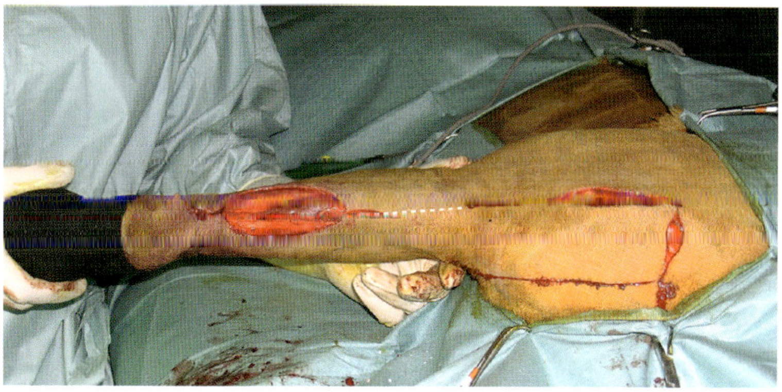

Closure (See Plate 43.5F)

F) The transposed flap and donor site are closed in two layers with a simple continuous suture pattern using monofilament absorbable suture material in the subcutis (i) and either skin staples or an interrupted (ii) or continuous suture pattern (iii) using monofilament nonabsorbable suture material in the skin.

Postoperative Management

1) Multimodal analgesia
2) Elizabethan collar
3) ± Closed suction drain management, if placed, for 2–5 days
4) ± Soft padded bandage

Complications – Dogs [2] (See Plate 43.5G)

- Overall: 100%
- Partial- or full-thickness necrosis of the distal aspect of the flap (G) (51%)
- Incisional dehiscence (44%)
- Seroma (31%)
- Flap edema (19%)

References

1 Pavletic, M.M. (2018). Axial pattern skin flaps. In: *Atlas of Small Animal Wound Management*, 4e (ed. M.M. Pavletic), 417–462. Hoboken: Wiley Blackwell.

2 Villedieu, E., Nolff, M.C., Del Magno, S. et al. (2022). Outcome of superficial brachial axial pattern flaps used to close skin defects in dogs: 16 cases (1996-2019). *J. Small Anim. Pract.* 63 (2): 136–141.

Plate 43.5

Superficial Brachial Axial Pattern Flap *continued*

F-i)

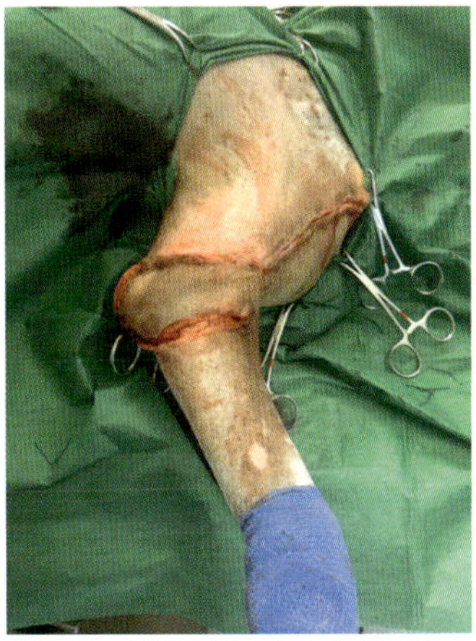

Courtesy of Dr. Maurizio Annoni

F-ii)

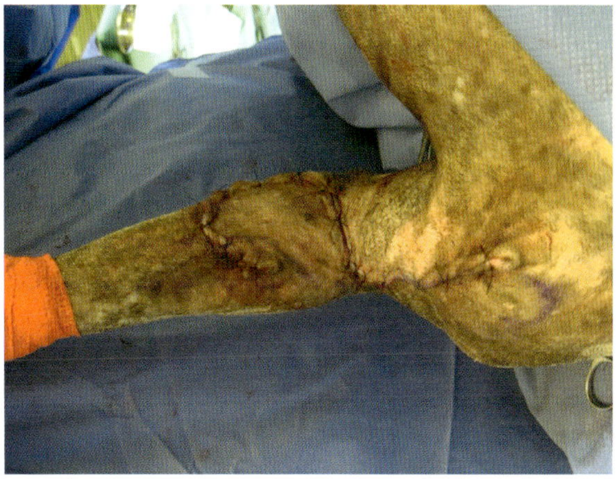

Courtesy of Dr. Ben Clarke

F-iii)

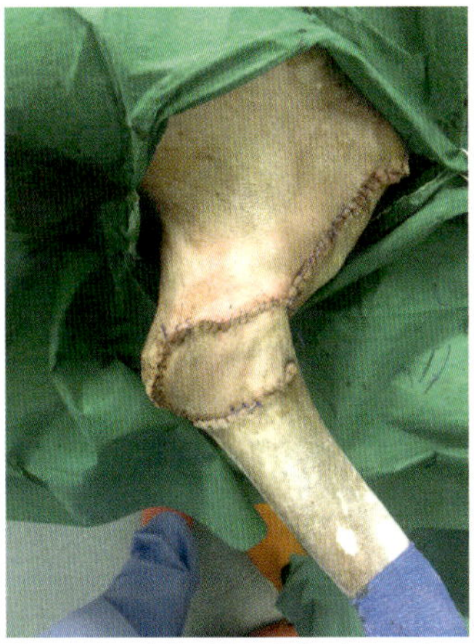

Courtesy of Dr. Maurizio Annoni

G)

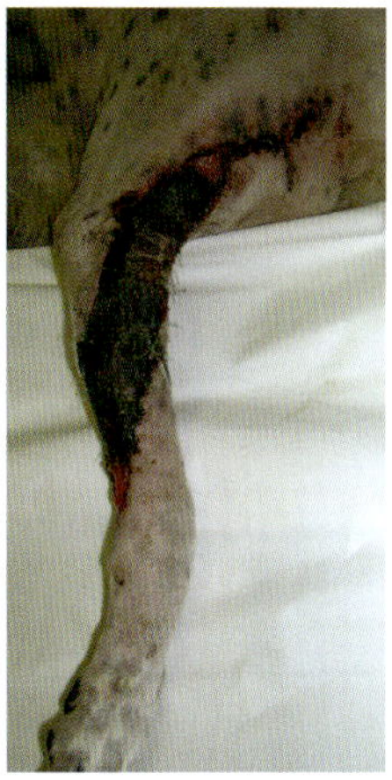

43.6 Latissimus Dorsi Muscle and Myocutaneous Flaps

General Considerations

The latissimus dorsi muscle is a type V muscle with a dominant pedicle and secondary segmental pedicles providing the blood supply to the muscle. This type of muscle can survive if either of the two vascular systems remains intact. In both dogs and cats, the dominant vascular pedicle has been identified as the thoracodorsal artery and vein.

Indications

1) Reconstruction of chest wall defects after chest wall resection for the treatment of primary rib neoplasia (see *14. Chest Wall Resection and Reconstruction*) [1, 2]
2) Reconstruction of abdominal wall, triceps brachii muscle, scapular, and esophageal defects has also been reported [3–6]

Patient Positioning

The patient is positioned in lateral recumbency with the affected side uppermost.

Surgical Technique (See Plate 43.6A–C)

A) If the latissimus dorsi muscle is not adhered to or invaded by the rib tumor, then this muscle can be used for later reconstruction of the chest wall defect. The ventral border of the latissimus dorsi muscle (i) is dissected free from its fascial attachments using blunt dissection or a vessel sealing device (ii). The caudal border of the muscle inserts on the 13th rib; this insertion should be released with sharp dissection or a vessel sealing device (ii). The dorsal border of the latissimus dorsi muscle, extending from the caudal border of the triceps muscle to the head of the 13th rib, is dissected free from its fascial attachments using blunt dissection or a vessel sealing device. If using a myocutaneous flap, then these same landmarks are also used for the skin overlying the latissimus dorsi muscle.
B) Once freed of its ventral, caudal, and dorsal attachments, the latissimus dorsi muscle is raised (i), progressively ligating and dividing perforating intercostal vessels, reflected cranially (ii, latissimus dorsi muscle flap; iii, latissimus dorsi myocutaneous flap), and protected with moistened laparotomy sponges (iv).
C) After chest wall resection, the latissimus dorsi muscle flap (i) is rotated into the defect and sutured ventrally to the pectoral muscles, cranially to either the rib or musculature along the cranial border of the chest wall defect, and caudally to either the rib or musculature along the caudal border of the chest wall defect (ii). Monofilament absorbable suture material is used in either an interrupted or simple continuous suture pattern. The same closure method is used for a latissimus dorsi myocutaneous flap, with the additional steps of closing the cutaneous trunci muscle, subcutaneous layer, and skin (iii).

Color Atlas of Canine and Feline Surgical Oncology, First Edition. Julius M. Liptak, Paolo Buracco, William T. N. Culp, and Nicholas J. Bacon.

Plate 43.6

Latissimus Dorsi Muscle and Myocutaneous Flaps

A-i)

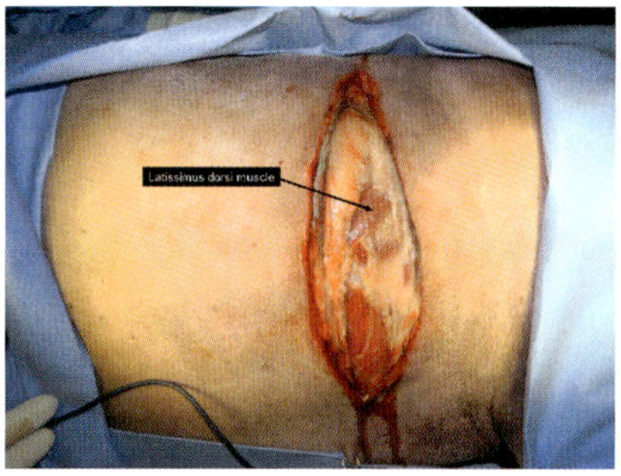

A-ii)

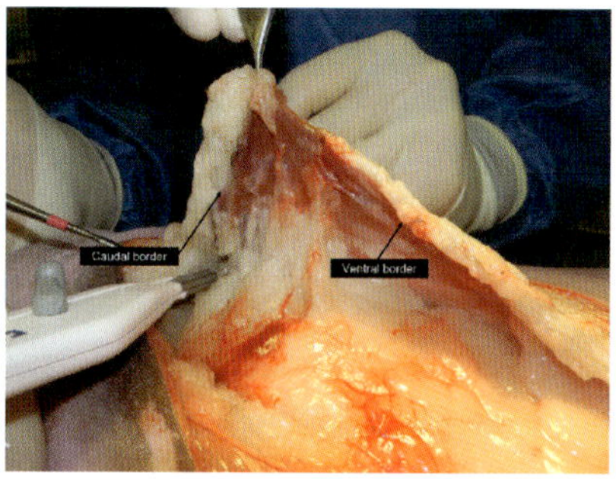

B-i)

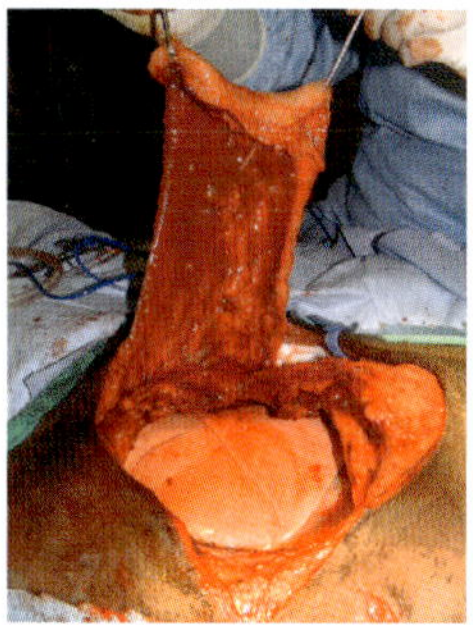

B-ii)

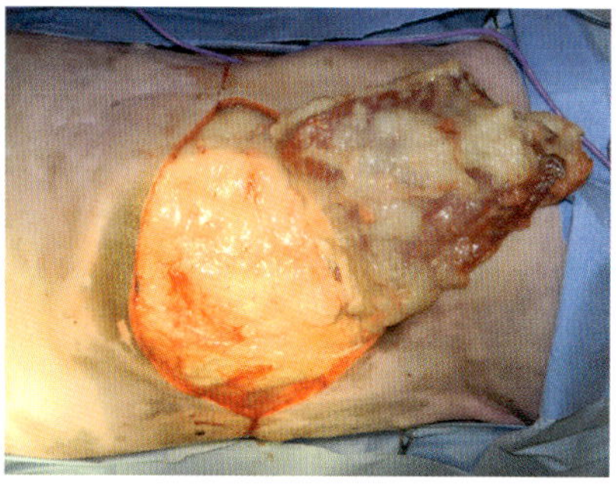

B-iii)

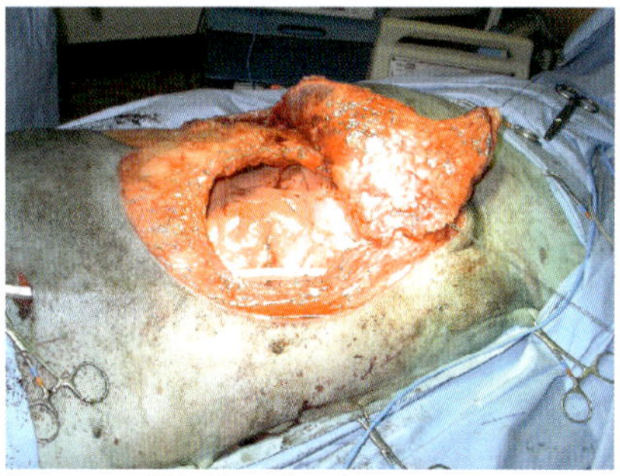

Courtesy of Dr. Dan Brockman

B-iv)

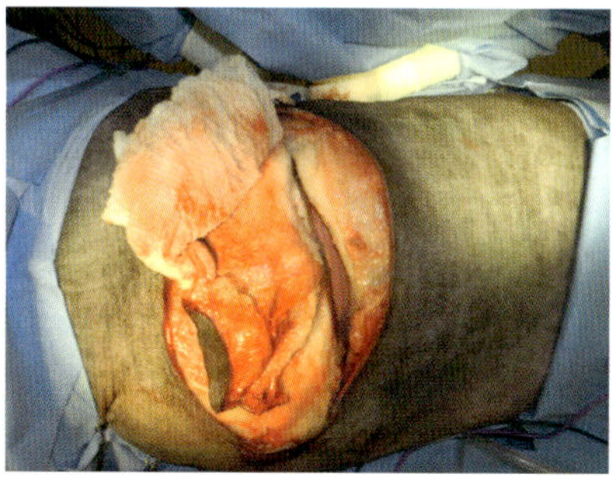

C-i)

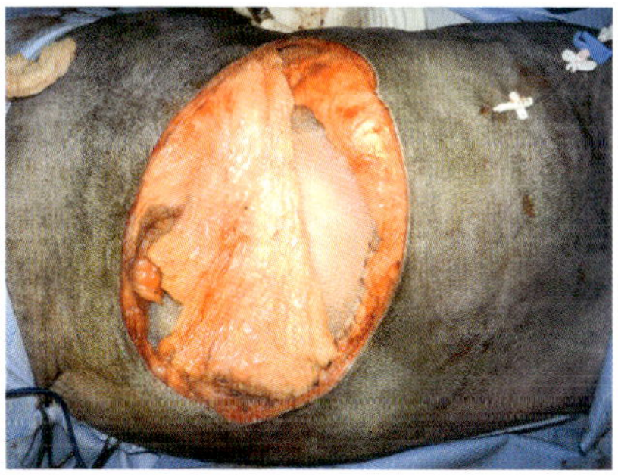

C-ii)

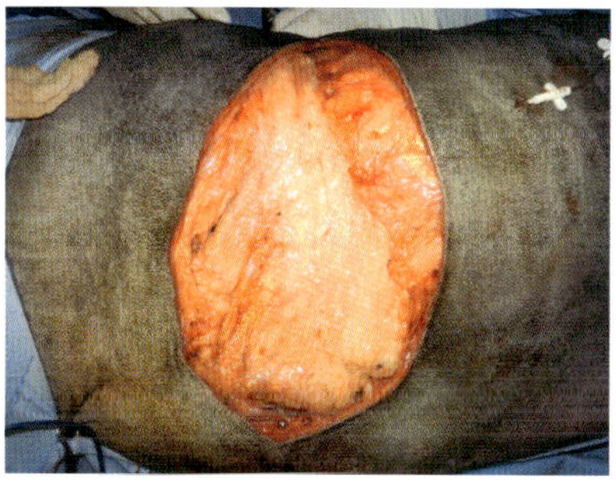

C-iii)

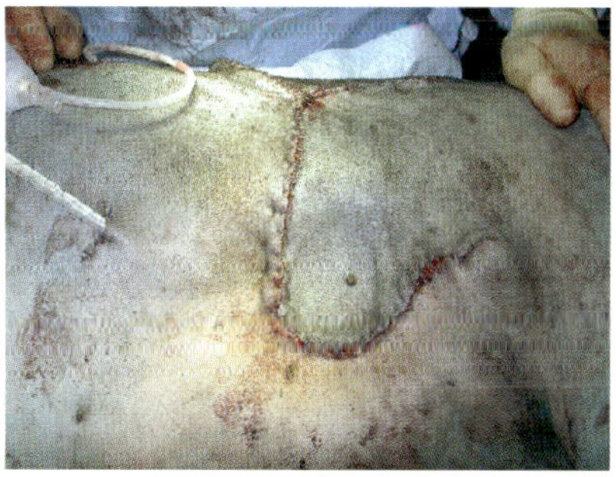

Courtesy of Dr. Dan Brockman

Postoperative Management

See *14. Chest Wall Resection and Reconstruction*.

Complications

See *14. Chest Wall Resection and Reconstruction*.

References

1 Liptak, J.M., Dernell, W.S., Rizzo, S.A. et al. (2008). Reconstruction of chest wall defects after rib tumor resection: a comparison of autogenous, prosthetic, and composite techniques in 44 dogs. *Vet. Surg.* 37 (5): 479–487.

2 Halfacree, Z.J., Baines, S.J., Lipscomb, V.J. et al. (2007). Use of a latissimus dorsi myocutaneous flap for one-stage reconstruction of the thoracic wall after en bloc resection of primary rib chondrosarcoma in five dogs. *Vet. Surg.* 36 (6): 587–592.

3 Feng, Y.C., Chen, K.S., and Chang, S.C. (2016). Reconstruction with latissimus dorsi, external abdominal oblique and cranial sartorius muscle flaps for a large defect of abdominal wall in a dog after surgical removal of infiltrative lipoma. *J. Vet. Med. Sci.* 78 (11): 1717–1721.

4 Pavletic, M.M., Kalis, R., Tribou, P. et al. (2015). Triceps brachii muscle reconstruction with a latissimus dorsi muscle flap in a dog. *J. Am. Vet. Med. Assoc.* 246 (2): 226–230.

5 Yamataka, A., Wang, K., Kobayashi, H. et al. (2000). Tubed latissimus dorsi musculocutaneous flaps for esophageal replacement in puppies: long-term follow-up. *J. Pediatr. Surg.* 35 (11): 1623–1625.

6 Canapp, S.O., Mann, F.A., Henry, C.J. et al. (2001). The use of a latissimus dorsi muscle flap for scapular reconstruction in a cat following fibrosarcoma excision. *J. Am. Anim. Hosp. Assoc.* 37 (3): 283–289.

43.7 Caudal Superficial Epigastric Axial Pattern Flap

Indication

1) The primary indication is reconstruction of defects on the caudal abdomen and inguinal region, pelvic limb, flank, perineum, and prepuce [1–3]. The caudal superficial epigastric flap can extend to the metatarsus in cats and tibia in dogs [4, 5]. Bilateral superficial epigastric axial pattern flaps can be raised simultaneously if necessary [6, 7].

Patient Positioning

The patient is positioned in dorsal recumbency. For wounds located on the limb, the limb is hung to allow for the limb to be mobilized as required during the surgical procedure.

Surgical Technique (See Plate 43.7A–D)

A) The caudal superficial epigastric axial pattern flap is based on the caudal superficial epigastric artery and vein at the level of the inguinal canal [3]. A sterile marker pen should be used to indicate the medial (M), lateral (L), and cranial (Cr) borders of the caudal superficial epigastric axial pattern flap. The caudal base is at the level of the last mammary gland in female dogs and the base of the prepuce in male dogs. In cats, the caudal extent is located at the inguinal ring [4]. The medial border is along the ventral midline, the lateral border is parallel to the medial border and equidistant from the medial border to the nipples (double-ended arrows), and the cranial border is dependent on the length of flap needed with the cranial extent between the first and second mammary glands in dogs [2] and to the level of the second nipple in cats [4].
B) Skin incisions are made along the marked medial, lateral, and cranial borders (i). The incisions are continued deep to the supramammary muscle but above the abdominal oblique musculature (ii).
C) The flap is carefully undermined deep to the supramammary muscle to preserve the direct cutaneous artery and vein.
D) The flap is transposed into the wound defect either directly if the donor site is adjacent to the wound defect or via a bridging incision (ii, dashed line) if the wound defect is not adjacent to the donor site. Alternatively, if there is a marked distance between the caudal superficial epigastric axial pattern flap donor site and the defect, then the caudal superficial epigastric axial pattern flap can be tubed rather than creating a long bridging incision (iii–v).
E) Consider placement of a closed suction drain (see D – i).

Color Atlas of Canine and Feline Surgical Oncology, First Edition. Julius M. Liptak, Paolo Buracco, William T. N. Culp, and Nicholas J. Bacon.

Plate 43.7

Caudal Superficial Epigastric Axial Pattern Flap

A)

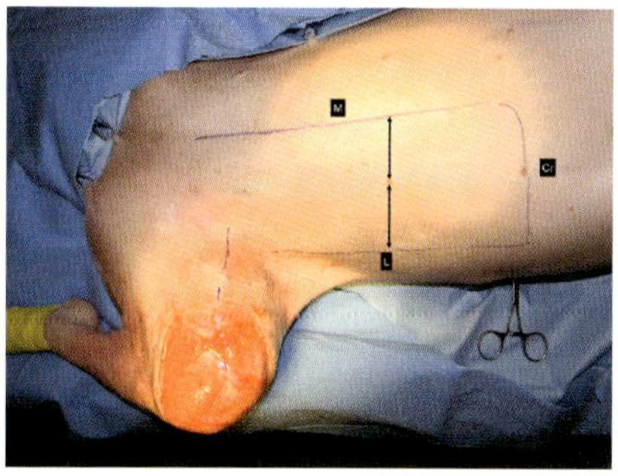

B-i)

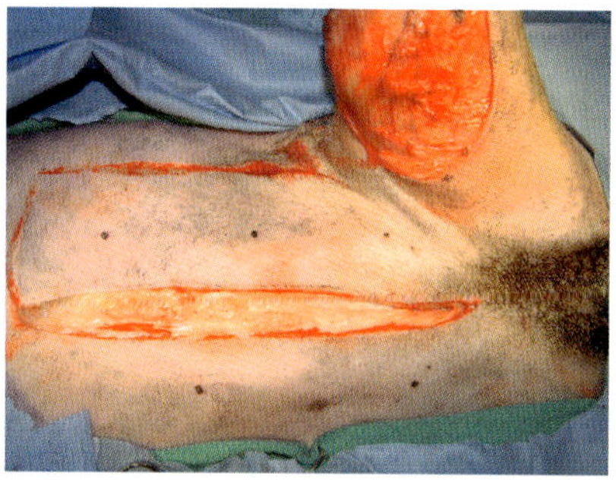

B-ii)

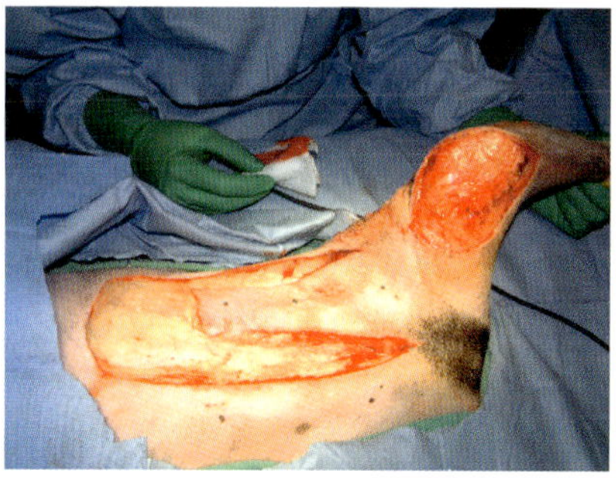

C)

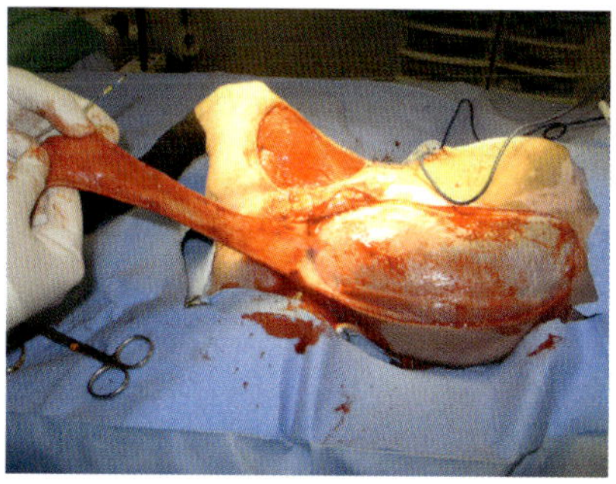

D-i)

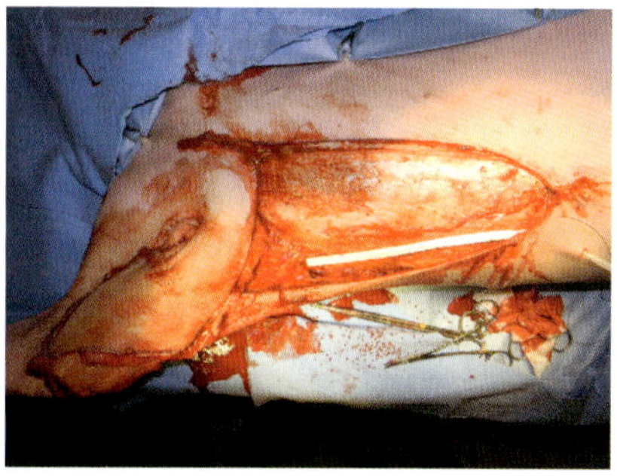

D-ii)

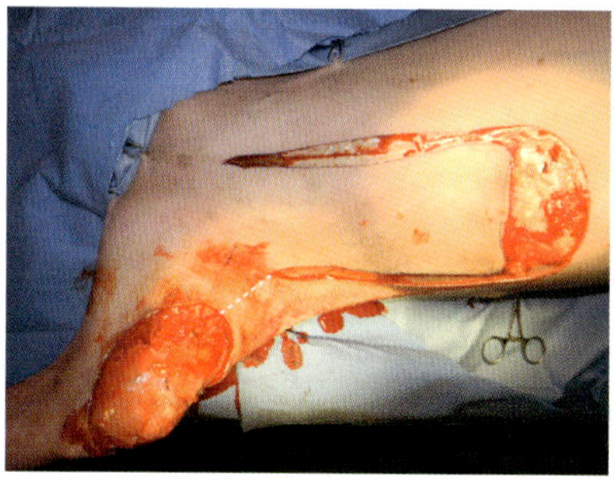

D-iii)

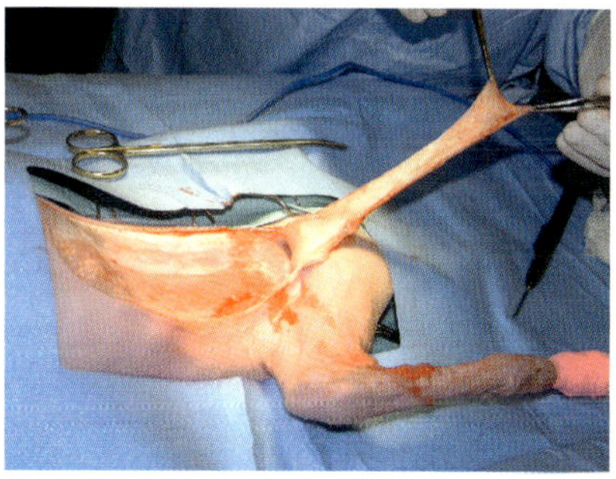

D-iv)

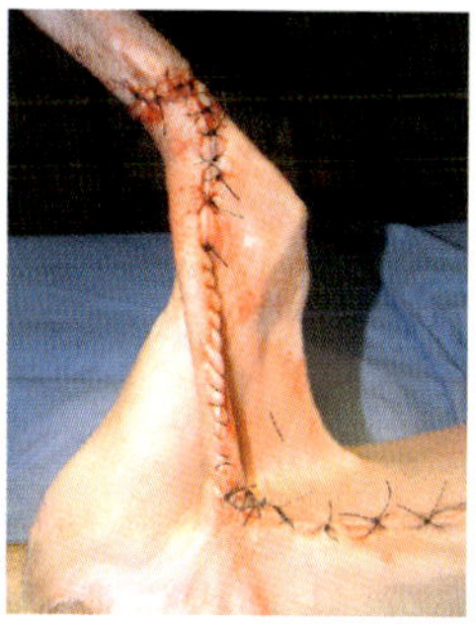

D-v)

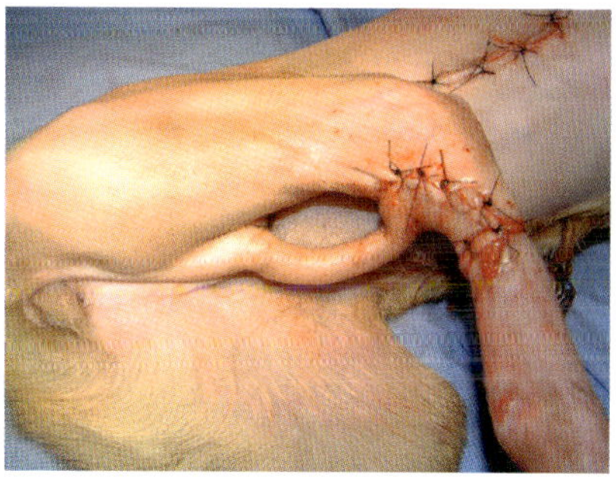

Closure (See Plate 43.7F, G)

The transposed flap (F – i) and donor site (F – ii) are closed in two layers with a simple continuous suture pattern using monofilament absorbable suture material in the subcutis and either skin staples or an interrupted or continuous suture pattern using monofilament nonabsorbable suture material in the skin. If a tubed caudal superficial epigastric axial pattern flap has been used, then the tube is resected after 3 or more weeks (G – i, ii). The proximal and distal transection sites of the tubed flap are closed routinely.

Postoperative Management

1) Multimodal analgesia
2) Elizabethan collar
3) ± Closed suction drain management, if placed, for 2–5 days
4) ± Soft padded bandage for up to 10 days

Complications – Dogs (See Plate 43.7H)

- Overall: 67% with 59% classified as minor and 8% as major [8]
  - Flap edema or swelling (H) (90%) [2]
  - Incisional dehiscence (30%–31%) [2, 8]
  - Partial necrosis of the distal extent of the flap (10%–29%) [2, 8]
  - Seroma (25%–30%) [2, 8]
  - Surgical-site infection (0%–16%) [2, 8]

Complications – Cats [8]

- Overall: 53% with 47% classified as minor and 5% as major
  - Incisional dehiscence (26%)
  - Partial necrosis of the distal extent of the flap (16%)
  - Surgical-site infection (5%)

References

1 Massari, F., Montinaro, V., Buracco, P. et al. (2018). Combined caudal-superficial-epigastric axial pattern flap and full-thickness buccal mucosa graft for single-stage preputial reconstruction in six dogs. *J. Small Anim. Pract.* 59 (7): 415–421.

2 Aper, R.L. and Smeak, D.D. (2005). Clinical evaluation of caudal superficial epigastric axial pattern flap reconstruction of skin defects in 10 dogs (1989-2001). *J. Am. Anim. Hosp. Assoc.* 41 (3): 185–192.

3 Pavletic, M.M. (1990). Axial pattern flaps in small animal practice. *Vet. Clin. North Am. Small Anim. Pract.* 20 (1): 105–125.

4 Remedios, A.M., Bauer, M.S., and Bowen, C.V. (1989). Thoracodorsal and caudal superficial epigastric axial pattern skin flaps in cats. *Vet. Surg.* 18 (5): 380–385.

5 Pavletic, M.M. (1982). Misapplication of subcutaneous pedicle flaps in the dog. *Vet. Surg.* 1 (1): 18–22.

6 Woods, S., de Marques, A.I.C., and Yool, D.A. (2009). Simultaneous bilateral caudal superficial epigastric skin flaps in a cat. *Vet. Rec.* 164 (14): 434–435.

7 Mayhew, P.D. and Holt, D.E. (2003). Simultaneous use of bilateral caudal superficial epigastric axial pattern flaps for wound closure in a dog. *J. Small Anim. Pract.* 44 (12): 534–538.

8 Forster, K., Cutando, L.S., Ladlow, J. et al. (2022). Outcome of caudal superficial epigastric axial pattern flaps in dogs and cats: 70 cases (2007-2020). *J. Small Anim. Pract.* 63 (2): 128–135.

Plate 43.7

Caudal Superficial Epigastric Axial Pattern Flap *continued*

F-i)

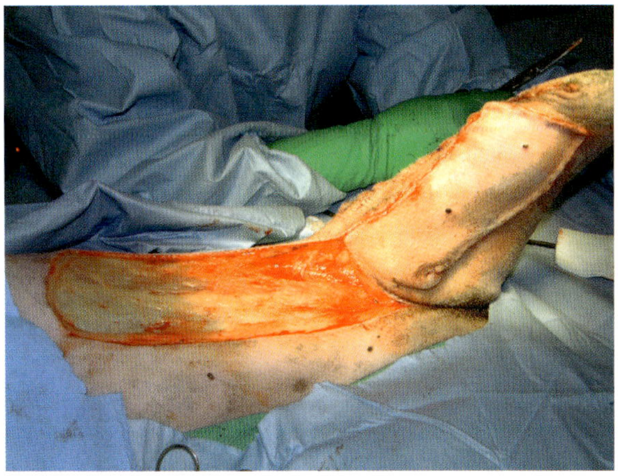

F-ii)

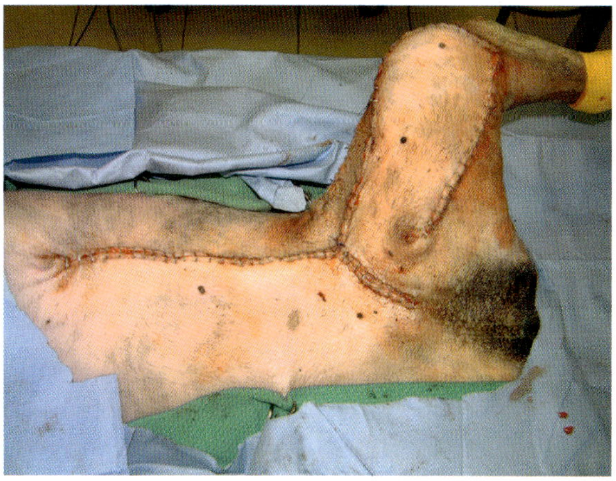

G-i)

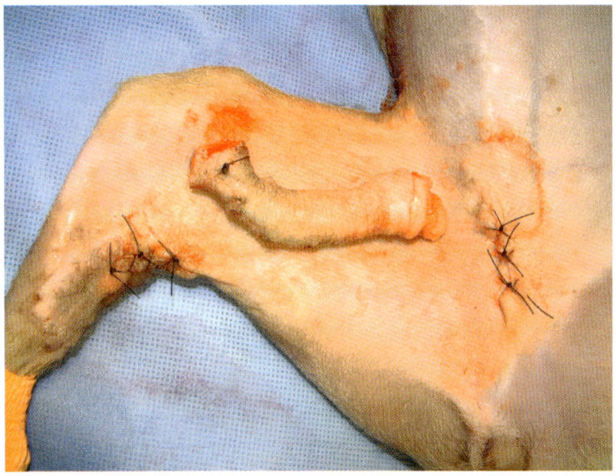

G-ii)

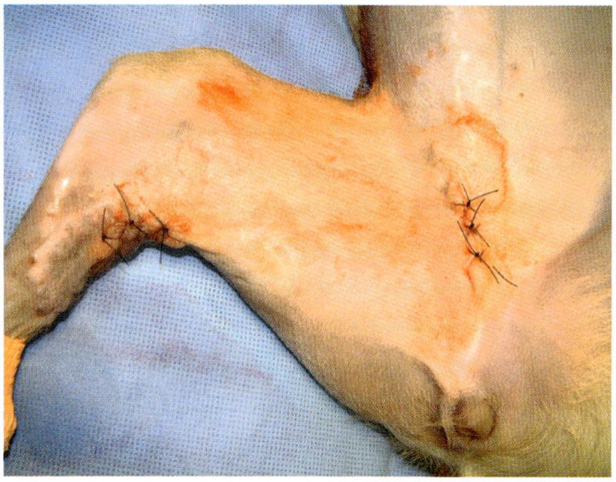

H)

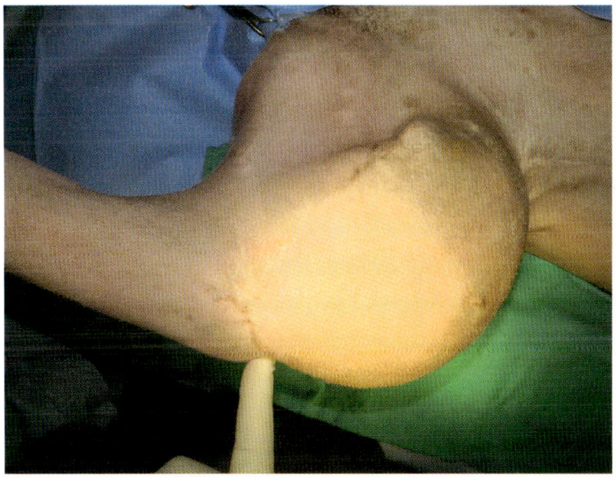

43.8 Deep Circumflex Iliac Axial Pattern Flap (Dorsal and Ventral Branches)

General Considerations

The deep circumflex iliac artery and vein are branches directly of the aorta and caudal vena cava, respectively. These vessels perforate the abdominal wall and can be found cranioventral to the wing of the ilium. There are major dorsal and ventral branches, and both can be used as the direct cutaneous blood supply for cutaneous flap usage.

After raising these flaps, both can be used as peninsula flaps to cover defects in the 180-degree arc of rotation. The deep circumflex iliac axial pattern flap based on its ventral branch can also be used as an island flap, and the deep circumflex iliac axial pattern flap based on its dorsal branch has been used in an L configuration [1–3].

Indication

1) Reconstruction of defects on the thorax, lateral abdominal wall, flank, and lateral thigh and hip [1]

Patient Positioning

The patient is positioned in lateral recumbency. For wounds located on the limb, the limb is hung to allow for the limb to be mobilized as required during the surgical procedure.

Surgical Technique – Dorsal Branch [1] (See Plate 43.8A, D)

A) A sterile marker pen should be used to indicate the cranial (Cr), caudal (Ca), and dorsal (D) borders of the dorsal branch of the deep circumflex iliac axial pattern flap. The caudal border originates at a point midway between the cranial edge of the wing of the ilium and the greater trochanter. The cranial border is parallel to the caudal incision and is an equal distance cranially from the edge of the wing of the ilium as the distance from the wing of the ilium to the caudal incision. The dorsal border connects the cranial and caudal borders on the dorsal midline.
B) Skin incisions are made along the marked cranial, caudal, and dorsal borders.
C) The flap is carefully undermined starting at the dorsal incision. The flap should be undermined deep to the cutaneous trunci muscle to preserve the direct cutaneous artery and vein. The flap is then elevated.
D) The flap is transposed into the wound defect either directly (pictured) if the donor site is adjacent to the wound defect or via a bridging incision if the wound defect is not adjacent to the donor site.

Color Atlas of Canine and Feline Surgical Oncology, First Edition. Julius M. Liptak, Paolo Buracco, William T. N. Culp, and Nicholas J. Bacon.

Plate 43.8

Deep Circumflex Iliac Axial Pattern Flap (Dorsal and Ventral Branches)

A)

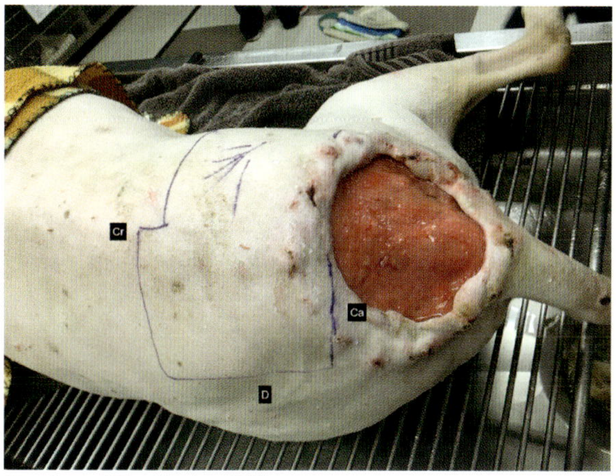

Courtesy of Dr. Stephen Bilbrey

B)

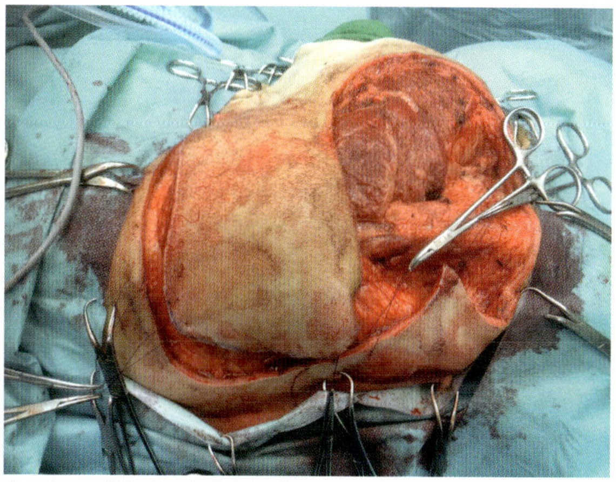

Courtesy of Dr. Lucinda Van Stee

C)

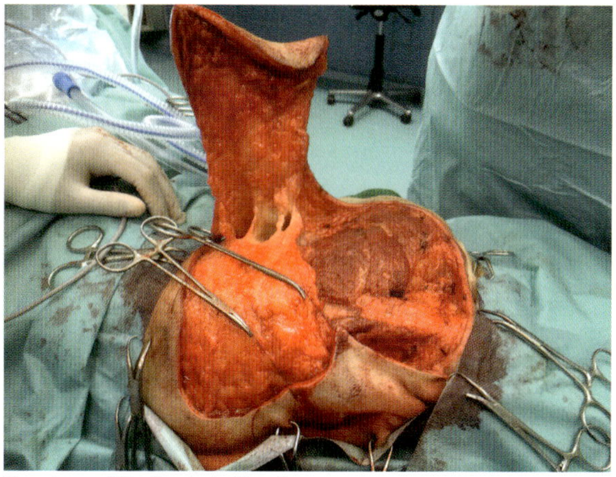

Courtesy of Dr. Lucinda Van Stee

D)

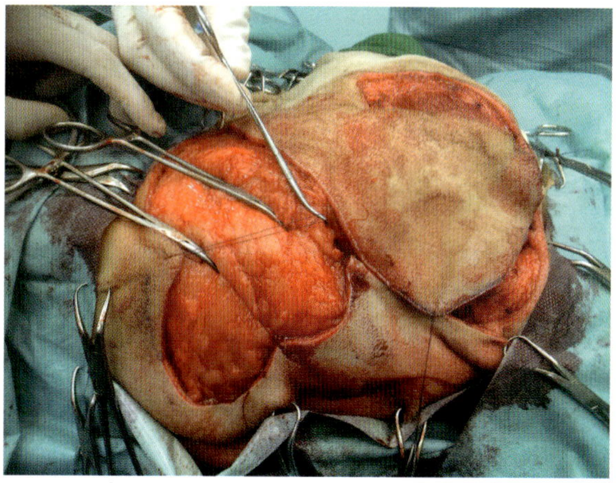

Courtesy of Dr. Lucinda Van Stee

Surgical Technique – Ventral Branch [1] (See Plate 43.8E, H, I)

E) A sterile marker pen should be used to indicate the cranial (Cr), caudal (Ca), and ventral (V) borders of the dorsal branch of the deep circumflex iliac axial pattern flap. Unlike the flap using the dorsal branch of the deep circumflex iliac artery, the cranial incision is extended distally, cranial to the long axis of the femur. The cranial border is parallel to the caudal incision and is an equal distance cranially from the edge of the wing of the ilium as the distance from the wing of the ilium to the caudal incision. The ventral border connects the cranial and caudal borders dorsal to the patella.
F) Skin incisions are made along the marked cranial, caudal, and ventral borders.
G) The flap is carefully undermined starting at the ventral border. The flap should be undermined deep to the cutaneous trunci muscle to preserve the direct cutaneous artery and vein. The flap is then elevated.
H) Alternatively, this flap can be raised as an island flap. To do this, an incision is made connecting the cranial and caudal incisions dorsally. This should be done carefully to preserve the direct cutaneous artery and vein. This flap can be rotated dorsally to cover defects on the dorsum [2, 3].
I) The flap is transposed into the wound defect either directly (see G) if the donor site is adjacent to the wound defect or via a bridging incision if the wound defect is not adjacent to the donor site.

Closure (See Plate 43.8J)

J) The transposed flap and donor site are closed in two layers with a simple continuous suture pattern using monofilament absorbable suture material in the subcutis and either skin staples or an interrupted or continuous suture pattern using monofilament nonabsorbable suture material in the skin (see steps D and I for the closure of the dorsal branch and ventral branch of the deep circumflex iliac axial pattern flap, respectively). Pictured is the island variation of the deep circumflex iliac axial pattern flap 2 weeks postoperatively.

Postoperative Management

1) Multimodal analgesia
2) Elizabethan collar
3) ± Closed suction drain management, if placed, for 2–5 days
4) ± Soft padded bandage for up to 10 days

Complications

No case series have reported the complications and outcomes after reconstruction with a deep circumflex iliac axial pattern flap. The following complications are for all axial pattern flaps.

Complications – Dogs [4]

- Overall: 92%
  - Incisional dehiscence (50%)
  - Partial necrosis of the distal extent of the flap (46%)
  - Edema or swelling of the axial pattern flap (43%)
  - Surgical-site infection (27%)
  - Seroma (23%)
  - Incisional discharge (14%)

Plate 43.8

Deep Circumflex Iliac Axial Pattern Flap (Dorsal and Ventral Branches) *continued*

E)

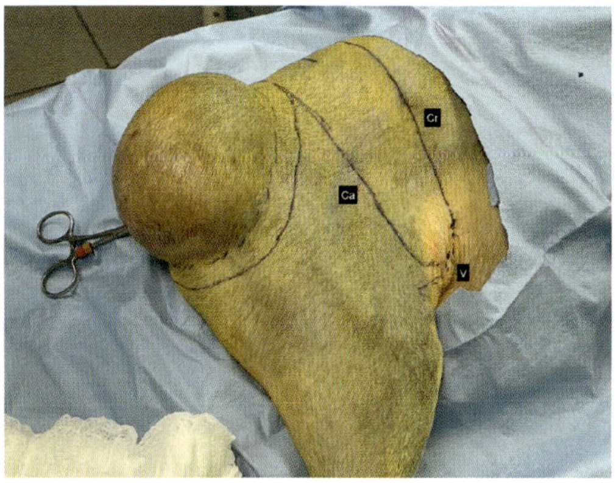

Courtesy of Dr. Rodrigo Rosa

F)

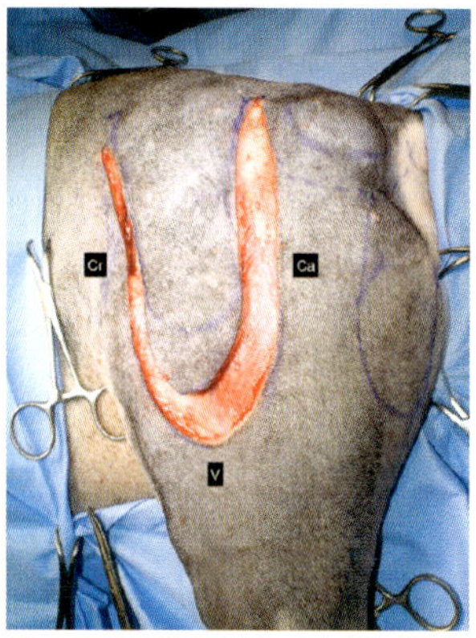

Courtesy of Dr. Laurent Findji

G)

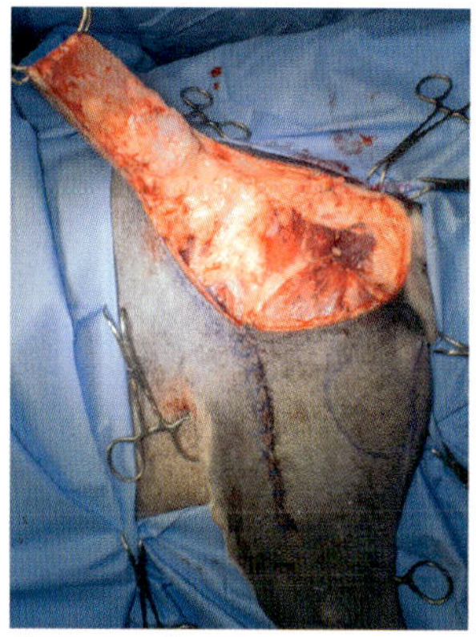

Courtesy of Dr. Laurent Findji

H-i)

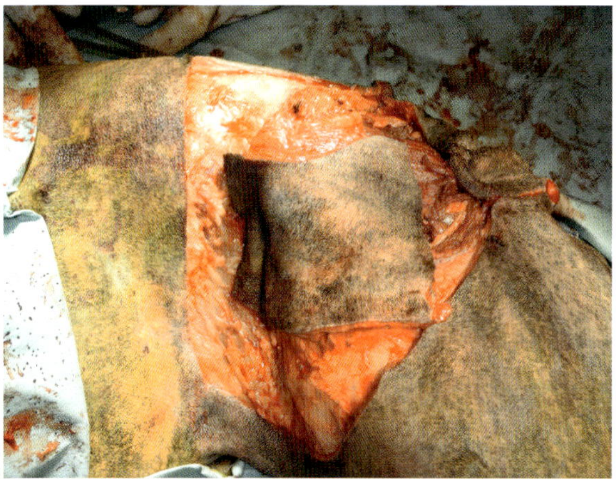

H-ii)

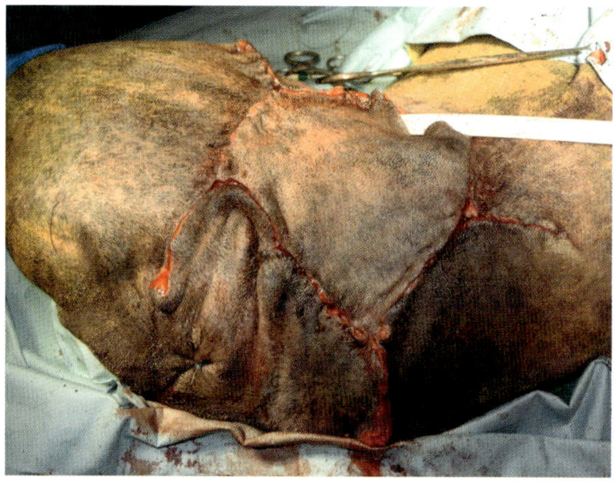

I)

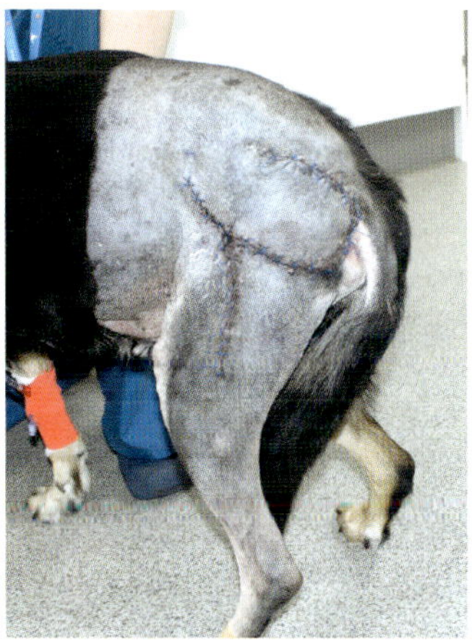

Courtesy of Dr. Laurent Findji

J)

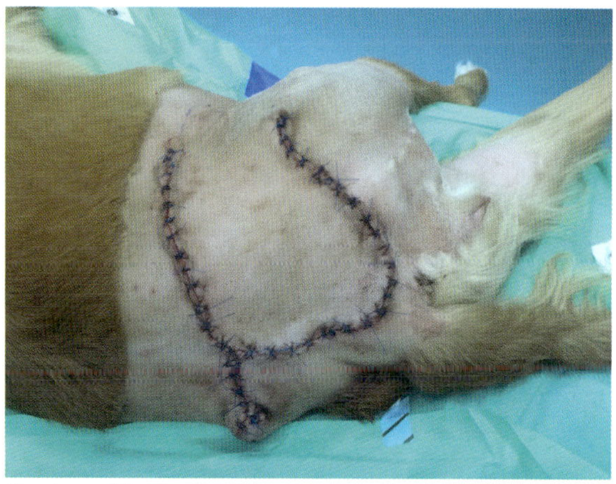

Courtesy of Dr. Stephen Bilbrey

Complications – Cats [4]

- Overall: 83%
  - Incisional dehiscence (75%)
  - Edema or swelling of the axial pattern flap (50%)
  - Incisional discharge (45%)
  - Surgical-site infection (40%)
  - Seroma (20%)
  - Partial necrosis of the distal extent of the flap (15%)

References

1 Pavletic, M.M. (1981). Canine axial pattern flaps, using the omocervical, thoracodorsal, and deep circumflex iliac direct cutaneous arteries. *Am. J. Vet. Res.* 42 (3): 391–406.

2 Jackson, A.H., Degner, D.A., Jackson, I.T. et al. (2003). Deep circumflex iliac cutaneous free flap in cats. *Vet. Surg.* 32 (4): 341–349.

3 Teunissen, B.D., Walshaw, R., Hauptman, J.G. et al. (2004). Evaluation of primary critical ischemia time for the deep circumflex iliac cutaneous flap in cats. *Vet. Surg.* 33 (5): 440–445.

4 Field, E.J., Kelly, G., Pleuvry, D. et al. (2015). Indications, outcome and complications with axial pattern skin flaps in dogs and cats: 73 cases. *J. Small Anim. Pract.* 56 (12): 698–706.

43.9 Genicular Axial Pattern Flap

Indication (See Plate 43.9 – 1)

1) Reconstruction of cutaneous defects on the lateral and medial surfaces of the tibia [1]

Patient Positioning

The patient is positioned in lateral recumbency with the affected limb uppermost.

Surgical Technique [1] (See Plate 43.9A–D)

A) The genicular artery and vein are branches of the saphenous artery and medial saphenous vein, respectively. A sterile marker pen should be used to indicate the cranial (Cr), caudal (Ca), and dorsal (D) borders of the genicular axial pattern flap. The base of the flap is located over the stifle joint, approximately 1 cm proximal to the patella cranially and 1–2 cm proximal to the tibial tuberosity laterally. The caudal border is 1–2 cm caudal to the long axis of the femur, the cranial border is parallel to the caudal border and equidistant from the caudal border to the femur, and the dorsal border connects the cranial and caudal border at the level of the greater trochanter.
B) Skin incisions are made along the marked cranial, caudal, and dorsal borders.
C) The flap is carefully undermined starting at the dorsal incision. The flap should be undermined deep to the cutaneous trunci muscle to preserve the direct cutaneous artery and vein (i). The flap is then elevated (ii).
D) The flap is transposed into the wound defect either directly if the donor site is adjacent to the wound defect (pictured) or via a bridging incision if the wound defect is not adjacent to the donor site.

Color Atlas of Canine and Feline Surgical Oncology, First Edition. Julius M. Liptak, Paolo Buracco, William T. N. Culp, and Nicholas J. Bacon.

Plate 43.9

Genicular Axial Pattern Flap

1)

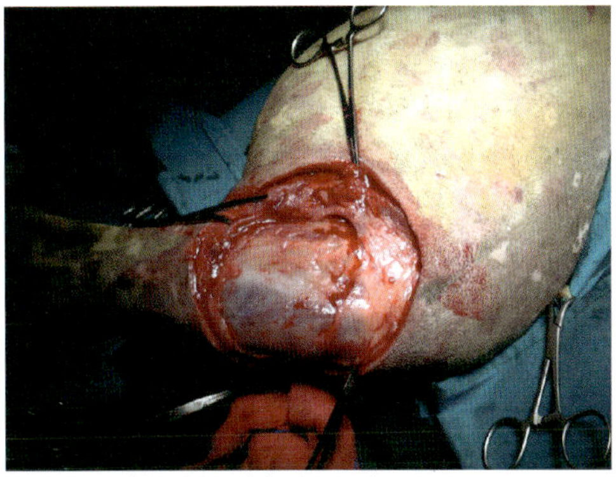

Courtesy of Dr. Maurizio Annoni

A)

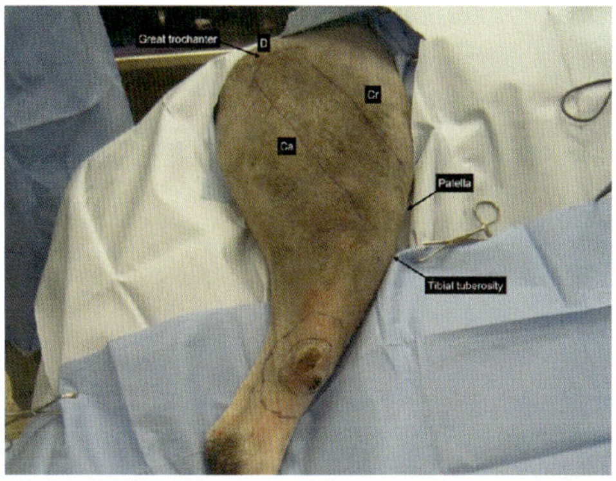

Courtesy of Dr. Pierre Amsellem

B)

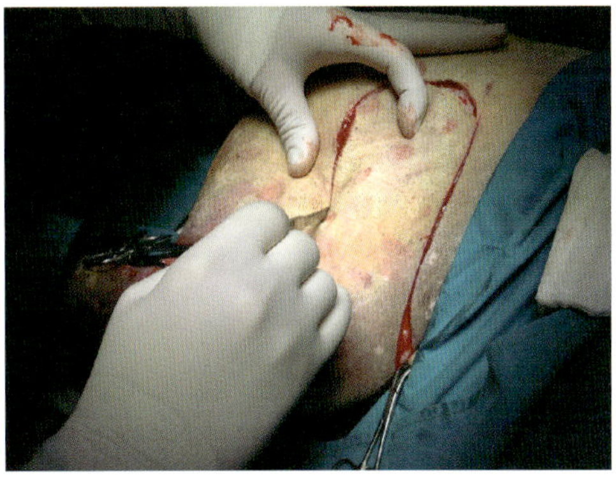

Courtesy of Dr. Maurizio Annoni

C-i)

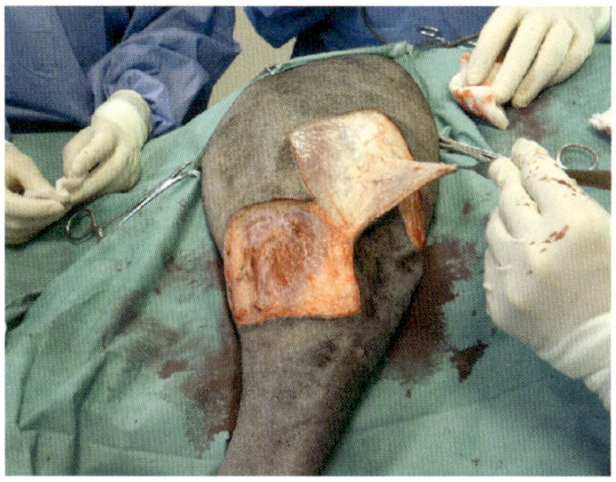

Courtesy of Dr. Rosario Vallefuoco

C-ii)

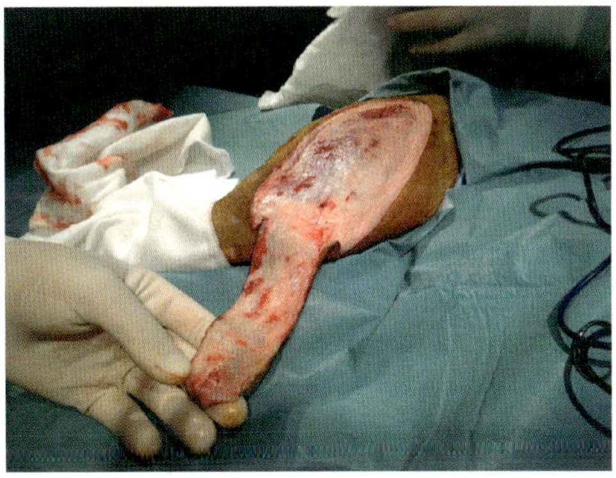

Courtesy of Dr. James Simcock

D)

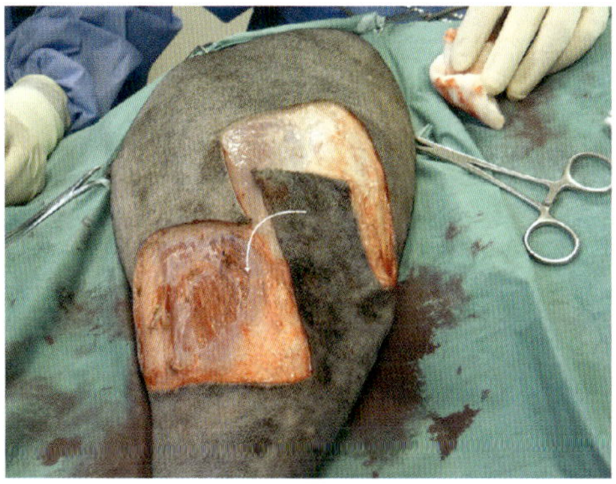

Courtesy of Dr. Rosario Vallefuoco

Closure (See Plate 43.9E)

E) The transposed flap and donor site are closed in two layers with a simple continuous suture pattern using monofilament absorbable suture material in the subcutis (i) and either skin staples or an interrupted or continuous suture pattern using monofilament nonabsorbable suture material in the skin (ii; iii, appearance of the genicular axial pattern flap 3 months postoperatively).

Postoperative Management

1) Multimodal analgesia
2) Elizabethan collar
3) ± Closed suction drain management, if placed, for 2–5 days
4) ± Soft padded bandage

Complications – Dogs

- Overall: 68% with 55% classified as minor and 14% as major [2]
- Incisional dehiscence (25%–36%) [1, 2]
- Partial necrosis of the distal extent of the flap (9%–11%) [1, 2]
- Seroma (9%) [2]
- Surgical-site infection (5%) [2]

References

1 Kostolich, M. and Pavletic, M.M. (1987). Axial pattern flap based on the genicular branch of the saphenous artery in the dog. *Vet. Surg.* 16 (3): 217–222.

2 Emmerson, T., de la Puerta, B., and Polton, G. (2019). Genicular artery axial pattern flap for reconstruction of skin defects in 22 dogs. *J. Small Anim. Pract.* 60 (9): 529–533.

Plate 43.9

Genicular Axial Pattern Flap *continued*

E-i)

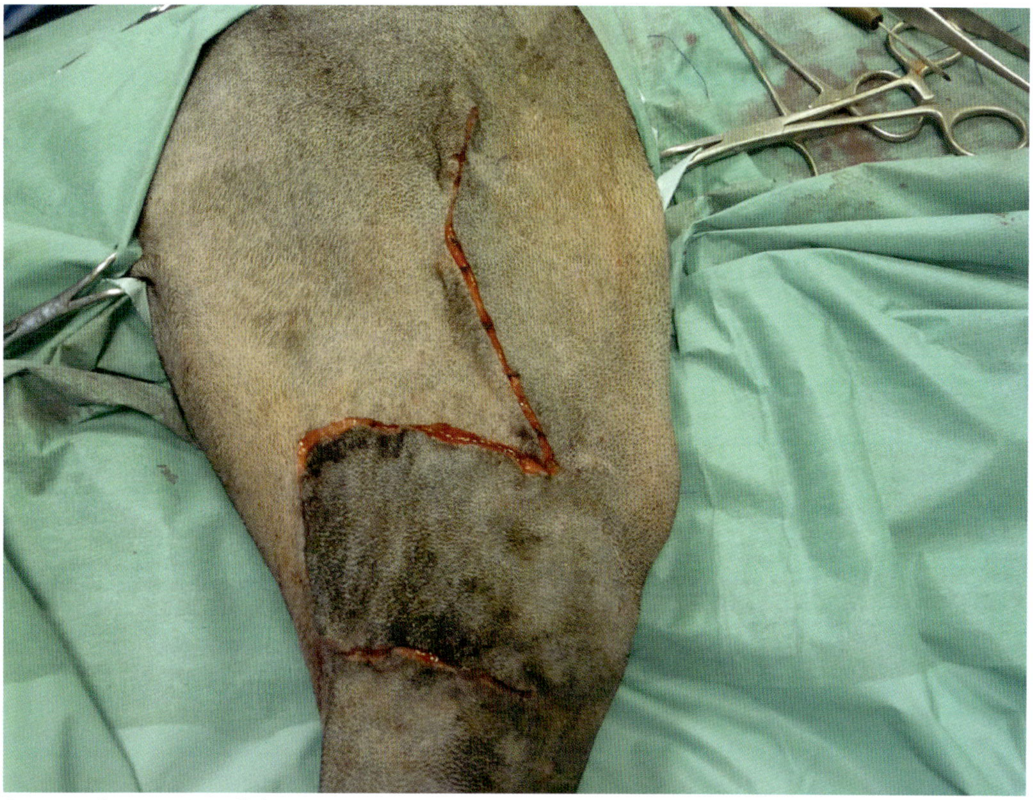

Courtesy of Dr. Rosario Vallefuoco

E-ii)

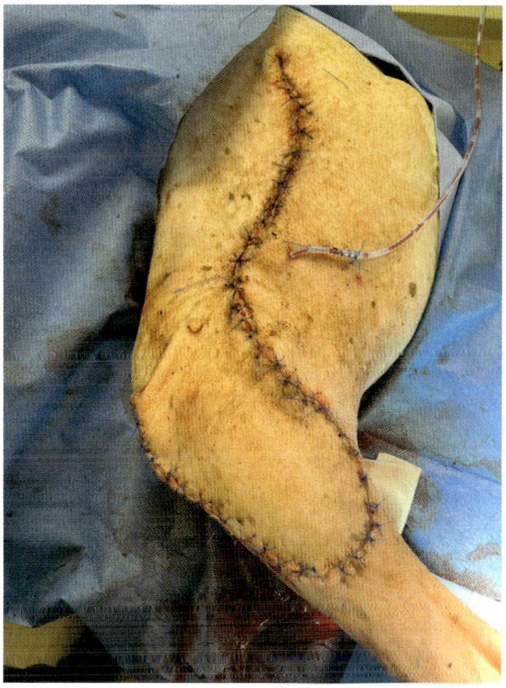

Courtesy of Dr. Dan Linden

E-iii)

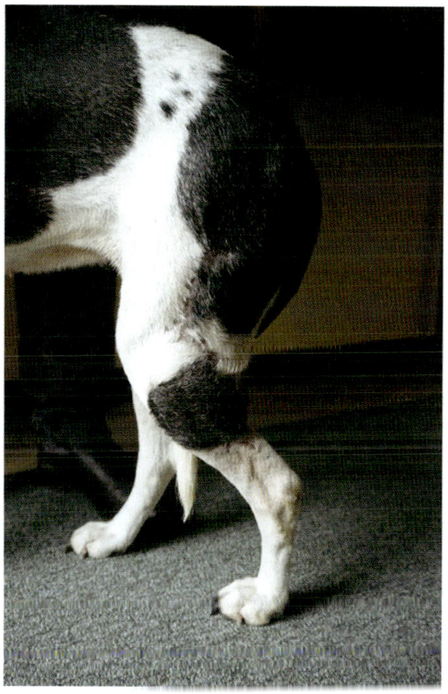

43.10 Reverse Saphenous Conduit Flap

General Considerations

The reverse saphenous conduit flap is not considered a true axial pattern flap because its blood supply of the flap is based on reverse flow in the arterial and venous systems [1]. Multiple anastomotic connections exist between the saphenous artery and vein and other arteries and veins in the limb, allowing for ligation of the saphenous artery and vein at their branching point off the femoral artery and vein.

Indication

1) Reconstruction of cutaneous defects at or distal to the tarsus (pictured, wound on plantar aspect of the metatarsal region resulting from a failed free-meshed skin graft reconstruction) [2]

Patient Positioning

The patient is positioned in lateral recumbency with the affected limb down.

Surgical Technique [1–4] (See Plate 43.10A–D)

A) A sterile marker pen should be used to indicate the cranial (Cr), caudal (Ca), and proximal (P) borders of the reverse saphenous conduit flap. The proximal border is perpendicular to the long axis of the limb at or immediately proximal the level of the patella. The cranial and caudal borders are parallel to the long axis of the tibia starting at the cranial and caudal extent of the proximal border and extending distally to immediately proximal to the level of the medial malleolus.
B) The proximal incision is performed initially. Using blunt and sharp dissection, the saphenous artery and vein are identified (i, ii, arrow). The saphenous artery and vein are ligated after branching from the femoral artery and vein, respectively. The cranial and caudal incisions are then made along their marked borders (iii).
C) The flap is raised deep to the saphenous artery and vein (pictured), and a section of the medial gastrocnemius fascia is maintained to prevent damage to the caudal branch of the saphenous artery and medial saphenous vein [3, 4].
D) The flap is transposed into the wound defect either directly if the donor site is adjacent to the wound defect or via a bridging incision (pictured, dashed line) if the wound defect is not adjacent to the donor site. The flap is frequently rotated 180 degrees from the donor site; care should be taken not to kink the vasculature during rotation and closure.

Color Atlas of Canine and Feline Surgical Oncology, First Edition. Julius M. Liptak, Paolo Buracco, William T. N. Culp, and Nicholas J. Bacon.

Plate 43.10

Reverse Saphenous Conduit Flap

1)

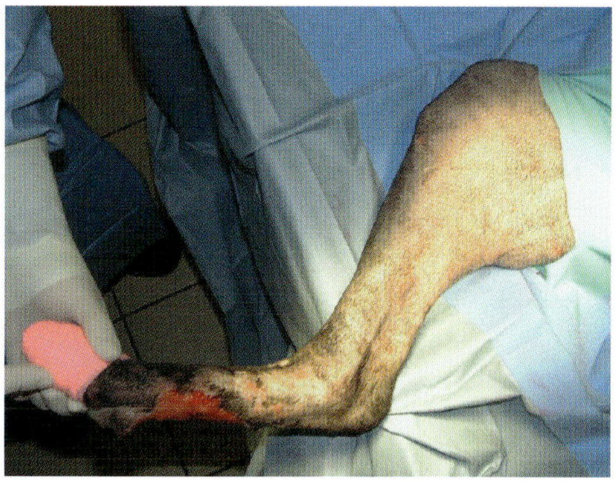

A)

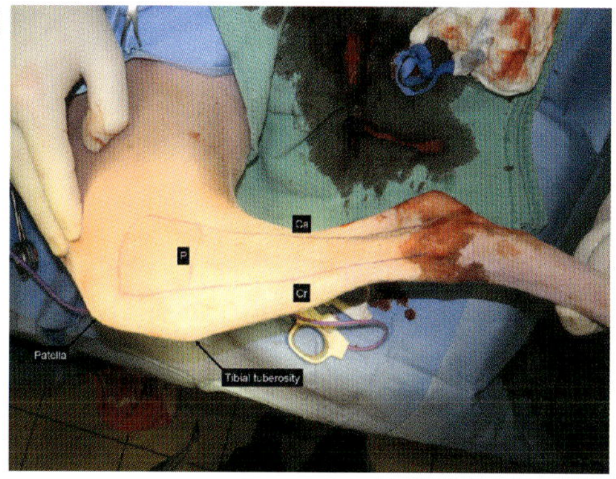

B-i)

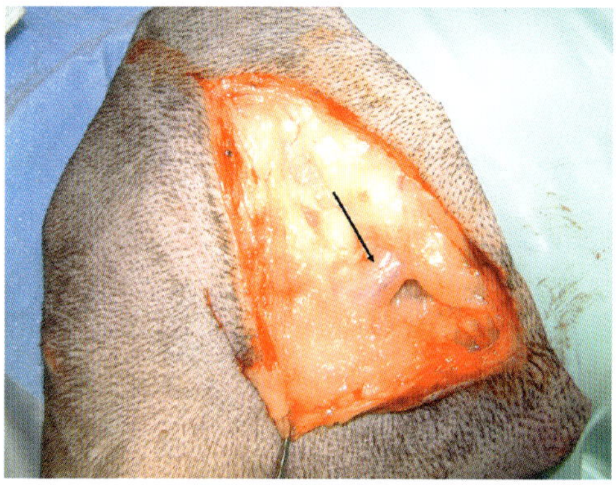

B-ii)

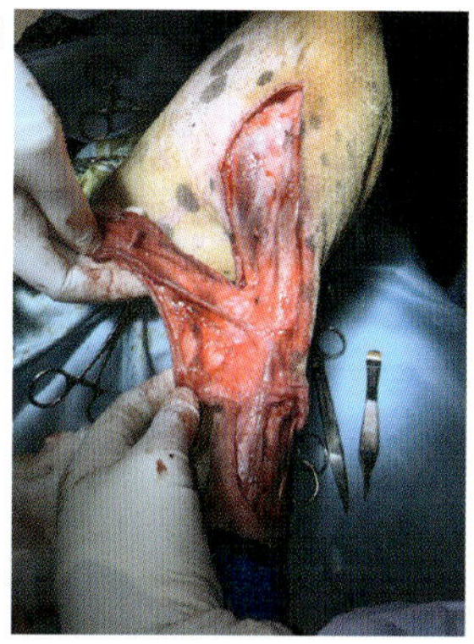

B-iii)

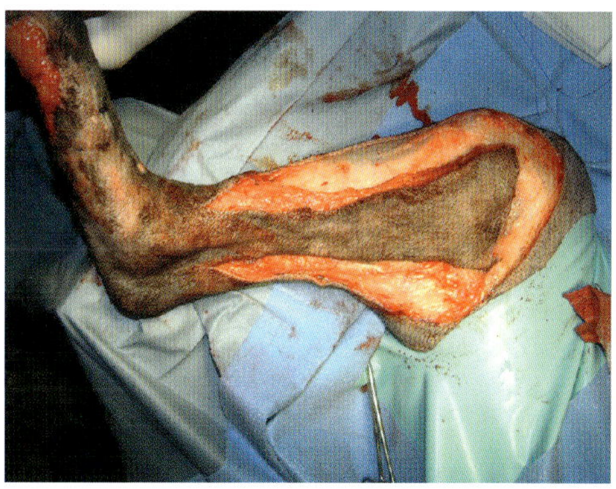

C)

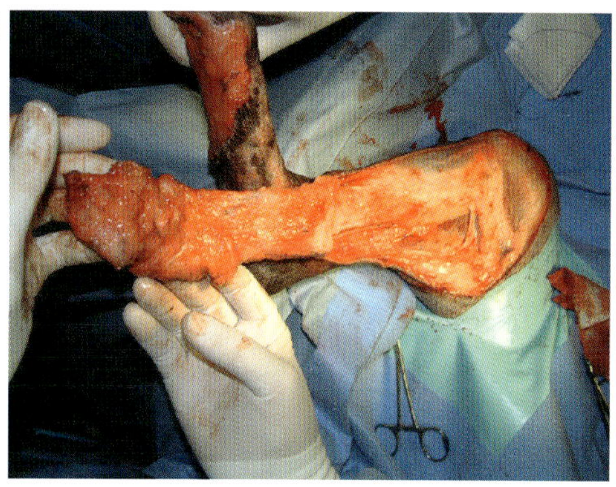

D)

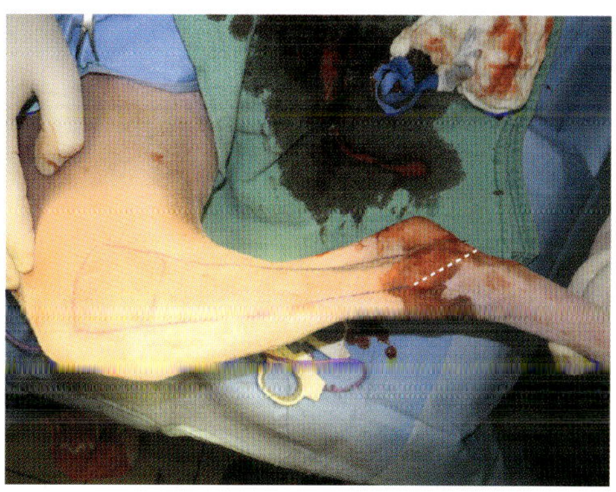

Closure (See Plate 43.10E)

E) The transposed flap and donor site are closed in two layers with a simple continuous suture pattern using monofilament absorbable suture material in the subcutis and either skin staples or an interrupted or continuous suture pattern using monofilament nonabsorbable suture material in the skin (i, ii, medial and lateral views after reconstruction of a wound resulting from resection of a cutaneous hemangioma; iii, iv, medial and plantar views after reconstruction of a wound resulting from wide soft tissue sarcoma resection and subsequent failure of a free-meshed skin graft reconstruction).

Postoperative Management

1) Multimodal analgesia
2) Elizabethan collar
3) ± Soft padded bandage

Complications – Dogs [5] (See Plate 43.10F, G)

- Overall: 30% with 30% classified as minor and 0% as major
  - Incisional dehiscence (25%)
  - Partial necrosis of the distal extent of the flap (F) (46%)
  - Edema or swelling of the axial pattern flap (G) (5%)
  - Transient flap discoloration [3, 4]
  - Superficial sloughing [3]

References

1 Cornell, K., Salisbury, K., Jakovljevic, S. et al. (1995). Reverse saphenous conduit flap in cats: an anatomic study. *Vet. Surg.* 24 (3): 202–206.

2 Pavletic, M.M., Watters, J., Henry, R.W. et al. (1983). Reverse saphenous conduit flap in the dog. *J. Am. Vet. Med. Assoc.* 182 (4): 380–389.

3 Elliott, R.C. (2014). Reverse saphenous conduit flap in small animals: clinical applications and outcomes. *J. South Afr. Vet. Med. Assoc.* 85 (1): 1038.

4 Murdoch, A.P., Greenaway, S.N., Owen, L.J. et al. (2016). Evaluation of an axial pattern flap based on the cranial cutaneous branch of the saphenous artery: a cadaveric perfusion study. *Vet. Surg.* 45 (7): 922–928.

5 Cavalcanti, J.V.J., Barry, S.L., Lanz, O.I. et al. (2018). Reverse saphenous conduit flap in 19 dogs and 1 cat. *J. Am. Anim. Hosp. Assoc.* 54 (4): 213–218.

Plate 43.10

Reverse Saphenous Conduit Flap *continued*

E-i)

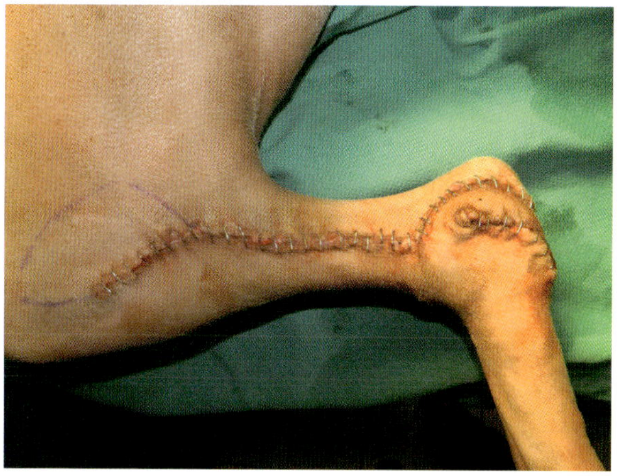

E-ii)

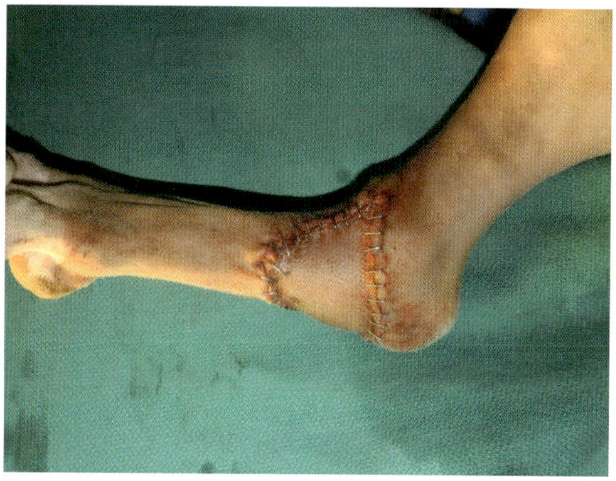

E-iii)

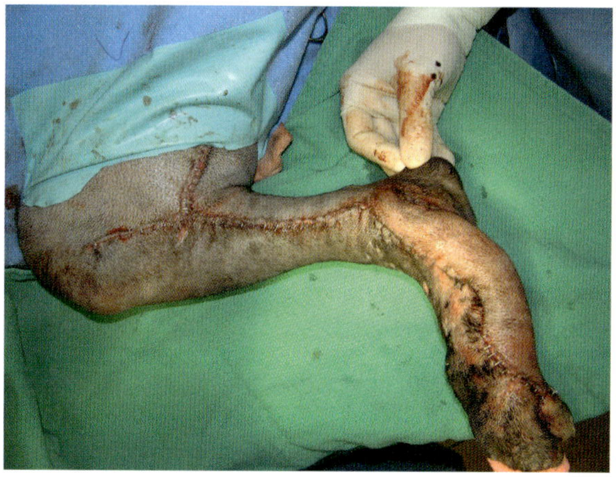

E-iv)

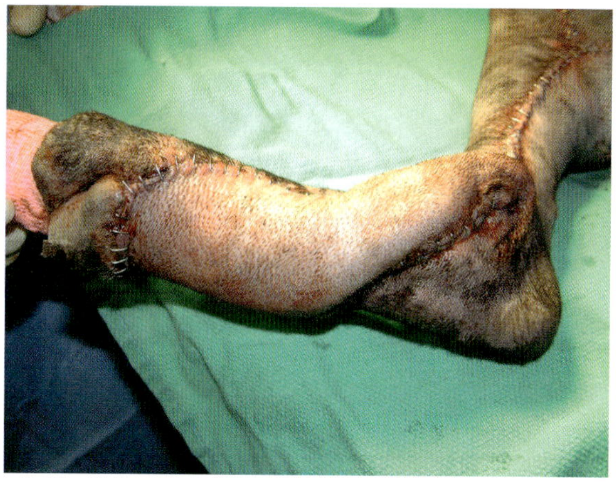

F)

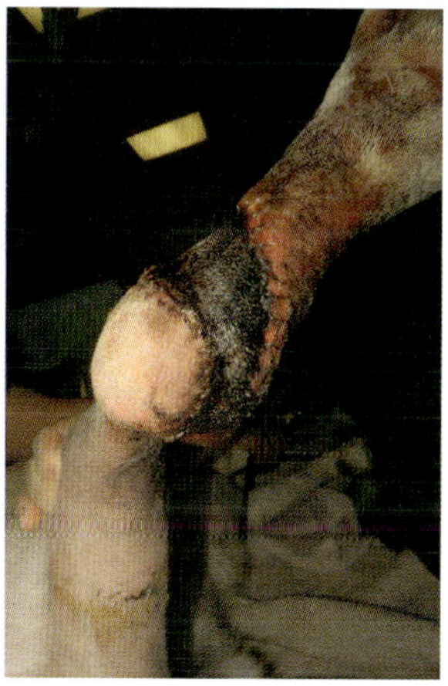

G)

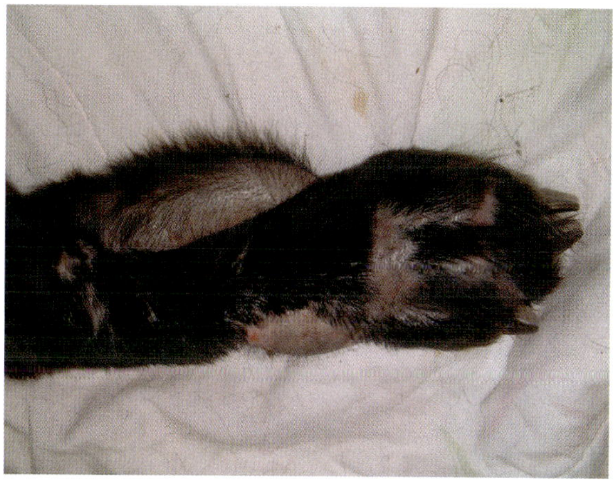

43.11 Lateral Caudal Axial Pattern Flap

Indications

1) Reconstruction of cutaneous defects in the gluteal, perineal, and dorsal tail base regions [1]
2) The lateral caudal axial pattern flap is combined with a tail amputation (see *38. Tail Amputation*)

Patient Positioning

The patient is positioned in sternal recumbency.

Surgical Technique [1] (See Plate 43.11A–H)

A) The paired lateral caudal arteries are branches (arrows) from the caudal gluteal arteries that provide the blood supply to the skin of the tail.
B) For reconstruction of a dorsal defect (after wide resection of a basal cell carcinoma), an incision is made along the dorsal midline of the tail.
C) For reconstruction of lateral (after wide resection of a soft tissue sarcoma) or ventrolateral perineal defects, an incision is made along the ventral midline of the tail.
D) The skin and subcutaneous tissue are dissected away from the deep caudal fascia of the tail (i, ii), which allows for preservation of the left and right lateral caudal arteries and veins (iii, arrow).
E) A full-thickness circumferential incision is made through the skin of the tail to the desired length of the flap (arrow).
F) The tail is amputated proximally, either by disarticulation or osteotomy (i) of the caudal vertebrae, usually at the level of the second to fourth caudal vertebrae (see *38. Tail Amputation*). The tail is removed from the surgical field (ii).

Plate 43.11

Lateral Caudal Axial Pattern Flap

A)

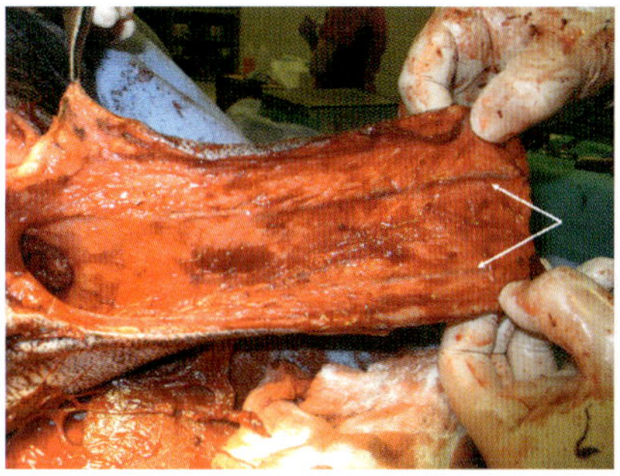

B)

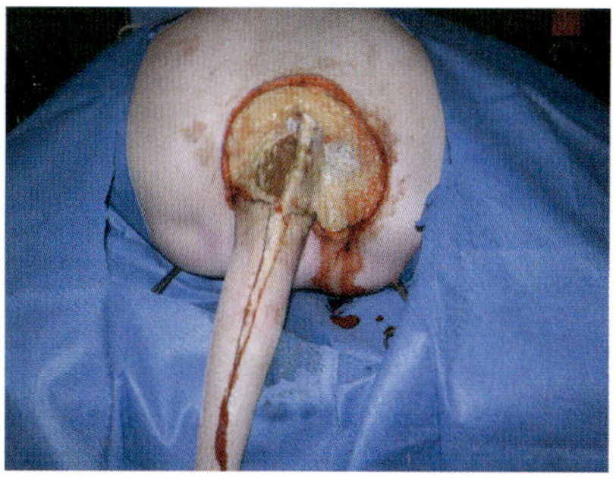

C)

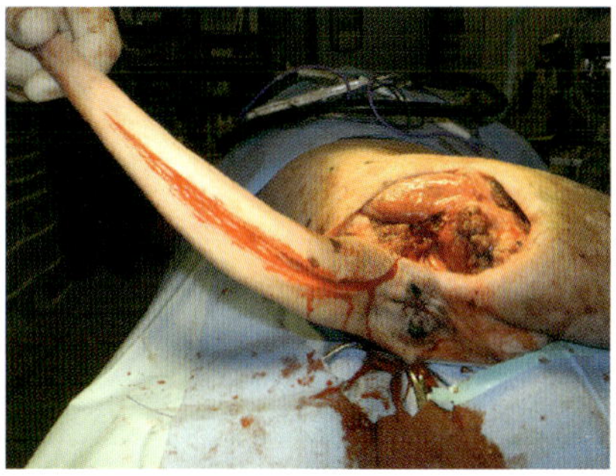

D-i)

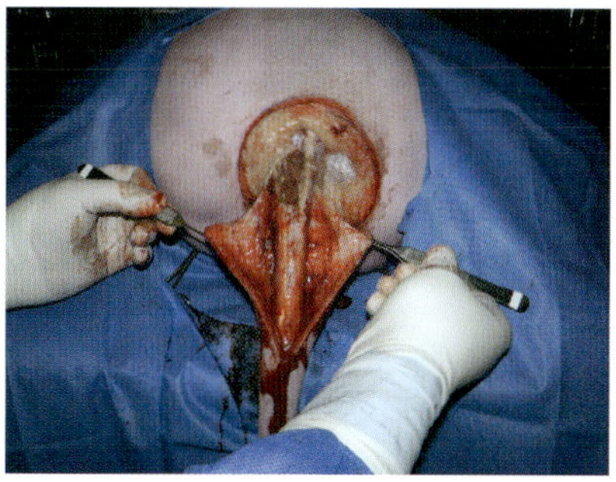

D-ii)

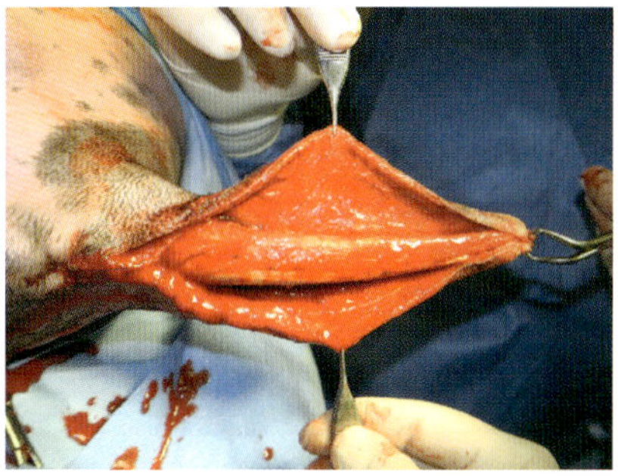

D-iii)

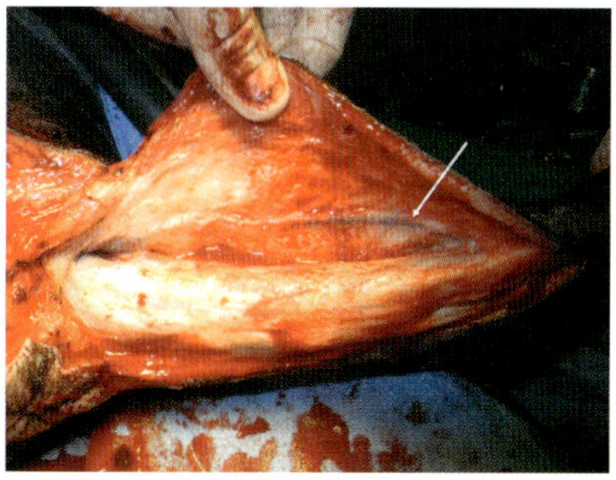

E)

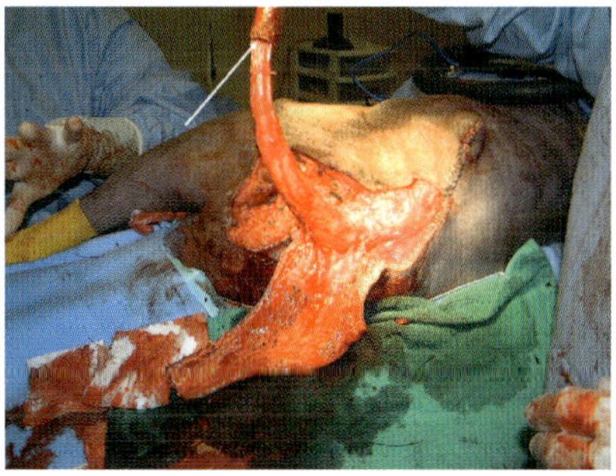

F-i)

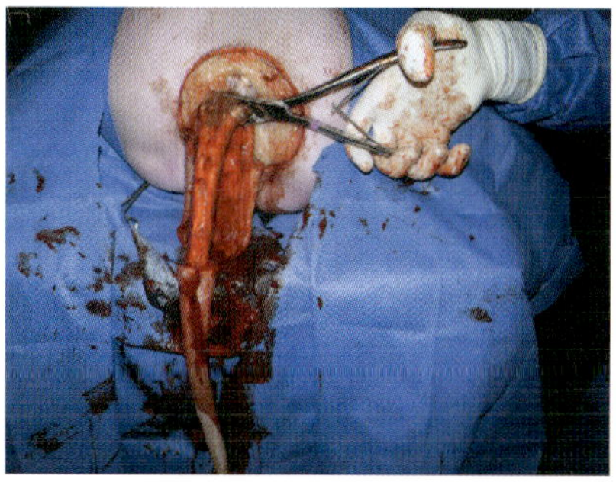

F-ii)

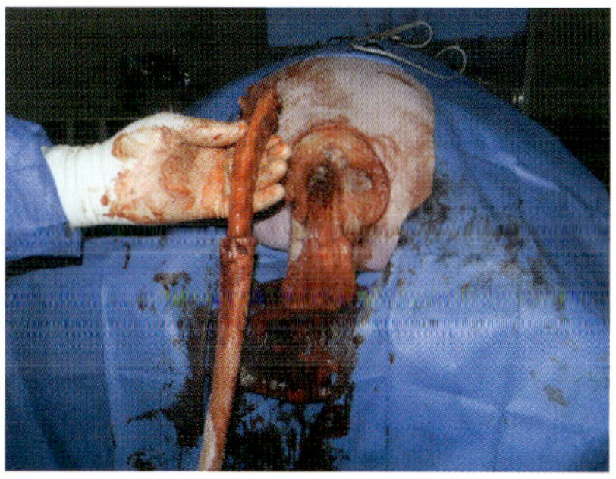

Surgical Technique [1] (See Plate 43.11A–H) *continued*

G) Consider placement of a closed suction drain.
H) The flap is transposed into the wound defect either directly if the donor site is adjacent to the wound defect (i; see step G) or via a bridging incision if the wound defect is not adjacent to the donor site (ii, dashed line; iii).

Plate 43.11

Lateral Caudal Axial Pattern Flap *continued*

G)

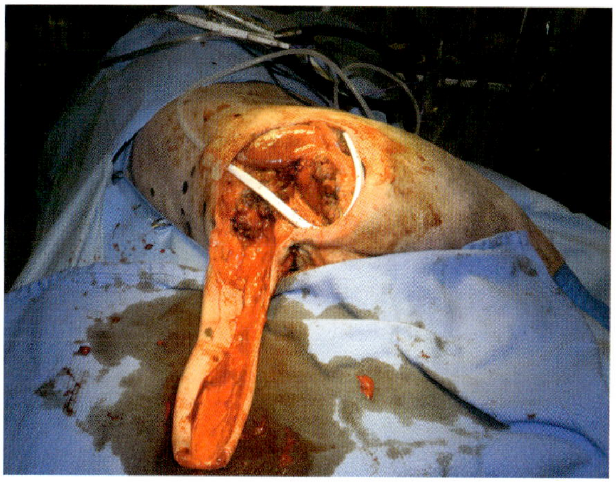

H-i)

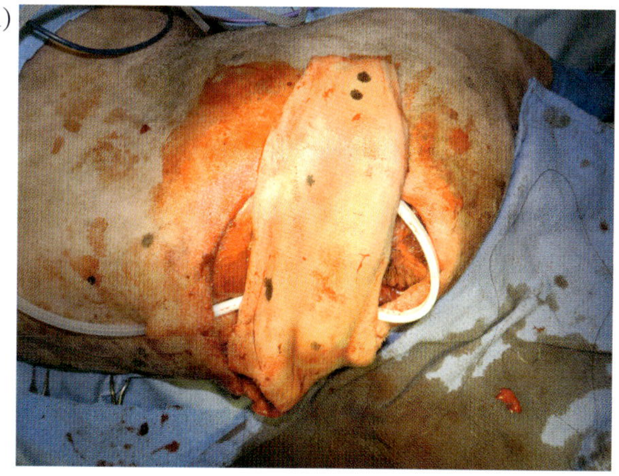

H-ii)

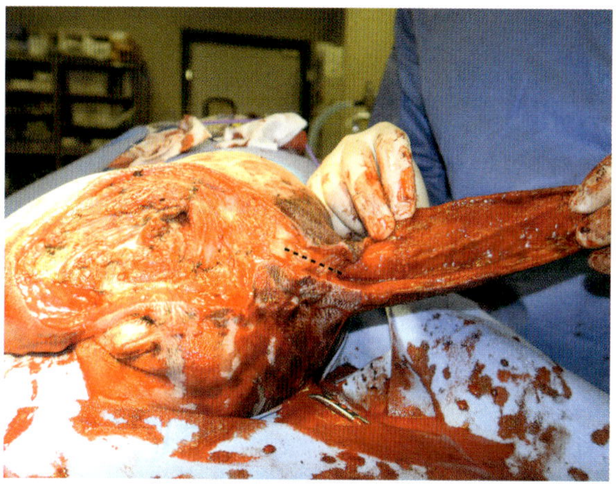

H-iii)

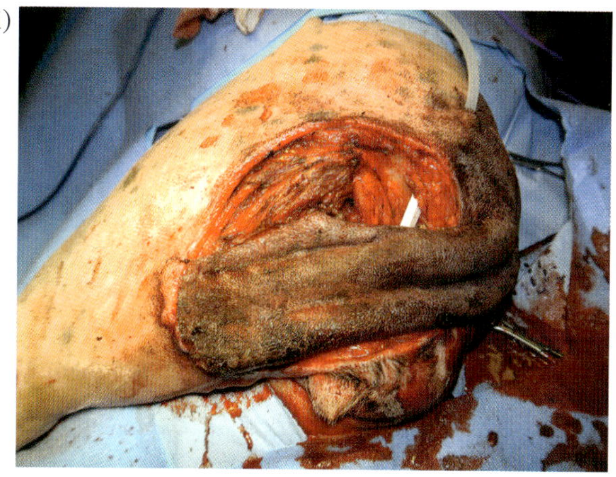

Closure (See Plate 43.11I)

I) The transposed flap and donor site are closed in two layers with a simple continuous suture pattern using monofilament absorbable suture material in the subcutis and either skin staples or an interrupted or continuous suture pattern using monofilament nonabsorbable suture material in the skin (i–iii, immediately postoperatively; iv–vi, 2 weeks postoperatively).

Postoperative Management

1) Multimodal analgesia
2) Elizabethan collar
3) ± Closed suction drain management, if placed, for 2–5 days

Complications – Dogs [1] (See Plate 43.11J)

- Overall: 31% with 15% classified as minor and 15% as major [1]
  - Incisional dehiscence (J) (15%)
  - Partial necrosis of the distal extent of the flap (15%)
  - Surgical-site infection (8%)

Reference

1 Montinaro, V., Massari, F., Vezzoni, L. et al. (2015). Lateral caudal axial pattern flap in 13 dogs. *Vet. Surg.* 44 (5): 642–647.

Plate 43.11

Lateral Caudal Axial Pattern Flap *continued*

I-i)

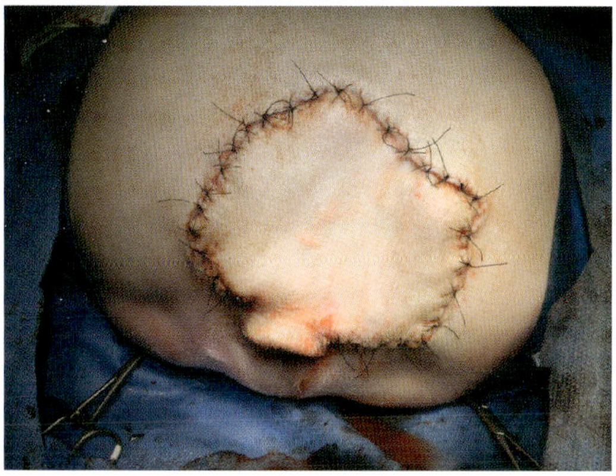

I-ii)

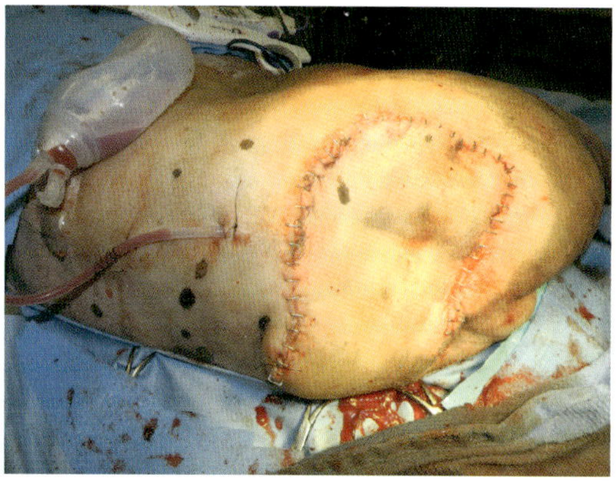

I-iii)

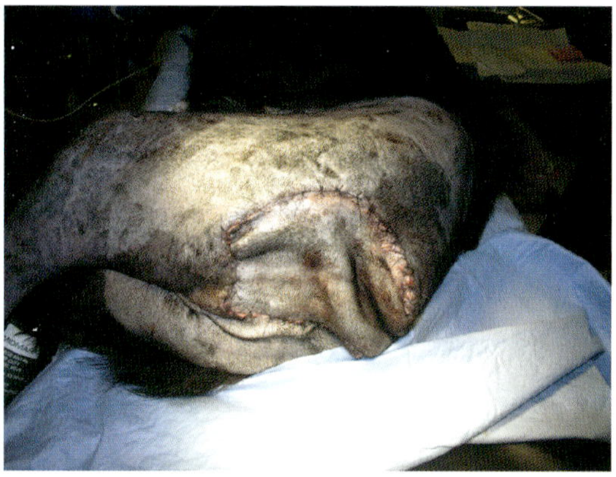

I-iv)

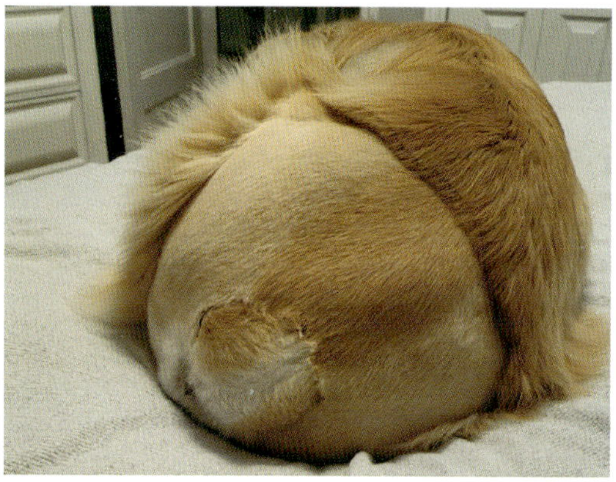

I-v)

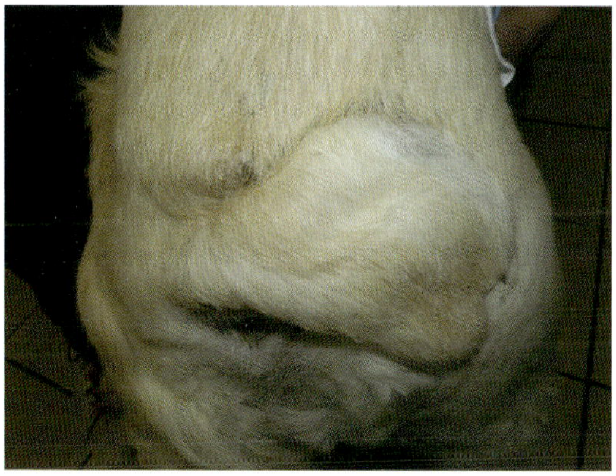

I-vi)

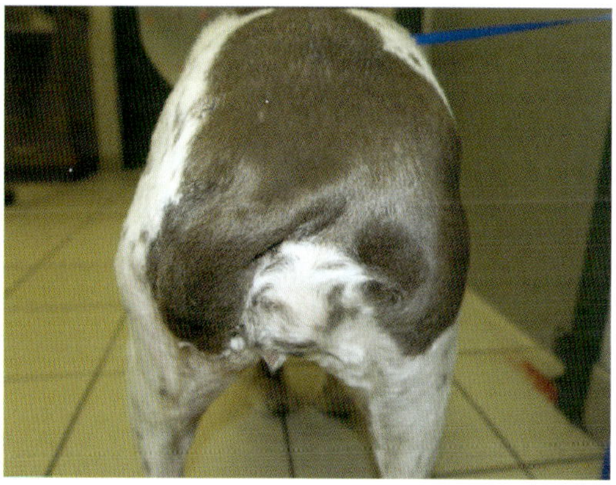

J)

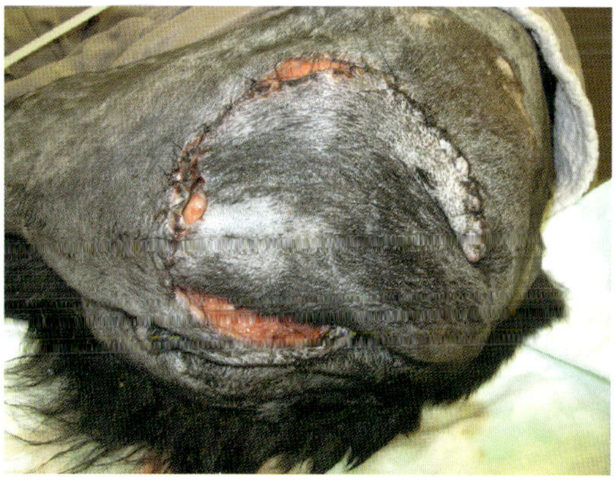

Chapter 44: Distant Indirect Flap

44.1 Distant Direct Flaps – Pouch Flaps

Indication

1) Reconstruction of defects on the mid-to-distal aspects of the thoracic and pelvic limbs

Patient Positioning

The patient is positioned in lateral recumbency with the affected limb uppermost.

Surgical Technique [1] (See Plate 44.1A–F)

A) The affected thoracic or pelvic limb is elevated (i), and the level of the defect on the limb is indicated with a sterile marker pen on the lateral thoracic or abdominal wall (ii).
B) Two parallel incisions are made in the lateral thoracic or abdominal wall at the site indicated by the sterile marker pen (i). The distance between the two parallel incisions is equivalent to the length of the defect on the limb. The length of the incisions should be adequate to allow passage of the paw through the bipedicle flap. The subcutaneous tissue between the two incisions is undermined (ii).
C) The paw is passed through the bipedicle flap (i, ii). The pouch flap can be closed in two layers with a simple continuous suture pattern using monofilament absorbable suture material in the subcutis and either an interrupted or continuous suture pattern using monofilament nonabsorbable suture material in the skin. Alternatively, these flaps can be closed in a single layer using either an interrupted or continuous suture pattern using monofilament nonabsorbable suture material in the skin. The cranial incision of the bipedicle flap is sutured to the proximal aspect of the defect on the thoracic limb or distal aspect of the defect on the pelvic limb (iii, iv). The caudal incision of the bipedicle flap is sutured to the distal aspect of the defect on the thoracic limb (iii, iv) or proximal aspect of the defect on the pelvic limb.

Color Atlas of Canine and Feline Surgical Oncology, First Edition. Julius M. Liptak, Paolo Buracco, William T. N. Culp, and Nicholas J. Bacon.

Plate 44.1

Distant Direct Flaps – Pouch Flaps

A-i)

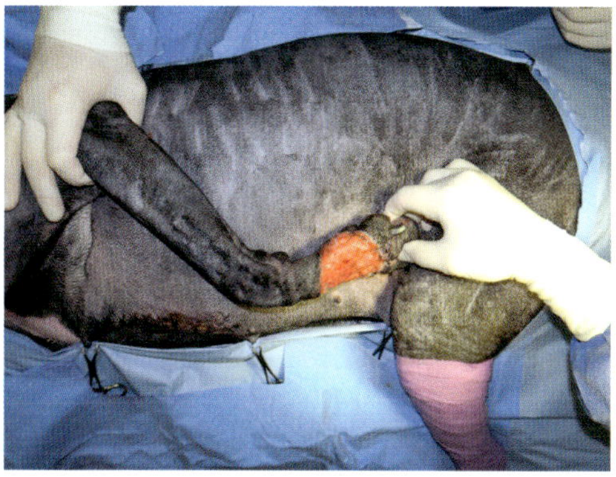

A-ii)

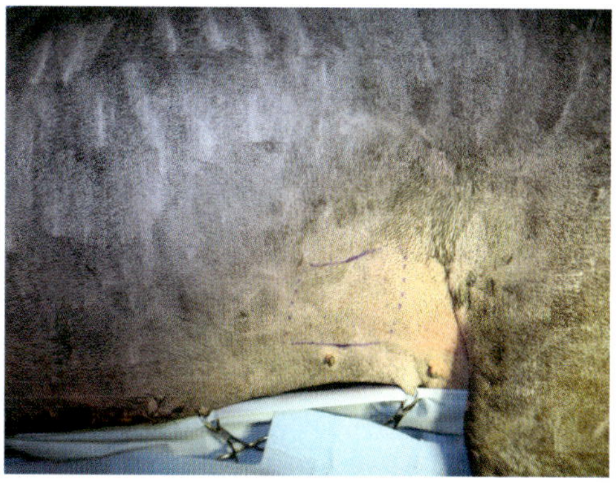

B-i)

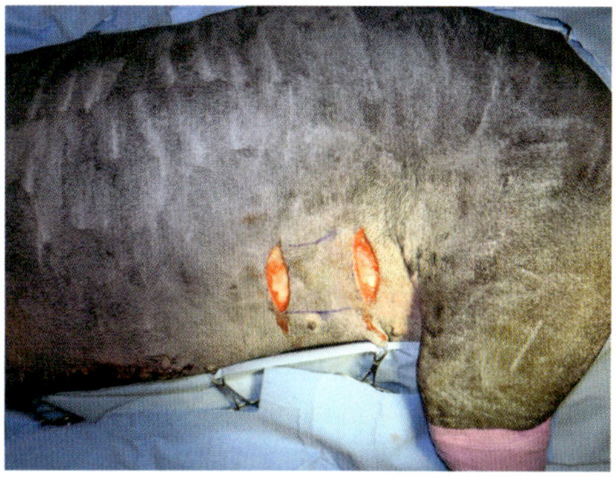

B-ii)

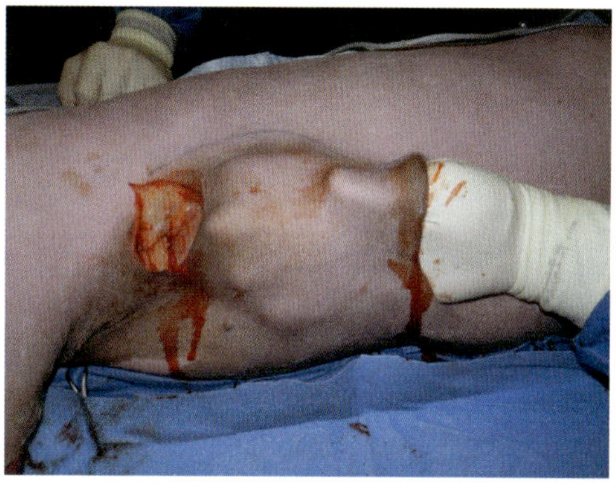

C-i)

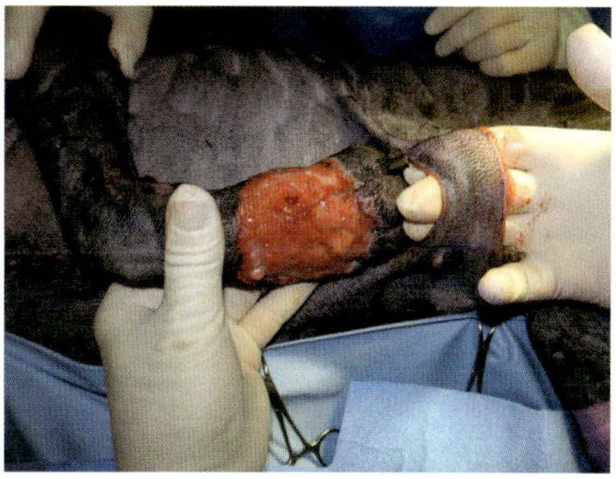

C-ii)

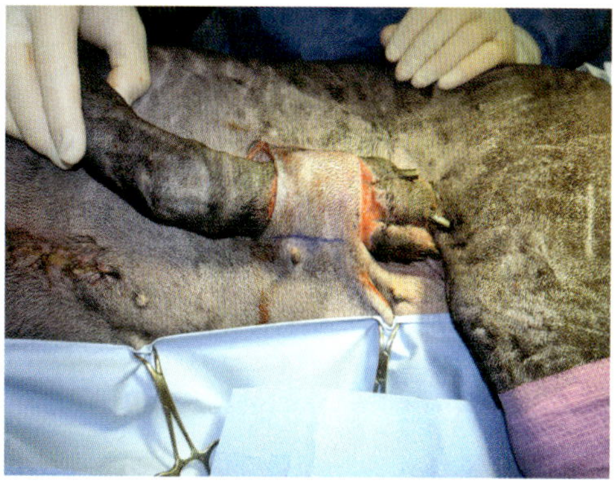

C-iii)

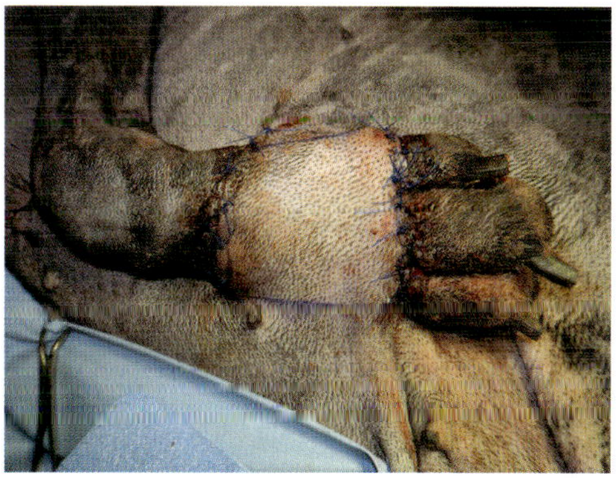

C-iv)

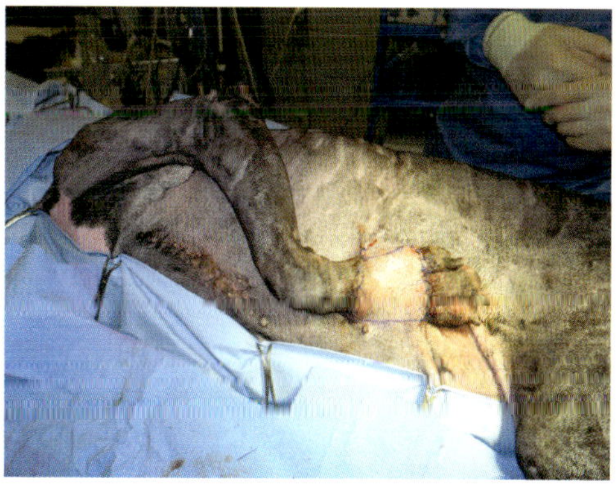

Surgical Technique [1] (See Plate 44.1A–F) *continued*

D) The limb is bandaged to the thoracic and abdominal wall with a soft padded bandage for 3 weeks.

E) The pouch flap can be released after a minimum of 3 weeks (i). The release procedure involves incisions along the dorsal (ii, iii) and ventral aspects of the flap with adequate additional skin either ventrally and/or dorsally to reconstruct any remaining open portions of the limb defect (iv, v). This can be done in one (pictured) to three procedures. If done in more than one procedure, a third to a half of the flap is released and then resutured to its original location. Subsequent procedures are repeated in 7-day intervals. Multiple release procedures are intended to maximize flap survival because of the delay phenomenon; however, one study showed no difference in flap survival between single and multiple release procedures [1].

Plate 44.1

Distant Direct Flaps – Pouch Flaps *continued*

D)

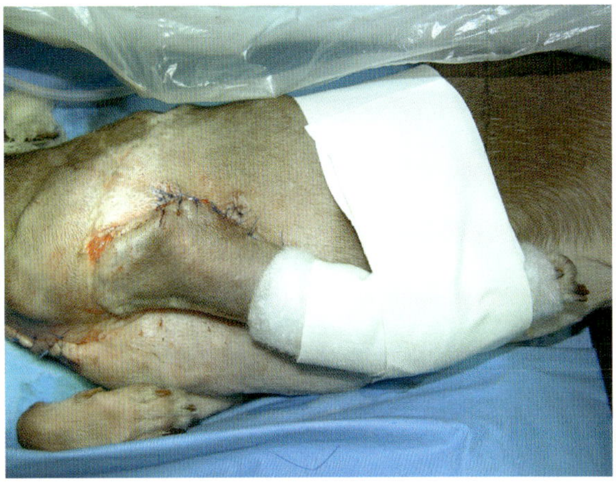

E-i)

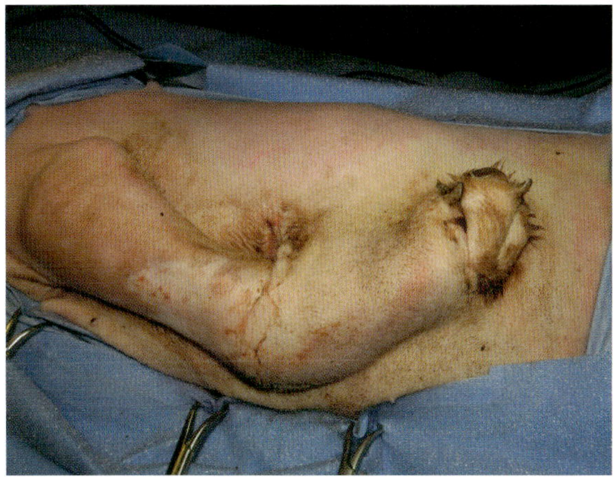

E-ii)

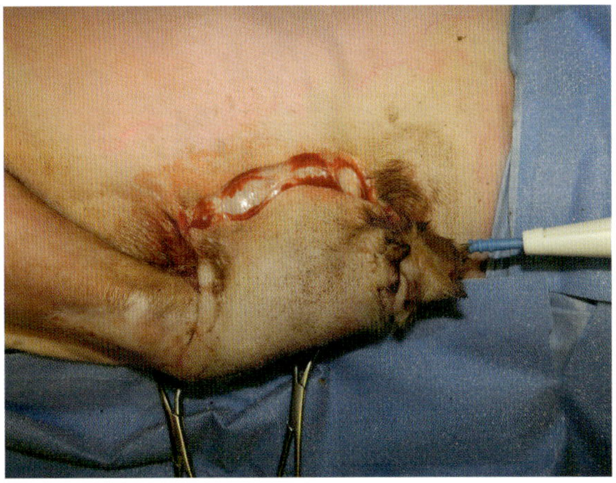

E-iii)

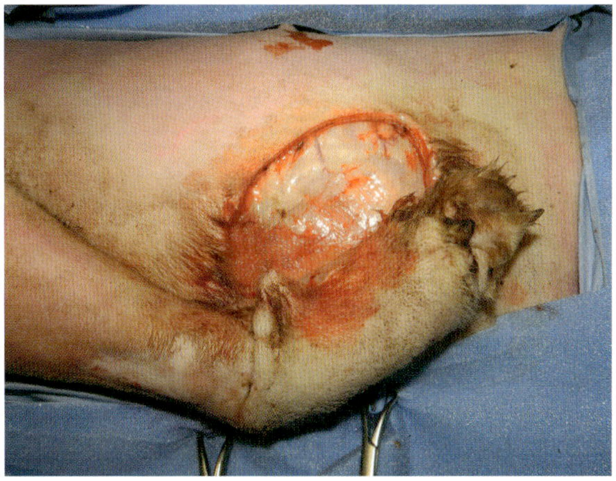

E-iv)

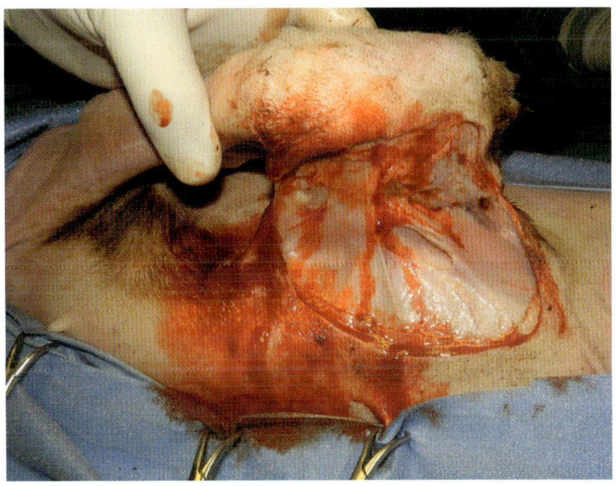

E-v)

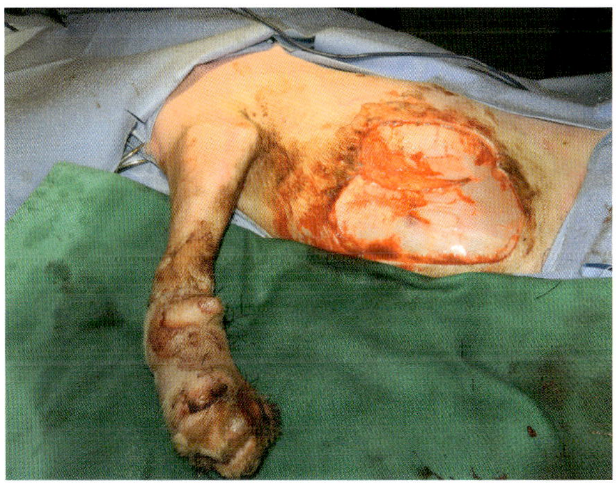

Surgical Technique [1] (See Plate 44.1A–F) *continued*

F) The defect resulting from release of the flap (i) and suturing of the flap to the limb defect can be closed in two layers with a simple continuous suture pattern using monofilament absorbable suture material in the subcutis and either an interrupted or continuous suture pattern using monofilament nonabsorbable suture material in the skin (ii, immediately postoperatively; iii, 2 weeks postoperatively; iv, 79 days postoperatively).

Postoperative Management

1) Multimodal analgesia
2) Elizabethan collar
3) Soft padded bandage to secure the limb to the body wall for 21 days
4) Exercise restriction for 21 days between the flap and release surgical procedures, and for 10–14 days after the flap is released

Complications – Dogs and Cats [1] (See Plate 44.1G)

- Overall: 79%
- Surgical-site infection (43%)
- Partial incisional dehiscence (G, arrow) (36%)
- Partial- or full-thickness necrosis of the distal aspect of the flap (29%)
- Decubital ulcer formation (14%)
- Moisture dermatitis between the limb and body wall
- Mild disuse muscle atrophy
- Carpal contracture
- Poor tolerance of limb immobilized against body wall for prolonged periods

Reference

1 Lemarie, R.J., Hosgood, G., Read, R.A. et al. (1995). Distant abdominal and thoracic pedicle skin flaps for treatment of distal limb skin defects. *J. Small Anim. Pract.* 36 (6): 255–261.

Plate 44.1

Distant Direct Flaps – Pouch Flaps *continued*

F-i)

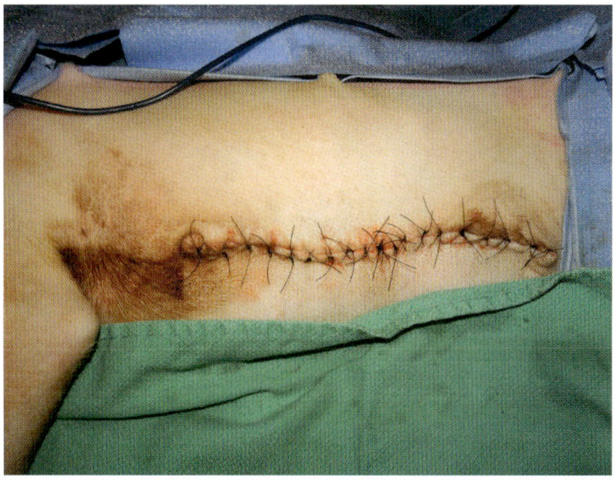

F-ii)

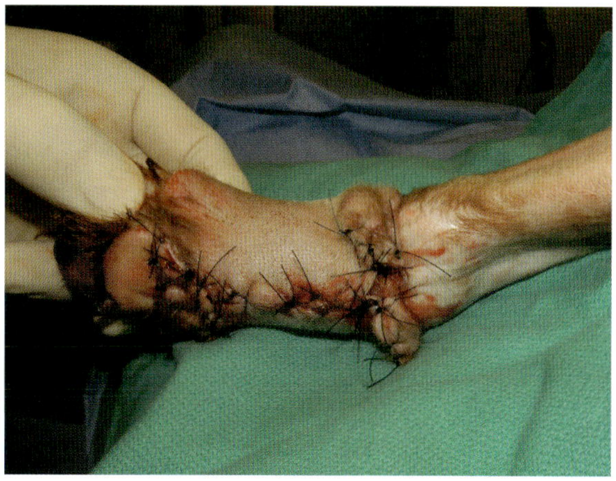

F-iii)

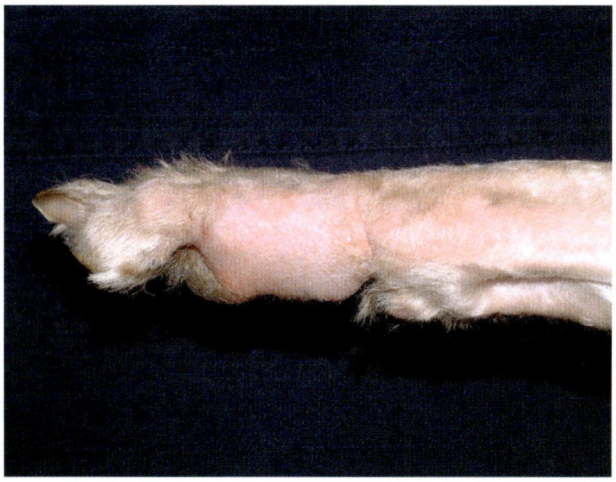

F-iv)

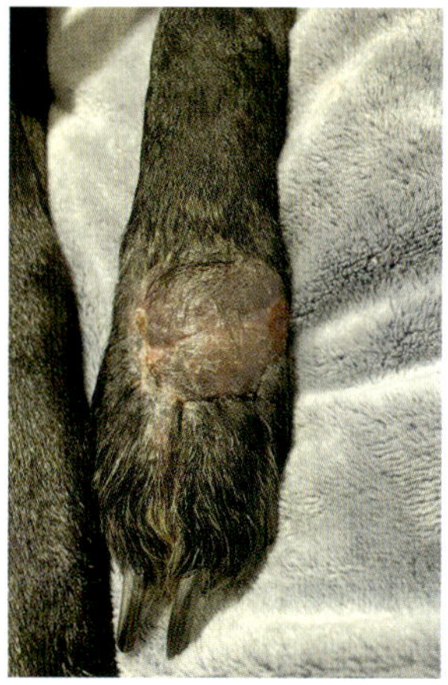

G)

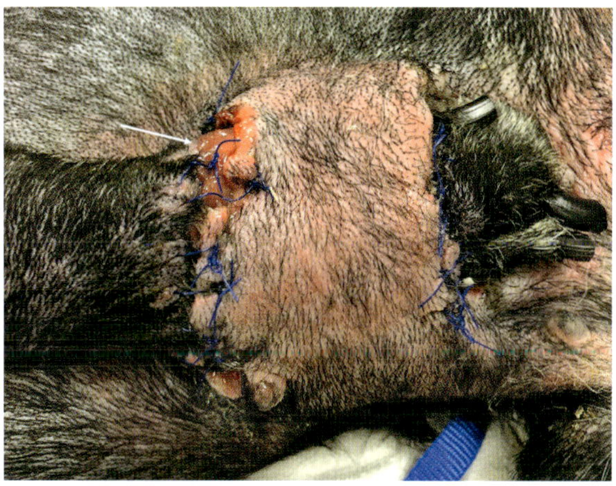

44.2 Distant Direct Flaps – Hinge Flaps

Indication

1) Reconstruction of defects on the mid-to-distal aspects of the thoracic and pelvic limbs

Patient Positioning

The patient is positioned in lateral recumbency with the affected limb uppermost.

Surgical Technique [1] (See Plate 44.2A–F)

A) The affected thoracic or pelvic limb is elevated (i), and the level of the defect on the limb is indicated with a sterile marker pen on the lateral thoracic or abdominal wall (ii).
B) Two parallel incisions are made in the lateral thoracic or abdominal wall at the site indicated by the sterile marker pen (i). The distance between the two parallel incisions is equivalent to the length of the defect on the limb. The length of the incisions is approximately equivalent to half of the circumference of the limb at the level of the defect. The parallel incisions are connected with a ventral or dorsal incision (i), as dictated by the location of the defect. The single pedicle flap is carefully undermined to preserve the subdermal plexus and elevated (ii).
C) The defect on the limb is positioned over the hinge flap site (i). The hinge flap can be closed in two layers with a simple continuous suture pattern using monofilament absorbable suture material in the subcutis (ii) and either an interrupted or continuous suture pattern using monofilament nonabsorbable suture material in the skin (iii). Alternatively, these flaps can be closed in a single layer using either an interrupted or continuous suture pattern using monofilament nonabsorbable suture material in the skin. The cranial aspect of the single pedicle flap is sutured to the proximal aspect of the defect on the thoracic limb or distal aspect of the defect on the pelvic limb (iii–v). The caudal aspect of the single pedicle flap is sutured to the distal aspect of the defect on the thoracic limb or proximal aspect of the defect on the pelvic limb (iii–v). The hinge flap donor site is closed in two layers with a simple continuous suture pattern using monofilament absorbable suture material in the subcutis and either an interrupted or continuous suture pattern using monofilament nonabsorbable suture material in the skin (iv, v).

Color Atlas of Canine and Feline Surgical Oncology, First Edition. Julius M. Liptak, Paolo Buracco, William T. N. Culp, and Nicholas J. Bacon.

Plate 44.2

Distant Direct Flaps – Hinge Flaps

A-i)

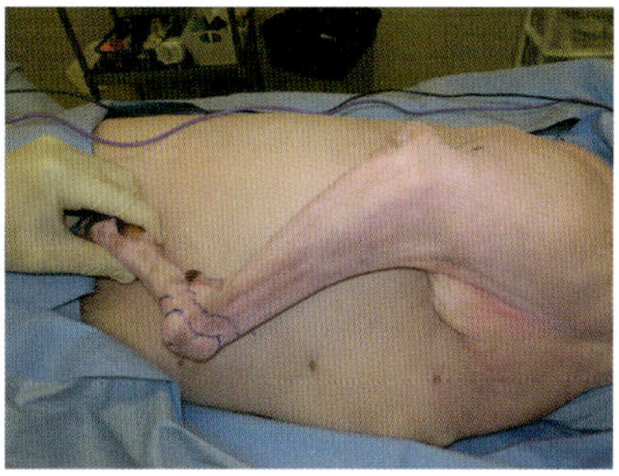

A-ii)

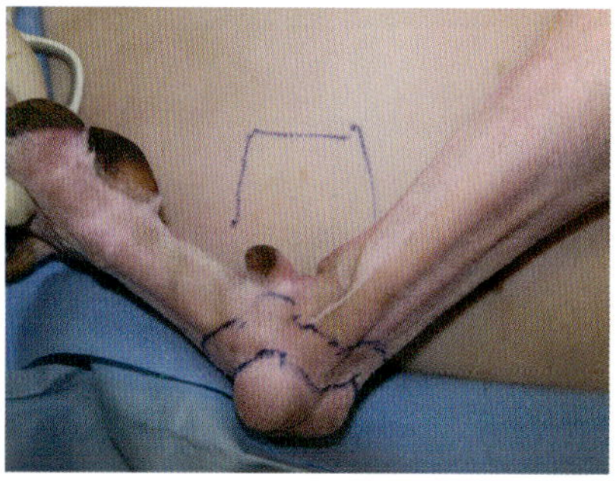

B-i)

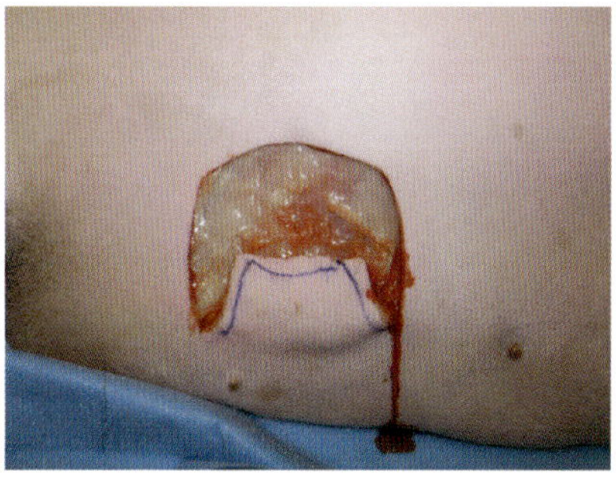

B-ii)

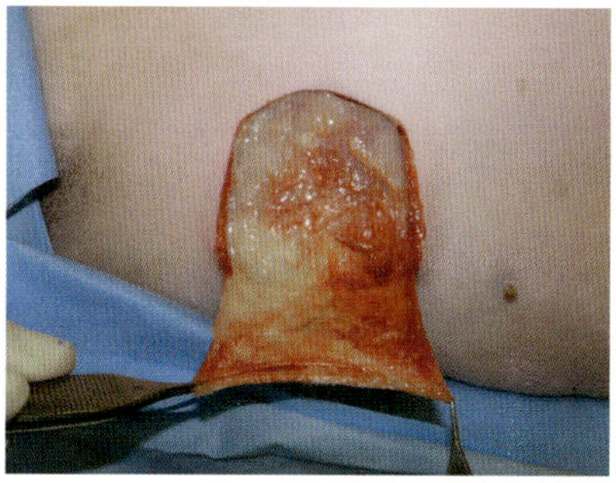

C-i)

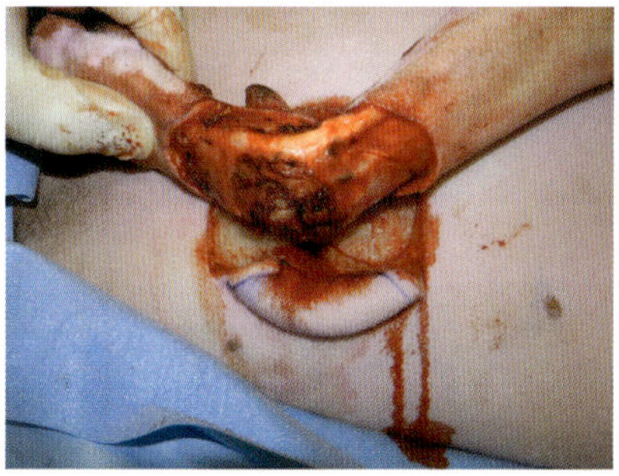

C-ii)

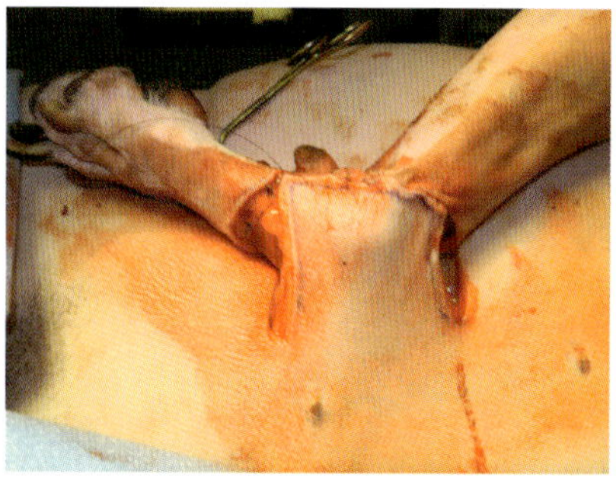

C-iii)

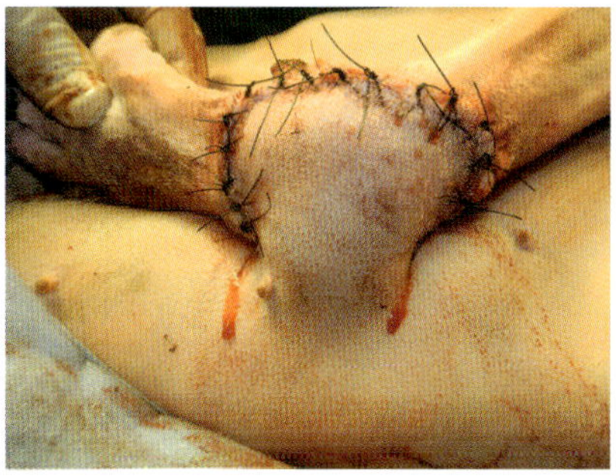

C-iv)

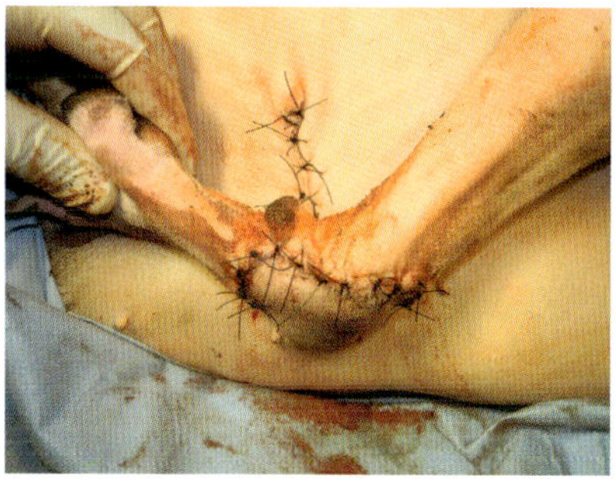

C-v)

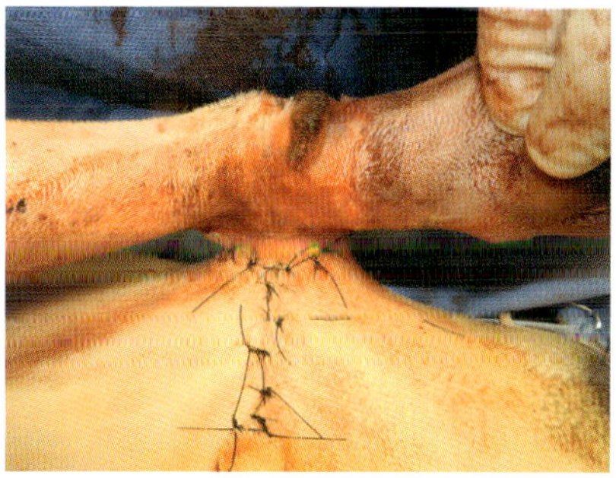

Surgical Technique [1] (See Plate 44.2A–F) *continued*

D) The limb is bandaged to the thoracic and abdominal wall with a soft padded bandage for 3 weeks.
E) The hinge flap can be released after a minimum of 3 weeks (i). The release procedure involves incisions along the dorsal and ventral aspects of the flap with adequate additional skin either ventrally and/or dorsally to reconstruct any remaining open portions of the limb defect (ii, iii). This can be done in one (pictured) to three procedures. If done in more than one procedure, a third to half of the flap is released and then resutured to its original location. Subsequent procedures are repeated in 7-day intervals. Multiple release procedures are intended to maximize flap survival because of the delay phenomenon; however, one study showed no difference in flap survival between single and multiple release procedures [1].
F) The defect resulting from release of the flap and suturing of the flap to the limb defect can be closed in two layers with a simple continuous suture pattern using monofilament absorbable suture material in the subcutis and either an interrupted or continuous suture pattern using monofilament nonabsorbable suture material in the skin.

Postoperative Management

1) Multimodal analgesia
2) Elizabethan collar
3) Soft padded bandage to secure the limb to the body wall for 21 days
4) Exercise restriction for 21 days between the flap and release surgical procedures, and for 10–14 days after the flap is released

Complications – Dogs and Cats [1] (See Plate 44.2G)

- Overall: 79%
- Surgical-site infection (43%)
- Partial incisional dehiscence (36%)
- Partial- or full-thickness necrosis of the distal aspect of the flap (G) (29%)
- Decubital ulcer formation (14%)
- Moisture dermatitis between the limb and body wall
- Mild disuse muscle atrophy
- Carpal contracture
- Poor tolerance of limb immobilized against body wall for prolonged periods

Reference

1 Lemarie, R.J., Hosgood, G., Read, R.A. et al. (1995). Distant abdominal and thoracic pedicle skin flaps for treatment of distal limb skin defects. *J. Small Anim. Pract.* 36 (6): 255–261.

Plate 44.2

Distant Direct Flaps – Hinge Flaps *continued*

D

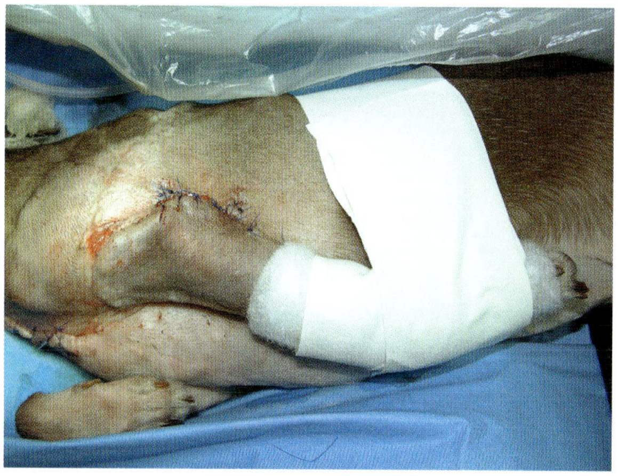

E-i)

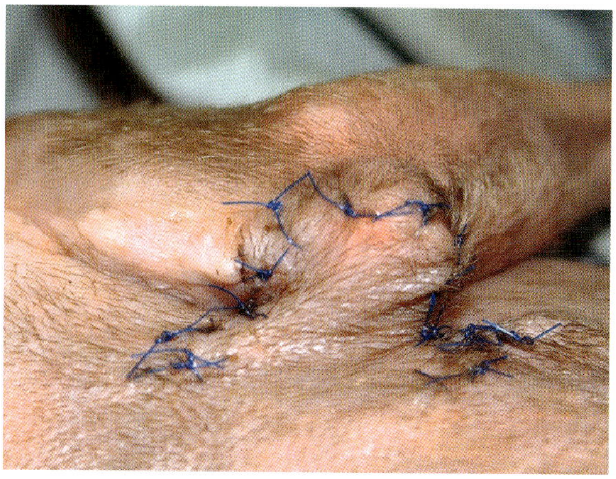

E-ii)

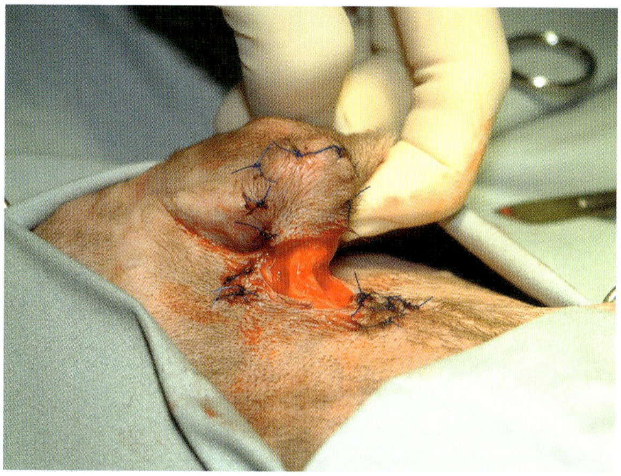

E-iii)

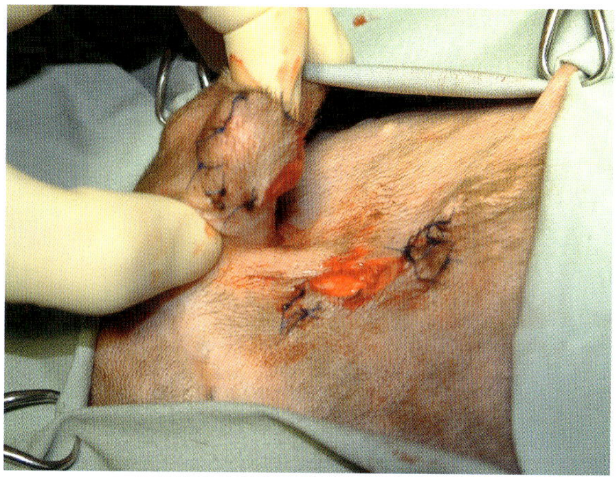

F)

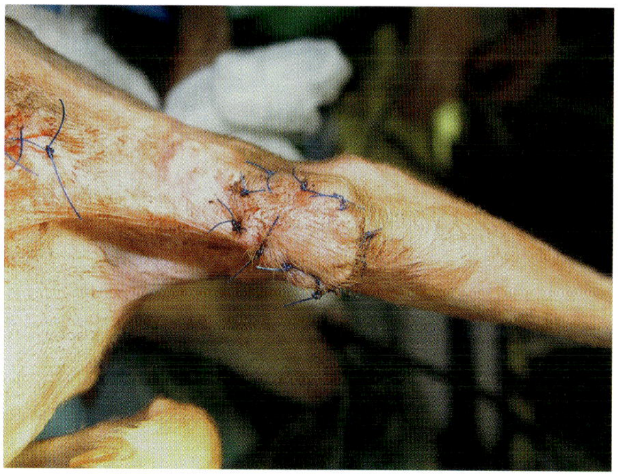

G)

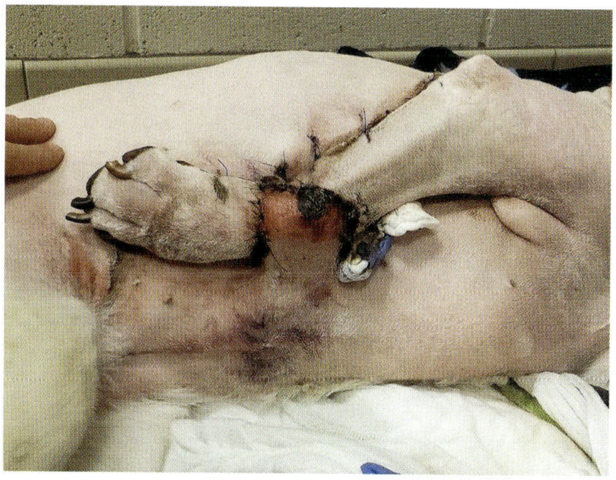

Chapter 45: Skin Grafts

45.1 Free-Meshed Skin Grafts

Indications

1) Reconstruction of full-thickness skin defects that cannot be closed primarily. Although theoretically plausible in any location, skin grafts are typically used to reconstruct wounds located below the elbow or stifle because of the requirement for rigid immobility of the skin graft in the immediate postoperative period. There is no difference in skin graft survival rates between grafts placed directly over a healthy granulation bed or freshly exposed muscle after tumor resection [1].
2) Free-meshed skin grafts can be combined with wide surgical resection of benign and malignant skin and subcutaneous tumors (see *1. Surgical Resection of Cutaneous and Subcutaneous Tumors*).

Patient Positioning

Patient positioning is dependent on the location of the skin defect. For wounds on the cranial, lateral, or caudal aspect of the limb, the patient is typically positioned with the affected limb uppermost. For wounds on the medial aspect of the limb, the patient is typically positioned in dorsal recumbency. In both cases, the donor bed also needs to be clipped and draped within the surgical field. The donor bed is typically located on the proximal limb, lateral thorax, or ventral abdomen, depending on patient positioning.

Surgical Technique (See Plate 45.1A, C, D, F–H)

A) The primary tumor is widely resected according to oncologic principles (see *1. Surgical Resection of Cutaneous and Subcutaneous Tumors*), including a deep fascial plane. If resection and grafting are being performed in a single session, then the wound bed ideally should be on healthy muscle (i). If there is exposed bone, tendon sheath, or fibrous connective tissue, then consider a staged procedure with open wound management until the wound is filled with healthy granulation tissue and then placing the free-meshed skin graft (ii) [2].
B) The surgical or granulated wound bed is covered with saline-soaked swabs to maintain a moist wound surface while the skin graft is being prepared (not pictured), and gloves and instruments are changed to minimize the risk of seeding the donor site with tumor cells.
C) A sterile gauze swab (i) or drape material (ii) is placed over the graft and a template cut with suture scissors to exactly fit the shape of the wound.
D) This template is then transferred to the donor site (i), and a sterile surgical marker is used to draw around the shape on the donor site (ii). The template is then removed from the surgical field (iii).

Color Atlas of Canine and Feline Surgical Oncology, First Edition. Julius M. Liptak, Paolo Buracco, William T. N. Culp, and Nicholas J. Bacon.

Plate 45.1

Free-Meshed Skin Grafts

A-i)

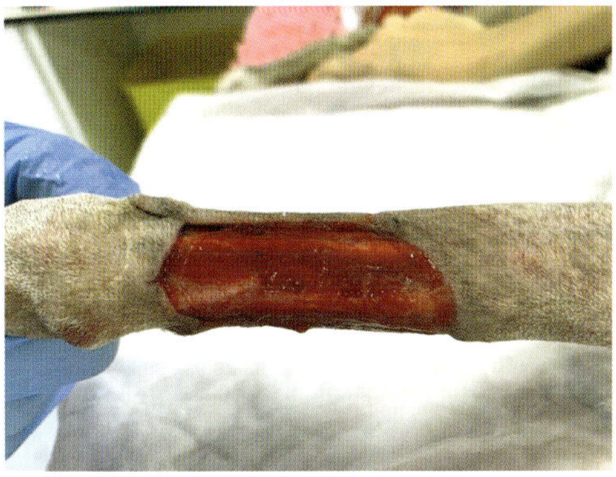

A-ii)

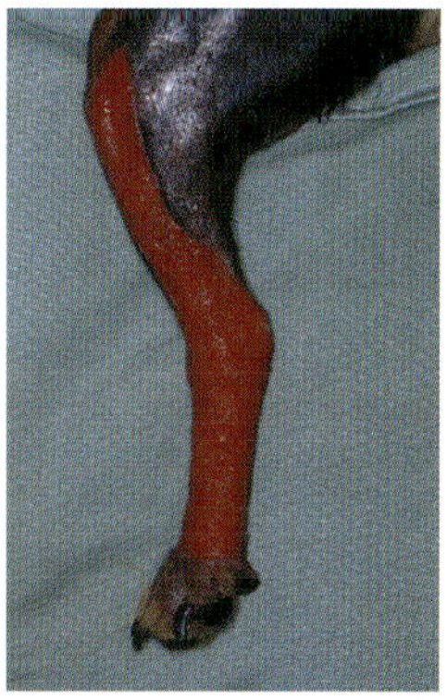

C-i)

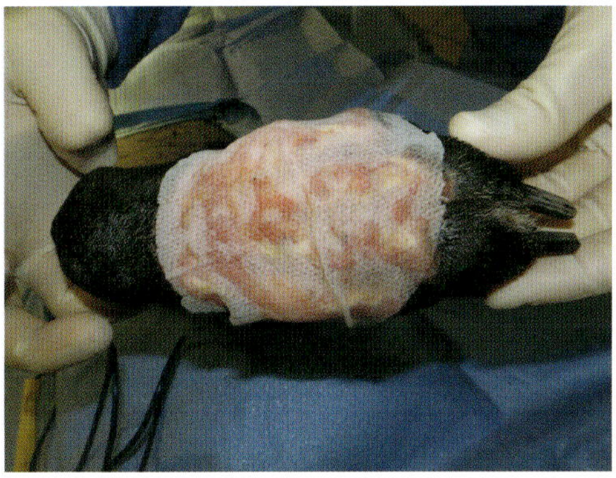

C-ii)

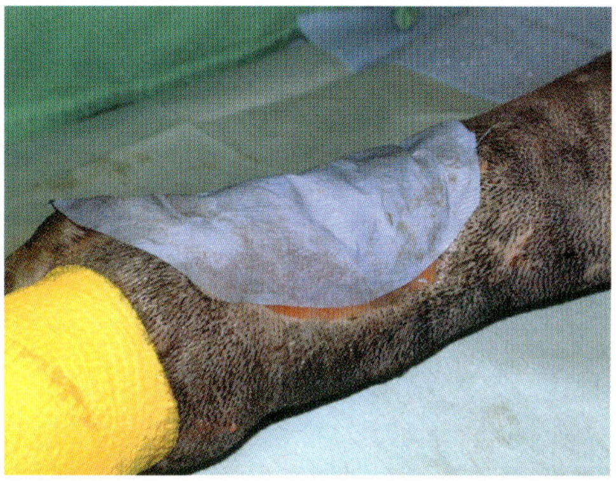

D-i)

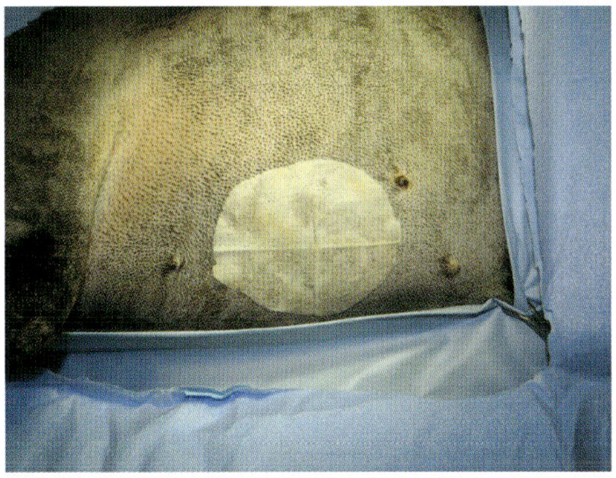

D-ii)

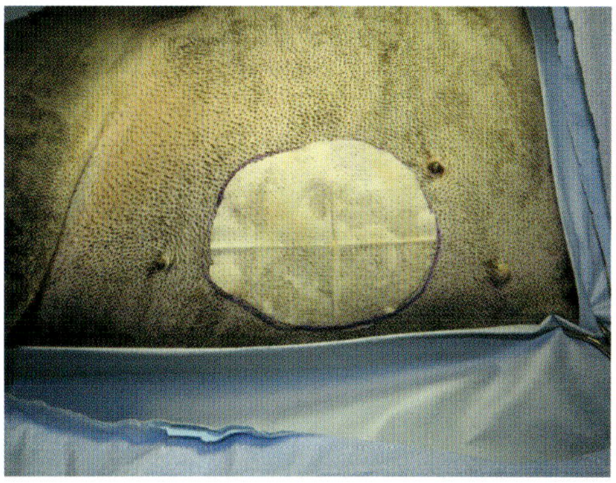

D-iii)

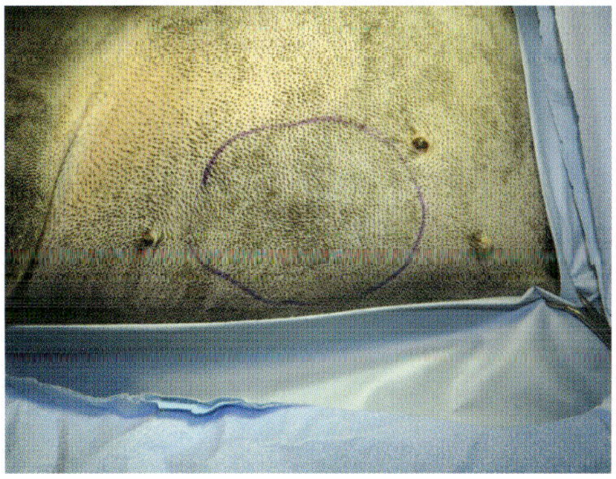

Surgical Technique (See Plate 45.1A, C, D, F–H) *continued*

E) Before harvesting the graft, the edges of the traced recipient site are digitally opposed to ensure primary wound closure of the donor site is feasible (not pictured). If not, then an alternative site should be used with more mobile skin to allow primary wound closure of the donor site.
F) A scalpel blade is used to incise along the traced template borders at the donor site (i). The skin graft is often elevated with the deeper cutaneous trunci muscle; however, as little extraneous tissue as possible should be raised with the graft. The donor site (ii) is covered with saline-soaked swabs to maintain a moist wound surface while the skin graft is being prepared.
G) There are many techniques to prepare the graft and the technique described herein is preferred by one of the authors. The graft is kept moist throughout preparation. The graft is folded over the index finger of the nondominant hand, skin side down. Curved Metzenbaum scissors (curve up) are then laid flat against the underside of the graft and, through repeated small cutting actions, the underlying soft tissues, namely, muscle and fat, are gently shaved away (i). Whenever excess soft tissue accumulates on the blades of the scissors, they are quickly washed in a bowl of sterile saline (ii), which also helps keep the graft moist. This action is continued until the roots of the hair follicles begin to become apparent on the underside of the graft (iii). The skin graft is continuously repositioned over the back of the finger to allow for all areas to be debrided in this fashion. Intermittently, a new no. 10 scalpel blade can be used to brush excess fat off the underside of the graft.
H) When the entire graft is prepared and the follicles are visible in all areas, the graft is placed over a metal or plastic bowl, skin side up (i), and multiple fenestrations are made across the entire graft (ii). These are typically 5–10 mm in length in staggered rows, depending on the overall area of the graft. The fenestrations allow the graft to contour to the wound better, allow for drainage of the wound bed, and increase the surface area of the graft, ensuring the graft is more than an adequate size for coverage of the wound defect.

Closure (See Plate 45.1I)

I) The graft is laid skin side up over the recipient and anchored to the defect with 2-0 to 3-0 monofilament nonabsorbable material in a simple interrupted pattern around the periphery of the graft to the skin margin (i). These can be placed 3–5 mm apart. The skin graft can also overlap the edges of the recipient site with any nonviable tissue sloughing off without the requirement for further surgical intervention. In uneven wound beds or large defects, tacking sutures can be placed in the center of the graft to anchor the graft to the underlying tissues (ii, arrows).
J) The graft site is protected with saline-soaked swabs, while the subcutaneous tissue and skin layers are closed routinely at the donor site (not pictured).

Plate 45.1

Free-Meshed Skin Grafts *continued*

F-i)
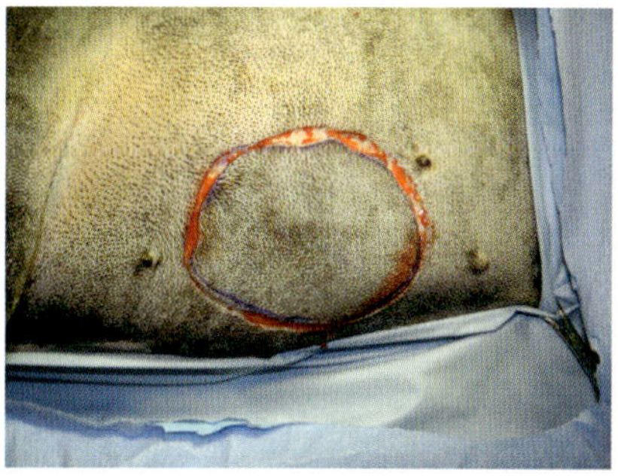

F-ii)
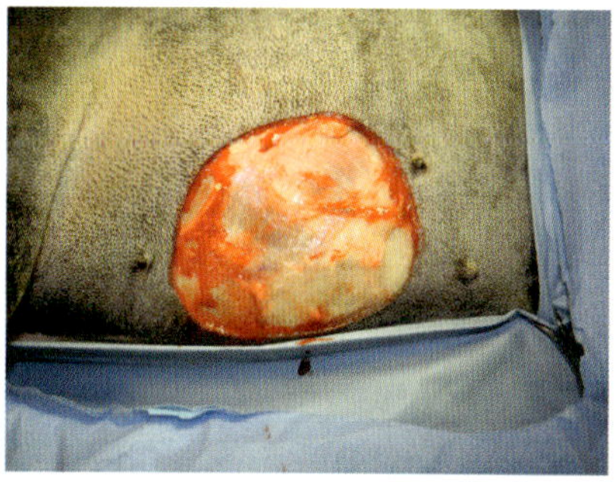

G-i)
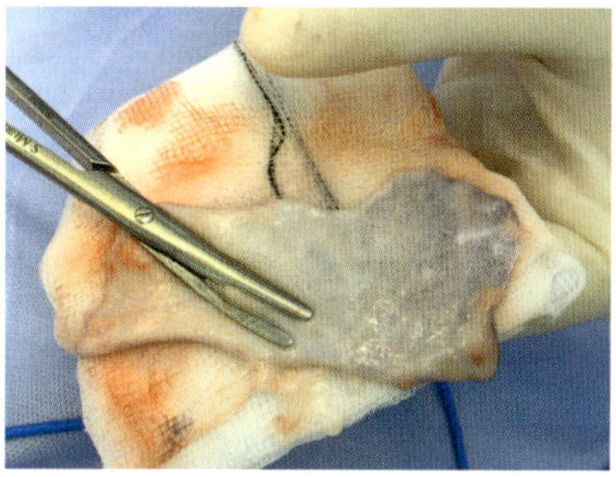

G-ii)
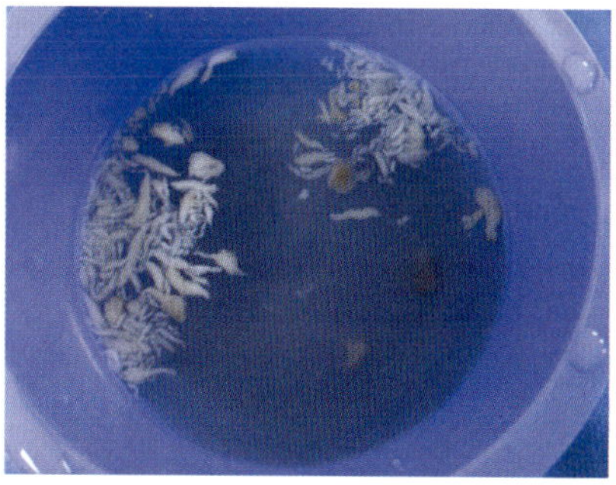

G-iii)
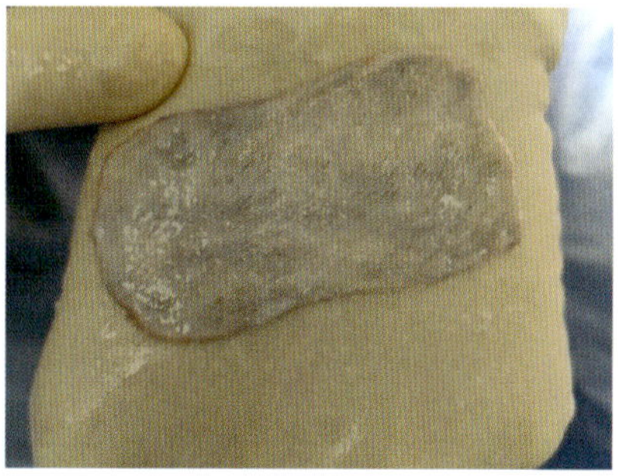

H-i)
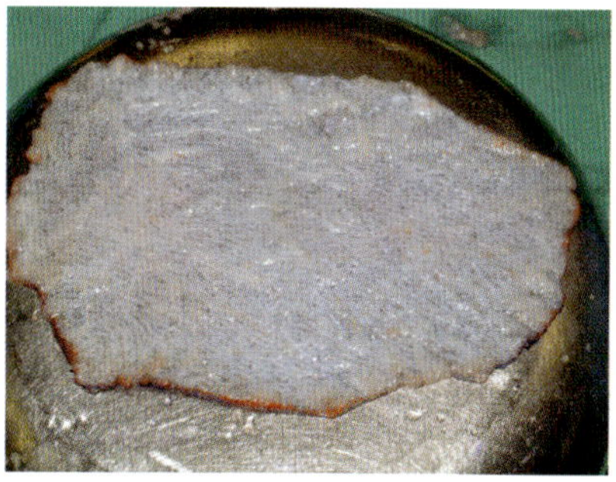

H-ii)
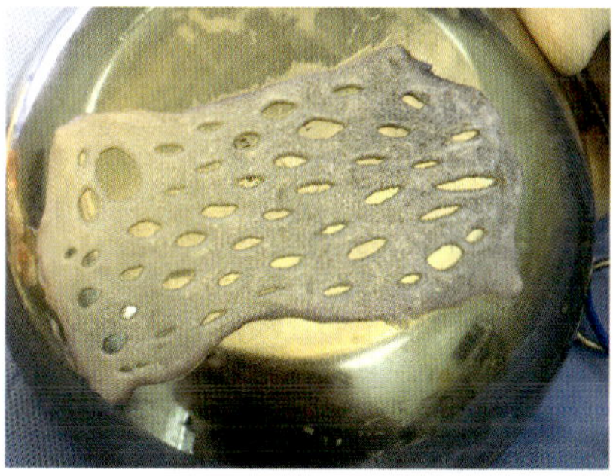

I-i)
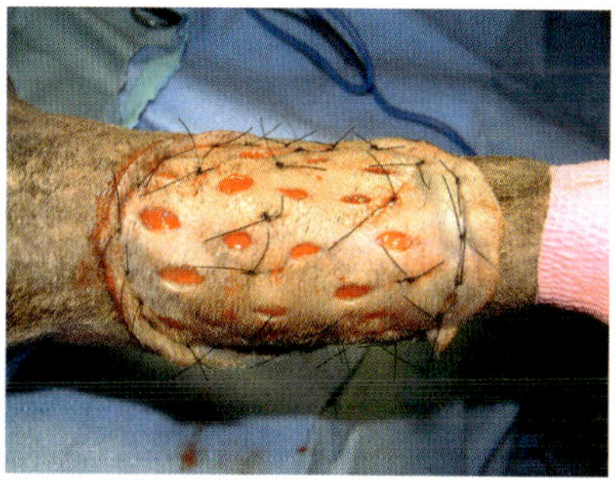

I-ii)
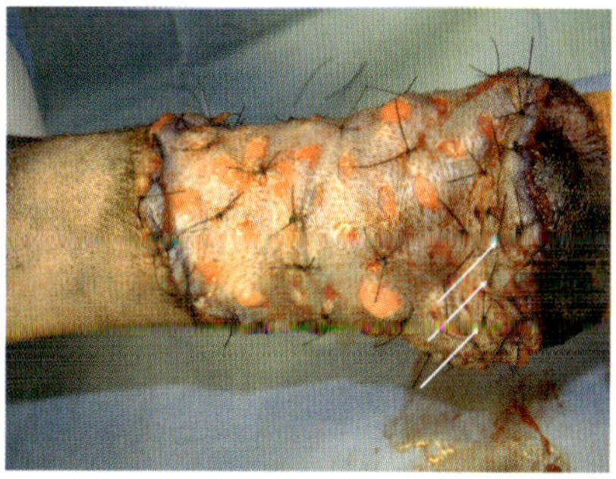

Postoperative Management (See Plate 45.1K, L, N, O)

K) The graft is then bandaged. The priority is to provide a nonadherent moist environment that does not allow the graft to move. One of the authors prefers the following:
  i) A primary layer of silicone dressing (e.g. Mepitel) that completely covers the graft and, if need be, the distal limb circumferentially
  ii) A secondary layer of paraffin-impregnated gauze (e.g. Jelonet) covering the entire graft and surrounding skin
  iii) A tertiary layer of a foam dressing (e.g. Allevyn)
  iv) Outer layers of soft padded wrap, conforming bandage, and then an elasticated outer (e.g. Vetrap); a splint is recommended if the skin graft is near or around a distal joint

L) Other bandaging protocols are available, including vacuum-assisted closure therapy (pictured), to immobilize the free-meshed skin graft [3].

M) The patient is hospitalized and cage rested for 6–8 days. If the outer layers are soiled, then they should be replaced in a sterile fashion under anesthesia because immobility of the graft is the utmost priority for success of the grafting procedure.

N) Although protocols vary, one of the authors prefers to change the bandage every 3–4 days under heavy sedation or, preferably, general anesthesia. The outer layers of the bandage can be removed in a nonsterile manner until the foam dressing is reached. The remaining layers are changed using an aseptic technique. Each layer is gently lifted from the underlying bandage layers as the external bandage layer is copiously lavaged at the area being elevated and while gentle counter pressure is applied with sterile forceps onto the wound to avoid the graft being lifted with the bandage material. The same technique is used to elevate the silicone dressing from the graft, with the underlying graft gently being immobilized with forceps. The wound is then cleaned and any exudate or debris is gently removed. The skin graft can appear red to purple and even almost black in areas (i, ii); however, a white-colored graft is a cause for concern (iii). The skin graft should not be debrided at this stage.

Plate 45.1

Free-Meshed Skin Grafts *continued*

K-ii)

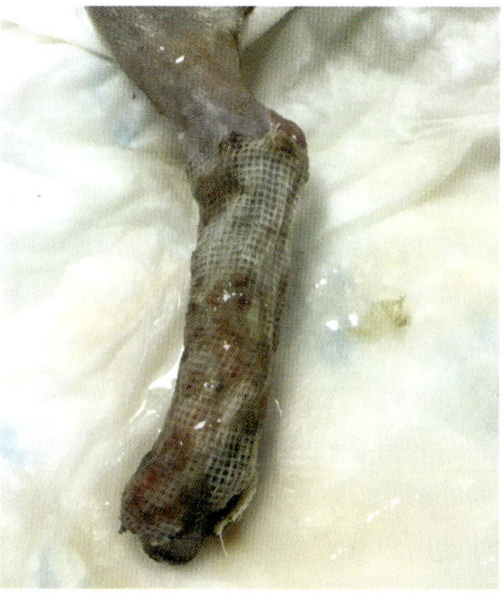

K-iv)

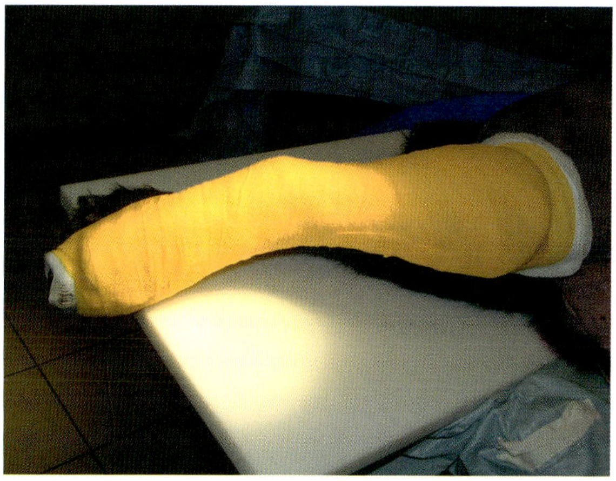

L)

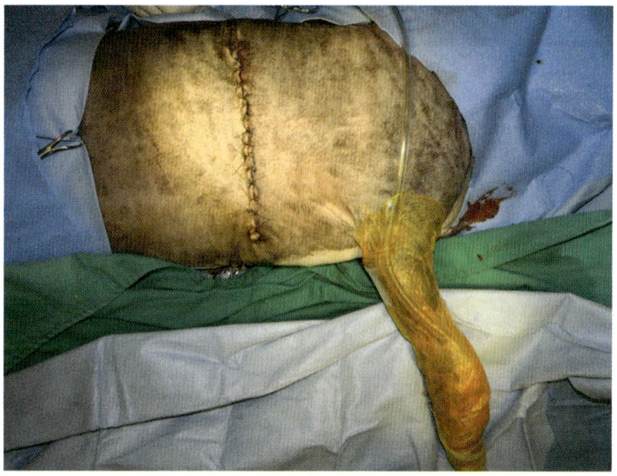

N-i)

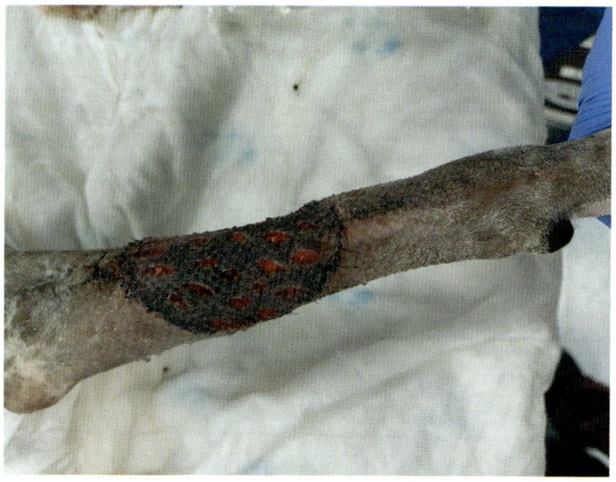

N-ii)

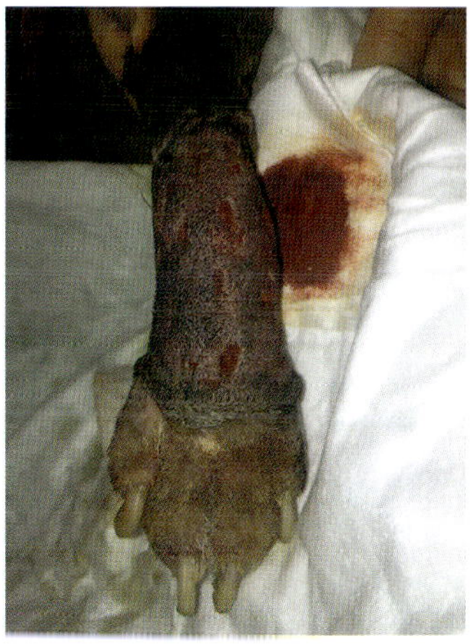

N-iii)

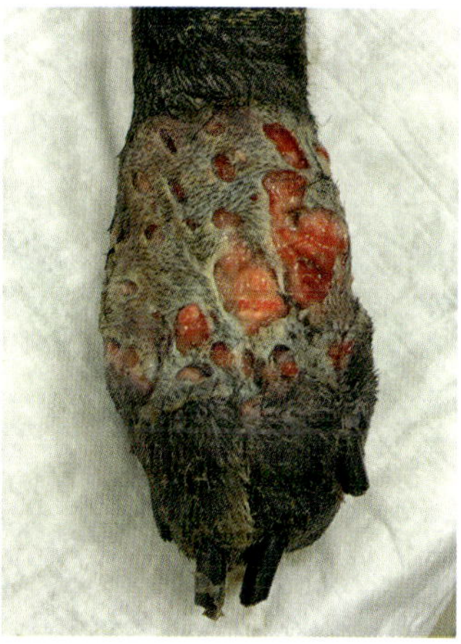

Postoperative Management (See Plate 45.1K, L, N, O) *continued*

O) The graft is then rebandaged as described in step K, and the patient is hospitalized for a further 3–4 days until the second bandage change. The bandage is changed as described in step N. A third bandage change using similar materials may be required. Once successful graft take is expected (typically in 8–12 days), the sutures can be removed, the bandage can be down-staged to a light dressing (e.g. Primapore), and the wound inspected every 3–4 days until it can be left uncovered (postoperative appearance of a free-meshed skin graft on the caudal aspect of the proximal antebrachium after single-session soft tissue sarcoma resection and free-meshed skin graft reconstruction: i, 10 days; ii, 18 days; iii, 25 days; iv, 50 days; v, 75 days).

Complications (See Plate 45.1P)

- Graft failure (≥75% full-thickness graft viability): 23% in cats and 62% in dogs (P and see N – iii) [4]
- Prolonged healing with staged procedures (median, 51 days) compared with single-session procedures (median, 30 days) [1]
- Surgical-site infection, incisional dehiscence, or seroma formation at the donor site

References

1 Bonaventura, N.C. and Ganjei, J.B. (2021). Comparison of outcomes for single-session and delayed full-thickness applications of meshed skin grafts used to close skin defects after excision of tumors on the distal aspects of the limbs in dogs. *J. Am. Vet. Med. Assoc.* 258 (4): 387–394.

2 Tong, T. and Simpson, D.J. (2012). Free skin grafts for immediate wound coverage following tumour resection from the canine distal limb. *J. Small Anim. Pract.* 53 (9): 520–525.

3 Miller, A.J., Cashmore, R.G., Marchevsky, A.M. et al. (2016). Negative pressure wound therapy using a portable single-use device for free skin grafts on the distal extremity in seven dogs. *Aust. Vet. J.* 94 (9): 309–316.

4 Riggs, J., Frazer Jennings, J.L., Friend, E.J. et al. (2015). Outcome of full-thickness skin grafts used to close skin defects involving the distal aspects of the limbs in cats and dogs: 52 cases (2005-2012). *J. Am. Vet. Med. Assoc.* 247 (9): 1042–1047.

Plate 45.1

Free-Meshed Skin Grafts *continued*

O-i)

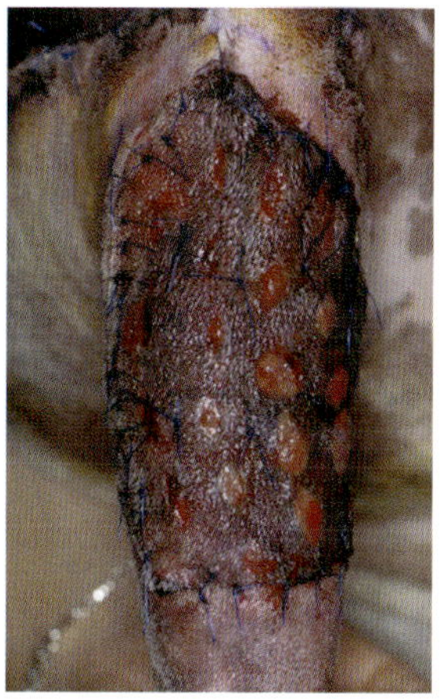

O-ii)

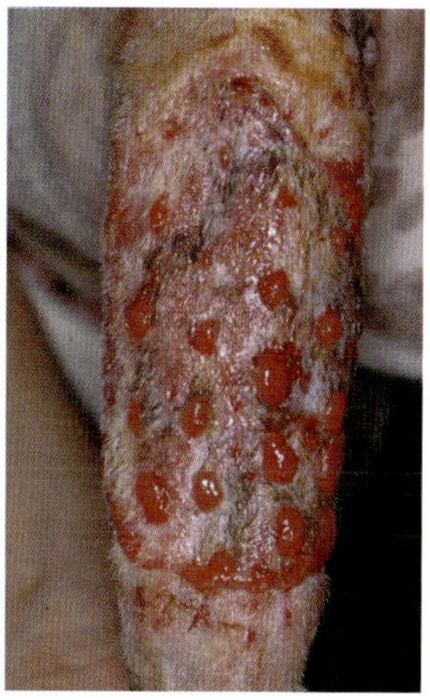

O-iii)

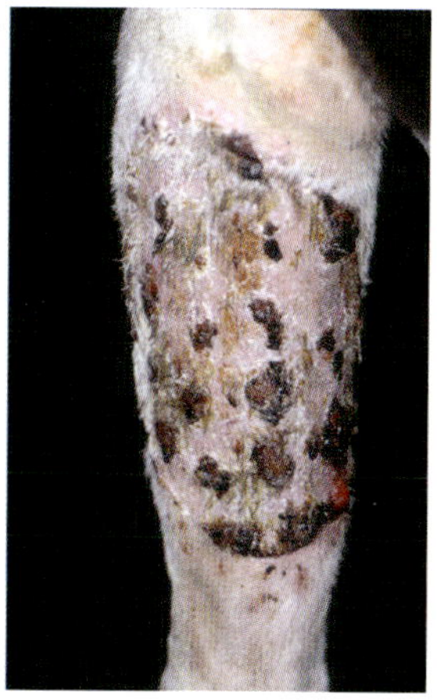

O-iv)

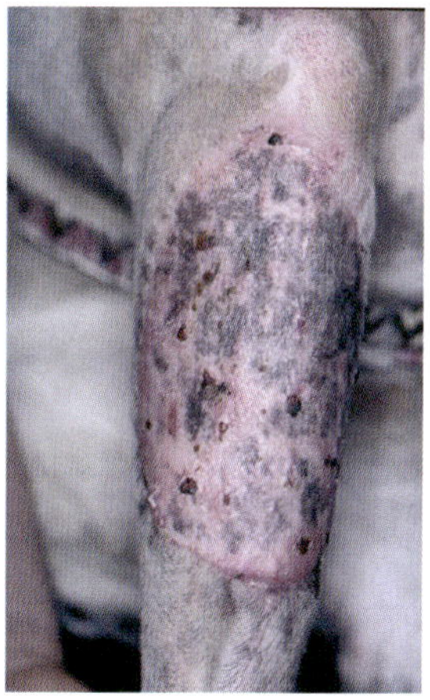

O-v)

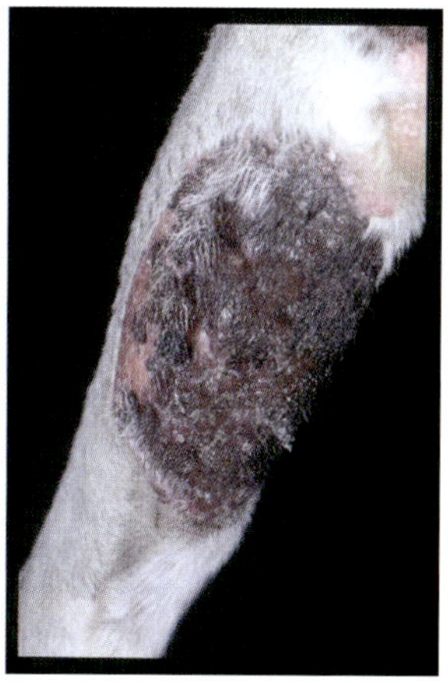

P)

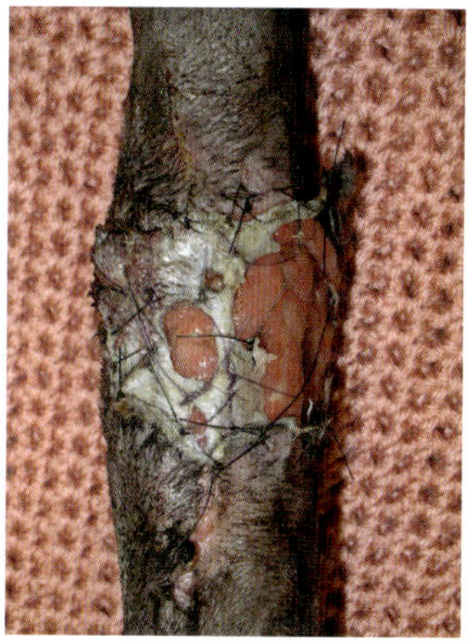

45.2 Punch Grafts

Indications (See Plate 45.2 – 1)

1) Reconstruction of full-thickness skin defects that cannot be closed primarily. Although theoretically plausible in any location, punch grafts are typically used to reconstruct wounds located below the elbow or stifle because of the requirement for rigid immobility of the skin graft in the immediate postoperative period. Punch grafts are often used for full-thickness skin defects where wound healing has stalled after open wound management and second intention healing (pictured).
2) Punch grafts can be combined with wide surgical resection of benign and malignant skin and subcutaneous tumors (see *1. Surgical Resection of Cutaneous and Subcutaneous Tumors*); however, bleeding from a fresh wound bed can displace punch grafts.

Patient Positioning

Patient positioning is dependent on the location of the skin defect. For wounds on the cranial, lateral, or caudal aspect of the limb, the patient is typically positioned with the affected limb uppermost. For wounds on the medial aspect of the limb, the patient is typically positioned in dorsal recumbency. In both cases, the donor bed also needs to be clipped and draped within the surgical field. The donor bed is typically located on the proximal limb, lateral thorax, or ventral abdomen, depending on patient positioning. Many surgeons are comfortable performing punch grafts in the induction area if the punch grafts are being placed into a fully granulated wound bed.

Surgical Technique [1] (See Plate 45.2A–F)

A) For 24–48 hours before punch graft placement, the granulation bed is prepared by covering it with a wet-dry dressing or daily gentle surface debridement with a no. 10 scalpel blade. Punch grafts are harvested from the donor site using a 6-mm skin punch to procure discs of skin from the donor bed.
B) The underlying fat of the punch graft is then gently removed with Metzenbaum scissors (I, dashed line) down to the firmer dermal layer to create a thin, flat disc of skin (ii).
C) A 4-mm skin punch (i) should then be used to remove a smaller disc of granulation tissue from the center of the recipient bed, a few millimeters deep (ii).
D) Once bleeding is controlled from the punch biopsy site in the recipient bed (i, with cotton swabs in this case), punch graft is pushed into this defect with the skin side up (ii). Gentle pressure is applied to the punch graft with a moist swab to seat the punch graft into the smaller punch biopsy site. The punch graft surface may be level with or slightly below the surface of the granulation bed.

Color Atlas of Canine and Feline Surgical Oncology, First Edition. Julius M. Liptak, Paolo Buracco, William T. N. Culp, and Nicholas J. Bacon.

Plate 45.2

Punch Grafts

1)

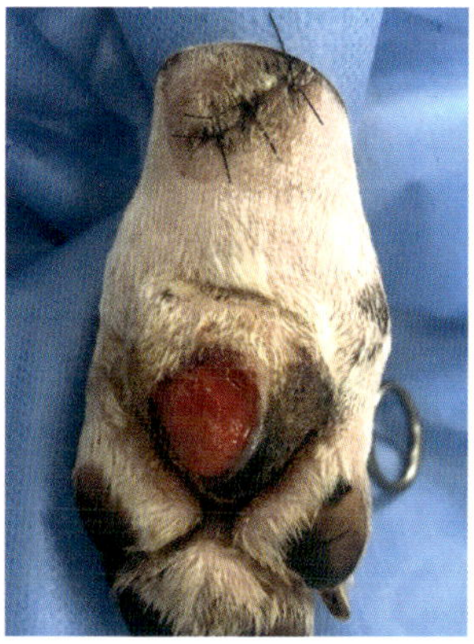

A)

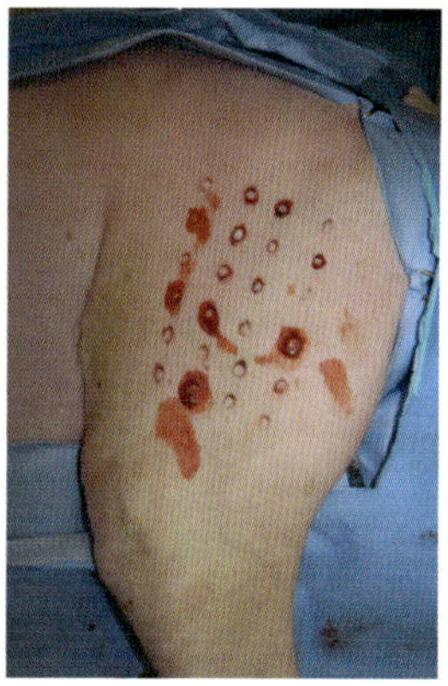

B-i)

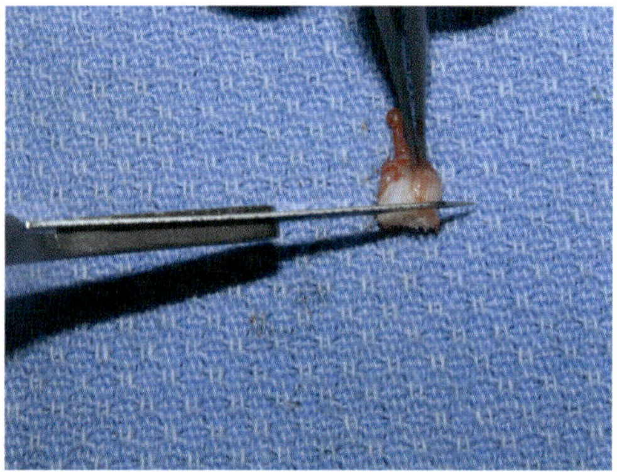

B-ii)

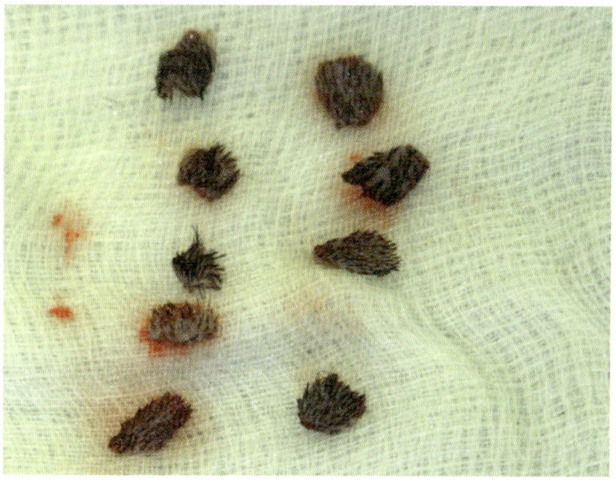

C-i)

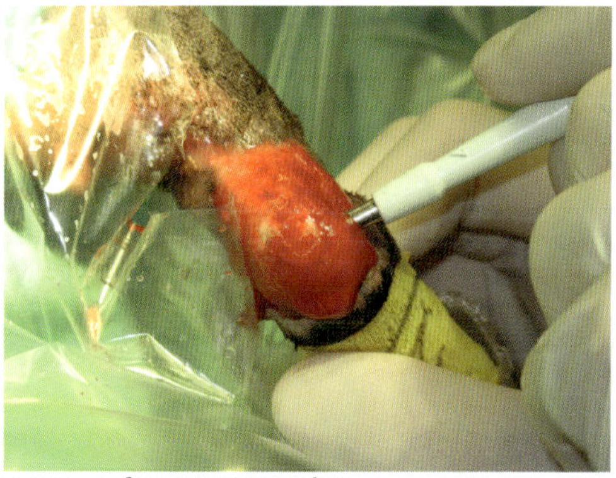

Courtesy of Dr. Martin Kessler

C-ii)

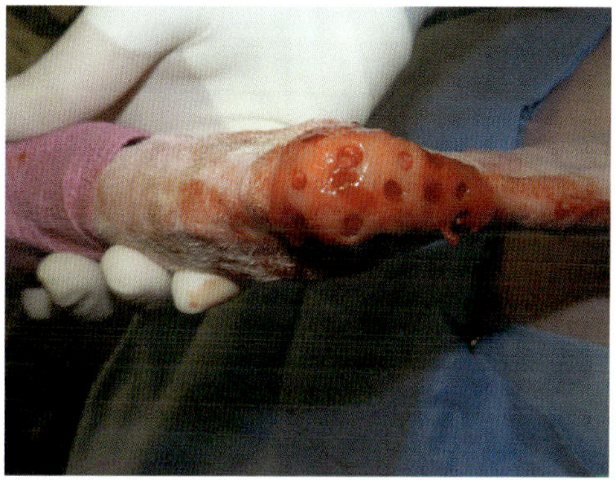

D-i)

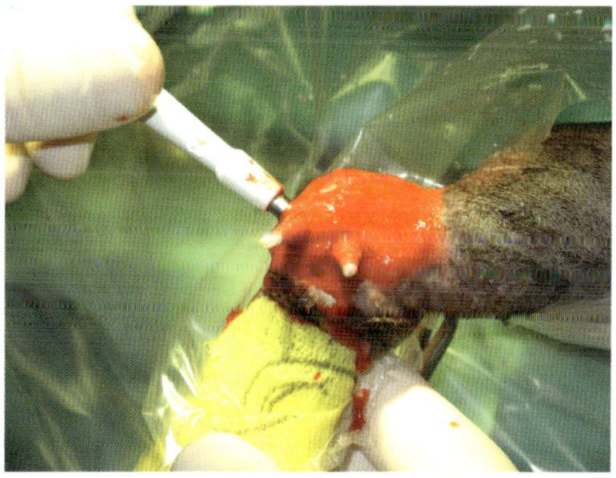

Courtesy of Dr. Martin Kessler

D-ii)

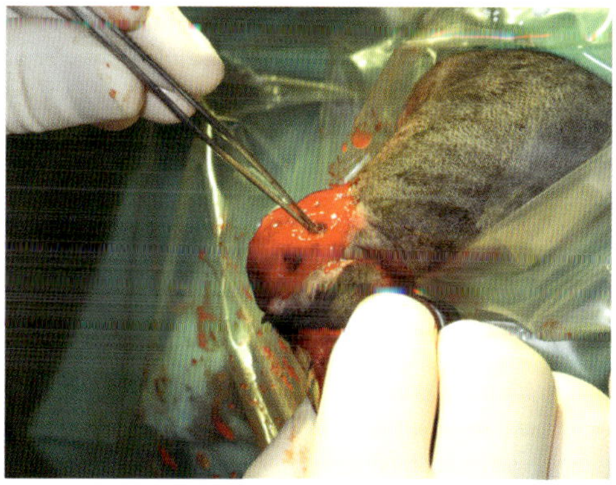

Courtesy of Dr. Martin Kessler

Surgical Technique [1] (See Plate 45.2A–F) *continued*

E) This process is repeated until the recipient wound bed is covered with punch grafts placed approximately 2–4 mm apart.
F) Each of the punch graft donor sites are sutured with a single simple interrupted suture of 3-0 to 4-0 nonabsorbable monofilament suture material.

Postoperative Management

G) The graft is then bandaged. The priority is to provide a nonadherent moist environment that does not allow the graft to move. One of the authors prefers the following:
   i) A primary layer of silicone dressing (e.g. Mepitel) that completely covers the graft and, if need be, the distal limb circumferentially
   ii) A secondary layer of paraffin-impregnated gauze (e.g. Jelonet) covering the entire graft and surrounding skin
   iii) A tertiary layer of a foam dressing (e.g. Allevyn)
   iv) Outer layers of soft padded wrap, conforming bandage, and then an elasticated outer layer (e.g. Vetrap); a splint is recommended if the skin graft is near or around a distal joint
H) Other bandaging protocols are available, including vacuum-assisted closure therapy.
I) The patient is hospitalized and cage rested for 6–8 days. If the outer layers are soiled, then they should be replaced in a sterile fashion under anesthesia because immobility of the graft is the utmost priority for success of the grafting procedure.
J) Although protocols vary, one of the authors prefers to change the bandage every 3–4 days under heavy sedation or, preferably, general anesthesia. The outer layers of the bandage can be removed in a nonsterile manner until the foam dressing is reached. The remaining layers are changed using an aseptic technique. Each layer is gently lifted from the underlying bandage layers as the external bandage layer is copiously lavaged at the area being elevated and while gentle counter pressure is applied with sterile forceps onto the wound to avoid the punch grafts being lifted with the bandage material. The same technique is used to elevate the silicone dressing from the grafted wound. The wound is then cleaned, and any exudate or debris is gently removed.
K) The graft is then rebandaged as described in step G, and the patient is hospitalized for a further 3–4 days until the second bandage change. The bandage is changed as described in step J. A third bandage change using similar materials may be required. Once successful graft take is expected (typically in 8–12 days), the sutures can be removed, the bandage can be down-staged to a light dressing (e.g. Primapore), and the wound inspected every 3–4 days until it can be left uncovered.

Complications

- Graft failure (rare)
- Epidermal inclusion cyst at recipient site (13%)

Reference

1 Crowley, J.D., Hosgood, G., and Appelgrein, C. (2020). Seed skin grafts for reconstruction of distal limb defects in 15 dogs. *J. Small Anim. Pract.* 61 (9): 561–567.

Plate 45.2

Punch Grafts *continued*

E)

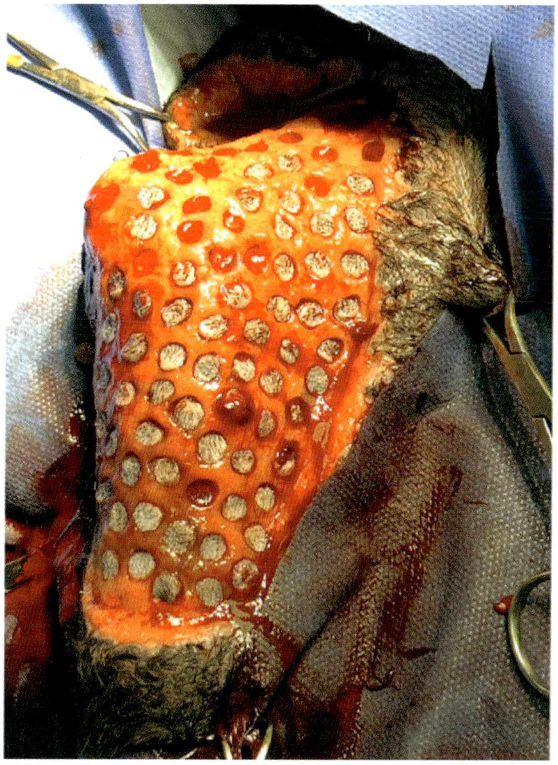

F)

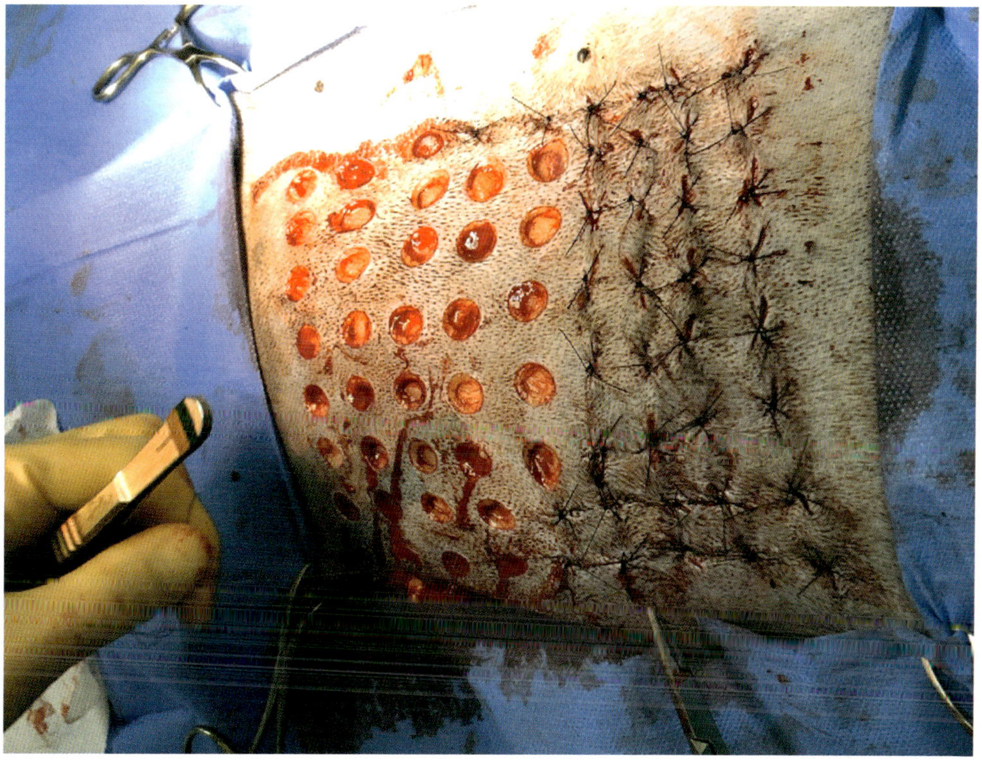

Chapter 46: Second Intention Healing

Indications

1) Elective management of open wounds after tumor resection
2) Management of open wounds after failure of primary wound closure or other reconstructive procedures

Suggested Diagnostic Workup

- Local wound and systemic assessment for any comorbid conditions that may negatively impact wound healing, such as culture and sensitivity for infection

Management (See Plate 46A–D)

A) The wound should be bandaged, if possible, to protect the wound and maintain a moist wound environment. A soft padded bandage can be used for wounds on the limbs and body wall, and a tie-over bandage (i, pictured) can be used in other locations (ii, 1 day; iii, 5 days; iv, 15 days; v, 42 days).

Color Atlas of Canine and Feline Surgical Oncology, First Edition. Julius M. Liptak, Paolo Buracco, William T. N. Culp, and Nicholas J. Bacon.

Plate 46

Second Intention Healing

A-i)

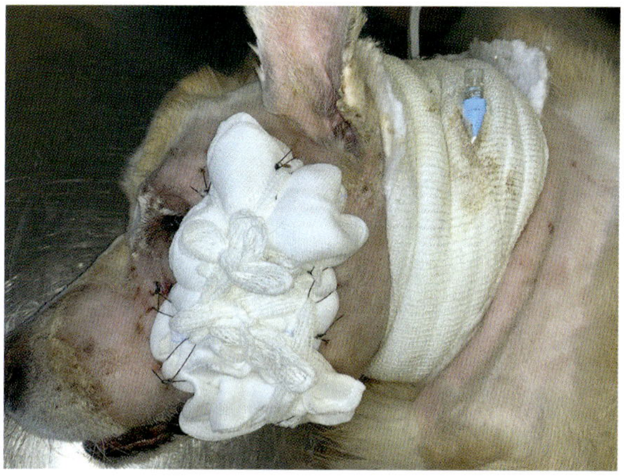

A-ii)

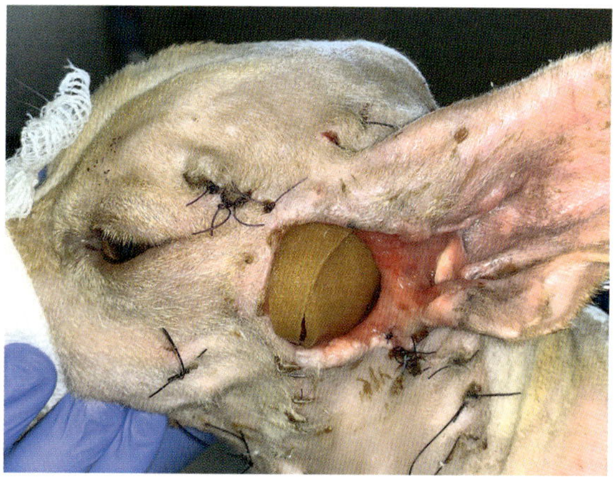

A-iii)

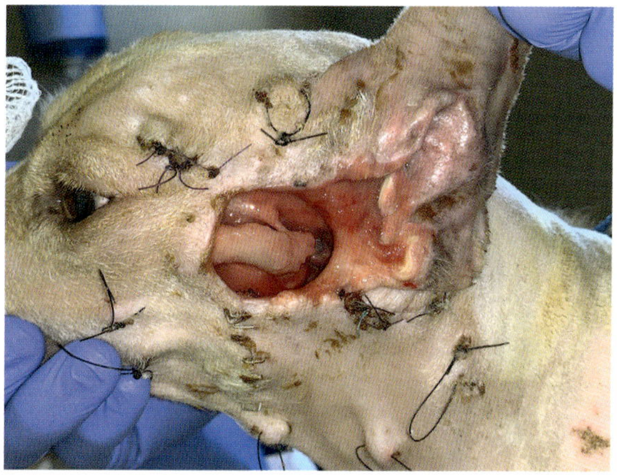

A-iv)

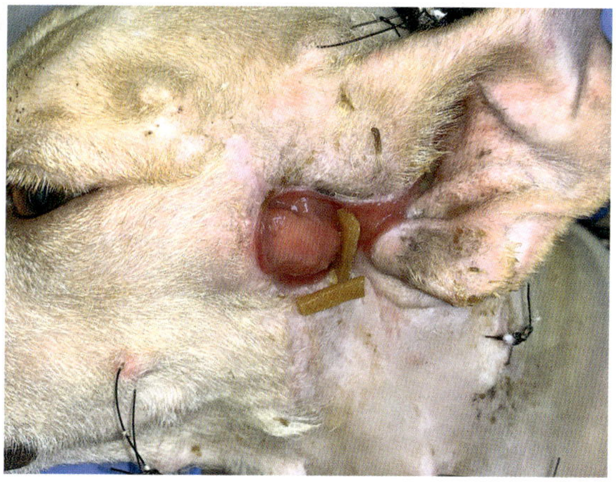

A-v)

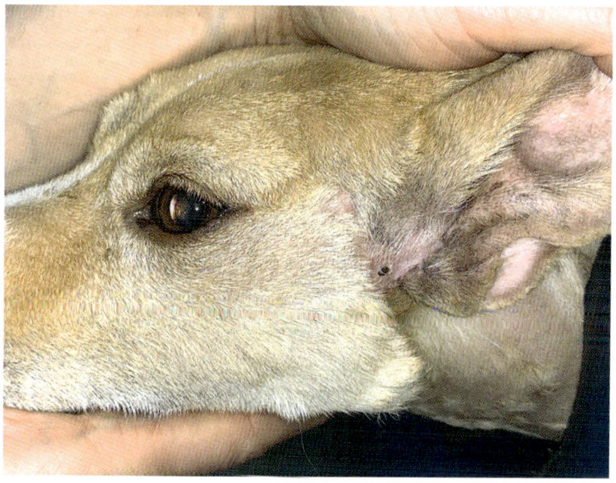

Management (See Plate 46A–D) *continued*

B) The contact layer of the bandage changes and is dependent on the phase of healing of the wound (i, 1 day; ii, 14 days; iii, 21 days; iv, 24 days; v, 42 days; vi, 58 days). An adherent dressing, such as a wet-to-dry dressing, or vacuum-assisted closure therapy is used for contaminated wounds. A petroleum-based or calcium alginate dressing is used for wounds transitioning to granulation tissue. A nonadherent, nonocclusive dressing (e.g. Telfa) is used for wounds with early granulation tissue formation. Nonadherent, occlusive dressings (e.g. hydrogels, hydrocolloids) are used for wounds with a good granulation tissue bed and epithelialization.

Plate 46

Second Intention Healing *continued*

B-i)

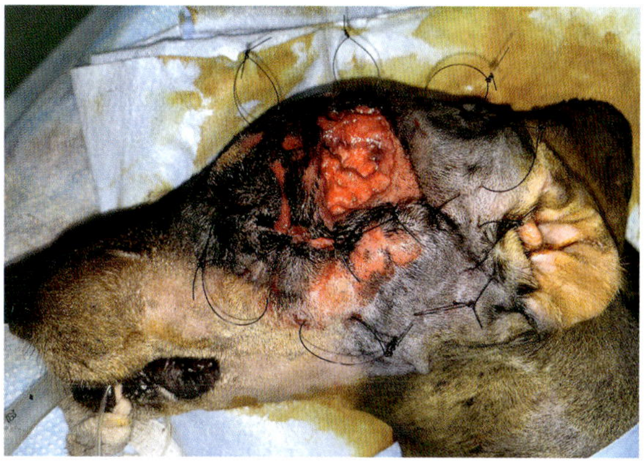

B-ii)

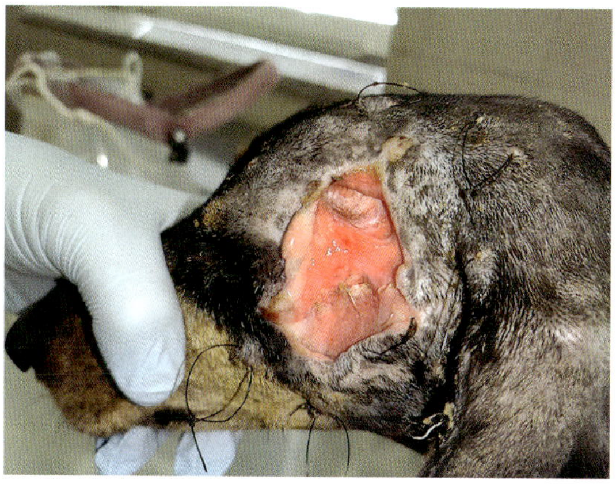

B-iii)

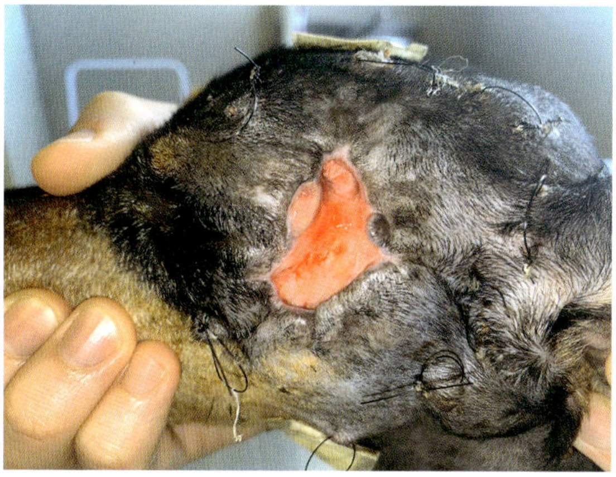

B-iv)

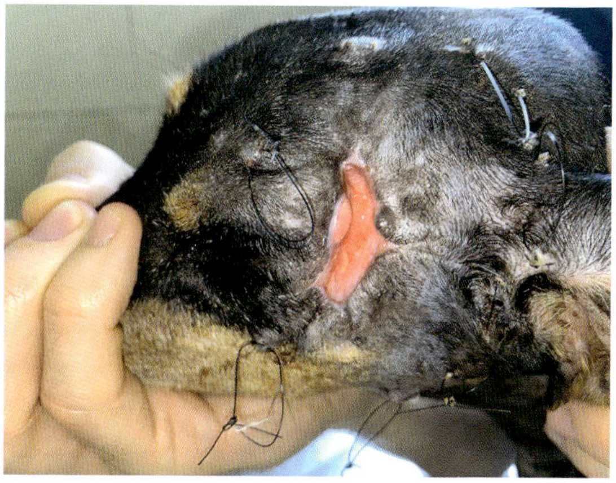

B-v)

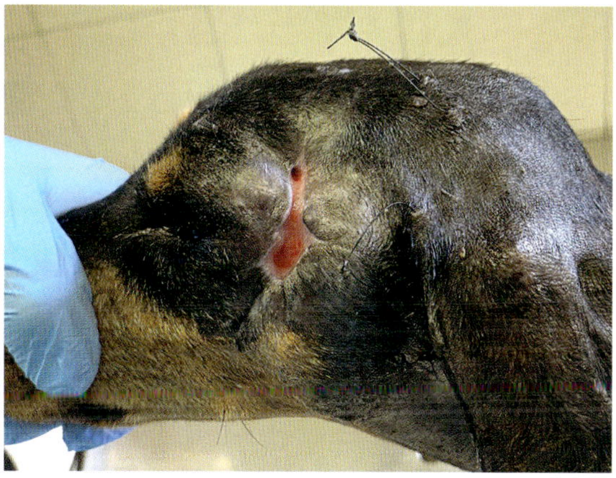

B-vi)

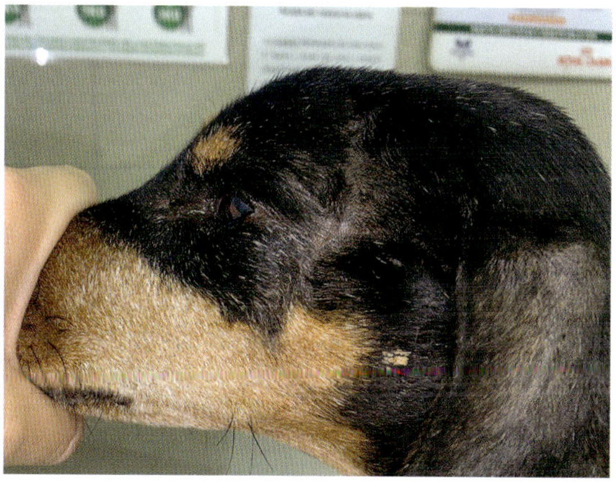

Management (See Plate 46A–D) *continued*

C) The frequency of bandage changes is dependent on the phase of wound healing (i, 1 day; ii, 7 days; iii, 14 days; iv, 19 days; v, 23 days; vi, 30 days) and the contact layer being used. Adherent dressings are changed every 12–24 hours; petroleum-based dressings are changed every 24 hours; Telfa pads are changed every 24–48 hours, and hydrogels and hydrocolloids are changed every 3–5 days.

Plate 46

Second Intention Healing *continued*

C-i)

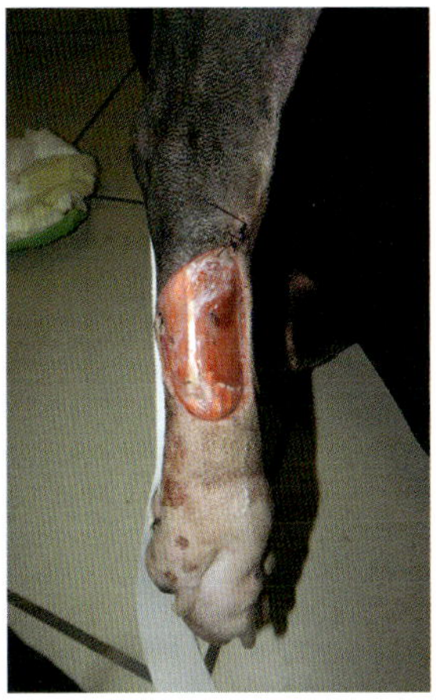

C-ii)

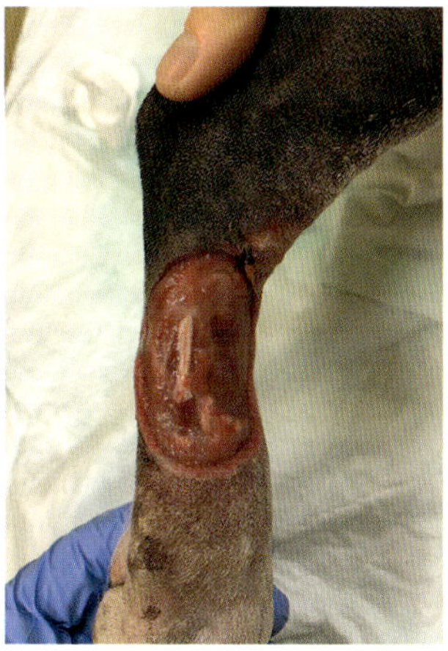

C-iii)

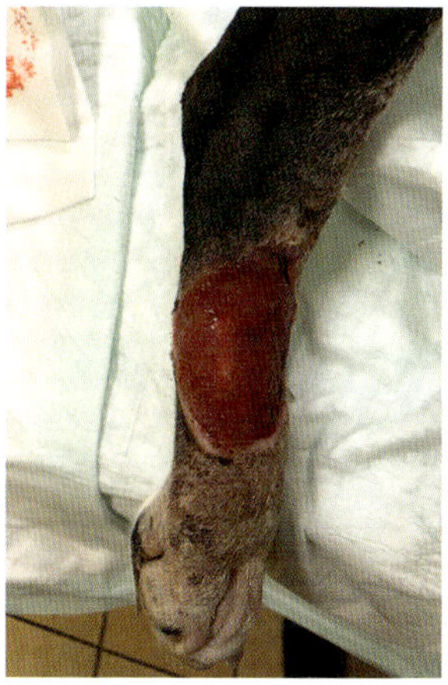

C-iv)

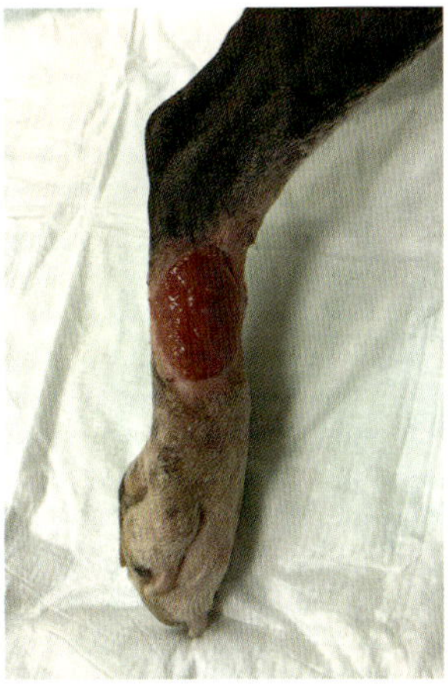

C-v)

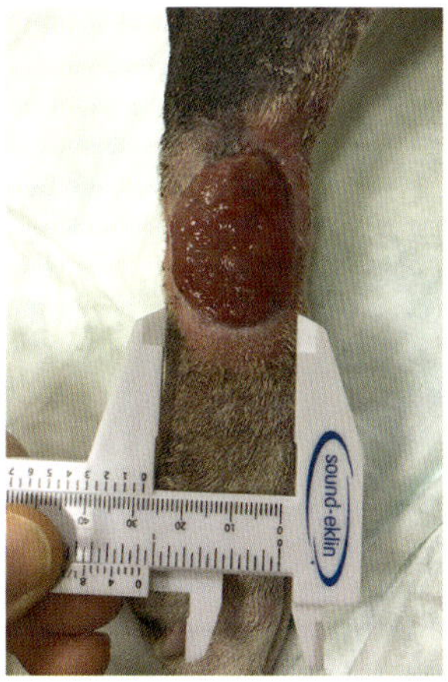

C-vi)

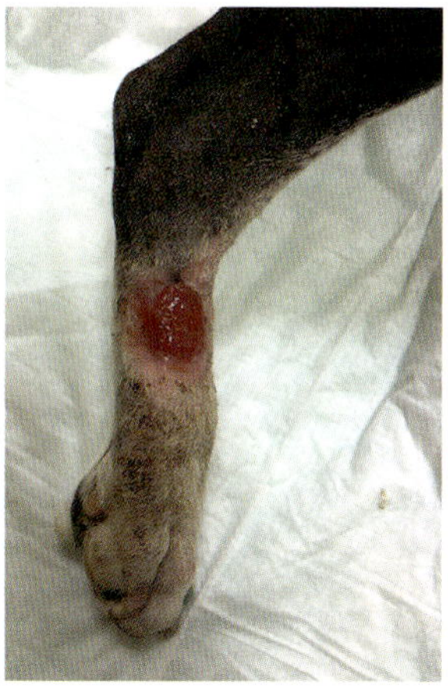

C-vii)

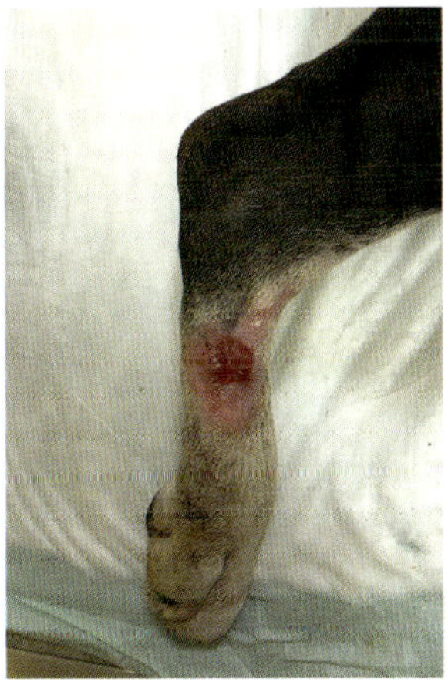

C-viii)

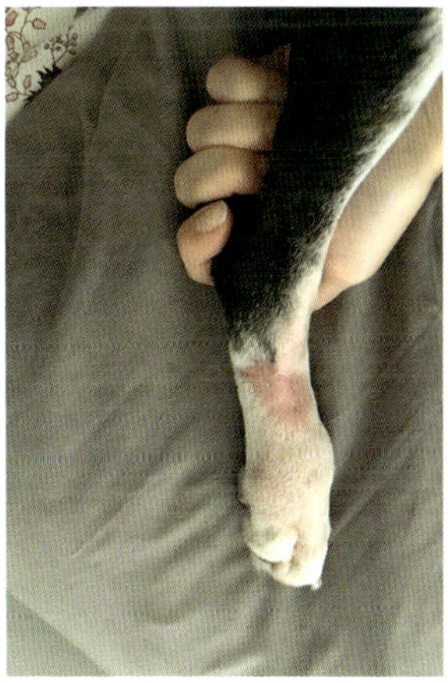

Management (See Plate 46A–D) *continued*

D) Systemic antibiotics should be used only in select cases with documented infection (i, 0 days; ii, 4 days; iii, 26 days; iv, 40 days; v, 104 days).

Cases

- Second intention healing of an infected wound after tissue debridement and flushing with sterile saline; bandage management included honey patches and a tie-over bandage (see step A)
- Second intention healing of a wound dehiscence after tissue debridement and flushing with sterile saline; a tie-over bandage was used (see step B)
- Elective second intention healing after wide surgical resection of a low-grade cutaneous mast cell tumor (see step C)
- Second intention healing after self-trauma to an inguinal flank fold flap (due to a paraesthesia) after wide surgical resection of a subcutaneous soft tissue sarcoma (see step D)

Outcomes [1]

- 94% of wounds resulting from wide resection of soft tissue sarcomas healed by second intention
- Median time to healing was 53 days (range, 25–179 days)

Complications [1]

Short-Term Complications (During Second Intention Healing)

- Overall: 23%
- Infection (13%)
- Incomplete wound healing (6%)
- Bleeding from the wound bed (3%)
- Transient swelling of the distal part of the limb (3%)

Long-Term Complications (After Completion of Second Intention Healing)

- Overall: 26%
- Intermittent traumatic disruption of the epidermis (16%)
- Wound contracture with decreased range of motion of the carpus (10%)

Reference

1 Prpich, C.Y., Santamaria, A.C., Simcock, J.O. et al. (2014). Second intention healing after wide local excision of soft tissue sarcomas in the distal aspects of the limbs in dogs: 31 cases (2005-2012). *J. Am. Vet. Med. Assoc.* 244 (2): 187–194.

Plate 46

Second Intention Healing *continued*

D-i)

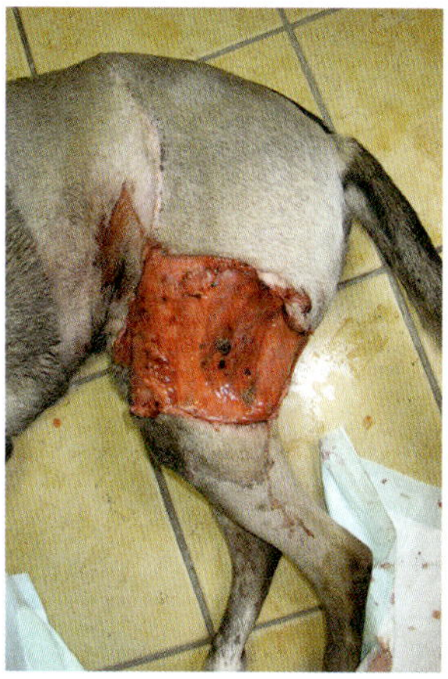

D-ii)

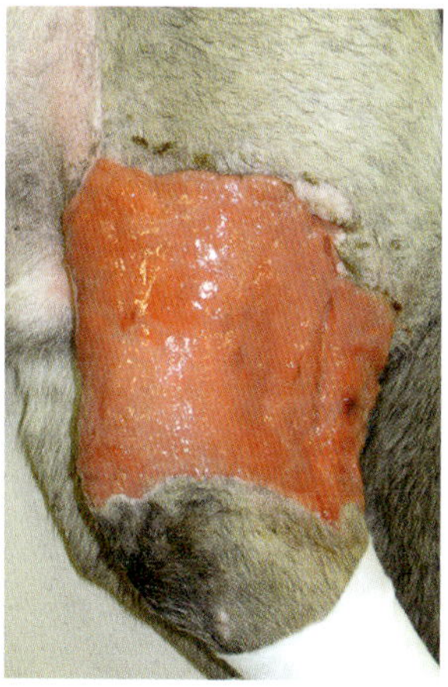

D-iii)

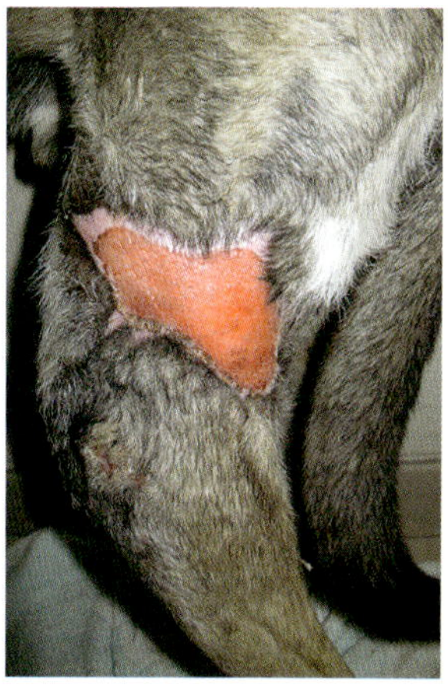

D-iv)

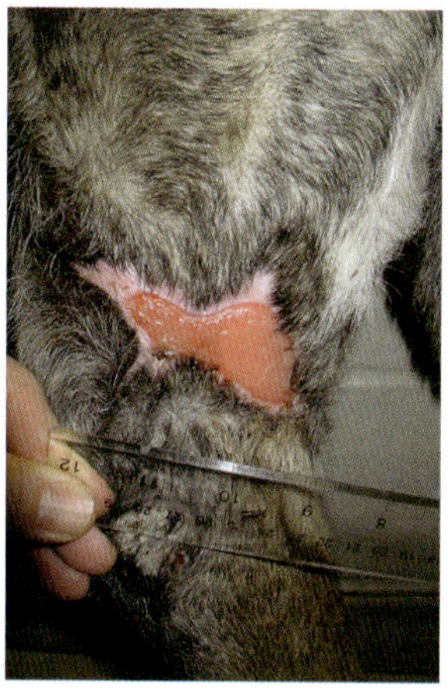

D-v)

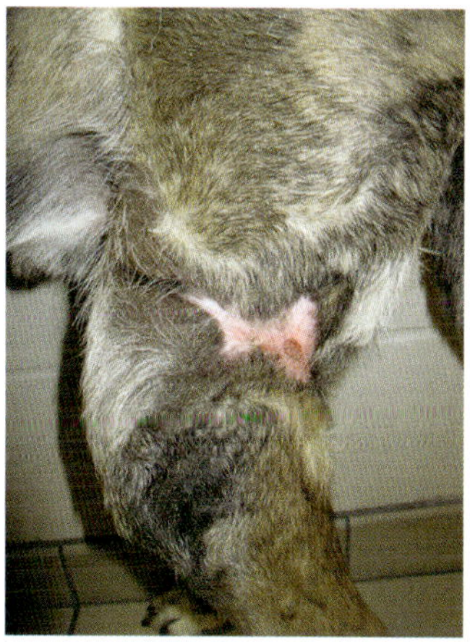

Section 9

Interventional Radiology

Chapter 47: Stenting

47.1 Tracheal Stenting

Indications

1) Palliative management of nonresectable tracheal tumors, tracheal tumors poorly responsive to chemotherapy, or when owners are reluctant to pursue local therapies such as surgery and/or radiation therapy [1–3]
2) Management of nononcologic airway conditions, such as tracheal collapse [3]

Suggested Diagnostic Workup and Clinical Staging

- Complete blood count, serum biochemistry, and urinalysis
- Fine-needle aspirate cytology
- ± Regional lymph node fine-needle aspirate cytology
- Three-view thoracic radiographs or thoracic computed tomography scan for assessment of lung metastasis
- Tracheoscopy

Patient Positioning

The patient is positioned in lateral recumbency.

Procedural Technique (See Plate 47.1B–F)

A) A mouth gag is placed to hold the mouth open (not pictured).
B) A 0.035-inch hydrophilic guidewire is introduced into the esophagus, and a catheter with markers of known length is passed over the guidewire to account for magnification during measurements (i, arrow). A 0.035-inch hydrophiiic guidewire is then passed either through the working channel of the endoscope or next to the endoscope (ii, arrow) into the trachea past the tumor.
C) Tracheoscopy is performed to assess the location of the mass and the extent of obstruction. In addition, the endoscope can be used to direct guidewire passage into the trachea to be sure that the guidewire is passing through the tumor to the lower airways.
D) The endotracheal tube is pulled cranially until the most caudal extent is sitting at the most cranial extent of the trachea. Positive pressure ventilation is performed to determine maximum tracheal diameter (pictured, 7.9 mm) and the length of trachea affected by the tumor. This will allow for stent sizing. A stent should be oversized to the maximally dilated tracheal diameter by 10%–20%. The stent length should be at least 1 cm longer than the region affected by the tumor on each side of the tumor.

Color Atlas of Canine and Feline Surgical Oncology, First Edition. Julius M. Liptak, Paolo Buracco, William T. N. Culp, and Nicholas J. Bacon.

Plate 47.1

Tracheal Stenting

B-i)

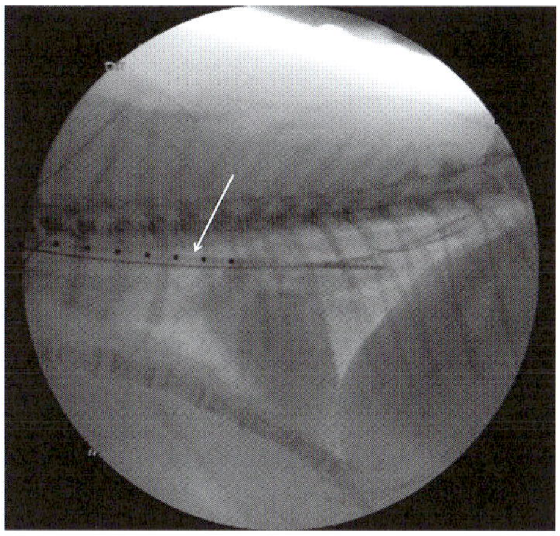

B-ii)

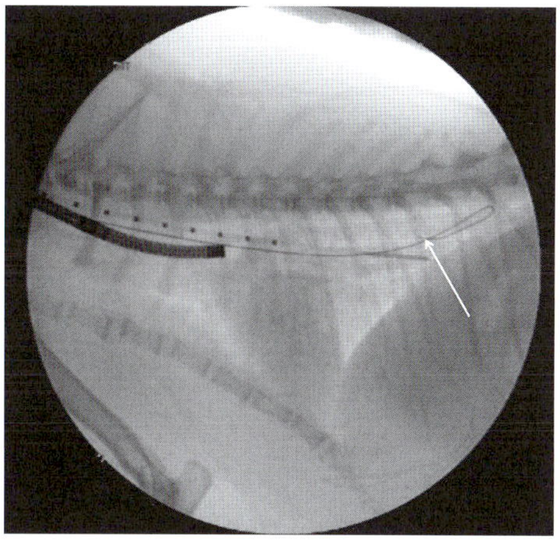

C)

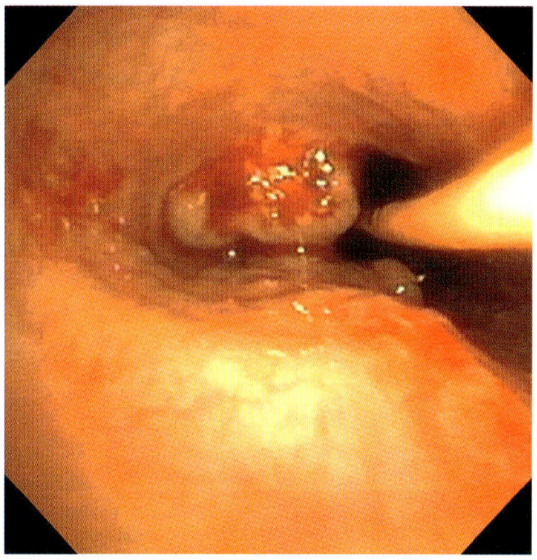

D)

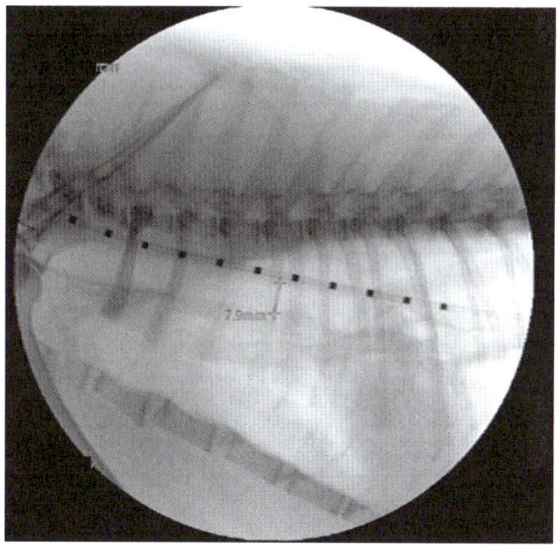

Procedural Technique (See Plate 47.1B–F) *continued*

E) The stent is introduced into the trachea over the guidewire (i, arrow) and deployed using a combination of endoscopic and fluoroscopic guidance (ii, arrow).
F) Endoscopy is performed after stent placement to confirm that the stent is well seated against the tracheal wall and the tracheal lumen has been opened sufficiently to allow for air passage.
G) The equipment is removed with fluoroscopic guidance to be sure that the stent position is not altered. The patient can be reintubated through the stent if necessary or immediately recovered.

Postoperative Management

1) Analgesia may not be necessary because this procedure is relatively minimally invasive; however, each patient should be assessed individually.
2) Supplemental oxygen may be necessary in the immediate poststent placement period.

Complications – Dogs [4]

Note that the complications summarized in the following sections are for treatment of tracheal collapse with tracheal stents rather than neoplastic obstruction of the trachea.

Intraoperative Complications

- Inadequate stent length requiring second stenting (5%)

Perioperative Complications

- Overall: 55%
- Pneumonia or tracheal infection (52%)
- Respiratory distress or dyspnea (7%)
- Regurgitation (3%)

Short-Term Complications (<45 days)

- Overall: 21% with 12% classified as minor and 9% as major
- Pneumonia or tracheal infection (16%)
- Stent fracture (4%)
- Repeat collapse (4%)
- Stent migration (2%)

Intermediate-Term Complications (45–180 days)

- Overall complications not reported, but 18% of complications were classified as minor and 9% as major
- Tissue ingrowth (18%)
- Pneumonia or tracheal infection (4%)
- Stent fracture (4%)
- Repeat collapse (2%)

Plate 47.1

Tracheal Stenting *continued*

E-i)

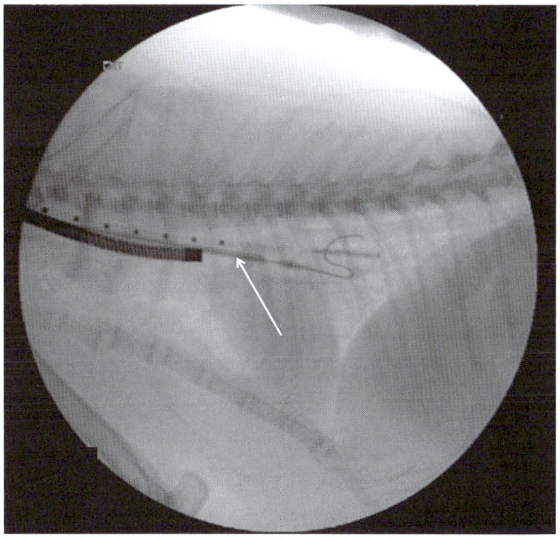

E-ii)

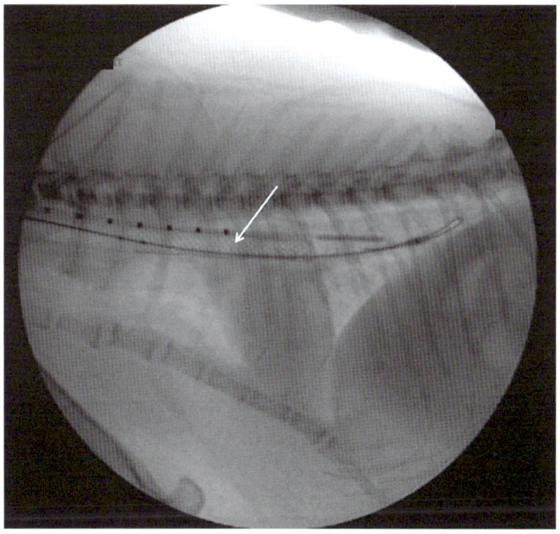

F)

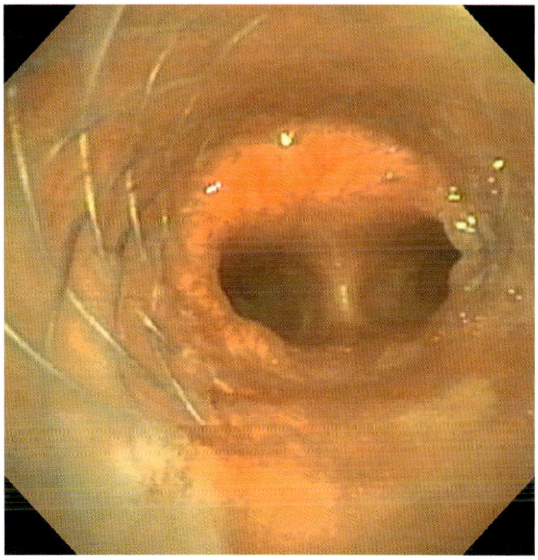

Long-Term Complications (>180 days)

- Overall complications not reported, but 66% of complications were classified as minor and 48% as major
- Pneumonia or tracheal infection (58%)
- Tissue ingrowth (44%)
- Stent fracture (18%)
- Repeat collapse (8%)

References

1 Hawley, M.M., Johnson, L.R., Johnson, E.G. et al. (2015). Endoscopic treatment of an intrathoracic tracheal osteochondroma in a dog. *J. Am. Vet. Med. Assoc.* 247 (11): 1303–1308.
2 Queen, E.V., Vaughan, M.A., and Johnson, L.R. (2010). Bronchoscopic debulking of tracheal carcinoma in 3 cats using a wire snare. *J. Vet. Intern. Med.* 24 (4): 990–993.
3 Culp, W.T., Weisse, C., Cole, S.G., and Solomon, J.A. (2007). Intraluminal tracheal stenting for treatment of tracheal narrowing in three cats. *Vet. Surg.* 36 (2): 107–113.
4 Weisse, C., Berent, A., Violette, N. et al. (2019). Short-, intermediate-, and long-term results for endoluminal stent placement in dogs with tracheal collapse. *J. Am. Vet. Med. Assoc.* 254 (3): 380–392.

47.2 Ureteral Stenting

Indications

1) Palliative management of malignant ureteral obstructions to reestablish ureteral patency and urine flow from the kidney to the bladder
2) Management of nononcologic ureteral obstructions, such as ureteral uroliths
3) Ureteral stenting can be combined with urethral stenting (see *47.3. Urethral Stenting*) in dogs and cats with concurrent urethral obstruction

Suggested Diagnostic Workup and Clinical Staging

- Complete blood count, serum biochemistry, and urinalysis
- Urine sediment cytology
- Cadet BRAF mutation urine test
- Abdominal ultrasound or precontrast and postcontrast computed tomography (CT) scan of the abdomen for assessment of location and extent of the ureteral mass and intra-abdominal metastasis
- Three-view thoracic radiographs or thoracic CT scan for assessment of lung metastasis

Patient Positioning

Dogs undergoing percutaneous ureteral stenting are positioned in lateral recumbency with the affected side uppermost. Cats undergoing ureteral stenting via a ventral midline celiotomy are positioned in dorsal recumbency.

Surgical Technique – Percutaneous Ureteral Stenting in Dogs [1] (See Plate 47.2A–F)

A) A stab incision is made in the skin over the affected kidney, and a 16- to 18-gauge over-the-needle catheter is directed into the renal pelvis using ultrasound guidance (i). Urine is extracted to decrease the volume of fluid within the renal pelvis and to potentially allow for a urine culture to be submitted. A T-port is attached to the catheter, and a 50–50 mixture of iodinated contrast agent and saline is injected to perform a nephroureterogram (ii).
B) The T-port is disconnected and a 0.035-inch × 260 cm long guidewire is introduced into the renal pelvis through the catheter (i). The guidewire is manipulated down the ureter and into the bladder (ii). The guidewire is then passed out of the urethra (iii) and grasped on both ends (i.e. from the kidney and urethra sides) with fingers or hemostats.
C) A 6 French (Fr) dilator/sheath combination is introduced into the urethra over the through-and-through guidewire (i, arrow). The dilator and sheath are passed into the ureter to within a few centimeters of the renal pelvis (ii), and the dilator is removed (iii).

Color Atlas of Canine and Feline Surgical Oncology, First Edition. Julius M. Liptak, Paolo Buracco, William T. N. Culp, and Nicholas J. Bacon.

Plate 47.2

Ureteral Stenting

A-i)

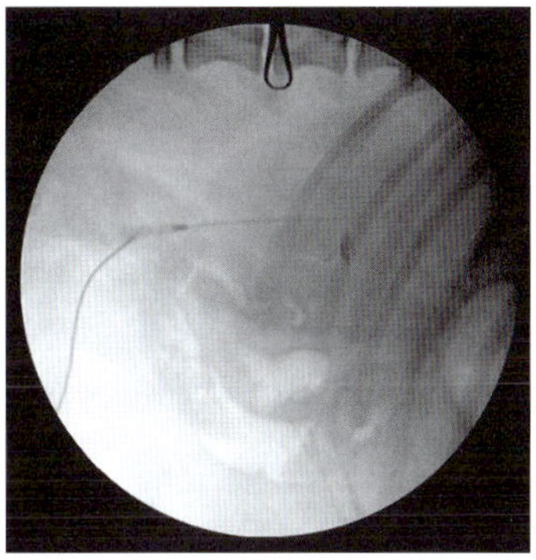

A-ii)

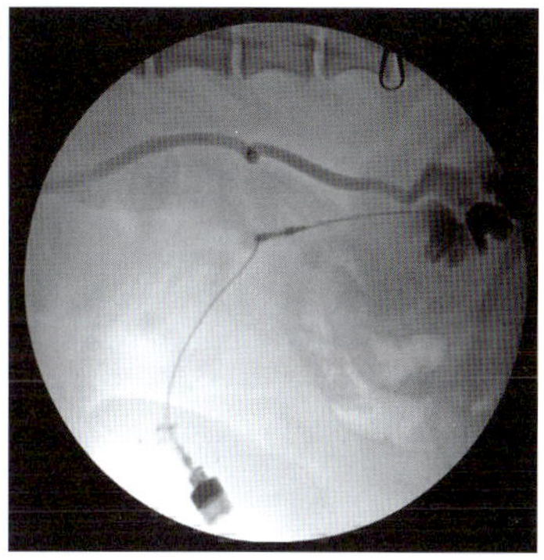

B-i)

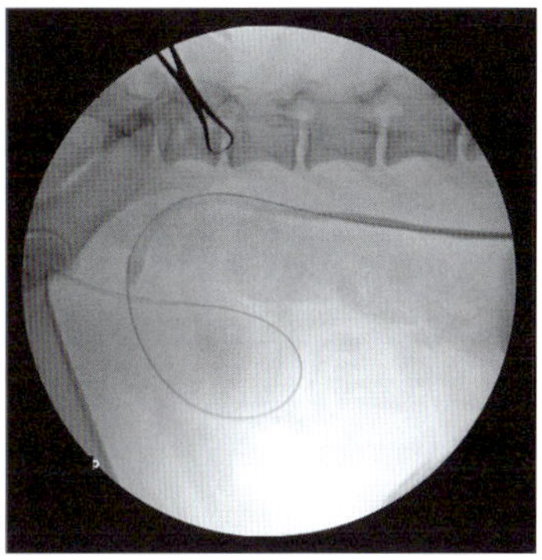

B-ii)

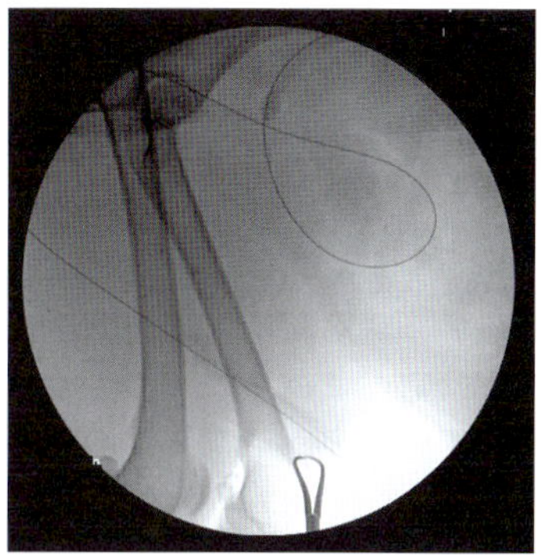

B-iii)

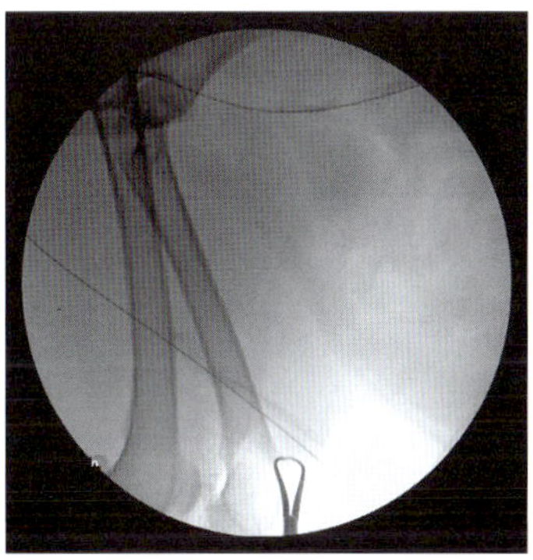

C-i)

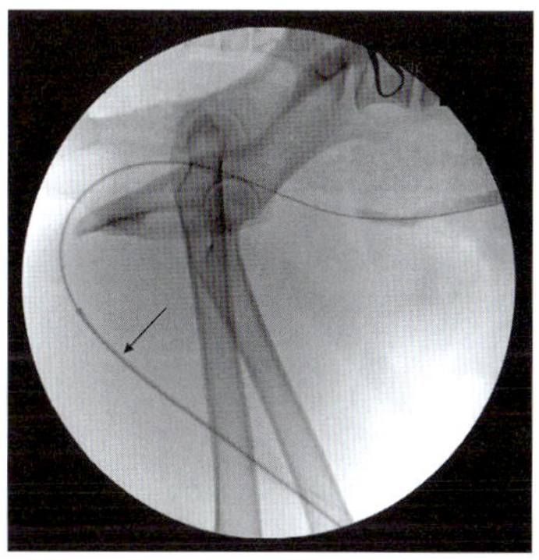

C-ii)

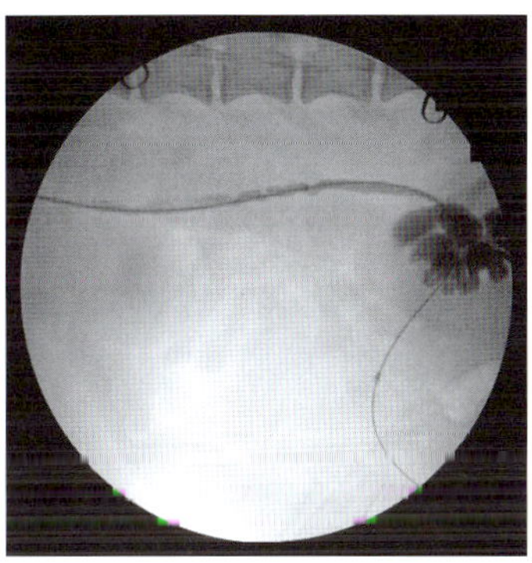

C-iii)

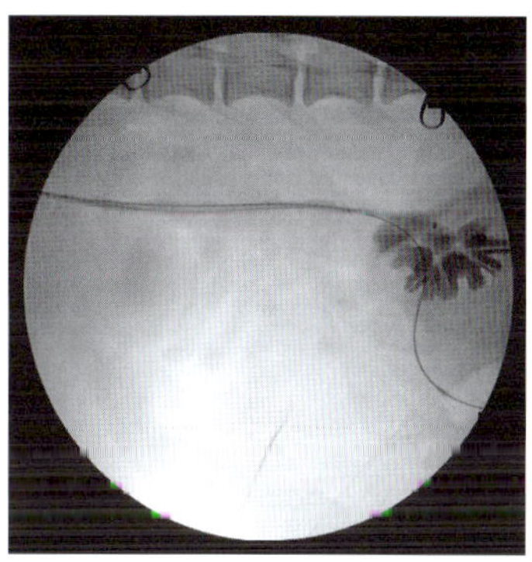

Surgical Technique – Percutaneous Ureteral Stenting in Dogs [1] (See Plate 47.2A–F) *continued*

D) A second 0.035-inch guidewire (180 cm in length) is then placed through the 6 Fr catheter into the renal pelvis. The 6 Fr sheath is removed off the through-and-through guidewire, the dilator is reintroduced into the sheath, and the combination is passed over the second guidewire (not the through-and-through guidewire) into the renal pelvis.

E) The ureteral stent length is selected based on placement of a marker catheter in the colon to account for fluoroscopic magnification. Alternatively, all medium- to giant-breed dogs will have a 6 Fr by 23-cm stent placed. This long length of stent allows for the tumor in the bladder to be bypassed to minimize the chance of neoplastic obstruction. The dilator is removed, and the ureteral stent is introduced through the 6 Fr sheath over the guidewire and into renal pelvis. The guidewire is slowly removed, allowing the cranial pigtail of the stent to curl in the renal pelvis (i, ii).

F) The 6 Fr sheath is slowly removed off the stent and used to gently push the caudal pigtail into the bladder (i–iii). After confirmation of appropriate placement, all guidewires and sheaths are removed.

G) A single simple interrupted or cruciate suture or skin glue is used to close the stab incision (not pictured).

Surgical Technique – Ureteral Stenting in Cats (Not Pictured) [1]

H) A ventral midline celiotomy is performed (see *15.1. Ventral Midline Celiotomy*) with the incision extending to the pubic brim.

I) The affected kidney is identified, and perirenal fat is dissected free from the kidney to expose the greater curvature of the kidney. The kidney is grasped and a 22-gauge over-the-needle catheter is inserted into the greater curvature of the kidney (equidistant dorsoventrally) and farther into the renal pelvis. When urine is obtained from the over-the-needle catheter, the needle is removed leaving the catheter in the renal pelvis. A T-port that had been primed with a 50–50 mixture of saline and iodinated contrast is attached to the catheter, and the renal pelvis is filled under fluoroscopic guidance to perform a nephroureterogram.

J) A 0.018-inch hydrophilic guidewire is introduced into the catheter and passed normograde down the ureter into the bladder. A stab incision is created in the bladder away from the tumor allowing the guidewire to be grasped from the bladder and passed externally (out of the bladder). Alternatively, the technique described earlier for dogs can be attempted, where the guidewire is passed out of the urethra. Steps should continue as described previously for dogs, except a 3 or 4 Fr sheath and dilator is preferred in cats.

K) The catheter is removed over the guidewire. A 0.032-inch dilator is passed normograde over the guidewire into the renal parenchyma and through the ureter until it passes through the ureterovesicular junction. The dilator is then removed, and a 2 Fr diameter ureteral stent is placed. The length of the ureter is measured from the renal pelvis to the urinary bladder to determine stent length.

L) The ureteral stent is passed over the guidewire. The cranial pigtail of the stent is located within the renal pelvis using fluoroscopic guidance. When placement is confirmed, the guidewire is removed in a normograde direction allowing the caudal pigtail to form in the bladder. The stab incision in the bladder is closed with 4-0 or 3-0 monofilament absorbable suture.

M) The linea alba, subcutaneous tissue, and skin are closed as described in *15.1. Ventral Midline Celiotomy*.

Postoperative Management

1) Multimodal analgesia
2) Elizabethan collar

Complications [1]

Intraoperative Complications

- Inability to be able to bypass the ureteral obstruction with the instrumentation (particularly the guidewire)
- Puncture of the renal pelvis, ureter, bladder, or urethra (8%)

Plate 47.2

Ureteral Stenting *continued*

D)

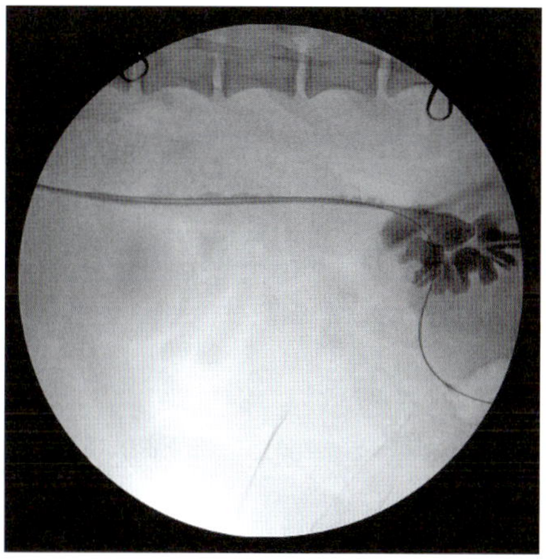

E-i)

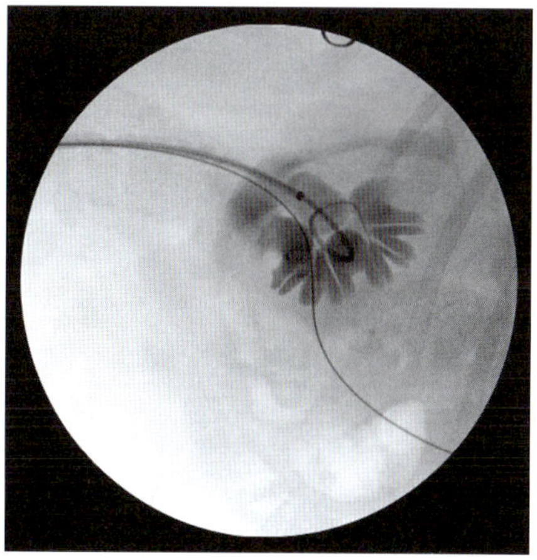

E-ii)

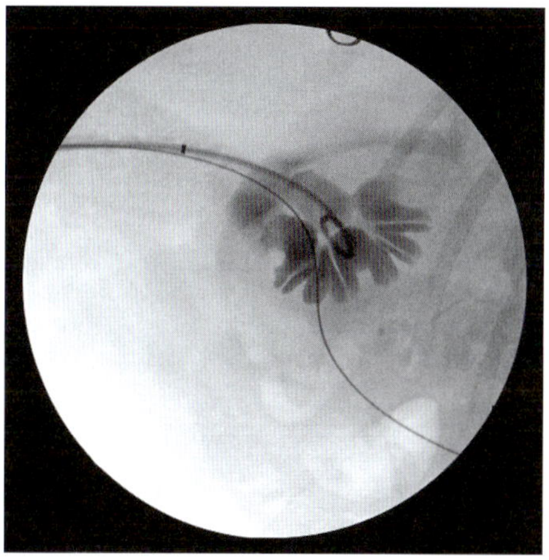

F-i)

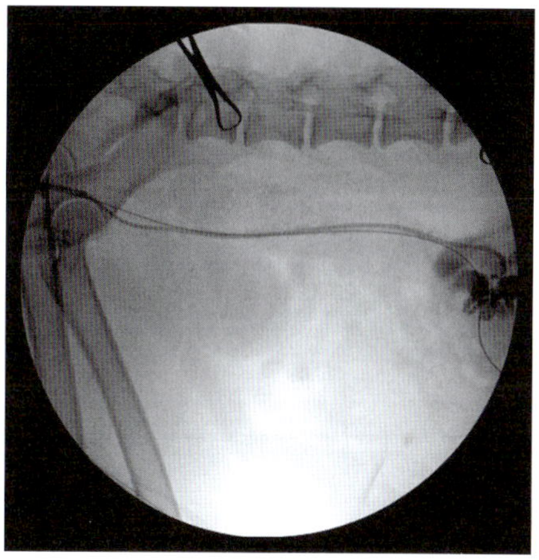

F-ii)

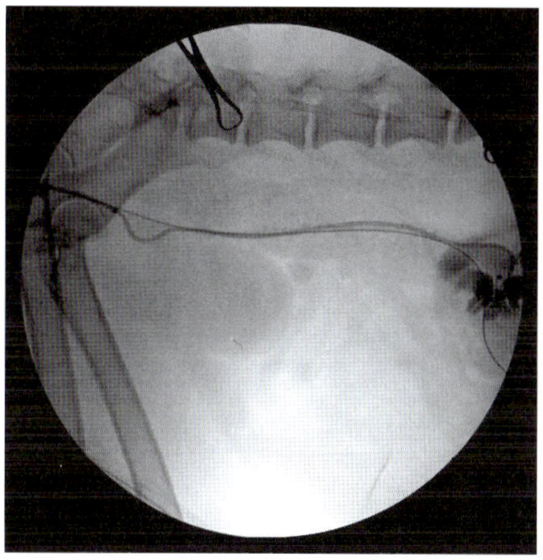

F-iii)

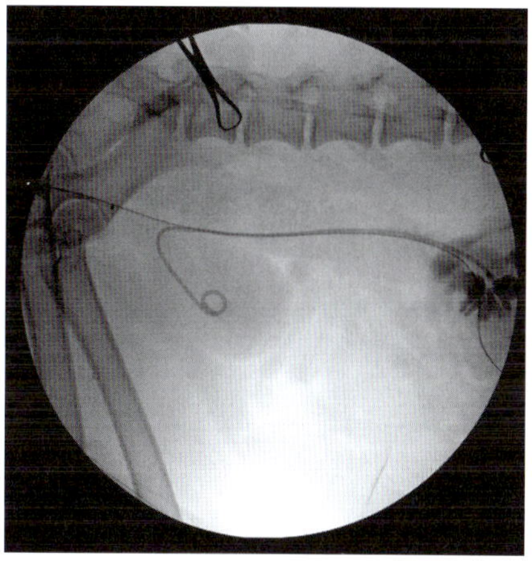

Postoperative Complications

- Ureteral stent migration
- Malignant obstruction of ureteral stent

Suggested Adjuvant Treatments

- Nonsteroidal anti-inflammatory drug [2, 3]
- ± Chemotherapy [2, 3]
- ± Intensity-modulated radiation therapy in dogs with local recurrence [4]

Prognosis and Oncologic Outcome [1]

Median survival time in one study of 12 dogs treated with ureteral stenting for palliation of neoplastic ureteral obstruction was 57 days. No dog died as a result of repeat urethral obstruction.

References

1 Berent, A.C., Weisse, C., Beal, M.W. et al. (2011). Use of indwelling, double-pigtail stents for treatment of malignant ureteral obstruction in dogs: 12 cases (2006-2009). *J. Am. Vet. Med. Assoc.* 238 (8): 1017–1025.
2 Marvel, S.J., Séguin, B., Dailey, D.D. et al. (2017). Clinical outcome of partial cystectomy for transitional cell carcinoma of the canine bladder. *Vet. Comp. Oncol.* 15 (4): 1417–1427.
3 Griffin, M.A., Culp, W.T.N., Giuffrida, M.A. et al. (2020). Lower urinary tract transitional cell carcinoma in cats: clinical findings, treatments, and outcomes in 118 cases. *J. Vet. Intern. Med.* 34 (1): 274–282.
4 Nolan, M.W., Kogan, L., Griffin, L.R. et al. (2012). Intensity-modulated and image-guided radiation therapy for treatment of genitourinary carcinomas in dogs. *J. Vet. Intern. Med.* 26 (4): 987–995.

47.3 Urethral Stenting

Indications

1) Palliative management of malignant urethral obstructions to reestablish urethral patency and urine flow
2) Urethral stenting can be combined with ureteral stenting (see *47.2. Ureteral Stenting*) in dogs and cats with concurrent ureteral obstruction

Suggested Diagnostic Workup and Clinical Staging

- Complete blood count, serum biochemistry, and urinalysis
- Urine sediment cytology
- Cadet BRAF mutation urine test
- ± Urethrocystoscopy for assessment and biopsy of the urethra and urinary bladder
- Abdominal ultrasound or precontrast and postcontrast computed tomography (CT) scan of the abdomen for assessment of location and extent of the urethral mass and intra-abdominal metastasis
- Three-view thoracic radiographs or thoracic CT scan for assessment of lung metastasis

Patient Positioning

The patient is positioned in lateral recumbency.

Surgical Technique – Urethral Stenting in Male Dogs (See Plate 47.3A–E)

A) A 4 or 5 French (Fr) marker catheter is inserted into the colon over a guidewire or inside a lubricated red rubber catheter (arrow). The marker catheter accounts for fluoroscopic magnification when determining urethral stent length and size.
B) A 0.035-inch × 180 cm guidewire is introduced into the urethra (arrow). A 6–8 Fr vascular access sheath is placed over the guidewire and sutured to the preputial skin. The dilator is then removed.
C) A 4 Fr angled catheter is introduced over the guidewire, through the sheath, and advanced into the bladder. The guidewire is removed. The bladder is filled with a 50–50 mixture of iodinated contrast agent and saline. A cystourethrogram (pictured) is performed by pulling the angled catheter out of the bladder and along the urethra under fluoroscopic guidance.
D) Measurements of the urethral diameter region of the urethra and bladder affected by the tumor are obtained. Urethral diameter is determined by measuring the height of the urethra in a region just caudal to the tumor that is not affected by the tumor. The diameter of the stent is slightly larger or the same as the measurement of normal urethral diameter, because the tumor will engage the stent interstices preventing migration. Once the diameter of the stent is determined, a stent that is approximately 1 cm longer cranially and 1 cm longer caudally than the obstructed region of the urethra is selected.

Plate 47.3

Urethral Stenting

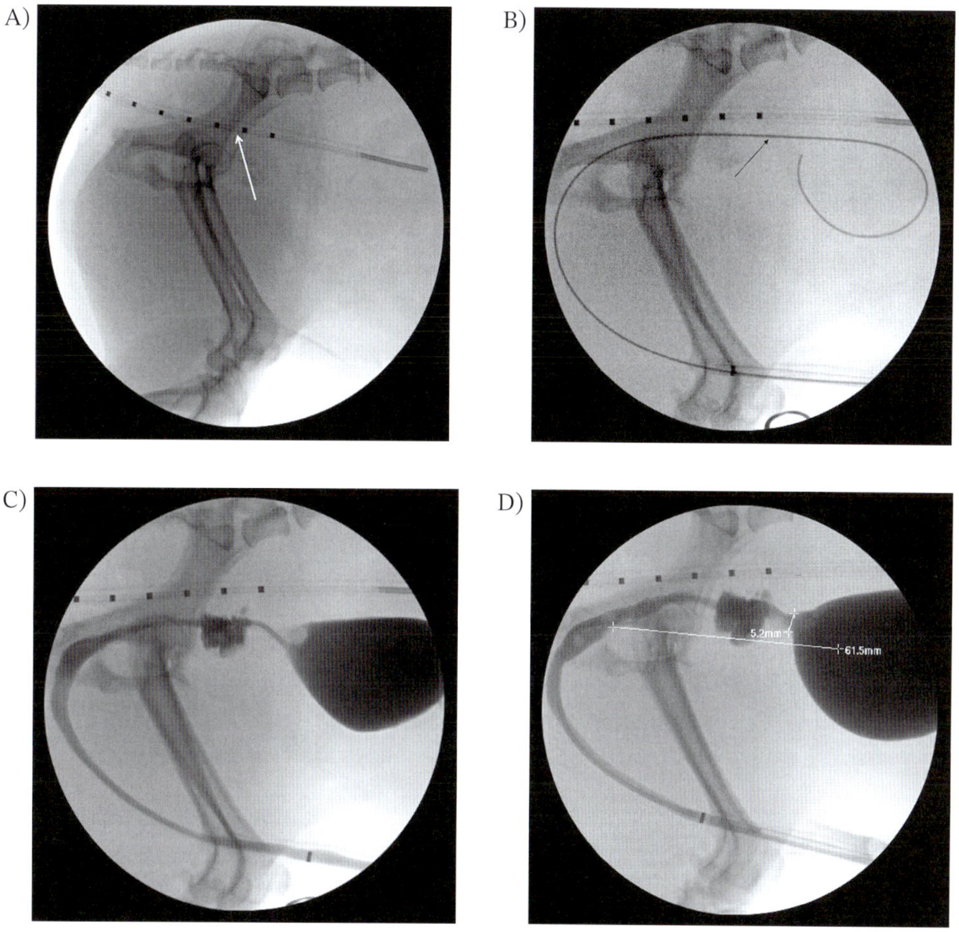

Surgical Technique – Urethral Stenting in Male Dogs (See Plate 47.3A–E) *continued*

E) The guidewire is reintroduced into the bladder through the angled catheter. The angled catheter is removed, the stent (arrow) is introduced into the bladder over the guidewire, and the stent is deployed. The delivery system is removed over the guidewire. The angled catheter is placed over the guidewire, and a contrast cystourethrogram is performed to confirm patency of the urethra (pictured). In addition, the ability to manually express the patient can be evaluated.

Surgical Technique – Female Dogs, Female Cats, and Male Cats with a Perineal Urethrostomy (See Plate 47.3F–I)

F) A 4 or 5 Fr marker catheter (arrow) is inserted into the colon over a guidewire or inside a lubricated red rubber catheter. The marker catheter accounts for fluoroscopic magnification when determining urethral stent length and size. A 0.035-inch × 180 cm long guidewire is introduced into the urethra and coiled in the bladder (dotted arrow). A 6 Fr vascular access sheath and dilator combination is placed over the guidewire and advanced into the urethra and into the bladder. The dilator is removed.

G) The bladder is filled with a 50–50 mixture of iodinated contrast agent and saline. Once complete filling of the bladder has been achieved, the sheath is slowly retracted out of the bladder and out of the urethra (over the guidewire) while injecting through the sidearm of the sheath to perform a contrast cystourethrogram. Urethral diameter is determined by measuring the height of the urethra in a region just caudal to the tumor that is not affected by the tumor. The diameter of the stent is slightly larger or the same as the measurement of normal urethral diameter, because the tumor will engage the stent interstices preventing migration. Once the diameter of the stent is determined, a stent that is approximately 1 cm longer cranially and 1 cm longer caudally than the obstructed region of urethra is selected.

H) The dilator is reintroduced into the sheath, and the sheath is advanced back into the bladder. The dilator is then removed. The stent is introduced into the bladder over the guidewire (i), and the stent is deployed (ii, iii). The stent delivery system is removed over the guidewire.

I) A contrast cystourethrogram is performed through the sheath or angled catheter to confirm patency of the urethra; in addition, the ability to manually express the patient can be evaluated.

Plate 47.3

Urethral Stenting *continued*

E)
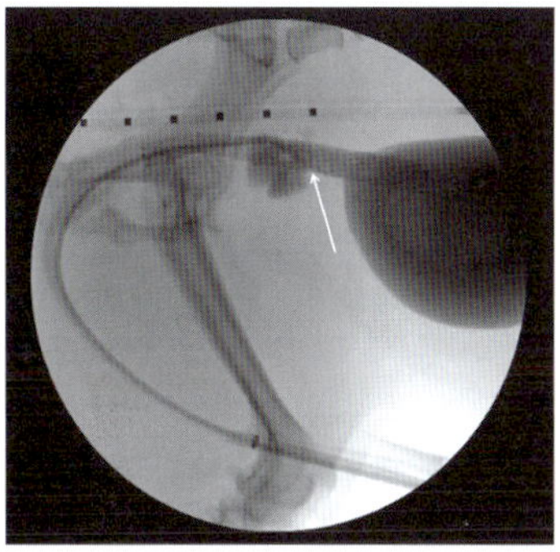

F)
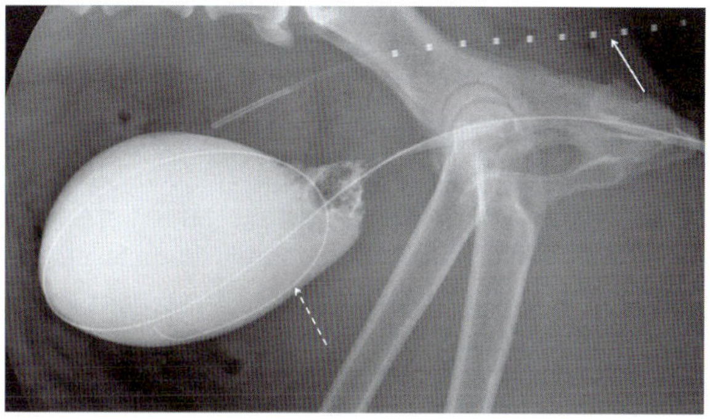

G)
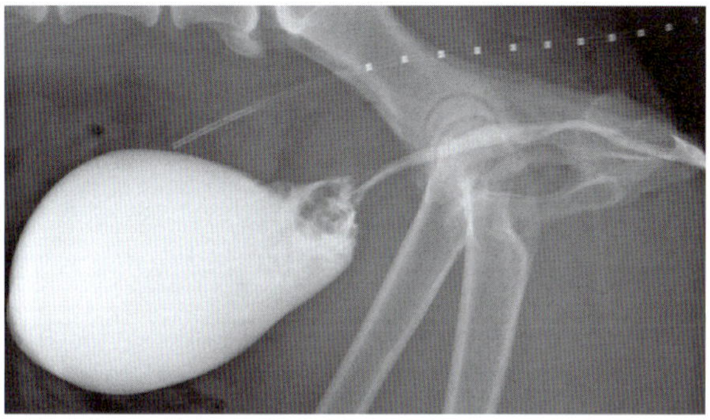

H-i)
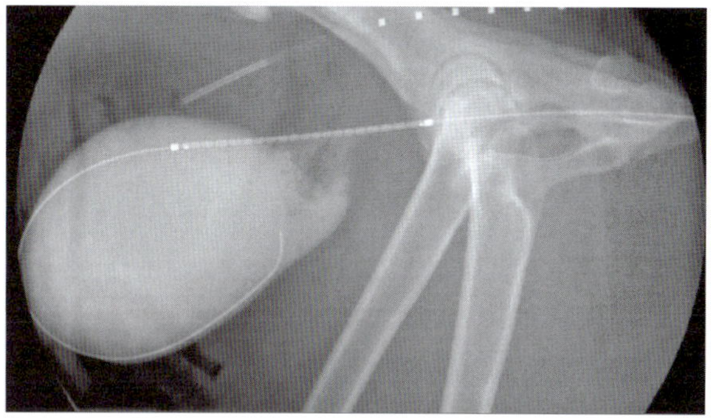

H-ii)
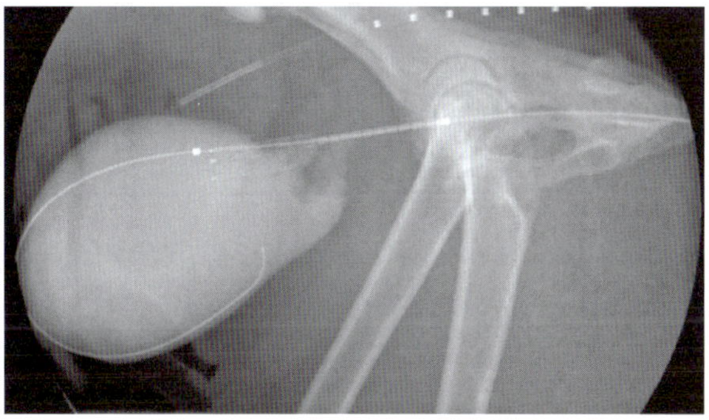

H-iii)
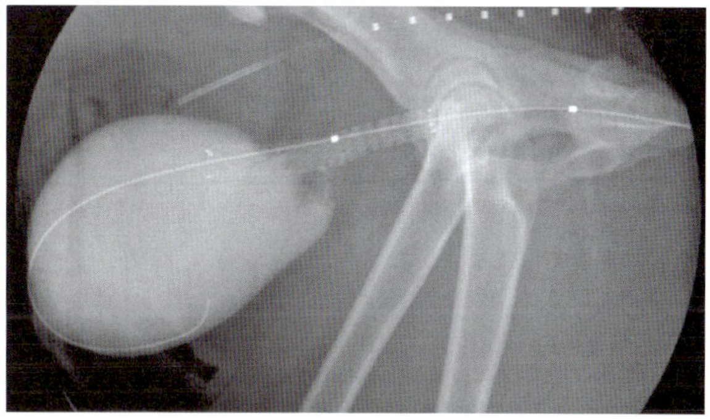

I)
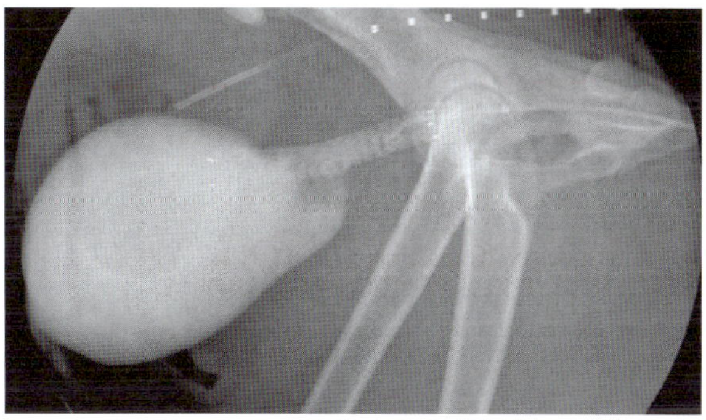

Surgical Technique – Male Cats (Not Pictured)

J) In male cats that have not previously undergone a perineal urethrostomy, the urethral opening is likely not large enough to perform a retrograde (or incisionless) urethral stenting procedure due to the size of the stent delivery system. First, a 4 or 5 Fr marker catheter is inserted into the colon over a guidewire or inside a lubricated red rubber catheter. The marker catheter accounts for fluoroscopic magnification when determining urethral stent length and size.

K) A small caudal ventral midline celiotomy is performed (see *15.1. Ventral Midline Celiotomy*) to expose the urinary bladder, and the procedure is performed in normograde fashion. A 6 Fr sheath is introduced directly into the urinary bladder, and the contrast cystourethrogram is performed directly through the sheath by injecting a 50–50 mixture of iodinated contrast agent and saline into the sidearm.

L) Urethral diameter is determined by measuring the height of the urethra in a region just caudal to the tumor that is not affected by the tumor. The diameter of the stent is slightly larger or the same as the measurement of normal urethral diameter, because the tumor will engage the stent interstices preventing migration. Once the diameter of the stent is determined, a stent that is approximately 1 cm longer cranially and 1 cm longer caudally than the obstructed region of urethra is selected.

M) The stent is introduced over the guidewire through the sheath and delivered in a normograde direction. Removal of the stent delivery system is performed over the guidewire.

N) The stab incision in the bladder is closed with 4-0 or 3-0 monofilament absorbable suture in a cruciate or simple interrupted pattern. The linea alba, subcutaneous tissue, and skin are closed as described in *15.1. Ventral Midline Celiotomy*.

Postoperative Management

1) Multimodal analgesia
2) Elizabethan collar

Complications – Dogs

Intraoperative Complications

- Unsuccessful stenting because of either extensive tumor preventing stenting or inadequate relief of obstruction (11%) [1]
- Inadequate stent length requiring second stenting (5%) [2]

Postoperative Complications

- Urinary incontinence (26%–64%) [1–3]
- Stranguria (38%–50%) [2, 3]
- Repeat obstruction (16%–22%) [1–3]
- Stent migration (2%–10%) [1–3]
- Tenesmus (7%) [2]

Complications – Cats [4]

Intraoperative Complications

- Inadequate relief of obstruction requiring second stent placement (25%)

Postoperative Complications

- Urinary tract infection (25%)

Suggested Adjuvant Treatments

- Nonsteroidal anti-inflammatory drug [2, 5]
- Chemotherapy [2, 5, 6]
- ± Intensity-modulated radiation therapy in dogs with local recurrence [7]

Prognosis and Oncologic Outcome – Dogs [1–3]

	Local Recurrence Rate	Metastatic Rate	Disease-Free Interval (d)	Median Survival Time (d)	1-Year Survival Rate	2-Year Survival Rate
Overall	–	5%%–21% [1, 2]	–	20–78 [1–3]	–	–
Neoadjuvant and adjuvant treatment [2]						
Neoadjuvant NSAID for minimum of 4 wk and adjuvant chemotherapy	–	–	–	251	–	–
No neoadjuvant or adjuvant treatment	–	–	–	43	–	–
Neoadjuvant NSAID only	–	–	–	70	–	–
Adjuvant chemotherapy only	–	–	–	90	–	–

NSAID, Nonsteroidal anti-inflammatory drug.

Prognosis and Oncologic Outcome – Cats

Median survival time for eight cats with urethral stenting for obstructive diseases other than urethral uroliths was not reached. Outcomes were subjectively assessed as excellent in three cats, good in one cat, fair in two cats, and poor in two cats [4].

References

1 McMillan, S.K., Knapp, D.W., Ramos-Vara, J.A. et al. (2012). Outcome of urethral stent placement for management of urethral obstruction secondary to transitional cell carcinoma in dogs: 19 cases (2007-2010). *J. Am. Vet. Med. Assoc.* 241 (12): 1627–1632.

2 Blackburn, A.L., Berent, A.C., Weisse, C.W. et al. (2013). Evaluation of outcome following urethral stent placement for the treatment of obstructive carcinoma of the urethra in dogs: 42 cases (2004-2008). *J. Am. Vet. Med. Assoc.* 242 (1): 59–68.

3 Weisse, C., Berent, A., Todd, K. et al. (2006). Evaluation of palliative stenting for management of malignant urethral obstructions in dogs. *J. Am. Vet. Med. Assoc.* 229 (2): 226–234.

4 Brace, M.A., Weisse, C., and Berent, A. (2014). Preliminary experience with stenting for management of non-urolith urethral obstruction in eight cats. *Vet. Surg.* 43 (2): 199–208.

5 Marvel, S.J., Séguin, B., Dailey, D.D. et al. (2017). Clinical outcome of partial cystectomy for transitional cell carcinoma of the canine bladder. *Vet. Comp. Oncol.* 15 (4): 1417–1427.

6 Griffin, M.A., Culp, W.T.N., Giuffrida, M.A. et al. (2020). Lower urinary tract transitional cell carcinoma in cats: clinical findings, treatments, and outcomes in 118 cases. *J. Vet. Intern. Med.* 34 (1): 274–282.

7 Nolan, M.W., Kogan, L., Griffin, L.R. et al. (2012). Intensity-modulated and image-guided radiation therapy for treatment of genitourinary carcinomas in dogs. *J. Vet. Intern. Med.* 26 (4): 987–995.

47.4 Colorectal Stenting

Indication

1) Palliative management of malignant colonic obstruction when owners do not elect surgery or surgery is not indicated

Suggested Diagnostic Workup and Clinical Staging

- Complete blood count, serum biochemistry, and urinalysis
- ± Colonoscopy
- Abdominal ultrasound or precontrast and postcontrast computed tomography (CT) scan of the abdomen for assessment of location and extent of the urethral mass and intra-abdominal metastasis
- ± Ultrasound- or CT-guided fine-needle aspirate cytology
- Three-view thoracic radiographs or thoracic CT scan for assessment of lung metastasis

Patient Positioning

The patient is positioned in lateral recumbency.

Surgical Technique (See Plate 47.4A–E)

A) A colonoscopy is performed to confirm the location and extent of the mass and to assist in stent sizing.
B) A 4 or 5 French (Fr) marker catheter is placed in the colon adjacent to the colonoscope (arrow). The colonoscope is positioned 1–2 cm cranial to the obstructed region, and a fluoroscopic image is obtained (with marker catheter included in the image). The colonoscope is then retracted caudally until it is positioned 1–2 cm caudal to the mass; an additional fluoroscopic image is obtained. A stent is chosen that is at least 1 cm longer cranially and 1 cm longer caudally than the obstructed region. The diameter of the colon is challenging to measure because this organ is highly distensible. In general, a 20- to 30-mm-diameter colonic stent is acceptable in most patients.
C) Once the stent size has been selected, a 0.035-inch hydrophilic guidewire is advanced into the colon and cranial to the mass under fluoroscopic guidance. The stent is introduced over the guidewire into the colon (arrow). The marker catheter and colonoscope are subsequently removed.
D) The stent is deployed using fluoroscopic guidance.
E) Positioning of the stent and opening of the obstructed region are confirmed with colonoscopy.

Color Atlas of Canine and Feline Surgical Oncology, First Edition. Julius M. Liptak, Paolo Buracco, William T. N. Culp, and Nicholas J. Bacon.

Plate 47.4

Colorectal Stenting

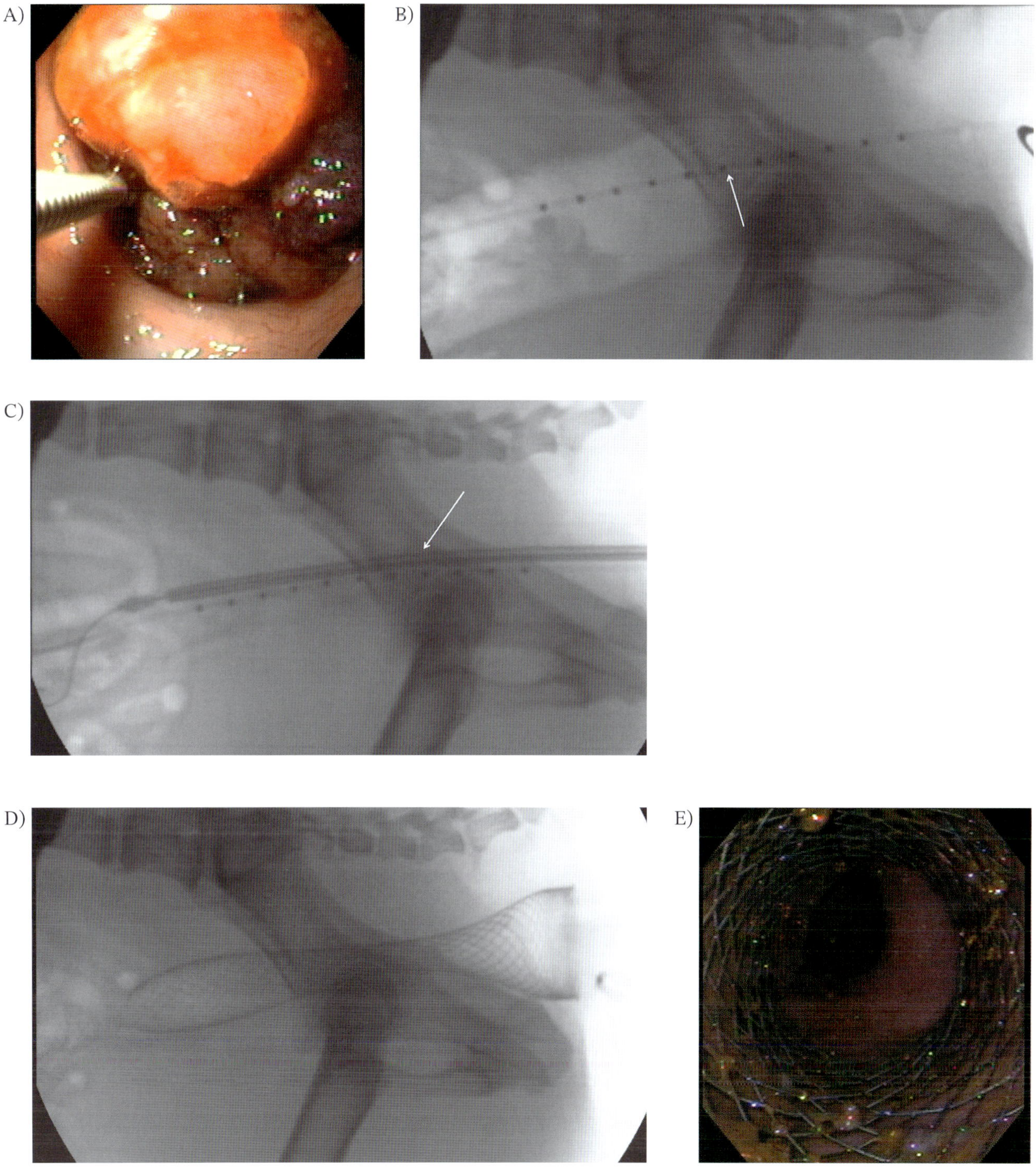

Postoperative Management

1) Multimodal analgesia

Complications

Intraoperative Complications

- Stent deployment partially outside of the anus; if a small amount of external deployment occurs, most stents can be manually pushed cranially so that the length of the stent outside the anus is pushed internally

Postoperative Complications

- Tenesmus
- Obstipation

Suggested Adjuvant Treatments

- Nonsteroidal anti-inflammatory drug
- ± Chemotherapy

Prognosis and Oncologic Outcome

Colonic stenting has been reported in two cats and one dog [1, 2]. Clinical signs improved in all animals. Both cats remained clinically improved at the time of euthanasia at 19 days (for pleural effusion secondary to carcinomatosis) and 274 days (for multiple distant metastases) [1, 2]. Clinical signs improved in the dog, but the dog was euthanized at 238 days because of recurrent obstipation [1].

References

1 Culp, W.T., Macphail, C.M., Perry, J.A. et al. (2011). Use of a nitinol stent to palliate a colorectal neoplastic obstruction in a dog. *J. Am. Med. Vet. Assoc.* 239 (2): 222–227.
2 Hume, D.Z., Solomon, J.A., and Weisse, C.W. (2006). Palliative use of a stent for colonic obstruction caused by adenocarcinoma in two cats. *J. Am. Med. Vet. Assoc.* 228 (3): 392–396.

Chapter 48: Embolization

48.1 Nasal Embolization

Indication

1) Palliative management of sinonasal tumors when owners decline radiation therapy; although not defined, nasal embolization is likely not indicated for patients with tumor penetration through the cribriform plate

Suggested Diagnostic Workup and Clinical Staging

- Complete blood count, serum biochemistry, and urinalysis
- Blind or rhinoscopic biopsy
- ± Regional lymph node fine-needle aspirate cytology
- Precontrast and postcontrast of the head and neck
- Three-view thoracic radiographs or thoracic computed tomography scan for assessment of lung metastasis

Patient Positioning

The patient is positioned in dorsal recumbency until selection of the maxillary artery, then the head of the patient is moved into lateral recumbency.

Procedural Technique (See Plate 48.1A–F)

A) The patient is placed in dorsal recumbency. The femoral artery is digitally palpated through the skin, and a 1- to 2-cm skin incision is made over the femoral artery (pictured). The subcutaneous tissue is dissected until the femoral artery is exposed. The fascia surrounding the femoral artery is dissected away allowing clear visualization. Two monofilament absorbable sutures are placed around the femoral artery. An 18-gauge over-the-needle catheter is introduced into the femoral artery and the needle is removed. A 0.035-inch and 180-cm-long guidewire is introduced into the femoral artery through the catheter. A 4–6 French vascular access sheath and dilator are introduced into the femoral artery over the guidewire. The dilator is then removed over the guidewire, and the guidewire is passed from the femoral artery through the external iliac artery to the abdominal aorta.

B) The guidewire is then passed cranially through the aorta to select the brachiocephalic trunk (BT). Once in the BT, the common carotid (CC) artery is selected.

C) A 4 French angled catheter is then placed into the vascular access sheath over the guidewire. Using the guidewire and angled catheter combination, the external carotid (EC) artery is selected. The guidewire is then removed from the vascular access sheath. A 50–50 iodinated contrast agent and saline mixture is drawn into a syringe, attached to the angled catheter, and injected under fluoroscopic guidance to visualize the vasculature of the nasal cavity (i). A microwire and microcatheter combination is then passed through the angled catheter into the maxillary (M) artery (ii).

Color Atlas of Canine and Feline Surgical Oncology, First Edition. Julius M. Liptak, Paolo Buracco, William T. N. Culp, and Nicholas J. Bacon.

Plate 48.1

Nasal Embolization

A)

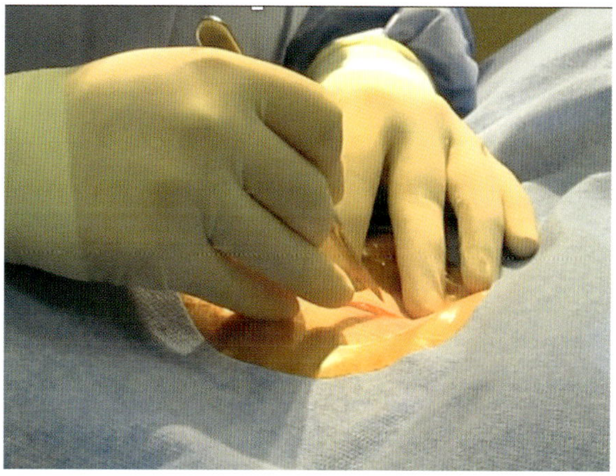

B)

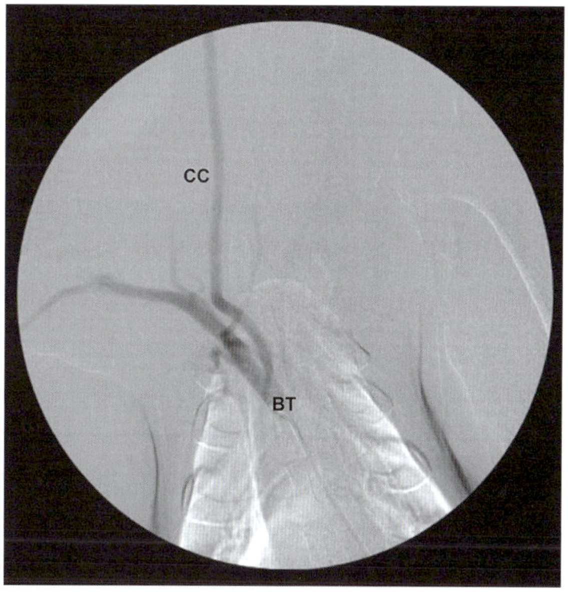

C-i)

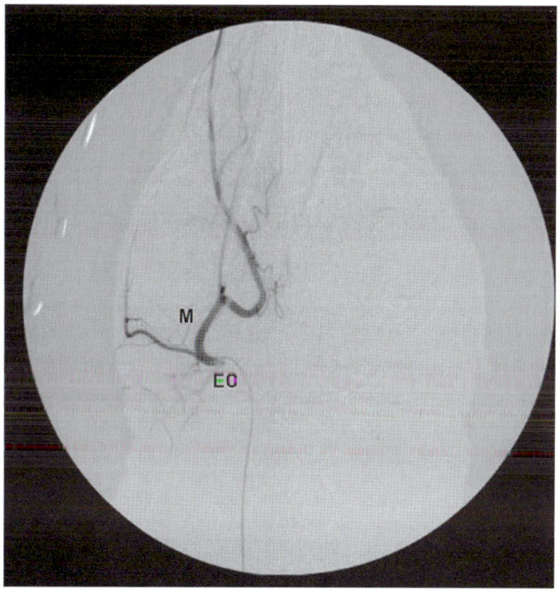

C-ii)

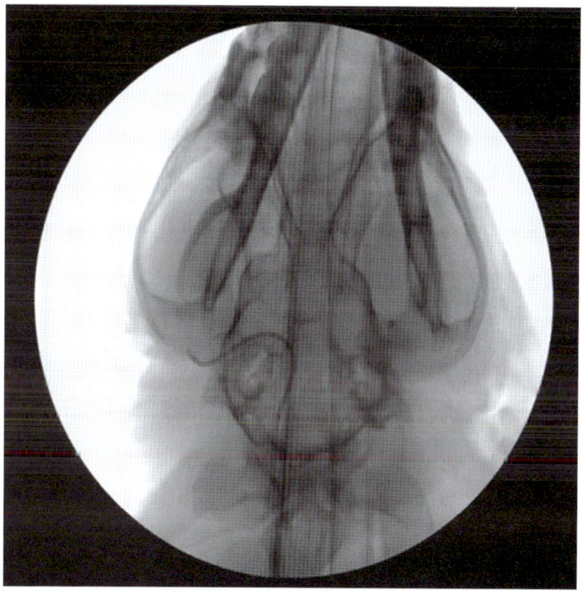

Procedural Technique (See Plate 48.1A–F) *continued*

D) The head of the patient is then rotated into lateral recumbency. An angiogram is performed. The infraorbital (I), sphenopalatine (SP), and major palatine (MP) arteries are identified (M, maxillary artery).
E) The microwire and microcatheter combination are used to select the sphenopalatine (SP) artery, and an arteriogram is performed to delineate the vascular supply to the nasal tumor (dashed line). A slurry of iodinated contrast agent, saline, and embolic agent is made and injected slowly under fluoroscopic guidance. The slurry is injected in short bursts, and the flow of the slurry through the vessel being embolized is monitored closely to prevent retrograde flow.
F) When cessation of blood flow is achieved, the injection is discontinued. Selective and nonselective arteriography is then performed to assess the efficacy of the procedure. In addition, arteriography is performed to ensure patency of the external ophthalmic artery and mandibular arteries (SP, sphenopalatine artery).
G) On completion of the arteriogram, the catheters are removed over a guidewire. The vascular access sheath is then removed from the femoral artery, and the artery is ligated (using previously placed encircling suture) or repaired. The subcutaneous tissue and skin are closed in a simple continuous pattern using 4-0 or 3-0 monofilament absorbable suture (SP, sphenopalatine artery).

Postoperative Management

1) Multimodal analgesia
2) Elizabethan collar

Complications

Intraoperative Complications

- Inability to select desired blood vessel
- Nontarget embolization
- Bleeding from the femoral artery

Postoperative Complications (0–14 Days)

- Tumor expulsion from nares

Postoperative Complications (>14 Days)

- Tumor abscessation
- Nasal cavity infection

Suggested Adjuvant Treatments

- ± Nonsteroidal anti-inflammatory drug
- ± Chemotherapy

Plate 48.1

Nasal Embolization *continued*

D)

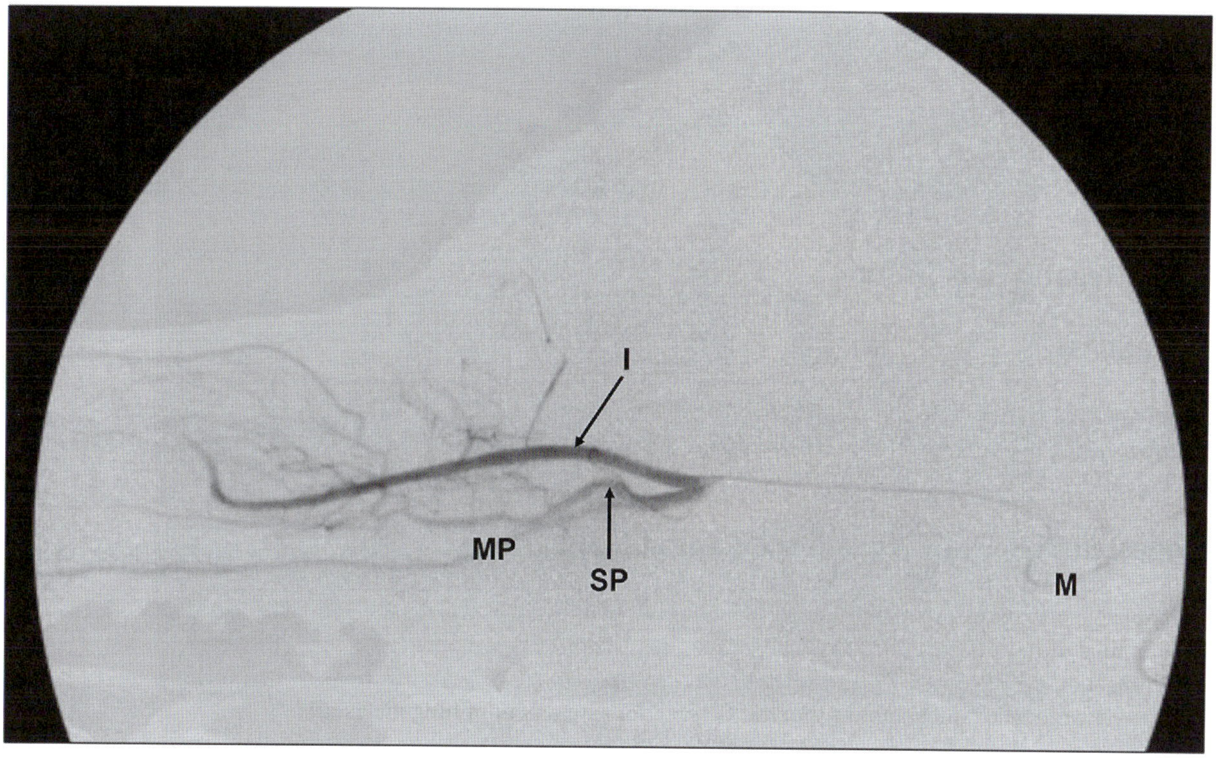

E)

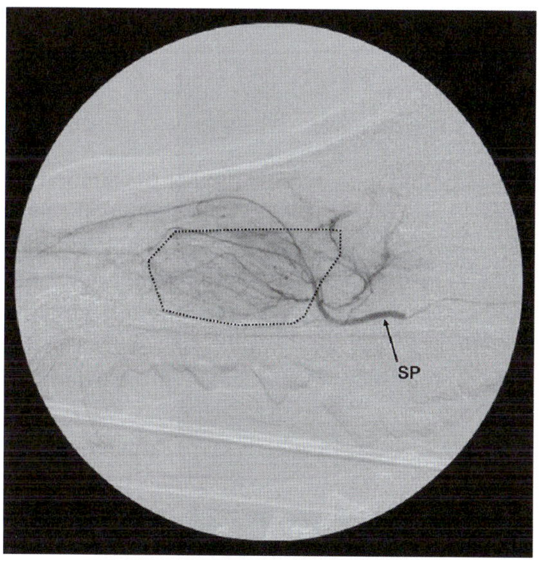

F)

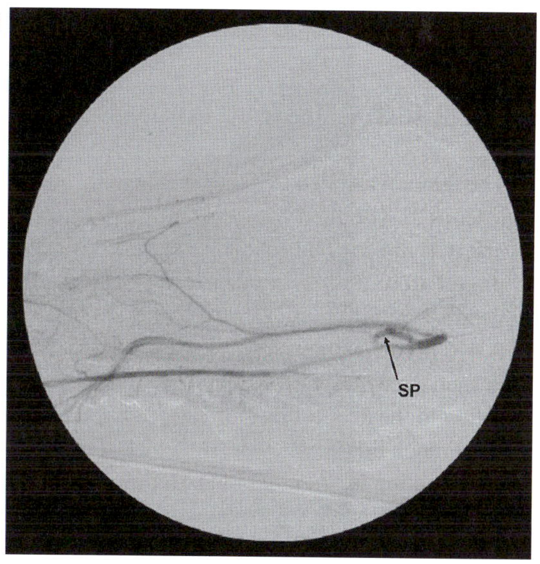

Surgical Technique (See Plate 48.2A–D) *continued*

C) A 50–50 mixture of iodinated contrast agent and saline is drawn into a syringe, attached to the hook catheter, and injected under fluoroscopic guidance into the hepatic artery to visualize both the normal blood supply and blood supply to the tumor (i, dashed line). A microwire–microcatheter combination is introduced into the hook catheter and used to select the tumoral (T) blood supply (ii). An iodinated contrast agent, saline, and embolic agent is made and injected slowly under fluoroscopic guidance. The slurry is injected in short bursts, and the flow of the slurry through the vessel being embolized is monitored closely to prevent retrograde flow. Alternatives to the above slurry can also be considered. Lipiodol can be used as both a contrast agent and an embolic agent for hepatic embolization. As an alternative to bland embolization, chemoembolization can be performed with the addition of chemotherapy to the slurry or in a drug-eluting bead form.
D) When cessation of blood flow is achieved, the injection is discontinued. An arteriogram is performed to determine whether another tumoral blood supply exists and can be treated. It is imperative not to perform the arteriogram through any catheters that have previously contained embolic agents unless those catheters have been cleared of those agents. Arteriography is performed to ensure patency of the main hepatic (H), celiac (C), and gastroduodenal (GD) arteries. On completion of the arteriogram, the instruments are removed from the vascular access sheath. The vascular access sheath is then removed from the femoral artery, and the artery is either ligated or repaired.
E) The incision is closed in two layers with a simple continuous suture pattern using monofilament absorbable suture material in the subcutis and either an interrupted or continuous suture pattern using monofilament nonabsorbable suture material in the skin.

Postoperative Management

1) Multimodal analgesia
2) Elizabethan collar

Complications

Intraoperative Complications

- Inability to select desired blood vessel
- Nontarget embolization
- Bleeding from the femoral artery

Postoperative Complications (0–14 Days)

- Embolization syndrome
- Mass rupture

Postoperative Complications (>14 Days)

- Tumor abscessation

Suggested Adjuvant Treatments

- ± Chemotherapy
- ± Intensity-modulated radiation therapy in dogs with local recurrence or progressive disease

Plate 48.2

Hepatic Embolization *continued*

C-i)

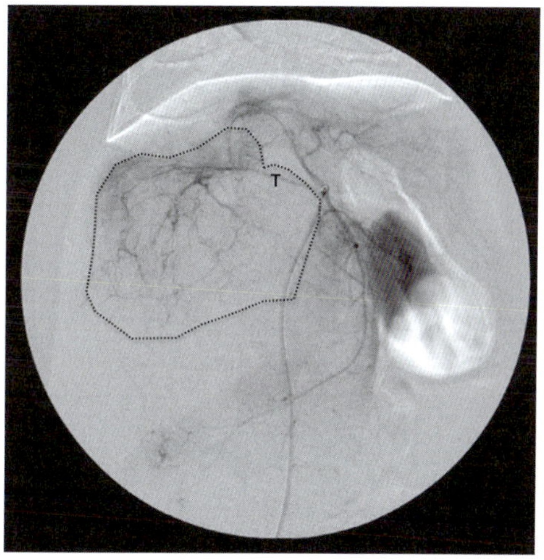

C-ii)

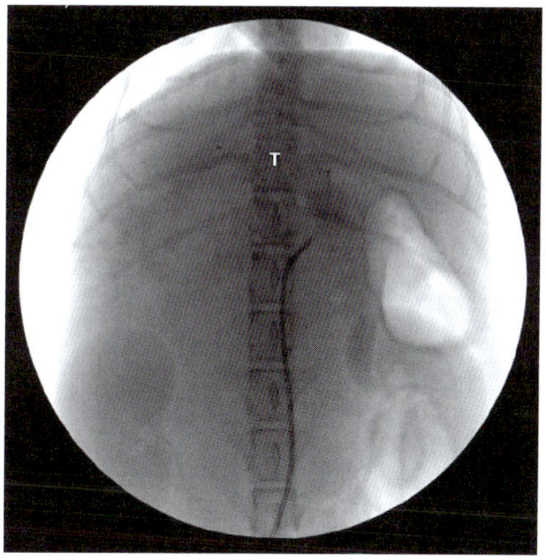

D)

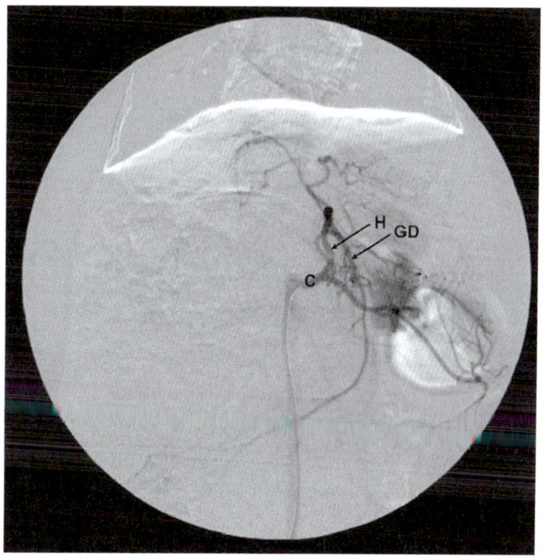

Prognosis and Oncologic Outcome

Liver embolization or chemoembolization has been described in four dogs and one cat [1–3]. Clinical improvement ± stable disease was documented in all four dogs, but progressive disease was noted by 3 months [1, 2]. In the cat, a partial response was noted at 71 days, and liver lobectomy of the down-staged tumor was performed 231 days after embolization [3].

References

1 Cave, T.A., Johnson, V., Beths, T. et al. (2003). Treatment of unresectable hepatocellular adenoma in dogs with transarterial iodized oil and chemotherapy with and without an embolic agent: a report of two cases. *Vet. Comp. Oncol.* 1 (4): 191–199.

2 Weisse, C., Clifford, C.A., Holt, D. et al. (2002). Percutaneous arterial embolization and chemoembolization for treatment of benign and malignant tumors in three dogs and a goat. *J. Am. Vet. Med. Assoc.* 221 (10): 1430–1436.

3 Iwai, S., Okano, S., Chikazawa, S. et al. (2015). Transcatheter arterial embolization for treatment of hepatocellular carcinoma in a cat. *J. Am. Vet. Med. Assoc.* 247 (11): 1299–1302.

48.3 Prostatic Embolization

Indications

1) Curative-intent treatment of benign and nonmetastatic malignant prostatic tumors
2) Palliative management of metastatic malignant prostatic tumors

Suggested Diagnostic Workup and Clinical Staging

- Complete blood count, serum biochemistry, and urinalysis
- Urine sediment cytology
- Cadet BRAF mutation urine test
- ± Urethrocystoscopy for assessment and biopsy of the urethra and urinary bladder
- Abdominal ultrasound or precontrast and postcontrast computed tomography (CT) scan of the abdomen for assessment of location and extent of the urethral mass and intra-abdominal metastasis
- Three-view thoracic radiographs or thoracic CT scan for assessment of lung metastasis

Patient Positioning

The dog is positioned in dorsal recumbency until selection of the internal iliac artery; then the pelvis of the dog is positioned into lateral recumbency.

Surgical Technique [1] (See Plate 48.3A–E)

A) A 1- to 2-cm skin incision (pictured) is made lateral to the cervical midline, approximately halfway between the trachea and jugular vein. The subcutaneous tissue is dissected until the carotid artery is exposed. The fascia surrounding the carotid artery is dissected away allowing clear visualization. Two monofilament absorbable sutures are placed around the carotid artery.
B) An 18-gauge over-the-needle catheter is introduced into the carotid artery (i) and the needle is removed. A 0.035-inch and 180-cm-long guidewire is introduced into the carotid artery through the catheter (ii). A 4–6 French (Fr) vascular access sheath and dilator are introduced into the carotid artery over the guidewire (iii). The dilator is then removed over the guidewire, and the guidewire is passed from the carotid artery to the distal aorta.

Color Atlas of Canine and Feline Surgical Oncology, First Edition. Julius M. Liptak, Paolo Buracco, William T. N. Culp, and Nicholas J. Bacon.

Plate 48.3

Prostatic Embolization

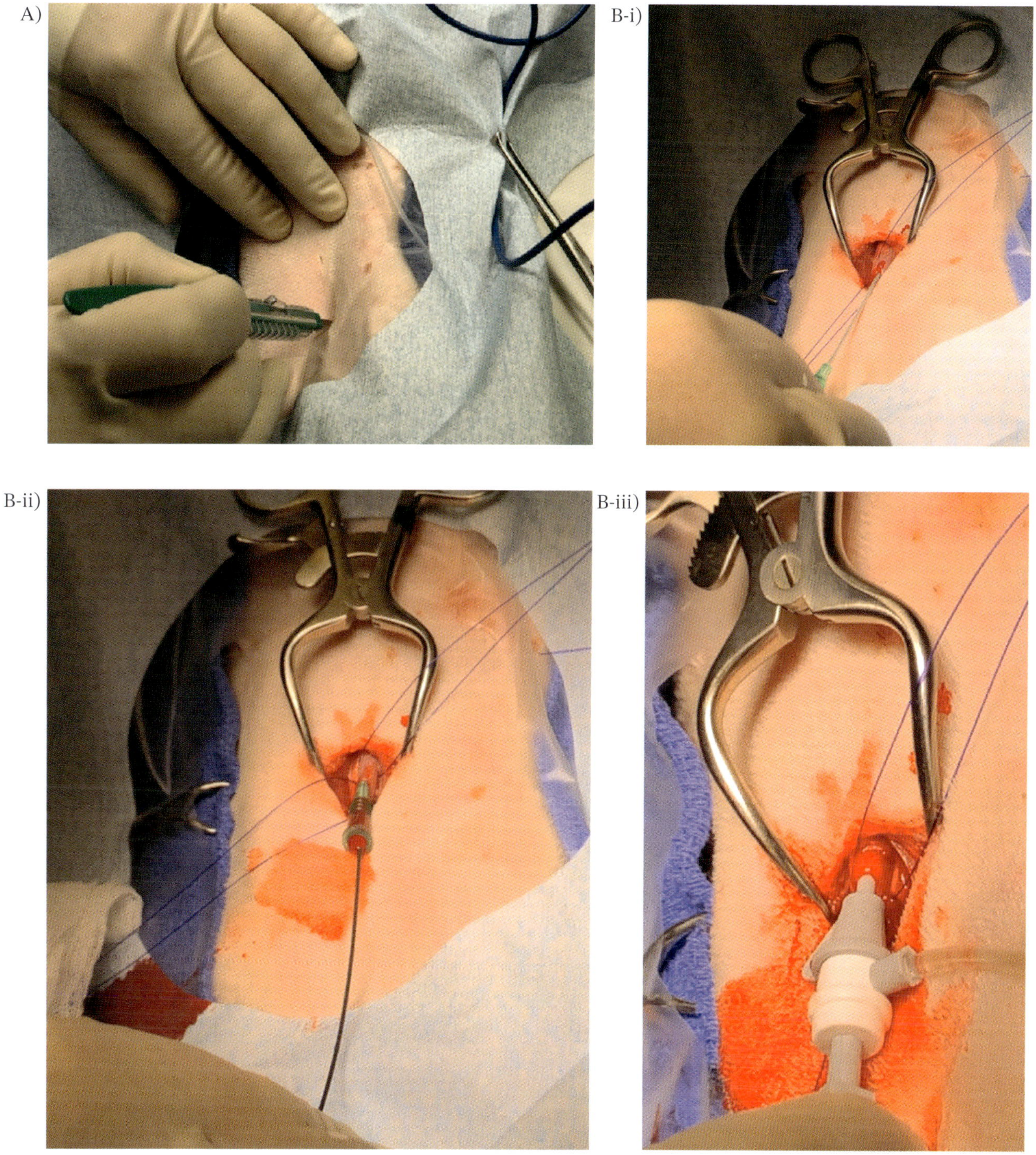

Surgical Technique [1] (See Plate 48.3A–E) *continued*

C) A 4 Fr angled catheter is then placed into the vascular access sheath over the guidewire, and an arteriogram at the level of the trifurcation of the aorta (A) is performed. A 50–50 mixture of iodinated contrast agent and saline is drawn into a syringe, attached to the angled catheter, and injected under fluoroscopic guidance to visualize the normal blood supply and blood supply to the tumor (dashed line). The goal of prostatic embolization is to treat the prostatic arterial supply bilaterally, so one internal iliac (II) artery is selected initially.
D) Once the angled catheter is in the internal iliac (II) artery, the pelvis is rotated into lateral recumbency. A microwire–microcatheter combination is introduced into the angled catheter and used to select the internal pudendal (IN) artery, then prostatic (P) artery, and finally, the specific tumoral (T) blood supply. Once the blood supply to the tumor (dashed line) has been confirmed (and the blood supply to the bladder can be avoided), a slurry of iodinated contrast agent, saline, and embolic agent is made and injected slowly under fluoroscopic guidance. The slurry is injected in short bursts, and the flow of the slurry through the vessel being embolized is monitored closely to prevent retrograde flow.
E) When cessation of blood flow is achieved, the injection is discontinued. An arteriogram is performed to determine whether another tumoral blood supply exists and can be treated. It is imperative not to perform the arteriogram through any catheters that have previously contained embolic agents unless those catheters have been cleared of those agents.
F) The procedure is repeated on the contralateral side. At the completion of the procedure, arteriography is performed to ensure complete stasis of blood flow to the prostate. On completion of the arteriogram, the instruments are removed from the vascular access sheath. The vascular access sheath is then removed from the carotid artery, and the artery is either ligated or repaired.
G) The incision is closed in two layers with a simple continuous suture pattern using monofilament absorbable suture material in the subcutis and either an interrupted or continuous suture pattern using monofilament nonabsorbable suture material in the skin.

Postoperative Management

1) Multimodal analgesia
2) Elizabethan collar

Complications – Dogs [1]

Intraoperative Complications

- Inability to select desired blood vessel
- Nontarget embolization
- Bleeding from the carotid artery

Suggested Adjuvant Treatments

- Nonsteroidal anti-inflammatory drugs [2]
- Chemotherapy [2, 3]
- ± Radiation therapy or intensity-modulated radiation therapy [4]

Plate 48.3

Prostatic Embolization *continued*

C)

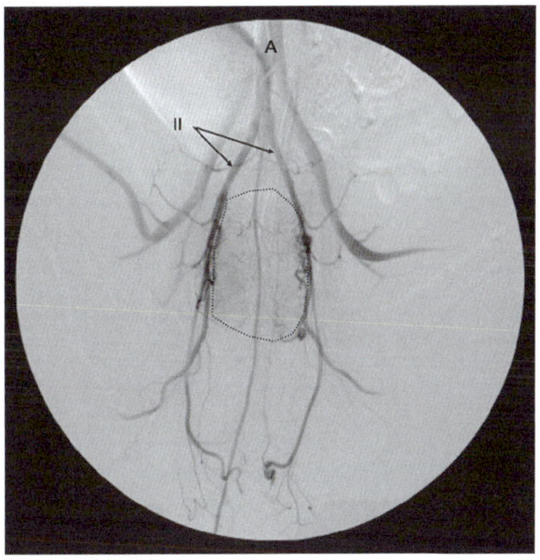

D)

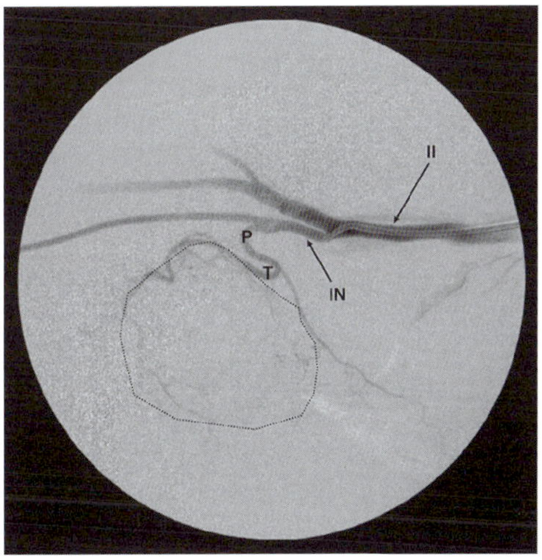

E)

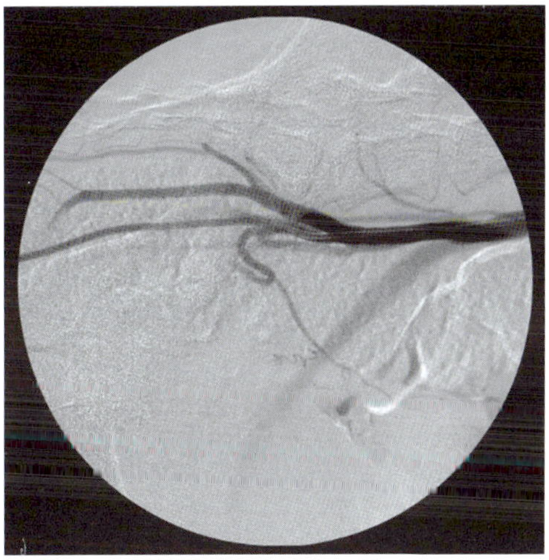

Prognosis and Oncologic Outcome [1]

- Significant reduction in stranguria (from 50% to 5%)
- Significant reduction in tenesmus (from 45% to 20%)
- Significant reduction in prostatic volume (from 21.7 to 14.8 cm^3) with median decrease in prostatic volume of 39%

References

1 Culp, W.T.N., Johnson, E.G., Giuffrida, M.A. et al. (2021). Procedural description and prospective evaluation of short-term outcome for the use of prostatic artery embolization in dogs with carcinoma of the prostate. *J. Am. Vet. Med. Assoc.* 259 (10): 1154–1162.

2 Ravicini, S., Baines, S.J., Taylor, A. et al. (2018). Outcome and prognostic factors in medically treated canine prostatic carcinomas: a multi-institutional study. *Vet. Comp. Oncol.* 16 (4): 450–458.

3 Clerc-Renaud, B., Gieger, T.L., Larue, S.M. et al. (2021). Treatment of genitourinary carcinoma in dogs using nonsteroidal anti-inflammatory drugs, mitoxantrone, and radiation therapy: a retrospective study. *J. Vet. Intern. Med.* 35 (2): 1052–1061.

4 Walz, J.Z., Desai, N., Van Asselt, N. et al. (2020). Definitive-intent intensity-modulated radiation therapy for treatment of canine prostatic carcinoma: a multi-institutional retrospective study. *Vet. Comp. Oncol.* 18 (3): 381–388.

Chapter 49: Pleural Port Placement

Indication

1) Drainage of fluid or air from the pleural space fluid or for the intracavitary administration of chemotherapy.

Patient Positioning

The patient is positioned in lateral recumbency with the affected side uppermost. An oblique positioning to the thorax with the dorsal aspect higher than the ventral aspect improves visualization of the thoracic cavity with fluoroscopy. The surgeon is positioned on the ventral side of the patient, and the monitor is across the table on the dorsum of the patient.

The intrathoracic catheter can be inserted through either a percutaneous approach or via either a mini-thoracotomy or thoracoscopic approach.

Surgical Technique – Percutaneous Intrathoracic Catheter Placement (See Plate 49A–D)

A) The ninth intercostal rib space is identified, and a stab incision is made at the ventral third of the thorax. An 18-gauge over-the-needle catheter is passed into the thorax (pictured).
B) An 0.035-inch × 150 cm hydrophilic guidewire is passed through the catheter and into the thorax (i). The wire is passed from the ipsilateral hemithorax, caudal to the heart, and into the contralateral hemithorax, which can be confirmed with fluoroscopy (ii).
C) A 9 French dilator and peel-away sheath are passed over the guidewire and into the thorax (i, ii). After confirming that the sheath has passed into the contralateral thorax, the dilator is withdrawn.
D) The 9 French intrathoracic catheter is passed through the introducer sheath, over the guidewire, and into the contralateral hemithorax while coursing through the ipsilateral hemithorax (i). Positioning is confirmed with fluoroscopy (ii).
E) The guidewire and peel-away sheath are withdrawn.

Color Atlas of Canine and Feline Surgical Oncology, First Edition. Julius M. Liptak, Paolo Buracco, William T. N. Culp, and Nicholas J. Bacon.

Plate 49

Pleural Port Placement

A)

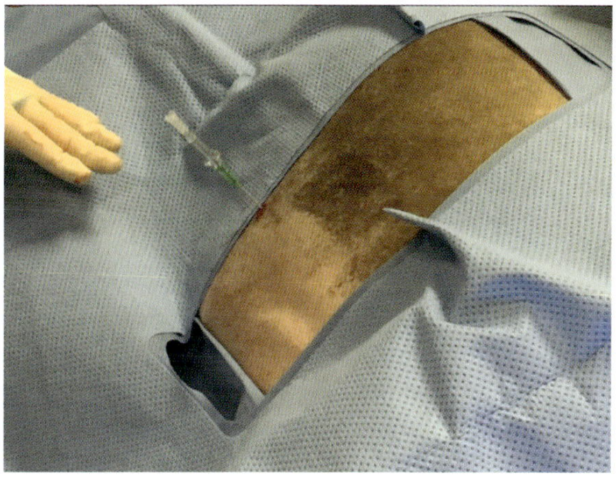

B-i)

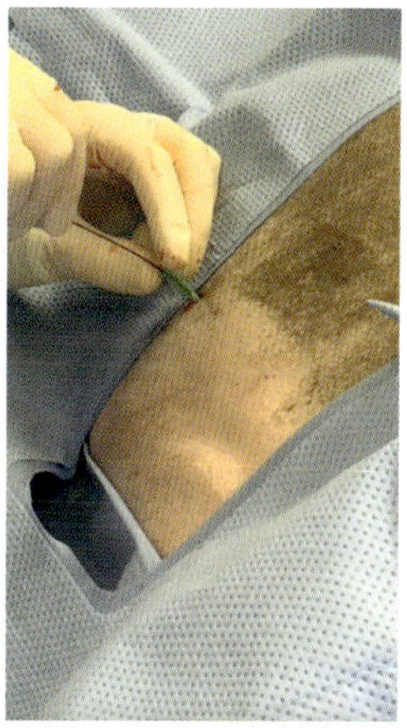

B-ii)

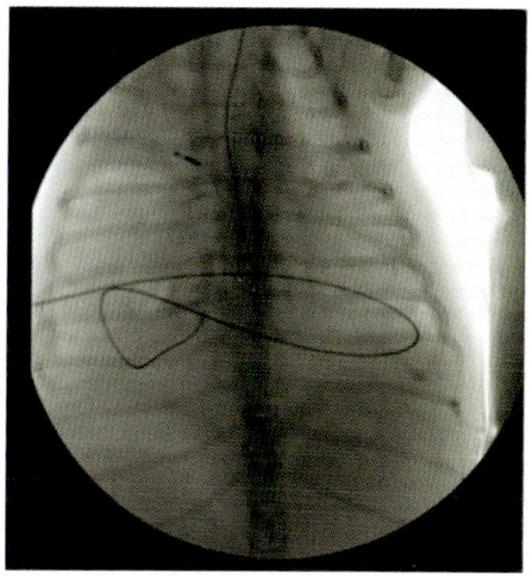

C-i)

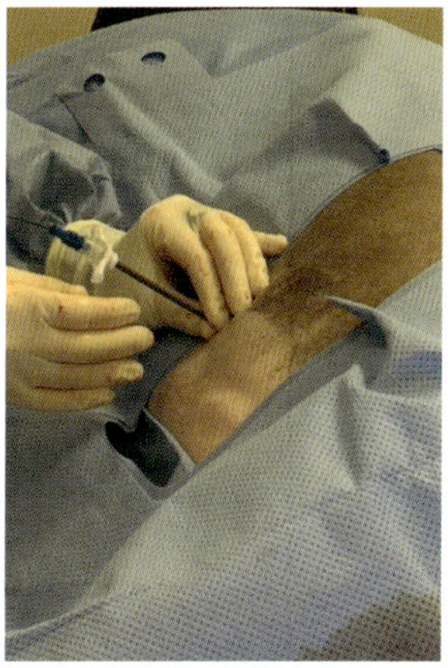

C-ii)

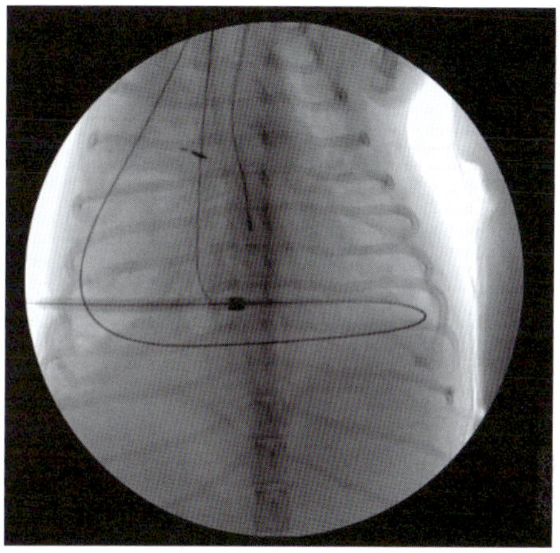

D-i)

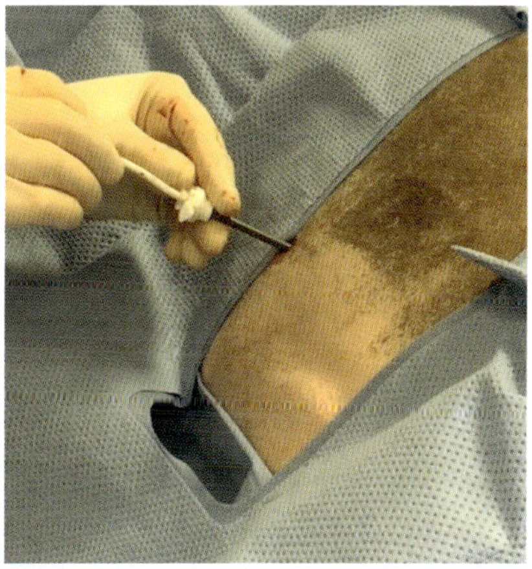

D-ii)

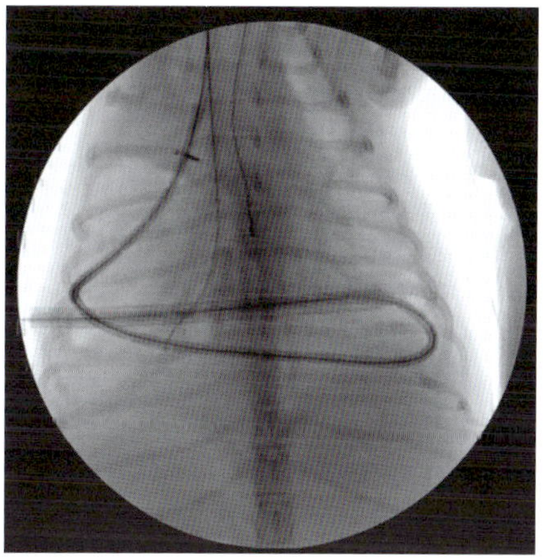

Surgical Technique – Surgical Intrathoracic Catheter Placement (See Plate 49F, G)

F) For the mini-thoracotomy approach, an incision large enough to fit the intrathoracic catheter is made, and the catheter is passed from the ipsilateral to the contralateral side of the thorax to ensure that the catheter is able to drain both hemithoraces.
G) For the thoracoscopic approach, a paraxiphoid port is established (see *10.3. Thoracoscopy*). Two instrument ports are established bilaterally between intercostal spaces 7 and 9. Through one instrument cannula, a thoracoscopic hemostat is introduced. The intrathoracic catheter is passed through the second instrument cannula. The catheter is grasped with the thoracoscopic hemostat, which can then be used to position the intrathoracic catheter in the desired location.

Surgical Technique – Subcutaneous Port Placement (See Plate 49H–K)

H) After placement of the intrathoracic catheter into the thorax, a skin incision is made on the dorsal third of the thoracic wall one to two intercostal spaces caudal to the entry point of the intrathoracic catheter into the thorax. The skin incision needs to be large enough for the subcutaneous port to be sutured to the underlying muscle.
I) The subcutaneous tissue is dissected to expose the underlying latissimus dorsi muscle. A hemostat is then passed through the subcutaneous tissue from the dorsal incision to the site where the intrathoracic catheter is exiting the thorax. The hemostat is used to grasp the end of the intrathoracic catheter, which is subsequently pulled subcutaneously into the port site.
J) The subcutaneous port is attached to the intrathoracic catheter (i). The subcutaneous port is sutured to the latissimus dorsi muscle with simple interrupted sutures of 2-0 monofilament nonabsorbable suture placed through the existing holes in the port (ii).
K) The subcutaneous port wound is closed in two layers with a simple continuous suture pattern using monofilament absorbable suture material in the subcutis and either an interrupted or continuous suture pattern using monofilament nonabsorbable suture material in the skin.

Postoperative Management

1) Multimodal analgesia
2) Supplemental oxygen therapy, if required
3) Elizabethan collar

Complications [1]

Intraoperative Complications

- Pneumothorax (10%)

Postoperative Complications

- Port obstruction (30%)

Suggested Adjuvant Treatments

- ± Chemotherapy depending on tumor type
- ± Intracavitary chemotherapy

Reference

1 Brooks, A.C. and Hardie, R.J. (2011). Use of the pleural port device for management of pleural effusion in six dogs and four cats. *Vet. Surg.* 40 (8): 935–941.

Plate 49

Pleural Port Placement *continued*

F)

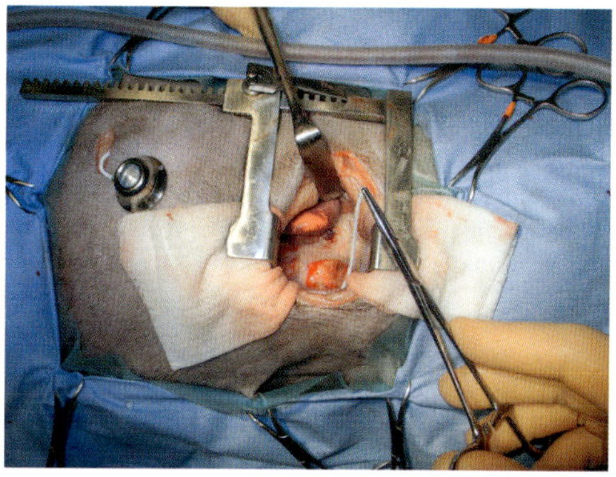

G)

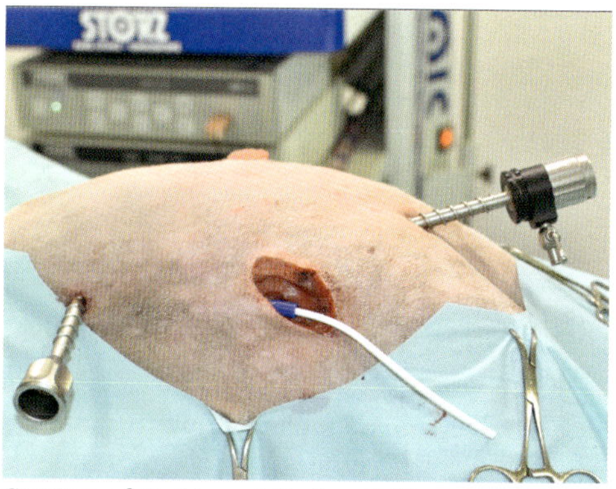

Courtesy of Dr. Manuel Jiménez Peláez

H)

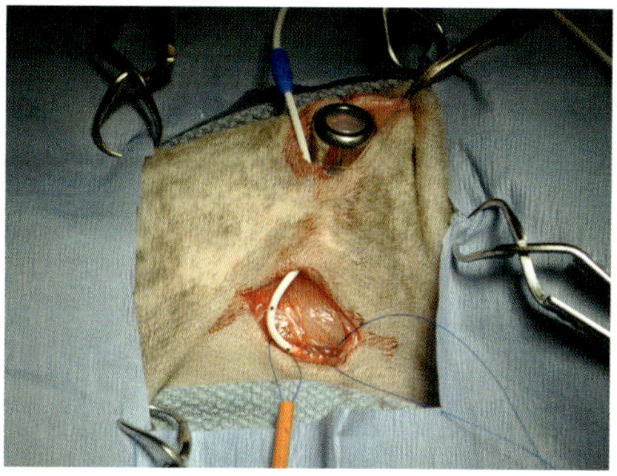

I)

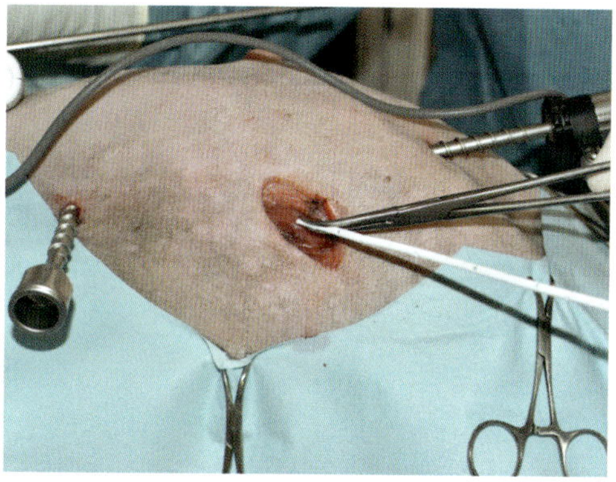

Courtesy of Dr. Manuel Jiménez Peláez

J-i)

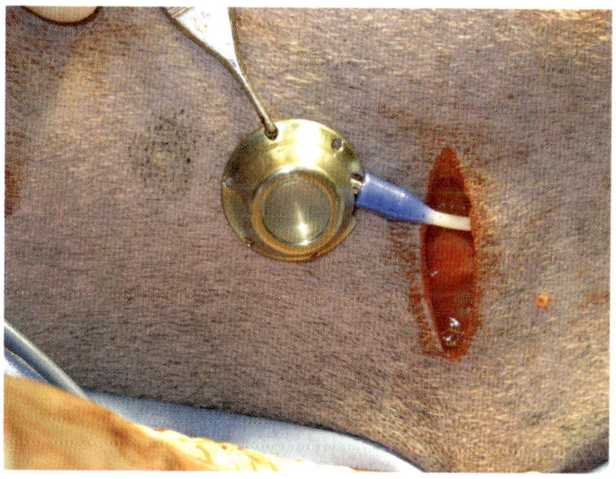

J-ii)

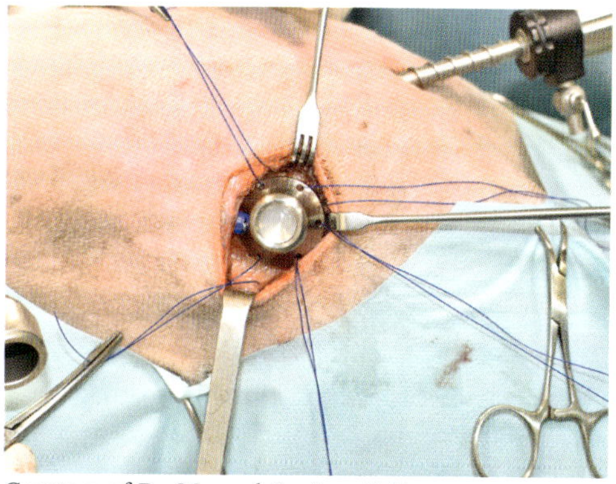

Courtesy of Dr. Manuel Jiménez Peláez

K)

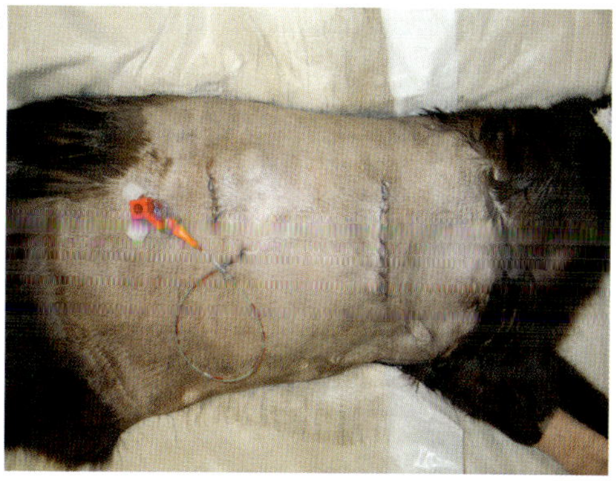

Section 10

Miscellaneous Procedures

Chapter 50: Lymph Node Excision

50.1 Sentinel Lymph Node Mapping

General Considerations (See Plate 50.1 – 1–6)

The sentinel lymph node (SLN) is an important concept in oncology and is based on the theory that the metastatic process occurs in an orderly progression within the lymphatic system with tumor cells draining into a specific lymph node (i.e. SLN) in a regional lymphatic field before draining into other regional lymph nodes [1]. The SLN is not specific for tumor type or location, but it is individual, changes from patient to patient, and is not the same as the regional anatomic lymph node [2, 3]. For instance, there is a wide variety of lymphatic drainage and SLN locations for normal canine mammary glands with the first and second mammary glands draining into the cranial sternal (1, arrow), axillary, and superficial cervical lymph nodes (2), and the fourth and fifth mammary glands draining into the superficial inguinal and medial iliac lymph nodes (3) [4]; however, there is much variability in the lymphatic drainage, and the presence of a tumor may change the lymphatic drainage pattern (4, preoperative SLN mapping radiograph of a dog with a mammary osteosarcoma of the fourth mammary gland showing the axillary lymph node [arrow] is the SLN). Similarly, malignant oral tumors can drain into the ipsilateral or contralateral mandibular, medial retropharyngeal, parotid, superficial cervical (5, preoperative SLN mapping of a cat with a lip squamous cell carcinoma), or even the minor buccal lymph nodes (6, preoperative SLN mapping of a cat with a lip malignant melanoma), but only the mandibular lymph nodes are palpable [5].

Conceptually, distant metastasis should not be present if the SLN does not have evidence of a tumor burden, but distant metastasis is possible if the SLN has histologic evidence of metastatic tumor cells. Hence the status of the SLN node may reflect the status of the entire regional lymphatic bed. Although not validated in cats and dogs, the probability that a non-SLN is positive for metastatic disease when the SLN is free of tumor is less than 0.1% in people [1].

In people and animals, identification of the SLN is important in the diagnosis of lymph node metastasis, early identification of patients requiring additional therapeutic options to manage metastatic disease (such as more extensive lymph node dissection and adjuvant chemotherapy or radiation therapy), and establishing a prognosis [2, 6].

The SLN mapping technique is more successful when both preoperative and intraoperative mapping techniques are used rather than a single technique. A number of SLN mapping techniques have been reported in both animals and people. Lymphoscintigraphy and indirect lymphography are the most commonly used preoperative SLN mapping techniques, and peritumoral injection of blue dye or indocyanine green (ICG) is the most commonly used intraoperative SLN mapping technique in animals.

Color Atlas of Canine and Feline Surgical Oncology, First Edition. Julius M. Liptak, Paolo Buracco, William T. N. Culp, and Nicholas J. Bacon.

Plate 50.1

Sentinel Lymph Node Mapping

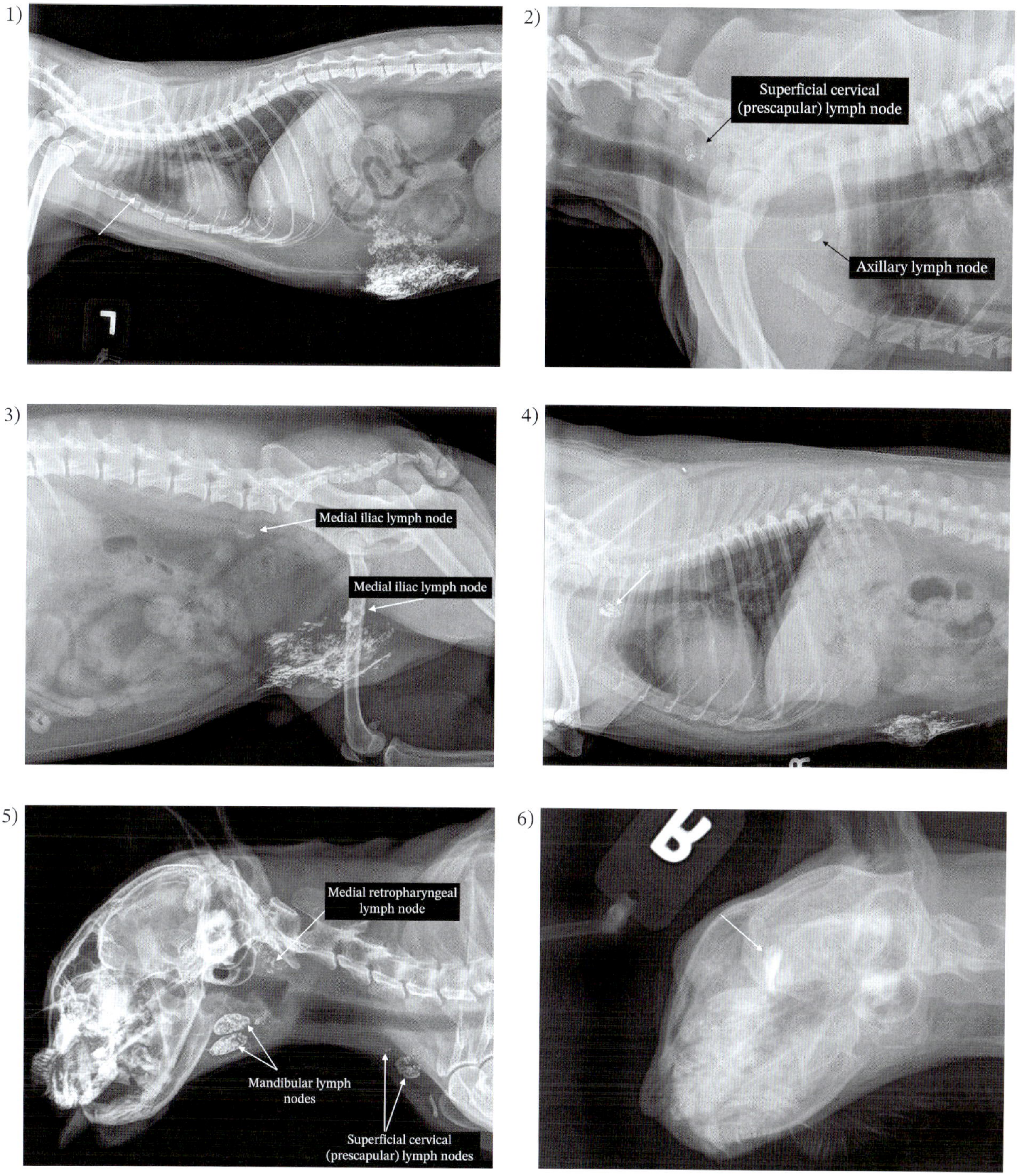

Preoperative Sentinel Lymph Node Mapping (See Plate 50.1A–C)

A) Indirect lymphography with iodinated contrast material [3, 7–11]
   i) A total of 0.25–1.0 ml of aqueous iodinated contrast material is injected subcutaneously and peritumorally in each of four quadrants around the edges of the tumor or 5–10 mm away from the edges of the tumor for known mast cell tumors, and the tumor is gently massaged for 10–15 seconds after peritumoral injection of the contrast material (a–d, dog with a high-grade cutaneous mast cell tumor).
   ii) Regional radiographs (a, contrast enhancement of the lymphatics draining the high-grade cutaneous mast cell tumor into the superficial inguinal lymph node [arrow]) or computed tomography (CT) scan (b, contrast enhancement of the right mandibular lymph node [arrow]) in a dog with a maxillary osteosarcoma) are done at 1 and 3–5 minutes after aqueous iodinated contrast material injection to identify the contrast-enhanced lymphatics and SLN, and repeated as necessary until the SLN is identified.
   iii) If the contrast material does not leave the tumor, then step Ai is repeated.

Plate 50.1

Sentinel Lymph Node Mapping *continued*

A-i, a)

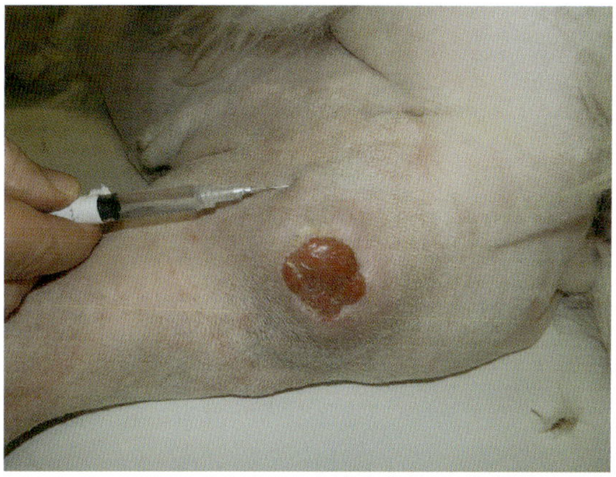

A-i, b)

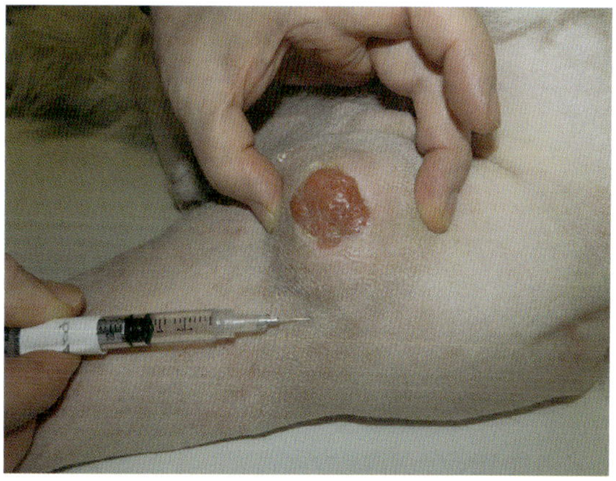

A-i, c)

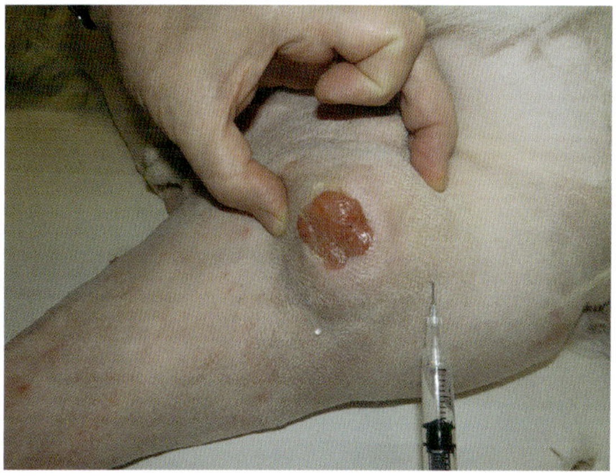

A-i, d)

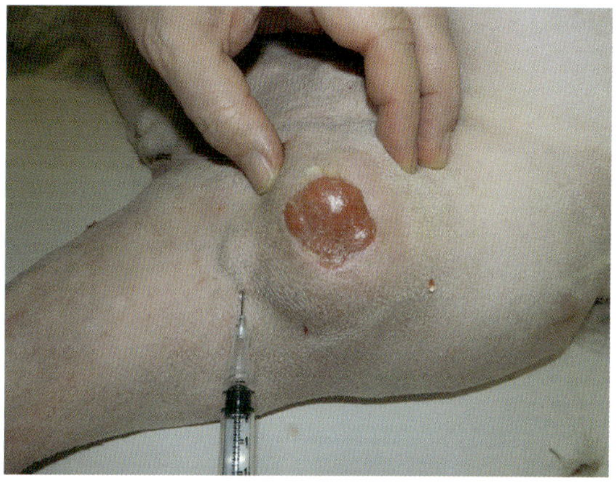

A-ii, a)

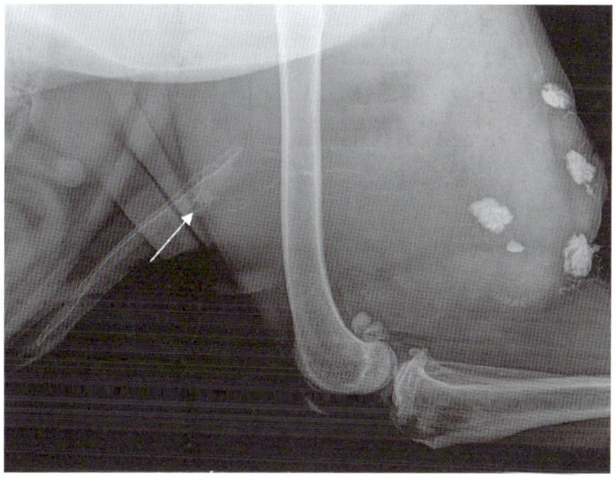

A-ii, b)

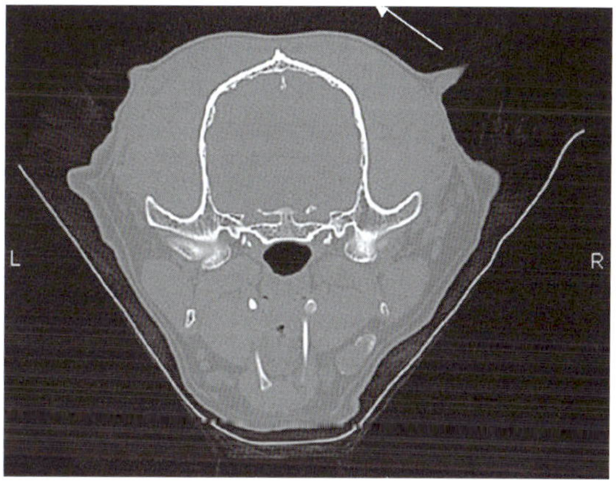

Preoperative Sentinel Lymph Node Mapping (See Plate 50.1A–C) *continued*

B) Indirect lymphography with Lipiodol [12]
   i) A total of 0.5 ml Lipiodol is injected subcutaneously and peritumorally in each of four quadrants around the edges of the tumor or 5–10 mm away from the edges of the tumor for known mast cell tumors (a–d, dog with a mucosal mast cell tumor of the upper lip).
   ii) Regional radiographs or CT scan are done 24 hours after Lipiodol injection to identify the contrast-enhanced SLN (pictured, contrast enhancement of the superficial cervical lymph node in a dog with a digit squamous cell carcinoma; also see earlier steps 1–6).

C) Lymphoscintigraphy (not pictured) [2]
   i) A total of 0.5 ml of 125 microcuries filtered technetium sulfur colloid is injected subcutaneously and peritumorally in four quadrants around the edges of the tumor.
   ii) A single-photon emission CT gamma camera is used to acquire images every 5 minutes until the SLN is identified.

Plate 50.1

Sentinel Lymph Node Mapping *continued*

B-i, a)

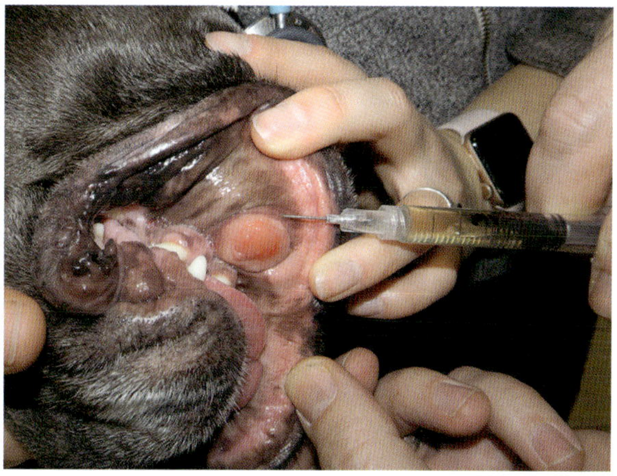

B-i, b)

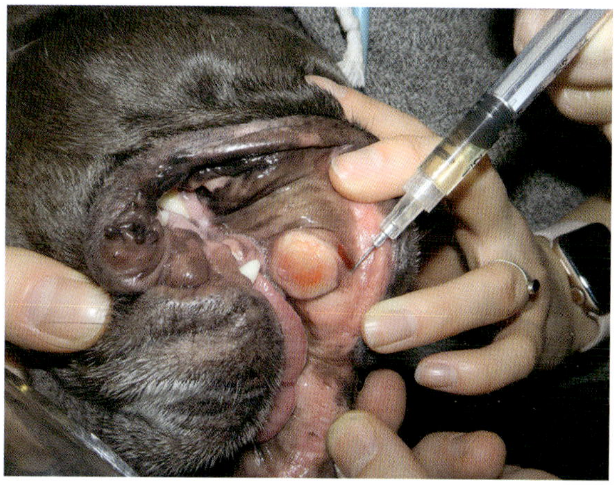

B-i, c)

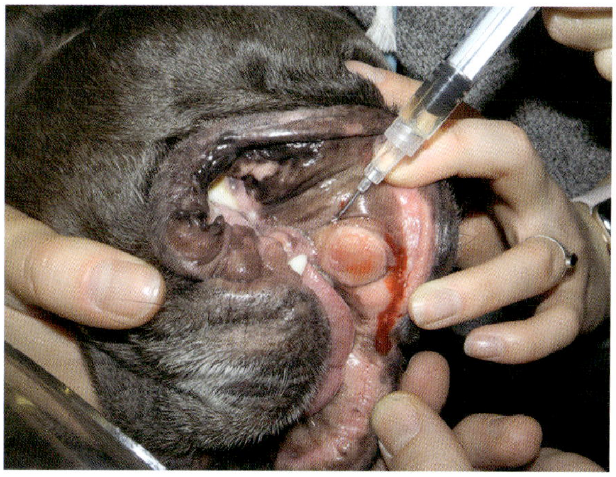

B-i, d)

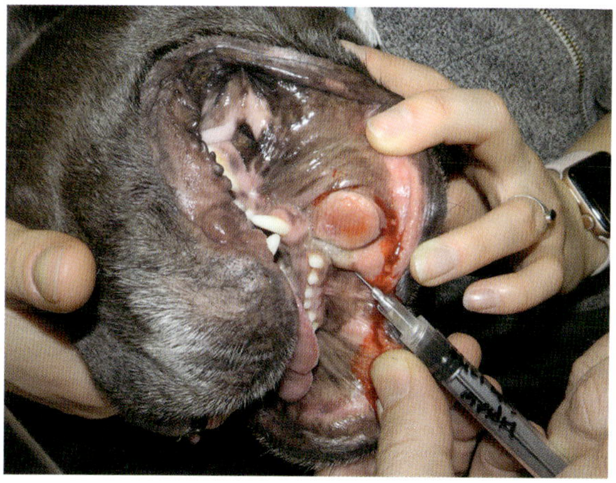

B-ii)

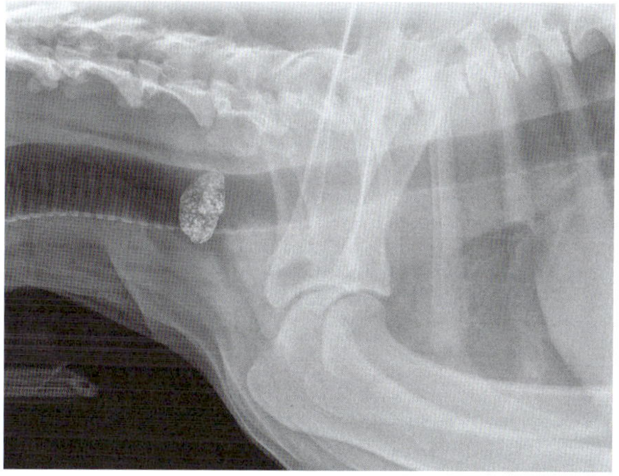

Intraoperative Sentinel Lymph Node Mapping (See Plate 50.1D, E)

D) Methylene blue [2, 3, 12]
  i) A sterile marker pen should be used to indicate the lateral surgical margins before peritumoral injection of methylene blue because the methylene blue will result in staining and can potentially obscure the tumor and its margins (see D – ii).
  ii) A total of 0.1–0.5 ml of methylene is injected subcutaneously in each of four quadrants around the edge of the tumor or 5–10 mm away from the edge of the tumor for known mast cell tumors (a–d). For dogs weighing less than 10 kg, methylene blue should be diluted 1:1 with a dextrose 5% solution.
  iii) If preoperative SLN mapping was not done, then the blue-colored afferent lymphatics are followed to the blue-colored SLN with the skin incision being performed 5 minutes after peritumoral injection of methylene blue to allow adequate time for lymphatic uptake of the blue dye (a, mandibular lymph node in a dog with a mandibular osteosarcoma; b, superficial inguinal lymph node in a cat with a mammary carcinoma; c, blue-colored lymphatics [arrowheads] coursing through the inguinal canal to the medial iliac lymph node [arrow]).
  iv) If preoperative SLN mapping was done, then a targeted approach is made to the lymph node identified as the SLN during the preoperative mapping procedure with the skin incision being performed 5 minutes after peritumoral injection of methylene blue to allow adequate time for lymphatic uptake of the blue dye (pictured, mandibular lymph node in a dog with a lip mast cell tumor).

E) ICG and near-infrared imaging [13]
  i) ICG powder is dissolved with 5 ml of sterile water to produce a 5 mg/ml solution, and then 0.5 ml of dissolved ICG is mixed with 4.5 ml of sterile water to produce a final ICGH concentration of 0.5 mg/ml.
  ii) A total of 0.1 ml of ICG is injected subcutaneously in each of four quadrants around the edge of the tumor.
  iii) A targeted approach is made to the lymph node identified as the SLN during the preoperative SLN mapping procedure with the skin incision being performed 5 minutes after peritumoral injection of ICG to allow adequate time for lymphatic uptake of the ICG.
  iv) Near-infrared fluorescence imaging is used to assess for fluorescence of the lymph node.

F) Handheld gamma probe (not pictured) [2]
  i) A handheld gamma probe and external collimator are used to obtain a background count at a location distant to the radioactive injection site.
  ii) The gamma probe is then moved at less than 1 cm/s over the lymphocentrum identified on the preoperative SLN mapping procedure.
  iii) A targeted approach is made over any lymph node with radioactive counts at least two times greater than the background count. After extirpation of the SLN, any additional lymph nodes in the region with radioactive counts ≥10% of the SLN should also be excised.

Complications

- Very rare [14]

Plate 50.1

Sentinel Lymph Node Mapping *continued*

D-ii, a)

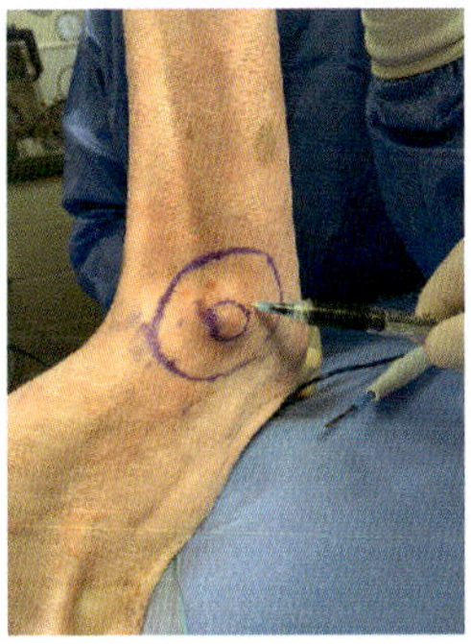

D-ii, b)

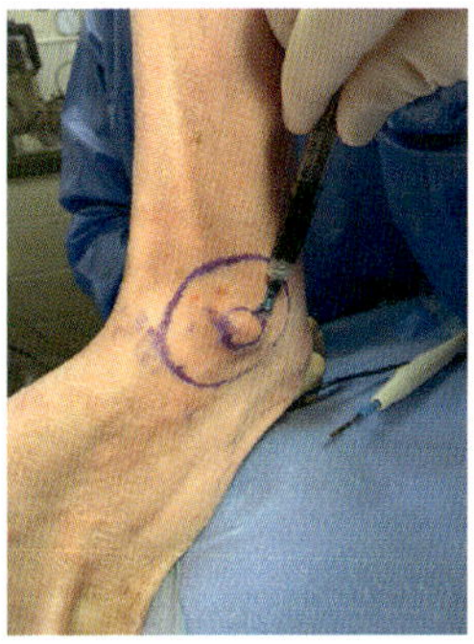

D-ii, c)

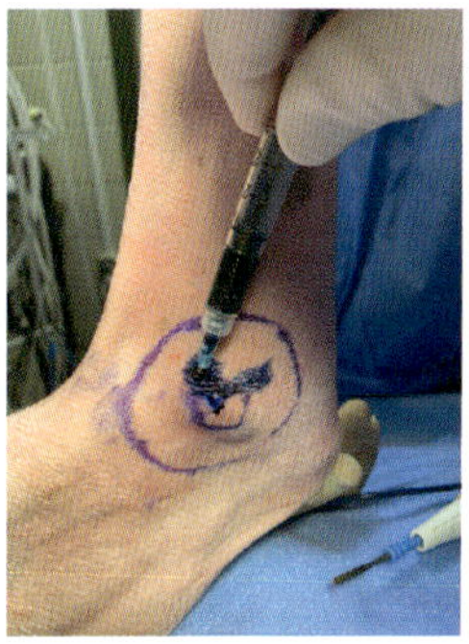

D-ii, d)

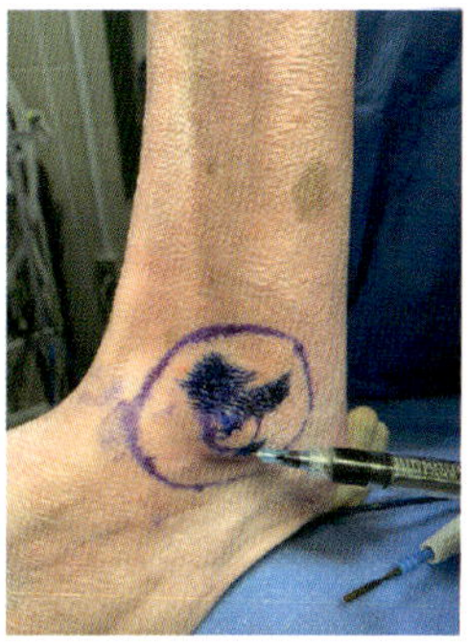

D-iii, a)

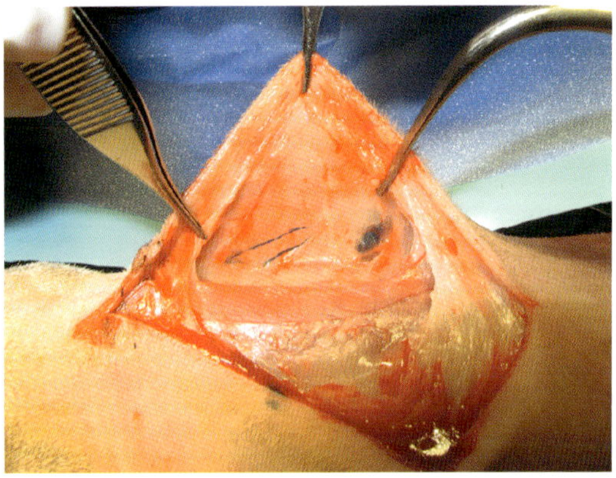

D-iii, b)

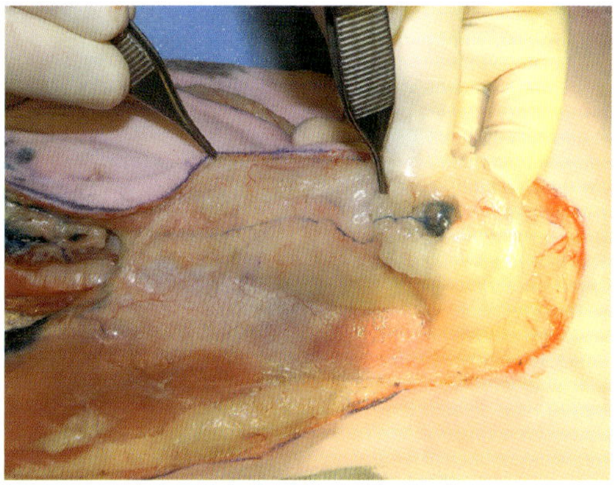

D-iii, c)

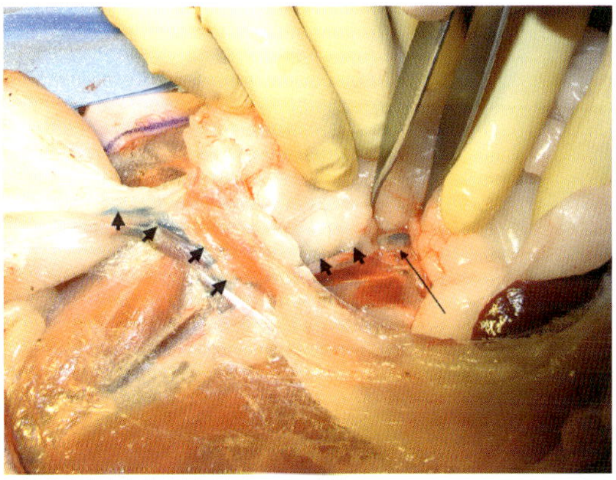

D-iv)

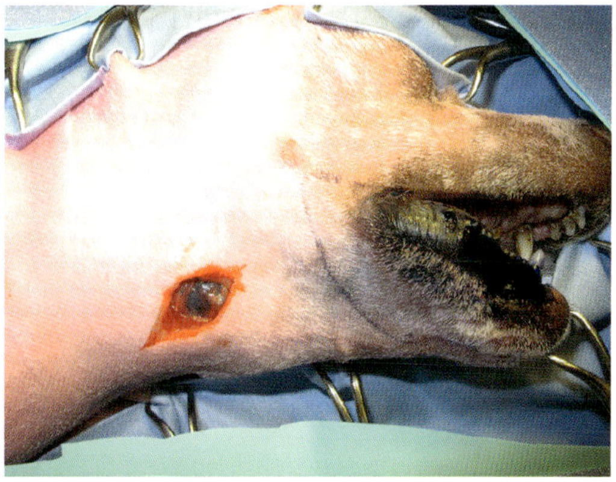

E-iv)

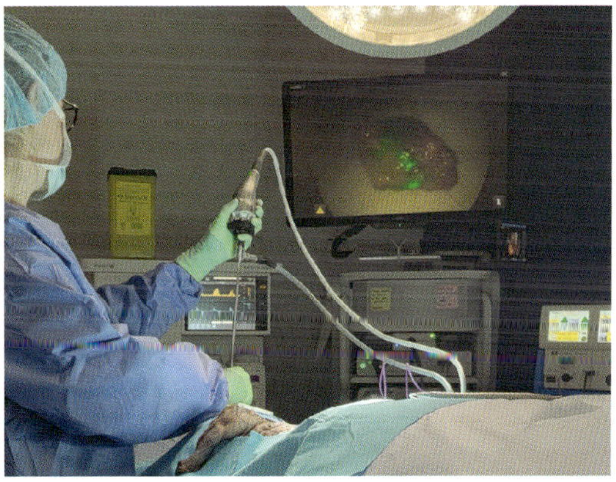

References

1 Balasubramanian, S.P. and Harrison, B.J. (2011). Systematic review and meta-analysis of sentinel node biopsy in thyroid cancer. *Br. J. Surg.* 98 (3): 334–344.

2 Worley, D.R. (2014). Incorporation of sentinel lymph node mapping in dogs with mast cell tumours: 20 consecutive procedures. *Vet. Comp. Oncol.* 12 (3): 215–226.

3 Ferraris, E.I., Olimpo, M., Giacobino, D. et al. (2023). Sentinel lymph node mapping with computed tomography lymphography for mast cell tumours and a comparison between regional and sentinel lymph node histological status: sixty-two cases. *Vet. Comp. Oncol.* 21 (2): 208–220.

4 Pereira, C.T., Marques, F.L.N., Williams, J. et al. (2008). 99m Tc-labeled dextran for mammary lymphoscintigraphy in dogs. *Vet. Radiol. Ultrasound* 49 (5): 487–491.

5 Herring, E.S., Smith, M.M., and Robertson, J.L. (2002). Lymph node staging of oral and maxillofacial neoplasms in 31 dogs and cats. *J. Vet. Dent.* 19 (3): 122–126.

6 Newman, L.A. (2004). Lymphatic mapping and sentinel lymph node biopsy in breast cancer patients: a comprehensive review of variations in performance and technique. *J. Am. Coll. Surg.* 199 (5): 804–816.

7 Soultani, C., Patsikas, M.N., Karayannopoulou, M. et al. (2017). Assessment of sentinel lymph node metastasis in canine mammary gland tumors using computed tomographic indirect lymphography. *Vet. Radiol. Ultrasound* 58 (2): 186–196.

8 Majeski, S.A., Steffey, M.A., Fuller, M. et al. (2017). Indirect computed tomographic lymphography for iliosacral lymphatic mapping in a cohort of dogs with anal sac gland adenocarcinoma: technique description. *Vet. Radiol. Ultrasound* 58 (3): 295–303.

9 Grimes, J.A., Secrest, S.A., Northrup, N.C. et al. (2017). Indirect computed tomography lymphangiography with aqueous contrast for evaluation of sentinel lymph nodes in dogs with tumors of the head. *Vet. Radiol. Ultrasound* 58 (5): 559–564.

10 Randall, E.K., Jones, M.D., Kraft, S.L. et al. (2020). The development of an indirect computed tomography lymphography protocol for sentinel lymph node detection in head and neck cancer and comparison to other sentinel lymph node mapping techniques. *Vet. Comp. Oncol.* 18 (4): 634–644.

11 Haas, S., Linden, D., Cole, R. et al. (2023). Indirect lymphography for sentinel lymph node detection in dogs with mast cell tumors. *Can. Vet. J.* 64 (2): 142–148.

12 Brissot, H.N. and Edery, E.G. (2017). Use of indirect lymphography to identify sentinel lymph node in dogs: a pilot study in 30 tumours. *Vet. Comp. Oncol.* 15 (3): 740–753.

13 Favril, S., Stock, E., Hernot, S. et al. (2019). Sentinel lymph node mapping by near-infrared fluorescence imaging and contrast-enhanced ultrasound in healthy dogs. *Vet. Comp. Oncol.* 17 (1): 89–98.

14 Chiti, L.E., Gariboldi, E.M., Stefanello, D. et al. (2022). Sentinel lymph node mapping and biopsy in cats with solid malignancies: an explorative study. *Animals* 12 (22): 3116.

50.2 Mandibular Lymph Node Excision

Indications

1) Nonselective lymphadenectomy for clinical staging of malignant head and neck tumors
2) Selective lymphadenectomy after sentinel lymph node mapping (see *50.1. Sentinel Lymph Node Mapping*)
3) Lymphadenectomy of a metastatic mandibular lymph node

Patient Positioning

The patient is positioned in lateral recumbency with the affected side uppermost for unilateral mandibular lymph node excision.

Surgical Technique (See Plate 50.2A–C)

A) A skin incision, either horizontal (pictured, dog with a cutaneous mast cell tumor) or vertical, is made immediately caudal to the caudal angle of the mandible over the palpable mandibular lymph node.
B) The mandibular lymphocentrum is located immediately caudal and ventral to the angle of the mandible (i, mandibular lymph node is blue because of intraoperative sentinel lymph node mapping with methylene blue), cranial to the mandibular salivary gland, and craniomedial to the bifurcation of the linguofacial vein into the lingual and facial veins (ii). The mandibular lymphocentrum includes between two and five lymph nodes (ii; iii, iv, arrows).

Color Atlas of Canine and Feline Surgical Oncology, First Edition. Julius M. Liptak, Paolo Buracco, William T. N. Culp, and Nicholas J. Bacon.

Plate 50.2

Mandibular Lymph Node Excision

A)

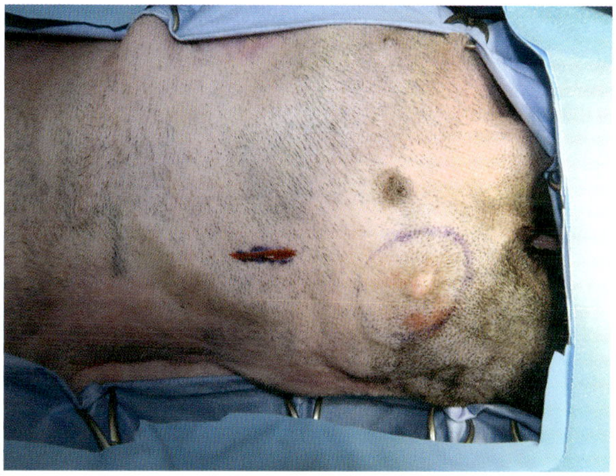

B-i)

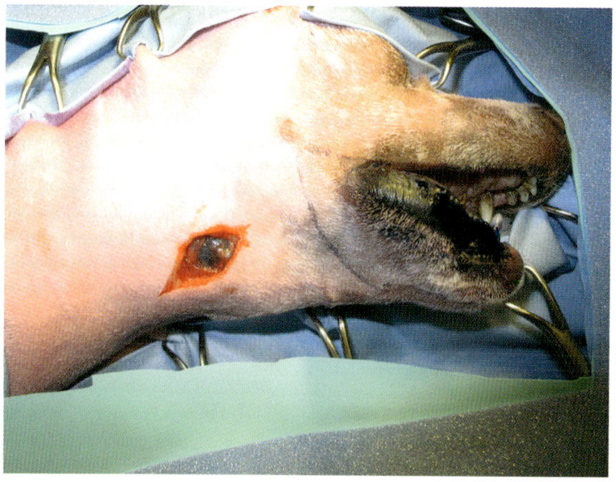

B-ii)

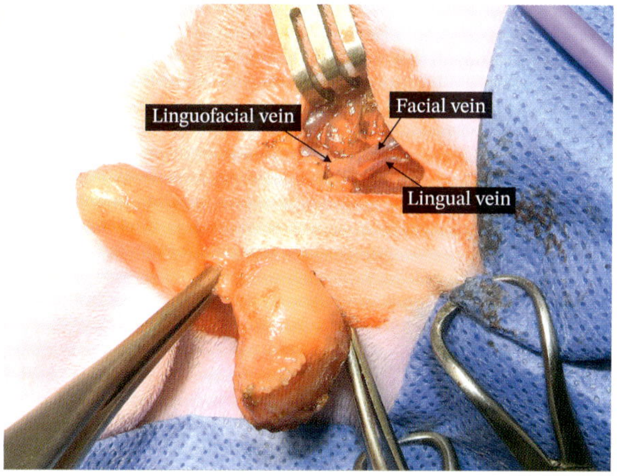

B-iii)

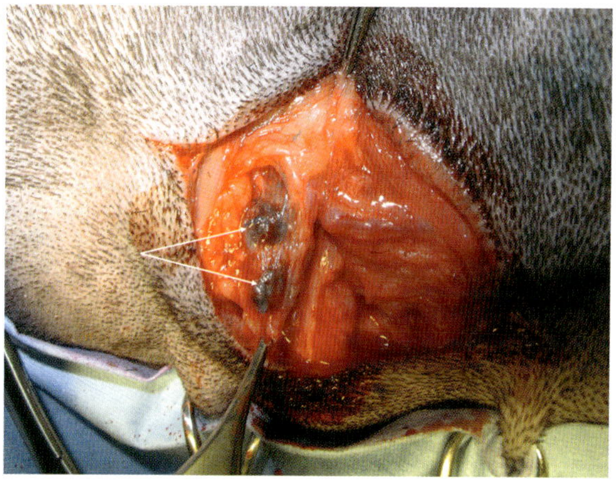

B-iv)

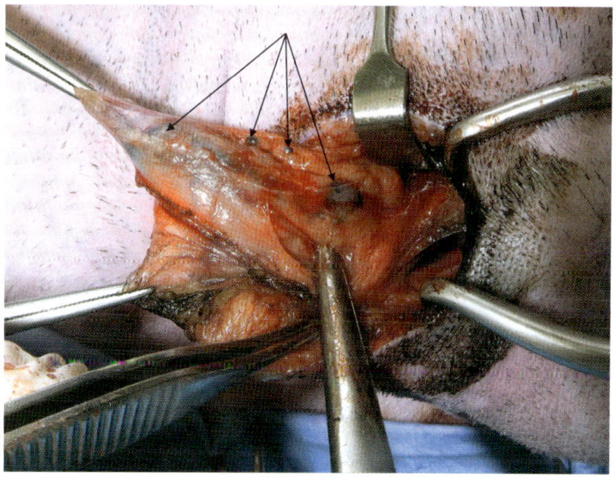

Surgical Technique (See Plate 50.2A–C) *continued*

C) The mandibular lymph nodes are excised using a combination of blunt and sharp dissection (i) or with a vessel sealing device (ii). The perinodal tissue should be grasped to manipulate the lymph node (iii) rather than directly grasping the lymph node because this will result in trauma to the lymph node. The facial vein courses medial to the mandibular lymph nodes; both the facial and lingual veins should be preserved (iv).

Closure (See Plate 50.2D)

D) The skin incision is closed routinely in two layers with a simple continuous suture pattern using monofilament absorbable suture material in the subcutis and either an interrupted or continuous (pictured) suture pattern using monofilament nonabsorbable suture material in the skin.

Postoperative Management

1) Multimodal analgesia
2) Elizabethan collar

Complications [1]

Intraoperative Complications

- None reported

Postoperative Complications

- Overall for all lymph node excisions: 21% with 19% being minor and 2% being major
- Lymphedema (11%)
- Seroma (10%)
- Hematoma (3%)
- Incisional dehiscence (1%)

Reference

1 Chiti, L.E., Gariboldi, E.M., Ferrari, R. et al. (2023). Surgical complications following sentinel lymph node biopsy guided by gamma-probe and methylene blue in 113 tumour-bearing dogs. *Vet. Comp. Oncol.* 21 (1): 62–72.

Plate 50.2

Mandibular Lymph Node Excision *continued*

C-i)

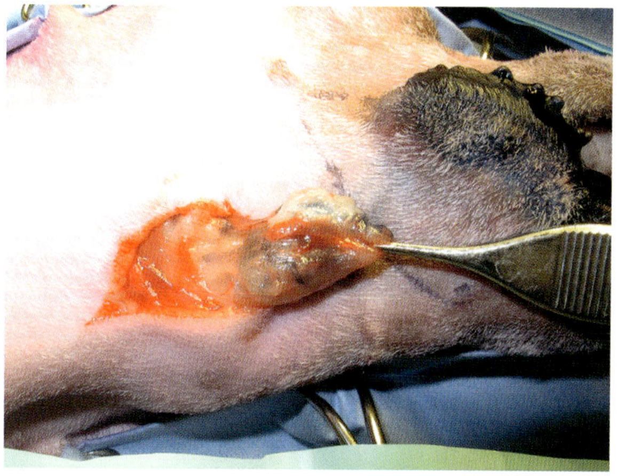

C-ii)

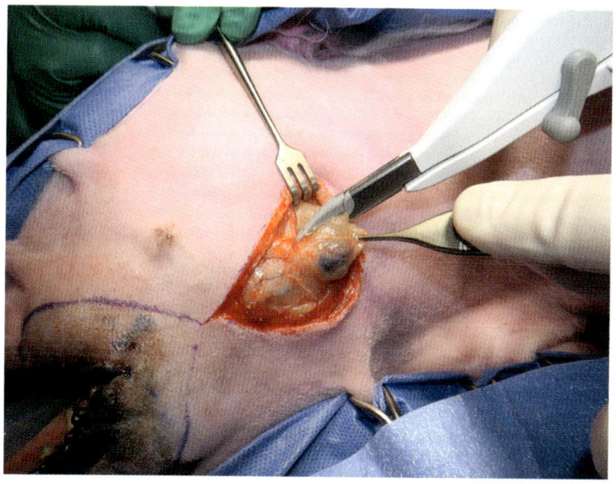

C-iii)

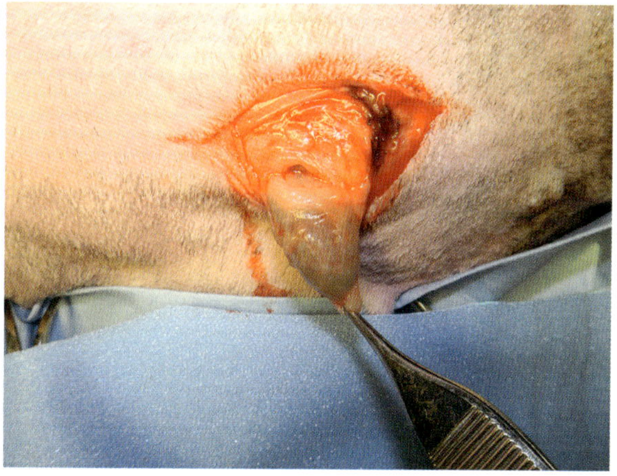

C-iv)

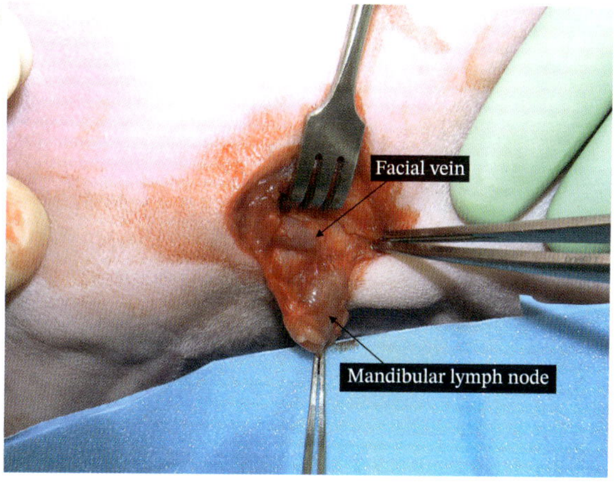

D)

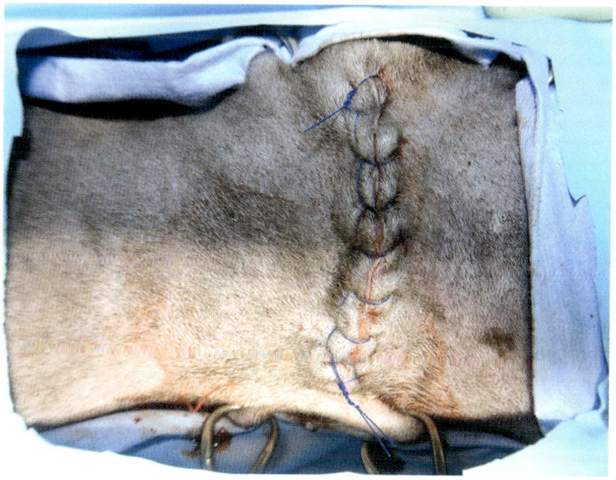

50.3 Combined Mandibular and Medial Retropharyngeal Lymph Node Excision

Indication

1) Nonselective lymphadenectomy for clinical staging of malignant head and neck tumors

Patient Positioning (See Plate 50.3A)

A) The patient is positioned in dorsal recumbency (pictured). A towel or sandbag can be placed under the neck to elevate the neck.

Surgical Technique [1, 2] (See Plate 50.3B–D)

B) A ventral midline incision is made through the skin (i) and platysma muscle (ii) from the caudal third of the mandible to the larynx.
C) The mandibular lymphocentrum, which includes two (i, arrows) to five lymph nodes on each side, is located ventral to the angle of the mandible and cranial to the mandibular salivary gland, at the bifurcation of the external jugular vein with the lingual and facial veins (ii, arrow). The mandibular lymph nodes are excised using a combination of blunt and sharp dissection (iii), preserving the lingual and facial veins and cauterizing the smaller vessels.
D) The mandibular salivary gland is retracted craniolaterally to identify the medial retropharyngeal node, which is located caudomedial to the mandibular salivary gland and ventral to the brachiocephalicus and sternocephalicus muscles (i). The medial retropharyngeal lymph node is excised using a combination of blunt and sharp dissection (ii), preserving the hypoglossal nerve medially and the carotid sheath containing the common carotid artery, vagus and sympathetic nerves, and internal jugular vein.

Color Atlas of Canine and Feline Surgical Oncology, First Edition. Julius M. Liptak, Paolo Buracco, William T. N. Culp, and Nicholas J. Bacon.

Plate 50.3

Combined Mandibular and Medial Retropharyngeal Lymph Node Excision

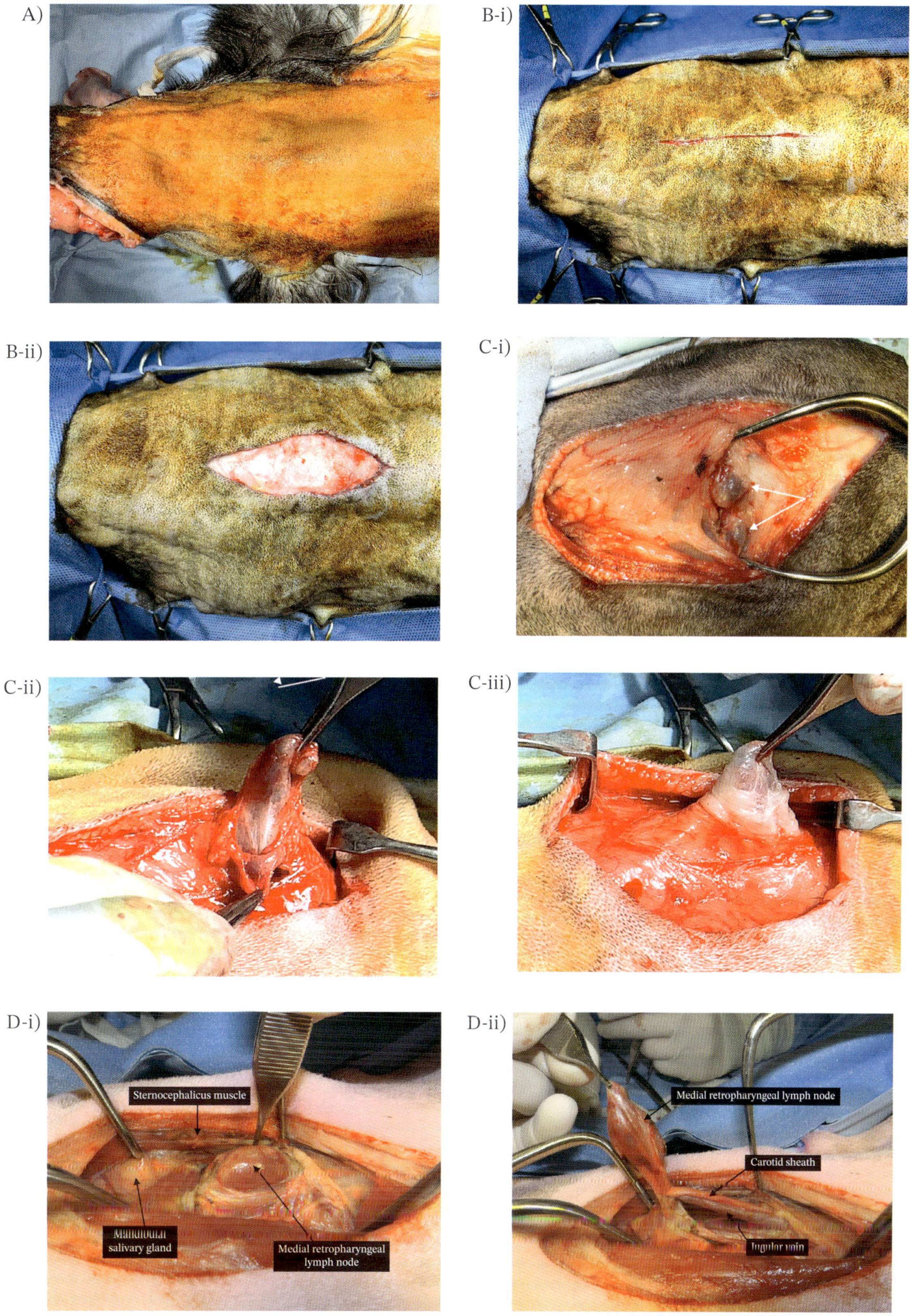

Closure (See Plate 50.3E)

E) The skin incision is closed routinely in two layers with a simple continuous suture pattern using monofilament absorbable suture material in the subcutis and either an interrupted or continuous suture pattern using monofilament nonabsorbable suture material in the skin (pictured).

Postoperative Management

1) Multimodal analgesia
2) Elizabethan collar

Complications [3]

Intraoperative Complications

- None reported

Postoperative Complications (See Plate 50.3F)

- Overall for all lymph node excisions: 21% with 19% being minor and 2% being major
- Lymphedema (F) (11%)
- Seroma (10%)
- Hematoma (3%)
- Incisional dehiscence (1%)

References

1 Green, K. and Boston, S.E. (2017). Bilateral removal of the mandibular and medial retropharyngeal lymph nodes through a single ventral midline incision for staging of head and neck cancers in dogs: a description of surgical technique. *Vet. Comp. Oncol.* 15 (1): 208–214.
2 Wainberg, S.H., Oblak, M.L., and Giuffrida, M.A. (2018). Ventral cervical versus bilateral lateral approach for extirpation of mandibular and medial retropharyngeal lymph nodes in dogs. *Vet. Surg.* 47 (5): 629–633.
3 Chiti, L.E., Gariboldi, E.M., Ferrari, R. et al. (2023). Surgical complications following sentinel lymph node biopsy guided by gamma-probe and methylene blue in 113 tumour-bearing dogs. *Vet. Comp. Oncol.* 21 (1): 62–72.

Plate 50.3

Combined Mandibular and Medial Retropharyngeal Lymph Node Excision *continued*

E)

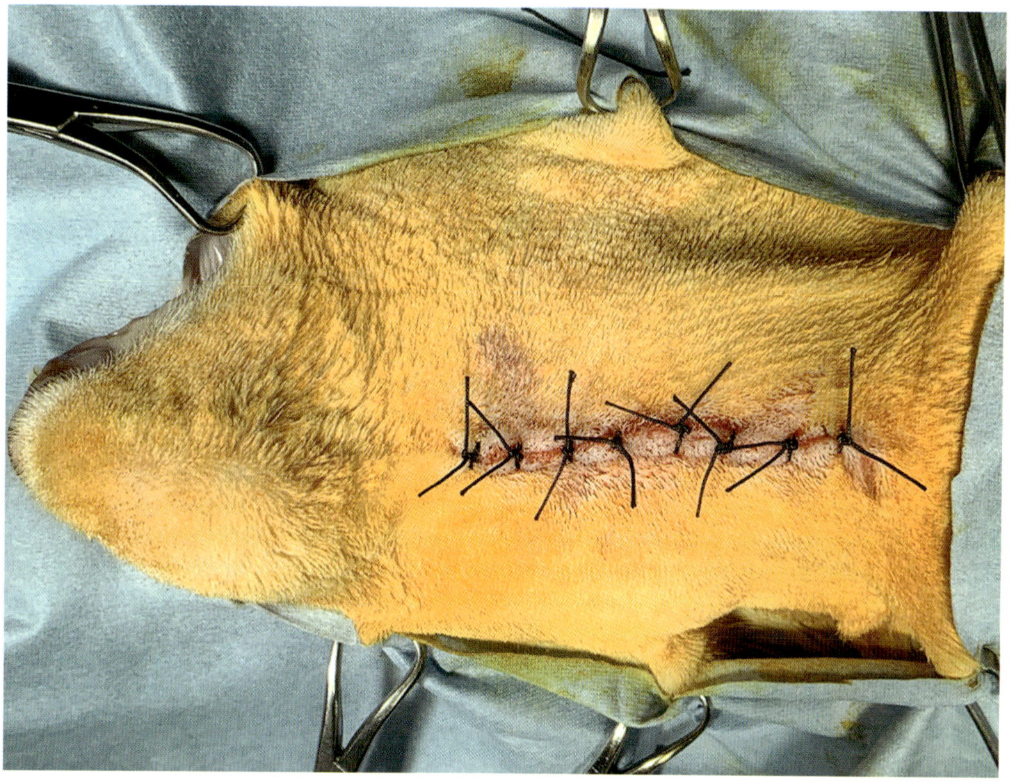

F)

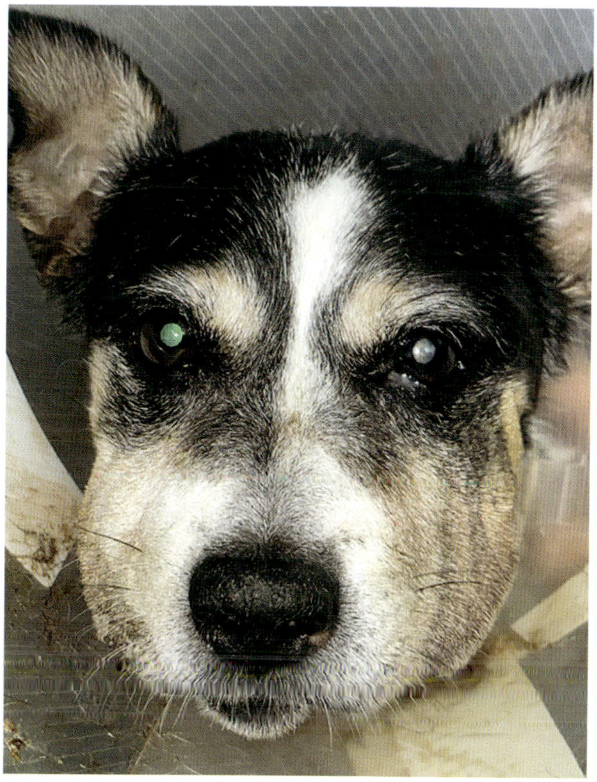

50.4 Combined Parotid, Mandibular, and Medial Retropharyngeal Lymph Node Excision

Indication

1) Nonselective lymphadenectomy for clinical staging of malignant head and neck tumors

Patient Positioning

The patient is positioned in lateral recumbency with the affected side uppermost.

Surgical Technique [1] (See Plate 50.4A–E)

A) A skin incision is made from the rostral aspect of the vertical ear canal, ventral to the zygomatic arch, to the bifurcation of the jugular vein.
B) The platysma and parotidoauricularis muscles are incised to expose the vertical ear canal and masseter muscle.
C) The parotid lymphocentrum, which includes one to three lymph nodes (i), is located on the rostral aspect of the parotid salivary gland at the ventral aspect of the zygomatic arch. The parotid lymph nodes are excised using a combination of blunt and sharp dissection or a vessel sealing device (ii).
D) The mandibular lymphocentrum (i, arrows), which includes two to five lymph nodes, is located ventral to the angle of the mandible and cranial to the mandibular salivary gland, at the bifurcation of the external jugular vein with the lingual and facial veins. The mandibular lymph nodes are excised using a combination of blunt and sharp dissection or vessel sealing device (ii), preserving the lingual and facial veins and cauterizing the smaller vessels.

Plate 50.4

Combined Parotid, Mandibular, and Medial Retropharyngeal Lymph Node Excision

A)

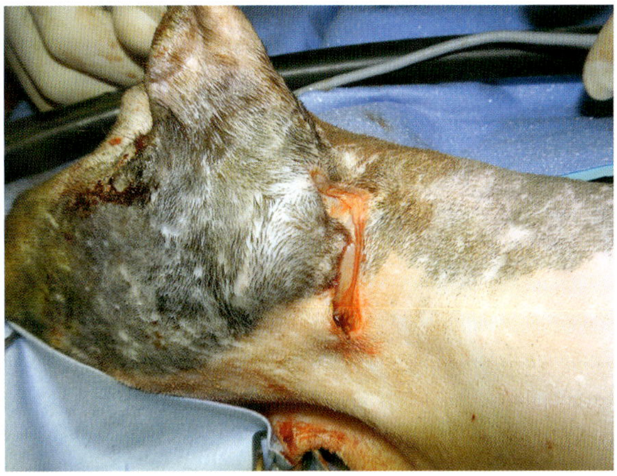

B)

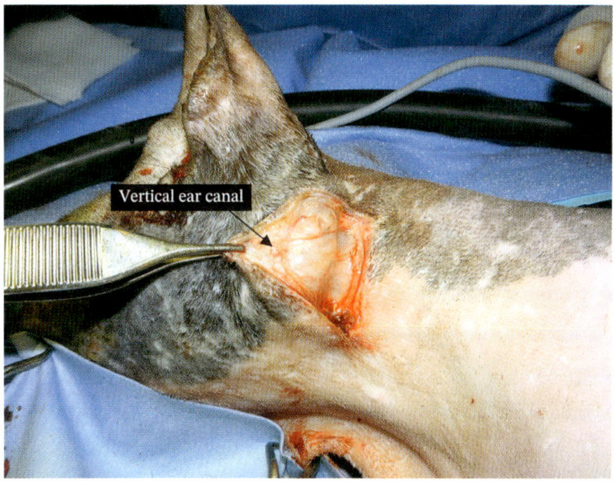

C-i)

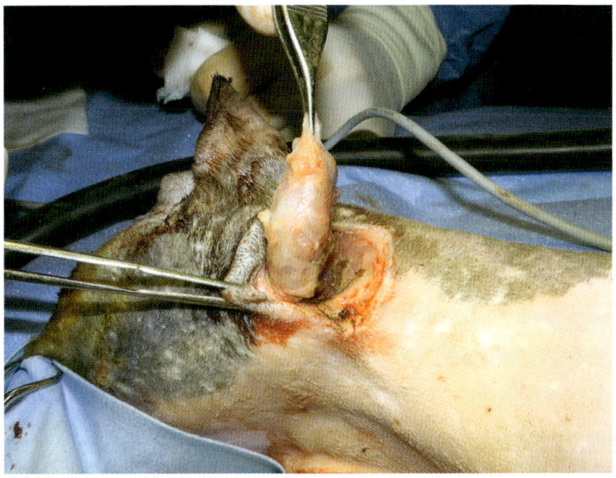

C-ii)

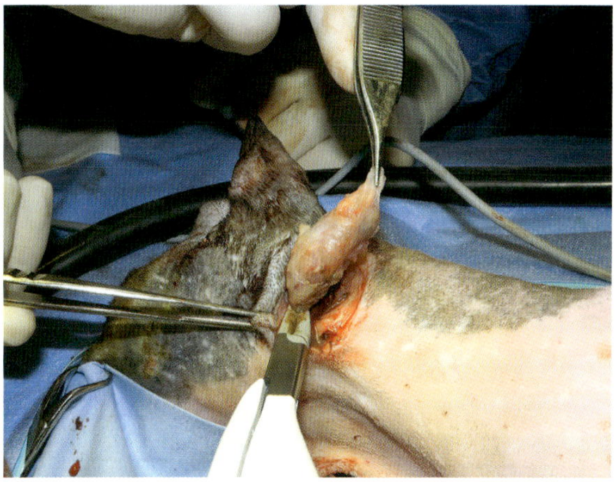

D-i)

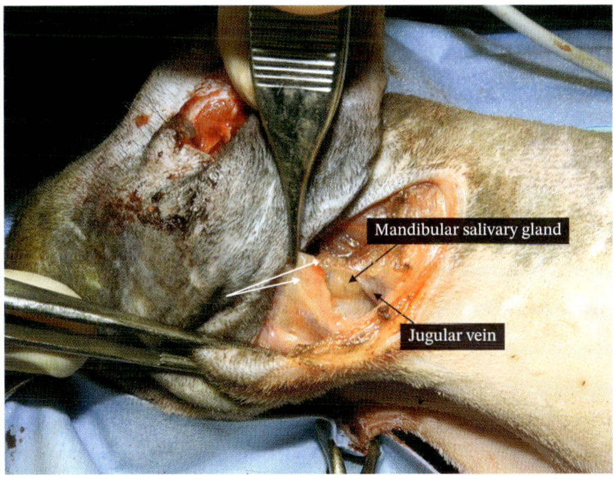

D-ii)

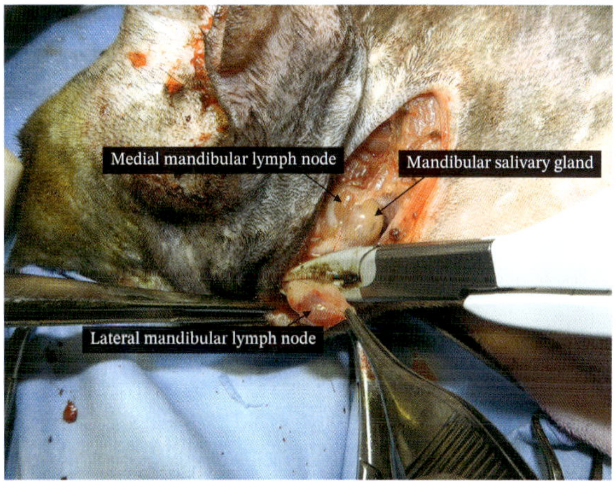

Surgical Technique [1] (See Plate 50.4A–E) *continued*

E) The mandibular salivary gland is retracted rostrally and the brachiocephalicus and sternocephalicus muscles are retracted dorsally to expose the medial retropharyngeal node (i, ii). The medial retropharyngeal lymph node is excised using a combination of blunt and sharp dissection or vessel sealing device (iii), preserving the hypoglossal nerve medially and the carotid sheath containing the common carotid artery, vagus and sympathetic nerves, and internal jugular vein.

Closure

The skin incision is closed routinely in two layers with a simple continuous suture pattern using monofilament absorbable suture material in the subcutis and either an interrupted or continuous suture pattern using monofilament nonabsorbable suture material in the skin (not pictured).

Postoperative Management

1) Multimodal analgesia
2) Elizabethan collar

Complications [2]

Intraoperative Complications

- None reported

Postoperative Complications

- Overall for all lymph node excisions: 21% with 19% being minor and 2% being major
- Overall for parotid, mandibular, and medial retropharyngeal lymph node excision: 29%
- Lymphedema (11%)
- Seroma (10%)
- Hematoma (3%)
- Incisional dehiscence (1%)

References

1 Smith, M.M. (1995). Surgical approach for lymph node staging of oral and maxillofacial neoplasms in dogs. *J. Am. Anim. Hosp. Assoc.* 31 (6): 514–518.
2 Chiti, L.E., Gariboldi, E.M., Ferrari, R. et al. (2023). Surgical complications following sentinel lymph node biopsy guided by gamma-probe and methylene blue in 113 tumour-bearing dogs. *Vet. Comp. Oncol.* 21 (1): 62–72.

Plate 50.4

Combined Parotid, Mandibular, and Medial Retropharyngeal Lymph Node Excision *continued*

E-i)

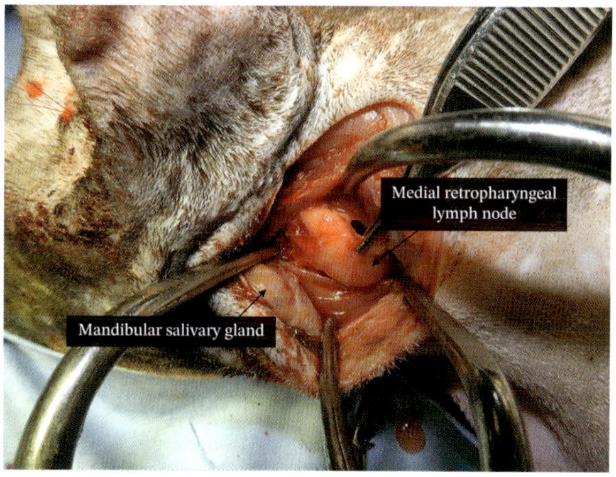

E-ii)

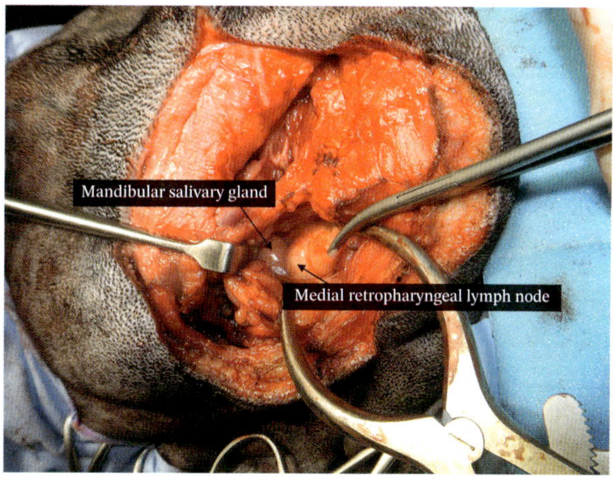

E-iii)

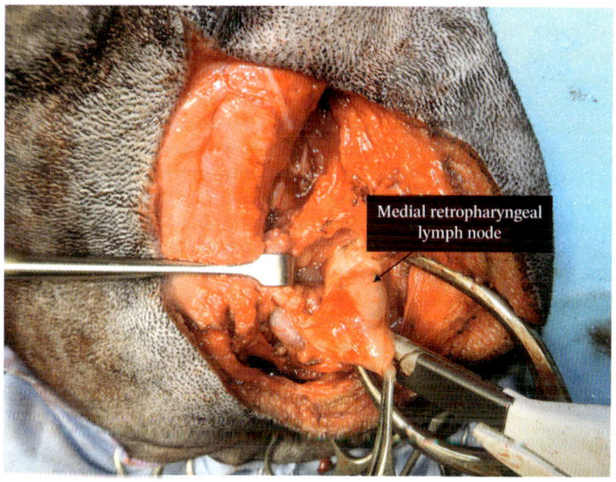

50.5 Superficial Cervical (Prescapular) Lymph Node Excision

Indications (See Plate 50.5 –2)

1) Nonselective lymphadenectomy for clinical staging of malignant head and neck tumors, especially tumors involving the pinna or ear canal
2) Selective lymphadenectomy after sentinel lymph node mapping (i, ii, preoperative sentinel lymph node mapping in a dog with a cutaneous mast cell tumor on the pinna, arrow) (see *50.1. Sentinel Lymph Node Mapping*)
3) Lymphadenectomy of a metastatic superficial cervical lymph node

Patient Positioning

The patient is positioned in lateral recumbency with the affected side uppermost and the thoracic limb either in a neutral position or pulled caudally.

Surgical Technique (See Plate 50.5A–C)

A) A skin incision is made cranial to the shoulder joint over the palpable superficial cervical lymph node (dashed line); however, the superficial cervical lymph node is not always easily palpable.
B) The superficial cervical lymphocentrum, which typically includes one or two lymph nodes but occasionally three or more lymph nodes, is located immediately cranial to the shoulder joint and medial to the omotransversarius and supraspinatus muscles. The subcutaneous fat can make visual identification of the lymph node difficult, but the lymph node is the only solid, rounded structure in this region.
C) The superficial cervical lymph node is excised using a combination of blunt and sharp dissection (i) or a vessel sealing device (ii). The perinodal tissue should be grasped to manipulate the lymph node (iii) rather than directly grasping the lymph node because this will result in trauma to the lymph node.

Closure

The skin incision is closed routinely in two layers with a simple continuous suture pattern using monofilament absorbable suture material in the subcutis and either an interrupted or continuous suture pattern using monofilament nonabsorbable suture material in the skin.

Color Atlas of Canine and Feline Surgical Oncology, First Edition. Julius M. Liptak, Paolo Buracco, William T. N. Culp, and Nicholas J. Bacon.

Plate 50.5

Superficial Cervical (Prescapular) Lymph Node Excision

2-i)

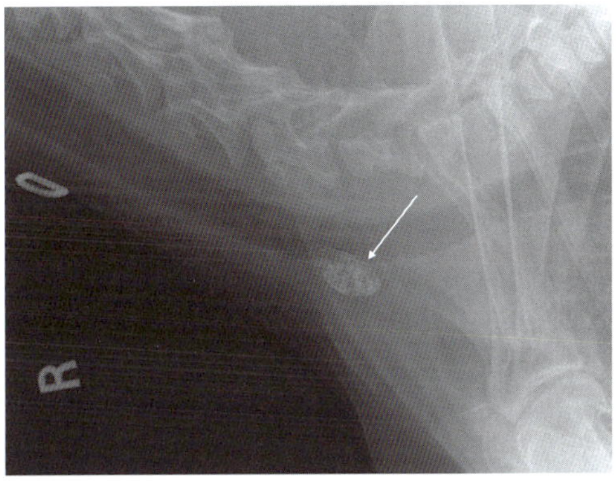

2-ii)

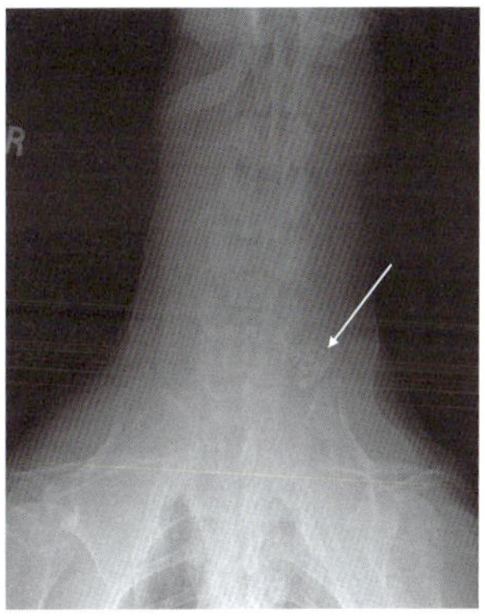

A)

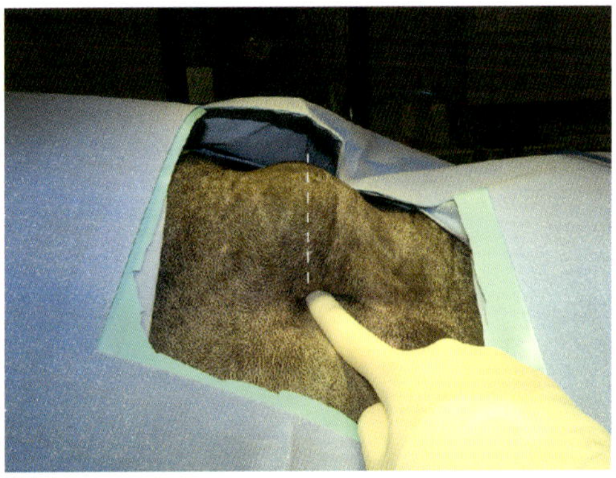

B)

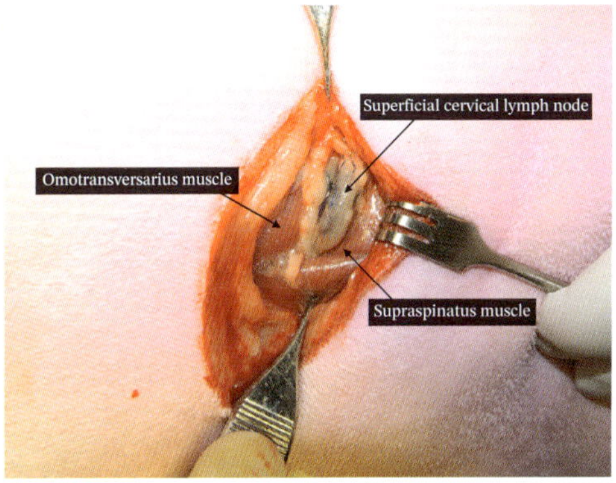

C-i)

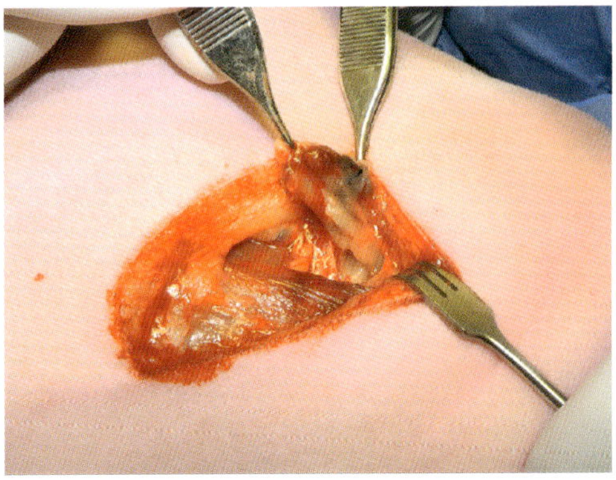

C-ii)

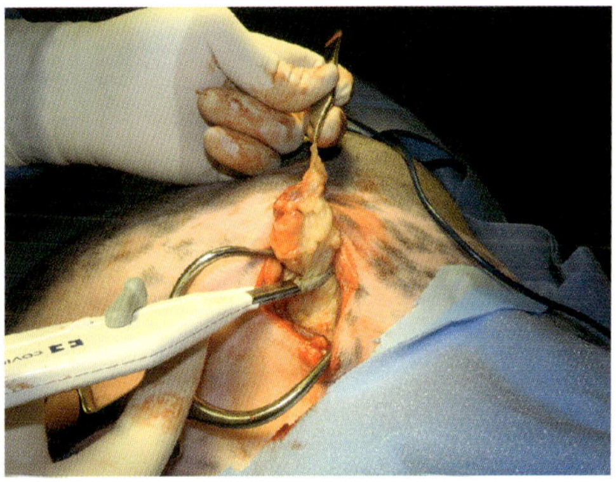

C-iii)

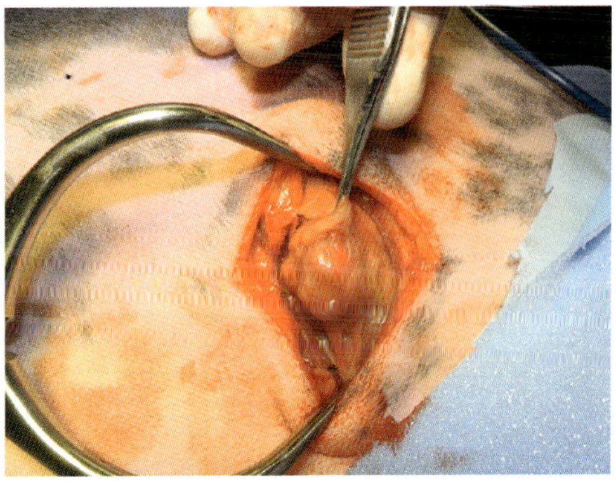

Postoperative Management

1) Multimodal analgesia
2) Elizabethan collar

Complications [1]

Intraoperative Complications

- None reported

Postoperative Complications

- Overall for all lymph node excisions: 21% with 19% being minor and 2% being major
- Overall for superficial cervical lymph node excision: 29%
- Lymphedema (11%)
- Seroma (10%)
- Hematoma (3%)
- Incisional dehiscence (1%)

Reference

1 Chiti, L.E., Gariboldi, E.M., Ferrari, R. et al. (2023). Surgical complications following sentinel lymph node biopsy guided by gamma-probe and methylene blue in 113 tumour-bearing dogs. *Vet. Comp. Oncol.* 21 (1): 62–72.

50.6 Axillary Lymph Node Excision

Indications (See Plate 50.6 – 2, 3)

1) Nonselective lymphadenectomy of the axillary node for clinical staging of malignant thoracic limb tumors
2) Selective lymphadenectomy after sentinel lymph node mapping (pictured, arrow) (see *50.1. Sentinel Lymph Node Mapping*)
3) Lymphadenectomy of a metastatic axillary lymph node (pictured, axillary lymph node metastasis [arrow] from a mammary carcinoma in a cat)

Surgical Technique 1 – Lateral Approach (See Plate 50.6A–G)

A) The patient is positioned in lateral recumbency with the affected side uppermost and the thoracic limb retracted cranially. The limb is tractioned until the costochondral junction of the first rib is easily palpable.
B) A longitudinal 4- to 6-cm curvilinear incision is made through the skin and subcutaneous tissue centered over the costochondral junction of the first rib, running from just caudal to the scapula ending just cranioventral to the costochondral junction of the first rib. Digital palpation of this bony landmark is used throughout the entire approach to orientate the surgeon.
C) The subcutaneous fat is retracted to reveal the latissimus dorsi muscle with the fibers running in a cranioventral direction.
D) A muscle window is made by splitting the fibers slightly cranial and dorsal to the underlying costochondral junction of the first rib.
E) Two self-retaining Gelpi retractors positioned perpendicularly are used to create a window in the latissimus dorsi muscle. Dissection of the underlying adipose tissue is continued dorsal to the deep pectoral muscle, craniodorsal to the costochondral junction, and directed cranially and ventrally into the axillary space. The axillary lymph node is typically cranial, dorsal, and superficial to the costochondral junction of the first rib. It is usually only a few millimeters deep and can be identified embedded in perinodal adipose tissue under the axillary fascia (i, ii). (The axillary lymph node is blue because of intraoperative sentinel lymph node mapping with methylene blue.)

Color Atlas of Canine and Feline Surgical Oncology, First Edition. Julius M. Liptak, Paolo Buracco, William T. N. Culp, and Nicholas J. Bacon.

Plate 50.6

Axillary Lymph Node Excision

2)

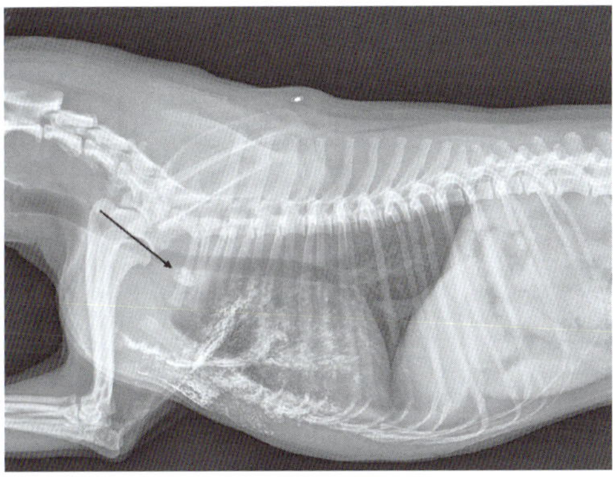

3)

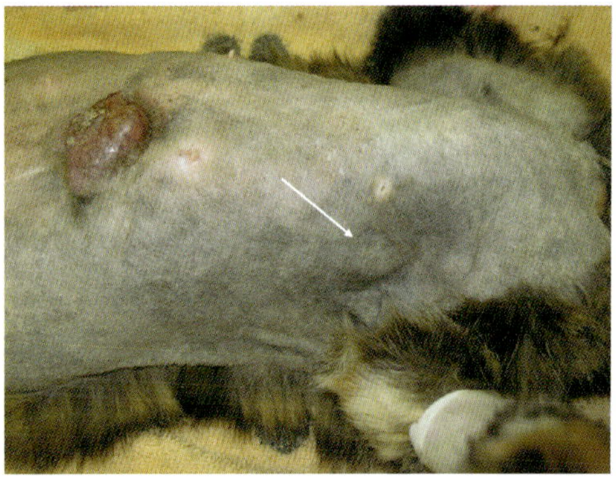

A)

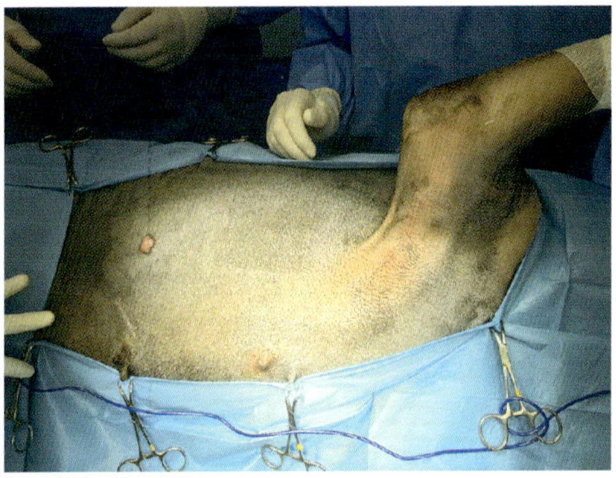

Courtesy of Dr. Dario Drudi

B)

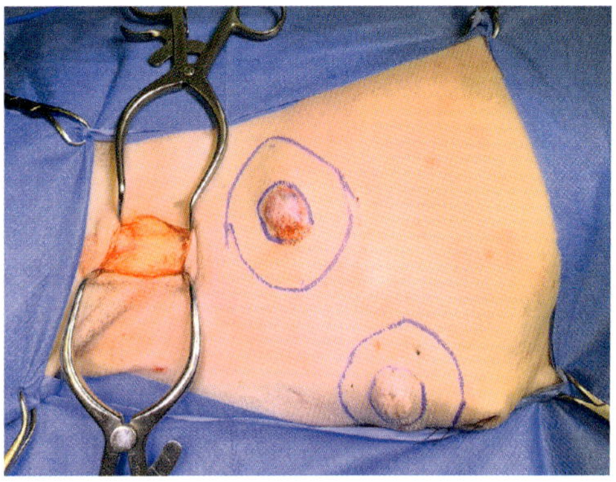

C)

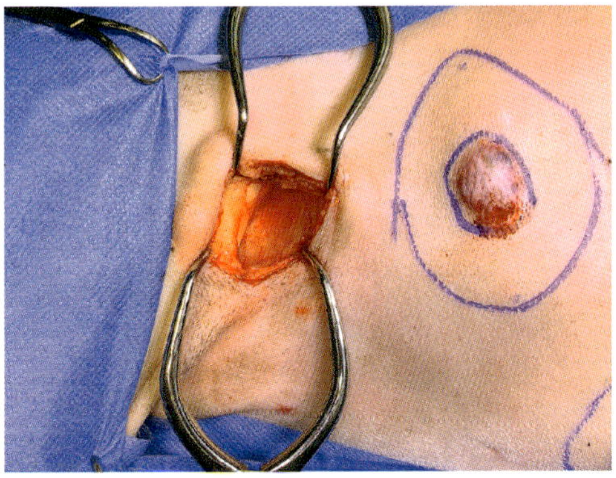

D)

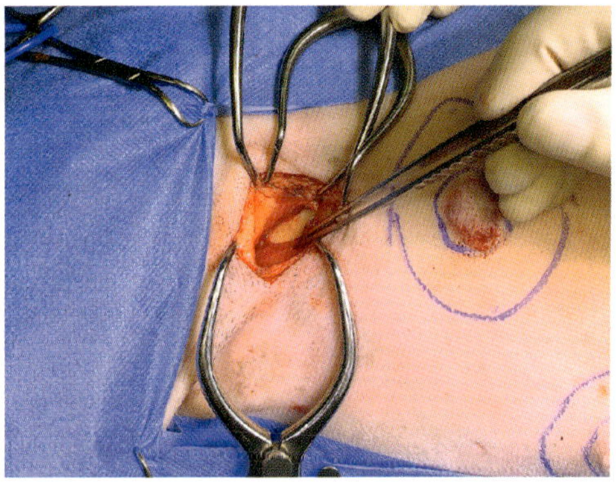

E-i)

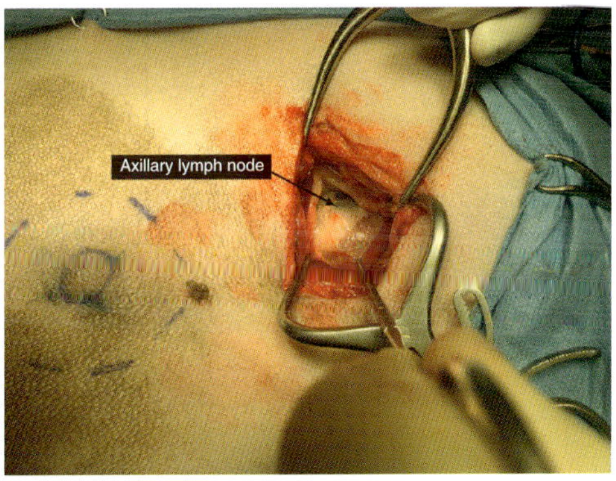

Courtesy of Dr. Maurizio Annoni

E-ii)

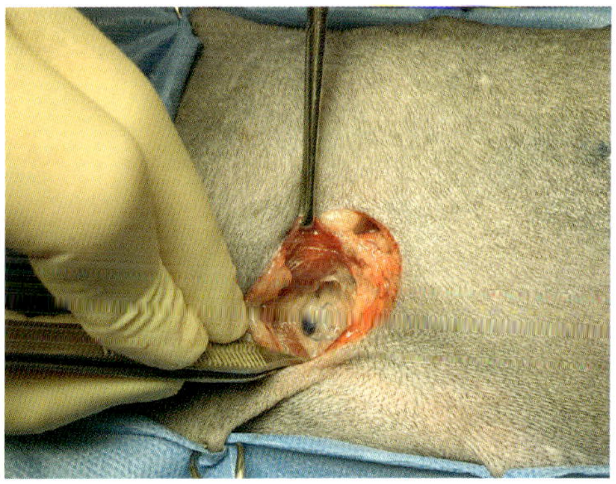

Courtesy of Dr. Maurizio Annoni

Surgical Technique 1 – Lateral Approach (See Plate 50.6A–G) *continued*

F) The node is excised with gentle blunt dissection. Care must be taken because of the proximity of the major vessels (especially the lateral thoracic artery and vein) located deep and cranial to the lymph node.
G) The latissimus dorsi muscle is closed in a simple continuous pattern with 0 to 3-0 monofilament absorbable suture material. The skin incision is closed routinely in two layers with a simple continuous suture pattern using monofilament absorbable suture material in the subcutis (pictured) and either an interrupted or continuous suture pattern using monofilament nonabsorbable suture material in the skin.

Surgical Technique 2 – Ventral Approach [1] (See Plate 50.6I–M)

H) The patient is positioned in dorsal recumbency with the thoracic limb retracted cranially (not pictured).
I) A cranial-to-caudal skin incision is made over the depression between the intersection of the pectoralis profundus and latissimus dorsi muscles. The cranial end of the incision starts at the caudal border of the humerus, and the caudal end of the incision extends to the second rib.
J) The subcutaneous tissue is dissected with Metzenbaum scissors to expose the border between the pectoralis profundus and latissimus dorsi muscles.
K) Blunt dissection is continued between these muscles and dorsally into the axillary space.
L) The axillary lymph node is located immediately caudal to the brachial vein. The axillary lymph node is excised using a combination of blunt and sharp dissection or with a vessel sealing device.
M) The lymphatic trunk at the caudal pole of the axillary lymph node is followed caudally with blunt dissection until the accessory axillary lymph node is identified deep to the lateral margin of the pectoralis profundus muscle. The accessory axillary lymph node is also excised using a combination of blunt and sharp dissection or with a vessel sealing device.
N) The skin incision is closed routinely in two layers with a simple continuous suture pattern using monofilament absorbable suture material in the subcutis and either an interrupted or continuous suture pattern using monofilament nonabsorbable suture material in the skin (not pictured).

Postoperative Management

1) Multimodal analgesia
2) Elizabethan collar or body suit

Complications [2]

Intraoperative Complications

- None reported

Postoperative Complications

- Overall for all lymph node excisions: 21% with 19% being minor and 2% being major
- Overall for axillary lymph node excision: 14%
- Lymphedema (11%)
- Seroma (10%)
- Hematoma (3%)
- Incisional dehiscence (1%)

References

1 Rehnblom, E.R., Skinner, O.T., Mickelson, M.A.S. et al. (2022). Axillary lymphadenectomy in dogs: a description of surgical technique. *Vet. Comp. Oncol.* 20 (3): 664–668.
2 Chiti, L.E., Gariboldi, E.M., Ferrari, R. et al. (2023). Surgical complications following sentinel lymph node biopsy guided by gamma-probe and methylene blue in 113 tumour-bearing dogs. *Vet. Comp. Oncol.* 21 (1): 62–72.

Plate 50.6

Axillary Lymph Node Excision *continued*

F)

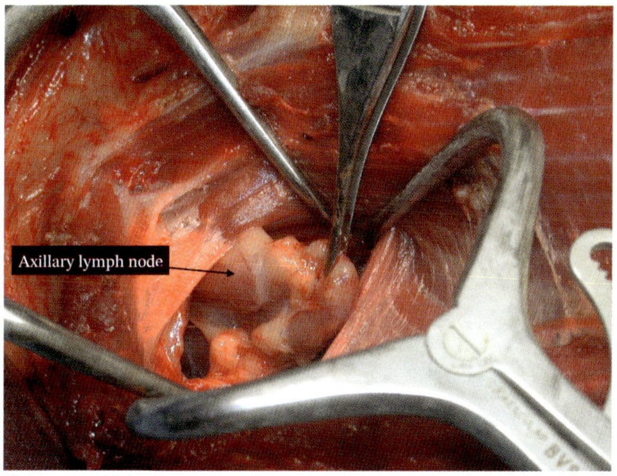

Courtesy of Dr. Dario Drudi

G)

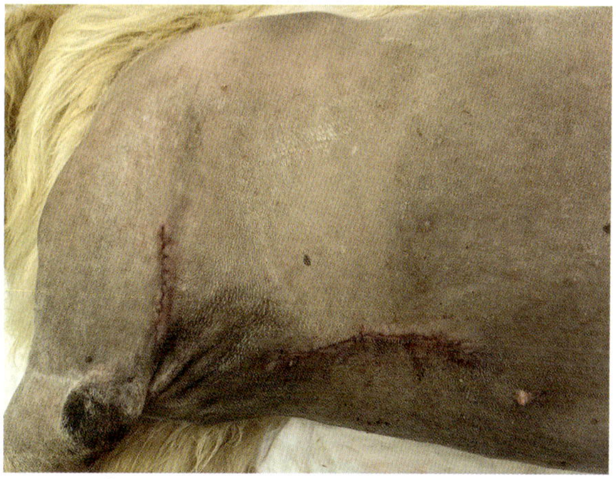

Courtesy of Dr. Maurizio Annoni

I)

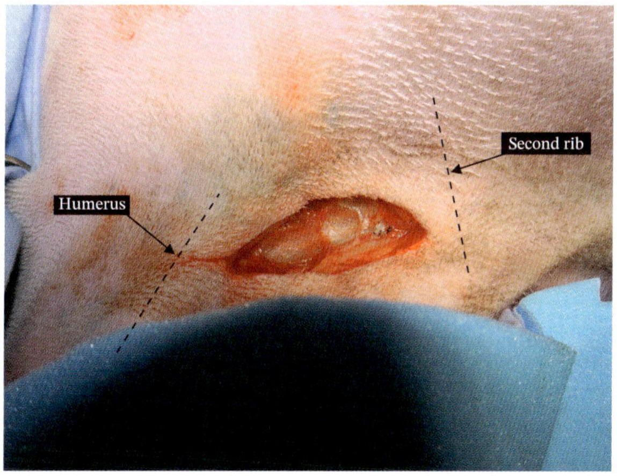

J/K)

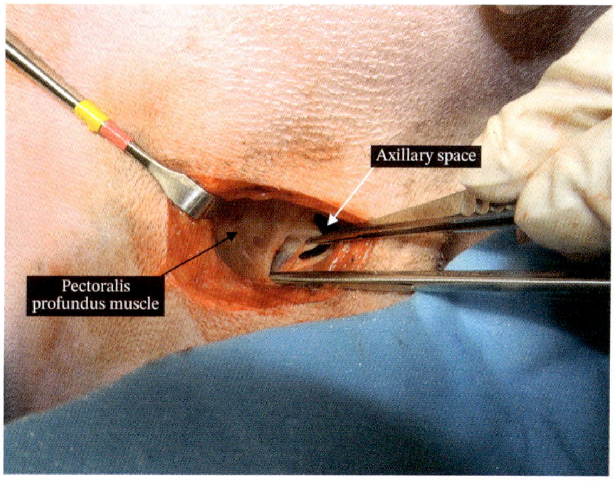

L)

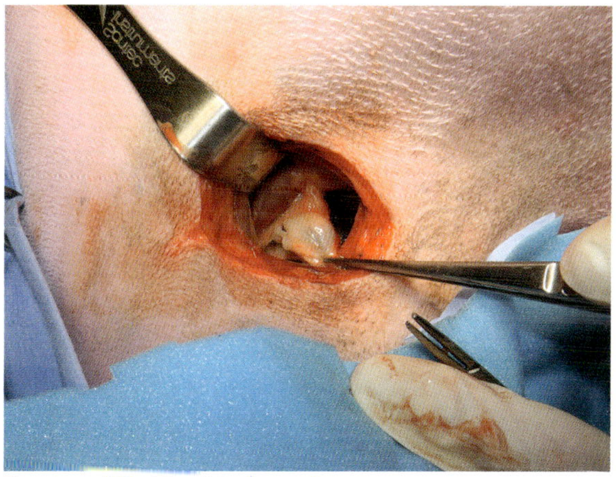

M)

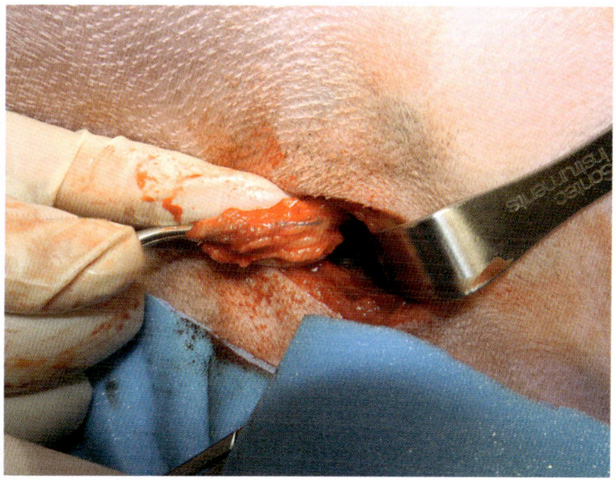

Courtesy of Dr. Maurizio Annoni

50.7 Superficial Inguinal Lymph Node Excision

Indications (See Plate 50.7 – 2)

1) Nonselective lymphadenectomy for clinical staging of malignant mammary or pelvic limb tumors
2) Selective lymphadenectomy after sentinel lymph node mapping (i, ii, preoperative sentinel lymph node mapping in a dog with a cutaneous mast cell tumor, arrow) (see *50.1. Sentinel Lymph Node Mapping*)
3) Lymphadenectomy of a metastatic superficial inguinal lymph node

Patient Positioning

The patient is positioned in dorsal recumbency.

Surgical Technique (See Plate 50.7A, B)

A) A skin incision is made immediately lateral and adjacent to the fifth mammary gland (i, female dog with a cutaneous mast cell tumor; ii, male dog with a preputial mast cell tumor; the superficial inguinal lymph node is blue because of intraoperative sentinel lymph node mapping with methylene blue).
B) The superficial inguinal lymphocentrum is located in the subcutaneous fat and inguinal fat pad along the caudal-to-caudolateral aspect of the caudal superficial epigastric vein. The superficial inguinal lymphocentrum includes one or more lymph nodes (i, arrows). Once the caudal superficial epigastric vein is identified (ii), the superficial inguinal lymph node is excised using a combination of blunt and sharp dissection (iii) or with a vessel sealing device (iv). The perinodal tissue should be grasped to manipulate the lymph node (v) rather than directly grasping the lymph node because this will result in trauma to the lymph node. The caudal superficial epigastrc vein should be preserved.

Color Atlas of Canine and Feline Surgical Oncology, First Edition. Julius M. Liptak, Paolo Buracco, William T. N. Culp, and Nicholas J. Bacon.

Plate 50.7

Superficial Inguinal Lymph Node Excision

2-i)

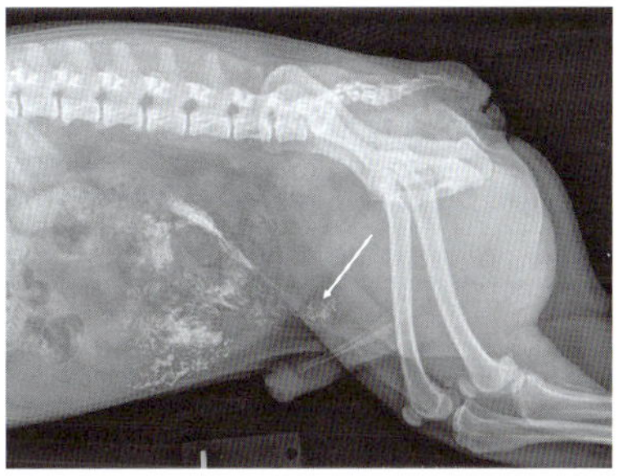

2-ii)

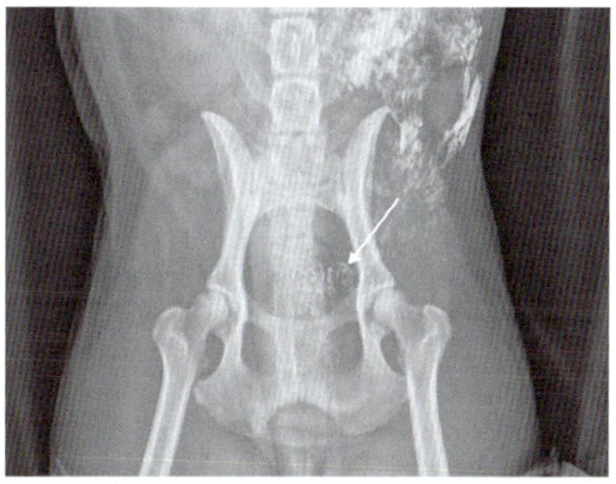

A-i)

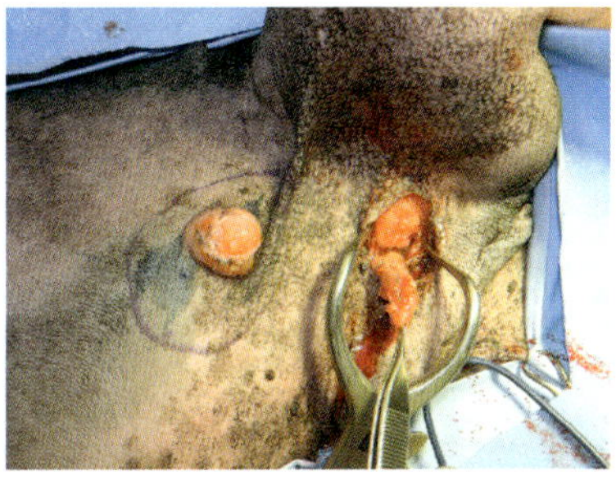

A-ii)

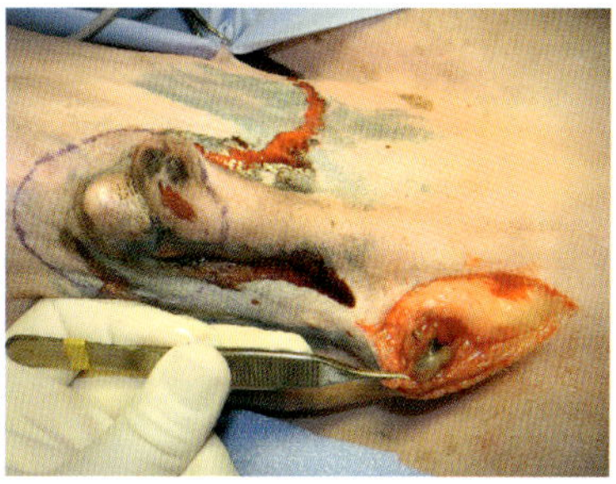

B-i)

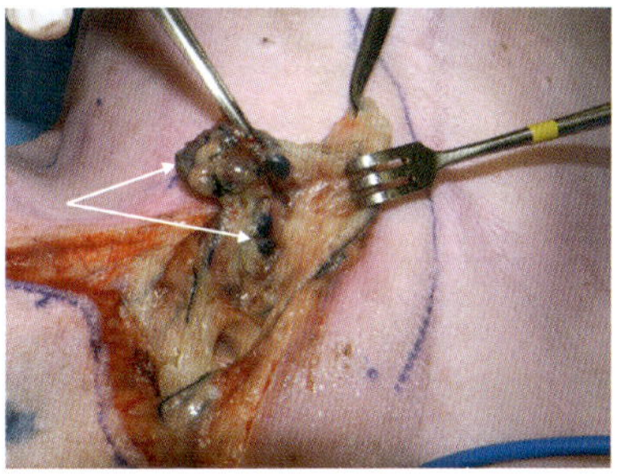

B-ii)

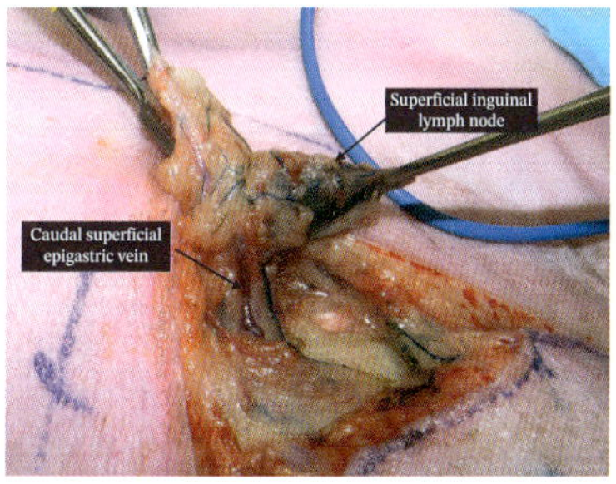

B-iii)

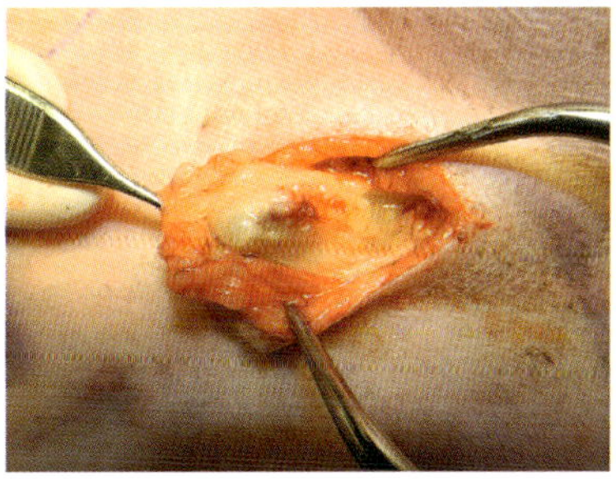

B-iv)

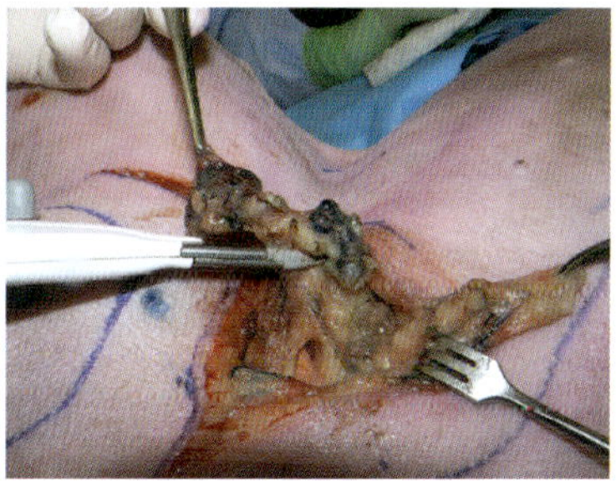

B-v)

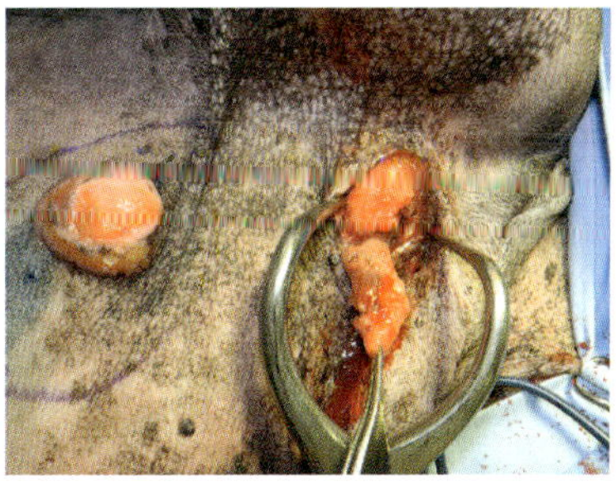

Closure (See Plate 50.7C)

C) The skin incision is closed routinely in two layers with a simple continuous suture pattern using monofilament absorbable suture material in the subcutis and either an interrupted (pictured) or continuous suture pattern using monofilament nonabsorbable suture material in the skin.

Postoperative Management

1) Multimodal analgesia
2) Elizabethan collar or body suit

Complications [1]

Intraoperative Complications

- None reported

Postoperative Complications

- Overall for all lymph node excisions: 21% with 19% being minor and 2% being major
- Overall for axillary lymph node excision: 21%
- Lymphedema (11%)
- Seroma (10%)
- Hematoma (3%)
- Incisional dehiscence (1%)

Reference

1 Chiti, L.E., Gariboldi, E.M., Ferrari, R. et al. (2023). Surgical complications following sentinel lymph node biopsy guided by gamma-probe and methylene blue in 113 tumour-bearing dogs. *Vet. Comp. Oncol.* 21 (1): 62–72.

Plate 50.7

Superficial Inguinal Lymph Node Excision *continued*

C)

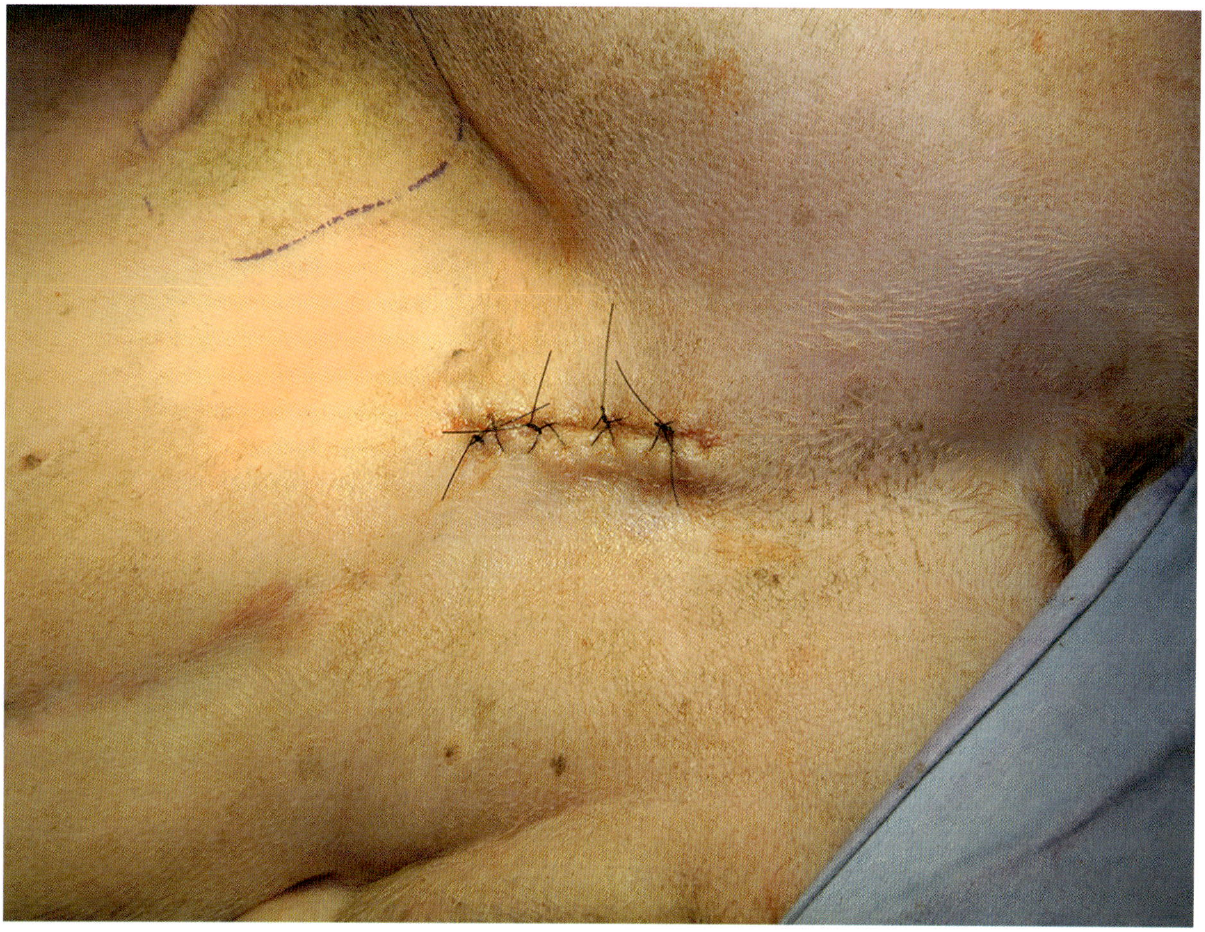

50.8 Popliteal Lymph Node Excision

Indications

1) Nonselective lymphadenectomy for clinical staging of malignant tumors at or distal to the stifle on the ipsilateral pelvic limb
2) Selective lymphadenectomy after sentinel lymph node mapping (see *50.1. Sentinel Lymph Node Mapping*)
3) Lymphadenectomy of a metastatic popliteal lymph node

Patient Positioning

The patient is positioned in lateral recumbency with the affected side uppermost.

Surgical Technique (See Plate 50.8A–C)

A) The popliteal lymph node is palpated in the popliteal fossa along the caudolateral aspect of the distal thigh (i) and a skin incision is made over the lymph node (ii).
B) The popliteal lymphocentrum, which typically includes a single lymph node but occasionally two lymph nodes, is located in the subcutaneous fat between the biceps femoris and semitendinosus muscles (i). The subcutaneous fat can make visual identification of the lymph node difficult (ii, arrow), but the lymph node is the only solid, rounded structure in this region (iii, arrow). The lateral saphenous vein courses over the cranial and lateral aspect of the popliteal lymph node and should be preserved.
C) The perinodal tissue should be grasped to manipulate the lymph node (i) rather than directly grasping the lymph node because this will result in trauma to the lymph node. The popliteal lymph node is excised using a combination of blunt and sharp dissection or a vessel sealing device (ii).

Closure (See Plate 50.8D)

D) The skin incision is closed routinely in two layers with a simple continuous suture pattern using monofilament absorbable suture material in the subcutis and either an interrupted or continuous suture pattern (pictured) using monofilament nonabsorbable suture material in the skin.

Color Atlas of Canine and Feline Surgical Oncology, First Edition. Julius M. Liptak, Paolo Buracco, William T. N. Culp, and Nicholas J. Bacon.

Plate 50.8

Popliteal Lymph Node Excision

A-i)

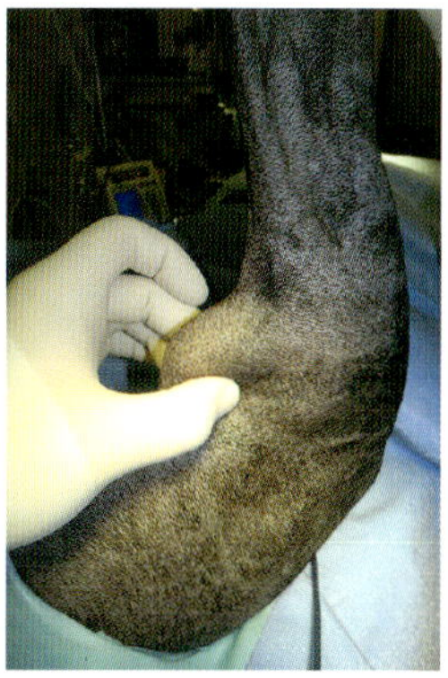

A-ii)

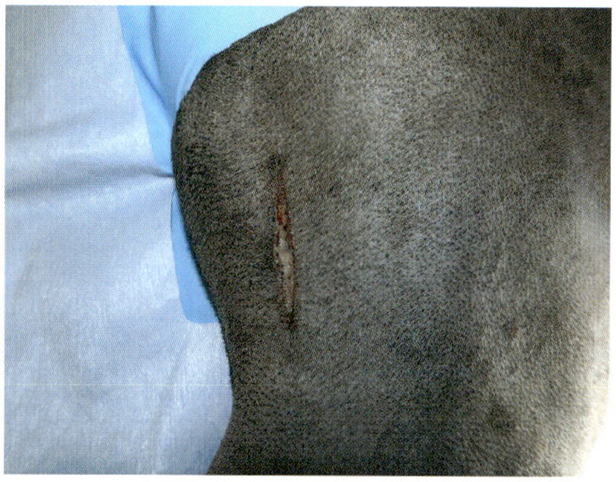

B-i)

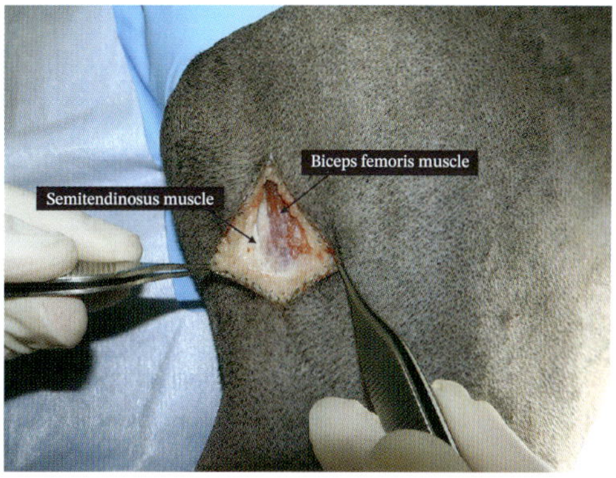

B-ii)

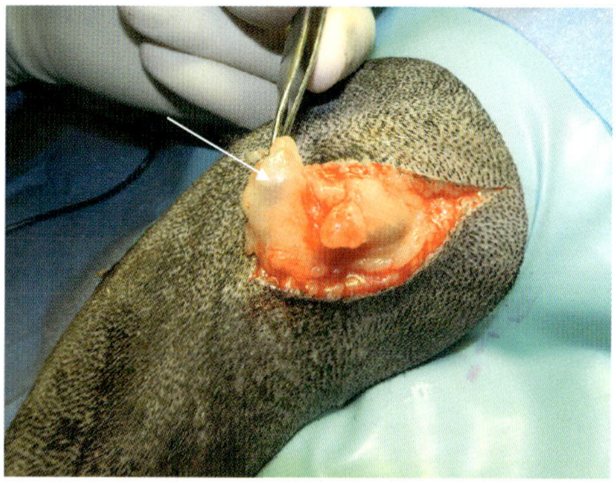

B-iii)

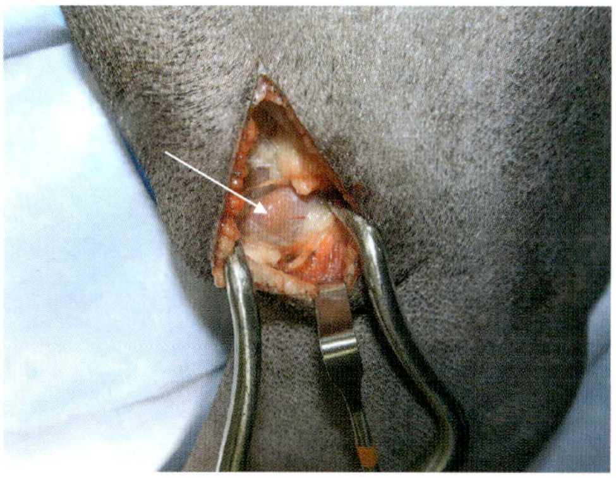

C-i)

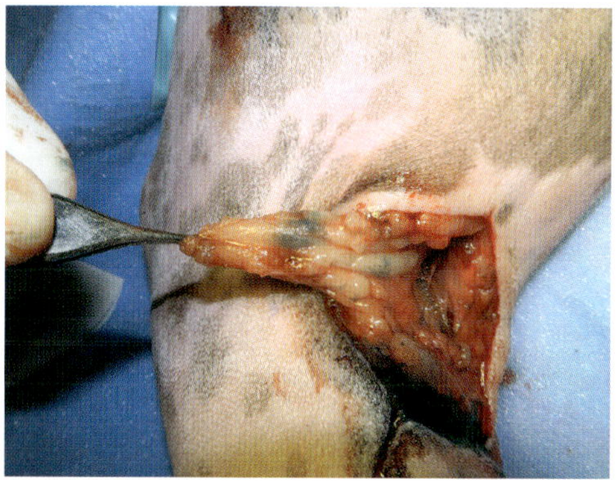

C-ii)

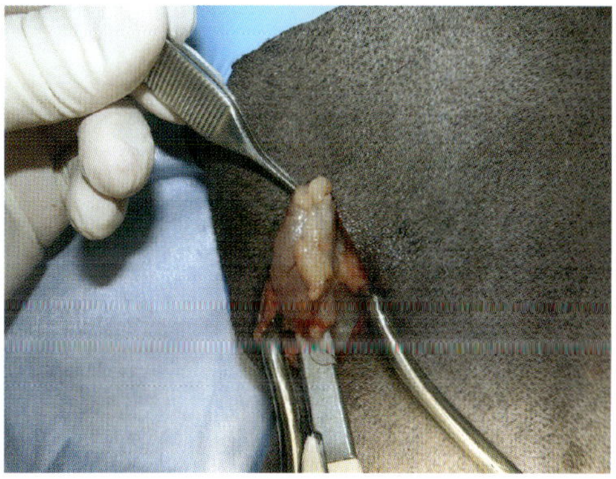

D)

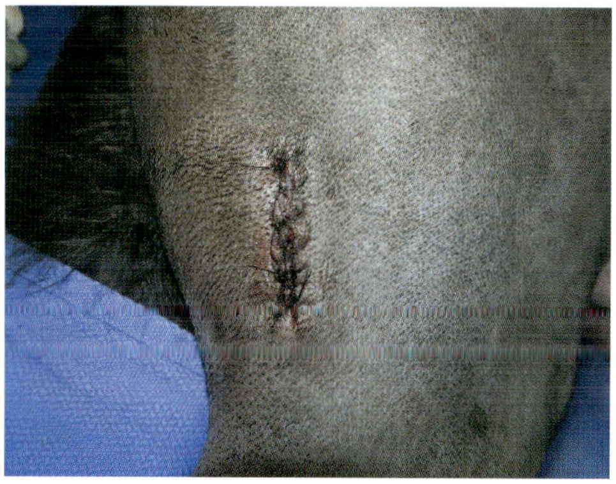

Postoperative Management

1) Multimodal analgesia
2) Elizabethan collar

Complications [1]

Intraoperative Complications

- None reported

Postoperative Complications

- Overall for all lymph node excisions: 21% with 19% being minor and 2% being major
- Overall for popliteal lymph node excision: 21%
- Lymphedema (11%)
- Seroma (10%)
- Hematoma (3%)
- Incisional dehiscence (1%)

Reference

1 Chiti, L.E., Gariboldi, E.M., Ferrari, R. et al. (2023). Surgical complications following sentinel lymph node biopsy guided by gamma-probe and methylene blue in 113 tumour-bearing dogs. *Vet. Comp. Oncol.* 21 (1): 62–72.

Chapter 51: Mastectomy

Mammary tumors can be resected using a spectrum of surgical doses, ranging from local to regional to unilateral to single-session or staged bilateral mastectomy. In dogs, the surgical dose does not result in an improvement in prognosis, and the type of mastectomy performed should be dependent on the location and number of mammary masses. In cats with malignant mammary carcinomas, survival times increase significantly as the surgical dose increases, and bilateral mastectomy is the preferred treatment, either in a single session or staged by 4–6 weeks. Ovariohysterectomy is recommended in intact female dogs to reduce the risk of further mammary tumor development [1, 2]. Although ovariohysterectomy is also recommended in intact female cats, the role of ovariohysterectomy in reducing further mammary tumor development is unknown.

Suggested Diagnostic Workup and Clinical Staging

- Complete blood count, serum biochemistry, and urinalysis
- ± Fine-needle aspirate, core aspirate, or needle-core biopsy
- ± Sentinel lymph node mapping or regional lymph node fine-needle aspirate cytology, dependent on tumor type
- ± Abdominal ultrasound or computed tomography (CT) scan, dependent on tumor type
- ± Three-view thoracic radiographs or thoracic CT scan for assessment of lung metastasis, dependent on tumor type

Suggested Adjuvant Treatments

- ± Chemotherapy depending on tumor type and histologic grade

Prognosis and Oncologic Outcome – Dogs

	Local Recurrence Rate	Metastatic Rate	Disease-Free Interval (d)	Median Survival Time (d)	1-Year Survival Rate	2-Year Survival Rate
			Mammary Carcinoma			
Overall [3]	–	–	1720	496	57%	38%
			Clinical stage[a] [4]			
Stage 1	–	–	–	1226	61%	61%
Stage 2	–	–	–	924	60%	60%
Stage 3	–	–	–	287	31%	10%
Stage 4	–	–	–	165	29%	14%
Stage 5	–	–	–	224	44%	29%

Color Atlas of Canine and Feline Surgical Oncology, First Edition. Julius M. Liptak, Paolo Buracco, William T. N. Culp, and Nicholas J. Bacon.

	Local Recurrence Rate	Metastatic Rate	Disease-Free Interval (d)	Median Survival Time (d)	1-Year Survival Rate	2-Year Survival Rate
			Clinical stage[b] [3]			
Stage 0	–	–	NR	1241	90%	–
Stage I	–	–	1720	813	83%	–
Stage II	–	–	NR	464	61%	–
Stage IIIA	–	–	423	213	35%	–
Stage IIIB	–	–	241	123	23%	–
			Tumor ulceration [4]			
No	–	–	–	443	53%	45%
Yes	–	–	–	118	11%	5%
			Perioperative desmopressin – grade 2 [5]			
No	–	–	85	351	–	–
Yes	–	–	>600	>600	–	–
			Perioperative desmopressin – grade 3 [5]			
No	–	–	26	35	–	–
Yes	–	–	>600	>600	–	–
			Surgical margins [4]			
Complete	–	–	–	872	56%	51%
Incomplete	–	–	–	70	15%	0%
			Lymphatic invasion [4]			
No	–	–	–	1098	66%	63%
Yes	–	–	–	179	29%	13%
			Extraskeletal Mammary Osteosarcoma [6]			
Overall	–	63%	–	90	–	–

[a] Modified TNM staging system [4].
[b] Modified histologic staging system [3].
NR, not reached.

Modified TNM Staging System [4]

Stage	Tumor Size	Nodal Metastasis	Distant Metastasis
1	<3 cm	Negative	Negative
2	3–5 cm	Negative	Negative
3	>5 cm	Negative	Negative
4	Any size	Positive	Negative
5	Any size	Negative or positive	Positive

Modified Histologic Staging System [3]

Stage	Invasiveness	Pathologic Tumor Size	Lymphovascular Invasion	Nodal Status
0	In situ	Any size	Negative	Negative or unknown
I	Invasive	pT1 ≤ 20 mm	Negative	Negative or unknown
II	Invasive	pT2 > 20 mm	Negative	Negative or unknown
IIIA	Invasive	pT1 ≤ 20 mm	Lymphovascular invasion positive and/or nodal metastasis positive	
IIIB	Invasive	pT2 > 20 mm	Lymphovascular invasion positive and/or nodal metastasis positive	

Prognosis and Oncologic Outcome – Cats

	Local Recurrence Rate	Metastatic Rate	Disease-Free Interval (d)	Median Survival Time (d)	1-Year Survival Rate	2-Year Survival Rate
Overall [7]	–	–	438	377	53%	30%
Clinical stage[a] [7]						
Stage 0	–	–	1484	999	72%	–
Stage I	–	–	496	545	67%	–
Stage II	–	–	366	355	48%	–
Stage IIIA	–	–	473	372	53%	–
Stage IIIB	–	–	237	175	21%	–
Surgical dose [8–10]						
Local/Regional mastectomy	–	86%	–	428	–	–
Unilateral mastectomy	47%	25% (lymph node) 38% (distant)	–	348–473	–	–
Bilateral mastectomy	13%–20%	33% (overall) 4% (lymph node) 33% (distant)	342 (local recurrence) 269 (metastasis)	1140–3145	67%	67%
Histologic grade [11]						
Grade 1	–	–	–	943	–	–
Grade 2	–	–	–	426	–	–
Grade 3	–	–	–	243	–	–
Chemotherapy – unilateral mastectomy only [12]						
Yes	–	–	–	1998	–	–
No	–	–	–	441	–	–
Development of metastatic disease [10]						
Yes	–	–	–	331	–	–
No	–	–	–	>2100	–	–

	Local Recurrence Rate	Metastatic Rate	Disease-Free Interval (d)	Median Survival Time (d)	1-Year Survival Rate	2-Year Survival Rate
			Site of metastasis [10]			
Lymph node	–	–	–	1543	–	–
Lungs	–	–	–	331	–	–
Pleura	–	–	–	188	–	–

[a] Modified histologic staging system [7].

Modified Histologic Staging System [7]

Stage	Invasiveness	Pathologic Tumor Size	Lymphovascular Invasion	Nodal Status
0	In situ	Any size	Negative	Negative or unknown
I	Invasive	pT1 $\leq$ 20 mm	Negative	Negative or unknown
II	Invasive	pT2 > 20 mm	Negative	Negative or unknown
IIIA	Invasive	pT1 $\leq$ 20 mm	Lymphovascular invasion positive and/or nodal metastasis positive	
IIIB	Invasive	pT2 > 20 mm	Lymphovascular invasion positive and/or nodal metastasis positive	

References

1 Sorenmo, K.U., Shofer, F.S., and Goldschmidt, M.H. (2000). Effect of spaying and timing of spaying on survival of dogs with mammary carcinoma. *J. Vet. Intern. Med.* 14 (3): 266–270.

2 Kristiansen, V.M., Nødtvedt, A.M., Breen, A.M. et al. (2013). Effect of ovariohysterectomy at the time of tumor removal in dogs with benign mammary tumors and hyperplastic lesions: a randomized controlled clinical study. *J. Vet. Intern. Med.* 27 (4): 935–942.

3 Chocteau, F., Abadie, J., Loussouarn, D. et al. (2019). Proposal for a histologic staging system of mammary carcinomas in dogs and cats. Part 1: canine mammary cancers. *Front. Vet. Sci.* 6: 388.

4 Tran, C.M., Moore, A.S., and Frimberger, A.E. (2016). Surgical treatment of mammary carcinomas in dogs with or without postoperative chemotherapy. *Vet. Comp. Oncol.* 14 (3): 252–262.

5 Hermo, G.A., Turic, E., Angelico, D. et al. (2011). Effect of adjuvant perioperative desmopressin in locally advanced canine mammary carcinoma and its relation to histologic grade. *J. Am. Anim. Hosp. Assoc.* 47 (1): 21–27.

6 Langenbach, A., Anderson, M.A., Dambach, D.M. et al. (1998). Extraskeletal osteosarcomas in dogs: a retrospective study of 169 cases (1986-1996). *J. Am. Anim. Hosp. Assoc.* 34 (2): 113–120.

7 Chocteau, F., Boulay, M.M., Besnard, F. et al. (2019). Proposal for a histologic staging system of mammary carcinomas in dogs and cats. Part 2: feline mammary cancers. *Front. Vet. Sci.* 6: 387.

8 Gemignani, F., Mayhew, P.D., Giuffrida, M.A. et al. (2018). Association of surgical approach with complication rate, progression-free survival time, and disease-specific survival time in cats with mammary adenocarcinoma: 107 cases (1991-2014). *J. Am. Vet. Med. Assoc.* 252 (11): 1393–1402.

9 Wood, C.J., Chu, M.L., Selmic, L.E. et al. (2021). Effect of perioperative desmopressin in cats with mammary carcinoma treated with bilateral mastectomy. *Vet. Comp. Oncol.* 19 (4): 724–734.

10 Novosad, C.A., Bergman, P.J., O'Brien, M.G. et al. (2006). Retrospective evaluation of adjunctive doxorubicin for the treatment of feline mammary gland adenocarcinoma: 67 cases. *J. Am. Anim. Hosp. Assoc.* 42: 110–120.

11 Mills, S.W., Musil, K.M., Davies, J.L. et al. (2015). Prognostic value of histologic grading for feline mammary carcinoma: a retrospective survival analysis. *Vet. Pathol.* 52 (2): 238–249.

12 McNeill, C.J., Sorenmo, K.U., Shofer, F.S. et al. (2009). Evaluation of adjuvant doxorubicin-based chemotherapy for the treatment of feline mammary carcinoma. *J. Vet. Intern. Med.* 23 (1): 123–129.

51.1 Local Mastectomy

Indications

1) The primary indication is resection of a centrally located benign or malignant mammary tumor involving a single mammary gland.
2) Local mastectomy can be combined with sentinel lymph node mapping (see *50.1. Sentinel Lymph Node Mapping*), axillary lymph node excision (see *50.6. Axillary Lymph Node Excision*), and/or superficial inguinal lymph node excision (see *50.7. Superficial Inguinal Lymph Node Excision*).
3) Local mastectomy should be combined with ovariohysterectomy in intact female dogs to reduce the risk of further de novo mammary tumor development [1, 2]. The effect of ovariohysterectomy on de novo mammary tumor development in cats has not been reported; however, ovariohysterectomy should be strongly considered in intact female cats. Ovariohysterectomy can be performed either before or after the local mastectomy is done.

Suggested Diagnostic Workup and Clinical Staging

See *51. Mastectomy*.

Patient Positioning

The patient is positioned in dorsal recumbency.

Surgical Technique (See Plate 51.1A–C)

A) A sterile marker pen can be used to mark a minimum of 1-cm lateral margins around the tumor (i), and skin incision is made along the marked margins (ii).
B) Dissection is continued deeply through the subcutaneous and mammary tissue perpendicular to the skin incision to the abdominal wall. The mammary glands are tightly adhered to the superficial pectoral muscles in the thoracic portion of the mammary glands, so partial pectoral muscle resection is often required en bloc during a local mastectomy of the first, second, or third mammary glands in dogs (i) and the first or second mammary glands in cats. For mammary tumors involving the third, fourth, or fifth mammary glands in dogs and the third or fourth mammary glands in cats, the external abdominal muscle fascia or partial- to full-thickness abdominal musculature deep to the mammary tumor, depending on the invasiveness of the mammary tumor, is resected en bloc with the local mastectomy for deep margins (ii).

Color Atlas of Canine and Feline Surgical Oncology, First Edition. Julius M. Liptak, Paolo Buracco, William T. N. Culp, and Nicholas J. Bacon.

Plate 51.1

Local Mastectomy

A-i)

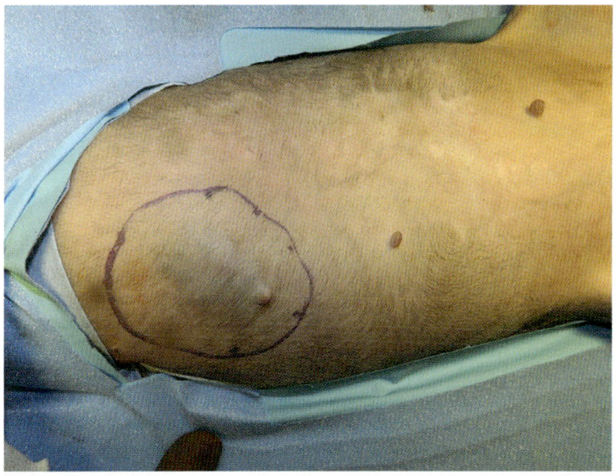

A-ii)

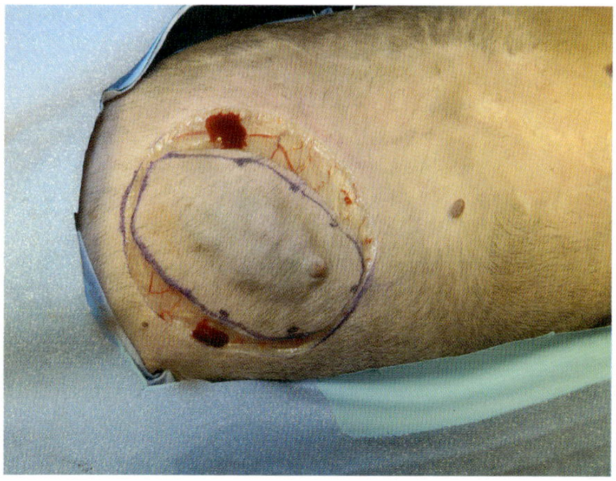

B-i)

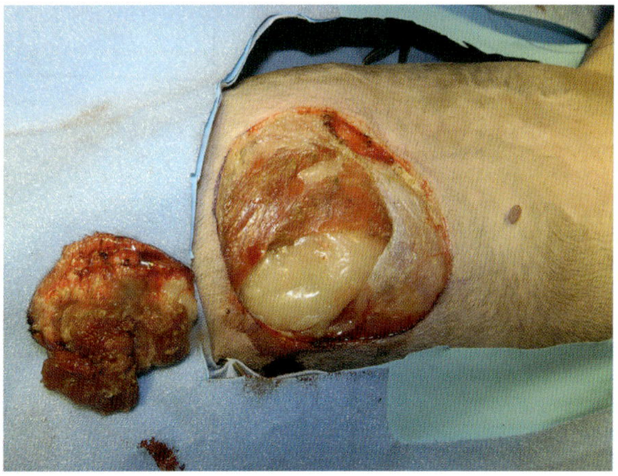

B-ii)

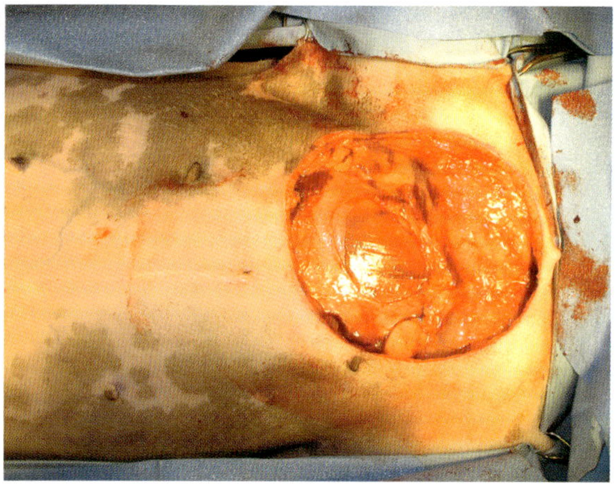

Surgical Technique (See Plate 51.1A–C) *continued*

C) For local mastectomies involving the caudal-most mammary gland (fifth in dogs and fourth in cats), the caudal superficial epigastric artery and vein should be ligated and divided or sealed and transected with a vessel sealing device. Instead of specifically dissecting the superficial inguinal lymph node in these cases, the inguinal fat pad can be resected en bloc with the regional mastectomy as the superficial inguinal lymph node is contained within the inguinal fat pad.

Closure (See Plate 51.1D)

D) Fascial or abdominal wall defects are closed with 0 to 2-0 absorbable monofilament suture material in a simple interrupted (i) or continuous suture pattern. The skin incision is closed routinely in two layers with a simple continuous suture pattern using monofilament absorbable suture material in the subcutis and either an interrupted or continuous suture pattern using monofilament nonabsorbable suture material in the skin (ii).

Postoperative Management

1) Multimodal analgesia
2) Elizabethan collar or body suit

Complications – Dogs

- Overall: 3%–12% [3, 4]
- Surgical-site infection (2%) [4]
- Seroma (7% overall for all types of mastectomies) [4]
- Incisional dehiscence (3% overall for all types of mastectomies) [4]

Suggested Adjuvant Treatments

- See *51. Mastectomy*.

Prognosis and Oncologic Outcome

- See *51. Mastectomy*.

References

1 Sorenmo, K.U., Shofer, F.S., and Goldschmidt, M.H. (2000). Effect of spaying and timing of spaying on survival of dogs with mammary carcinoma. *J. Vet. Intern. Med.* 14 (3): 266–270.

2 Kristiansen, V.M., Nødtvedt, A.M., Breen, A.M. et al. (2013). Effect of ovariohysterectomy at the time of tumor removal in dogs with benign mammary tumors and hyperplastic lesions: a randomized controlled clinical study. *J. Vet. Intern. Med.* 27 (4): 935–942.

3 Brooks, A., Evans, B.J., Holt, D.E. et al. (2021). Factors influencing complications following mastectomy procedures in dogs with mammary gland tumors: 140 cases (2009-2015). *J. Am. Vet. Med. Assoc.* 258 (3): 295–302.

4 Spåre, P., Ljungvall, I., Ljungvall, K. et al. (2021). Evaluation of post-operative complications after mastectomy peformed with and without perioperative antimicrobial prophylaxis in dogs. *Acta Vet. Scand.* 63 (1): 35.

Plate 51.1

Local Mastectomy *continued*

C)

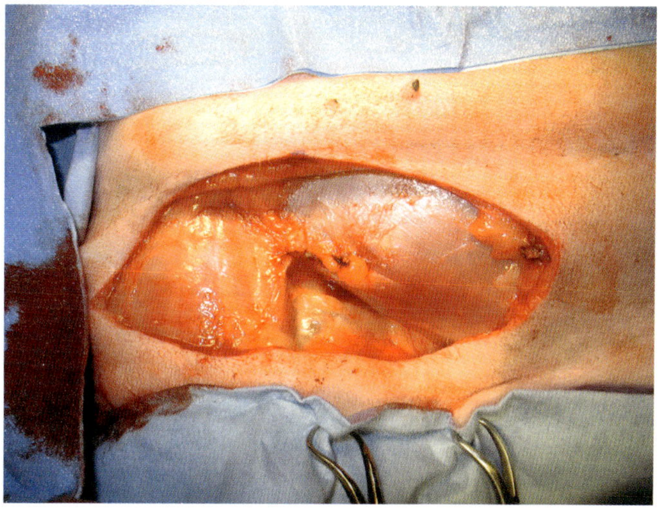

D-i)

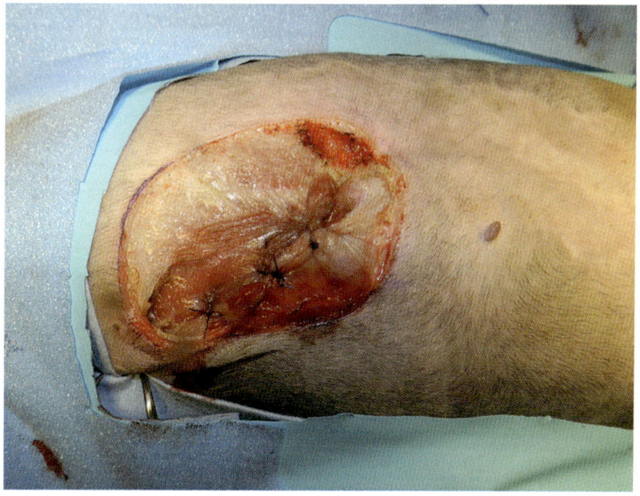

D-ii)

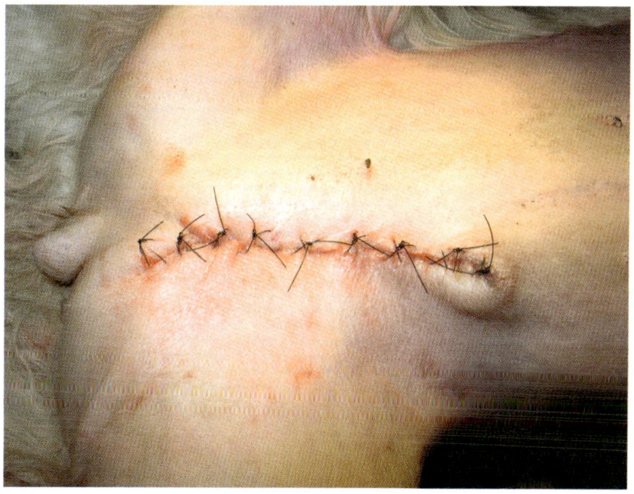

51.2 Regional Mastectomy

Indications (See Plate 51.2 – 1)

1) Resection of a single benign or malignant mammary mass involving two to three adjacent mammary glands (pictured, mammary carcinoma in a dog), or two or more benign or malignant mammary masses involving two to three adjacent mammary glands. Regional mastectomy has also been more specifically defined based on the regional blood supply and lymphatics as resection of either the first and second mammary glands or the fourth and fifth mammary glands in dogs.
2) Regional mastectomy can be combined with sentinel lymph node mapping (see *50.1. Sentinel Lymph Node Mapping*), axillary lymph node excision (see *50.6. Axillary Lymph Node Excision*), and/or superficial inguinal lymph node excision (see *50.7. Superficial Inguinal Lymph Node Excision*).
3) Regional mastectomy should be combined with ovariohysterectomy in intact female dogs to reduce the risk of further de novo mammary tumor development [1, 2]. The effect of ovariohysterectomy on de novo mammary tumor development in cats has not been reported; however, ovariohysterectomy should be strongly considered in intact female cats. Ovariohysterectomy can be performed either before or after the regional mastectomy is done.

Suggested Diagnostic Workup and Clinical Staging

- See *51. Mastectomy*.

Patient Positioning

The patient is positioned in dorsal recumbency.

Surgical Technique (See Plate 51.2A–C)

A) A sterile marker pen can be used to mark a minimum of 1-cm lateral margins around the tumor (i), and skin incision is made along the marked margins (ii).
B) Dissection is continued deeply through the subcutaneous and mammary tissue perpendicular to the skin incision to the abdominal wall. The mammary glands are tightly adhered to the superficial pectoral muscles in the thoracic portion of the mammary glands, so partial pectoral muscle resection is often required en bloc during a regional mastectomy of the first to third mammary glands in dogs and the first and second mammary glands in cats. For mammary tumors involving the third to fifth mammary glands in dogs and the third and fourth mammary glands in cats, the external abdominal muscle fascia or partial- to full-thickness abdominal musculature deep to the mammary tumor, depending on the invasiveness of the mammary tumor, is resected en bloc with the regional mastectomy for deep margins (pictured).

Color Atlas of Canine and Feline Surgical Oncology, First Edition. Julius M. Liptak, Paolo Buracco, William T. N. Culp, and Nicholas J. Bacon.

Plate 51.2

Regional Mastectomy

1)

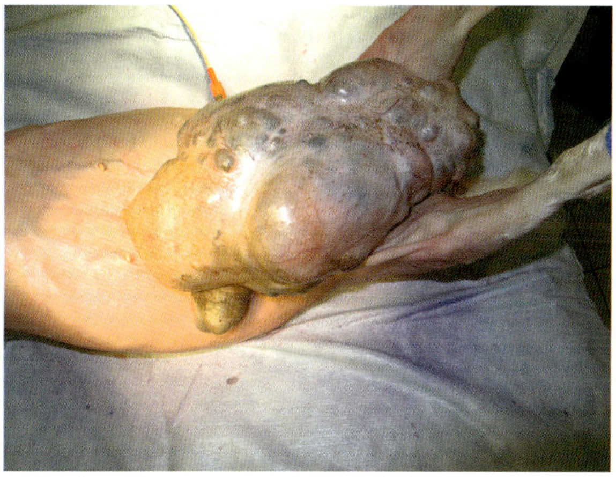

A-i)

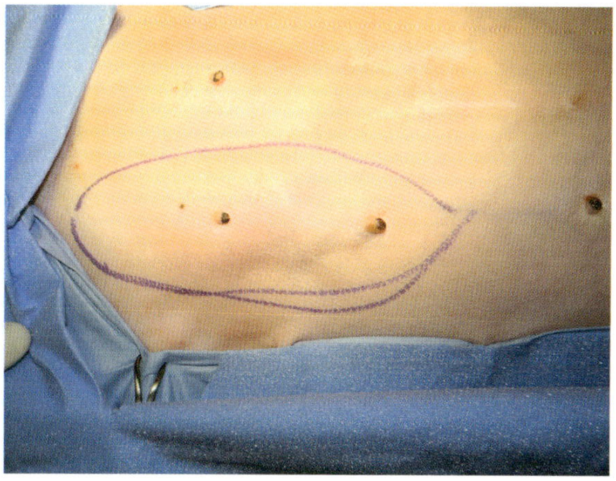

A-ii)

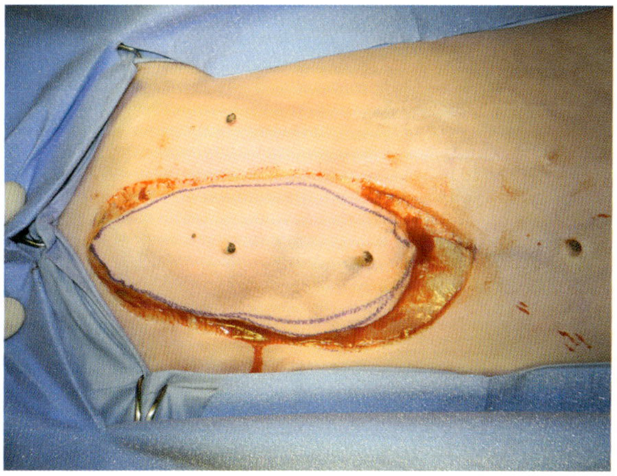

B)

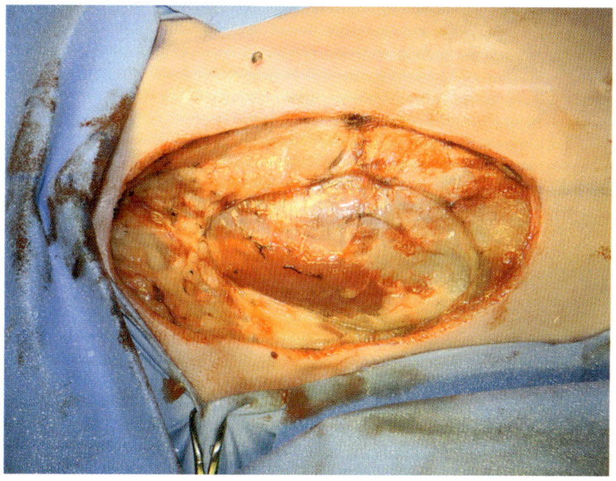

Surgical Technique (See Plate 51.2A–C) *continued*

C) For regional mastectomies involving the caudal-most mammary gland (fifth in dogs and fourth in cats), the caudal superficial epigastric artery and vein should be ligated and divided or sealed and transected with a vessel sealing device. Instead of specifically dissecting the superficial inguinal lymph node in these cases, the inguinal fat pad can be resected en bloc with the regional mastectomy as the superficial inguinal lymph node is contained within the inguinal fat pad.

Closure (See Plate 51.2D)

D) Fascial or abdominal wall defects are closed with 0 to 2-0 absorbable monofilament suture material in a simple interrupted (i) or continuous suture pattern. The skin incision is closed routinely in two layers with a simple continuous suture pattern using monofilament absorbable suture material in the subcutis and either an interrupted (ii) or continuous suture pattern using monofilament nonabsorbable suture material in the skin.

Postoperative Management

1) Multimodal analgesia
2) Elizabethan collar

Complications – Dogs

- Overall: 16%–39% [3, 4]
- Surgical-site infection (14%) [4]
- Seroma (7% overall for all types of mastectomy) [4]
- Incisional dehiscence (3% overall for all types of mastectomy) [4]

Suggested Adjuvant Treatments

- See *51. Mastectomy*.

Prognosis and Oncologic Outcome

- See *51. Mastectomy*.

References

1 Sorenmo, K.U., Shofer, F.S., and Goldschmidt, M.H. (2000). Effect of spaying and timing of spaying on survival of dogs with mammary carcinoma. *J. Vet. Intern. Med.* 14 (3): 266–270.

2 Kristiansen, V.M., Nødtvedt, A.M., Breen, A.M. et al. (2013). Effect of ovariohysterectomy at the time of tumor removal in dogs with benign mammary tumors and hyperplastic lesions: a randomized controlled clinical study. *J. Vet. Intern. Med.* 27 (4): 935–942.

3 Brooks, A., Evans, B.J., Holt, D.E. et al. (2021). Factors influencing complications following mastectomy procedures in dogs with mammary gland tumors: 140 cases (2009-2015). *J. Am. Vet. Med. Assoc.* 258 (3): 295–302.

4 Spåre, P., Ljungvall, I., Ljungvall, K. et al. (2021). Evaluation of post-operative complications after mastectomy peformed with and without perioperative antimicrobial prophylaxis in dogs. *Acta Vet. Scand.* 63 (1): 35.

Plate 51.2

Regional Mastectomy *continued*

C)

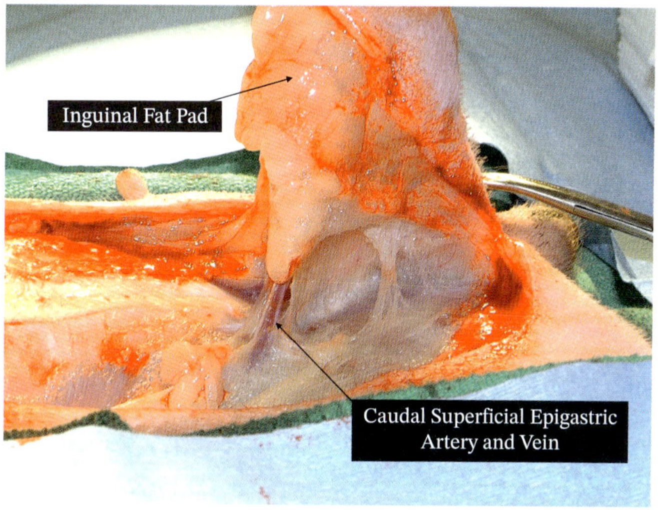

D-i)

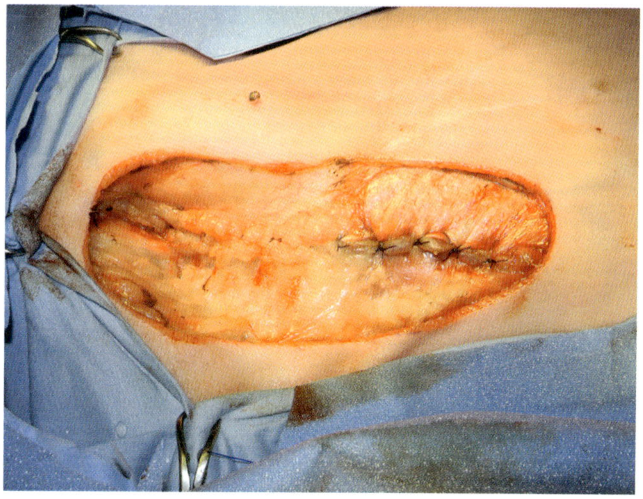

D-ii)

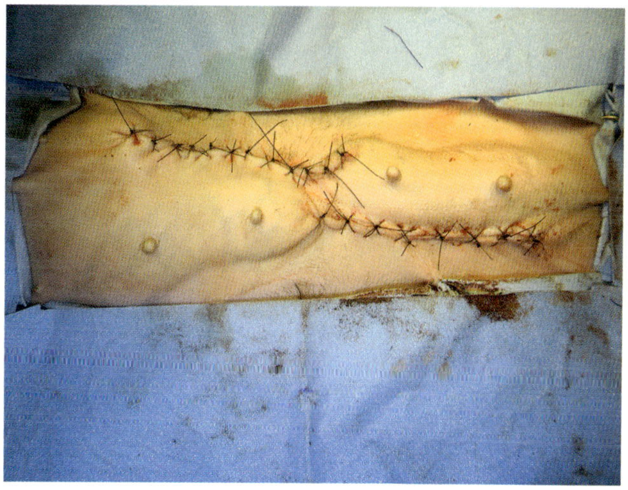

51.3 Unilateral Mastectomy

Indications (See Plate 51.3 – 5)

1) Resection of a single benign or malignant mammary mass involving more than three adjacent mammary glands.
2) Resection of multiple benign or malignant mammary masses involving an ipsilateral mammary chain.
3) Prophylactic resection of single or multiple benign or malignant mammary masses because up to 58% of mammary masses will develop further de novo mammary masses in the ipsilateral mammary chain [1]. Note that surgical dose was not prognostic for local tumor recurrence in a meta-analysis of canine mammary tumor studies [2].
4) Unilateral mastectomy can be combined with sentinel lymph node mapping (see *50.1. Sentinel Lymph Node Mapping*), axillary lymph node excision (see *50.6. Axillary Lymph Node Excision*), and/or superficial inguinal lymph node excision (see *50.7. Superficial Inguinal Lymph Node Excision*).
5) Unilateral mastectomy should be combined with ovariohysterectomy in intact female dogs to reduce the risk of further de novo mammary tumor development [3, 4]. The effect of ovariohysterectomy on de novo mammary tumor development in cats has not been reported; however, ovariohysterectomy should be strongly considered in intact female cats. Ovariohysterectomy can be performed either before or after (pictured) the unilateral mastectomy is done.

Suggested Diagnostic Workup and Clinical Staging

See *51. Mastectomy*.

Patient Positioning

The patient is positioned in dorsal recumbency.

Surgical Technique (See Plate 51.3A–D)

A) A sterile marker pen can be used to mark a minimum of 1-cm lateral margins around the tumor(s) and the first to fifth mammary glands in dogs or the first to fourth mammary glands in cats (i), and skin incision is made along the marked margins (ii).
B) Dissection is continued deeply through the subcutaneous tissue perpendicular to the skin incision to the abdominal and thoracic walls (i). The mammary glands are tightly adhered to the superficial pectoral muscles in the thoracic portion of the mammary glands, so partial pectoral muscle resection is often required en bloc during a unilateral mastectomy. The external abdominal muscle fascia (ii, arrow) or partial- (iii) to full-thickness (iv, arrow) abdominal musculature deep to the mammary tumor, depending on the location and invasiveness of the mammary tumor(s), is resected en bloc with the unilateral mastectomy for deep margins.

Color Atlas of Canine and Feline Surgical Oncology, First Edition. Julius M. Liptak, Paolo Buracco, William T. N. Culp, and Nicholas J. Bacon.

Plate 51.3

Unilateral Mastectomy

5)

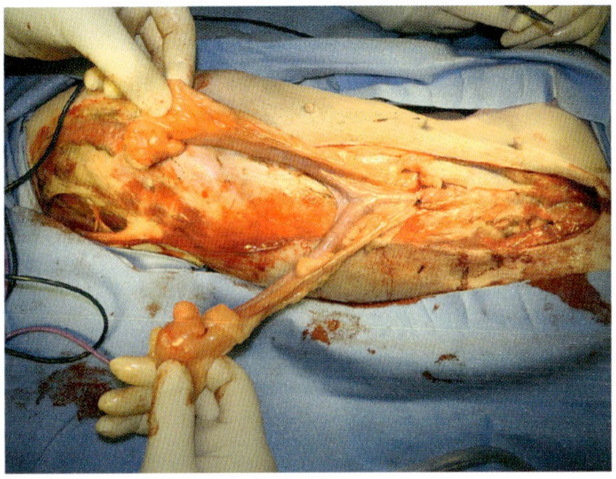

A-i)

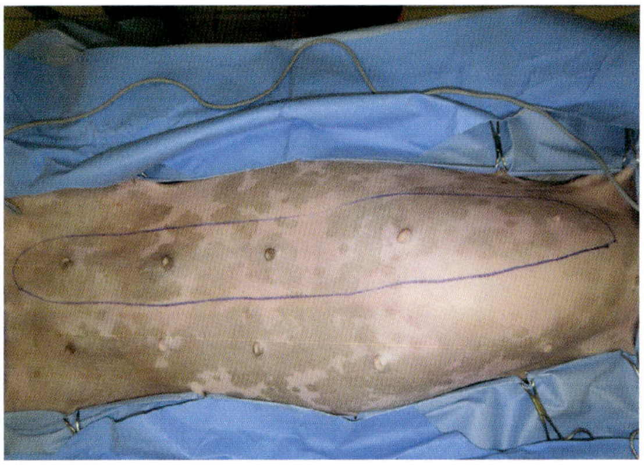

A-ii)

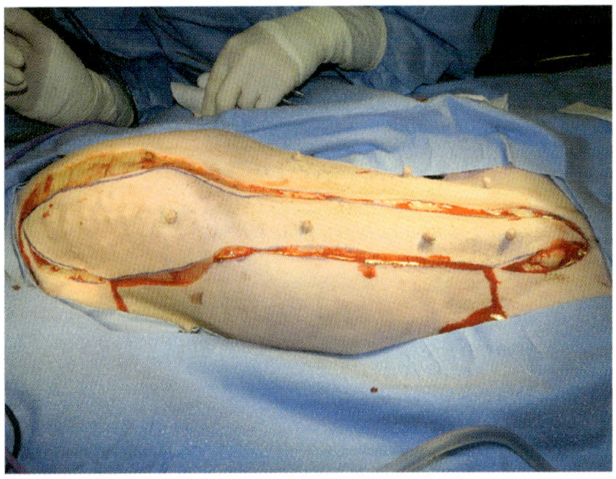

B-i)

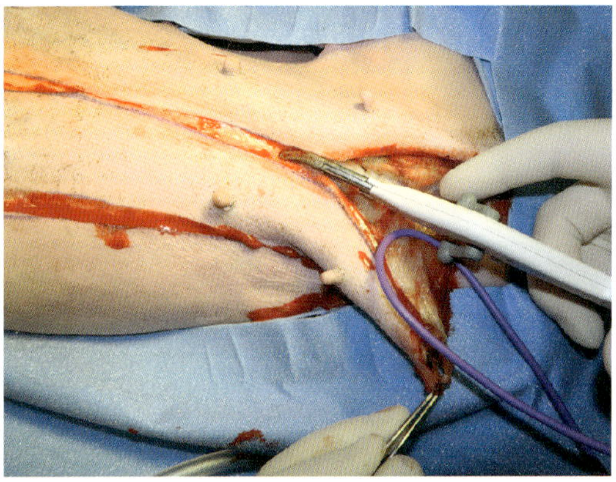

B-ii)

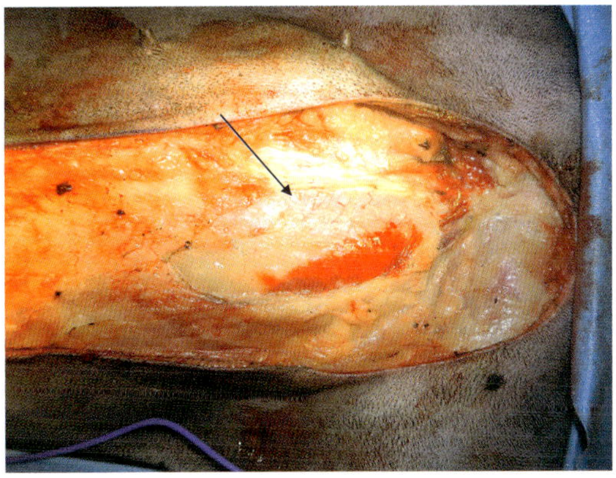

B-iii)

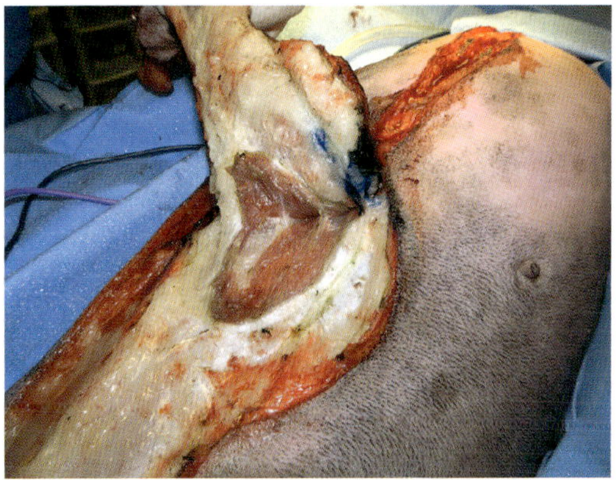

B-iv)

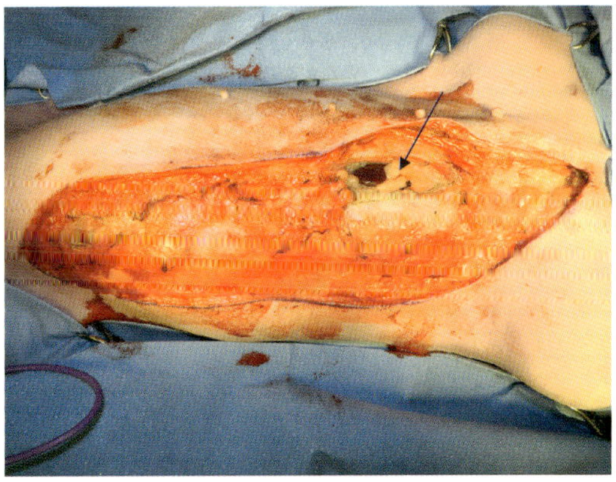

Surgical Technique (See Plate 51.3A–D) *continued*

C) The caudal superficial epigastric artery and vein should be ligated and divided or sealed and transected with a vessel sealing device.
D) The inguinal fat pad can be resected en bloc with the unilateral mastectomy as the superficial inguinal lymph node is contained within the inguinal fat pad.

Closure (See Plate 51.3E)

E) Fascial or abdominal wall defects are closed with 0 to 2-0 absorbable monofilament suture material in a simple interrupted (i, arrow) or continuous suture pattern. The skin incision is closed routinely in two layers with a simple continuous suture pattern using monofilament absorbable suture material in the subcutis and either an interrupted (ii) or continuous suture pattern using monofilament nonabsorbable suture material or skin staples (iii) in the skin.

Postoperative Management

1) Multimodal analgesia
2) Elizabethan collar

Complications – Dogs

- Overall: 37%–41% [5, 6]
- Surgical-site infection (17%) [6]
- Seroma (7% overall for all types of mastectomies) [6]
- Incisional dehiscence (3% overall for all types of mastectomies) [6]

Complications – Cats [7]

- Overall: 20%
- Surgical-site infection or incisional dehiscence (15%)
- Seroma (2%)
- Abdominal wall hernia (2%)
- Respiratory distress (2%)

Suggested Adjuvant Treatments

- See *51. Mastectomy*.

Prognosis and Oncologic Outcome

- See *51. Mastectomy*.

Plate 51.3

Unilateral Mastectomy *continued*

C)

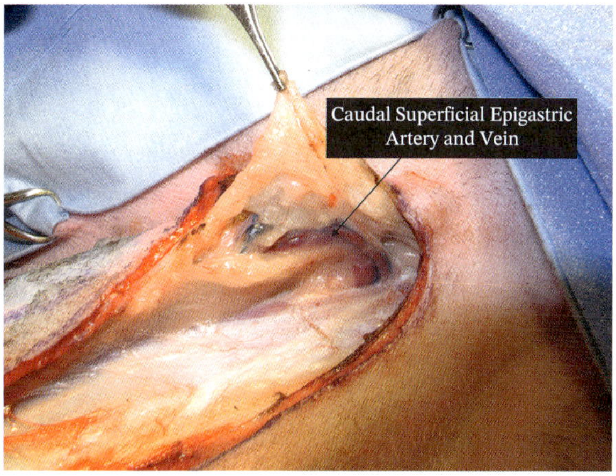

D)

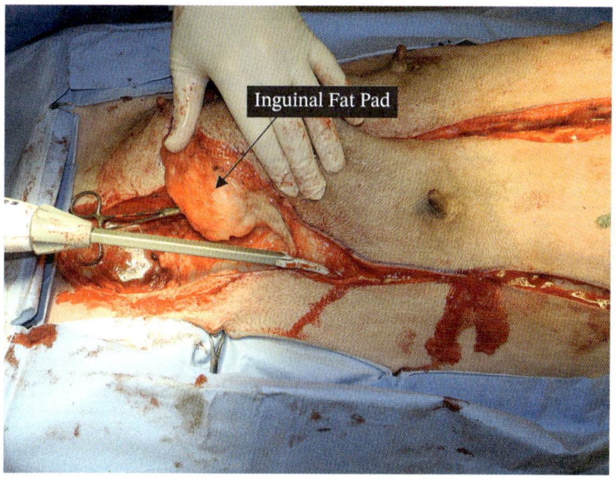

E-i)

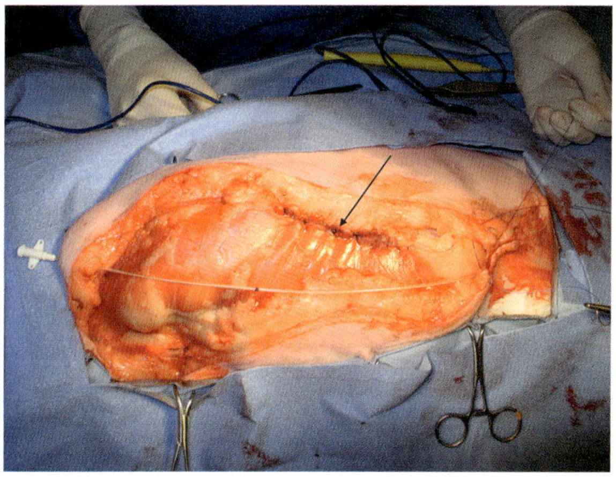

E-ii)

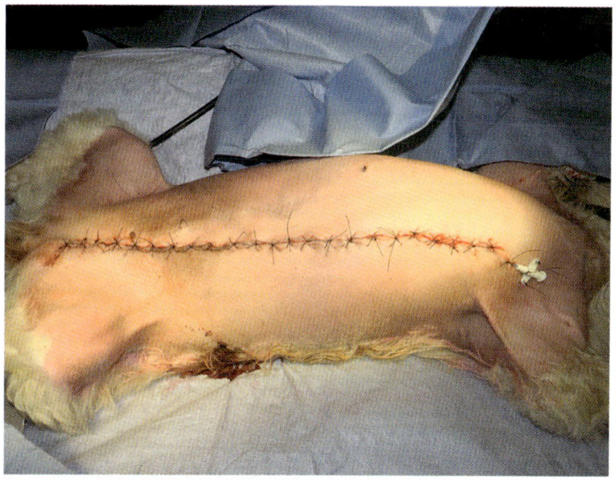

E-iii)

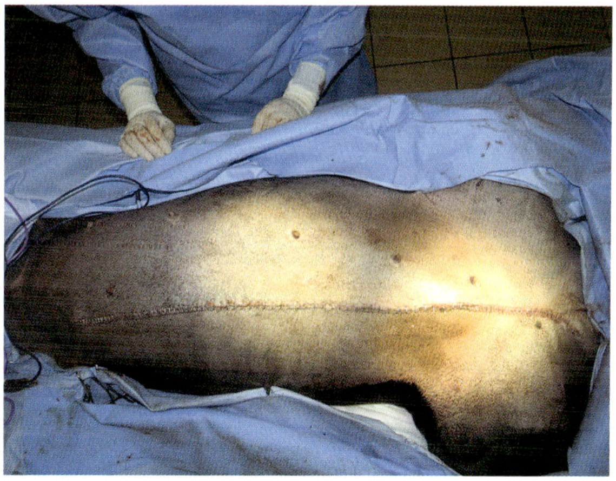

References

1 Stratmann, N., Failing, K., and Wehrend, A. (2008). Mammary tumor recurrence in bitches after regional mastectomy. *Vet. Surg.* 37 (1): 82–86.

2 Hörnfeldt, M.B. and Mortensen, J.K. (2023). Surgical dose and the clinical outcome in the treatment of mammary gland tumours in female dogs: a literature review. *Acta Vet. Scand.* 65 (1): 12.

3 Sorenmo, K.U., Shofer, F.S., and Goldschmidt, M.H. (2000). Effect of spaying and timing of spaying on survival of dogs with mammary carcinoma. *J. Vet. Intern. Med.* 14 (3): 266–270.

4 Kristiansen, V.M., Nødtvedt, A.M., Breen, A.M. et al. (2013). Effect of ovariohysterectomy at the time of tumor removal in dogs with benign mammary tumors and hyperplastic lesions: a randomized controlled clinical study. *J. Vet. Intern. Med.* 27 (4): 935–942.

5 Evans, B.J., Holt, D.E., Stefanovski, D. et al. (2021). Factors influencing complications following mastectomy procedures in dogs with mammary gland tumors: 140 cases (2009-2015). *J. Am. Vet. Med. Assoc.* 258 (3): 295–302.

6 Spåre, P., Ljungvall, I., Ljungvall, K. et al. (2021). Evaluation of post-operative complications after mastectomy peformed with and without perioperative antimicrobial prophylaxis in dogs. *Acta Vet. Scand.* 63 (1): 35.

7 Gemignani, F., Mayhew, P.D., Giuffrida, M.A. et al. (2018). Association of surgical approach with complication rate, progression-free survival time, and disease-sxpecific survival time in cats with mammary adenocarcinoma: 107 cases (1991-2014). *J. Am. Vet. Med. Assoc.* 252 (11): 1393–1402.

51.4 Single-Session Bilateral Mastectomy in Dogs

Indications (See Plate 51.4 – 1, 3)

1) The primary indication is resection of multiple benign or malignant mammary masses involving both mammary chains.
2) Bilateral mastectomy can be combined with sentinel lymph node mapping (see *50.1. Sentinel Lymph Node Mapping*), axillary lymph node excision (see *50.6. Axillary Lymph Node Excision*), and/or superficial inguinal lymph node excision (see *50.7. Superficial Inguinal Lymph Node Excision*).
3) Bilateral mastectomy should be combined with ovariohysterectomy in intact female dogs to reduce the risk of further de novo mammary tumor development [1, 2]. Ovariohysterectomy can be performed either before or after (pictured) the regional mastectomy is done.

Suggested Diagnostic Workup and Clinical Staging

- See *51. Mastectomy*.

Patient Positioning

The patient is positioned in dorsal recumbency.

Surgical Technique (See Plate 51.4A–D)

A) A sterile marker pen can be used to mark a minimum of 1-cm lateral margins around the tumor(s), then in a Y shape around the left and right third to fifth mammary glands, and then individually around the left first and second and right first and second mammary glands (i). A skin incision is then made along the marked margins (ii). It is important not to do an elliptical incision around both mammary chains because the subsequent defect will not be able to be closed primarily without causing significant respiratory compromise because of restriction of ventilation as a result of the inability to expand the thoracic wall during inspiration.
B) Dissection is continued deeply through the subcutaneous tissue perpendicular to the skin incision to the abdominal and thoracic walls (i). The mammary glands are tightly adhered to the superficial pectoral muscles in the thoracic portion of the mammary glands, so partial pectoral muscle resection is often required en bloc during the cranial portion of bilateral mastectomies. The external abdominal muscle fascia (ii, arrow) or partial- to full-thickness (iii, arrow) abdominal musculature deep to the mammary tumor, depending on the location and invasiveness of the mammary tumor(s), is resected en bloc with the bilateral mastectomy for deep margins.

Color Atlas of Canine and Feline Surgical Oncology, First Edition. Julius M. Liptak, Paolo Buracco, William T. N. Culp, and Nicholas J. Bacon.

Plate 51.4

Single-Session Bilateral Mastectomy in Dogs

1)

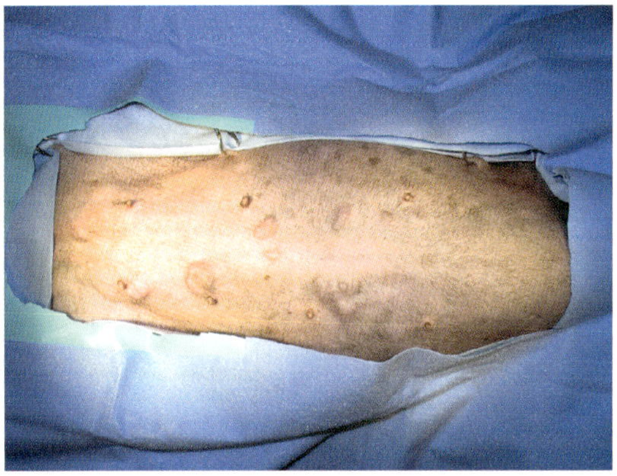

3)

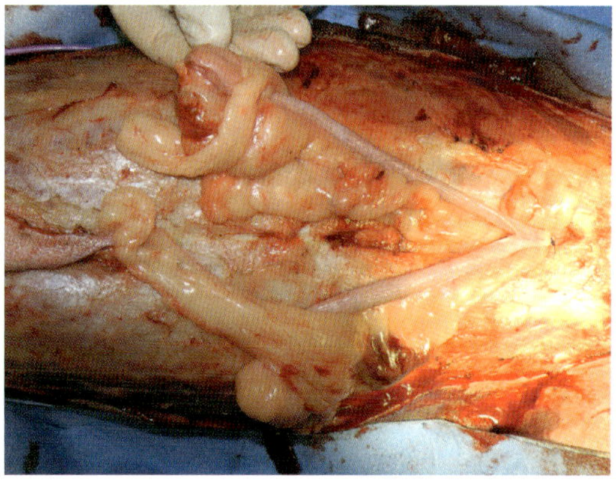

A-i)

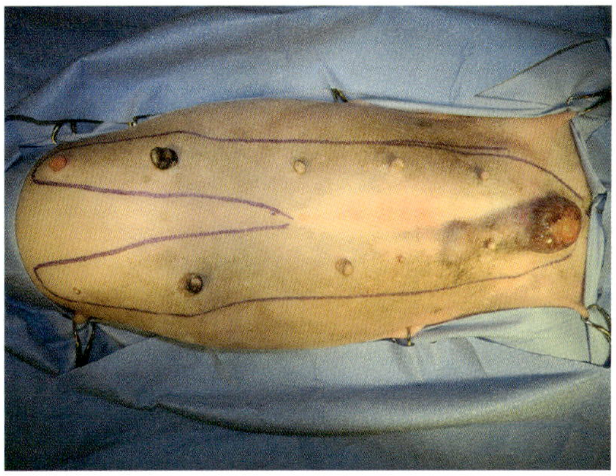

A-ii)

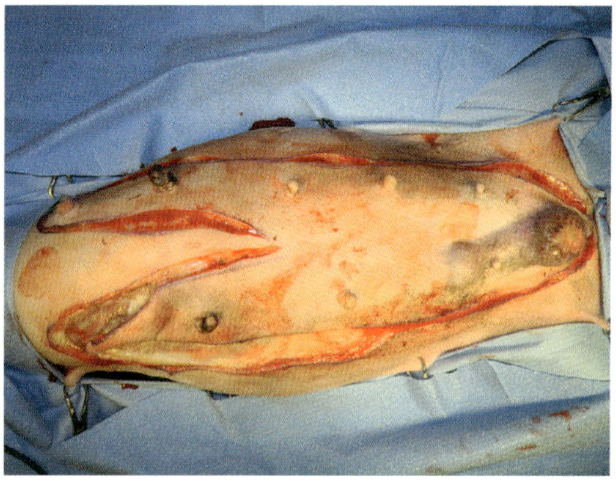

B-i)

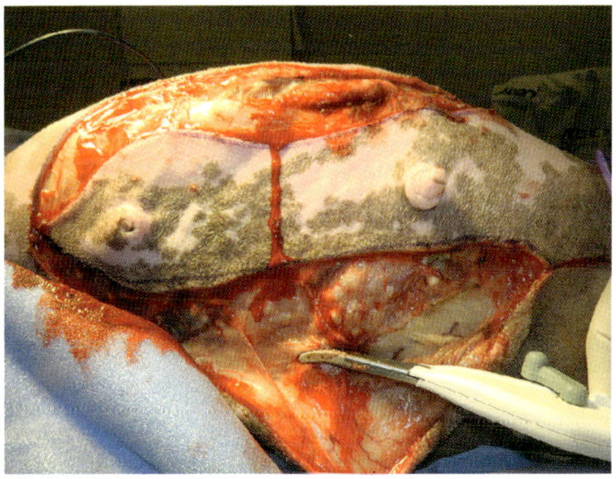

B-ii)

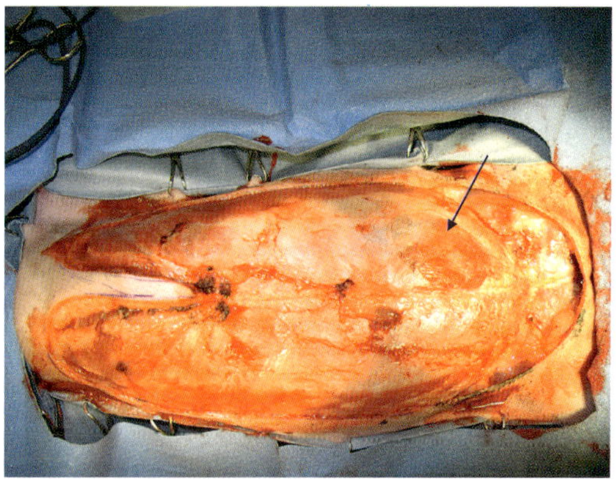

B-iii)

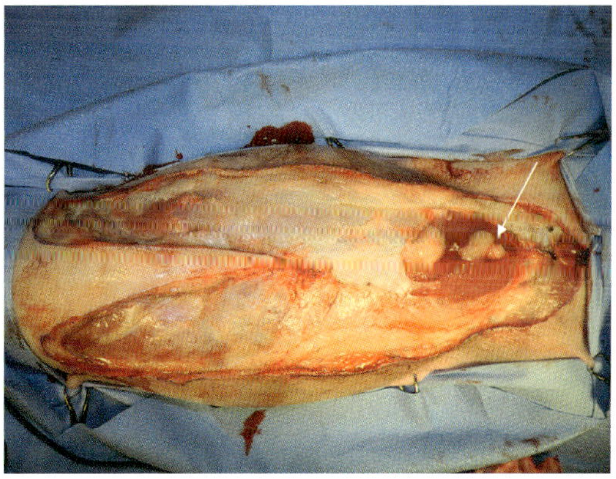

Surgical Technique (See Plate 51.4A–D) *continued*

C) The left and right caudal superficial epigastric arteries and veins should be ligated and divided (i, dashed lines) or sealed and transected with a vessel sealing device (ii).
D) The inguinal fat pads can be resected en bloc with the bilateral mastectomy because the superficial inguinal lymph nodes are contained within the inguinal fat pads.

Closure (See Plate 51.4E)

E) Fascial or abdominal wall defects are closed with 0 to 2-0 absorbable monofilament suture material in a simple interrupted or continuous suture pattern (i, arrow). The skin incision is closed routinely in two layers with a simple continuous suture pattern using monofilament absorbable suture material in the subcutis and either an interrupted (ii) or continuous suture pattern using monofilament nonabsorbable suture material or skin staples in the skin.

Postoperative Management

1) Multimodal analgesia
2) Elizabethan collar

Complications – Dogs

- Overall: 37%–41% [3, 4]
- Surgical-site infection (17%) [4]
- Seroma (7% overall for all types of mastectomies) [4]
- Incisional dehiscence (3% overall for all types of mastectomies) [4]

Suggested Adjuvant Treatments

- See *51. Mastectomy*.

Prognosis and Oncologic Outcome

- See *51. Mastectomy*.

References

1 Sorenmo, K.U., Shofer, F.S., and Goldschmidt, M.H. (2000). Effect of spaying and timing of spaying on survival of dogs with mammary carcinoma. *J. Vet. Intern. Med.* 14 (3): 266–270.

2 Kristiansen, V.M., Nødtvedt, A.M., Breen, A.M. et al. (2013). Effect of ovariohysterectomy at the time of tumor removal in dogs with benign mammary tumors and hyperplastic lesions: a randomized controlled clinical study. *J. Vet. Intern. Med.* 27 (4): 935–942.

3 Brooks, A., Evans, B.J., Holt, D.E. et al. (2021). Factors influencing complications following mastectomy procedures in dogs with mammary gland tumors: 140 cases (2009-2015). *J. Am. Vet. Med. Assoc.* 258 (3): 295–302.

4 Spåre, P., Ljungvall, I., Ljungvall, K. et al. (2021). Evaluation of post-operative complications after mastectomy peformed with and without perioperative antimicrobial prophylaxis in dogs. *Acta Vet. Scand.* 63 (1): 35.

Plate 51.4

Single-Session Bilateral Mastectomy in Dogs *continued*

C-i)

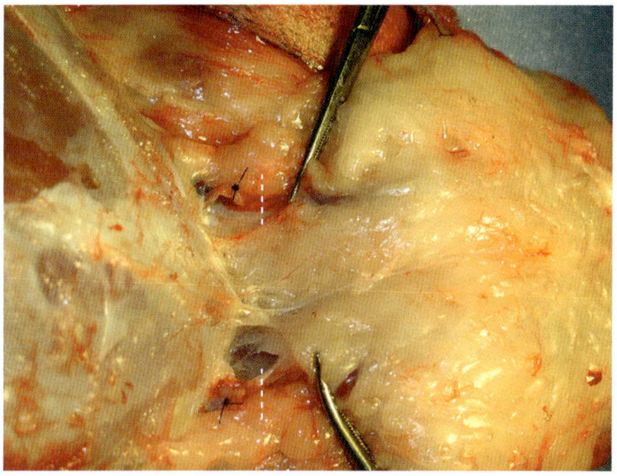

C-ii)

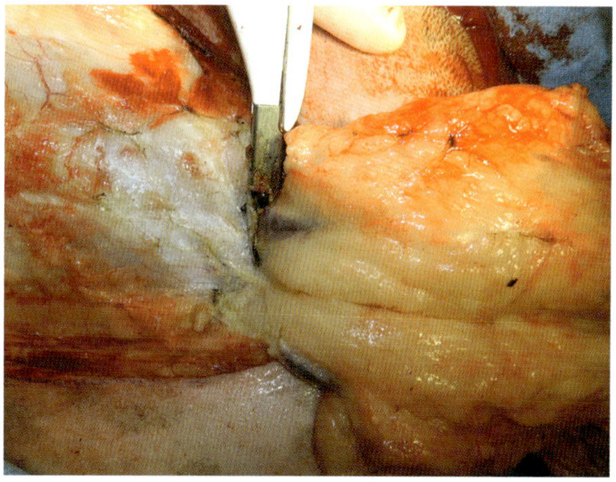

D)

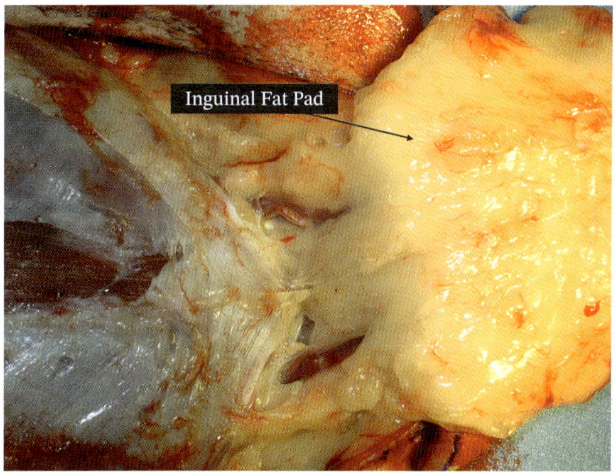

E-i)

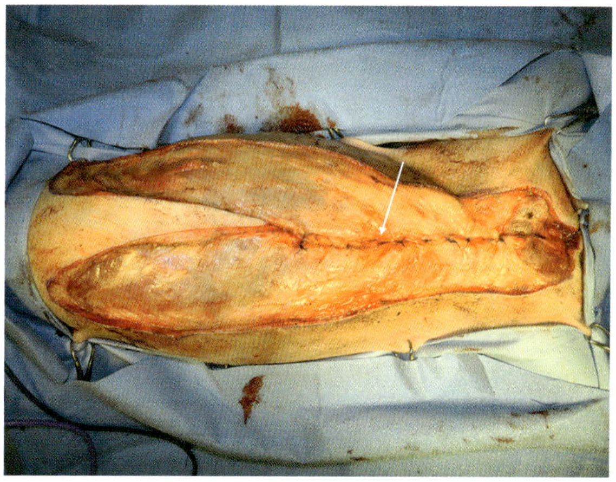

E-ii)

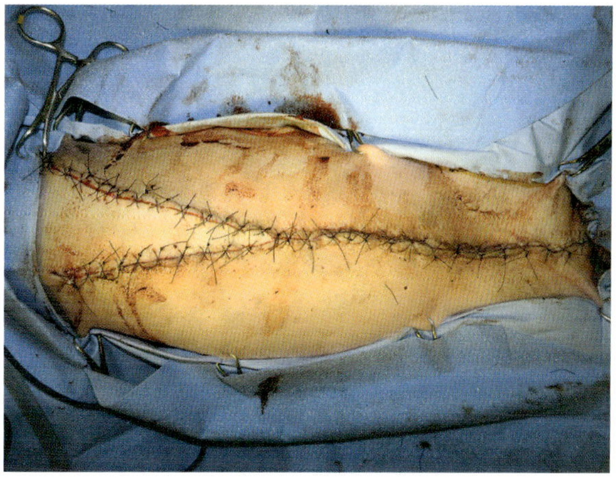

51.5 Single-Session Bilateral Mastectomy in Cats

Indications (See Plate 51.5 – 1, 2)

1) Resection of one (i) or more (ii) malignant mammary masses in cats. Survival outcomes are significantly better in cats with malignant mammary tumors treated with bilateral mastectomy compared with either unilateral or local mastectomy [1, 2]. Bilateral mastectomy can be done either as a single-session procedure or staged with two unilateral mastectomies performed 4–6 weeks apart.
2) Bilateral mastectomy can be combined with sentinel lymph node mapping (i, intraoperative peritumoral injection of methylene blue in four quadrants around the mammary carcinoma; ii, tracking the blue-colored lymphatics [arrows] to the sentinel lymph node; iii, blue-colored superficial inguinal lymph node is the sentinel lymph node; iv, blue-colored lymphatics [arrowheads] bypassed the superficial inguinal lymph node and entered through the inguinal canal into the abdominal cavity to the blue-colored medial iliac lymph node [arrow]) (see *50.1. Sentinel Lymph Node Mapping*), axillary lymph node excision (see *50.6. Axillary Lymph Node Excision*), and/or superficial inguinal lymph node excision (see *50.7. Superficial Inguinal Lymph Node Excision*).
3) The effect of ovariohysterectomy on de novo mammary tumor development in cats has not been reported; however, ovariohysterectomy should be strongly considered in intact female cats. Ovariohysterectomy can be performed either before or after the regional mastectomy is done.

Suggested Diagnostic Workup and Clinical Staging

See *51. Mastectomy*.

General Considerations (See Plate 51.5 – 4)

The clip is important in cats being treated with single-session bilateral mastectomy and should extend from the midneck to the caudal ischiatic tuberosities and almost circumferentially around the cat. The latter is important to avoid drawing hair into the surgical field during closure of the bilateral mastectomy defect.

For single-session bilateral mastectomy, it is important that the ability to close the defect with minimal tension is assessed before surgery, because excessive tension can cause significant respiratory compromise as a result of the inability to expand the thoracic wall during inspiration. Wound tension can be assessed by marking the left and right lateral margins after the cat has been anesthetized and clipped (4 – i), grasping these margins and apposing them in the midline (4 – ii). If the tension on the wound is likely to be minimal, which is the case in most cats other than grossly overweight cats, then a single-session bilateral mastectomy should be able to be performed safely. If the tension is likely to be excessive based on this evaluation, then staged bilateral mastectomies should be done instead.

Bilateral mastectomy is a painful procedure. Perioperative multimodal analgesia is imperative for a good outcome, including regional blocks administered preoperatively and possibly postoperatively, perioperative continuous rate infusions of ketamine and fentanyl, wound diffuser catheters, and oral postoperative analgesia, such as a nonsteroidal anti-inflammatory drug, gabapentin, and buprenorphine.

Color Atlas of Canine and Feline Surgical Oncology, First Edition. Julius M. Liptak, Paolo Buracco, William T. N. Culp, and Nicholas J. Bacon.

Plate 51.5

Single-Session Bilateral Mastectomy in Cats

1-i)

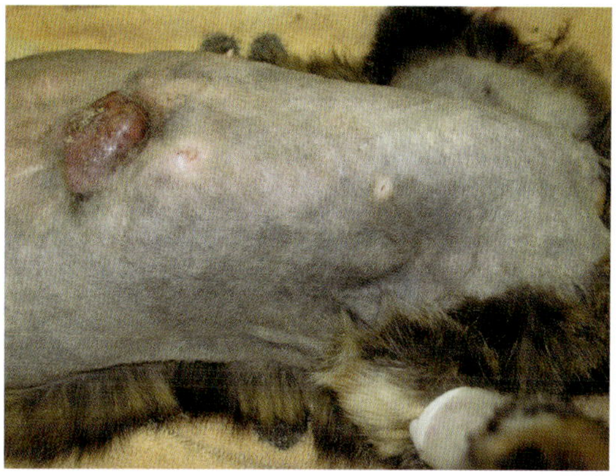

1-ii)

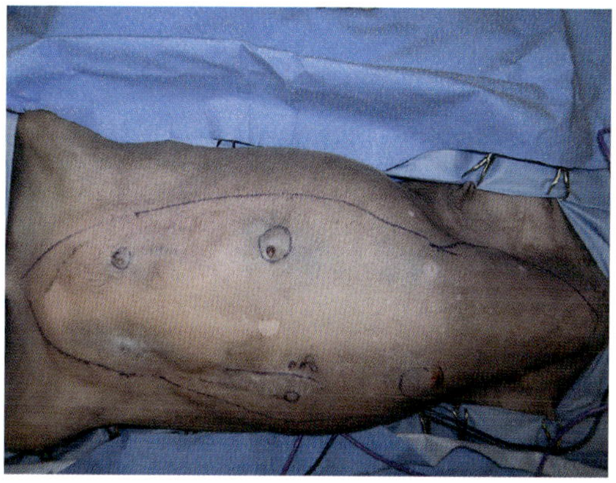

2-i)

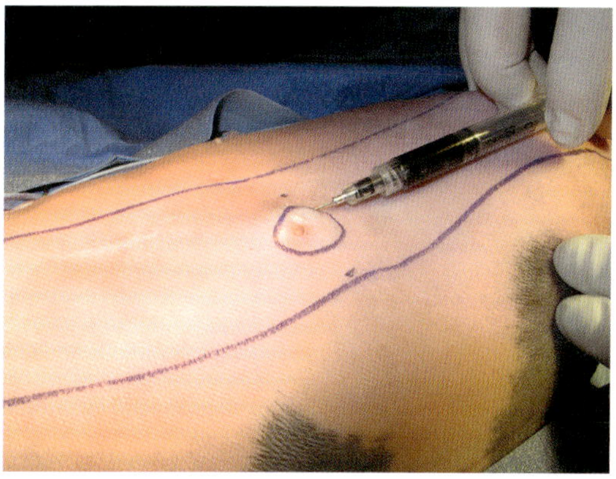

2-ii)

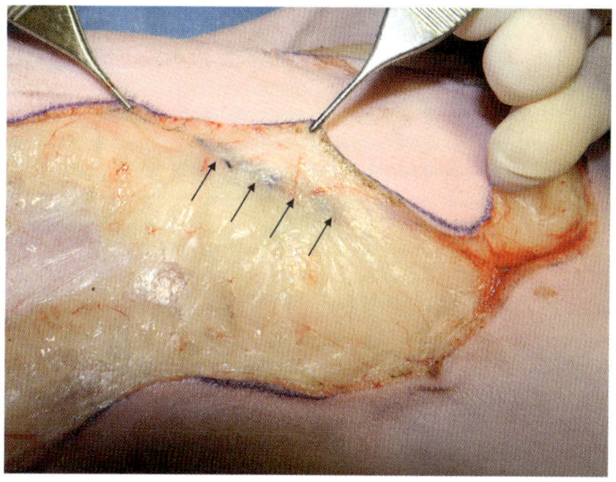

2-iii)

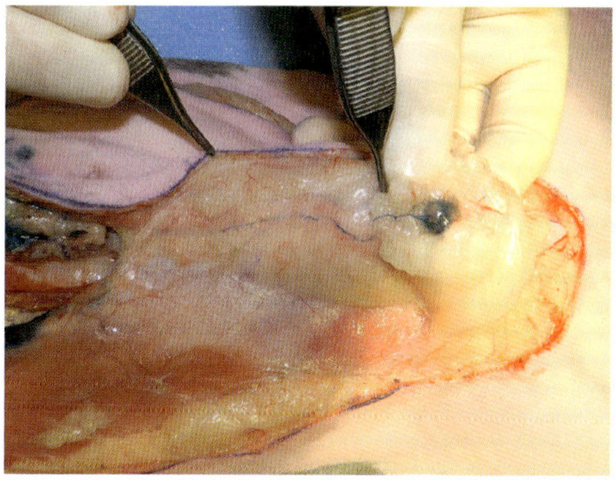

2-iv)

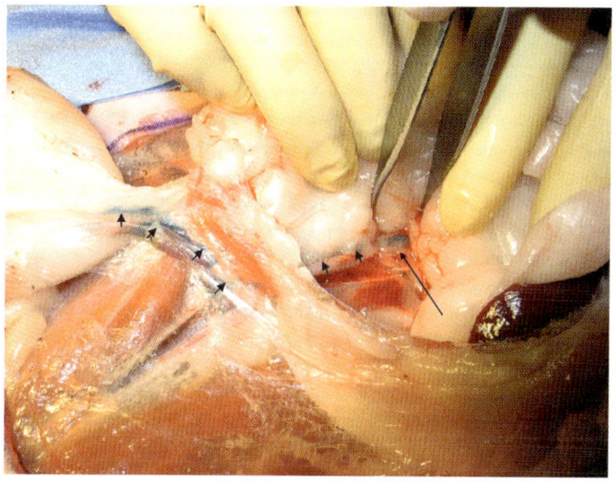

4-i)

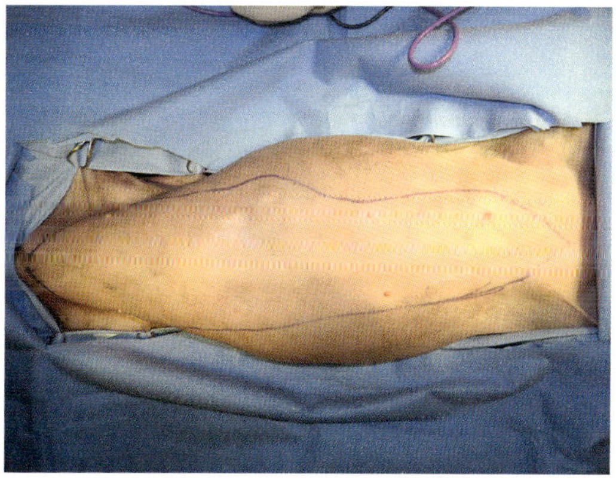

4-ii)

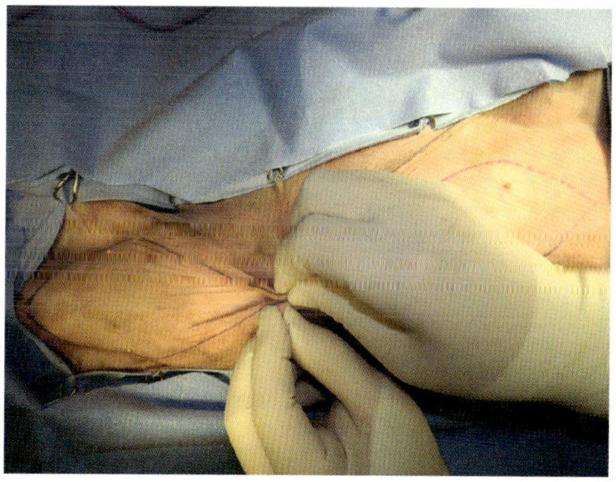

Patient Positioning

The patient is positioned in dorsal recumbency.

Surgical Technique (See Plate 51.5A–D)

A) A sterile marker pen can be used to mark a minimum of 1-cm lateral margins around the mammary tumor(s) and around both left and right first to fourth mammary glands (i), and a skin incision is then made along the marked margins (ii).
B) Dissection is continued deeply through the subcutaneous tissue perpendicular to the skin incision to the abdominal and thoracic walls. The mammary glands are tightly adhered to the superficial pectoral muscles in the thoracic portion of the mammary glands, so partial pectoral muscle resection is often required en bloc during the cranial portion of bilateral mastectomies (i). The external abdominal muscle fascia or partial- (ii) to full-thickness (iii) abdominal musculature deep to the mammary tumor, depending on the location and invasiveness of the mammary tumor(s), is resected en bloc with the bilateral mastectomy for deep margins.
C) The left and right caudal superficial epigastric arteries and veins should be ligated and divided or sealed and transected with a vessel sealing device.
D) The inguinal fat pads can be resected en bloc with the bilateral mastectomy as the superficial inguinal lymph nodes are contained within the inguinal fat pads.

Plate 51.5

Single-Session Bilateral Mastectomy in Cats *continued*

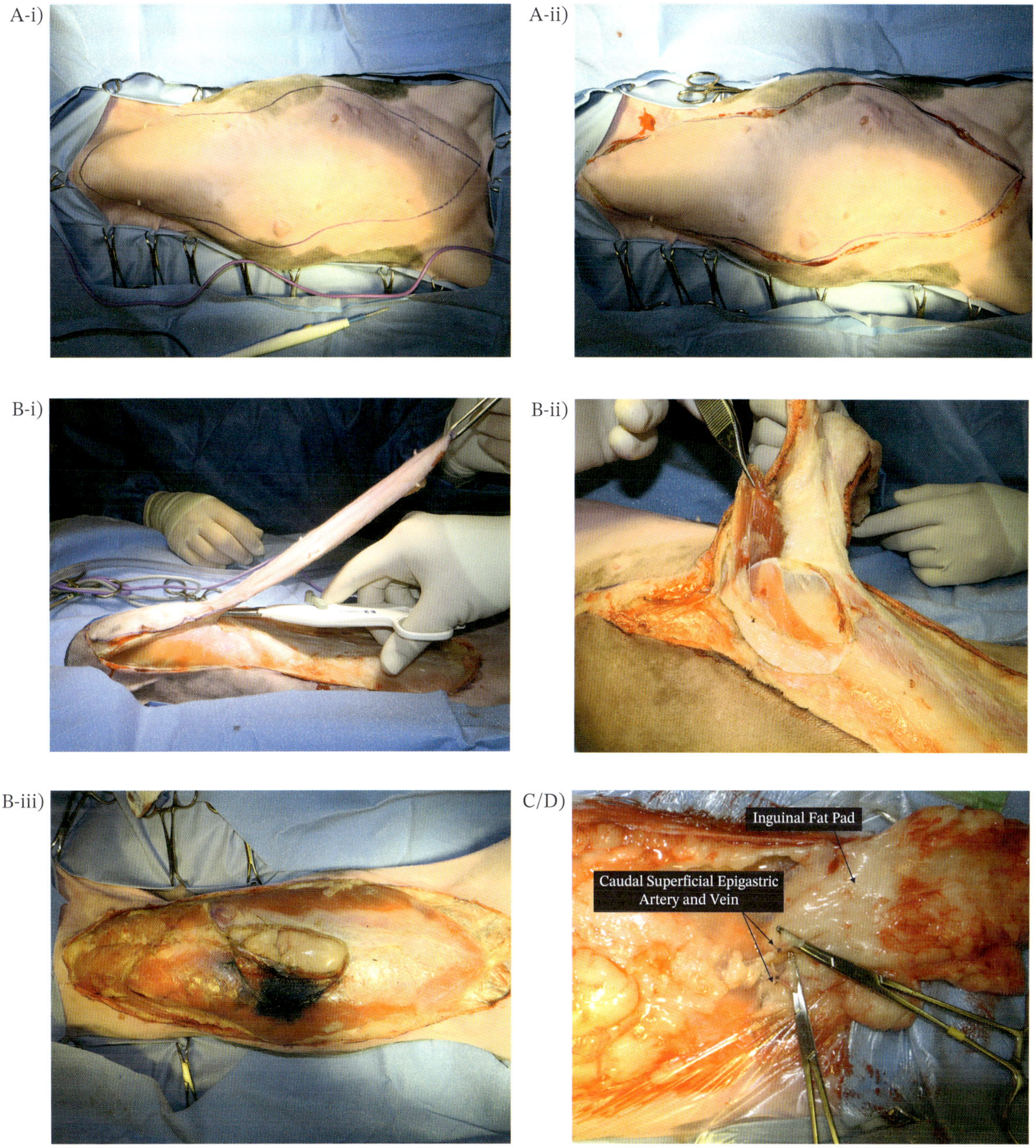

Closure (See Plate 51.5E)

E) Fascial or abdominal wall defects are closed with 2-0 absorbable monofilament suture material in a simple interrupted (i) or continuous suture pattern. The skin incision is closed routinely in two layers with a simple continuous suture pattern using monofilament absorbable suture material in the subcutis (ii) and either an interrupted (iii; note that occasionally, particularly when closing from a caudal-to-cranial direction, the cranial aspect of the incision needs to be closed in a small Y shape) or continuous suture pattern (iv) using monofilament nonabsorbable suture material or skin staples (v) in the skin.

Postoperative Management

1) Multimodal analgesia (see earlier General Considerations section)
2) Elizabethan collar or body suit

Complications – Staged Bilateral Mastectomy

- Overall: 23%–36% [1, 2]
- Surgical-site infection/incisional dehiscence or general wound (14%–23%) [1, 2]
- Seroma (7%) [1]

Complications – Single-Session Bilateral Mastectomy

- Overall: 38%–41% [1, 2]
- Surgical-site infection/incisional dehiscence or general wound (25%–36%) [1, 2]
- Seroma (9%) [1]
- Abdominal wall hernia (3%) [1]
- Respiratory distress (3%–11%) [1, 2]

Suggested Adjuvant Treatments

- See *51. Mastectomy*.

Prognosis and Oncologic Outcome

- See *51. Mastectomy*.

References

1 Gemignani, F., Mayhew, P.D., Giuffrida, M.A. et al. (2018). Association of surgical approach with complication rate, progression-free survival time, and disease-sxpecific survival time in cats with mammary adenocarcinoma: 107 cases (1991-2014). *J. Am. Vet. Med. Assoc.* 252 (11): 1393–1402.

2 Wood, C.J., Chu, M.L., Selmic, L.E. et al. (2021). Effect of perioperative desmopressin in cats with mammary carcinoma treated with bilateral mastectomy. *Vet. Comp. Oncol.* 19 (4): 724–734.

Plate 51.5

Single-Session Bilateral Mastectomy in Cats *continued*

E-i)

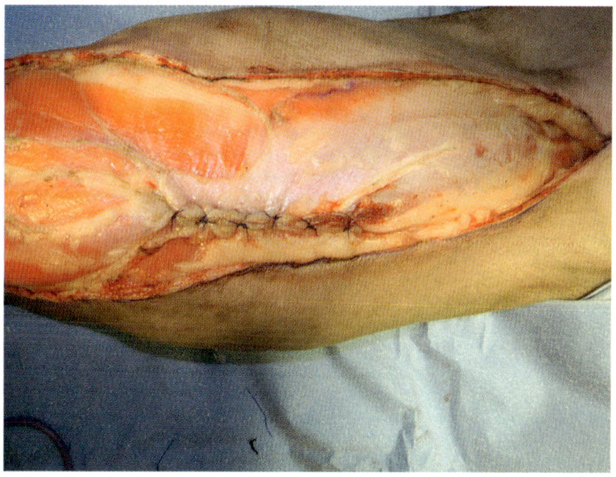

E-ii)

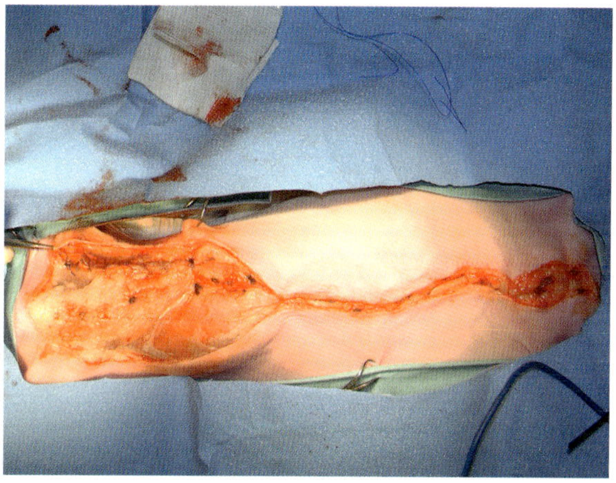

E-iii)

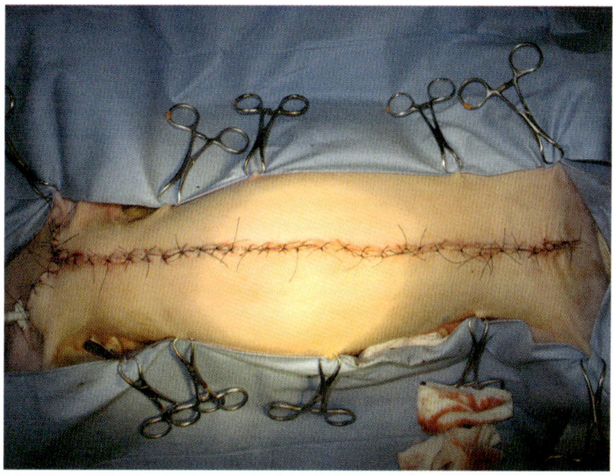

E-iv)

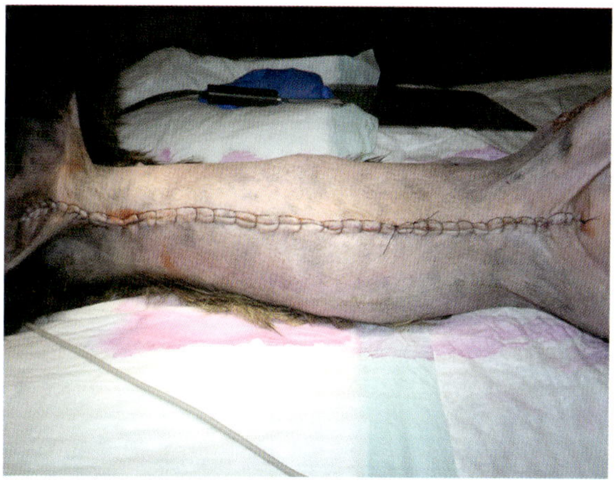

E-v)

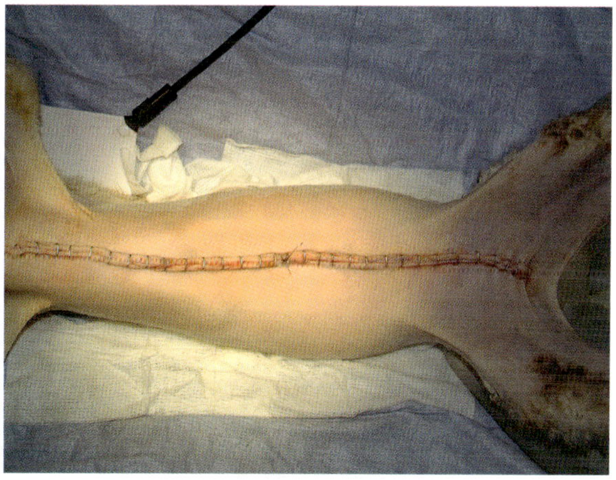

Chapter 52: Other Procedures

52.1 Intermuscular Lipoma Excision

Indication (See Plate 52.1 – 1)

1) Excision of intermuscular lipomas: Intermuscular lipomas are most commonly located between the semitendinosus and semimembranosus muscles but are also reported between the semitendinosus and biceps femoris muscles, biceps femoris and vastus lateralis muscles, deep to the sartorius muscle, and in the axillary region [1, 2].

Suggested Diagnostic Workup and Clinical Staging

- Complete blood count, serum biochemistry, and urinalysis
- Fine-needle aspirate cytology
- ± Computed tomography scan of the affected limb

Patient Positioning

The patient is positioned in either dorsal recumbency (preferred) or lateral recumbency with the affected limb uppermost.

Surgical Technique (See Plate 52.1A–E)

A) An incision is made along the caudal aspect of the thigh extending for the length of the swelling (i), and this incision is then continued deeply through the subcutaneous tissue (ii).
B) The fascia between the muscle bellies overlying the lipoma (i, arrow) is separated using a vessel sealing device (ii) or a combination of blunt and sharp dissection (iii).

Color Atlas of Canine and Feline Surgical Oncology, First Edition. Julius M. Liptak, Paolo Buracco, William T. N. Culp, and Nicholas J. Bacon.

Plate 52.1

Intermuscular Lipoma Excision

1)
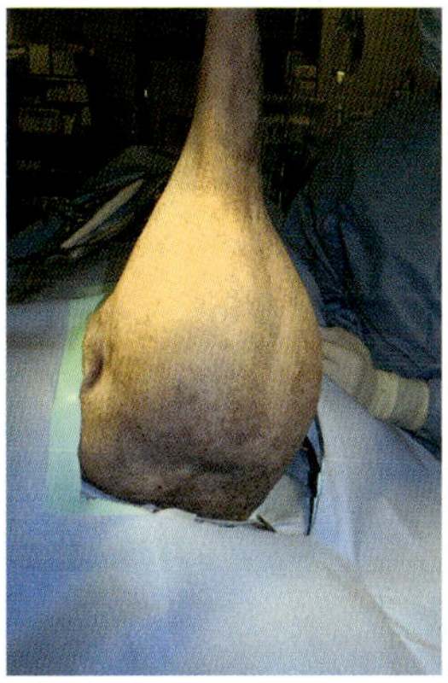

1)
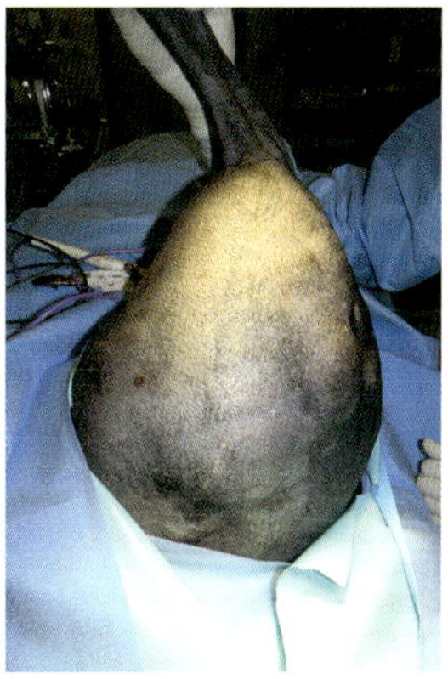

1)
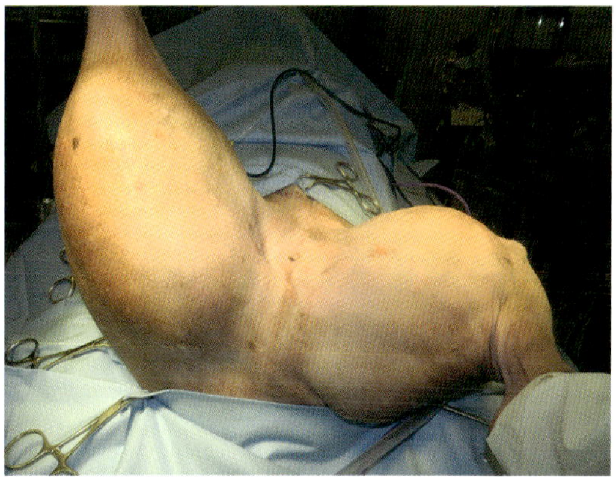

A-i)
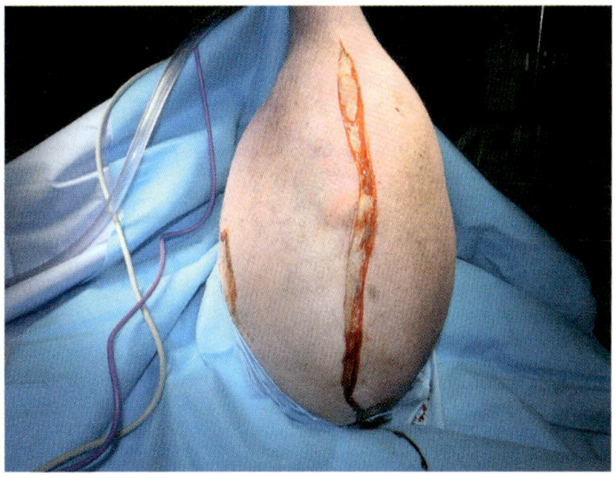

A-ii)
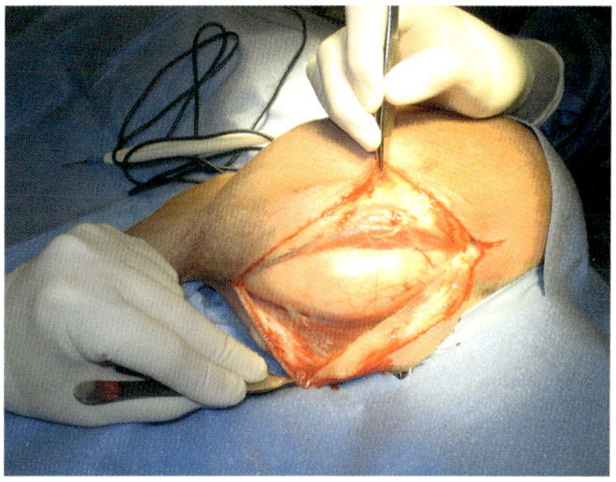

B-i)
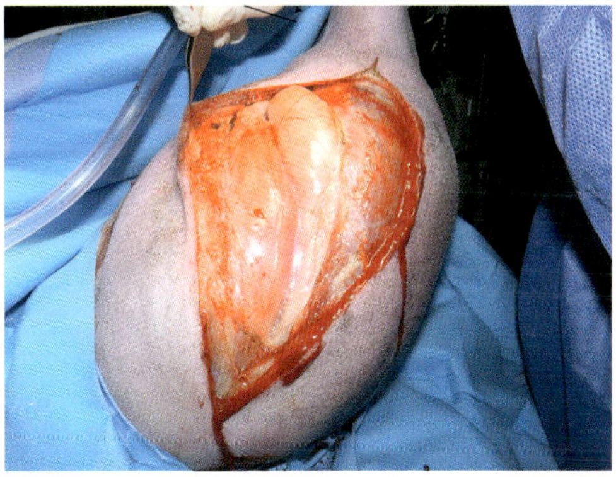

B-ii)
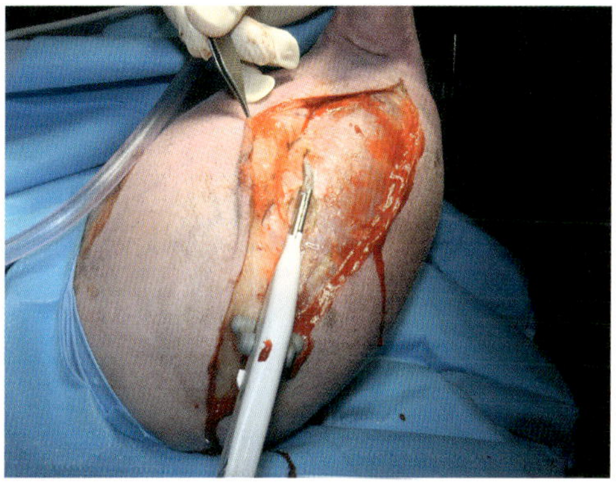

B-iii)
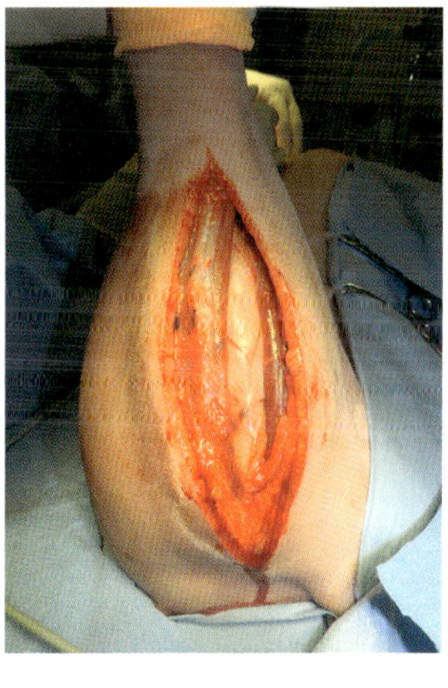

Surgical Technique (See Plate 52.1A–E) *continued*

C) The lipoma is then extirpated using a combination of blunt dissection and digital extrusion (i–iii) [1].

D) The sciatic nerve may be in either close proximity (i, ii) or course through the lipoma, and hence the sciatic nerve should be identified and carefully dissected away from the lipoma.

Plate 52.1

Intermuscular Lipoma Excision *continued*

C-i)

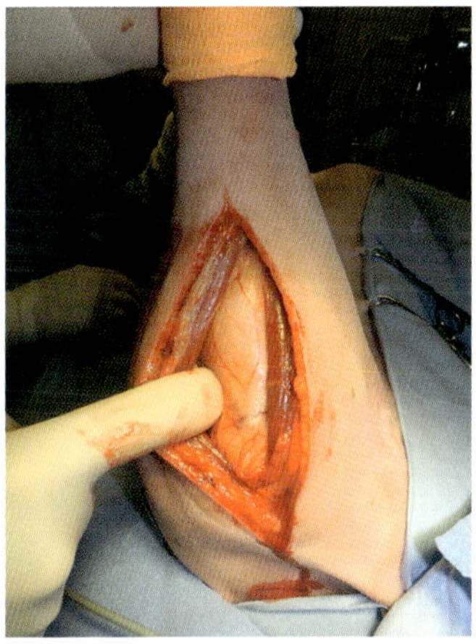

C-ii)

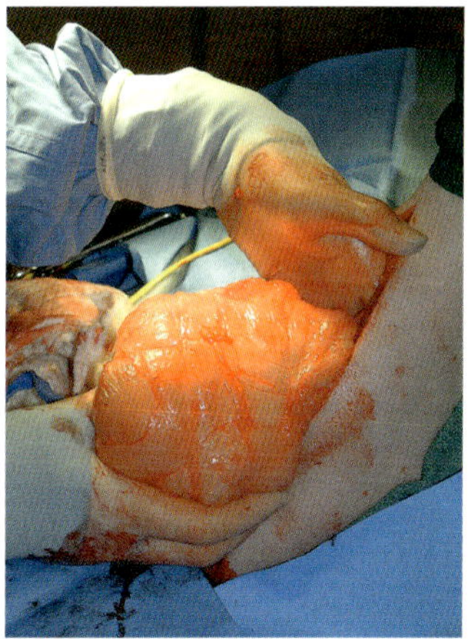

C-iii)

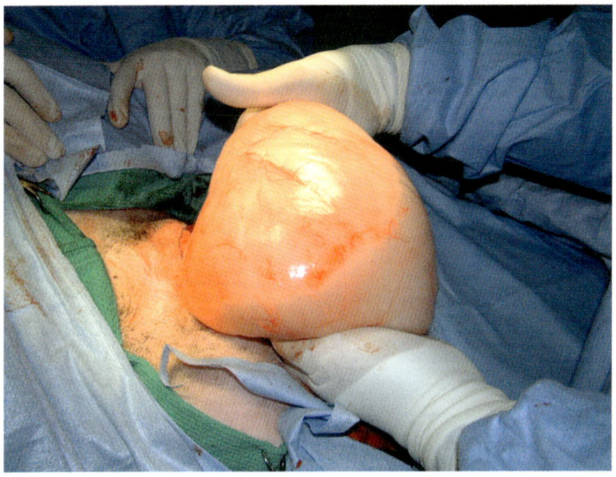

D-i)

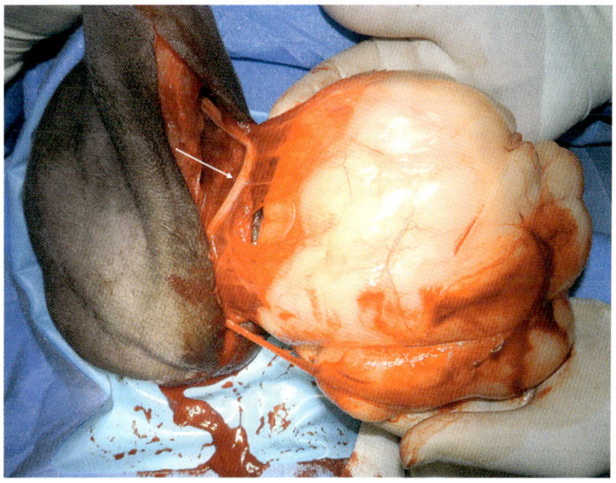

D-ii)

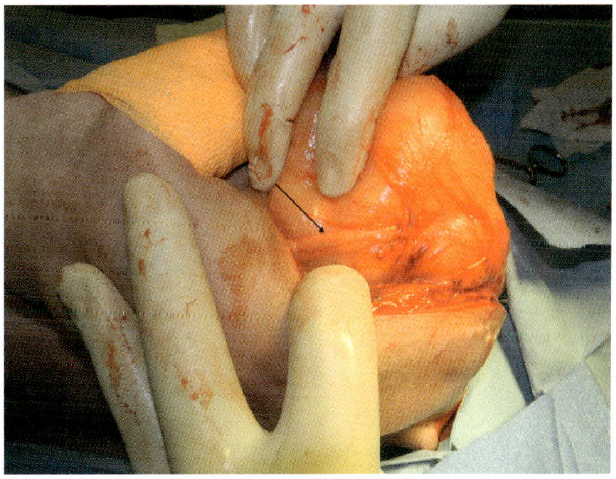

Surgical Technique (See Plate 52.1A–E) *continued*

E) Placement of a closed suction drain is recommended (i, ii) and preferred over a Penrose drain (iii).

Closure (See Plate 52.1F)

F) The skin incision is closed routinely in three layers with a simple continuous suture pattern using monofilament absorbable suture material to close the muscle bellies (i) and the subcutis and either an interrupted or continuous suture pattern using monofilament nonabsorbable suture material in the skin (ii). The Jackson-Pratt drain is secured with a horizontal mattress suture at the stoma and a Chinese finger trap suture pattern on the tubing (ii).

Postoperative Management

1) Multimodal analgesia
2) Elizabethan collar
3) Closed suction drain management for 2–5 days

Complications [1, 2]

Intraoperative Complications

- Bleeding [1]

Postoperative Complications

- Seroma (67% of dogs without a closed suction drain and 0% of dogs with a closed suction drain) [1]
- Surgical-site infection (6%) [2]

Suggested Adjuvant Treatments

- None

References

1 Thomson, M.J., Withrow, S.J., Dernell, W.S. et al. (1999). Intermuscular lipomas of the thigh region in dogs: 11 cases. *J. Am. Anim. Hosp. Assoc.* 35 (2): 165–167.

2 Case, J.B., MacPhail, C.M., and Withrow, S.J. (2012). Anatomic distribution and clinical findings of intermuscular lipomas in 17 dogs (2005-2010). *J. Am. Anim. Hosp. Assoc.* 48 (4): 245–249.

Plate 52.1

Intermuscular Lipoma Excision *continued*

E-i)
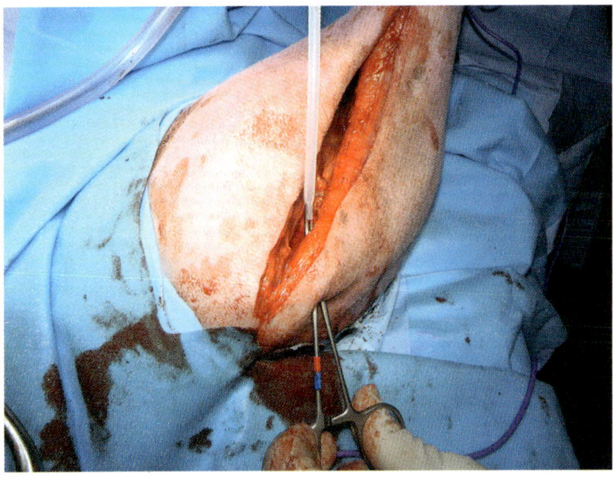

E-ii)
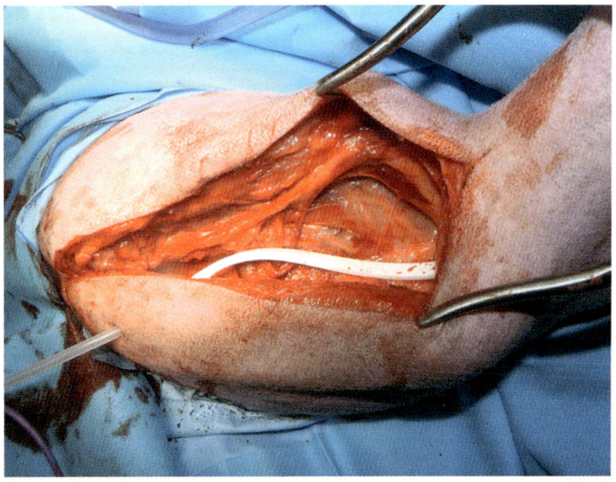

E-iii)
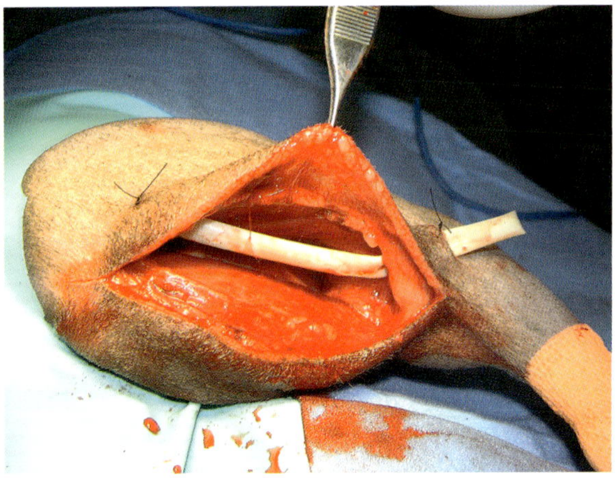

F-i)
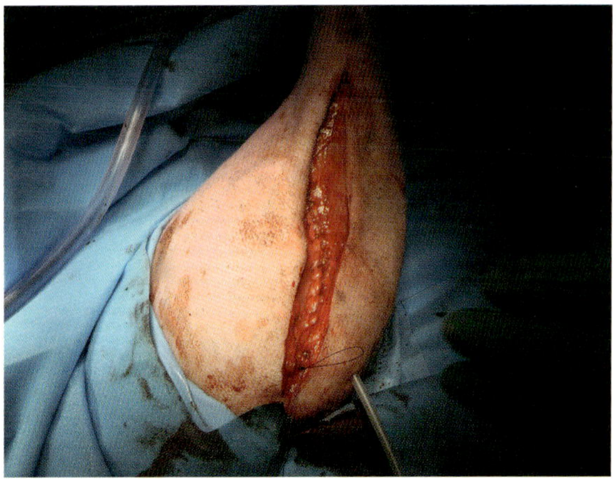

F-ii)
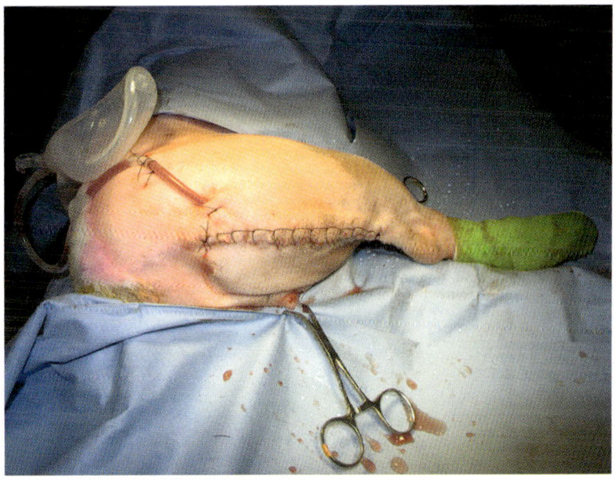

Index

a

b

Color Atlas of Canine and Feline Surgical Oncology, First Edition. Julius M. Liptak, Paolo Buracco, William T. N. Culp, and Nicholas J. Bacon.

t

W

Z